NEURORADIOLOGY
WITH
COMPUTED TOMOGRAPHY

RUTH G. RAMSEY, M.D.

Associate Professor of Radiology,
Rush Medical College; Associate
Attending, Section of Neuroradiology,
Rush-Presbyterian-St. Luke's Medical
Center, Chicago

1981

W. B. SAUNDERS COMPANY
Philadelphia London Toronto

W. B. Saunders Company: West Washington Square
Philadelphia, PA 19105

1 St. Anne's Road
Eastbourne, East Sussex BN21 3UN, England

1 Goldthorne Avenue
Toronto, Ontario M8Z 5T9, Canada

Library of Congress Cataloging in Publication Data

Ramsey, Ruth G

Neuroradiology with computed tomography.

1. Nervous system – Radiography. 2. Tomography.
I. Title. [DNLM: 1. Nervous system – Radiography.
2. Tomography, X-ray computed. WL 141 R183n]

RC349.R3R35 616.8′047572 78–65381

ISBN 0–7216–7444–5

Neuroradiology with Computed Tomography ISBN 0-7216-7444-5

Last digit is the print number: 9 8 7 6 5 4 3 2 1

To

Michael M. Ramsey

PREFACE

It was in 1918, after seeing Lockett's description of traumatic pneumocephalus, that Walter Dandy performed and reported the first air ventriculogram, which was soon followed by the first reported pneumoencephalogram. These were early special radiologic techniques that allowed accurate nonoperative localization of intracranial disease—an accomplishment not previously possible.

Cerebral angiography was introduced in 1927 by Egas Moniz. Contrast media and injection devices improved over the years, an important advance being the Seldinger technique of femoral catheterization in 1953. At the present time, arteriography poses little danger, carries a high degree of assurance and achieves readily reproducible results. The addition of radionuclide scanning further improved the diagnostic process.

In 1973, the introduction of Computed Tomography (CT) began to revolutionize neuroradiology totally. CT scanning uses ionizing radiation, but dosages are significantly lower than with other methods, and more information is provided. Furthermore, the CT scan is almost noninvasive and is performed with a minimum of discomfort to the patient. The study allows greater diagnostic accuracy than any other, and certain processes such as demyelinating diseases are detectable by CT that are not seen by other radiologic procedures. Contemporary scanners provide more information in less time and with less danger than was ever thought possible.

A significant point is that computed tomography has actually reduced the number of radiologic procedures needed to arrive at a correct diagnosis, for often it is the only examination necessary before appropriate treatment can be instituted. Consequently, there has been a precipitous drop in the number of pneumoencephalograms, thus eliminating a great deal of discomfort as well as a small but significant morbidity. The use of cerebral angiography has not decreased as sharply, but some patients are spared this procedure as well. CT scanning also directs attention to those patients who will benefit most from angiography.

This book has two complementary purposes. First, the broad field of neuroradiology is covered in sufficient depth to provide more than a primer on traditional neuroradiologic procedures. Second, students, residents and practicing radiologists need a modern description of the discipline of neuroradiology as it has been affected by computed tomography. For each neurologic disorder reviewed, CT scans are included whenever appropriate; in many instances, these are correlated with angiographic studies. Studies of the same patient are presented when available; otherwise, similar entities in different patients are illustrated. Evaluation of computed tomography both as an independent diagnostic tool and, more particularly, in comparison to older methods is thus made practical. Thus, readers may develop a base of knowledge in CT scanning either independent of or correlated with angiography.

The CT scans in this book are presented as if seen from above, looking downward at the patient's head. The patient's right side is to the right in the CT illustrations. Similarly, all myelographic studies are presented as if the patient is seen from behind. This convention simulates the operative approach. When scans are performed both before and after infusion of iodinated contrast material, they are appropriately labeled "Pre" and "Post" when necessary for clarity.

It was only after a great deal of thought and lengthy discussion that we elected to eliminate a separate chapter on pneumoencephalography. This chapter had, in fact, been written, but served only to reemphasize the merits of computed tomography and the fact that this new technique has essentially eliminated the need for pneumoencephalography. Therefore, it was decided to omit the chapter on pneumoencephalography as inappropriate to a modern text on neuroradiology.

Depending on their needs, readers may wish to review the entire contents of the book, study particular topics in detail or refer to the individual case examples for help with a special problem. Neuroradiology is both challenging and complicated, although computed tomography has made it easier to understand. An investment of time and effort in its study will be rewarded with an appreciation of its challenges and its limitless possibilities.

RUTH GODWIN RAMSEY, M.D.

ACKNOWLEDGMENTS

There are many individuals who have helped me with this project. My husband was a great encouragement to me from beginning to end. Our children, Thomas and Timothy, were equally encouraging and understanding. Dr. Michael S. Huckman assisted by providing a teaching file of cases for my use. Drs. Oscar Sugar and Glenn Dobben from the University of Illinois made their entire collection available to me. Dr. Justo Rodriquez from Cook County Hospital also provided interesting teaching cases. Dr. Richard E. Buenger made the necessary arrangements for the project to be carried out. Dr. Avrum (Josh) Epstein helped me with the research and the content of the entire text. Most important, my thanks to Dr. John Fennessy, who encouraged me to undertake a project like this in the first place.

Mr. Robert B. Walker, Jr. of our Photography Department worked closely with me throughout. Mr. Walker worked very hard to obtain photos of excellent technical quality—sometimes from original photographs that were far from optimal. His assistance is acknowledged and greatly appreciated. Elissa Ray kept track of all these materials; none were ever misplaced.

The special procedure technicians also deserve mention. Without them and their efforts, excellent radiographs could not be obtained. Outstanding among others are Tamara Shepard, Carlene Smith, Sharon Trammell, Sharon Johnson, Paula Knish and Ellen McNee.

The wonderful people at the W. B. Saunders Company also deserve mention. It is impossible to list all the people behind the scenes; however, I do appreciate their help. Special mention goes to John Hanley, Albert Meier, John Dyson, Kathy Pitcoff, Grace Gulezian and Walter Verbitski.

I can list only some of the many others who assisted me with this project: Gladys Nord, Eileen Tuttley, John Lobick, James Wilk, Michael Boxer, Charlene Sisco, Nora Sykes, Gladys Trice and Dolores W. Godwin.

Of course, the real reason for this text is to provide a source of information for students, residents and practicing physicians. Their interest and questions provided the true inspiration for this undertaking.

RUTH GODWIN RAMSEY, M.D.

CONTENTS

CONTENTS

CHAPTER 1

THE ORDER OF NEURORADIOLOGIC PROCEDURES

Selecting the most effective sequence of neuroradiologic procedures from the variety available today is not always an easy matter. A thoughtful approach to the problems unique to each individual patient is required. In some cases only one examination may be necessary before instituting therapy; others may require all of the several examinations if a correct diagnosis is to be determined.

In general, the work-up of a patient should begin with noninvasive studies. The patient's symptoms may serve as a guide, dictating the order of testing to a certain extent. Unfortunately, even patients with sizeable tumor masses may have minimal symptoms. Therefore, diagnostic acumen and judgment also contribute significantly to choosing the order of testing. Of course, all thorough diagnostic work must begin with a history of the present illness and significant past history and with a thorough physical and neurologic examination. Whether the patient's illness is acute or chronic is very important — particularly if alteration of mentation has occurred following head trauma.

SKULL RADIOLOGY

A routine skull examination will demonstrate the presence or absence of bony metastatic deposits, areas of reactive bone formation, intracranial calcification, skull fractures, sinusitis, changes in size of the sella turcica and such metabolic changes as those of Paget's disease, fibrous dysplasia or the hemoglobinopathies.

ELECTROENCEPHALOGRAPHY

A discussion of the electroencephalogram is beyond the scope of this book. This study can be helpful in certain patients, particularly those with a seizure disorder.

RADIONUCLIDE SCAN

The radionuclide brain scan has been a very helpful diagnostic tool, although since the introduction of the CT scan the indications for its use are less clear. The radionuclide angiogram may show decreased flow through the carotid arteries in a patient with suspected occlusive vascular disease. Following a stroke it may provide evidence of decreased perfusion in the area of infarction, which after several days will demonstrate an area of increased uptake secondary to breakdown of the blood-brain barrier. In the presence of an acute subdural hematoma the radionuclide angiogram may show an area of poor perfusion over the cerebral convexity, while the static scan is normal. With a chronic subdural hematoma the scan reveals a crescentic area of increased activity. Brain tumors demonstrate areas of increased activity on the scan, as do areas of abscess formation.

COMPUTED TOMOGRAPHY

BRAIN TUMORS

It is not unreasonable to say that the introduction of computed tomography of the brain has revolutionized our approach to the diagnosis of neurologic disorders. There is no better method than the CT scan for demonstrating intracranial pathology. The scan demonstrates the size of the lesion, its location, its configuration and its relationship to any surrounding edema. From its appearance on the scan we can tell whether the mass is solid or cystic, space-occupying or not, of CSF density or of a density equal to normal brain tissue (isodense) or of higher or lower density than normal brain. The CT scan also demonstrates any evidence of ventricular enlargement and/or cortical sulcus enlargement better than any other diagnostic test available. Additionally, the scan also demonstrates shift of the ventricles that may be secondary to cerebral edema or a mass lesion.

All patients with suspected brain metastases should have a CT examination both with and without infusion.

SUBARACHNOID HEMORRHAGE

Following subarachnoid hemorrhage, blood can be seen in the basilar cisterns, the interhemispheric fissure, over the cerebral cortex and occasionally within the ventricular system. The CT scan accurately reflects the presence of blood in the subarachnoid space in approximately 80 to 90 per cent of cases. Patients with severe headaches, photophobia, a stiff neck and an alteration in mental status without or with focal neurologic findings require a lumbar tap if the CT scan does not show evidence of a subarachnoid hemorrhage. The CT scan does not accurately demonstrate the presence of an aneurysm unless it is very sizeable (probably over 2 cm); therefore, angiography is necessary to establish or rule out aneurysm.

Angiography is necessary for the evaluation of patients with subarachnoid hemorrhage. None of the other ancillary tests will reveal the size and position of the aneurysm, nor whether there is or is not evidence of vascular spasm. In approximately 15 per cent of cases the cause of subarachnoid hemorrhage will not be found.

INTRACEREBRAL HEMATOMA

Intracerebral hematoma is readily demonstrated using the CT scan, and even small areas of hemorrhage can easily be identified. The areas of hemorrhage may be in any portion of the cerebral hemispheres, particularly in patients suffering from coagulopathies. Hypertensive hemorrhages occur most commonly in the region of the basal ganglia and cerebellum, but also may involve the brain stem. Often the CT scan will be the only examination to demonstrate these abnormalities.

Intracerebral hemorrhage may be associated with an element of intraventricular hemorrhage; thus, the clinical appearance of headache, photophobia, altered mental status and stiff neck may mimic that of a subarachnoid hemorrhage. The CT scan reveals the true nature of the problem, although at times an aneurysm may cause an intracerebral hematoma.

If an intracerebral hematoma is suspected, a CT scan is the examination of choice.

ATROPHY

When a possible diagnosis of atrophy is entertained, the CT scan is the examination of choice. The sizes of the lateral ventricle and cortical sulci are readily demonstrated. It appears that there is some increase in the size of both the ventricles and the cortical sulci with increasing age, but precise guidelines are not yet available. The CT scan also rules out the presence of an unsuspected brain tumor or chronic subdural hematoma.

TRAUMA

In the patient who has sustained head trauma the CT scan is also the procedure of choice. With acute head trauma and a change in mentation and/or focal physical findings an immediate scan should be performed. This can be performed with the patient sedated or, in the uncooperative patient, under general anesthesia. It cannot be over-emphasized that all efforts should be made to obtain a diagnostic examination so that prompt treatment can be instituted as needed. In acute subdural or epidural hematoma the neurosurgeon commonly undertakes an operative procedure without an angiogram or any other work-up. Indeed, in rare instances, a single scan through the mid-portion of the brain to confirm the existence of a hematoma, followed by rapid evacuation, may be a life-saving procedure. If computed tomography is not available, angiography may be necessary for evaluation.

ANGIOGRAPHY

In general, angiography is performed following the noninvasive examinations. Definitive morbidity and even mortality can follow angiography, and this examination should be performed only after adequate consideration.

Angiography is needed whenever the operating surgeon feels that it is necessary to outline the vascular supply to the tumor — and, just as important, to demonstrate the position and relationship of the major intracerebral vessels to the tumor mass. This is especially true of the cortical veins, which serve as markers for the surgeon as the surgical approach is planned.

If the tumor is a meningioma, the blood supply usually is from the external carotid artery, although the tentorial artery arises from the internal carotid artery and may supply a posterior fossa or tentorial meningioma.

At times posterior fossa tumors can be operated upon without the benefit of angiography. This is especially true of acoustic neurinomas.

GENERAL INDICATIONS FOR ANGIOGRAPHY

1. For evaluation of intracranial mass lesions identified by other diagnostic methods.
2. In patients with vascular abnormalities; e.g., arteriovenous malformations, subarachnoid hemorrhage, transient ischemic attacks, certain intracerebral hematomas and cerebral venous thrombosis.
3. With cerebral trauma when computed tomography is not available.

GENERAL (RELATIVE) CONTRAINDICATIONS TO ANGIOGRAPHY

1. Patients with "stroke in evolution" or a progressing stroke.
2. Inadequate equipment or technical personnel.
3. Untrained or inexperienced operators to perform the procedures without adequate supervision.
4. Allergy to contrast material.
5. Professional help should be available to deal with any abnormalities found in a way that will benefit the patient. Without such assistance, angiography should not be performed.

PNEUMOENCEPHALOGRAPHY

Since the introduction of computed tomography there has been a precipitous drop in the number of pneumoencephalograms performed. At the present time one indication for pneumoencephalography is to evaluate a mass lesion in the sella and its suprasellar extension. Even this indication has become less firm since the introduction of scanning units that allow visualization of the sella in the coronal or even the sagittal section. Recon-

component from an extra-axial tumor — both the anatomy around the sella sufficiently to eliminate any need for pneumoencephalogram.

A second indication is to aid in differentiating mass lesions in the posterior fossa, where it may at times be difficult to distinguish a brain stem tumor which has an exophytic component from an extra-axial tumor — both of which may have a similar angiographic appearance.

In a patient with persistent symptoms, a progressive hemiparesis or a confusing clinical picture, a repeat CT scan with infusion is indicated following a suitable period of medical management. This interval may range from one or two days to months or even a year.

CHAPTER 2

THE PLAIN SKULL FILM

INTRODUCTION

For many years the plain film examination of the skull served as one of the main diagnostic tools in the work-up of the patient with suspected intracranial pathology. Careful examination of the plain skull film may reveal important information that will be helpful in diagnosis. Skull fractures, intracranial air, intracranial calcification and alterations in the bony calvaria are only a few of the pathologic changes that can be seen on plain films. Even today, after the introduction of such diagnostic tools as pneumoencephalography, arteriography, radionuclide scanning and, most recently, computed tomography of the brain, plain skull films continue to be an important diagnostic tool, although the newer techniques are more informative and more accurate in their evaluation of intracranial pathology.

These developments led to a decreased emphasis on the skull film, and some clinicians have even suggested that there is no longer a need for the plain skull examination. While it is true that other diagnostic tools have added greatly to our ability to diagnose intracranial disorders, the plain skull examination continues to provide excellent data about the structure of the bony calvaria. It should not be discarded, and routine radiography should be correlated with other diagnostic tools.

DEFINITION

Routine radiographs of the skull are known as the "plain skull" examination, as opposed to roentgen examinations of the skull which are not "plain" but either involve the administration of contrast material or are altered in some other manner. The routine set of films varies from institution to institution, but most employ approximately the same set of standard films. The routine examination is set up in such a fashion that all the parts of the skull that are of interest in the case at hand are visualized on one or more films. In our department the routine set includes a right and left lateral, a Towne's view, a posteroanterior view with the internal auditory canal projected through the mid-portion of the orbit, and a submentovertex view of the skull. Each of these views provides a unique look at some area of the skull that is of particular interest and that is not as well visualized on the other views. Some departments routinely include a stereo lateral view of the skull for evaluation of intracranial calcifications or skull fractures. The Caldwell view also may be included as part of the routine series.

Although some authors have questioned the need for routine skull films since the advent of computed tomography of the brain, a more conservative approach would indicate that skull films can be of great value and generally should be obtained wherever intracranial pathology is suspected. They are particularly helpful in cases of head trauma. In addition, close examination of the series occasionally will reward the physician by providing diagnostic clues. If nothing else, they may be of importance in planning which examinations should be performed next in order to arrive at the diagnosis expeditiously.

When reviewing routine skull films it is helpful to have a brief but pertinent clinical history as a guide in reviewing the radiographic findings. In general, when reviewing the skull for evidence of trauma one is looking for a fracture. Particular attention should be paid to the area showing external signs of trauma when a clinical history or positive physical findings are not available. Lacking a history, "bright lighting" the film may give a clue to the area of interest by revealing a localized area of soft tissue swelling.

If a skull fracture is found, one should be aware of the possibility of an associated traumatic pneumocephalus (see Chapter 14). The sphenoid sinus should be checked for an air-fluid level indicating either blood or cerebrospinal fluid leakage into the sinus. When air-fluid levels are found secondary to trauma or sinusitis, skull radiography in the upright position is strongly suggested. If the patient is prone or supine these abnormalities may not be visualized. If the patient is too ill to sit upright for routine radiographs, lateral skull films with the patient supine may be obtained for initial evaluation (see Chapter 14).

POSTEROANTERIOR VIEW OF THE SKULL (FIGURE 2–1)

This view is obtained with the patient lying prone with the forehead closest to the film. The patient is positioned in such a way that the internal auditory canals are projected into the mid- or lower portion of the orbit. The central ray is angled 10° rostrally in relation to the anthropologic base line. This view is used to evaluate the internal auditory canals and for inspection of the orbits and the frontal bone. The lambdoid suture will be projected lower than the coronal suture in this view. The posterior parietal and upper portion of the occipital bone are also readily visualized with this position.

Figure 2–1. Posteroanterior view with internal auditory canals viewed through the orbit. 1 Internal auditory canal 2 Vestibule 3 Superior semicircular canal 4 Floor of sella turcica 5 Crista galli 6 Superior orbital fissure 7 Nasal septum 8 Roof of ethmoid sinus 9 Roof of orbit 10 Linea innominata 11 Zygomatic process of frontal bone 12 Arcuate eminence 13 Floor of posterior cranial fossa 14 Infraorbital canal 15 Anterior clinoid process 16 Foramen rotundum 17 Zygomatic arch 18 Maxillary sinus 19 Alveolar ridge of maxilla 20 Hard plate 21 Cribriform plate 22 Lateral wall of maxillary sinus 23 Medial wall of maxillary sinus

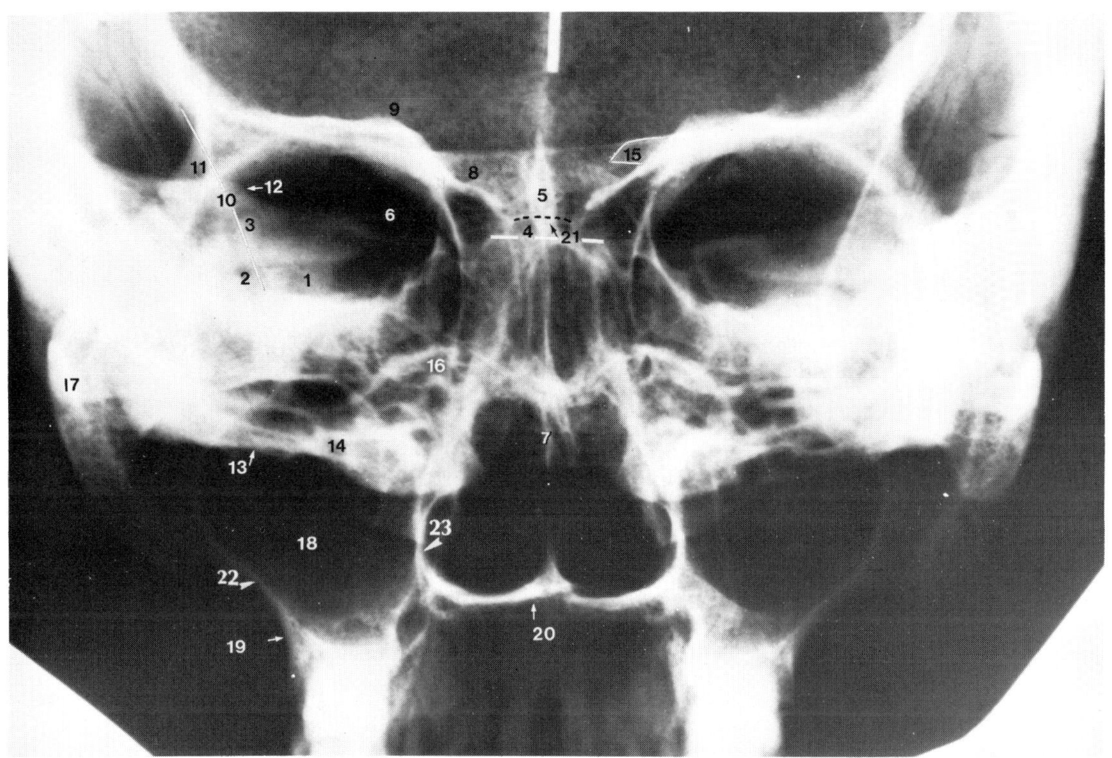

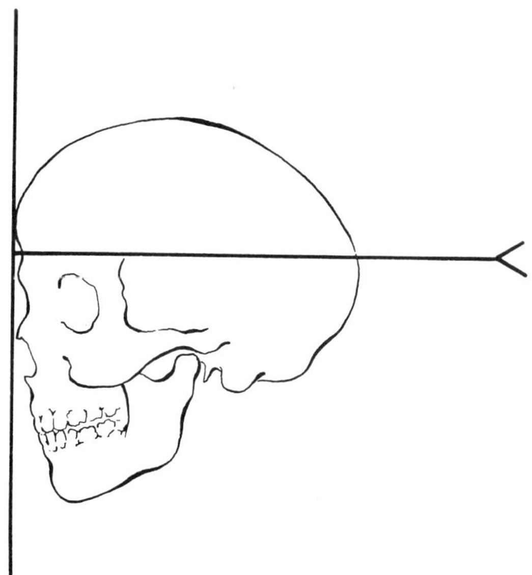

Figure 2–1. *See legend on the opposite page.*

OCCIPITAL OR TOWNE-CHAMBERLAIN VIEW (FIGURE 2–2)

The patient is placed in the prone position and the central ray is directed at an angle of 25 to 35° caudad with respect to the orbitomental line. This Towne's view of the skull provides the best view of the occipital bone. It also allows for evaluation and comparison of the size of the internal auditory canals, which are readily seen in this view. Evaluation of the petrous bones and mastoid air cells can also be made on the Towne's view. Lesions of the frontal lobes of the brain will be seen to project lower in the Towne's view than in the posteroanterior view; this may help to better localize a lesion that is visible only on anteroposterior or posteroanterior views. In addition, the orbits will also be projected more inferiorly on this view, allowing for visualization of the inferior orbital fissure. The zygomatic arches are frequently seen in silhouette on this view. If a base-of-skull fracture is suspected, careful inspection of the occipital bone on the Towne's view may reveal a linear fracture that extends forward to involve the temporal bone. The foramen magnum is well visualized on this view, and the dorsum sellae and the posterior clinoids should project into the foramen magnum in a well positioned Towne's view.

Figure 2–2. Towne's view. 1 Dorsum sellae 2 Posterior clinoid process 3 Posterior margin of foramen magnum 4 Internal occipital crest 5 Inferior orbital fissure 6 Nasal septum 7 Floor of middle cranial fossa 8 Zygomatic arch 9 Styloid process 10 Maxillary sinus 11 Internal auditory canal 12 Vestibule 13 Superior semicircular canal 14 Tip of mastoid process 15 Posterior wall of porus acusticus internus 16 Posterior surface of petrous pyramid 17 Frontal sinus 18 Nasal lacrimal duct canal

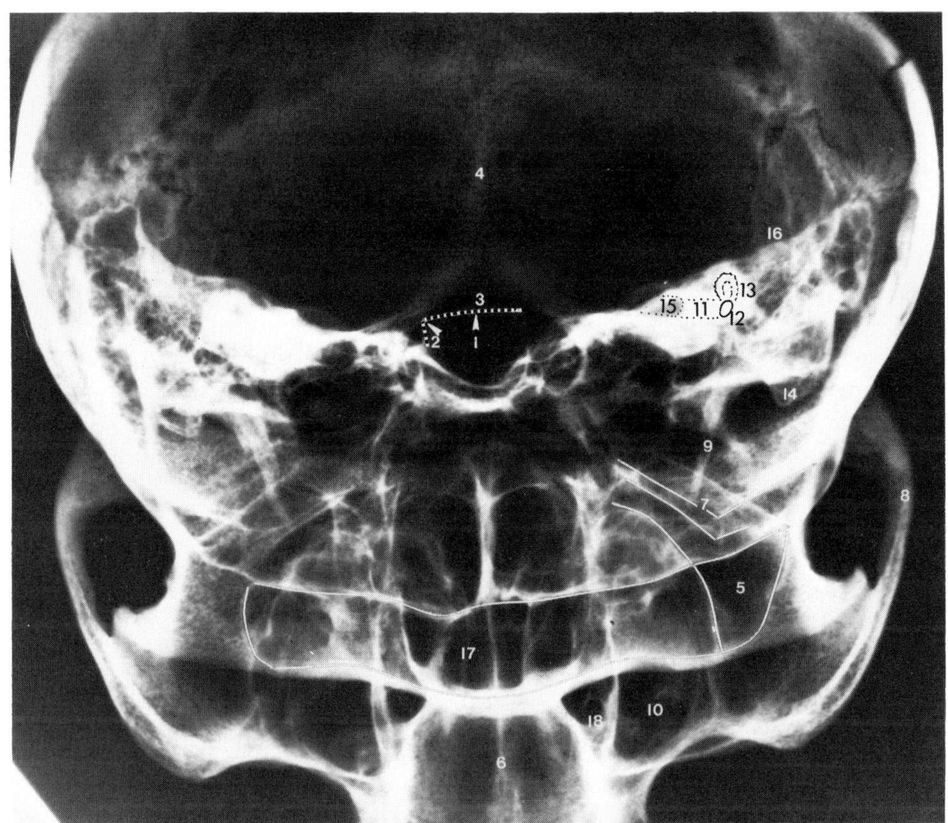

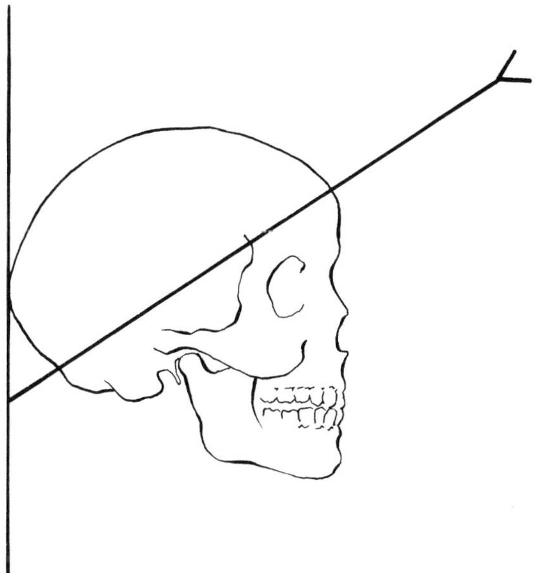

Figure 2–2. *See legend on the opposite page.*

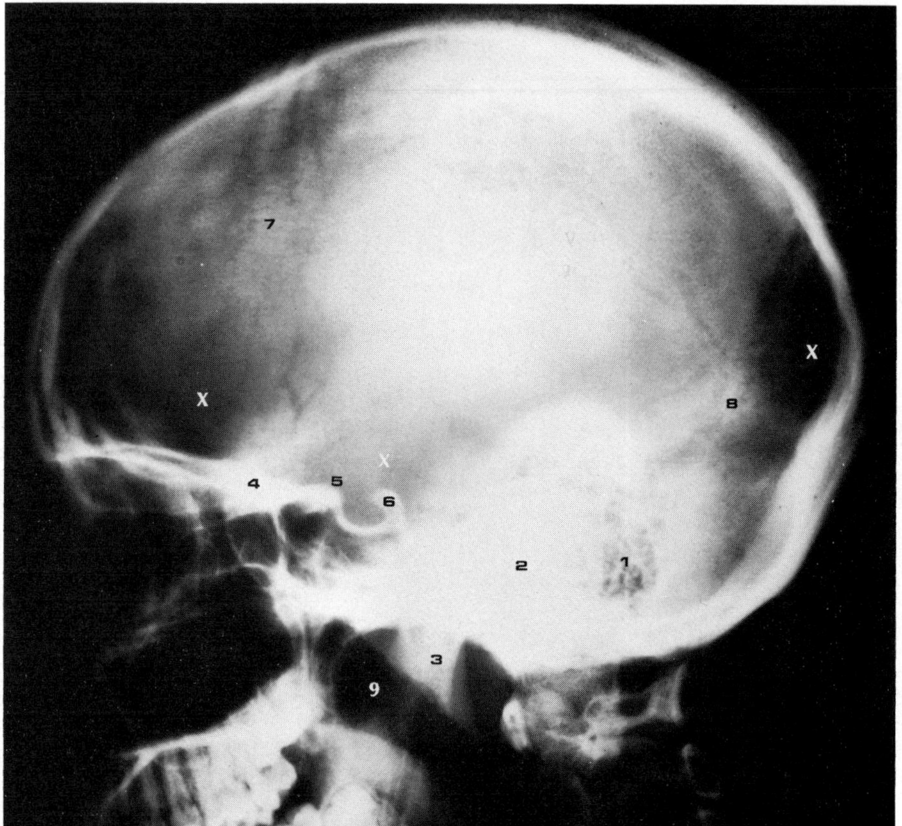

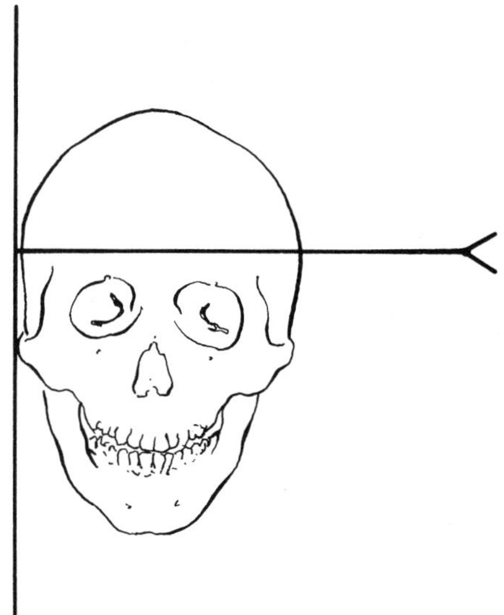

Figure 2–3. Lateral view. 1 Mastoid air cells 2 External auditory canal 3 Nasopharyngeal soft tissues 4 Roof of orbits 5 Tuberculum sellae 6 Posterior clinoids and dorsum sellae 7 Coronal suture 8 Lambdoid suture 9 Nasopharyngeal air shadow X Areas of physiologic thinning of the calvarium

LATERAL VIEW (FIGURES 2–3 and 2–4)

The right and left lateral views of the skull are obtained first with the patient's right side and then with the patient's left side closest to the film. It should be noted that the patient may be "off lateral" in one or two planes in the lateral projection. The patient may tilt the head to one side or the other, resulting in one orbital roof being higher than the other, or the patient may turn the head slightly to the right or the left, resulting in failure of superimposition of the greater wings on the sphenoid bone on the radiograph (see illustration). These "off lateral" positions can easily be evaluated by inspecting the radiograph. This is most important when the tilting of the head may give the false appearance of a double floor of the sella. The right and left lateral views are especially helpful in evaluating a possible skull fracture; i.e., if a linear skull fracture is present on the right side it will appear sharpest on the right lateral view of the skull. Conversely, inspection of the left lateral view will reveal that the fracture line is less distinct and appears wider because of the magnification that occurs through the width of the skull. Obviously the reverse will be true when a fracture is present on the left side.

Stereoscopic lateral views also may be helpful in this instance and in other cases where localization of an area of calcification is needed. Since CT became available we no longer obtain stereo views of the skull in our department.

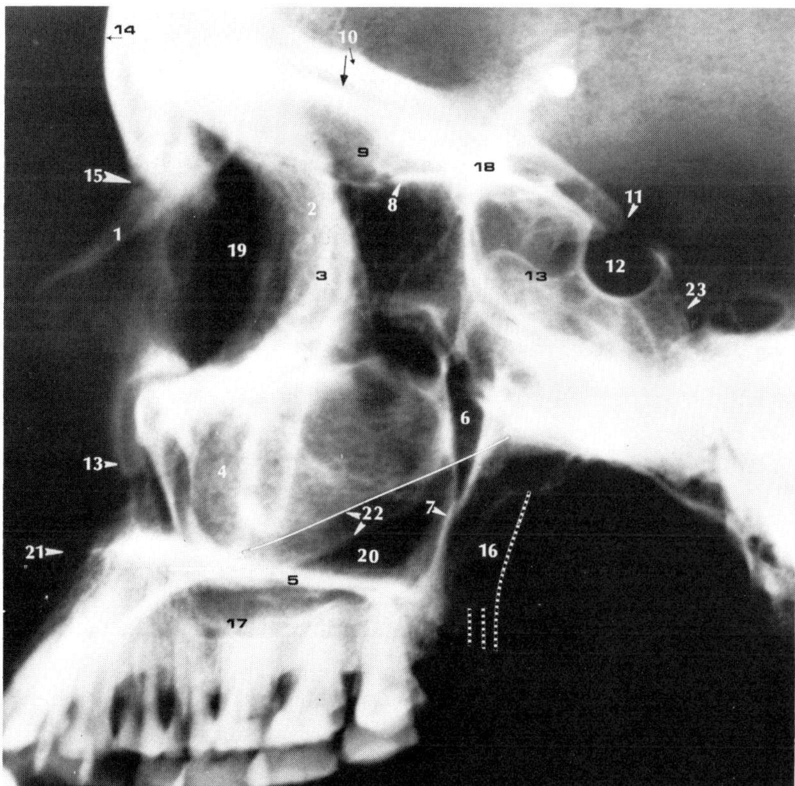

Figure 2–4. Lateral view of facial bones. 1 Nasal bone 2 Zygomatic process of frontal bone 3 Frontal process of zygomatic bone 4 Zygomatic recess of maxillary antrum 5 Hard palate 6 Pterygomaxillary space 7 Posterior wall of maxillary antrum 8 Cribriform plate 9 Roof of ethmoid sinuses 10 Roof of orbits 11 Anterior clinoid processes 12 Sella turcica 13 Anterior wall of maxillary antrum 14 Anterior wall of frontal sinus region 15 Nasofrontal suture 16 Pterygoid plates 17 Floor of maxillary antrum 18 Greater wing of sphenoid bone (anterior margin of middle cranial fossa) 19 Orbit 20 Maxillary sinus 21 Anterior maxillary spine 22 Inferior margin of zygomatic bones 23 Upper margin of clivus

SUBMENTOVERTEX OR BASE VIEW OF THE SKULL (FIGURE 2–5)

This view is obtained by placing a film at the top of the skull, hyperextending the patient's neck and angling the tube slightly toward the front of the head with the tube in front of the patient's chest. It should be noted that this view may be difficult to obtain in elderly patients, particularly in those with degenerative arthritis of the cervical spine, which limits mobility. This view may also be difficult or impossible to obtain in combative or unconscious patients.

The base view gives particularly excellent images of the clivis and of the multiple foramina at the base of the skull, which are not visible on any other projection. The pterygoid plates are also well seen (see illustration).

The three lines of the middle cranial fossa are also visualized on the base view. With this view one looks tangentially down the greater wing of the sphenoid bone, which forms a curvilinear line on either side of the skull outlining the anterior margin of the middle cranial fossa (13). The curvilinear line anterior to this, which will be seen to form an "S" configuration and to be continuous with the zygomatic bone laterally, is the bony margin of the back wall of the maxillary sinus (22). A mnemonic useful for remembering this is that the "*S*" line outlines the back wall of the sinus. This "S"-shaped line is to be differentiated from the straight line that forms the back wall of the orbit (23). This straight line will be seen to course from medial-posterior to lateral-anterior (see illustration).

The base view of the skull also provides an opportunity for an additional look at the maxillary sinuses when they are not well seen on the routine views and when it cannot be decided whether they are indeed normal or abnormal.

The submentovertex view is also particularly helpful when trying to evaluate varying degrees of asymmetry of the cranial vault. CT scans simulate the base position and can be correlated with the plain film base view. In addition, evaluation can be made of the internal auditory canals, the jugular foramen and the mastoid air cells. Since metastatic carcinoma and primary nasopharyngeal carcinomas often involve the base of the skull, the base view will be helpful to the oncologist or radiotherapist for evaluation of bony erosions. Indeed, radiographic tomographic studies of the base of the skull are often performed for the purpose of evaluating a metastatic lesion or local invasion of the base of the skull.

This view also lends itself well to oral and written certification examinations because of the multiple anatomic landmarks which are visible.

Figure 2–5. The submentovertex view. 1 Foramen magnum 2 Hypoglossal canal 3 Foramen ovale 4 Foramen spinosum 5 Internal auditory canal 6 External auditory canal 7 Clivus 8 Jugular foramen 9 Lateral pterygoid 10 Inferior portion of lateral pterygoid 11 Medial pterygoid 12 Nasal septum 13 Greater wing of sphenoid bone (anterior margin of middle cranial fossa) 14 Carotid canal 15 Bony portion of eustachian tube 16 Air cells of sphenoid sinus around sella turcica 17 Foramen lacerum 18 Cochlea 19 Vestibule 20 Medial wall of maxillary sinus 21 Zygomatic arch 22 Posterolateral wall of maxillary sinus 23 Posterior wall of orbit

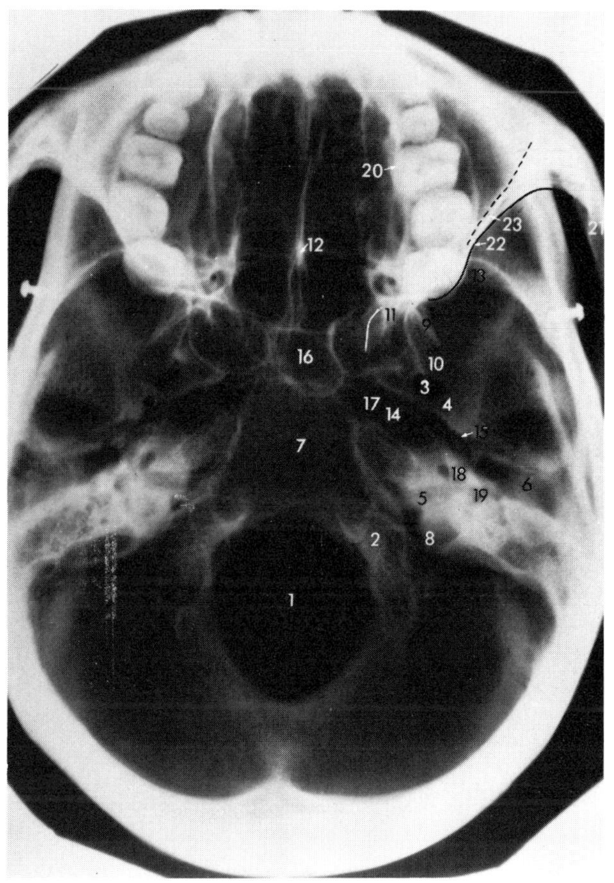

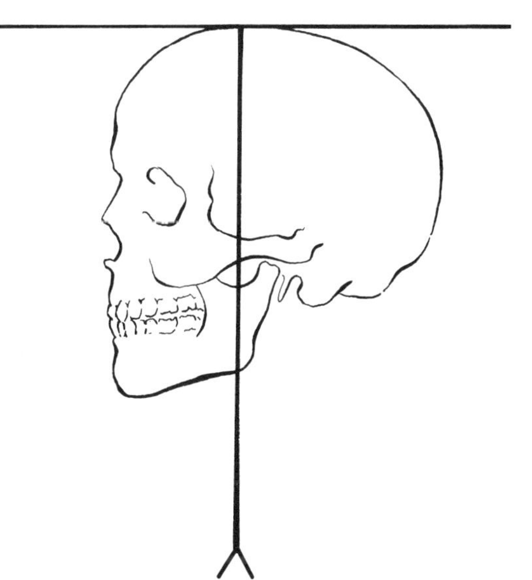

Figure 2–5. *See legend on the opposite page.*

NORMAL SELLA CONFIGURATION (FIGURES 2–6 and 2–7)

Figure 2–6 illustrates three separate lines of the posterior portion of the sella which frequently can be demonstrated in an individual case. These lines are the clivus, the anterior margin of the dorsum sellae and the anterior margin of the posterior clinoids which wrap forward around the sella and project anterior to the dorsum sellae.

The depth of the sella (Figure 2–7) is measured by drawing a line between the tuberculum sellae (*T*) and the dorsum sellae (*D*) and then dropping a perpendicular to this line at the deepest part of the sella. The depth of the sella should not exceed 14 mm.

The anteroposterior dimension of the sella is measured by drawing a line from the anterior margin of the sella turcica to the dorsum sellae at the longest part of the sella (A–P). This measurement should not be oblique and should not be taken from the tuberculum to the lowest portion of the dorsum sellae. The anteroposterior measurement should not exceed 17 mm.

Note that the posterior clinoid processes extend superior and anterior to the dorsum sellae.

The standard chest radiograph measures 14 × 17 inches — thus providing a good way to remember the upper limits of the size of the sella.

In actual fact, sellas even larger than these measurements are sometimes seen, and no detectable abnormality can be found in the patient. In these cases one can hypothesize an arrested pituitary adenoma, which was probably functioning at one time but is no longer active.

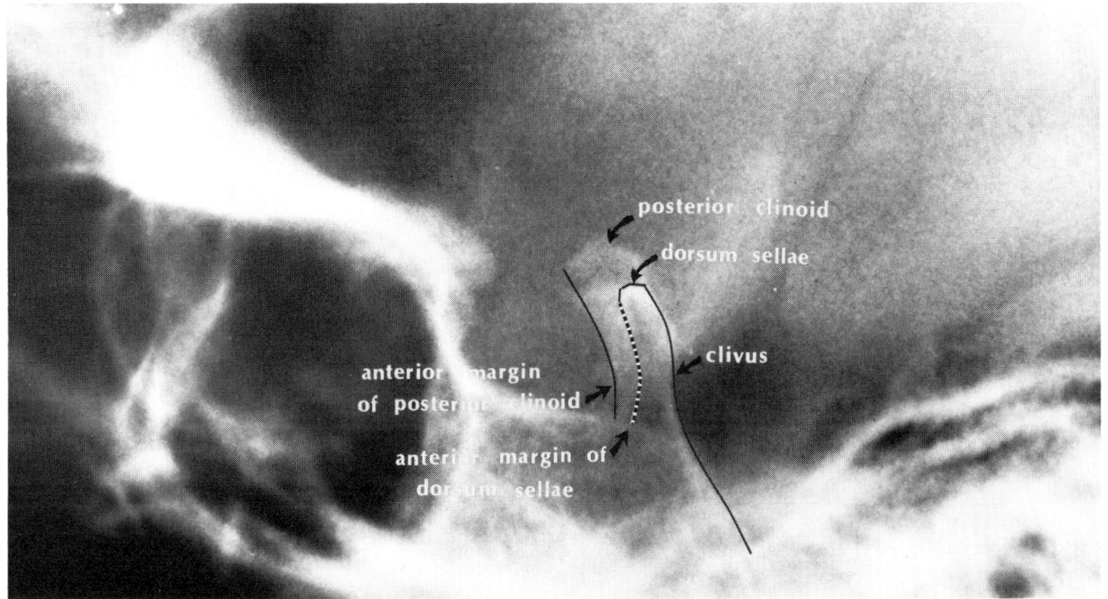

Figure 2–6

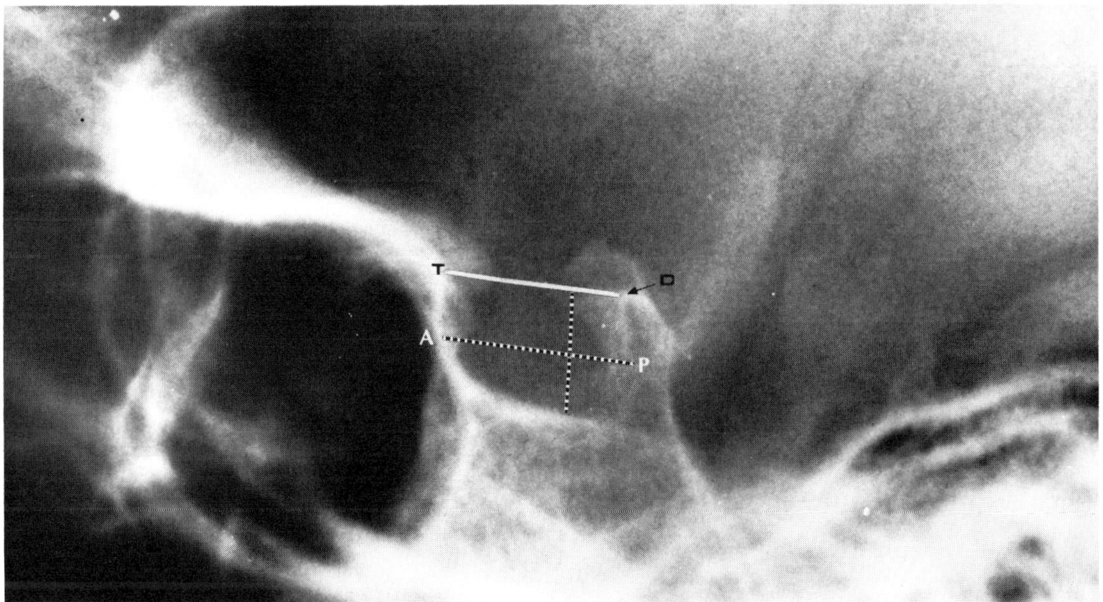

Figure 2–7

TABLE 2–1. IMPORTANT CRANIAL STRUCTURES AND FORAMINA

1. *Cavernous Sinus*
   a. Internal carotid artery
   b. Third cranial nerve (III)
   c. Fourth cranial nerve (IV)
   d. Ophthalmic branch of the fifth cranial nerve (V^1)
   e. Maxillary branch of the fifth cranial nerve (V^2)
   f. Sixth cranial nerve (VI)
   g. Internal carotid artery

2. *Superior Orbital Fissure*
   a. Superior ophthalmic vein
   b. Third cranial nerve (III)
   c. Fourth cranial nerve (IV)
   d. Sixth cranial nerve (VI)
   e. Ophthalmic branch of the fifth cranial nerve (V^1)

3. *Inferior Orbital Fissure*
   a. Maxillary branch of the fifth cranial nerve (V^2)
   b. Infraorbital artery and vein
   c. Sympathetic nerves

4. *Foramen Ovale*
   a. Mandibular branch of the fifth cranial nerve (V^3)

5. *Foramen Spinosum*
   a. Middle meningeal artery

6. *Foramen Rotundum*
   a. Maxillary branch of the fifth cranial nerve (V^2)

7. *Foramen Lacerum*
   a. Sympathetic nerves

8. *Carotid Canal*
   a. Carotid artery

9. *Jugular Foramen*
   a. Internal jugular vein
   b. Ninth cranial nerve
   c. Tenth cranial nerve
   d. Eleventh cranial nerve

10. *Internal Auditory Canal*
    a. Seventh cranial nerve
    b. Eighth cranial nerve

11. *Stylomastoid Foramen*
    a. Facial nerve

12. *Supraorbital Foramen*
    a. Ophthalmic division of the fifth cranial nerve (V^1)
    b. Supraorbital artery and vein

13. *Infraorbital Foramen*
    a. Infraorbital nerve (V^2)

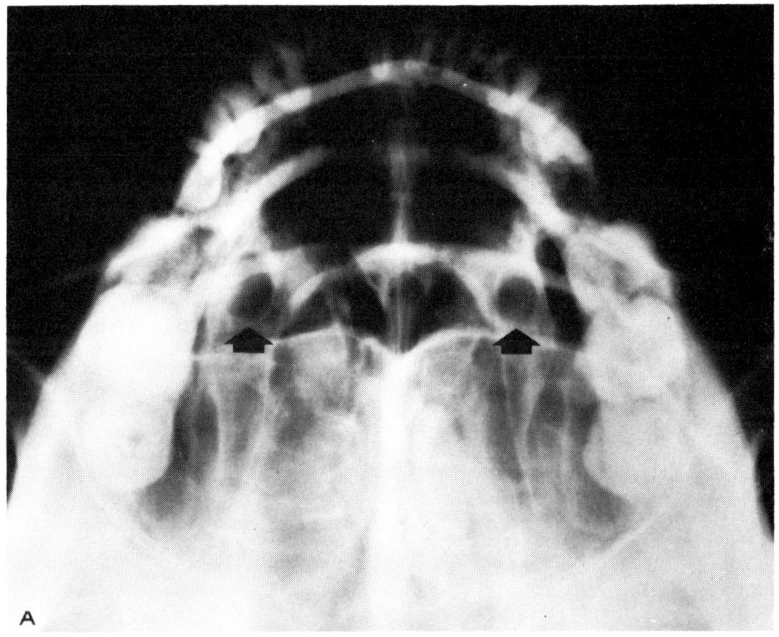

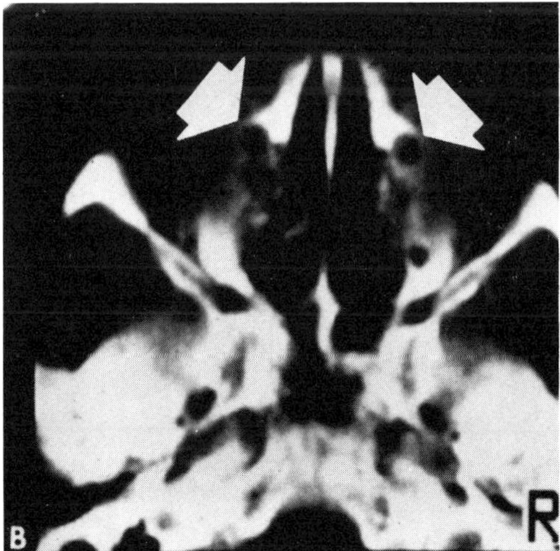

Figure 2–8. NASOLACRIMAL DUCT CANAL: This submentovertex view of the skull (*A*) demonstrates the nasolacrimal duct canal (*arrows*). They lie along the medial inferior margin of the orbit. The patient is positioned so that the nasolacrimal duct canal projects in a direct line with the aerated frontal sinus and just behind the mandible. The nasolacrimal canal also can be seen on the CT scan (*B*), where it appears as rounded foramina (*white arrows*).

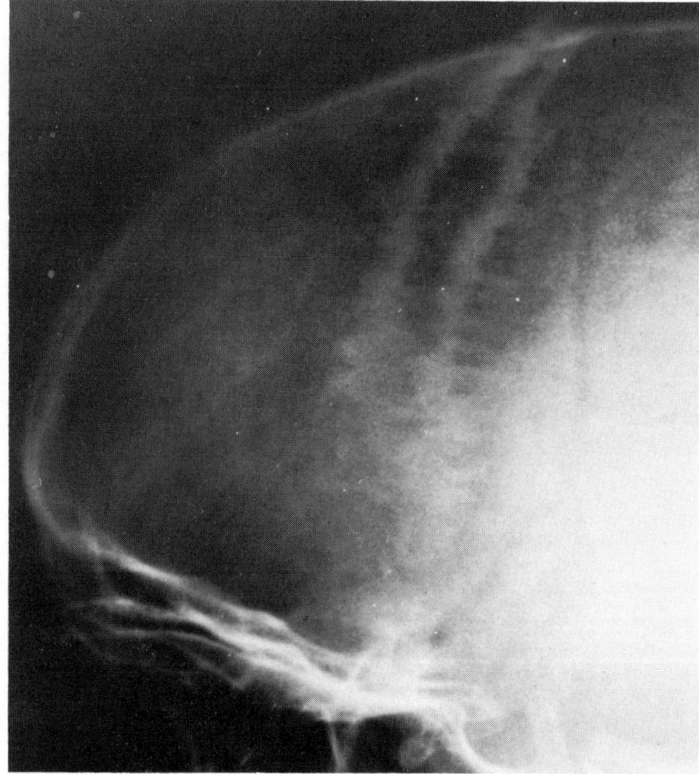

Figure 2–9. The suture lines as they fuse together frequently exhibit perisutural sclerosis, which gives the suture lines a very dense appearance. This patient is turned slightly so that each coronal suture is seen independently. The suture of the outer table of the skull exhibits large interdigitations, whereas the suture of the inner table is relatively straight.

PHYSIOLOGIC CALCIFICATION

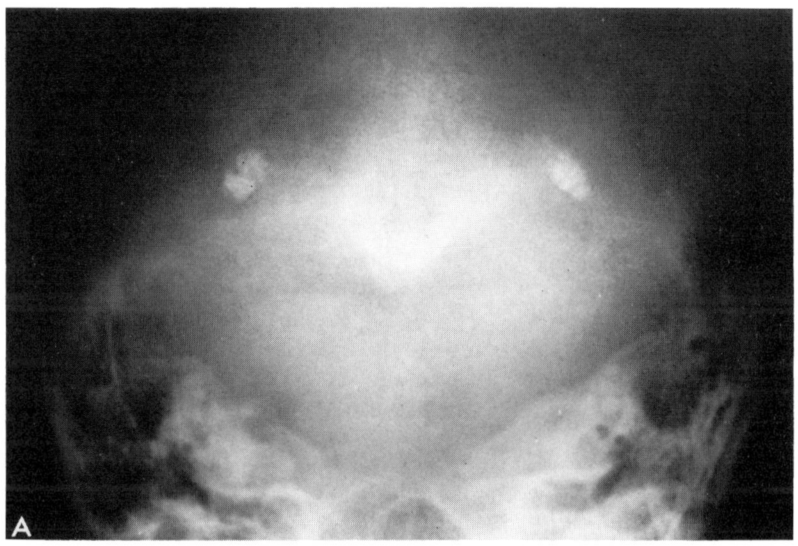

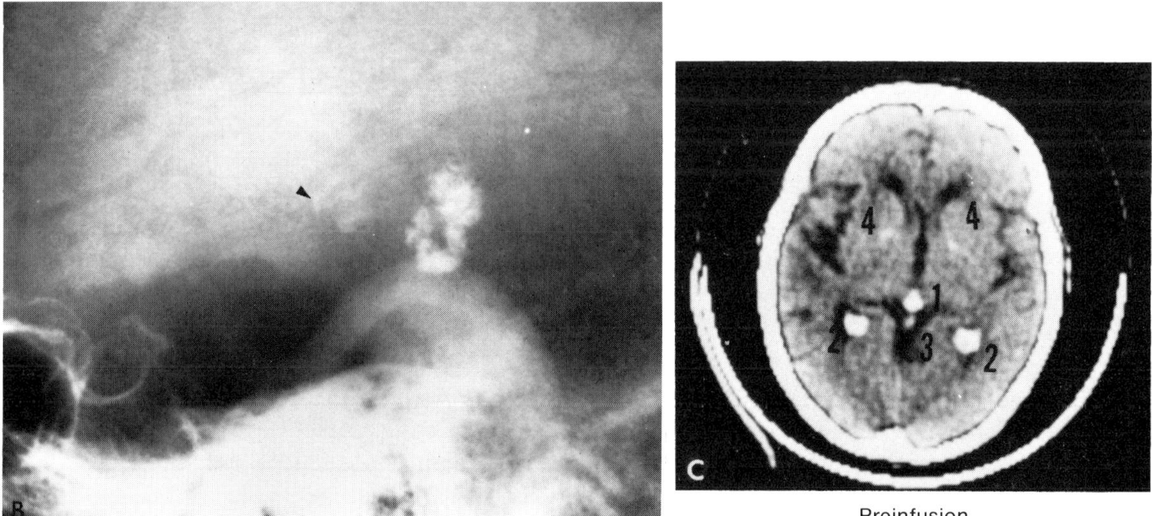

Preinfusion

Figure 2–10. HABENULAR COMMISSURE: The habenular commissure calcifies in its anterior margin and forms a curvilinear line convex posteriorly just anterior to the pineal gland (*black arrow* in *B*). The habenula may be mistaken for pineal calcification and may itself calcify without calcification of the pineal.

Legend continued on the following page.

Figure 2–10 *Continued.*

Pineal: The pineal gland is calcified in 55 per cent of white adults over the age of 20 years. The normal pineal may measure up to 15 mm in size. The gland may be evaluated for changes in its anteroposterior and superoinferior position by comparing its position radiographically with the anticipated normal position originally described by Vastine and Kinney. Various modifications of the Vastine-Kinney charts have been made since the original charts were described; however, recent advances in neuroradiologic techniques, especially CT scanning, have made these measurements less important than previously. The measurements are reliable only in the normally shaped skull; and, of course, not all masses create a displacement of the pineal gland.

On the other hand, the side-to-side displacement of the pineal is very useful in daily practice for rapid and convenient evaluation of the shift of midline structures. This is especially true of Emergency Room patients and others with head trauma, where rapid evaluation of the shift of the midline structures is necessary. (See Figure 2–11).

The anteroposterior view (*A*) demonstrates the calcifications in the glomus of the choroid plexus bilaterally. They are located in the atrium of the lateral ventricles. On the lateral view (*B*) the calcifications in the glomus of the choroid plexus project posterior to the pineal gland. The patient is tilted slightly for this examination so that the calcifications project one slightly higher than the other.

C, The CT scan reveals the calcified pineal gland (1) and the well calcified glomus in the atrium of the lateral ventricles bilaterally (2). The vein of Galen is also visualized because of the injection of contrast material; it projects just posterior to the pineal gland (3). Tiny areas of calcification are also present bilaterally in the basal ganglia. This small amount of basal ganglia calcification is not visible on plain skull films (4).

Figure 2–11. PINEAL GLAND MEASUREMENTS: Shift of the pineal gland from side to side is determined on the frontal views of the skull (*A*). A small dot is placed in the center of the pineal gland and the distance from this point to the outer table on one side is compared to the distance from this point to the outer table on the contralateral side. One half the difference between these two measurements represents the actual shift of the pineal gland i.e., ½ (A–B) = amount of shift. The pineal gland may be shifted up to 2 mm and still be considered to be within normal limits because the gland may calcify asymmetrically. Obviously, a noncalcified pineal is of no value for measurement, and symmetric, bilateral lesions will not cause a shift of the pineal gland.

If there is a question of possible intracranial pathology a CT scan should be obtained for evaluation. Indeed, the availability of CT scanning has greatly decreased the importance of all these measurements.

B and *C*, The CT scan demonstrates a large area of calcification which projects to the right of the midline. The calcification is actually in the tentorium, but could be mistaken for a shifted pineal gland on plain film examination. A tentorial calcification usually is flattened to follow the dura, whereas the pineal gland usually has a rounded configuration.

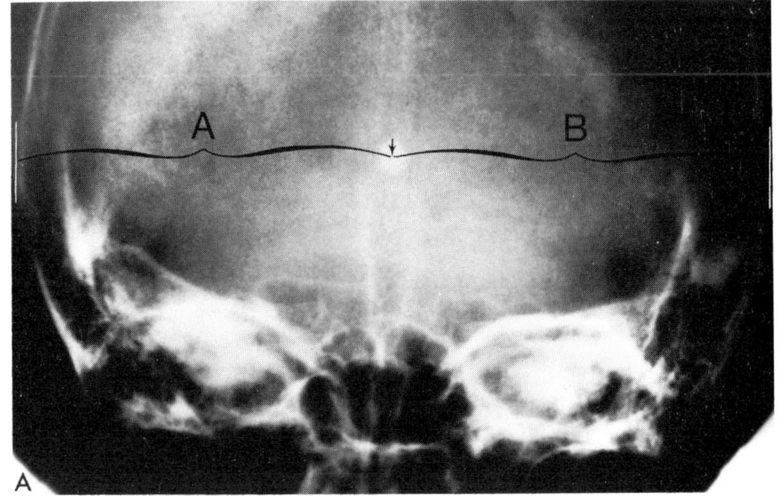

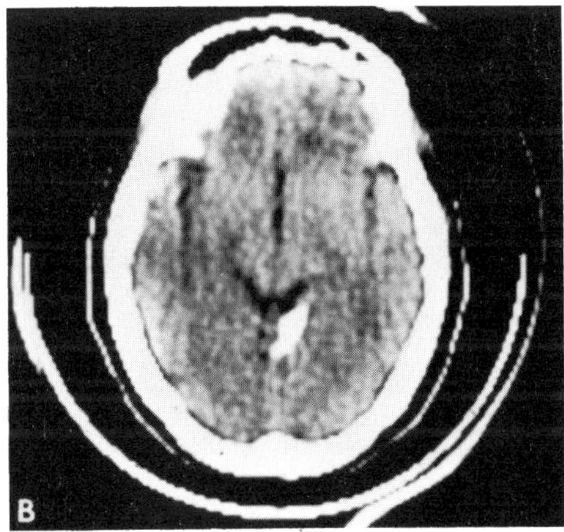

Preinfusion

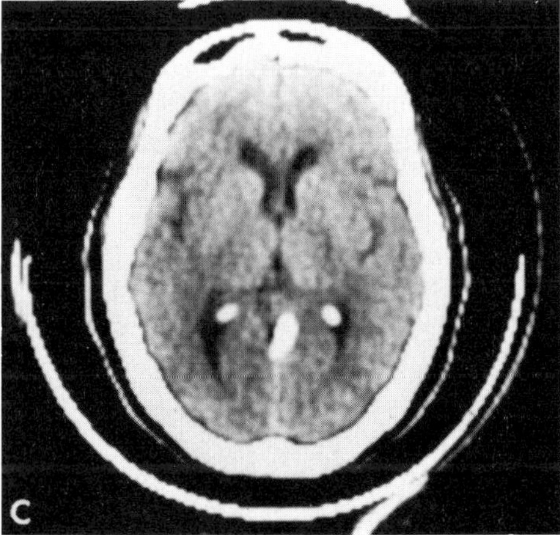

Preinfusion

Figure 2–11. *See legend on the opposite page.*

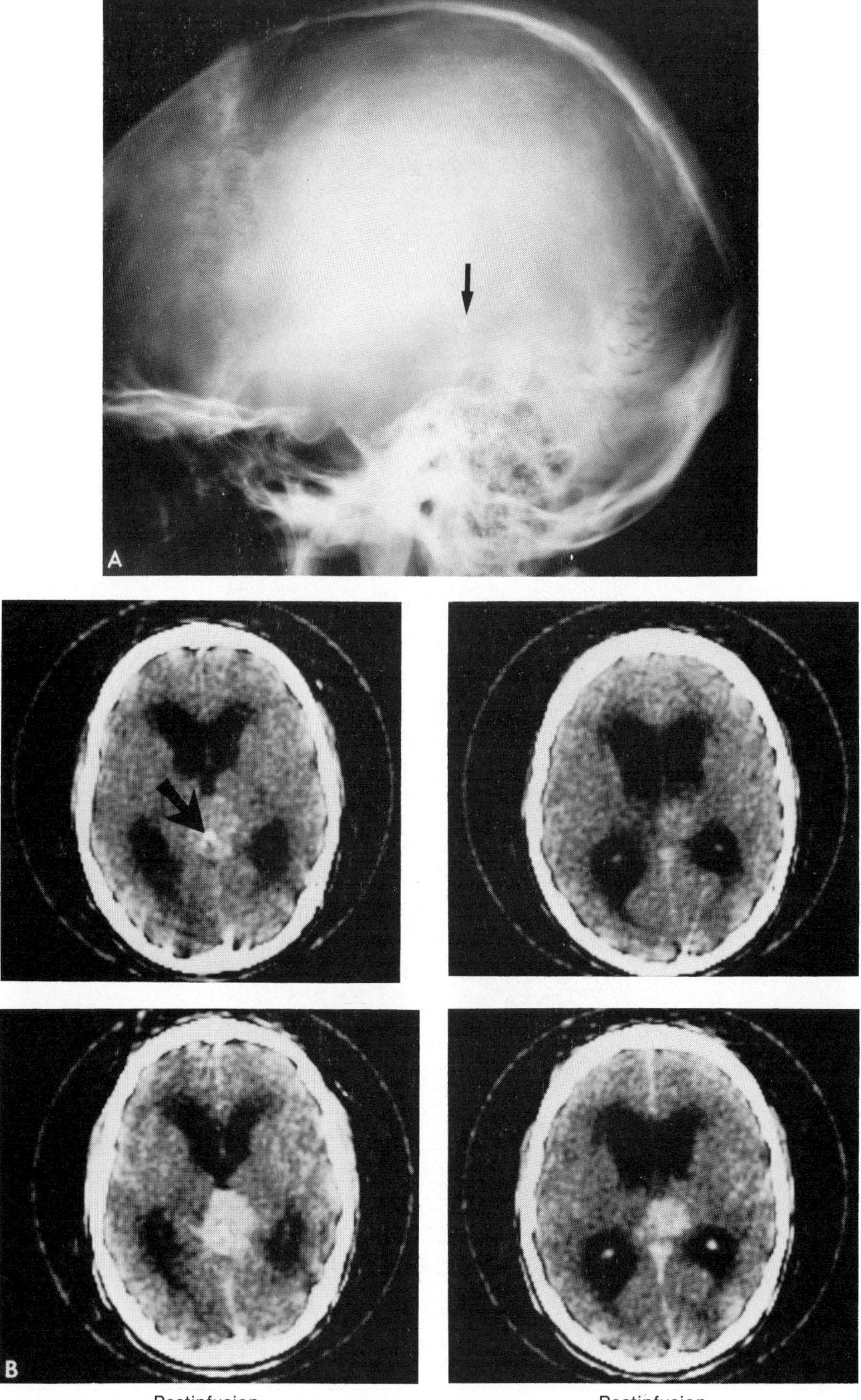

Figure 2–12. *See legend on the opposite page.*

Figure 2–12. PINEALOMA: The lateral view of the skull (*A*) reveals that the pineal gland is obviously displaced posteriorly and inferiorly (*arrow*). The sella turcica reveals truncation of the dorsum sellae and demineralization of the floor of the sella, particularly along the anterior inferior margin of the dorsum sellae.

The CT scan (*B*) reveals a mass in the region of the pineal gland that is of higher density than normal brain tissue; it also shows that the pineal gland (*arrow*) has calcified and has been displaced posteriorly and surrounded by the mass. The mass is slightly larger on the right side than on the left, and it flattens the posterior portion of the third ventricle. There is moderately severe obstructive hydrocephalus because the tumor blocks the outlet of the third ventricle and the aqueduct of Sylvius. The postinfusion scan reveals marked homogeneous enhancement of the tumor, which was found surgically to be a germinoma.

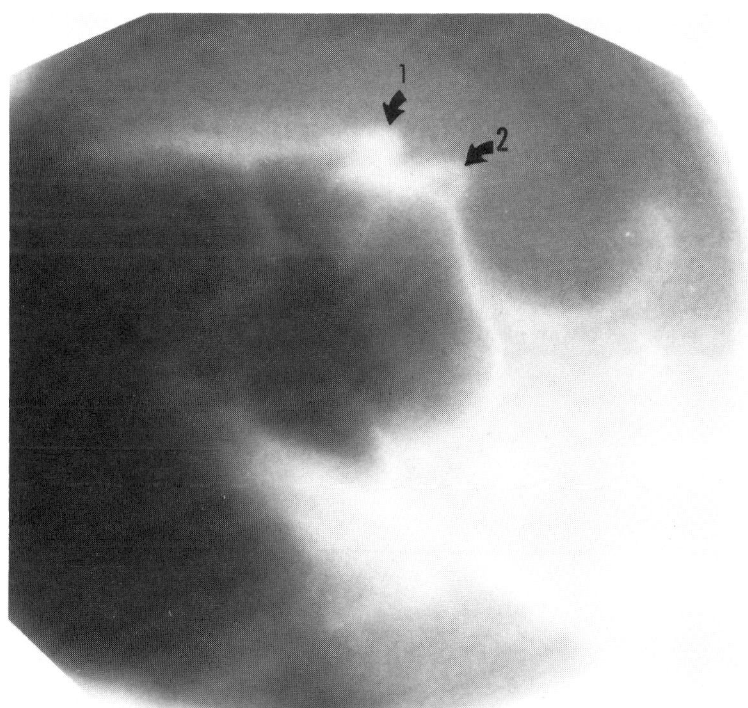

Figure 2–13. LIMBUS AND TUBERCULUM SELLAE: (1) The *limbus sphenoidalis* represents the most posterior extent of the planum sphenoidale. It is most commonly fused with and inseparable from the tuberculum sellae. However, as in this case, total fusion does not always occur. (2) The tuberculum sellae represents the actual anterior boundary of the pituitary fossa in the midline. The chiasmatic groove is of variable size and lies between the limbus and tuberculum; fusion of the two may result in flattening of the tuberculum sellae.

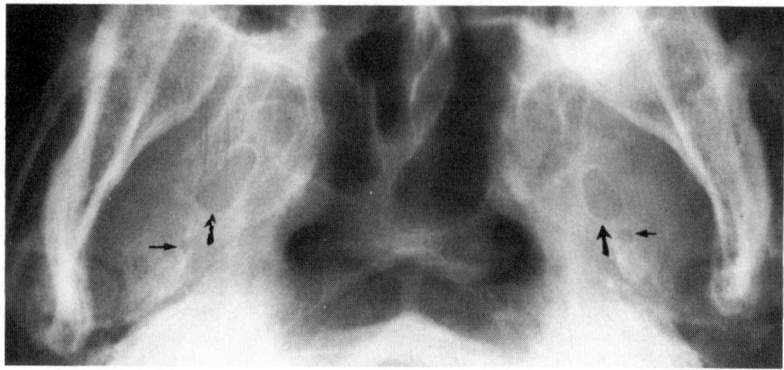

Figure 2–14. ASYMMETRIC FORAMEN OVALE: The mandibular branch of the fifth cranial nerve passes through the *foramen ovale*. The size of the foramen normally may vary from side to side, and may be divided by a calcified ligament (*large arrows*). In this case we see that the right foramen ovale is larger than the left and has a somewhat more oval configuration. This is a normal variation.

Foramen Spinosum: The middle meningeal artery passes through this foramen, which may also vary in size from side to side. In the presence of a meningioma the foramen spinosum may enlarge unilaterally to accommodate an enlarged middle meningeal artery, but this is not a reliable sign — particularly if other supporting evidence is lacking. In this case, the foramen spinosum is larger on the left side (*small arrows*) — a normal variation.

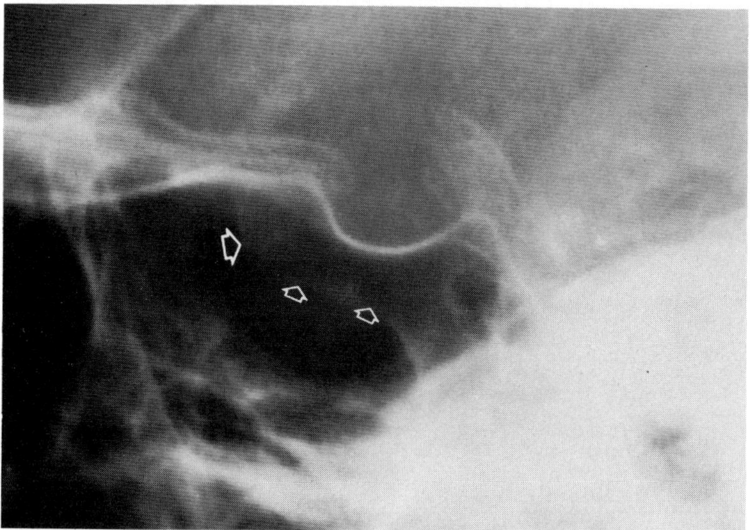

Figure 2–15. CAROTID GROOVE: The arrow heads mark the bony fossa which contains the carotid artery as it courses on either side of the sella turcica. If this groove is positioned higher it may be mistaken for a double floor of the sella. This is called the "pseudo-double floor" of the sella.

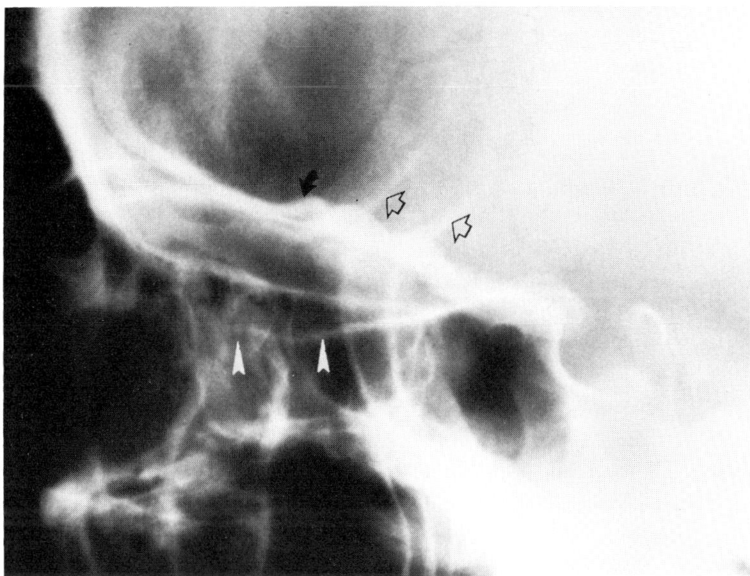

Figure 2–16. ANTERIOR CRANIAL FOSSA: The black arrow points to the irregular roofs of the orbits, which are superimposed in this view. The white arrow heads show the planum sphenoidale posteriorly and its anterior continuation, the cribriform plate. The cribriform plate is a very thin bone with multiple perforations; therefore, it is rarely seen on routine skull films and only infrequently demonstrated on tomograms. The tiny bony line between the orbital roofs and the planum sphenoidale/cribriform plate is the roof of the the ethmoid sinuses. The open arrow heads indicate the upper portions of the greater wings of the sphenoid bone bilaterally. In a true lateral projection these curvilinear lines will be superimposed.

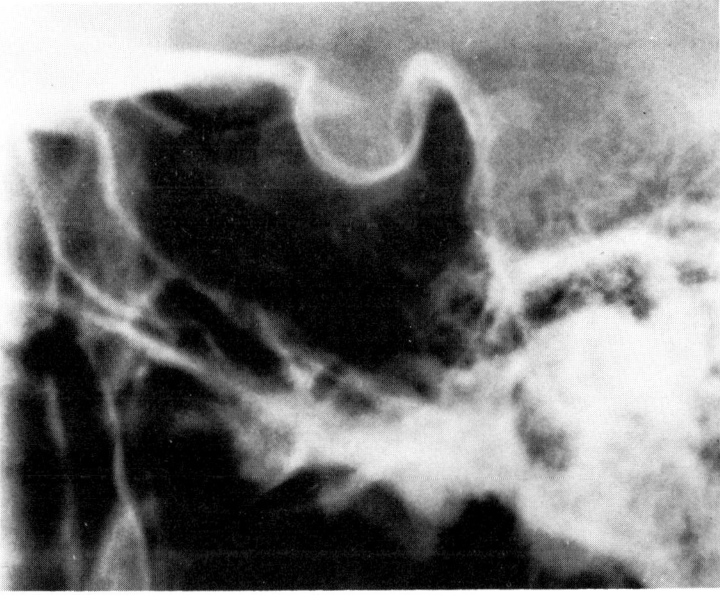

Figure 2–17. AERATED SPHENOID BONE: The entire sphenoid bone is aerated and surrounds the sella turcica.

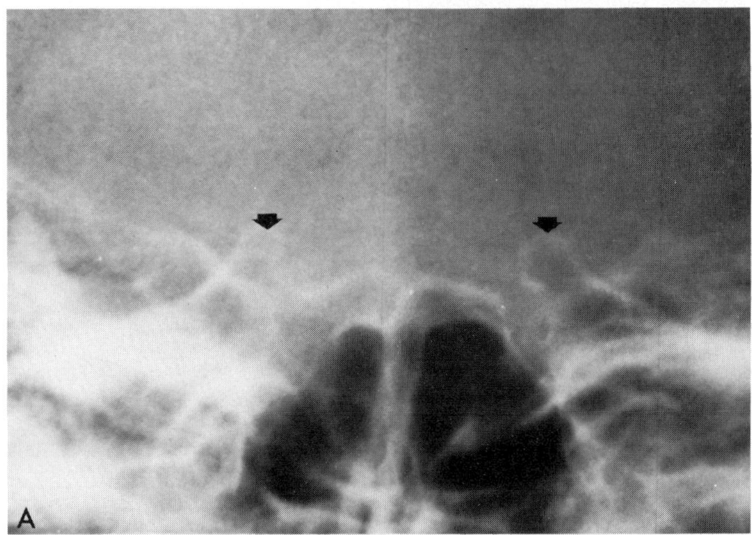

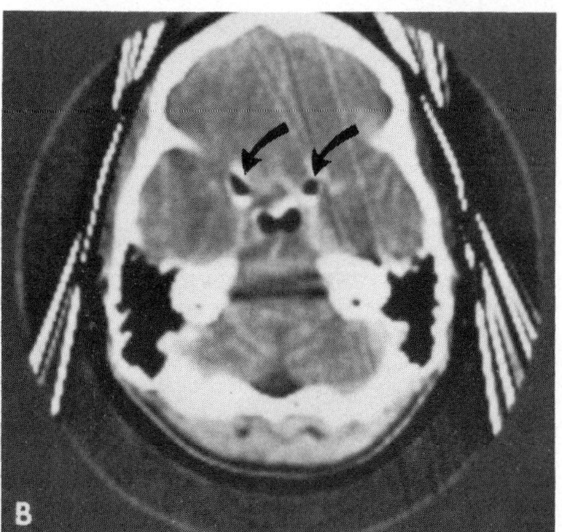

Figure 2–18. AERATED ANTERIOR CLINOIDS: The posteroanterior view of the skull (*A*) reveals the aerated anterior clinoids (*arrowheads*) bilaterally. The low cut of the CT scan (*B*) reveals both the aerated anterior clinoids (*arrows*) and the aerated dorsum sellae. Note that the mastoid air cells are particularly well developed and well aerated in this case.

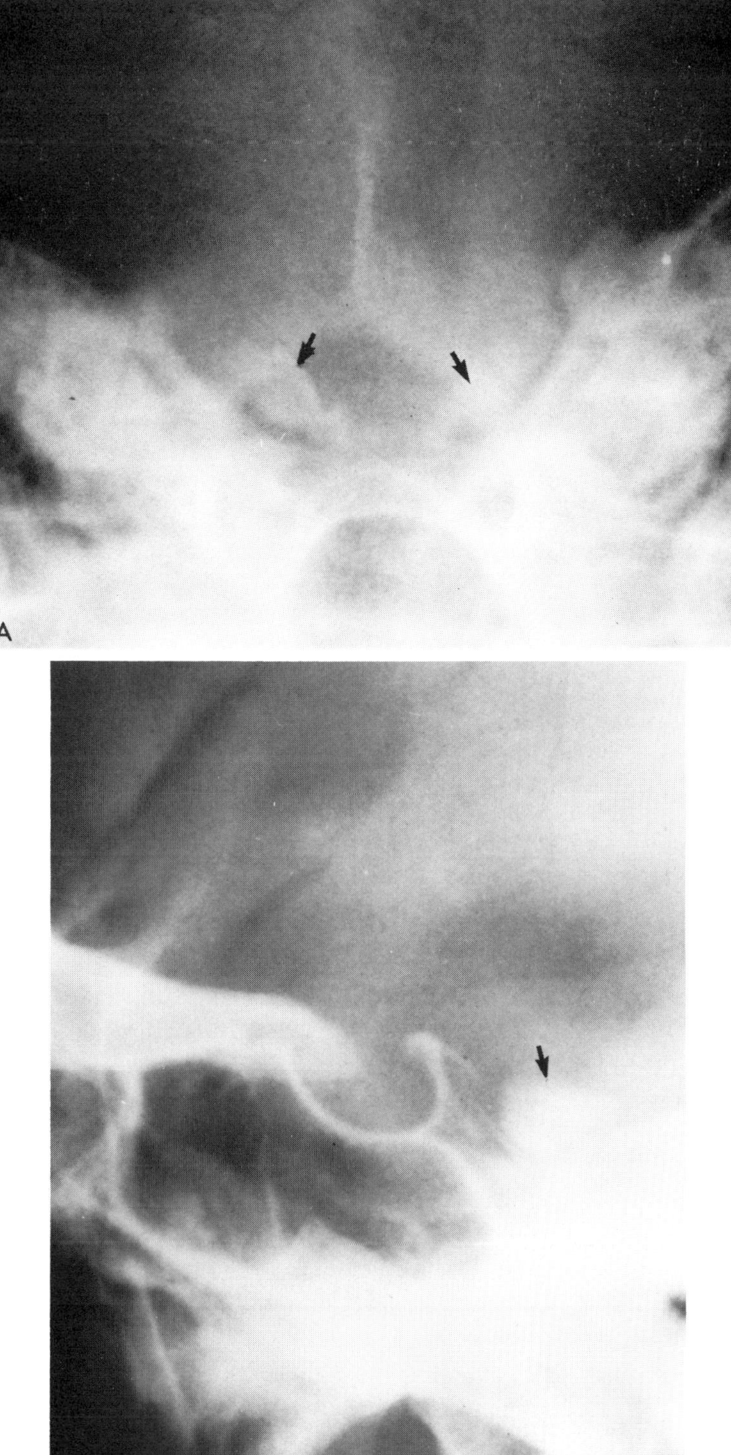

Figure 2–19. PETROCLINOID LIGAMENT: This dural reflection extends from the posterior clinoid process on each side posterolaterally to the petrous bone. It is frequently calcified and more commonly appears as a linear area of calcification. If the calcification takes on a globular appearance, it is known as "horsetail" calcification of the petroclinoid ligament. In the case shown, the horsetail calcification (*arrows*) is seen clearly on both the Towne's (*A*) and the lateral (*B*) views. A small area of linear calcification is seen on the lateral view just anterior to the larger globular area of calcification. The CT scan (*C*) also demonstrates the petroclinoid ligament calcification (*arrowheads*).

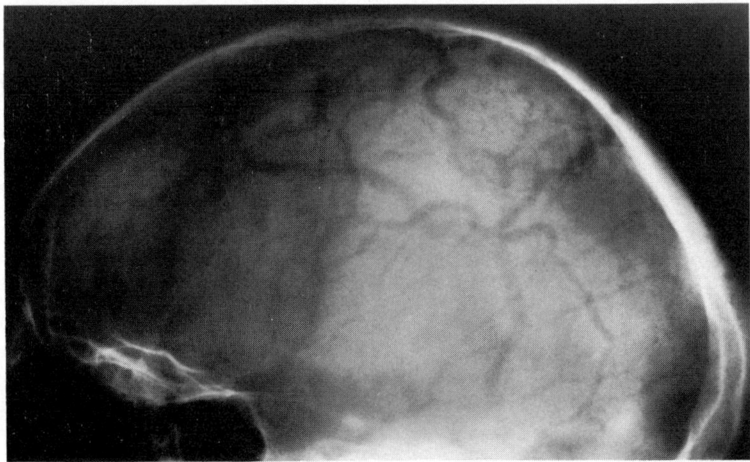

Figure 2–20. NORMAL PROMINENT VASCULAR PATTERN: The veins in the diploic space can appear very prominent in some cases. Extensive venous markings and multiple venous lakes, known as phlebectasia, are of no significance. At times it is difficult or impossible to differentiate these from multiple metastases.

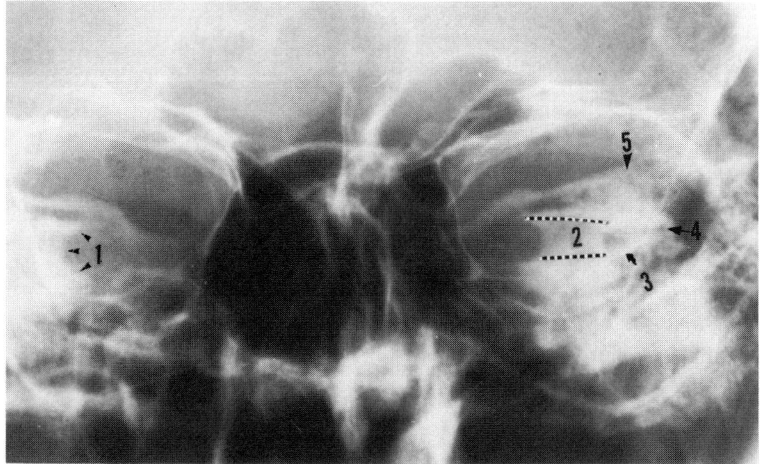

Figure 2–21. EAR STRUCTURES ON PLAIN FILM EXAMINATION: The normal ear structures are readily visualized on the standard posteroanterior skull films — particularly when the internal auditory canals (2) are projected through the center of the orbit. The posterior margin of the internal auditory canal is readily demonstrated (1). The internal auditory canal abuts on the vestibule (3), and the horizontal semicircular canal extends laterally from the vestibule (4). The superior (5) semicircular canal extends superiorly from the vestibule; it is frequently, but not always, located just below the arcuate eminence of the petrous bone.

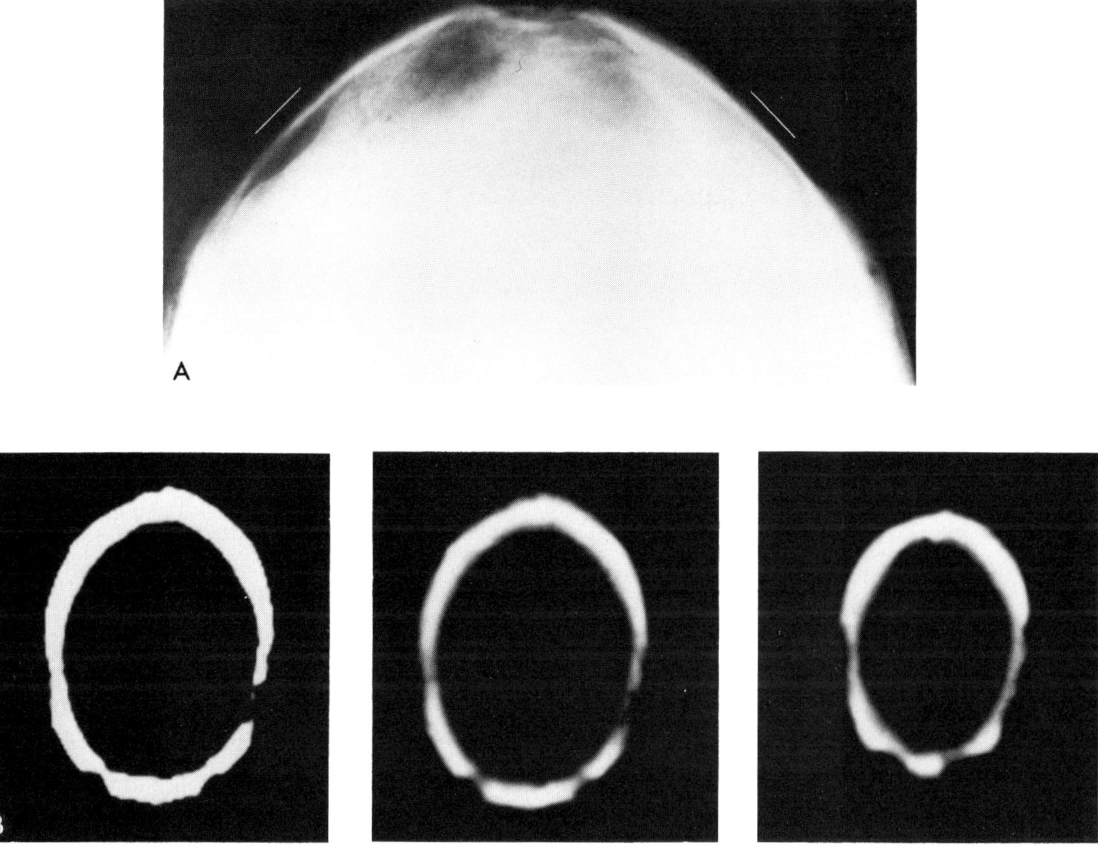

Figure 2–22. BIPARIETAL THINNING: Biparietal thinning affects the outer table of the skull; it is of no pathologic significance and its occurrence may be familial. (*A*) The plain skull film reveals bilateral thinning of the outer table of the skull. The white lines represent the anticipated position of the outer table of the skull. (*B*) CT scans of the bony calvaria demonstrate the thinning of the skull bilaterally. Note that this affects only the outer table and leaves the inner table intact.

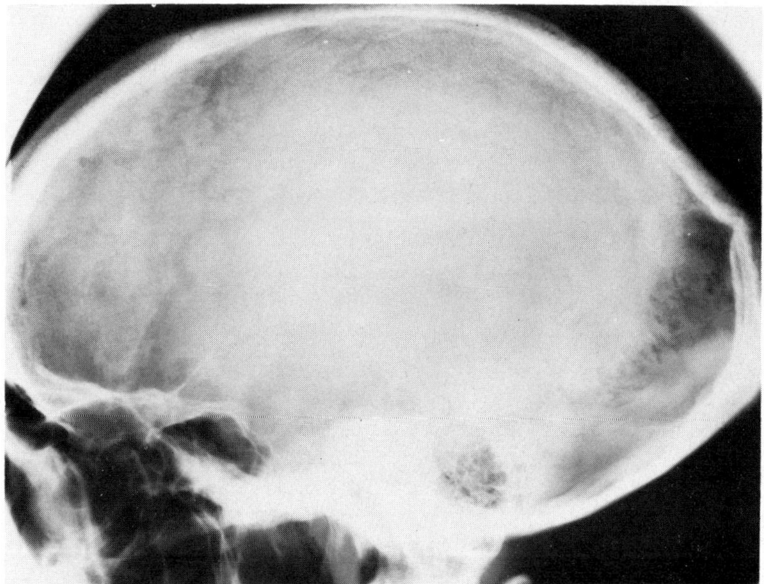

Figure 2–23. BATHROCEPHALY: The occipital bone is seen on the lateral view to protrude more posteriorly than the parietal bone at the level of the lambdoid suture. This is a normal anatomic variation.

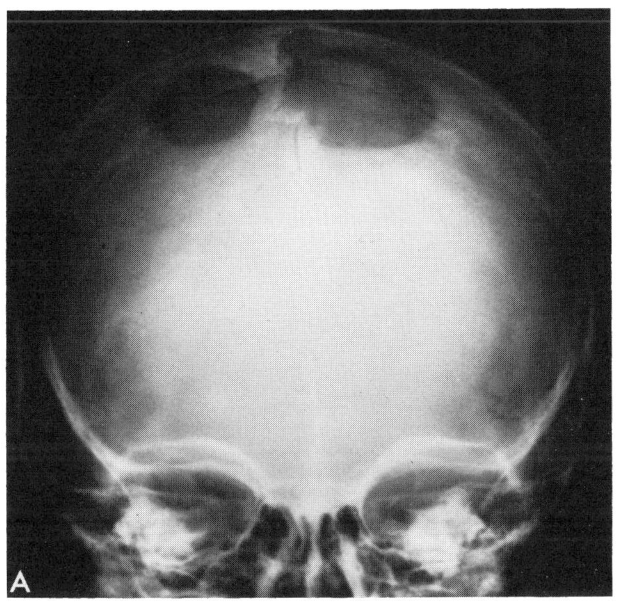

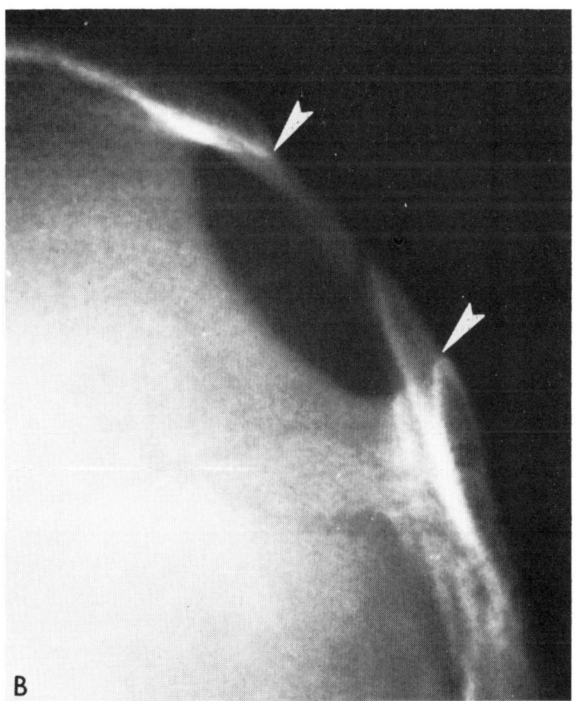

Figure 2–24, A and B. BIPARIETAL FORAMINA: These openings in the parietal region involve both the inner and outer tables of the skull. They vary in size from very small to large and are of no pathologic significance. The lateral view (*B*) demonstrates the foramina and also shows the point of meeting of the inner and outer tables of the skull (*arrows*). These foramina are also visible on CT scans.

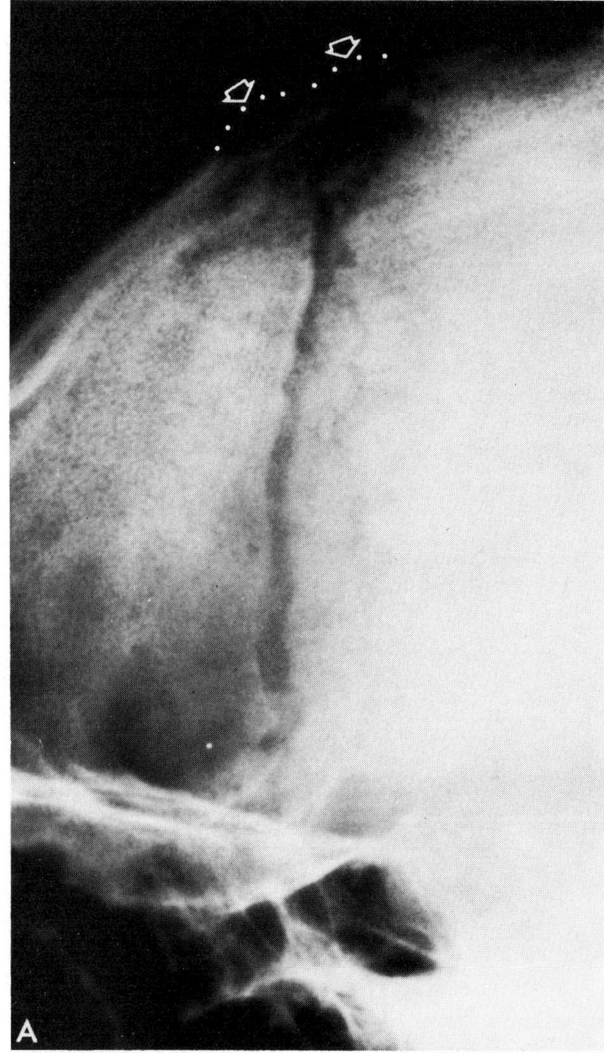

Figure 2–25. PACCHIONIAN GRANULATIONS: *A*, The arachnoid villi protrude through the dura and function to resorb the cerebrospinal fluid. These villi erode the inner table of the skull in a localized fashion (*arrows*). These areas of thinning usually are situated within 3 cm of the mid-sagittal plane in the frontal and parietal regions; they may at times be very prominent.

In the case shown, a large venous structure in the diploic space — the sphenoparietal sinus — is seen draining the pacchionian granulations in the posterior frontal region (*arrows*).

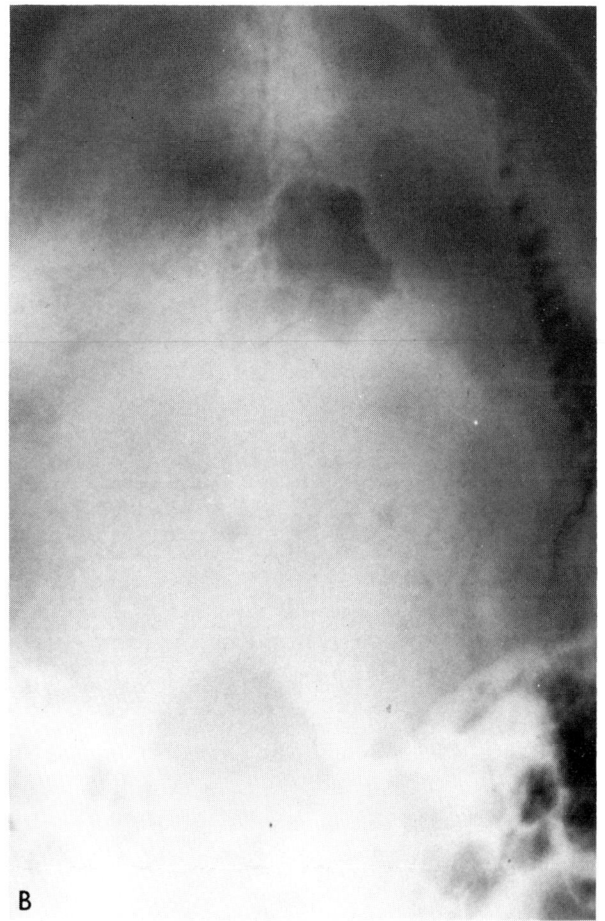

Figure 2–25 *Continued.*
B, Pacchionian granulations also may be seen in the region of the torcula, where they may be quite prominent.

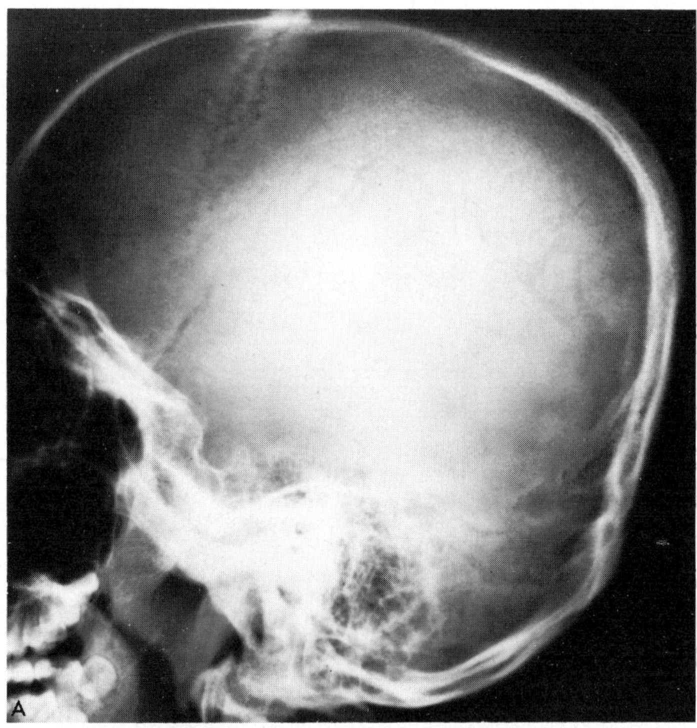

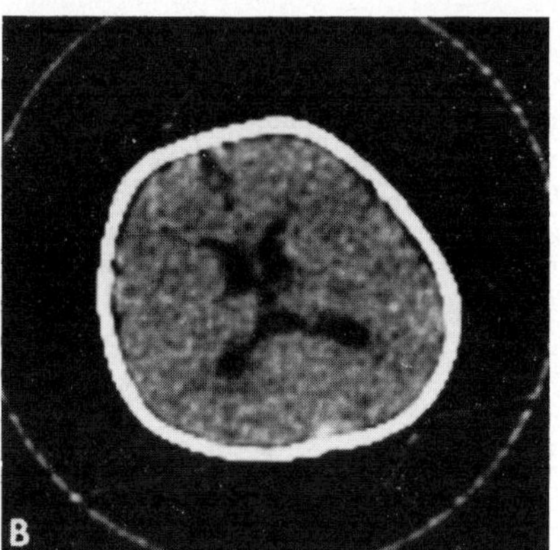

Preinfusion

Figure 2–26. BRACHIOCEPHALY: This malformation may be developmental or may be secondary to premature closure of the coronal or lambdoidal suture, which results in decreased anteroposterior length and increases in the width and height of the skull.

In this example (*A*), the head is short and wide, giving a brachiocephalic appearance; however, the back of the vault is flattened. The brachiocephalic appearance in this case, a mentally retarded patient, is secondary to prolonged periods spent lying supine.

The CT scan (*B*) is of a different patient whose brachiocephaly was developmental. Note that the cranial contents and the lateral ventricles are normal.

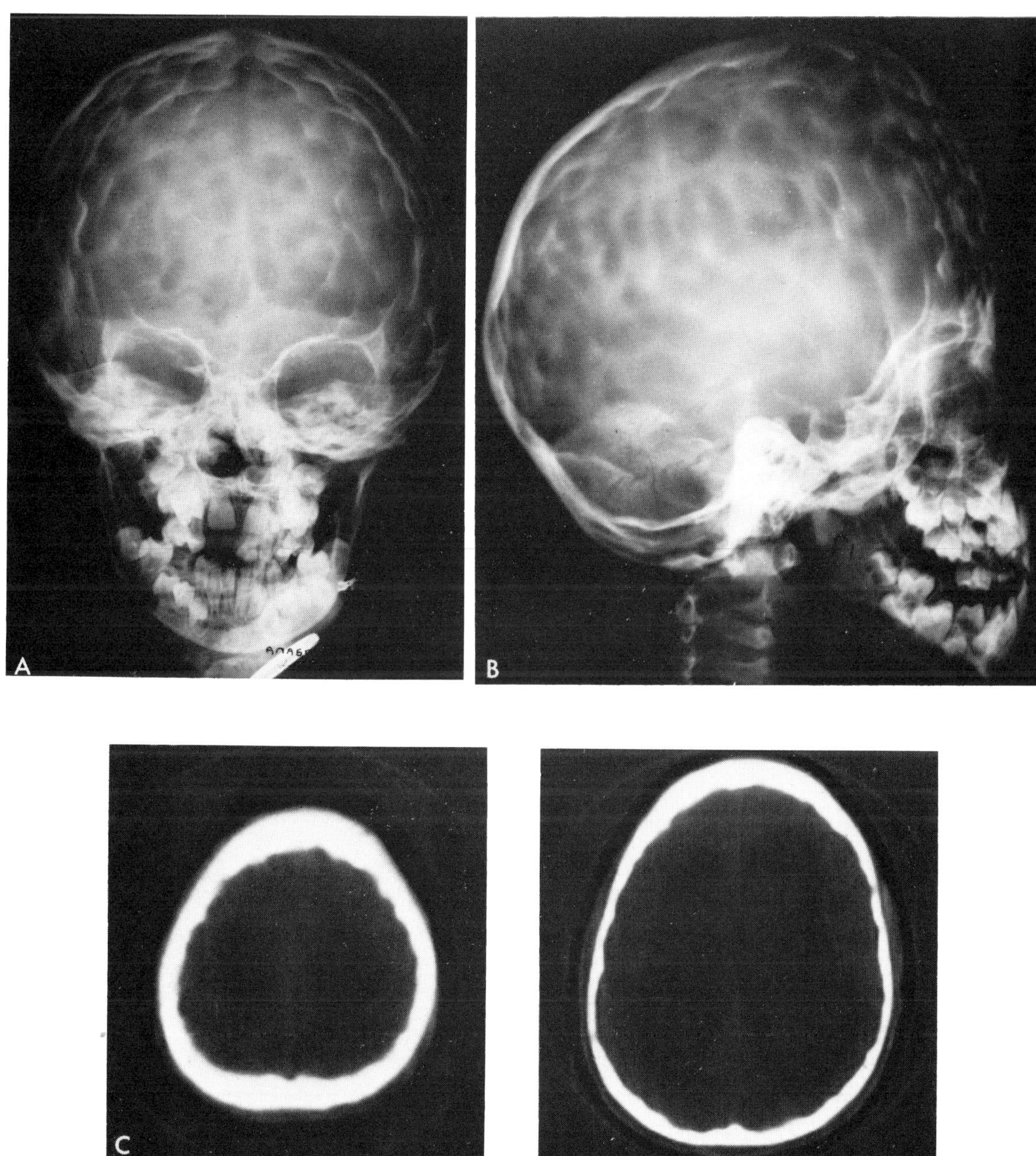

Preinfusion Preinfusion

Figure 2–27, A, B, C. TURRICEPHALY: Premature closure of the lambdoid suture causes a short, wide and high cranial vault. Note also the marked prominence of the digital markings of the skull. The CT scans (*C*) also demonstrate these pronounced digital markings.

Trigonocephaly results in a pointed appearance of the forehead. It is secondary to premature closure of the metopic suture. (No example shown.)

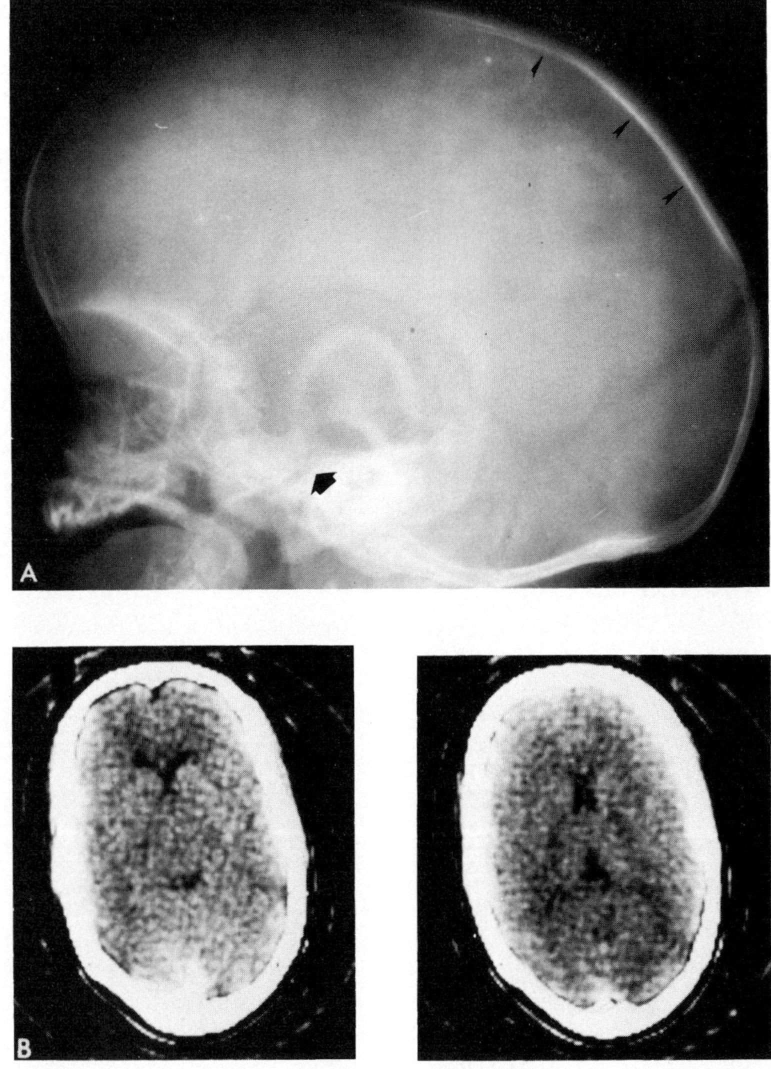

Figure 2–28. *A,* DOLICHOCEPHALY: Premature closure of the sagittal suture results in compensatory excessive growth of the sutures perpendicular to it (i.e., coronal and lambdoid). This results in an elongated but narrow skull: i.e., dolichocephalic craniostenosis. In some individuals a mild degree of dolichocephaly appears to be developmental, as there is no premature suture closure.

B, CT scans reflect the radiographic appearance of the bony calvaria, but the cranial contents otherwise appear to be normal.

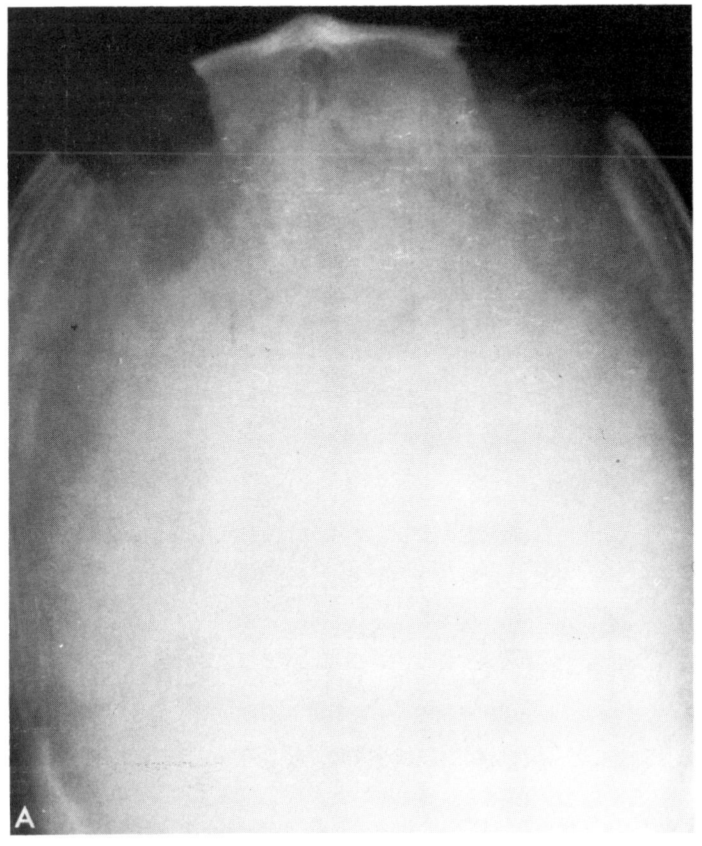

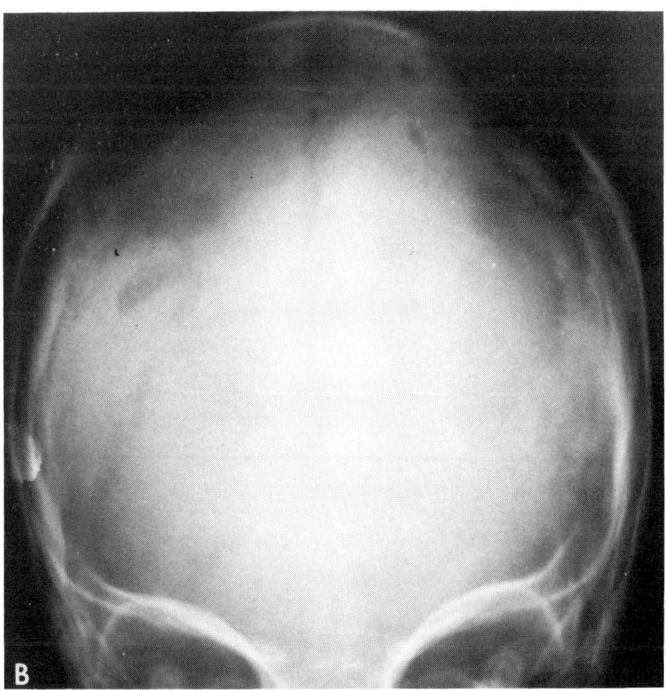

Figure 2–29. *A*, MORCELLATION PROCEDURE: The surgical treatment for dolichocephalic craniostenosis involves placement of long cuts in the skull in the parasagittal areas bilaterally. This allows the skull to grow in the transverse direction. A later film (*B*) demonstrates partial bony overgrowth of the surgical incisions. (Case courtesy of Drs. Oscar Sugar and Glen Dobben.)

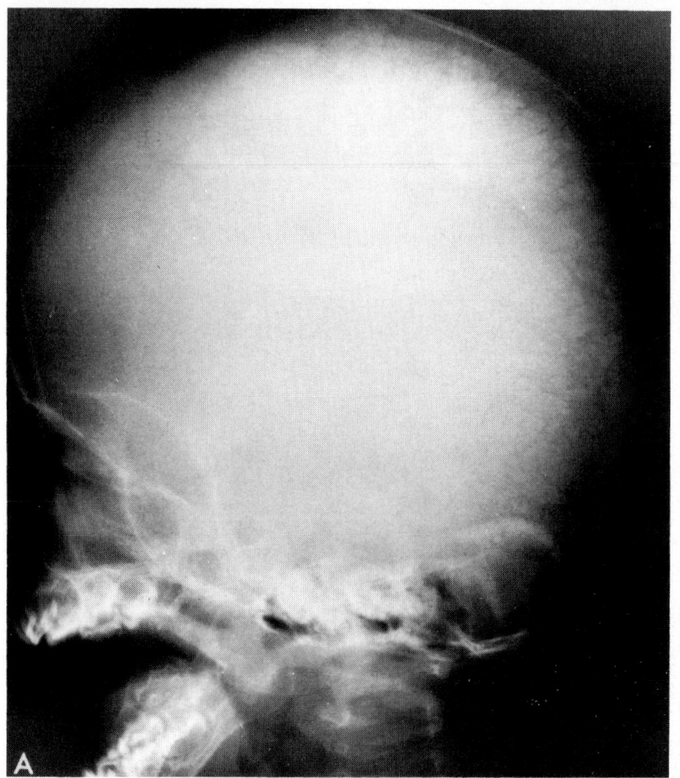

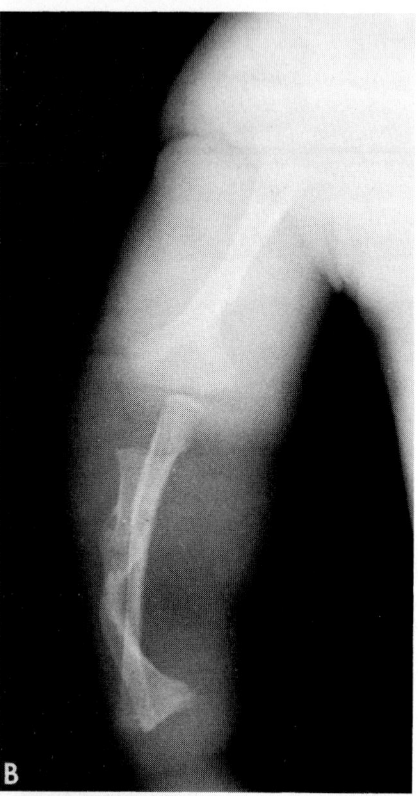

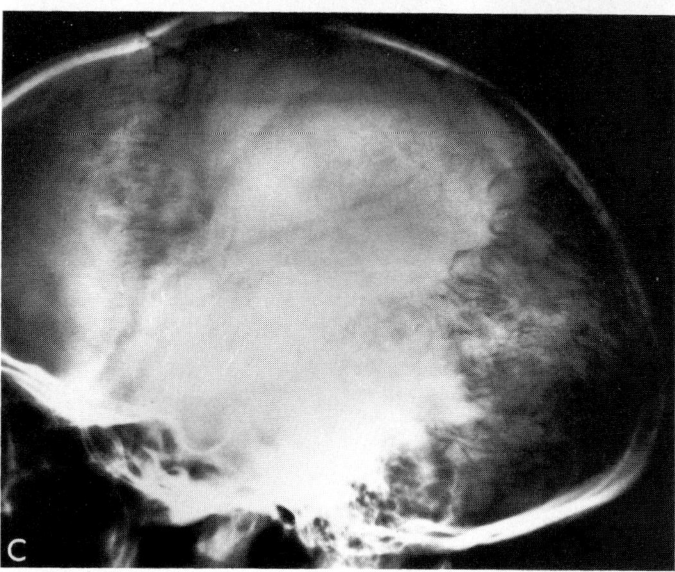

Figure 2–30. WORMIAN BONES: These intrasutural bones are small, irregular islands of bones that occur most commonly in the lambdoid suture. The number of bones is highly variable, and bones may be found in normal individuals. They are also found in other conditions such as cleidocranial dysostosis, cretinism, osteogenesis imperfecta and chronic hydrocephalus as well as less common disease processes.

A, In this example, the patient, in addition to multiple wormian bones, also has marked thinning of the bony calvaria secondary to osteogenesis imperfecta.

B, The same patient demonstrates multiple long bone fractures following minimal trauma.

C, Innumerable wormian bones are present in the coronal, sagittal, and lambdoid sutures. The etiology is unknown in this normal individual. (Case courtesy of Dr. Kenneth D. Schmidt.)

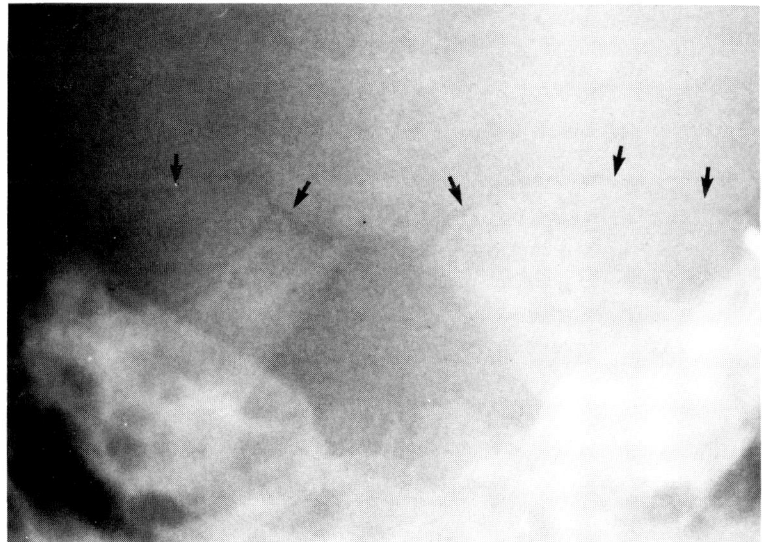

Figure 2–31. OCCIPITAL SYNCHONDROSIS: This Towne's view of a dry pediatric skull demonstrates the synchondrosis between the supra- and exoccipital portions of the occipital bone.

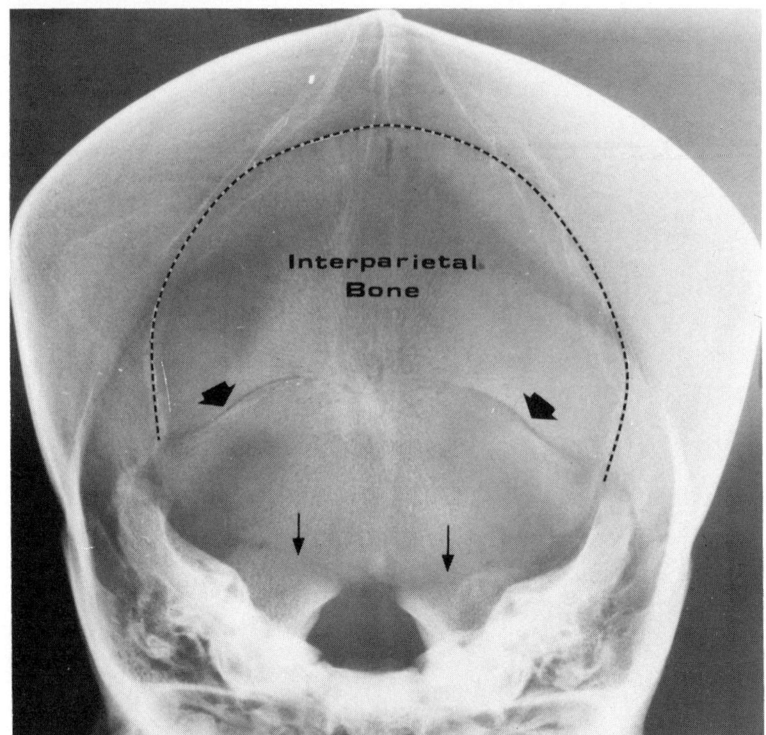

Figure 2–32. OCCIPITAL BONE: The dotted line follows the lambdoid suture. The large black arrowheads demonstrate the mendosal suture. The interparietal portion of the occipital bone develops in membranous bone; if the mendosal suture fails to fuse, this portion of the occipital bone becomes known as the interparietal bone. Beneath the mendosal suture the supraoccipital portion of the occipital bone is seen; it is separated from the exoccipital portion of the occipital bone by the synchondrosis between the two (*small arrows*). Both the synchondrosis and the mendosal suture may be mistaken for fractures. The mendosal suture may be present unilaterally, in which case differentiation from fracture may be quite difficult.

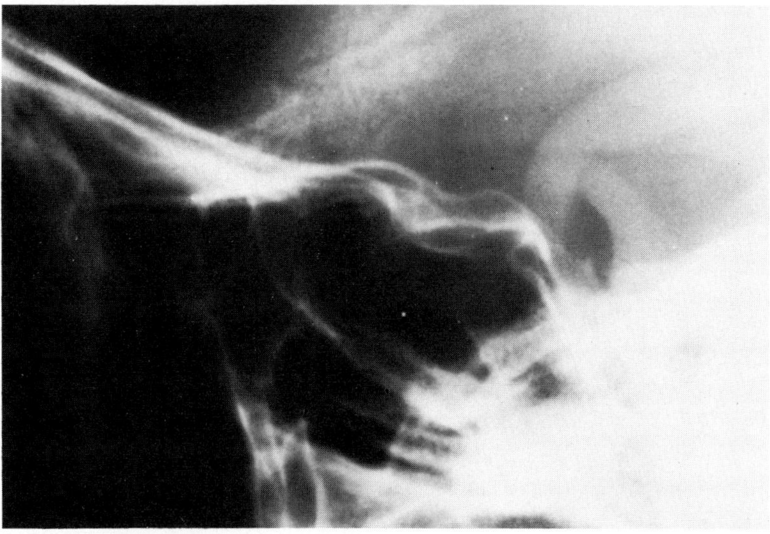

Figure 2–33. SMALL SELLA TURCICA: This patient demonstrates a developmentally small sella of no pathologic significance. In this case there is also calcification of the interclinoid ligament.

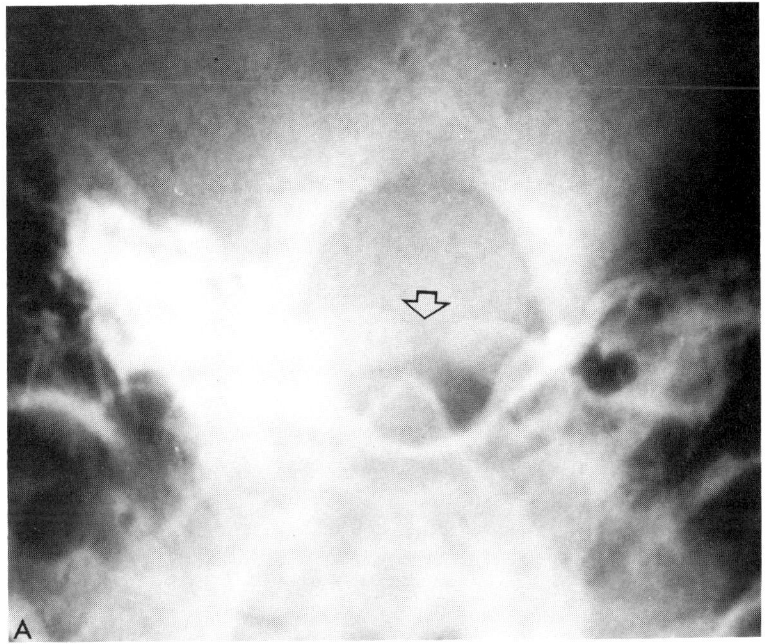

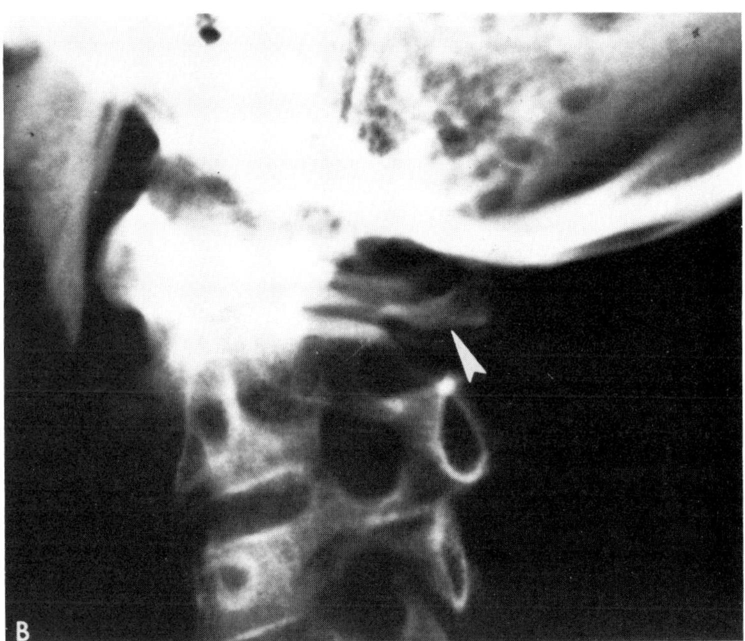

Figure 2–34. UNOSSIFIED POSTERIOR ARCH OF C_1: *A*, The Towne's view of the skull demonstrates the unossified mid-portion of the posterior arch of C_1. The posterior arch of C_2 can be seen just inferior to the arch of C_1. *B*, The lateral view in another patient demonstrates that the white line marking the point of fusion between the laminae of either arch is not present, owing to a failure of fusion of the posterior margin of the arch similar to that demonstrated in *A*. This is of no pathologic significance, and the visualized bony structures are held in place by fibrous bands.

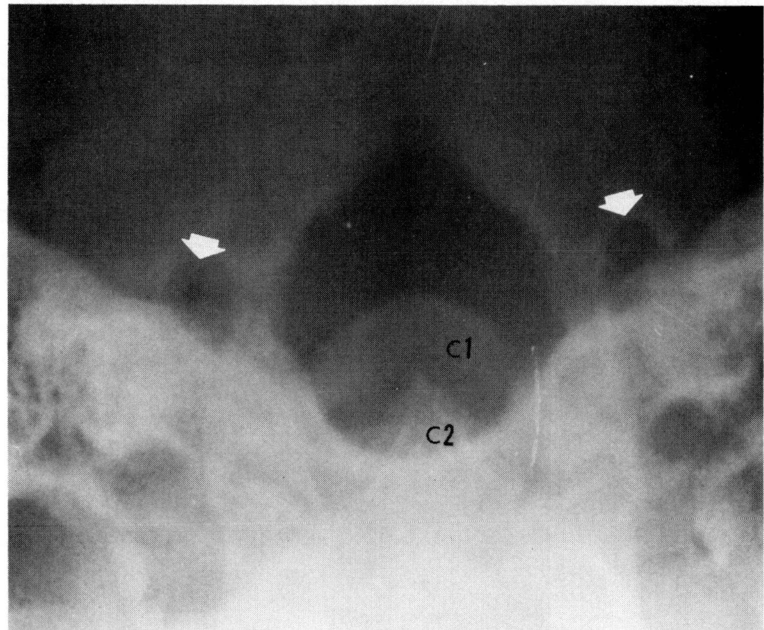

Figure 2–35. CONDYLOID FORAMEN: At the point where the atlas articulates with the occiput there is a fossa for the lateral masses of the atlas. In some cases (*arrows*) a foramen actually develops. The foramen is bridged by fibrous tissue and should not be mistaken for lytic lesions of the skull. The posterior arch of both C_1 and C_2 can be seen through the foramen magnum.

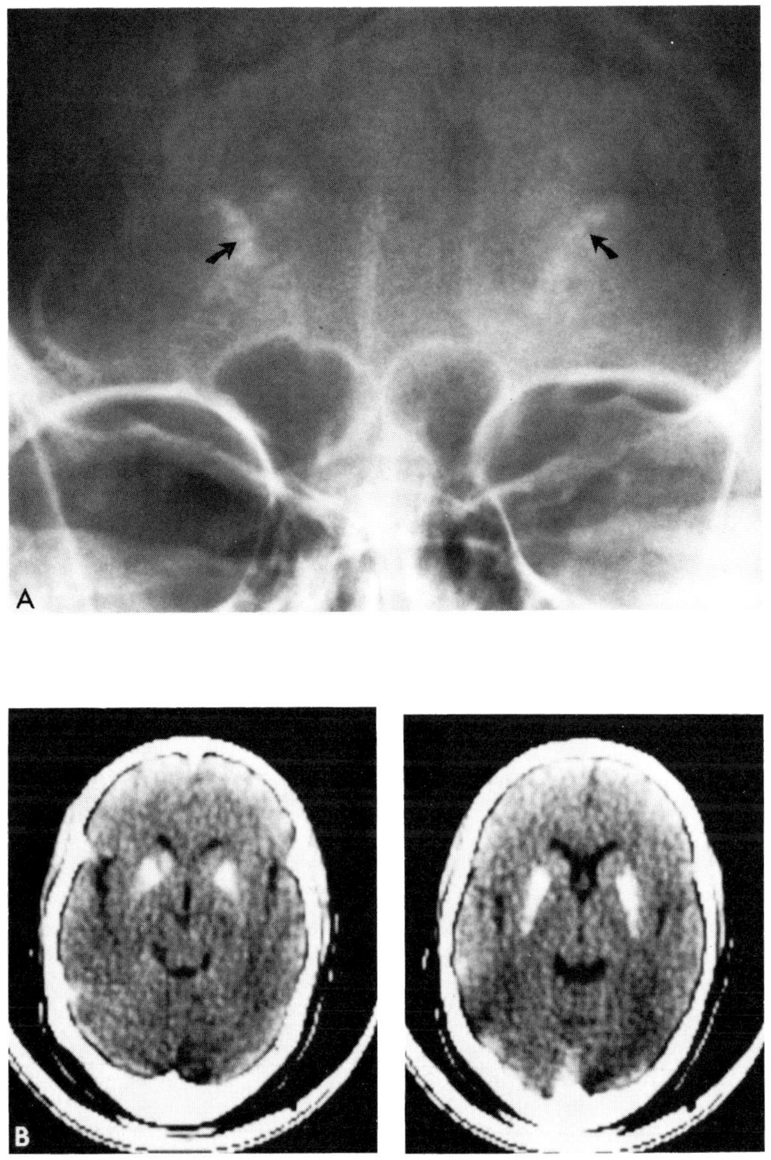

Figure 2–36. BASAL GANGLIA CALCIFICATION: *A*, These calcifications may be readily visible (*arrows*) or, more commonly, only faintly visible or invisible on skull radiographs. These areas of calcification may also present in the dentate nucleus of the cerebellum. *B*, The calcifications are readily visible on the CT scans — even when they are seen only faintly or not at all on plain film radiography. Basal ganglia calcifications may be seen with a variety of conditions, including: hypoparathyroidism; pseudohypoparathyroidism; Fahr's syndrome; Cockayne's syndrome and other less common diseases. It also may be idiopathic.

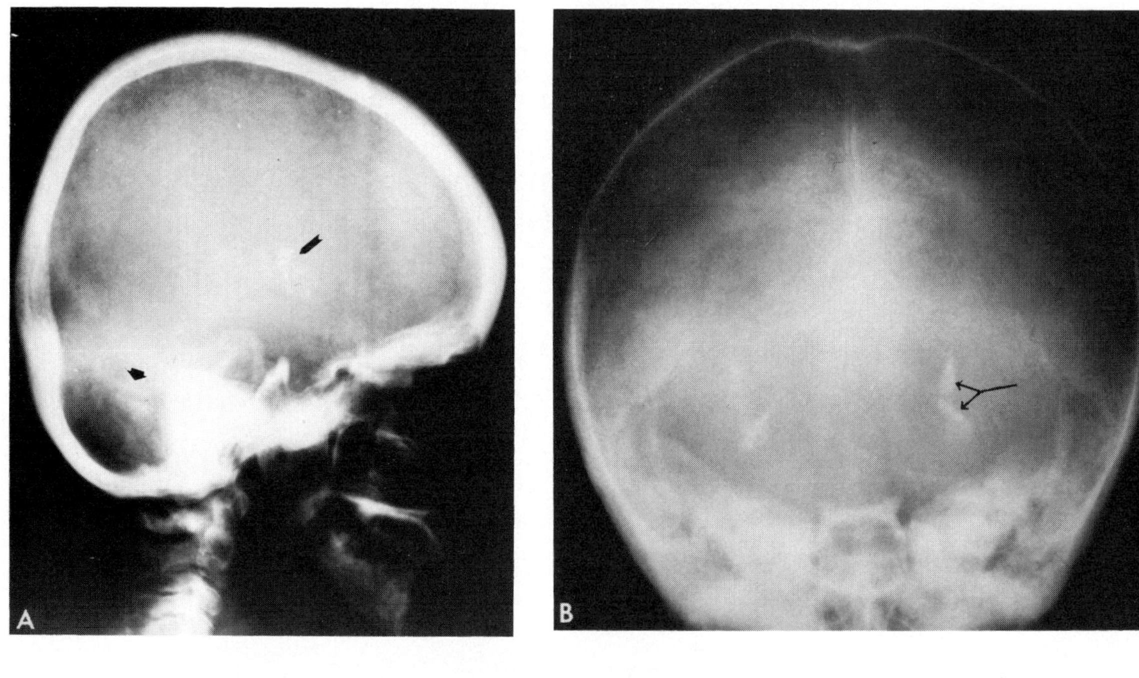

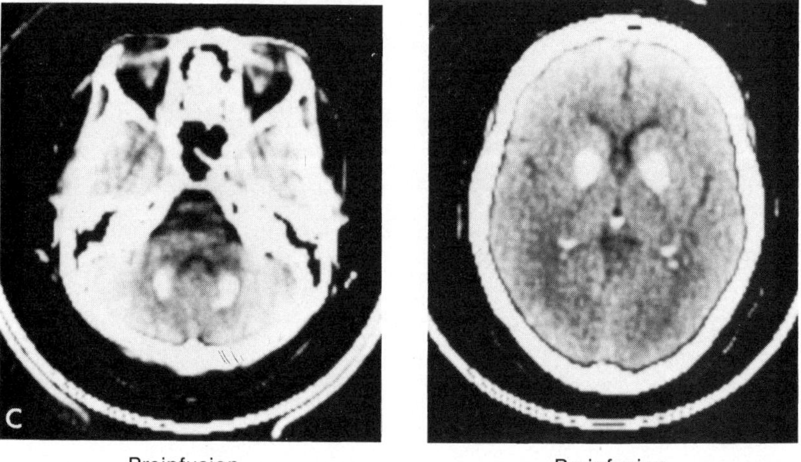

Figure 2–37. BASAL GANGLIA AND DENTATE NUCLEUS CALCIFICATION: *A*, The lateral view of the skull demonstrates readily visible basal ganglia and dentate nucleus calcification (*arrows*). *B*, The Towne's view of the skull reveals that the two areas of calcification are now superimposed (*double-headed arrows*). *C*, Small areas of calcification not apparent on the skull film may be demonstrated on the CT scan. At times, even relatively extensive areas of calcification may be present that are not readily apparent on skull films except, perhaps, in retrospect. The patient shown here had a clinical diagnosis of progeria.

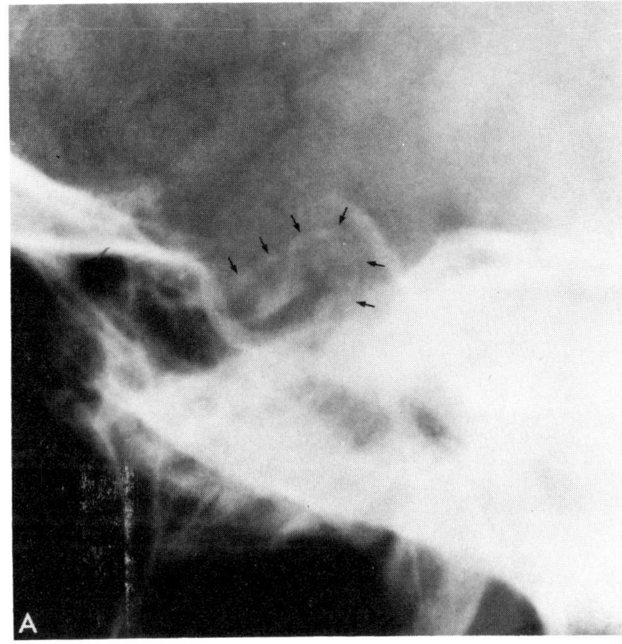

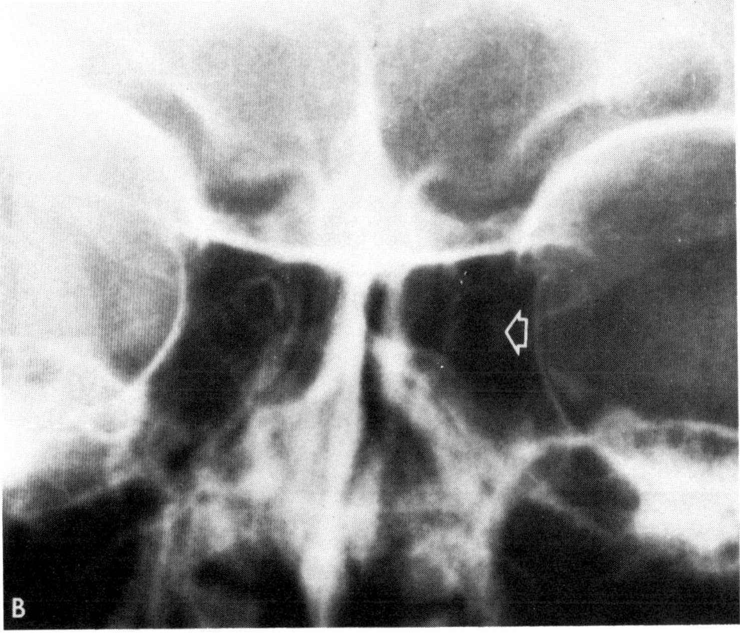

Figure 2–38. CALCIFIED CAVERNOUS CAROTID ARTERY: *A*, The curvilinear areas of calcification of the cavernous carotid artery are readily visualized in this example. *B*, On the posteroanterior views they are viewed end-on and appear as rounded circles of calcification — in this case seen bilaterally through the sphenoid sinus in the parasellar area (arrow is on the left-sided calcification).

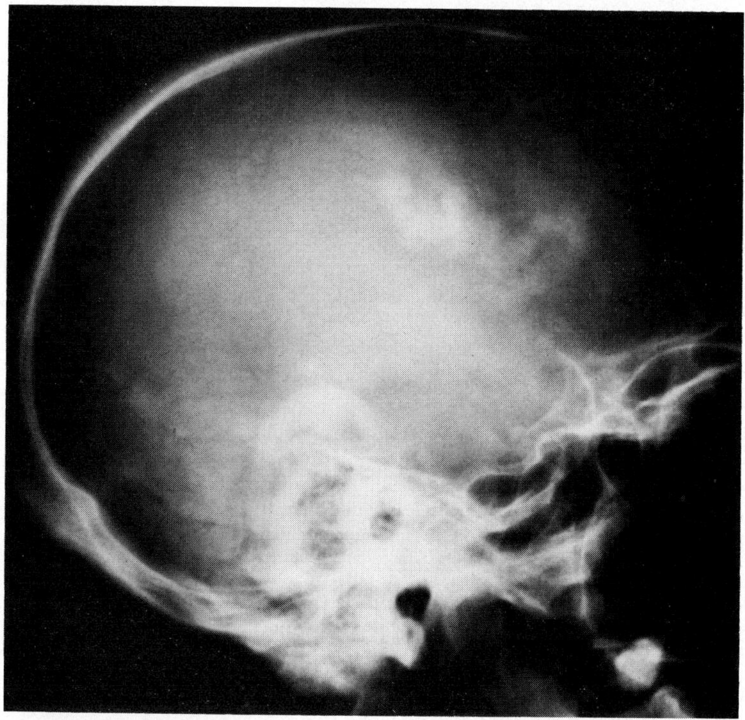

Figure 2–39. BRAIDS OF HAIR: Braided locks of hair may project over the skull and give the appearance of osteoblastic metastatic lesions. However, their appearance is changeable and not reproducible on multiple views, and close examination of the films reveals their true nature. These hair braids may be multiple, and better evaluation of the bony calvaria can be obtained if the hair is unbraided before radiography.

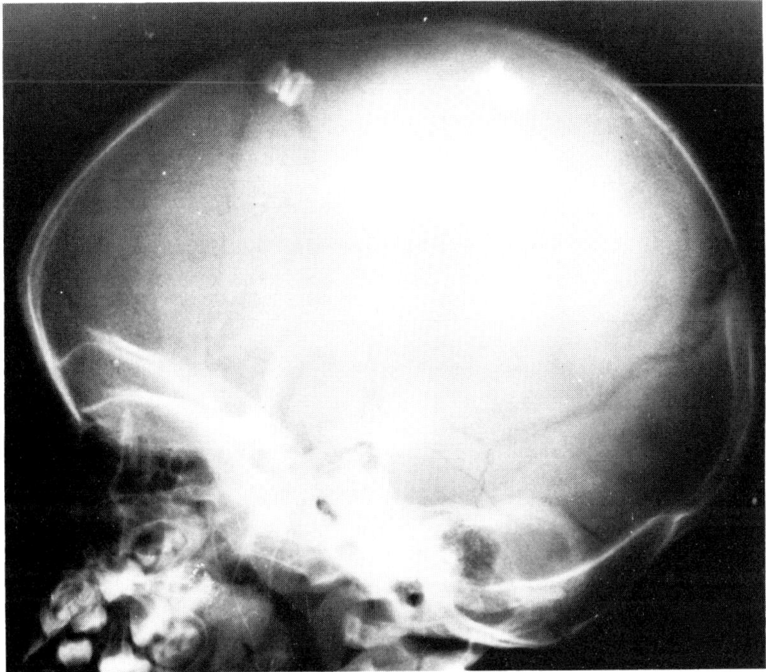

Figure 2–40. RUBBER BANDS: Rubber bands on the hair also may give the false appearance of metastatic lesions involving the bony calvaria.

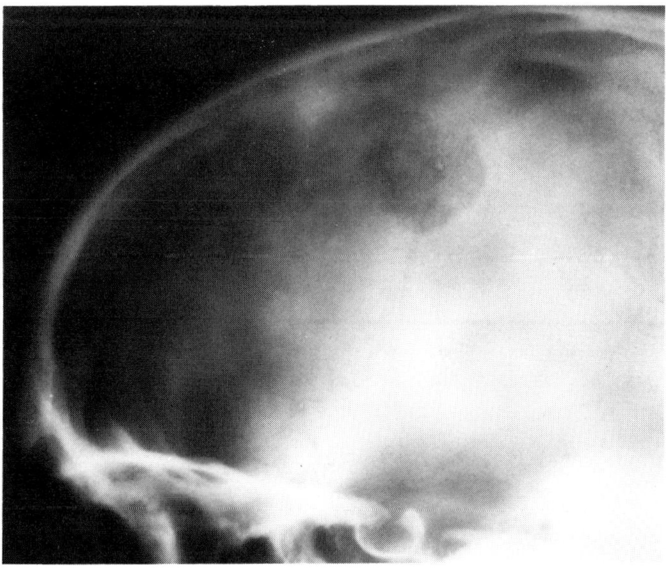

Figure 2–41. CAVERNOUS HEMANGIOMA: The lesion is lucent with a border that is smooth and well defined but not sclerotic. The area of lucency frequently has a granular or salt-and-pepper appearance. Hemangiomas may demonstrate a "spoke-wheel" appearance. These are benign lesions and vary greatly in size. There may be a vascular groove which drains away from the hemangioma.

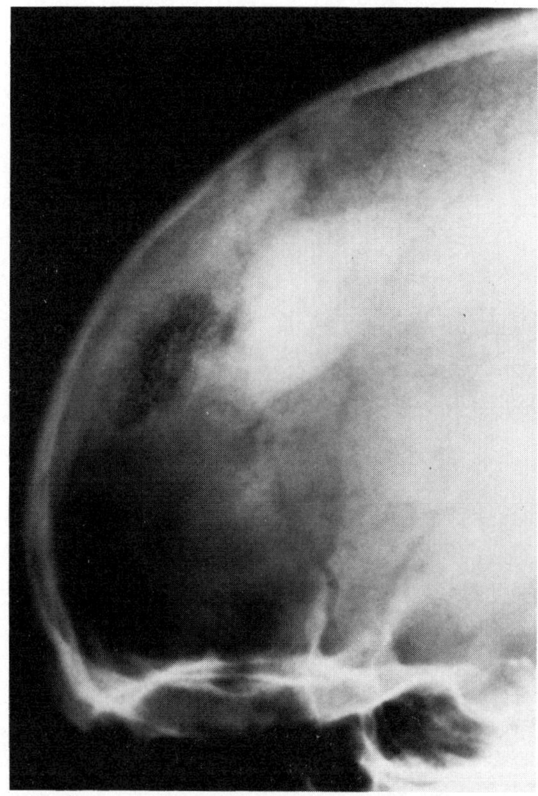

Figure 2–42. CAVERNOUS HEMANGIOMA AND OSTEOMA: There is a lucent defect in the midfrontal region with a well defined border and a granular appearance. In addition, there is an osteoma which involves the outer table of the skull just posterior to the hemangioma. The osteoma is typical in that the density is quite high and the border is well defined; however, it is not typical because the border is irregular — not rounded, as is usually the case.

Osteomas usually involve the outer table of the skull; they may involve the inner table and, rarely, the diploë. A tangential view may reveal a radiolucent line at the base of the osteoma. Osteomas are very dense, have a well defined margin and arise abruptly from the bony calvaria. An osteoma of the inner table may be difficult to differentiate from a meningioma without the aid of a CT scan.

The CT scan reveals a well defined high density bony lesion arising from the outer or inner table of the skull. Osteomas may also be identified in the diploë of the skull on the CT scan.

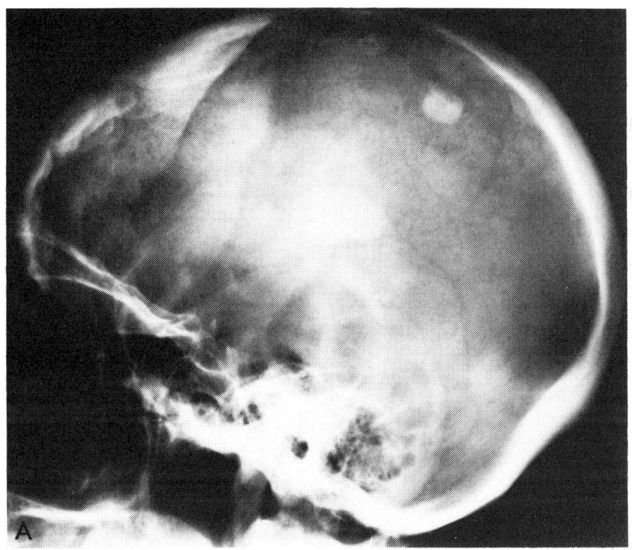

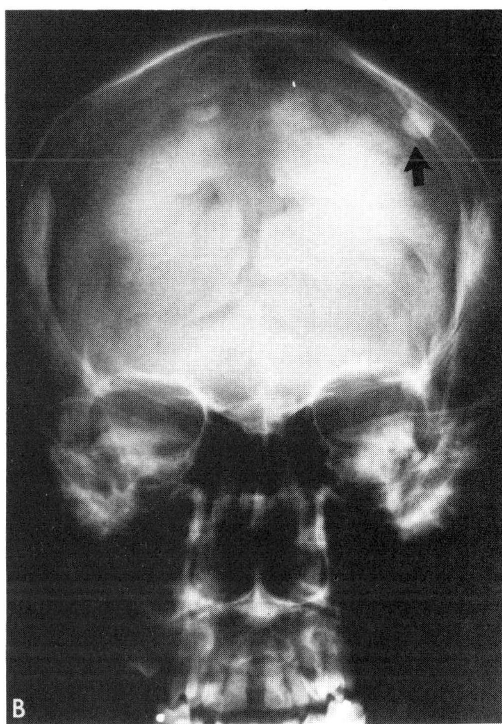

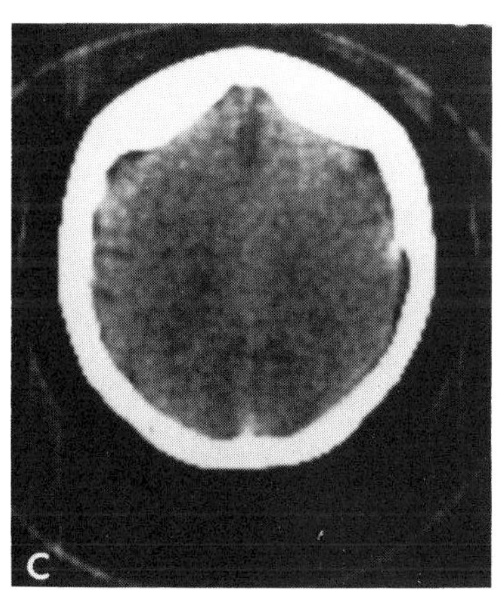

Preinfusion

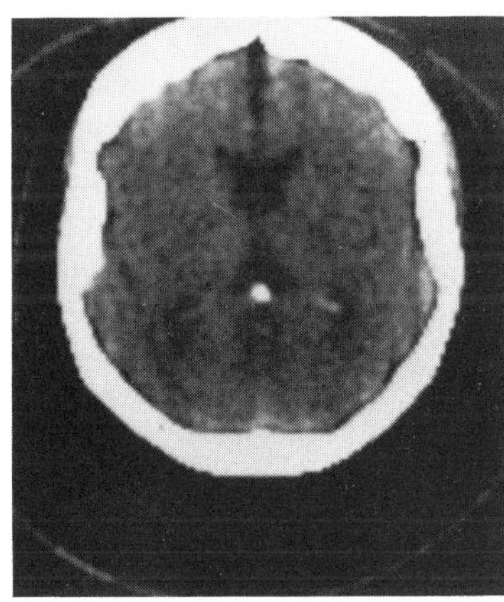

Preinfusion

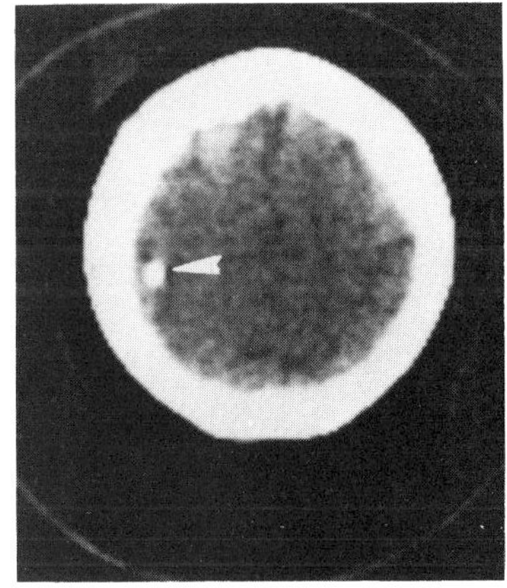

Preinfusion

Figure 2–43. OSTEOMA OF THE INNER TABLE OF THE SKULL AND DIFFUSE HYPEROSTOSIS: *A*, The plain skull film demonstrates a small osteoma in the midparietal region on the lateral view. *B*, The osteoma also can be seen arising from the inner table of the skull on the posteroanterior view. *C*, CT scans also reveal the osteoma high in the left parietal region *(arrow)*. The osteoma is of high density, is not associated with edema and does not change following the infusion of contrast material.

In addition to the osteoma there is marked thickening of the inner table of the skull in the frontal region bilaterally. Note that in the posteroanterior view the hyperostosis does not cross the midline. This is a typical appearance of "hyperostosis frontalis interna," a process that affects the inner table of the skull, has curvilinear margins and does not cross the midline because of the dural reflection of the falx. This process of hyperostosis is more common in older women and is most common in the frontal region. This process of hyperostosis may affect other areas of the skull — as seen in this case, where the parietal and temporal areas are involved along with the frontal region. If other areas are affected it should not be considered a separate process, but rather a process similar to that seen in the frontal region.

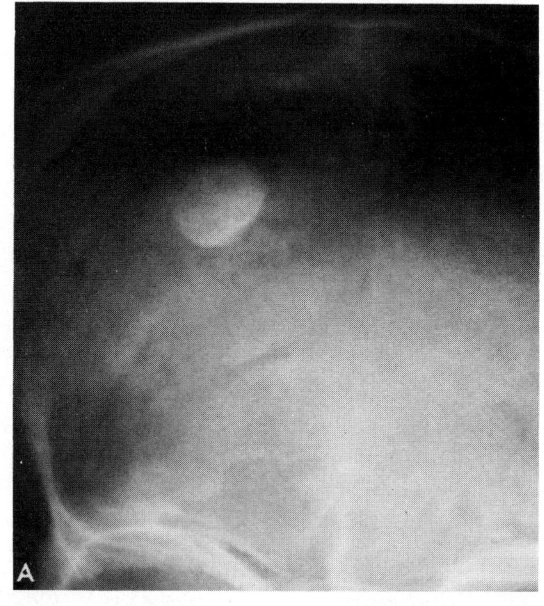

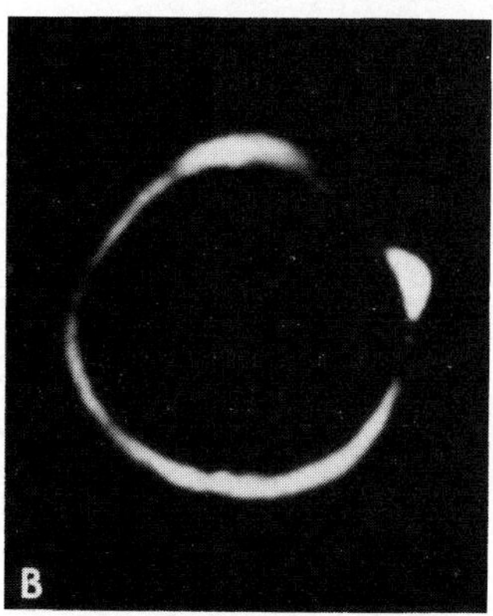

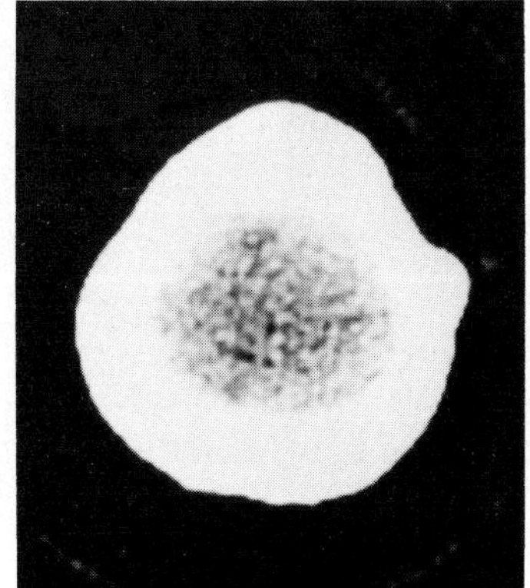

Figure 2–44. OSTEOMA: *A*, The plain skull film reveals a well defined area of bony density arising from the outer table of the skull. *B*, The osteoma is demonstrated on the CT scan in another patient.

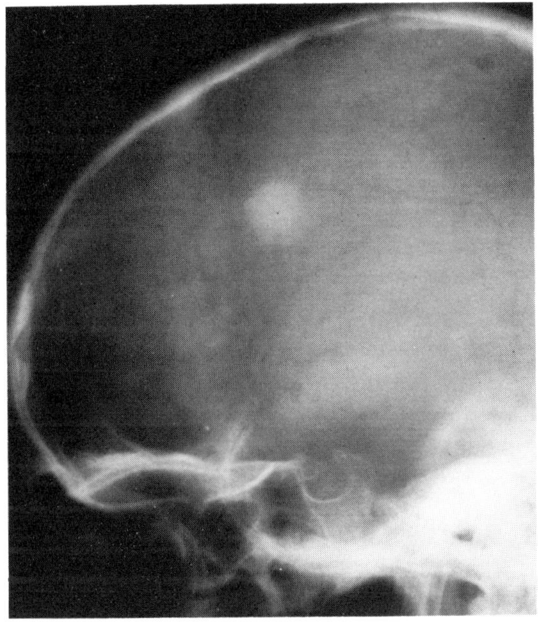

Figure 2–45. SEBACEOUS CYST: The plain skull series reveals a high density lesion; but the density is not that of bone, and the margins are rather indistinct. This is a sebaceous adenoma of the scalp. It could be readily palpated and moved with the skin of the scalp. It may be difficult to differentiate the two radiographically.

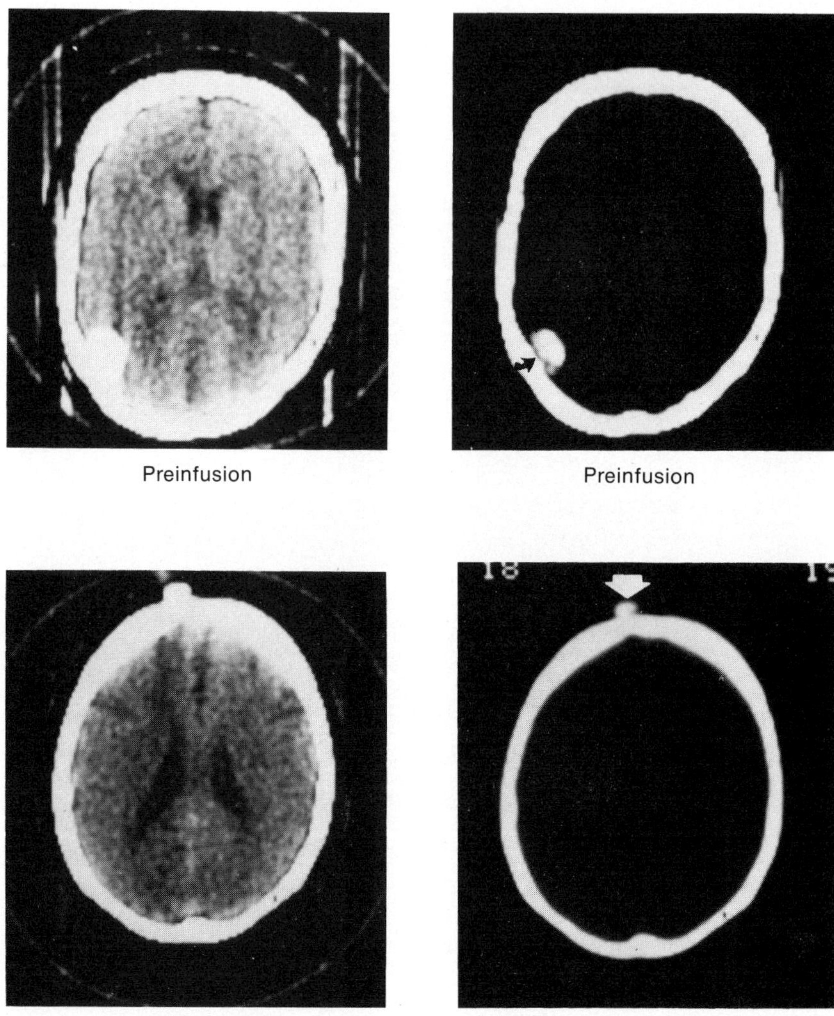

Figure 2–46. CT OF AN OSTEOMA: The osteoma *(arrowhead)* is of bone density, and the thin radiolucent line can be identified at the base of the lesion on the high window level views. The appearance is typical of an osteoma.

In these examples from different individuals, one osteoma arises from the inner table of the skull; another arises from the outer table.

Osteochondromas arise from the base of the skull, which develops from endochondral bone. They are rare and resemble osteochondromas found elsewhere. (No example shown.)

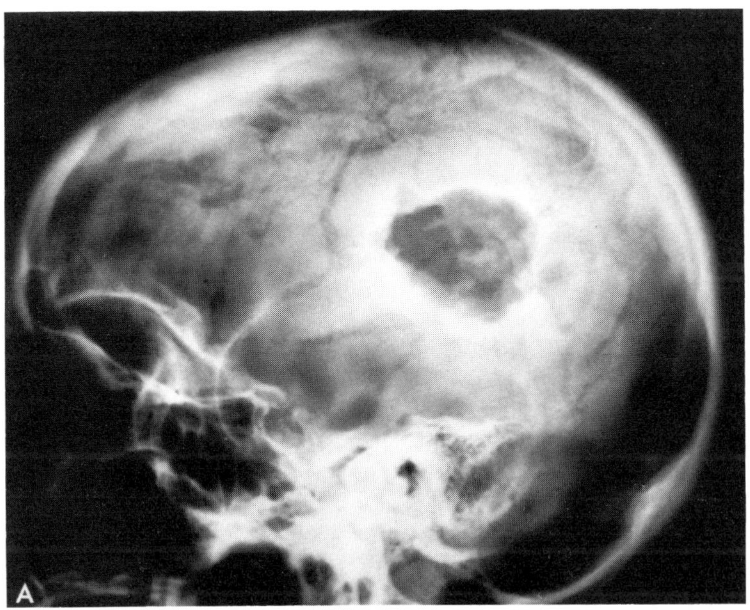

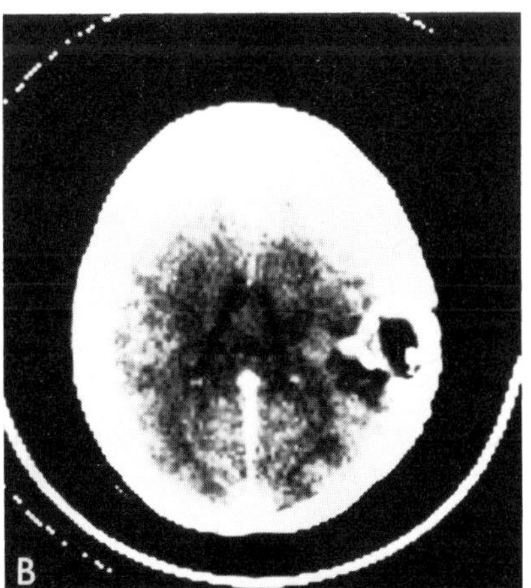

Figure 2–47. EPIDERMOID OF BONY CALVARIA: These present as lucent lesions *(A)* with well defined, scalloped margins that have a characteristic sclerotic appearance. They expand the diploë, contain desquamated dermal tissues, and may be called cholesteatomas of the skull. They are most common in the vault, but may occur in the orbital region.

The CT scan *(B)* demonstrates the lucent, low density expansile nature of the lesion, which tends to protrude more intracranially than extracranially. The sclerotic high density margin is also well demonstrated. (Case courtesy of Dr. Kenneth D. Schmidt.)

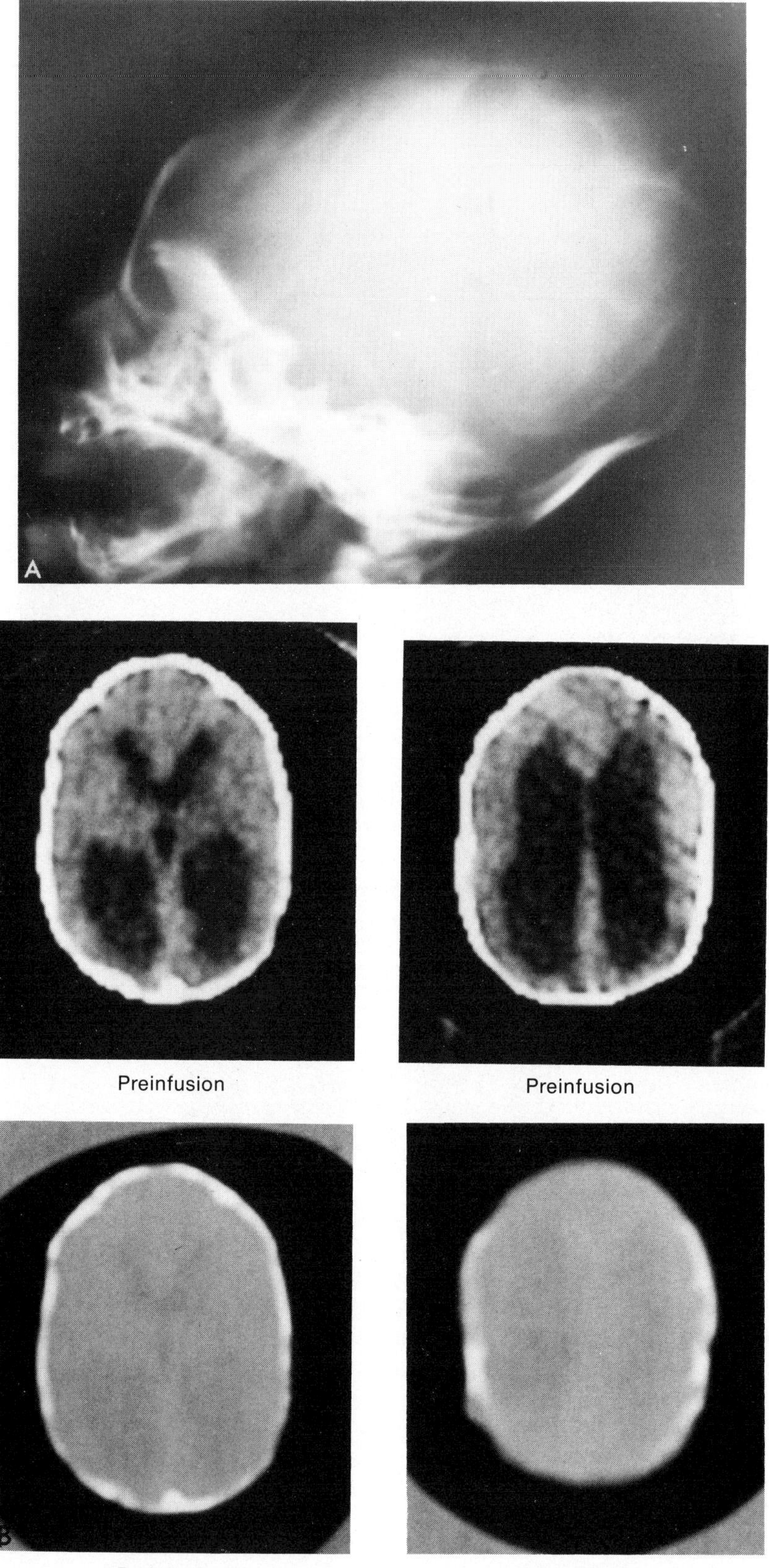

Figure 2–48. *See legend on the opposite page.*

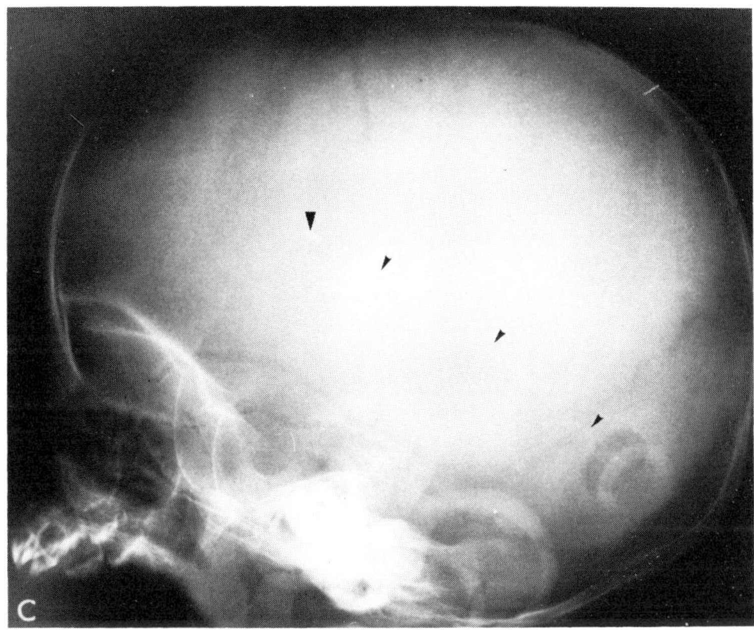

Figure 2–48. CRANIOLACUNIA (LÜCKENSCHÄDEL): *A,* This abnormal honeycomb appearance of the calvaria is caused by areas of dense bone separated by radiolucent areas of very thin or absent bone. This congenital abnormality is present at birth and is usually seen in patients who have a meningocele or meningoencephalocele. The etiology is unknown, but it may be related to increased intracranial pressure in utero. *B,* CT scans reveal the honeycomb appearance of the bony calvaria with multiple areas of bony thinning. In addition, there is hydrocephalus secondary to the obstruction of the aqueduct in this patient with an Arnold-Chiari II malformation. The patient demonstrates typical craniolacunia and had a meningomyelocele.

The abnormal appearance disappears soon after birth and is followed by changes of increased intracranial pressure. The craniolacunia disappear, the head enlarges and the sutures widen because of continued enlargement of the lateral ventricles. *C,* The skull film at 6 months of age reveals the enlarged skull with the widened suture and the absence of the craniolacunia. A shunt tubing device is in place (*arrows*).

Figure 2–49. MENINGOENCEPHALOCELE: A varying amount of meningeal and/or brain tissue may protrude through an abnormal opening in the bony calvaria—usually in the midline. If the protruding tissue is made up only of the meninges, it is called a meningocele; with both brain tissue and meninges it is a meningoencephalocele. *A,* The lateral arteriographic view reveals a large meningoencephalocele in the occipital region. The vertebral arteries *(arrows)* can be seen to supply the brain tissue that is outside the cranial vault.

B, CT scans in a different patient reveal a large occipital meningocele. The density of the material in the meningocele is of CSF density, and no brain tissue is present. In addition there is hypoplasia of the cerebellum with posterior fossa structures that appear to be abnormal. There is moderate hydrocephalus — probably secondary to aqueduct stenosis. The bony defect is readily identified at the midline in the posterior fossa.

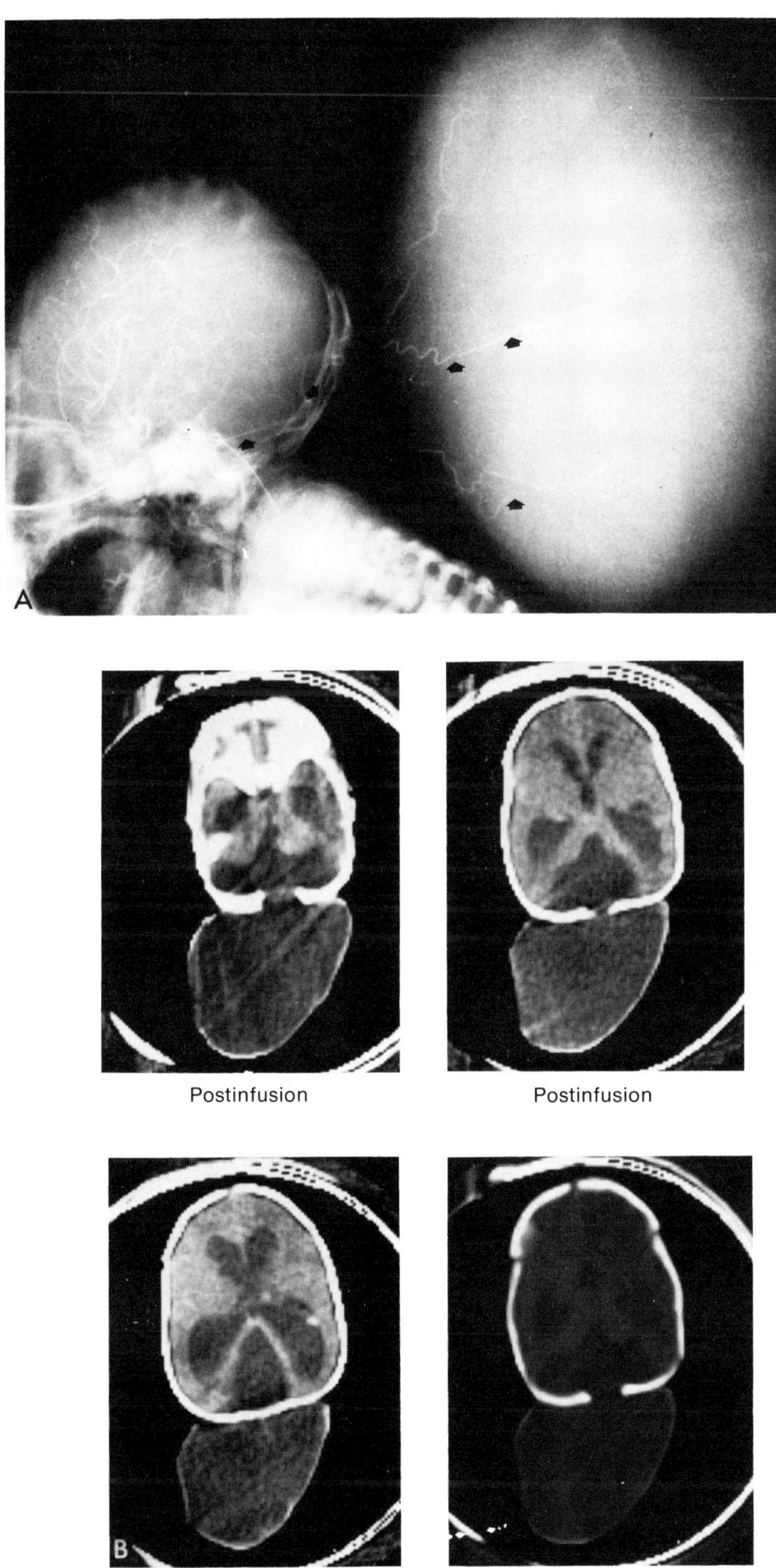

Figure 2–49. *See legend on the opposite page.*

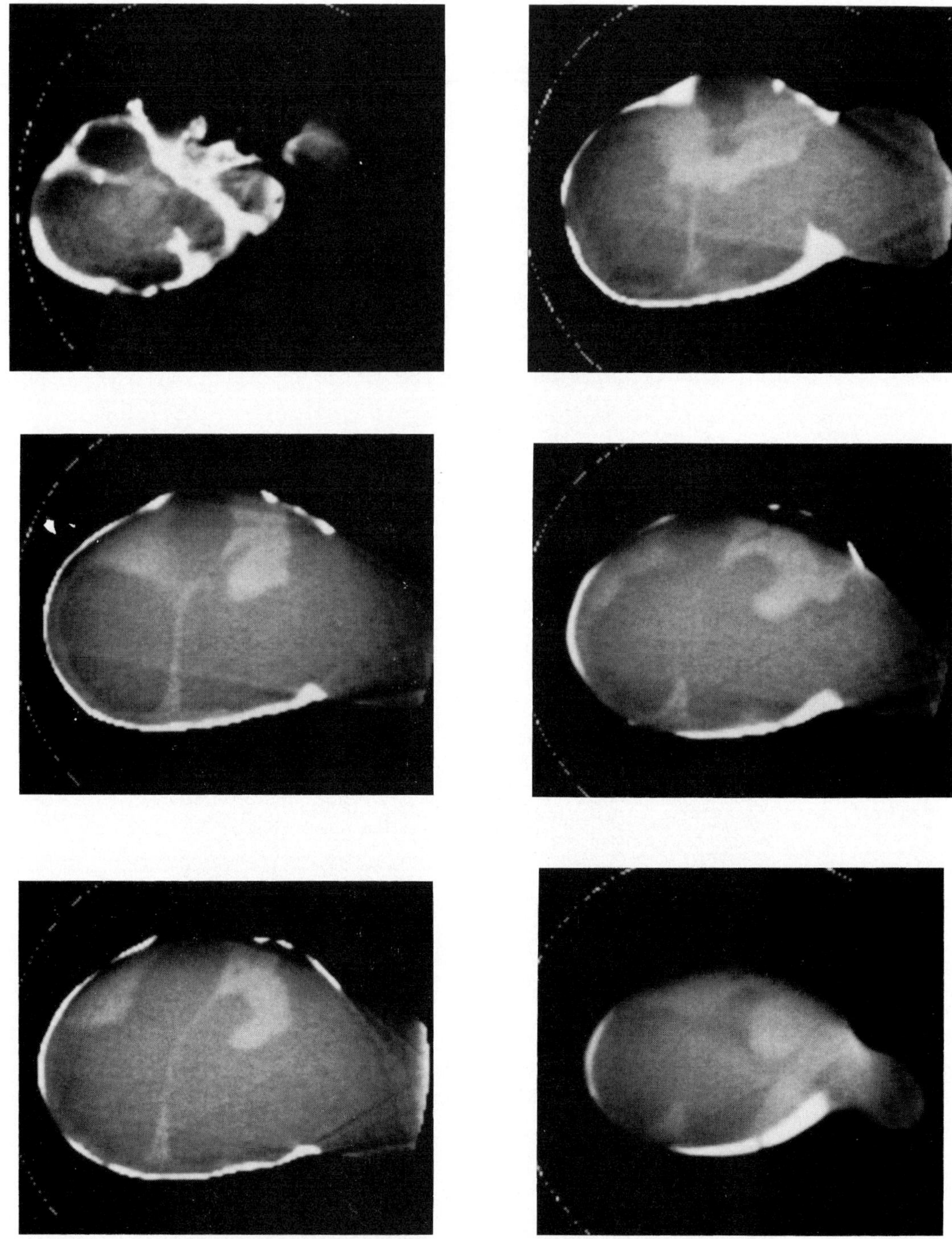

Figure 2–50. MENINGOENCEPHALOCELE: Clinically, this patient had a grossly misshapen cranial vault, and only one eye was identifiable. The CT scans reveal a large right frontal meningoencephalocele that communicates with the right lateral ventricle. In addition, there is severe hydrocephalus with deformity of the intracranial structures. A large bony defect is seen in the right lateral wall of the bony calvaria. Except for pathologic examination, the CT scan provides a much more accurate impression of the intracranial structures than is possible with any other neuroradiologic examination. In most cases of hydrocephalus, the only examination necessary before undertaking appropriate treatment is the CT scan of the cranial contents.

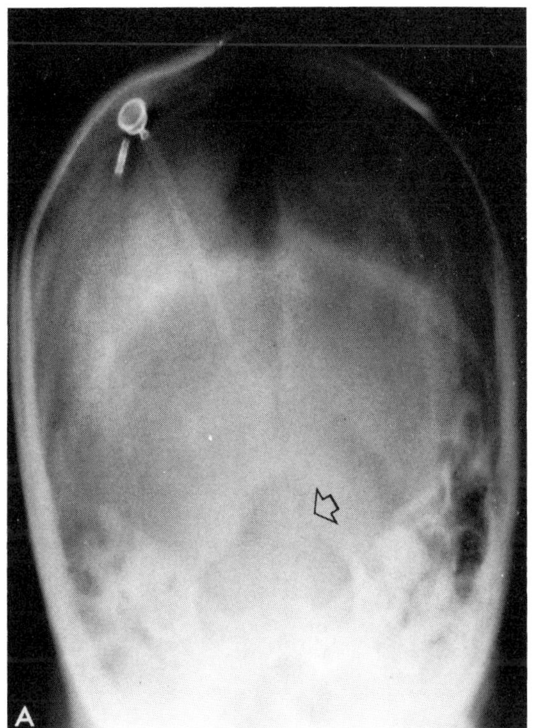

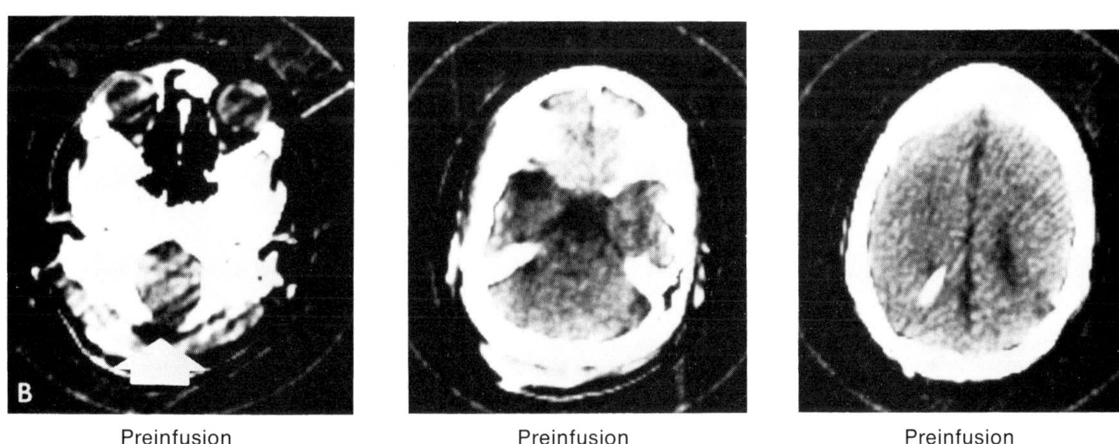

Figure 2–51. ARNOLD-CHIARI TYPE II: *A*, There is downward displacement of the posterior fossa structures into the upper cervical region; because of this, there is enlargement of the foramen magnum *(arrow)* to accommodate the additional structures. Because there is also an associated aqueduct stenosis, the patient developed hydrocephalus, and a shunt tubing device can be seen in place on the right side.

B, CT scans on the same patient demonstrate the large foramen magnum. The posterior margin is actually intact, but because of the projection of the cut appears to be open posteriorly. The fourth ventricle is never seen because it is positioned down in the cervical region. The upper cuts reveal the shunt tubing device in place and adequate decompression of the lateral ventricles.

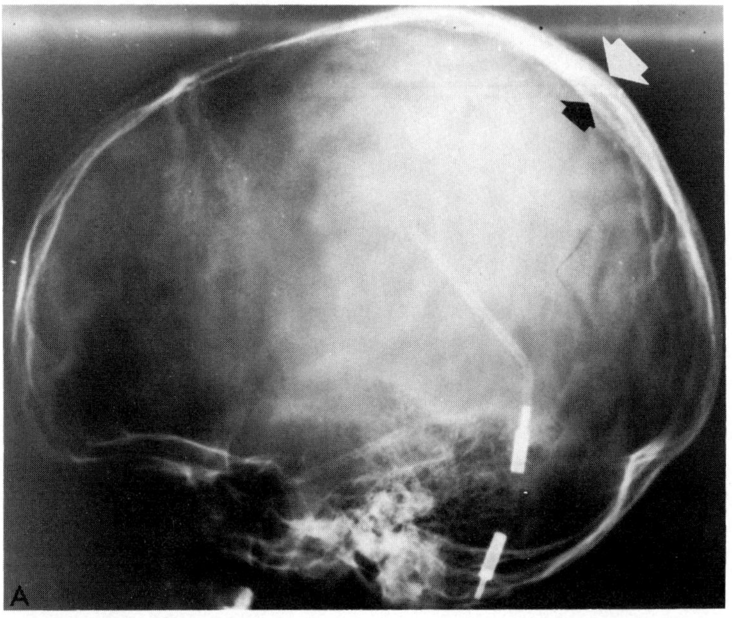

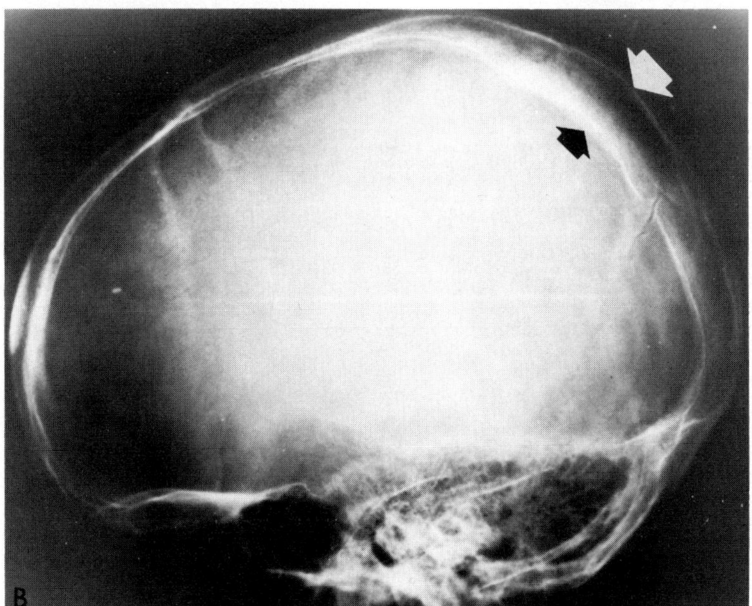

Figure 2–52. POST-SHUNTING CHANGES: With increased intracranial pressure secondary to hydrocephalus, widening of the sutures occurs that is most marked in the coronal and sagittal sutures. The lambdoid suture is frequently spared. There may also be an increase in the digital markings.

Post-shunting the sutures will no longer be widened; in response to a decrease in the intracranial pressure on the cranial vault there may be an increase in the thickness of the bony calvaria. *A,* The early skull film reveals a shunt in place and a mild increase in the thickness of the cranial vault secondary to the initial shunting procedure. *B,* After additional shunt revisions, a skull film obtained at a later date shows a marked increase in the thickness of the bone in the parietal and occipital regions *(arrows).* (Case courtesy of Drs. O. Sugar and G. Dobben.)

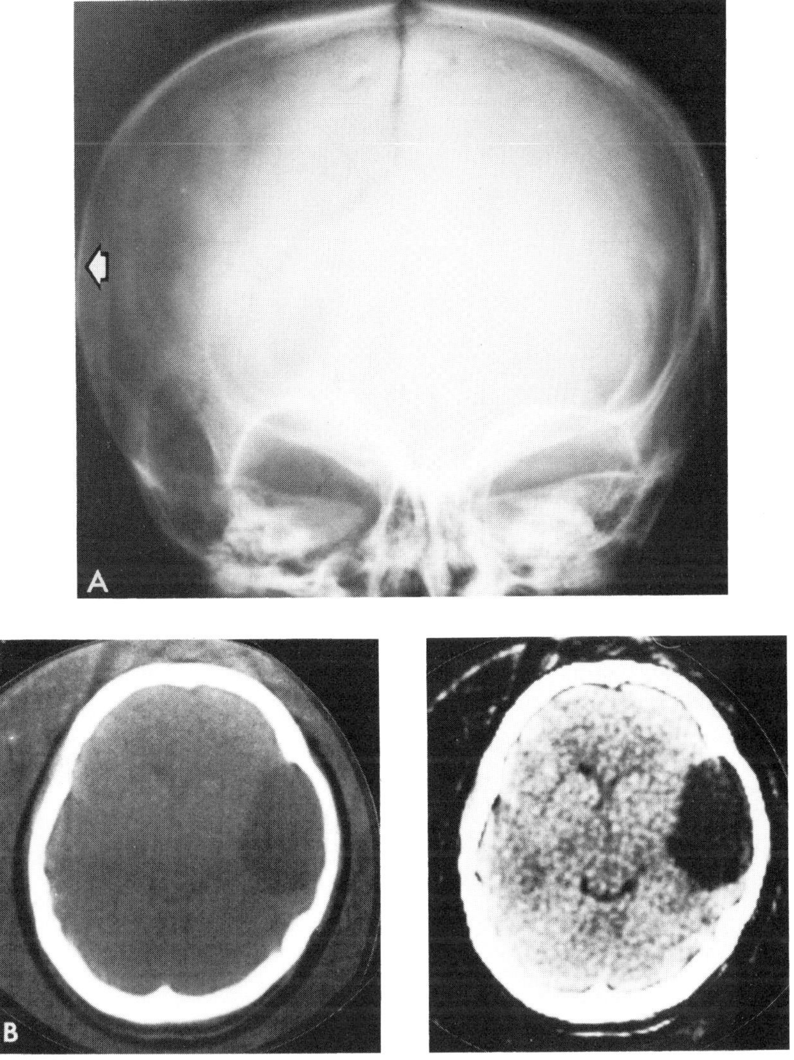

Figure 2–53. PORENCEPHALY: Frequently the skull will be normal. There may be areas of thinning of the bone over the porencephalic cysts because they appear to exert some pressure on the bony calvarium. The CT scan demonstrates these areas to excellent advantage, and, in fact, the areas of bone thinning seen on the CT scan may not be appreciated on the skull series.

By definition, a porencephalic cyst is lined by ependyma and is an outpouching from the lateral ventricles. Through the years this definition has been broadened to include cystic lesions that communicate with the lateral ventricle, the subarachnoid space, or a "closed" porencephalic cyst that lies deep within the cerebral substance and does not communicate with either.

Porencephaly in a general sense implies any lesion of cerebrospinal fluid density that is nonmalignant. These lesions may be caused by germ plasm abnormalities, birth trauma, anoxia, hemorrhage, vascular thrombosis or embolism, both postinflammatory and postsurgical.

A, The skull film demonstrates an area of bony expansion and thinning over a porencephalic cyst. This PA view demonstrates bulging of the skull in the right temporal and parietal regions with thinning of the bone. These changes are of long standing and are secondary to an underlying cyst. The cyst may be a porencephalic cyst or a temporal arachnoid cyst. (Case courtesy of Drs. O. Sugar and G. Dobben.)

B, The CT scan demonstrates a well defined, cerebrospinal fluid-containing lesion that has caused a thinning of the overlying bony calvaria. This example is of a temporal arachnoid cyst, not a porencephalic cyst. At times, as in this case, it is difficult to differentiate between the two. These arachnoid cysts are lined by an arachnoid-like membrane.

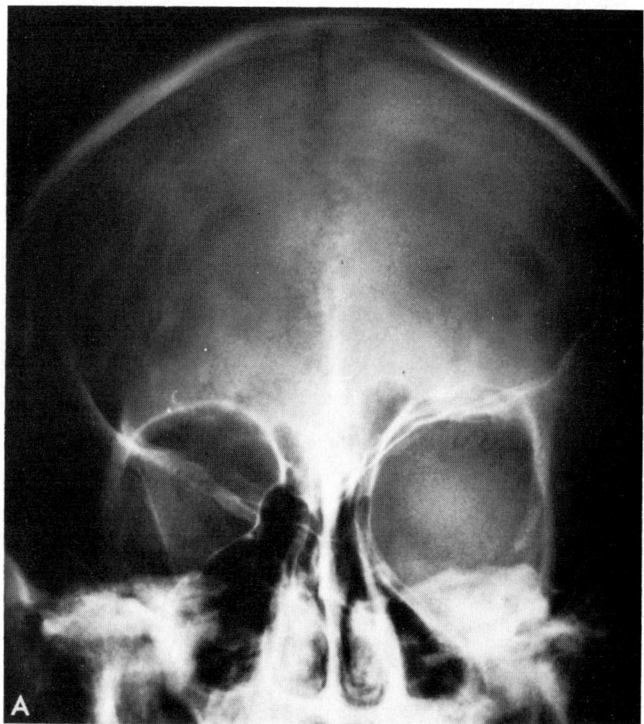

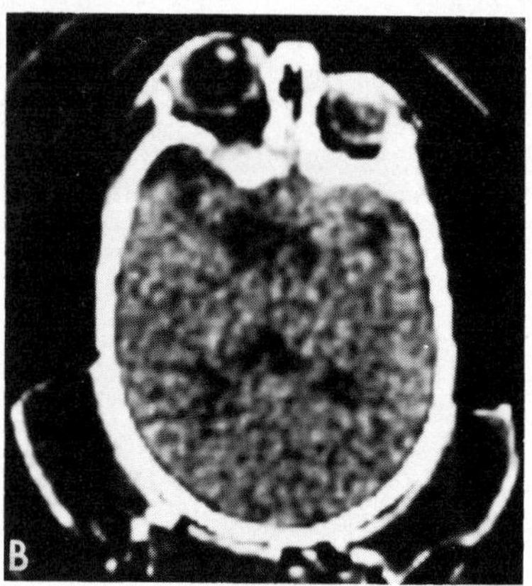

Preinfusion

Figure 2–54. NEUROFIBROMATOSIS: This disease is characterized by developmental abnormalities of mesenchymal tissues, even in the absence of soft tissue neurofibromas. Skull films frequently demonstrate changes secondary to orbital and middle cranial fossa dysplasias. The sella turcica may be enlarged. The developmental abnormality that affects the sphenoid wings results in elevation of the orbital roof and absent or marked thinning of the greater wing of the sphenoid. This is a mesenchymal abnormality and is not related to the presence of a neurofibroma. The orbit appears "empty" on the skull films *(A)* — the "harlequin eye." Exophthalmos may be present on the affected side. The entire orbit may be enlarged, as it is in this case.

The CT scan *(B)* reflects these changes, but does not demonstrate a mass lesion.

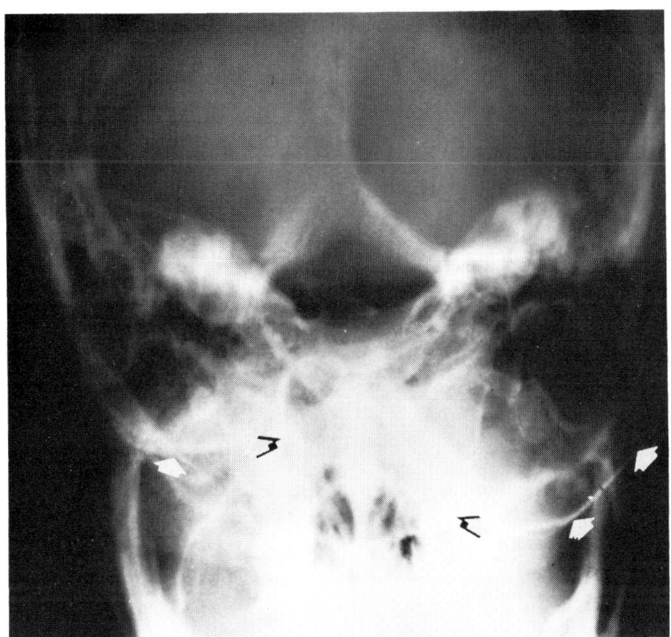

Figure 2–55. MIDDLE CRANIAL FOSSA DYSPLASIA OF NEUROFIBROMATOSIS: The Towne's view of the skull reveals a normal middle cranial fossa on the right side and an enlarged and ballooned middle cranial fossa on the left side *(arrowheads)*.

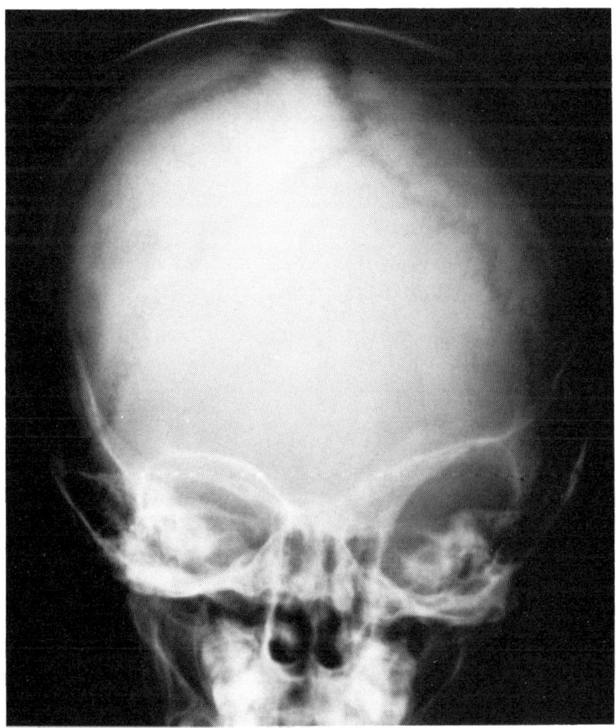

Figure 2–56. PLAGIOCEPHALY: This irregularly shaped deformity of the cranial vault is often due to unilateral premature closure of the coronal or lambdoidal suture. It may also be seen with generalized premature craniostenosis.

Premature closure of one coronal suture elevates the roof of the orbit on the ipsilateral side, creating an appearance similar to that seen in hemiatrophy or in dysplasias secondary to neurofibromatosis. Note that the hemicranium on the left side demonstrates a sloping cranial vault because the entire left hemicranium is smaller than the right, secondary to premature suture closure.

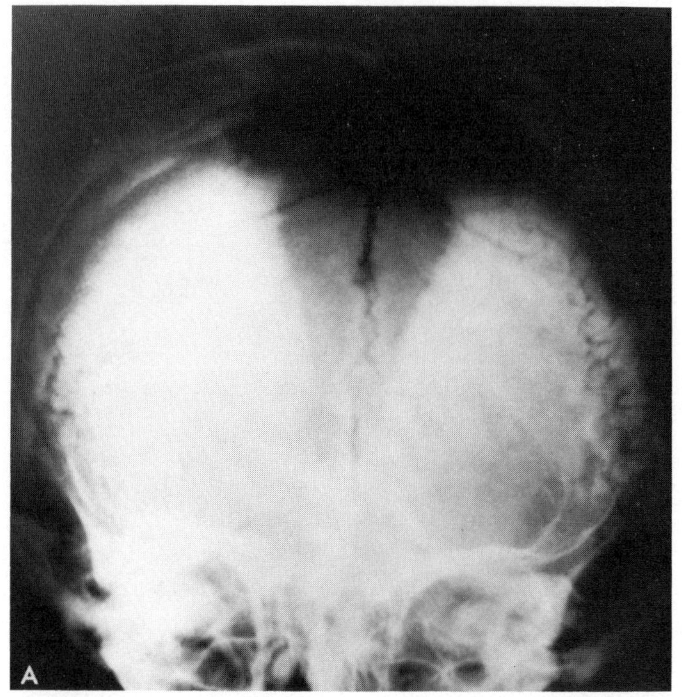

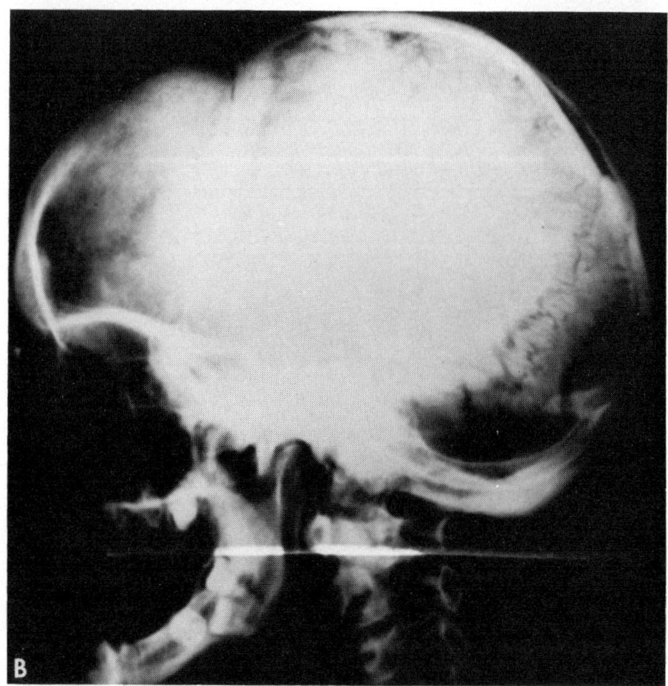

Figure 2–57. *See legend on the opposite page.*

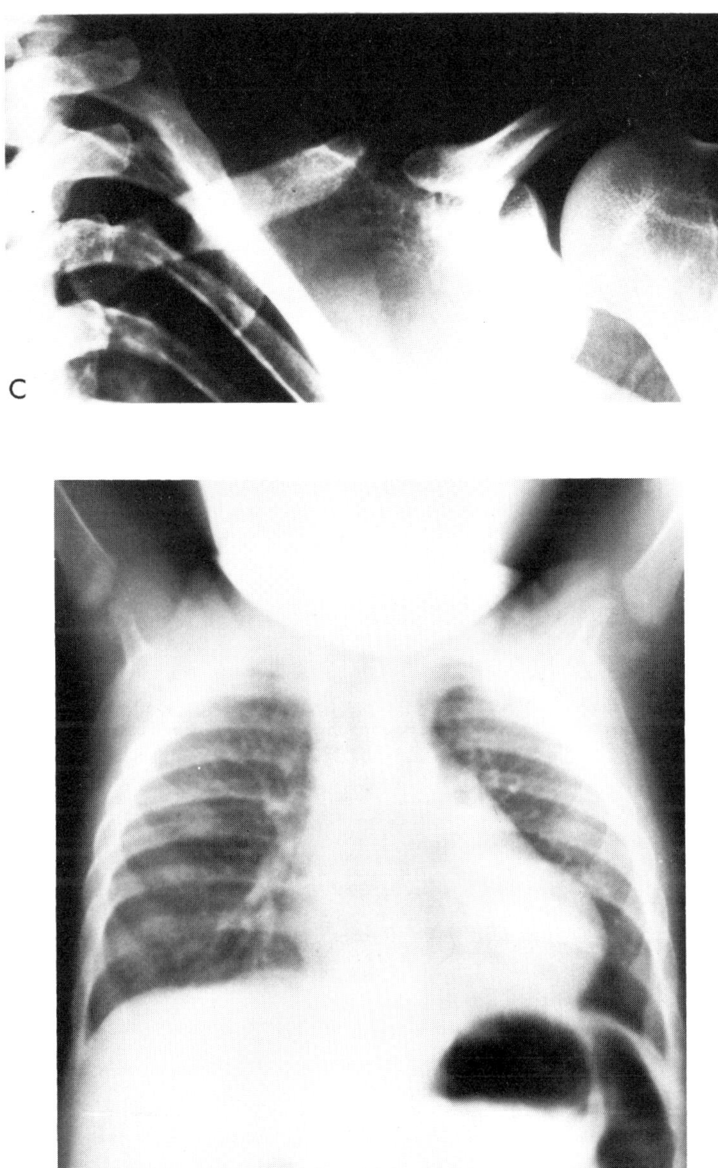

Figure 2–57. CLEIDOCRANIAL DYSOSTOSIS: *A*, and *B*, The skull abnormalities include midline defects with wide sutures and numerous wormian bones. There is delayed closure of the fontanelles. All these findings are present in this case. In addition, dental abnormalities are a major part of this syndrome. There are multiple defects of the teeth, with retention of deciduous teeth, delayed eruption and enamel defects. Note the retained teeth in the mandible and maxilla.

As the name suggests, there are congenital ossification defects in the clavicles that may be partly *(C)* or completely absent *(D)*. These patients may be intellectually intact. (Case courtesy of Drs. Glen Dobben and Oscar Sugar.)

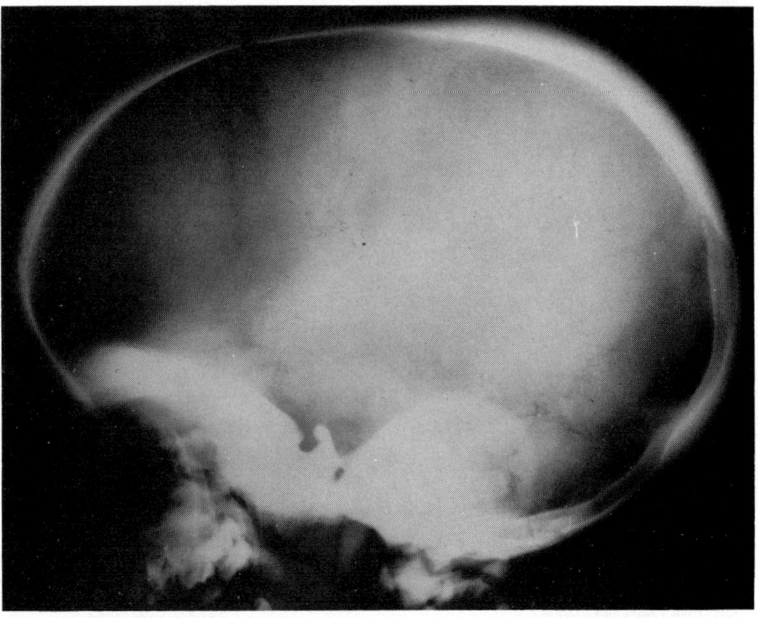

Figure 2–58. OSTEOPETROSIS: There is an increased density of all the bones of the body including the bones of the base of the skull. This may result in encroachment upon the foramina of the base of the skull and may result in visual problems, including blindness when it involves the optic foramina.

Figure 2–59. PAGET'S DISEASE (OSTEITIS DEFORMANS, OSTEOPOROSIS CIRCUMSCRIPTA): The initial phases of Paget's disease of the skull may reveal a diffuse osteolysis of a large, well defined area of the calvarium (*A*). This process usually begins in the frontal-parietal and occipital areas, while the vertex appears of normal density. The area of demineralization is often large, with a well defined but irregular border that crosses the sutures.

B, With time, osteoporosis circumscripta or the lytic phase of Paget's disease may be combined with the productive or blastic phase of the disease, resulting in biphasic Paget's disease *(B).*

With the biphasic form of Paget's disease there is thickening of the skull with widening of the diploic space. This process preferentially involves the outer table and diploë, but, less frequently, the inner table also may be involved. The calvarium becomes involved with rounded areas of increased and decreased density in a patchy distribution described as the "cotton-wool" appearance.

The incidence of bony metastases to the calvaria is decreased in the presence of Paget's disease. For a long time this was felt to be caused by rapid blood flow with arteriovenous shunting. However, it has been shown recently that A-V shunting does *not* take place in Paget's disease, and the reason for the decreased incidence of metastases is unknown.

An increased incidence of osteogenic sarcoma is associated with Paget's disease of the bone.

C, As a result of softening of the base of the skull, basilar invagination (basilar impression) may develop. Note the upward tilting (*arrowheads*) of the medial ends of the petrous bones.

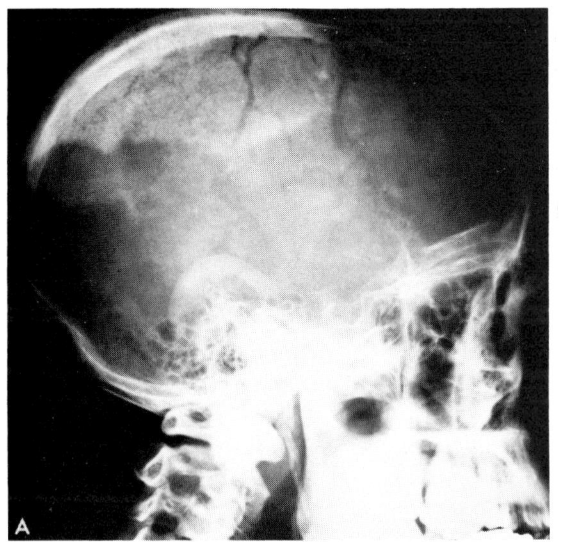

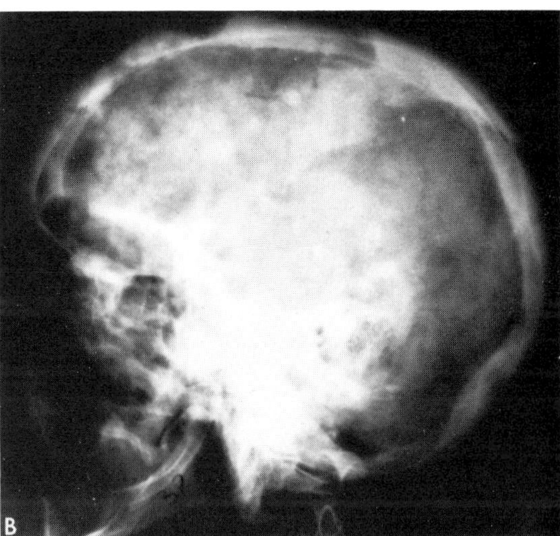

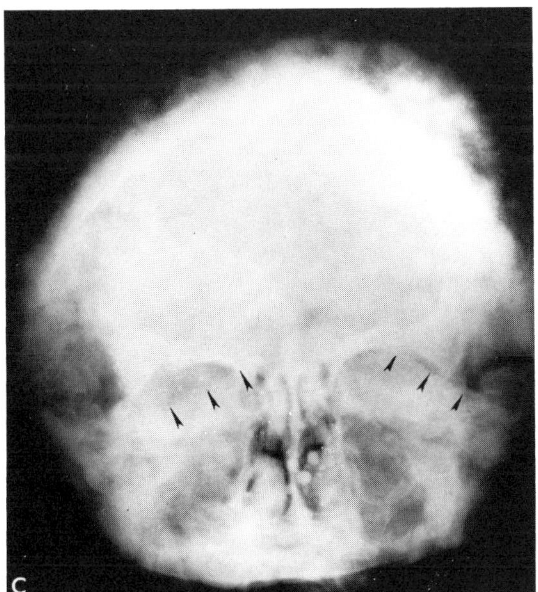

Figure 2–59. *See legend on the opposite page.*

The presence of basilar impression can be judged by measurements taken from the plain skull film using the lateral view (see Fig. 2–60). These measurements are known as Chamberlain's line and McGregor's line. In some cases, notably the normal, Chamberlain's line and McGregor's line are superimposed; in others they are widely separated.

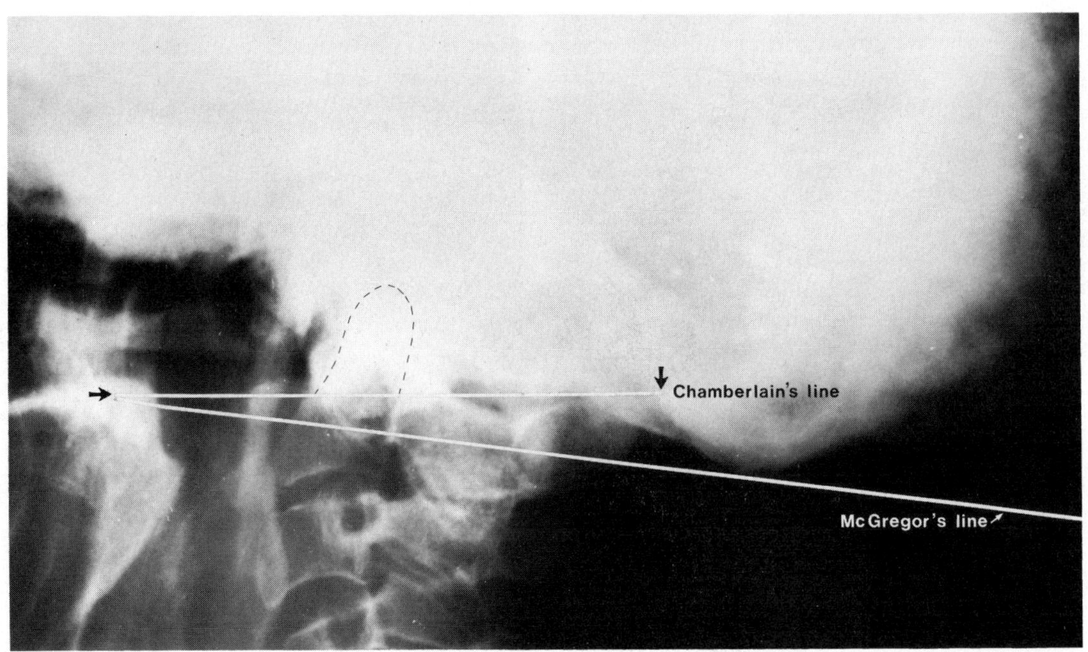

Figure 2–60. CHAMBERLAIN'S LINE: When a line connecting the posterior margin of the hard palate to the posterior margin of the foramen magnum is drawn, basilar impression is present if one half or more of the odontoid projects above this line. This upward displacement of the odontoid reflects elevation of the posterior portion of the base of the skull. Basilar impression can be seen with atlanto-occipital fusion, which is a congenital deformity, or with acquired conditions such as Paget's disease (as in this case), osteogenesis imperfecta, hyperparathyroidism and osteomalacia. It reflects a softening and pliability of the bones of the base of the skull. Basilar impression may be present congenitally in patients with the Arnold-Chiari malformation.

McGregor's Line. When a line is drawn from the posterior margin of the hard palate to the most inferior margin of the occipital squama, the odontoid should not extend more than 4 to 5 mm above this line. If the odontoid protrudes farther than 4 to 5 mm, basilar impression is present.

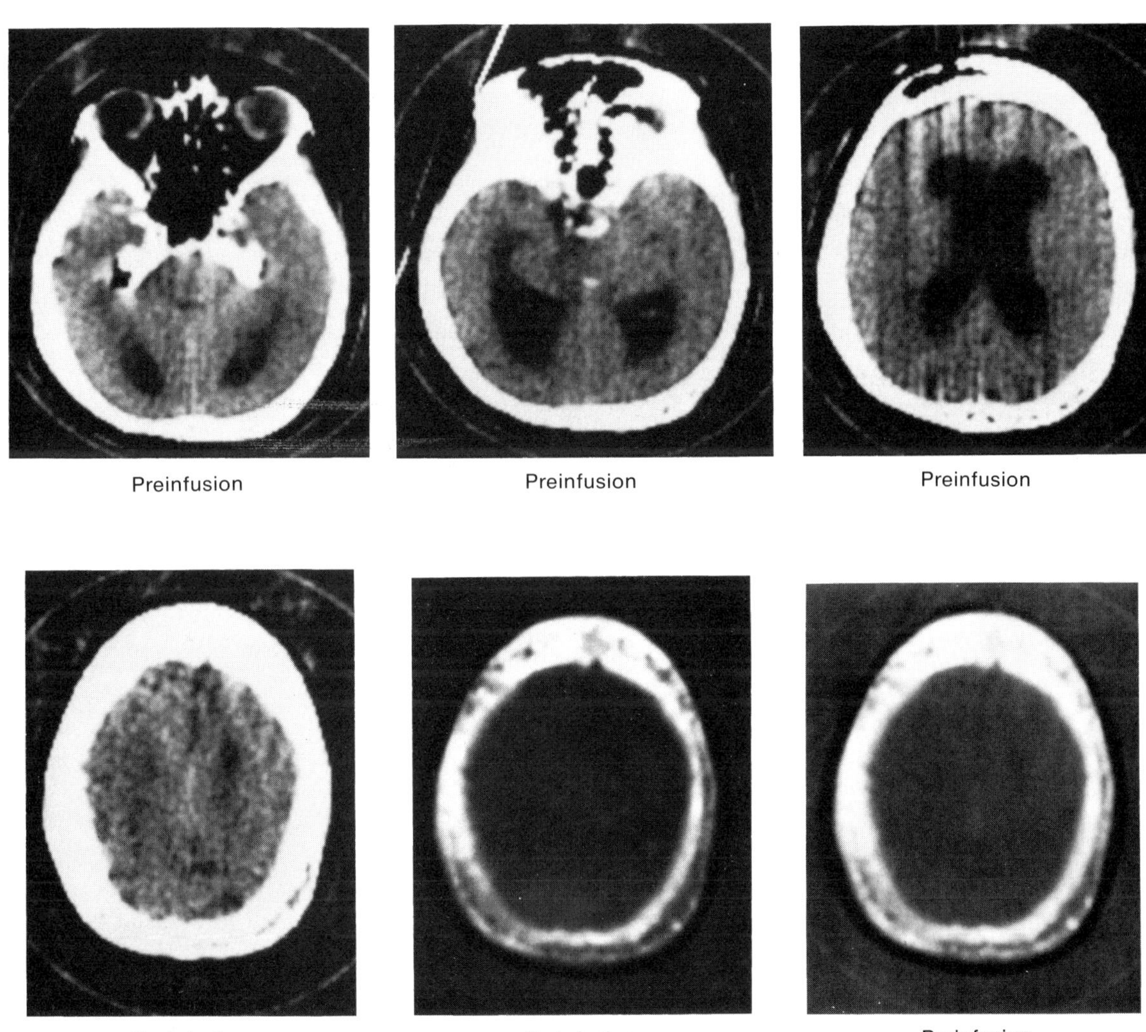

Figure 2–61. PAGET'S DISEASE WITH BASILAR IMPRESSION AND OBSTRUCTIVE HYDROCEPHALUS: CT scans reveal that the petrous apices are displaced superiorly and are visualized on the same cut with the sella. Because they are pushed so high, the occipital horns of lateral ventricles are also seen on the same cut. There is thickening of the bony calvaria that involves mainly the outer table and the diploë but also compromises the inner table. The typical cotton-wool appearance is also apparent on CT scans at high window widths and window levels.

There is dilatation of the lateral ventricles because of the obstruction of the ventricular system that results when the basiocciput is elevated and the cerebellar tonsils become impacted in the foramen magnum, thus preventing free flow of cerebrospinal fluid out of the foramina of Magendie and Luschka.

Platybasia. Platybasia (not illustrated) is an entity entirely different from basilar impression. Platybasia refers to the basal angle of the skull. The basal angle is measured by connecting the nasion to the tuberculum sellae and then to the anterior margin of the foramen magnum. The angle formed is normally 125° to 143°. If the angle is greater than 143° there is flattening of the base of the skull or platybasia. If the angle formed is less than 125° there is basilar kyphosis.

Platybasia may be congenital, may occur in association with the Arnold-Chiari malformation and may be acquired following suboccipital craniectomy in childhood.

Platybasia and basilar impression may be seen in association with one another.

Figure 2–62. ATLANTO-OCCIPITAL FUSION: The atlas may fuse with the base of the skull. This results in upward displacement of the odontoid into the foramen magnum, causing basilar impression and compromise of the size of the foramen magnum.

There may be partial or complete fusion of the atlas. The anterior arch of C_1 becomes incorporated into the clivus. The lateral mass is fused to the base of the skull on either side of the foramen magnum, and the posterior arch of the atlas fuses to the squama of the occiput. Because the vertebral artery normally lies in a groove along the upper margin of C_1 before entering the foramen magnum, a separate foramen must be formed to allow the artery to enter the cranial vault.

Because of the narrowing of the spinal canal at the level of the foramen magnum, pressure may be exerted on the spinal cord and medulla. The patient may develop symptoms simulating multiple sclerosis, amyotrophic lateral sclerosis, syringomyelia and other neurologic disorders.

A, The lateral view of the cervical spine reveals that C_1 is fused *(white arrow)* to the base of the skull, and the second cervical vertebrae and the odontoid process are displaced superiorly. In addition, there is narrowing of the disk space at C_3–C_4, and degenerative changes are present. This is probably secondary in part to the abnormal relationship of C_1 to the base of the skull.

B, The midline lateral tomogram reveals that the odontoid process rests *above* the level of the foramen magnum, with its tip resting at the inferior margin of the medulla and markedly narrowing the foramen magnum *(arrow).*

C, The AP tomogram reveals that the lateral mass of C_1 is fused to the base of the skull and is actually incorporated into the base of the skull *(large arrowhead).* In addition, the foramen for the vertebral artery is also visible in this projection *(small arrow).*

D, A tomogram through the lateral masses of C_1 and C_2 reveals that C_1 is incorporated into the base of the skull, and the foramen *(open arrowhead)* for the vertebral artery is readily demonstrated. The degenerative changes are also seen at the C_3–C_4 level.

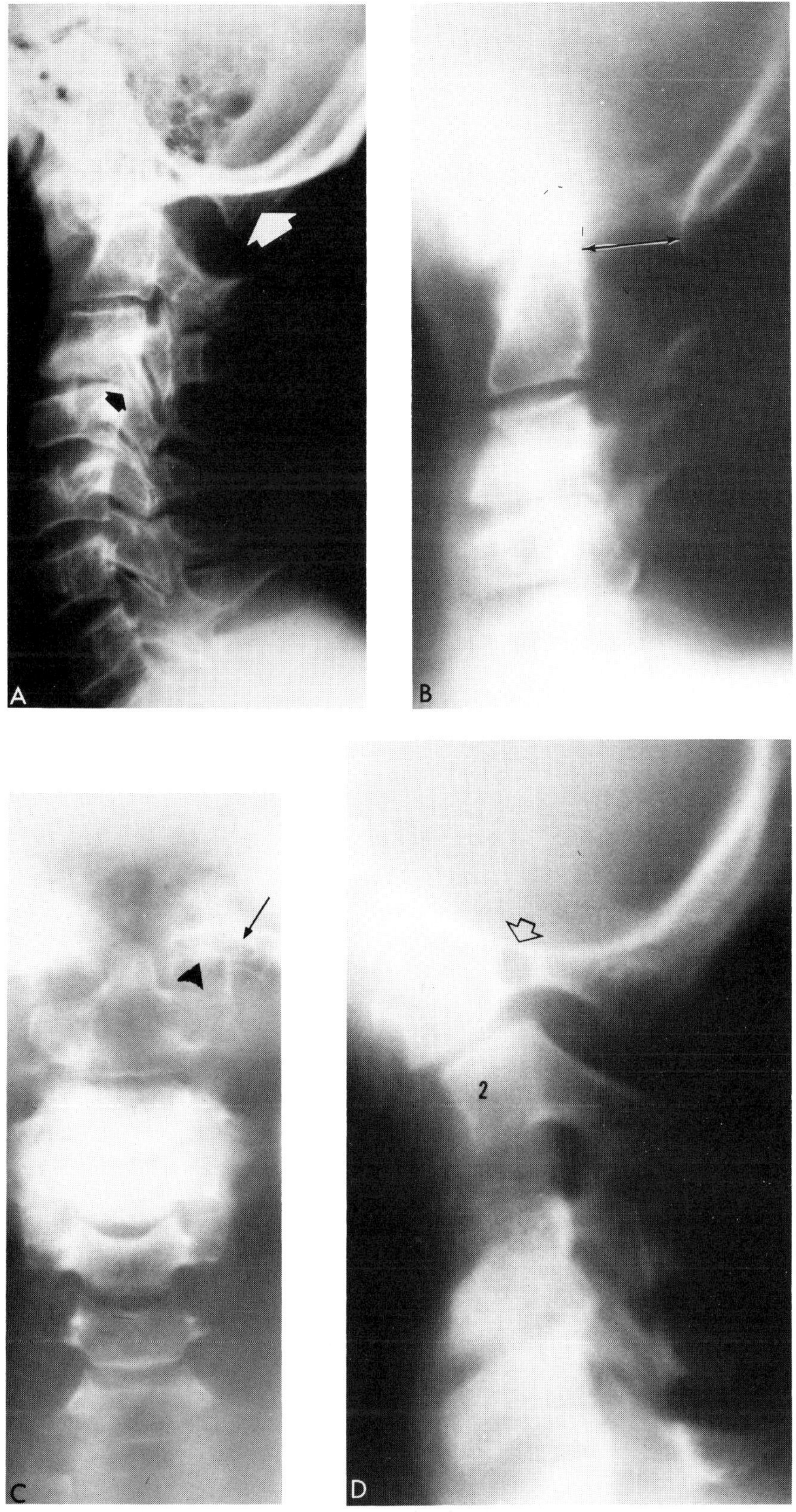

Figure 2–62. *See legend on the opposite page.*

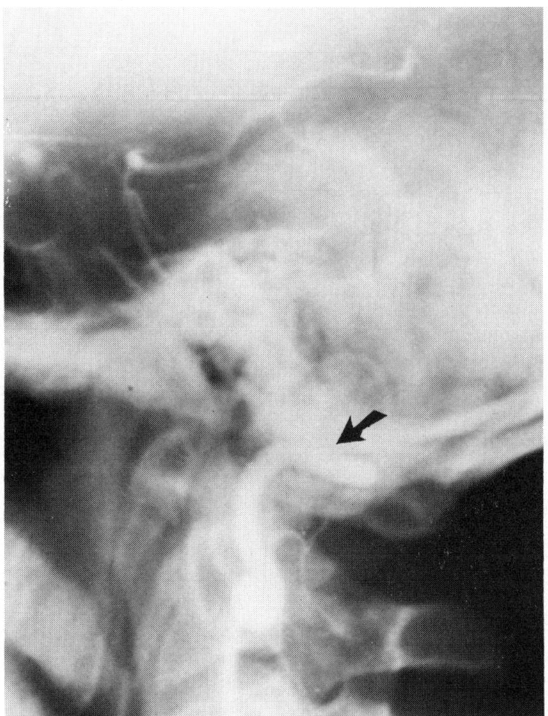

Figure 2-63. VERTEBRAL ARTERIOGRAM IN ATLANTO-OCCIPITAL FUSION: In a different case, the posterior arch of C_1 is fused to the base of the skull and the vertebral artery passes through a separate foramen as it enters the cranial vault *(arrow)*.

Figure 2-64. JUVENILE ANGIOFIBROMA: These patients are almost always in the second decade of life; they present clinically with recurrent epistaxis; marked male predominance.

A, Radiographs demonstrate a soft tissue mass in the nasopharynx with marked forward bowing of the posterior wall of the maxillary sinus *(arrows)*. The pterygomaxillary space is present only on the contralateral side; it has been destroyed on the side of the mass.

The blood supply is via the internal maxillary artery and its branches. The highly vascular mass frequently feeds from both external carotid arteries.

B, The lateral arterial film of a selective external carotid arteriogram reveals a markedly vascular tumor which fed primarily from the internal maxillary artery. This appearance is very typical.

A choanal polyp may have a similar soft tissue appearance on the plain radiographs, but demonstrates only minimal vascularity with arteriography.

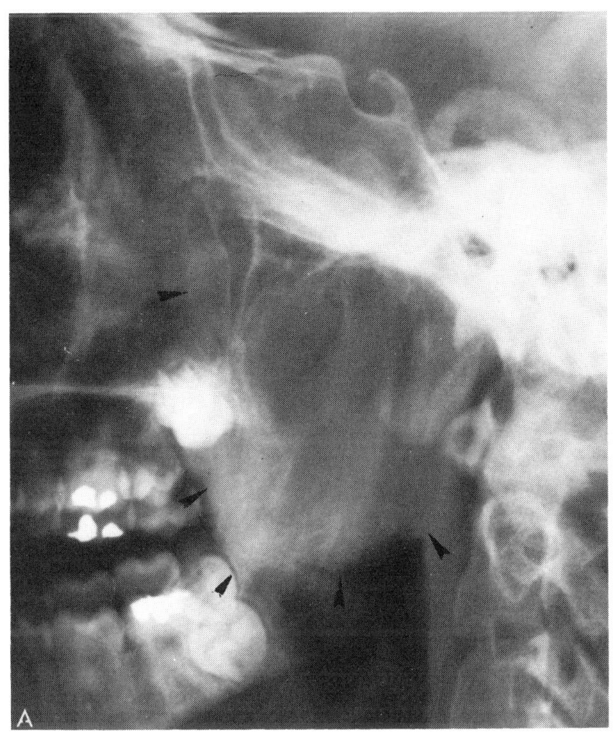

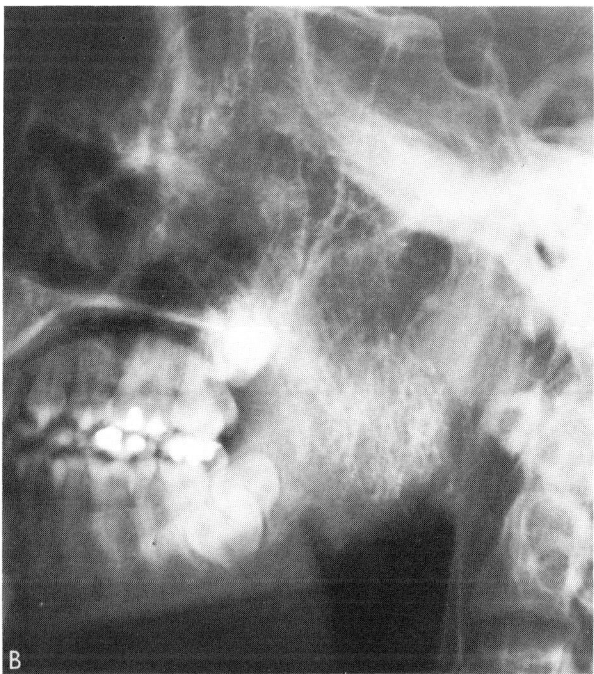

Figure 2–64. *See legend on the opposite page.*

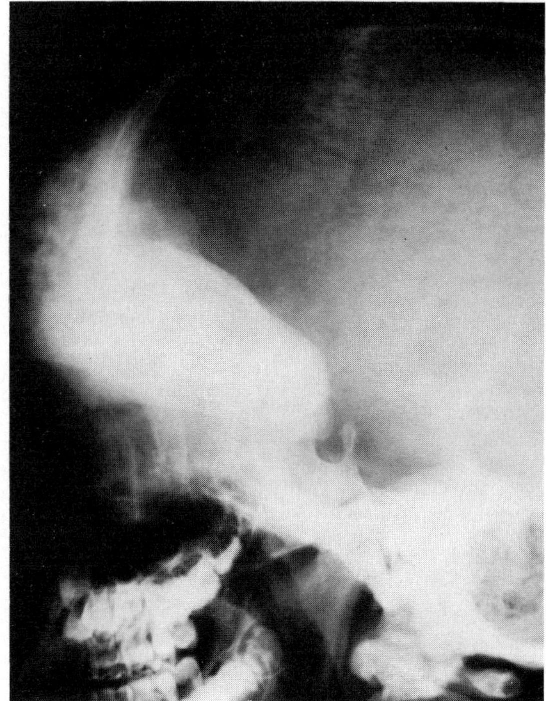

Figure 2–65. FIBROUS DYSPLASIA: This entity may present in many forms. A purely sclerotic form frequently involves the orbits and the base of the skull (see illustration). The clinical picture is that of "lion-like facies" because of the involvement and thickening of the bony structures of the face. The extensive homogeneous increase in density is typical of fibrous dysplasia, although lesser degrees of involvement may be impossible to differentiate from the reactive sclerosis secondary to a meningioma. If other bones are involved, as in polyostotic fibrous dysplasia, differentiation from meningioma is easier.

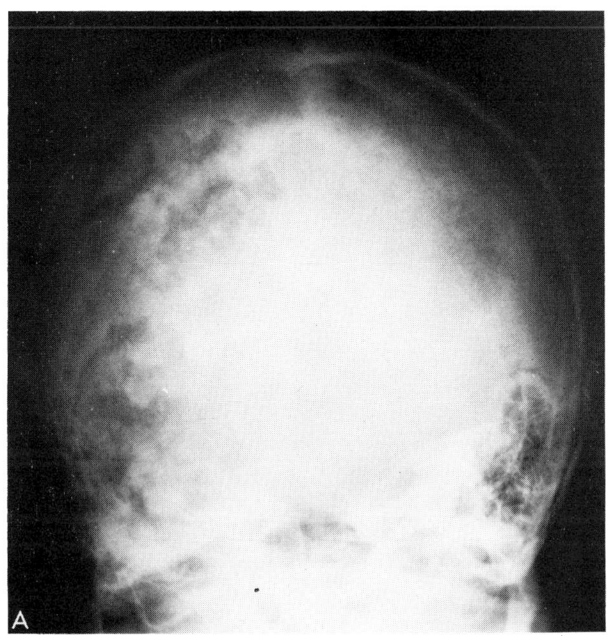

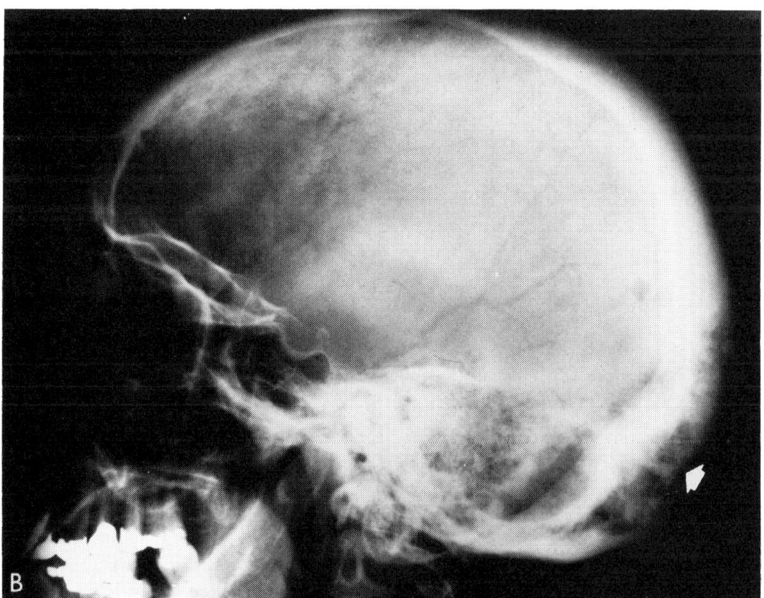

Figure 2–66. *A* and *B*, The mixed sclerotic and radiolucent type of fibrous dysplasia is more common in the cranial vault than in the long bones. This gives the "soap bubble" appearance typical of fibrous dysplasia. This type of fibrous dysplasia may be mistaken for Paget's disease.

Fibrous dysplasia can present a variety of appearances, and perhaps should be mentioned in the differential diagnosis of any obscure skull lesion.

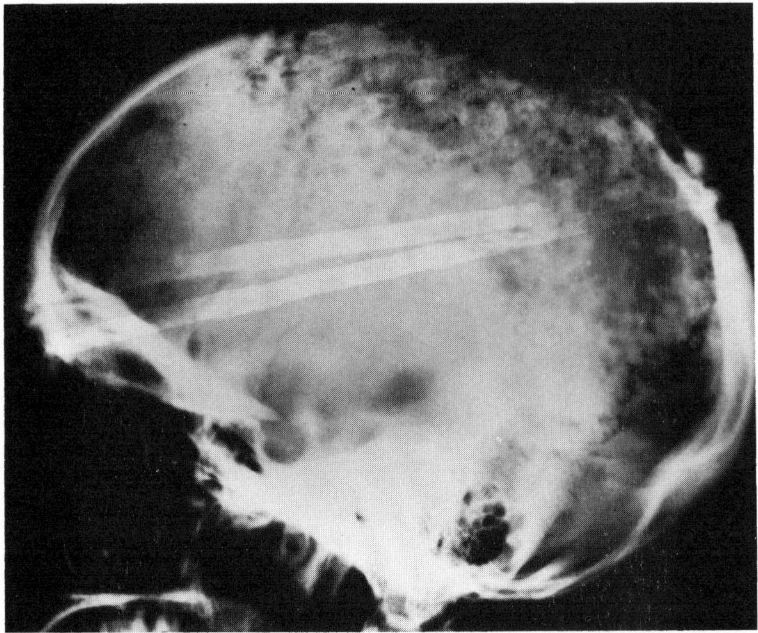

Figure 2–67. OSTEOMYELITIS: The entire parietal bone as well as portions of the frontal and occipital bones are involved with a diffuse osteolytic process that presents as multiple lucent areas with poorly defined margins. A history of an infected scalp wound is frequently obtained in these patients. In addition, osteomyelitis can be seen following a severe frontal sinusitis.

Figure 2–68. POSTOPERATIVE OSTEOMYELITIS: This patient had an operative procedure for removal of a sphenoid wing meningioma. *A,* Immediately postoperatively, the skull films reveal a craniotomy flap with well defined margins. The patient developed a wound infection and the follow-up skull films 6 weeks later *(B)* reveal that the anterior inferior margin of the flap is now poorly defined. The bone on either side of the craniotomy line is also poorly defined and has a mottled appearance *(arrows)* — findings consistent with osteomyelitis. The skull films may not reveal the true extent of the bony involvement, and wide surgical excision is necessary to remove the affected bone.

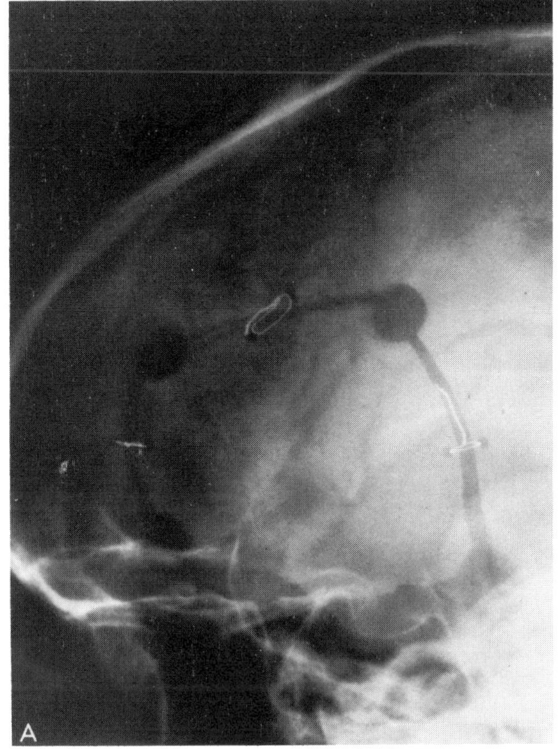

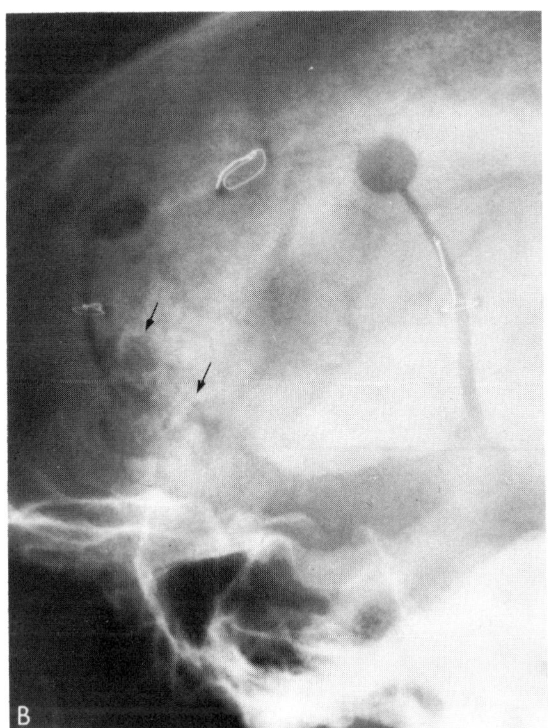

Figure 2–68. *See legend on the opposite page.*

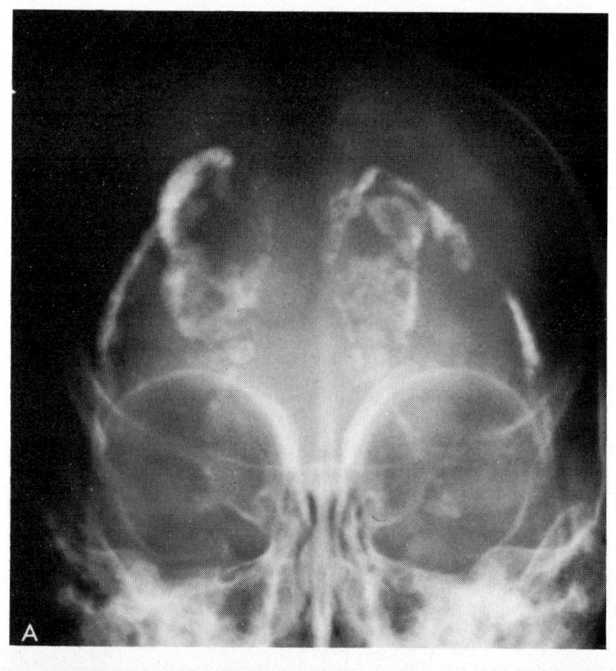

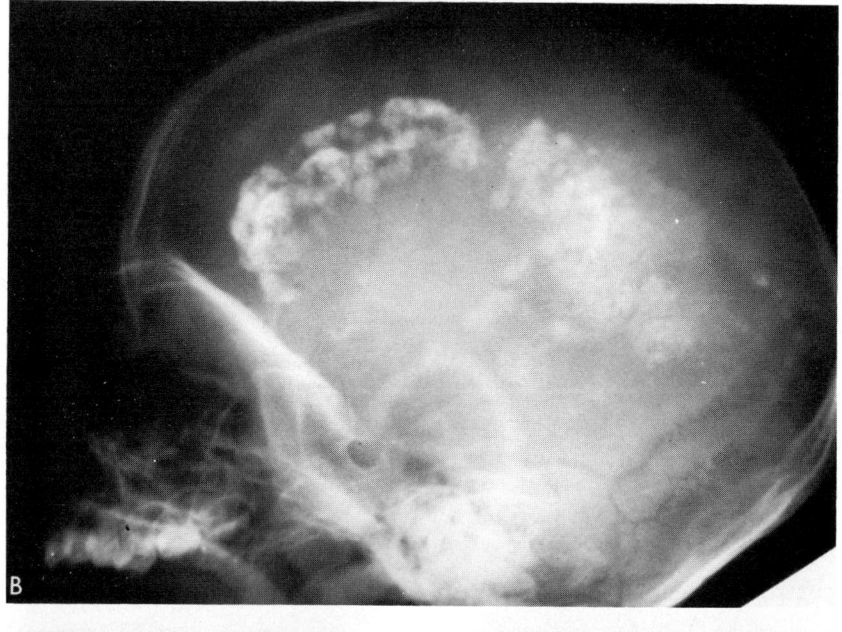

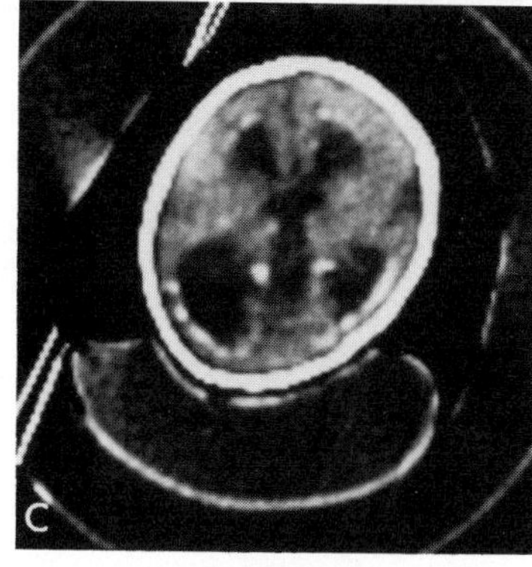

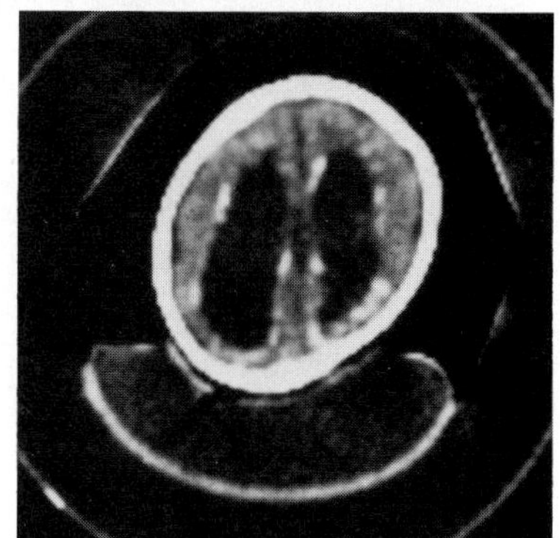

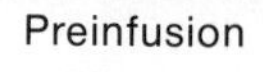

Preinfusion

Figure 2–69. *See legend on the opposite page.*

Figure 2–69. CYTOMEGALIC INCLUSION DISEASE: This disease is caused by a cytomegalovirus from the herpes family. The disease is often subclinical, and may be acquired in utero. The skull films *(A* and *B)* reveal multiple intracranial periventricular calcifications. The infection results in destruction of the cerebral tissues and microcephaly secondary to loss of cerebral substance. It is associated with enlargement of the lateral ventricles.

The calcifications may be periventricular or may occur in any portion of the brain substance. Differentiation from toxoplasmosis by radiography is impossible. The CT scan *(C)* reveals multiple periventricular calcifications associated with microcephaly and ventricular dilatation. Both the microcephaly and the ventricular dilatation are secondary to loss of brain substance. (The skull films are courtesy of Drs. O. Sugar and G. Dobben.)

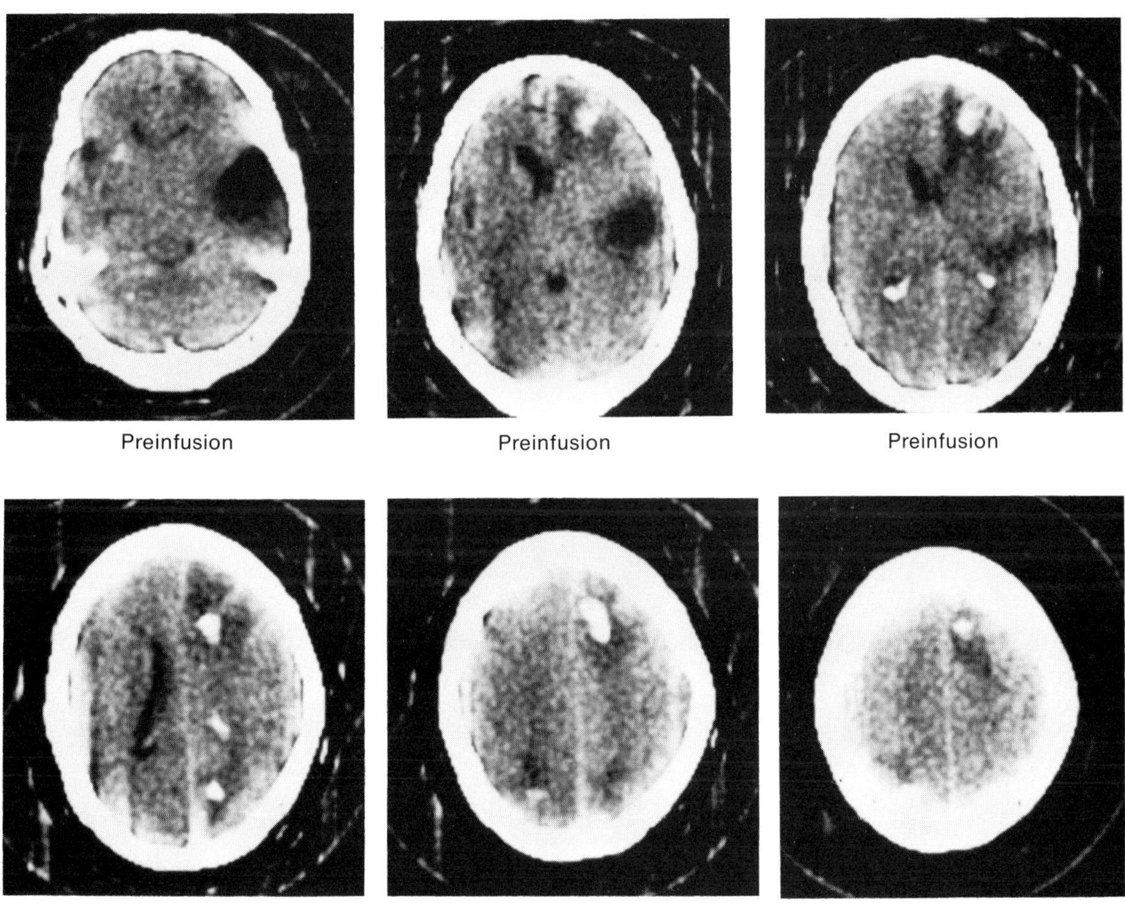

Figure 2–70. CYSTICERCOSIS: This disease results from the ingestion of eggs of the pork tapeworm, *Taenia solium*. The larvae become encysted in muscles and brain and cause multiple areas of calcification. The pig is the usual host, with man the intermediate host following ingestion of poorly cooked pork. However, when sanitation is poor, man becomes the primary host.

Skull films (not illustrated) show multiple small scattered intracranial calcifications. The CT scans reveal similar findings. In this case the areas of calcification are surrounded by edema. There is also a cystic lesion in the right temporal region.

Diagnosis rests on a strong clinical history or tissue diagnosis. The disease is prevalent in Latin America, Mexico and the West Indies.

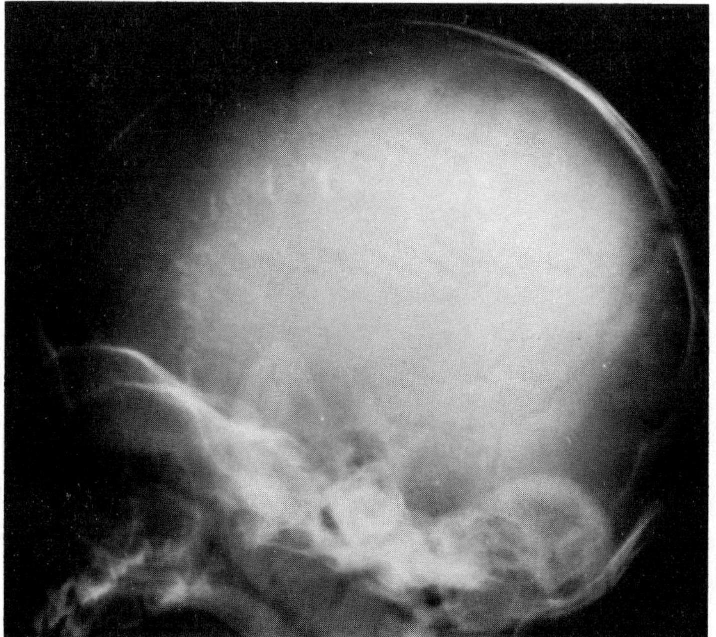

Figure 2–71. TOXOPLASMOSIS: This encephalitis is secondary to a protozoan infestation seen in utero or in early life. Radiographs reveal calcifications scattered throughout the parenchyma; these form within areas of necrosis and granuloma formation. The radiologic appearance cannot be differentiated from that of cytomegalic inclusion disease. The calcifications may be periventricular in distribution, as demonstrated in this case. Because of brain destruction there is associated microcephaly and enlargement of the lateral ventricles.

The CT scan (not shown) readily demonstrates these areas of calcification.

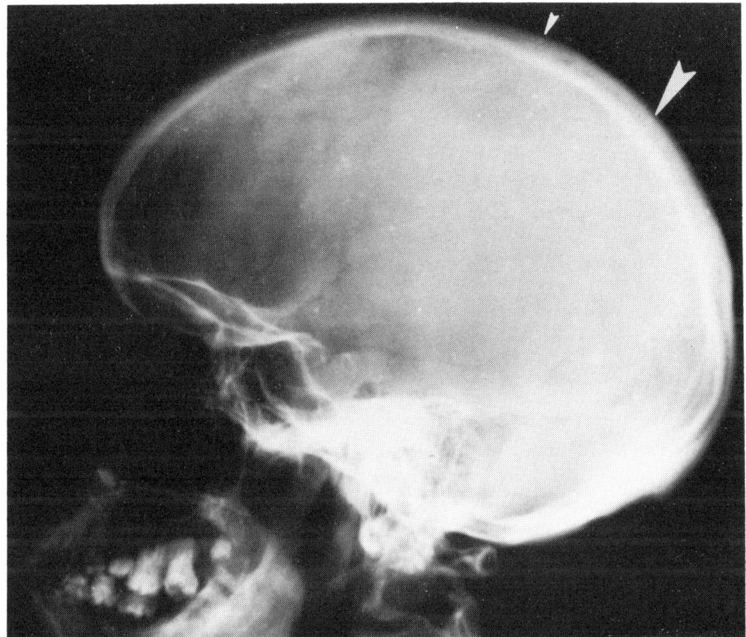

Figure 2–72. CEILING PLASTER IN THE HAIR: Multiple high density areas of varying size project over the calvaria. Close inspection reveals that many of the densities project outside the bony calvaria *(arrows)*, and the history establishes that a plaster ceiling had fallen on the patient's head and that small fragments of the plaster were trapped by the patient's hair. This possibly could be mistaken for intracranial calcification.

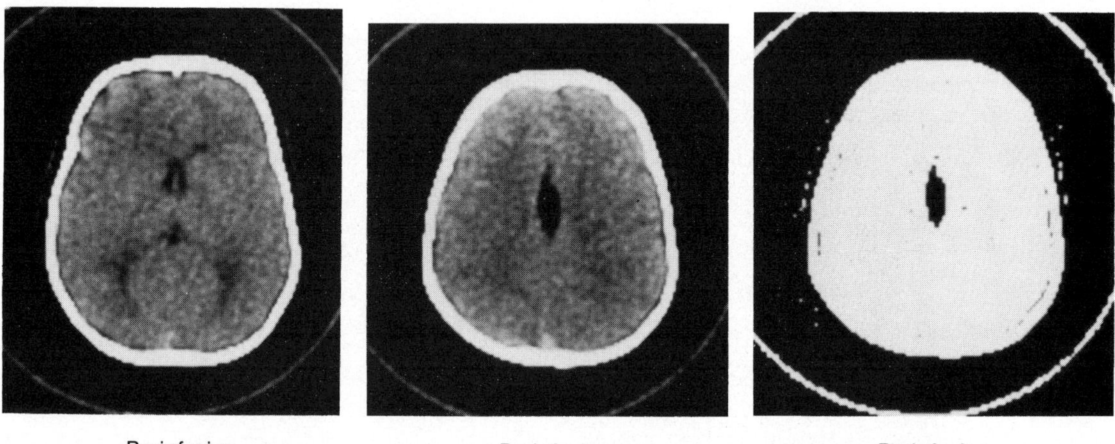

Figure 2–73. LIPOMA: These tumors arise in the corpus callosum and separate the lateral ventricles. Most probably they are not visible radiographically; but, if they are identified, they reveal a low density area that may be outlined by peripheral calcification. These tumors are readily demonstrated on the CT scan, and may have density numbers as low as −100 Hounsfield units. The lipomas are of varying sizes and may or may not contain areas of calcification. The tumors are incidental findings in some cases.

Lipomas are readily demonstrated on the CT scan even when not visible on the plain skull radiograph. The CT scans of this asymptomatic patient demonstrate a small oval lipoma of the corpus callosum. There is a well defined low density lesion in the midline that measures in the range of the density of fat. This is well demonstrated on the measure mode (at right). Skull films of this patient were normal.

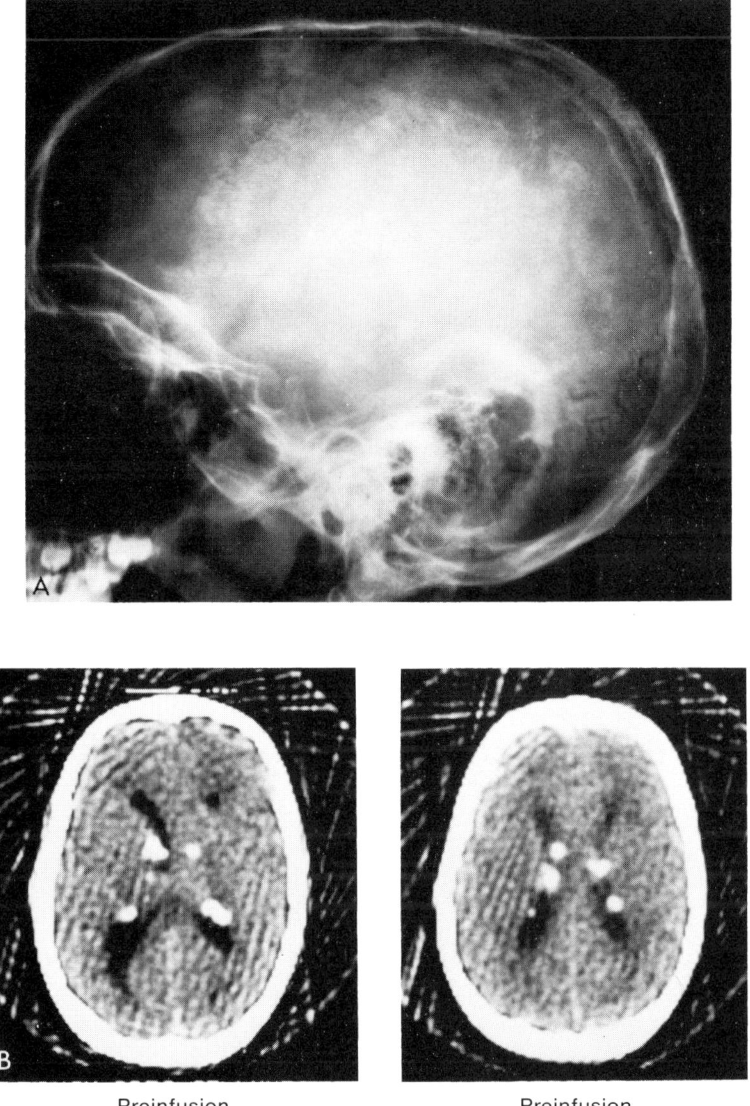

Figure 2–74. TUBEROUS SCLEROSIS (Bourneville's Disease): Skull films demonstrate multiple scattered calcifications in a periventricular distribution. Scattered random intracranial calcifications also may occur. The subependymal periventricular calcifications are associated with giant glial cells and subependymal astrocytomas, which frequently degenerate into glioblastomas. The calcifications usually appear after two years of age.

Localized areas of increased or decreased density also occur in the bony calvaria in a large percentage of cases, and differentiation from intracranial calcification may be difficult *(A)*. Computed tomography *(B)* readily demonstrates the periventricular areas of calcification and any degeneration into gliomas.

Cystic changes may occur in the hand; hamartomas (angiomyolipomas) may be present in the kidneys. Hamatomas also may occur in the liver.

The clinical syndrome is that of mental retardation, seizures and sebaceous adenomas of the face with a "butterfly" distribution.

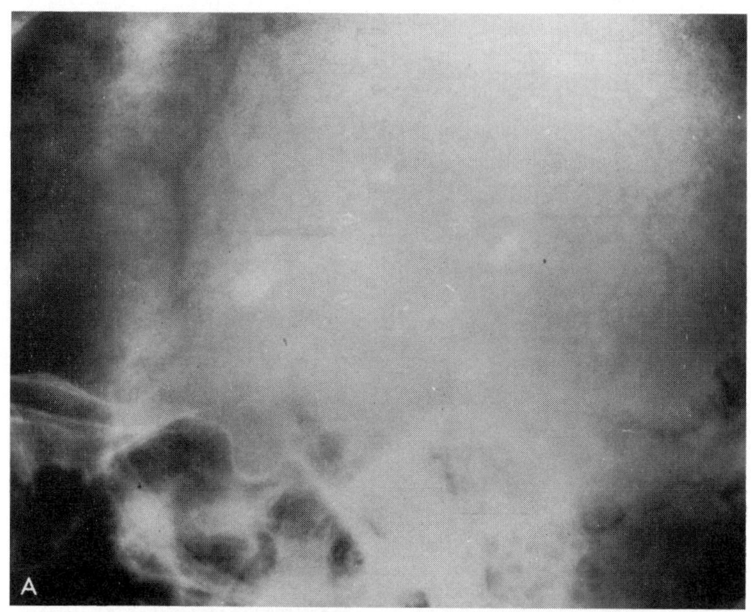

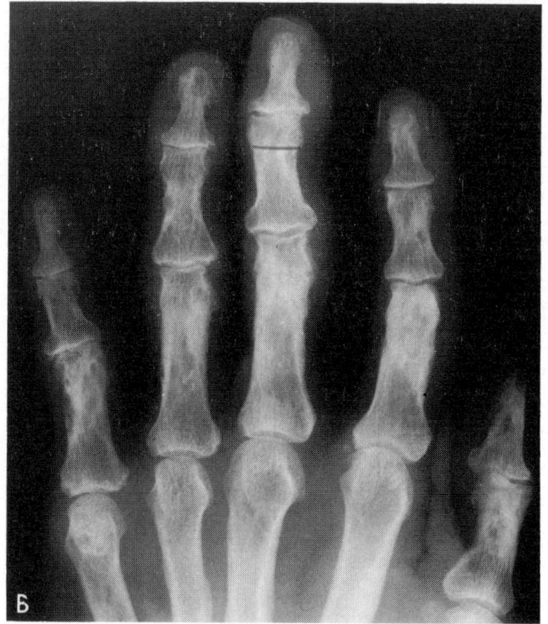

Figure 2–75. *A*, The lateral view of a patient with tuberous sclerosis reveals multiple intracranial calcifications in a periventricular distribution.

B, Multiple small cystic lesions are scattered throughout the phalanges.

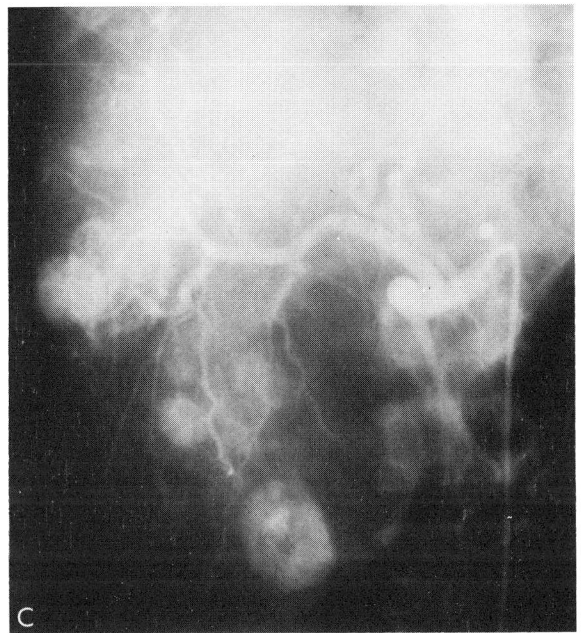

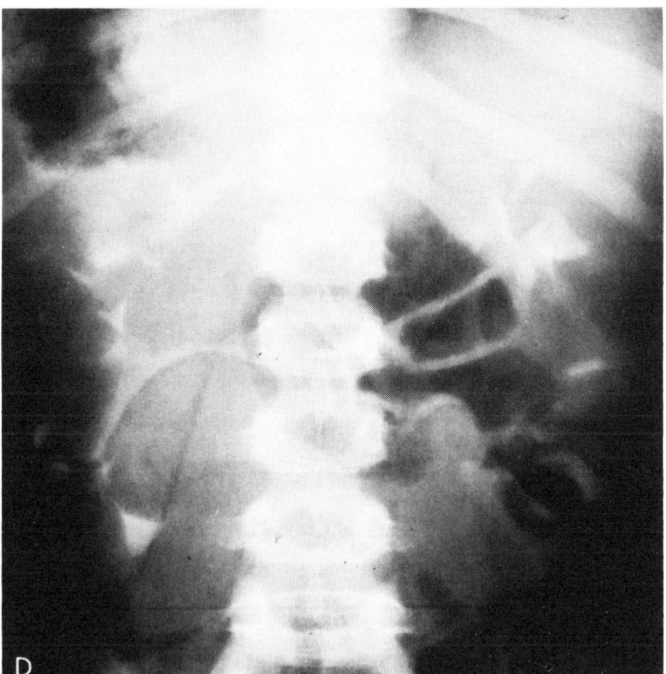

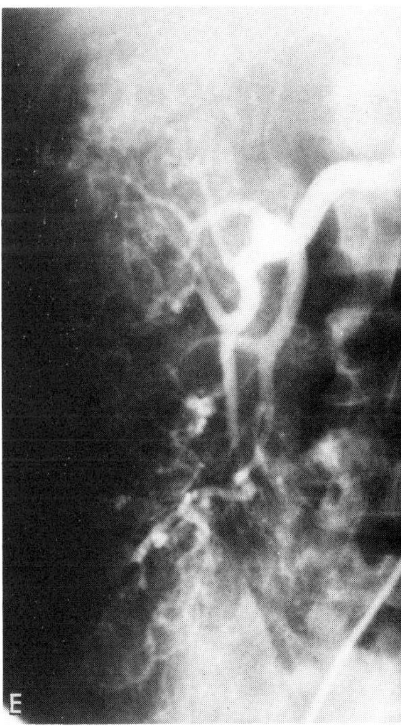

Figure 2–75 *Continued.* *C,* The selective hepatic arteriogram demonstrates hepatomegaly with multiple hypervascular, nodular hamartomas of the liver.

D, The intravenous pyelogram reveals marked enlargement of the kidney bilaterally. The calices are distorted and splayed apart. The infundibula are elongated.

E, The renal arteriogram demonstrates intrinsically abnormal blood vessels supplying multiple vascular hamartomas throughout the greatly enlarged kidney.

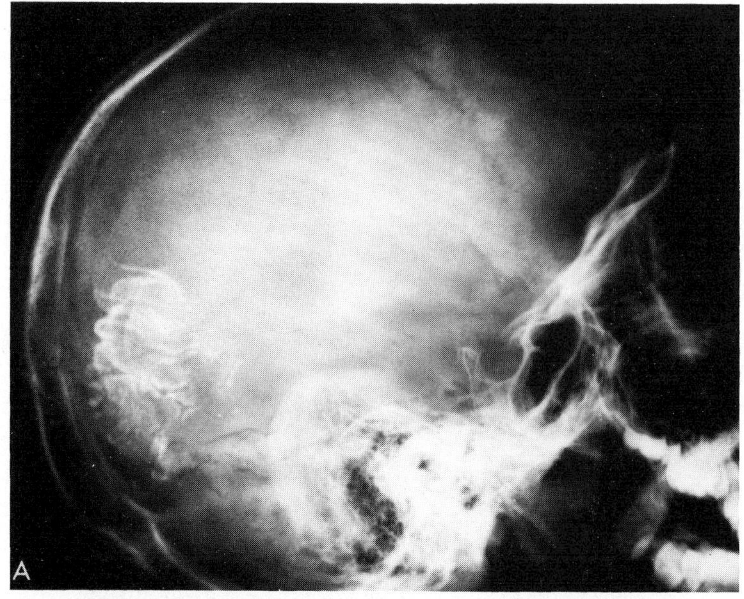

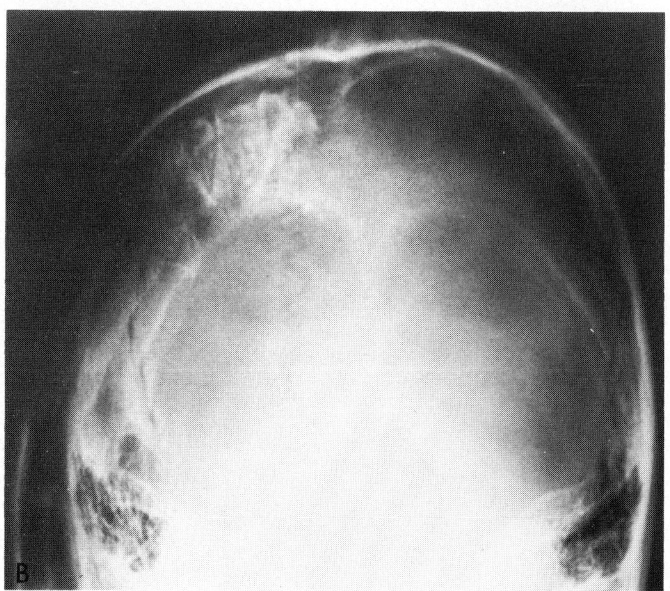

Figure 2–76. STURGE-WEBER SYNDROME: This entity is one of the neurocutaneous syndromes, which include von Recklinghausen's disease (neurofibromatosis), tuberous sclerosis, von Hippel-Lindau's disease, Sturge-Weber syndrome and ataxia telangiectasia.

Sturge-Weber is associated with a hemangioma in the ophthalmic distribution of the 5th cranial nerve, mental retardation, hemiatrophy of the skull on the same side as the facial hemangioma, and intracranial calcification — usually in the occipital region and also on the same side. The calcifications are in a venous angioma of the brain and usually are described as railroad-track calcifications because the curvilinear lines are paired and run parallel to one another.

The hemiatrophy (*A* and *B*) is characterized by a sloping hemicranial elevation of the petrous bone and greater wing of the sphenoid bone, enlargement of the frontal sinus on the side of the atrophy and tilting of the crista galli toward the atrophic side. The hemiatrophy picture was originally described by Davidoff and Dyke in patients with chronic relapsing subtemporal hematomas.

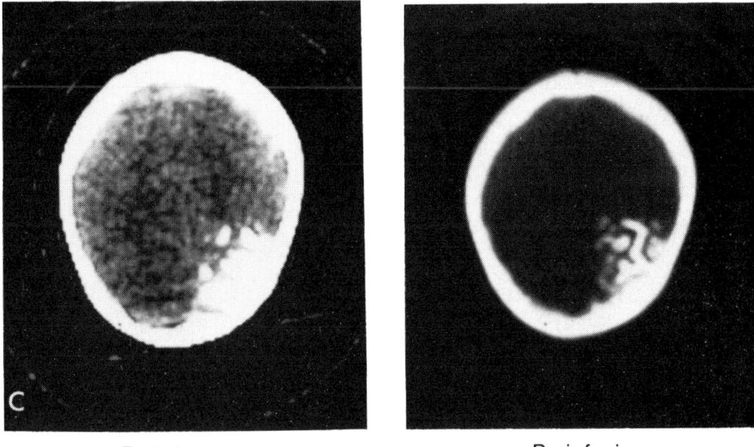

Figure 2–76. *Continued.* The CT scan *(C)* in the same patient demonstrates the asymmetry of the cranial vault, with fattening of the posterior portion of the right hemicranium. Curvilinear areas of calcification deep in the substance of the brain correspond to the plain skull findings.

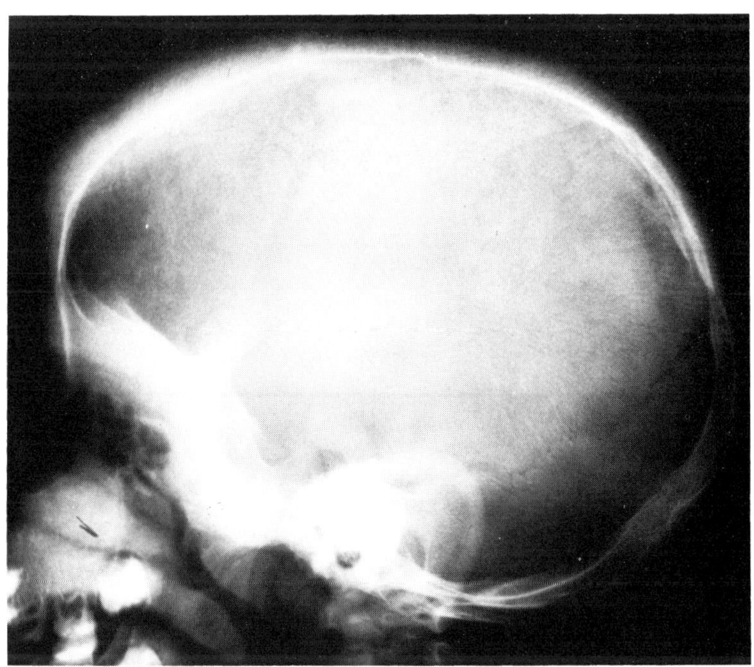

Figure 2–77. THALASSEMIA: The appearance is similar to sickle cell disease, with expansion of the diploic space and a "hair-on-end" appearance of the bony spicules. With thalassemia, however, there may be involvement of the maxillary sinuses and mastoid regions with hematopoiesis — not seen in sickle cell anemia.

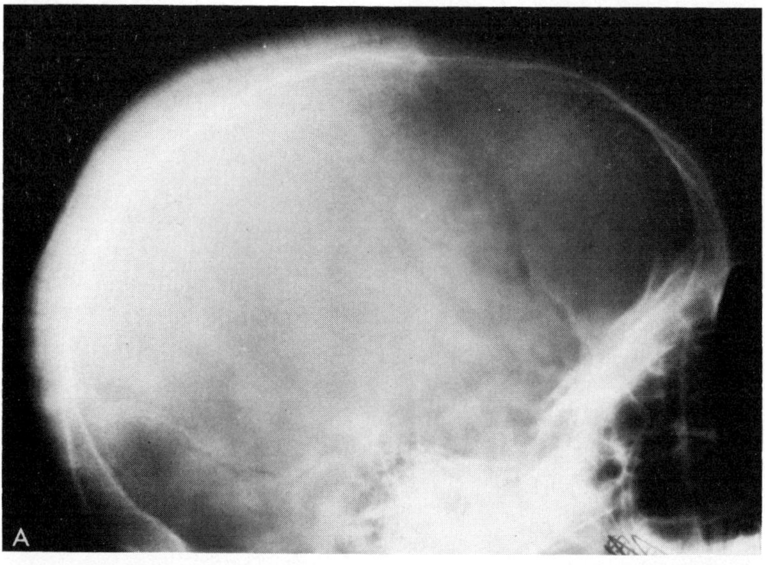

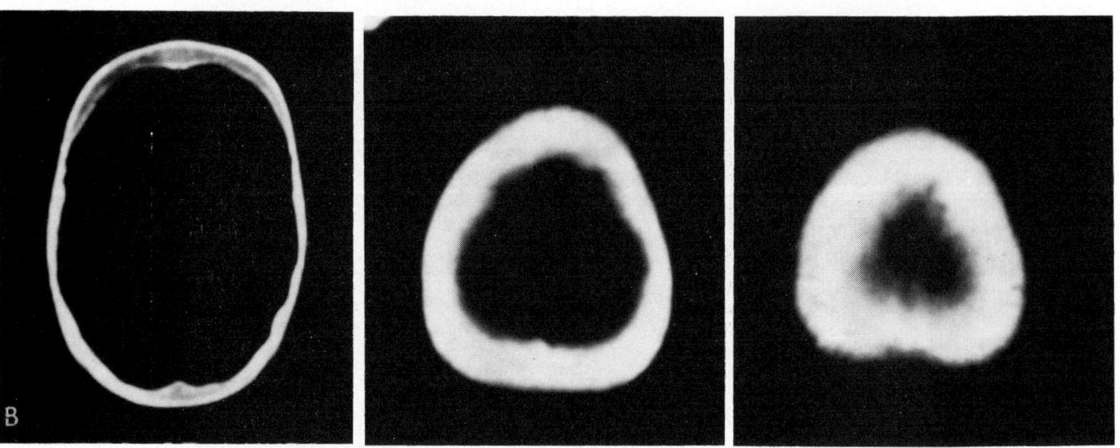

Figure 2–78. SICKLE CELL ANEMIA: *A*, Because of hyperplasia of the bone marrow, there is expansion of the diploic space. The spicules of bone are arranged in a radial pattern perpendicular to the inner table — apparently in an attempt to support the diploic space and outer table, which are weakened and thinned. *B*, These changes are also apparent on CT scans of the bony calvaria.

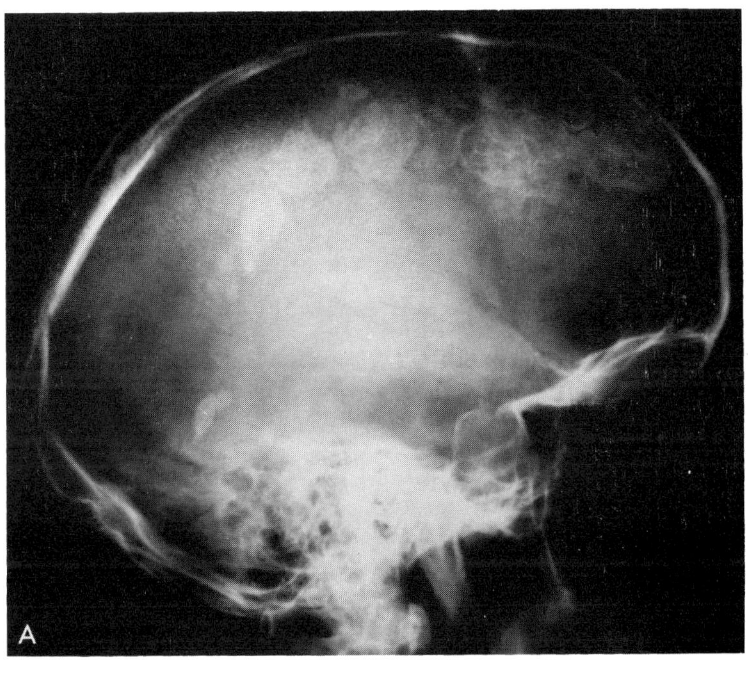

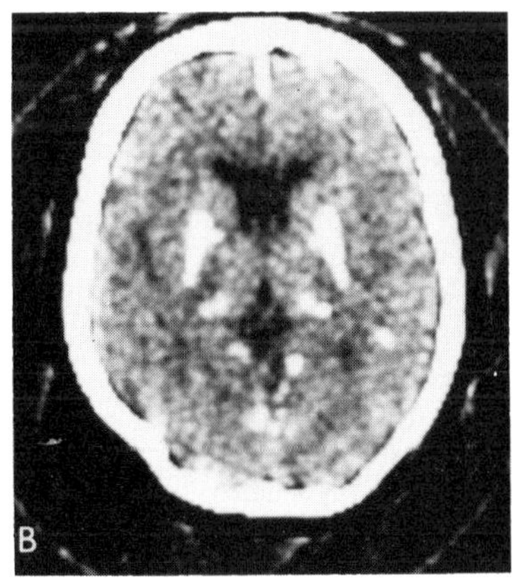

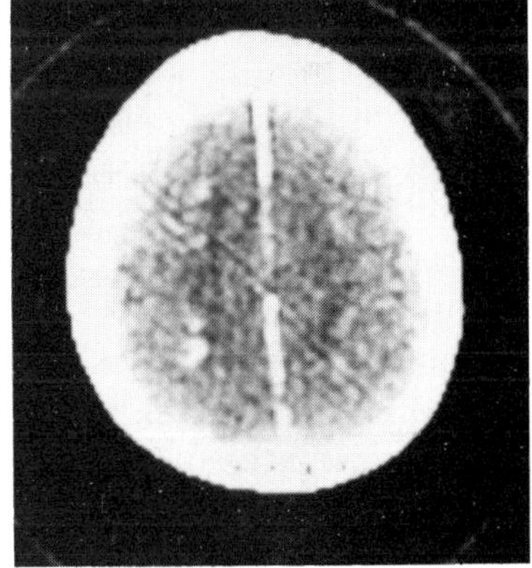

Preinfusion Preinfusion

Figure 2–79. SECONDARY HYPERPARATHYROIDISM: The plain skull lateral view (*A*) demonstrates diffuse deossification of the bony calvaria. In addition, there is extensive calcification of the falx cerebri and tentorium cerebelli.

The CT scan (*B*) also demonstrates the falx and tentorial calcification. In addition, extensive calcification of the basal ganglia and thalamus is seen, which is not visible on the plain films. The calcium deposition is typical of *secondary* hyperparathyroidism.

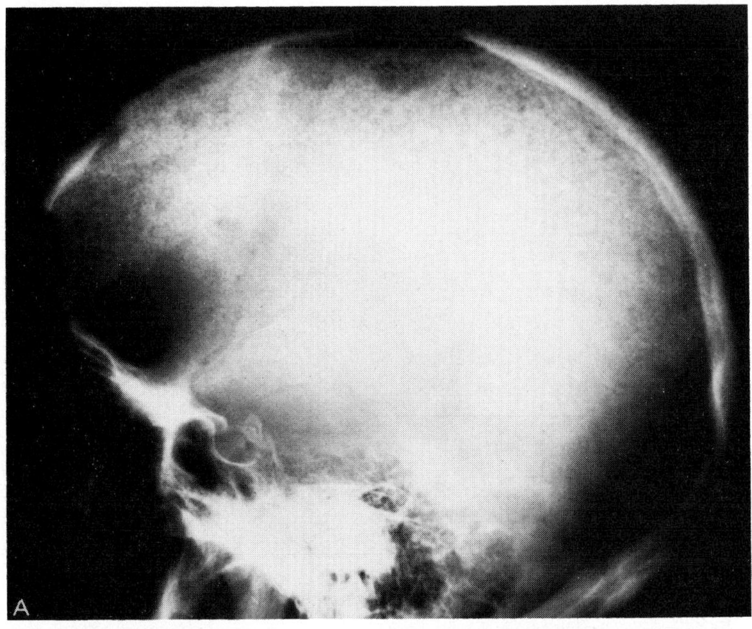

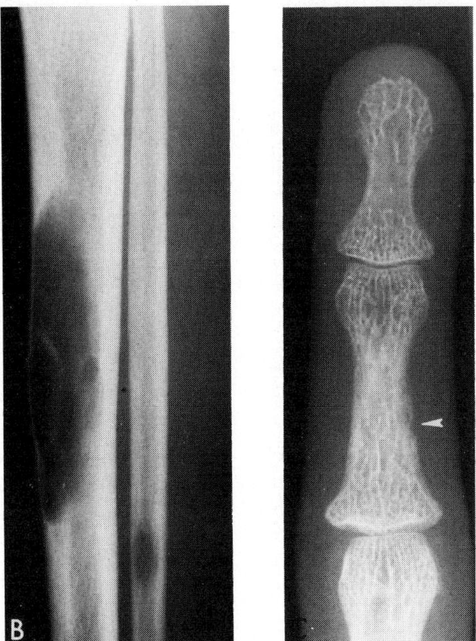

Figure 2–80. PRIMARY HYPERPARATHYROIDISM: The skull may develop a diffuse granular (*A*) "salt and pepper" appearance because of a combination of bone production and destruction. In addition, cystic brown tumors may also involve the bony calvaria. Demonstration of brown tumors in the long bones (*B*) and subperiosteal bony resorption along the radial side of the phalanges (*C*) also substantiate the diagnosis of hyperparathyroidism. The changes in this patient are secondary to a functioning parathyroid adenoma. Laboratory data are necessary for complete evaluation.

THE ABNORMAL SELLA

General Appearance. In thc abscncc of trauma, plain skull evaluation is generally done to demonstrate the presence of primary or metastatic disease to the bony calvaria or cranial contents, metabolic disease, pituitary tumor or evidence of sellar erosion.

Erosion of the sella secondary to increased intracranial pressure can be demonstrated quite early by plain film examination. The earliest signs of erosion secondary to increased intracranial pressure are erosion of the anterior inferior aspect of the dorsum sellae and demineralization of the dorsum sellae. Over a period of time these changes of demineralization will come to involve the entire sella and may even affect the planum sphenoidale. With time, there will not only be demineralization of the floor sella but also thinning and truncation of the uppermost portion of the dorsum sellae and the posterior clinoids. These changes are secondary to nonspecific changes of increased intracranial pressure; they do not necessarily indicate a tumor adjacent to the sella itself. Indeed, the tumor may be quite remote from the region of the sella.

Even more remote changes may be seen, but are found less frequently in today's practice, because patients seek medical care earlier in the course of their illness and do not suffer from this increased intracranial pressure long enough to exhibit these marked changes. In addition, better diagnostic techniques make early diagnosis of intracranial lesions possible.

On the other hand, the changes seen in the sella may be secondary to continued erosion by the anterior recesses of a dilated third ventricle as the transmitted pulsations of both respiration and heart beat produce erosion of the very top of the dorsum sellae, resulting in truncation of the dorsum as well as demineralization.

This type of change is seen in the presence of a space occupying lesion that leads to the production of hydrocephalus secondary to obstruction at or below the level of the posterior portion of the third ventricle. Most commonly, this is secondary to a posterior fossa mass lesion, a pineal tumor or, occasionally, to adult onset of symptoms of aqueduct stenosis.

In the pediatric age group the changes of increased intracranial pressure are reflected in splitting the sutures, usually without changes in the sella turcica. After 10 to 12 years of age, thc sutures become functionally closed, and the changes of increased pressure are reflected in alterations of the sella turcica. Between the ages of 1 year and 10 to 12 years the sutures should not be more than 2 mm wide.

In the presence of changes of increased intracranial pressure, other findings will be helpful and may suggest a diagnosis; e.g., if the pineal gland is shifted, the lateralization of a supratentorial tumor mass may be possible (see Fig. 2–11).

Care must be taken in measuring the shift of the midline structures, and the use of a measure ruler rather than trusting the eye is strongly suggested. Because of possible asymmetric calcification of the pineal, a shift of the pineal of up to 2 mm is considered within normal limits.

Other diagnostic clues are the presence of tumor calcification secondary to pinealoma, oligodendroglioma, astrocytoma, dermoid, cholesteatoma, aneurysm, calcified granuloma and a variety of other disorders. There may likewise be localized areas of hyperostosis secondary to the presence of a meningioma. Again, a pertinent clinical history may be helpful.

Evaluation of the absolute size of the sella should be made during the course of the skull examination. This is not only because the sella may be enlarged secondary to increased intracranial pressure, but also because the presence of intrasellar tumors will lead to an enlarged sellae. Depending on the age group, the pituitary tumor is probably the most common cause of sellar enlargement. There are, however, multiple other causes of enlargement of the sella. These include:

1. Pituitary adenoma:
   A. Chromophobe adenomas
   B. Eosinophilic adenomas
2. Carotid artery aneurysms
3. Meningiomas adjacent to the sella
4. Teratoma
5. Craniopharyngioma
6. Optic glioma
7. Increased intracranial pressure
8. Empty sella syndrome.

This list of relatively common and some less common causes of sellar enlargement should be committed to memory. In addition, there are other more obscure and more rare lesions that also lead to similar changes in the sella.

EMPTY SELLA SYNDROME

The empty sella syndrome is a clinical entity that has been associated with enlargement of the sella and subsequent demonstration of the entrance of air or contrast material into the enlarged sella. There appears to be absence or incompetence of the diaphragma sellae. These patients may be symptomatic, complaining of visual difficulties — apparently because the optic nerves are able to "fall" into the empty sella. Commonly, headache is their main complaint. This syndrome has been seen more often in women than in men, and it has been postulated that the sella may enlarge following swelling of the pituitary gland in response to pregnancy. This initial swelling later shrinks, leaving the "empty sella."

AMIPAQUE CISTERNOGRAPHY

The recent introduction of Amipaque has led to a new method for the diagnosis of a suprasellar mass lesion or even for the evaluation of the empty sella syndrome. Additional clinical experience and expertise may eliminate the need for pneumoencephalography for lesions around the sella.

Amipaque can be introduced into the lumbar subarachnoid space using 6 cc of a 180 mg/ml concentration. The patient is placed immediately in the strongly head-down position and the contrast medium is allowed to flow cephalad and to accumulate in the basilar cisterns. With the patient in the 15° head-down position, the scan is then performed. If a sellar tumor with suprasellar extension is present, there will be a lucent defect — the tumor — surrounded by the higher density Amipaque in the suprasellar cistern. With an "empty sella," the Amipaque will be identified within the confines of the sella.

With thin section tomography a fairly accurate estimate of the size of the lesions can be made. In addition, the patient can be scanned using coronal sections for direct visualization of the size of the tumor. This is frequently unsatisfactory because metallic fillings in the teeth will interfere with the scanning device and degrade the image.

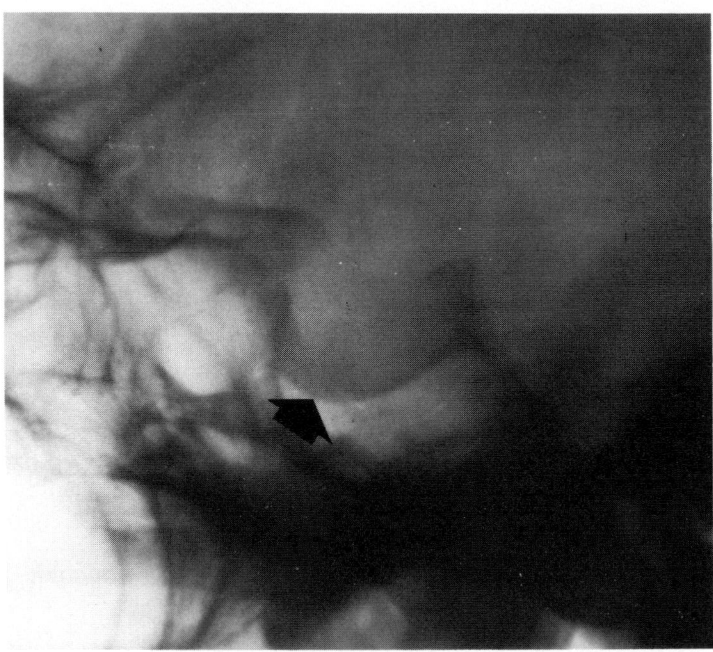

Figure 2–81. DEMINERALIZATION OF THE DORSUM SELLAE SECONDARY TO INCREASED INTRACRANIAL PRESSURE: There is marked demineralization of the floor of the sella, especially in its anterior, inferior margin (*arrow*). The sella is also minimally expanded.

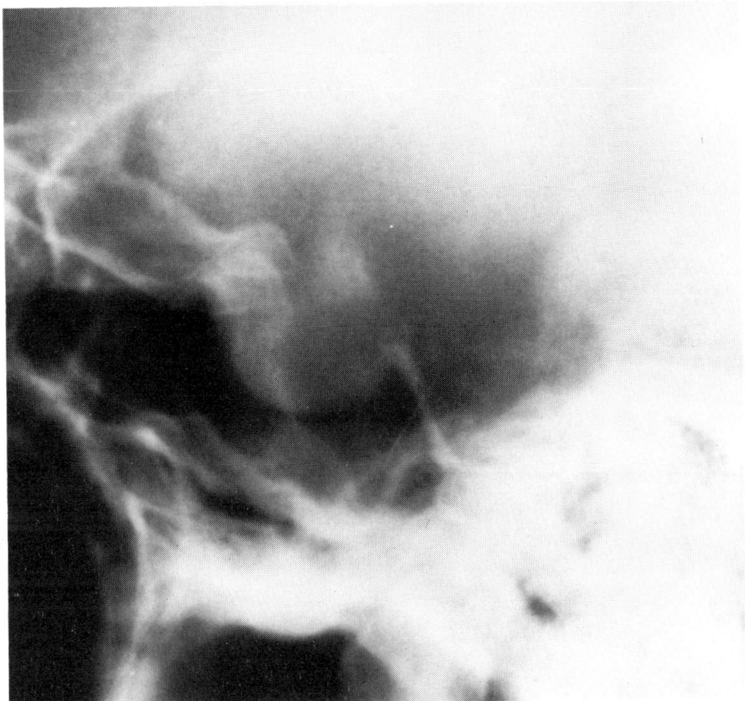

Figure 2–82. MARKED SELLA CHANGES SECONDARY TO CHRONIC INCREASED INTRACRANIAL PRESSURE: There is almost complete dissolution of the floor of the sella; the dorsum sellae is truncated, and the posterior clinoids are markedly demineralized and almost completely destroyed. These changes are secondary to an enlarged, dilated third ventricle protruding into the sella. (Case courtesy of Dr. Gregory I. Shenk; see also Chapter 11.)

PITUITARY ADENOMAS

Chromophobe Adenoma. Of the pituitary adenomas the chromophobe adenoma causes the greatest amount of sellar enlargement and may even progress to cause total destruction of the sella. Massive destructive changes of the sella may be present, with complete erosion of the dorsum sellae and posterior clinoids. These tumors may extend downward through the floor of the sella, eroding the sphenoid sinus and causing a nasopharyngeal mass. Calcification of these tumors is very rare. The clinical syndrome is usually that of panhypopituitarism secondary to pressure obliteration of the remainder of the gland, and the classic physical finding is the presence of a bitemporal hemianopia secondary to pressure on the optic chiasm.

CT scanning of these tumors may be helpful for diagnosis, and scans obtained in coronal section and/or reconstruction tomography is also helpful for better evaluation of the suprasellar extent of the mass. Such studies eventually may obviate the need for pneumoencephalography for sellar lesions. At the present time, however, it appears that CT scanning does not totally evaluate the presence or absence of suprasellar extension, nor, in the presence of detectable suprasellar extension, does it always adequately outline the upper margin of the pituitary mass. More important, for a pituitary mass confined to the sella or with only a small amount of suprasellar extension, the CT scan may not detect the tumor at all. This is because of the close proximity of the bony margins of the sella, which create a partial volume effect with the contents of the sella and interfere with the detection of small changes in density within the sella. If a pituitary tumor is suspected, a pneumoencephalogram may be needed for complete evaluation. This is particularly true with cystic pituitary tumors, where contrast enhancement of the tumor cannot be demonstrated.

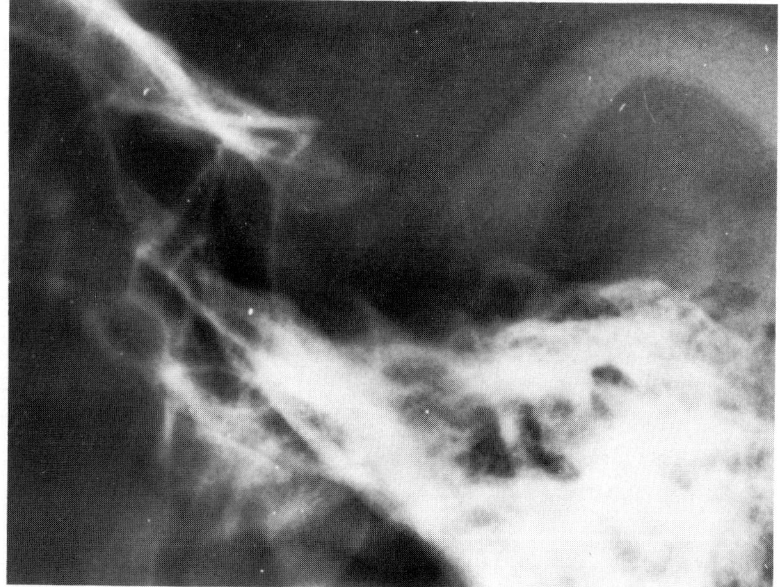

Figure 2–83. CHROMOPHOBE ADENOMA: The sella is greatly enlarged, and there is destruction of the dorsum sellae and posterior clinoids. There is "undercutting" of the anterior clinoids, which also demonstrate a pointed appearance secondary to the expansion of an intrasellar adenoma — in this case a chromophobe adenoma.

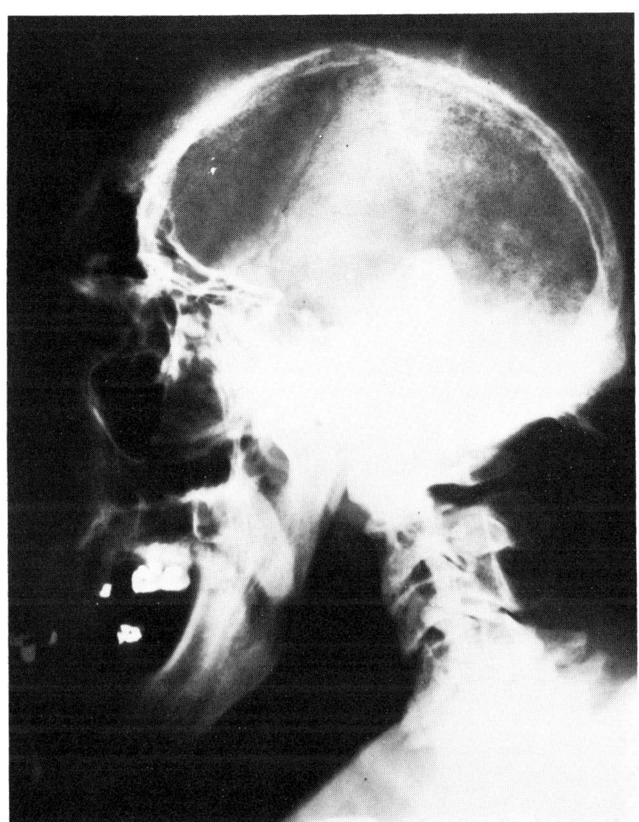

Figure 2–84. ACROMEGALY (Eosinophilic adenoma): In acromegaly there may or may not be enlargement of the sella turcica secondary to an eosinophilic tumor of the pituitary. There may be a diffuse increase in calvarial thickness, or the process may be confined to the frontal region — as opposed to hyperostosis frontalis interna, which spares the midline. This hyperostosis crosses the midline. One may also detect enlargement of the frontal sinuses and of the external occipital protuberance, and an increase in the angle of the jaw, with prognathism and enlarged spaces between the teeth. This case demonstrates all these findings; in addition, there is an increase in the degenerative changes in the spine — a finding also seen with acromegaly. Other changes that may be detected include enlargement of the ungual tufts of the fingers and accentuation of the dorsal kyphosis of the spine.

In the younger age groups, excess secretion of growth hormone results in pituitary gigantism.

Basophilic Adenoma. Basophilic adenomas of the pituitary gland rarely cause sellar enlargement. The clinical picture is that of Cushing's disease. The one exception to this would be following lateral adrenalectomy, when the sella may enlarge secondary to an ACTH-producing tumor. Changes in the sella with this rare disease may be only those seen with Cushing's disease — i.e., diffuse demineralization.

In actual fact, any cell type of pituitary adenoma may demonstrate any of the clinical syndromes, and there is a great deal of crossover between the various types of tumors.

A variety of brain tumors and inflammatory processes may lead to intracranial calcification. Table 2–2 lists most of the causes of intracranial calcification. Examples of these calcifications are given in the illustrations that follow.

TABLE 2–2. INTRACRANIAL CALCIFICATIONS

1. Meningioma	16. Dermoid
2. Astrocytoma	17. Epidermoid
3. Oligodendroglioma	18. Tuberous sclerosis
4. Glioblastoma	19. Cytomegalic inclusion disease
5. Abscess	20. Toxoplasmosis
6. Infarct	21. Rubella
7. Arteriovenous malformation	22. Herpes simplex
8. Aneurysm	23. Parasite infestations:
9. Basal ganglia calcification	(a) cysticercosis
10. Hematoma	(b) paragonimiasis
11. Granuloma	(c) *Trichinella spiralis*
12. Gumma	24. Sturge–Weber syndrome
13. Ependymoma	25. Craniopharyngioma
14. Pinealoma	26. Pituitary adenoma (rare)
15. Teratoma	27. Aneurysm of the vein of Galen

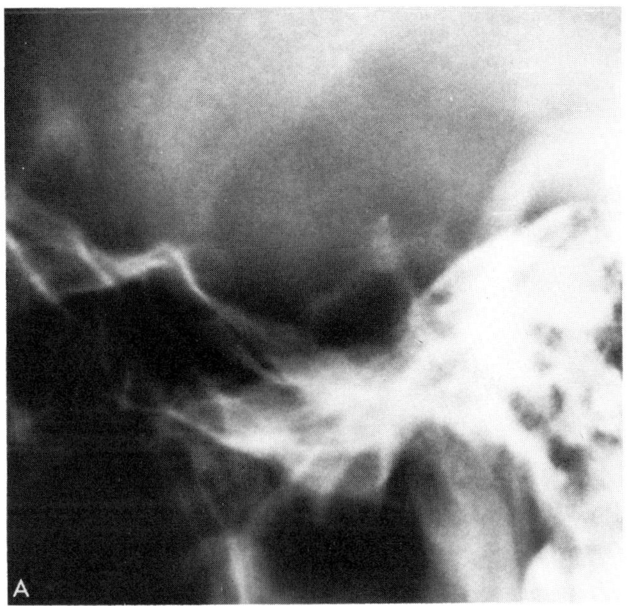

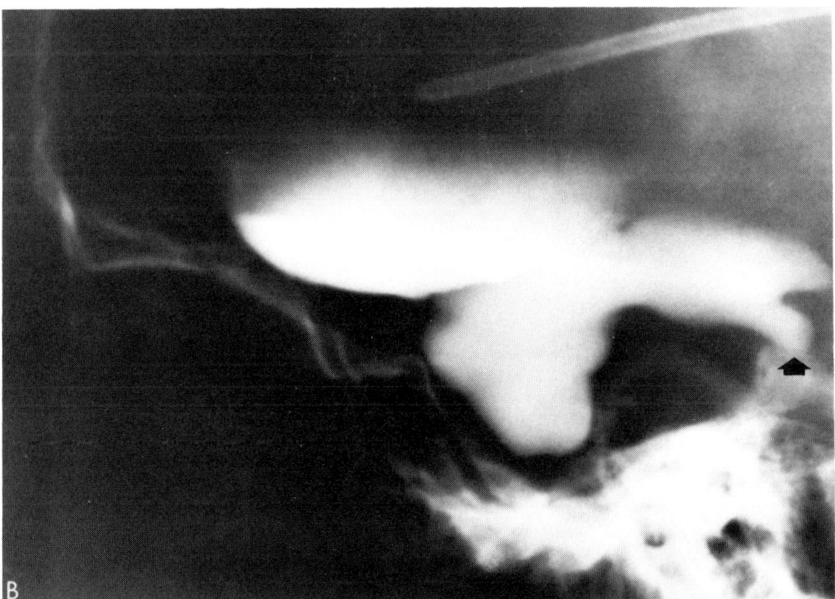

Figure 2–85. ENLARGED SELLA SECONDARY TO DILATED THIRD VENTRICLE: *A*, The sella is greatly enlarged, especially in its posterior inferior portion, and is markedly demineralized throughout. The dorsum sellae is thinned and displaced posteriorly.

B, The Conray ventriculogram demonstrates dilatation of the lateral and third ventricles and obstruction of the dilated aqueduct (*arrowhead*). The dilated third ventricle exactly conforms to the abnormal shape of the sella.

This patient was an adult with aqueduct obstruction.

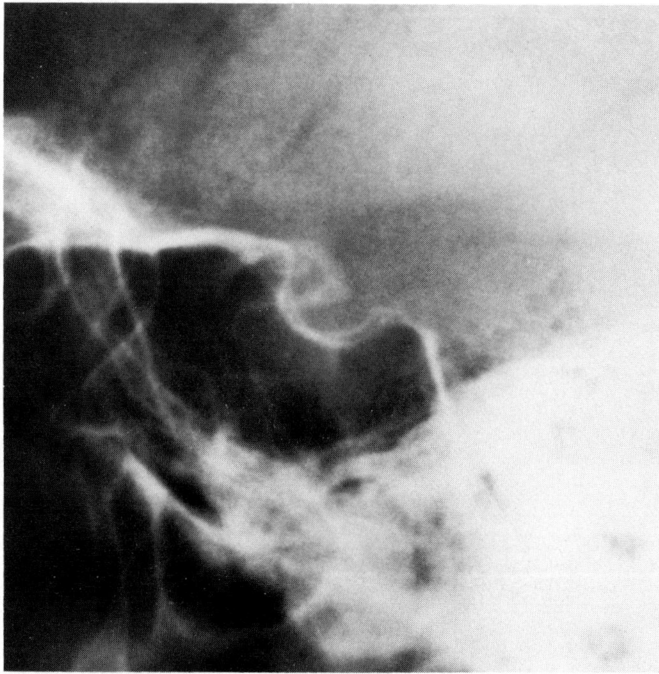

Figure 2–86. AMPUTATION OF DORSUM SELLAE: Because of the nonspecific changes of chronic increased intracranial pressure, there is total amputation of the dorsum sellae and the posterior clinoid processes. Note that the size of the sella is otherwise unchanged in this example.

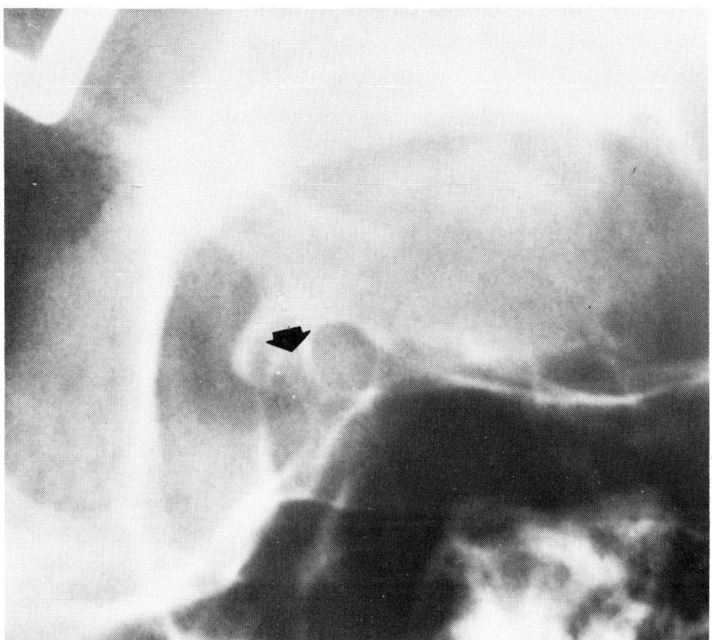

Figure 2–87. OPTIC CANAL: The optic canal is oval in a vertical dimension on the orbital side, round in the midportion and oval in a horizontal dimension on the brain side. The optic canal points laterally at degrees from the straight anteroposterior plane. The optic canals should never exceed 7 mm in diameter. The maximum difference between the two sides should not exceed 2 mm.

The optic canal may be enlarged by such processes as an optic glioma or chronic increased intracranial pressure or decreased in size secondary to optic atrophy or encroachment by osteopetrosis.

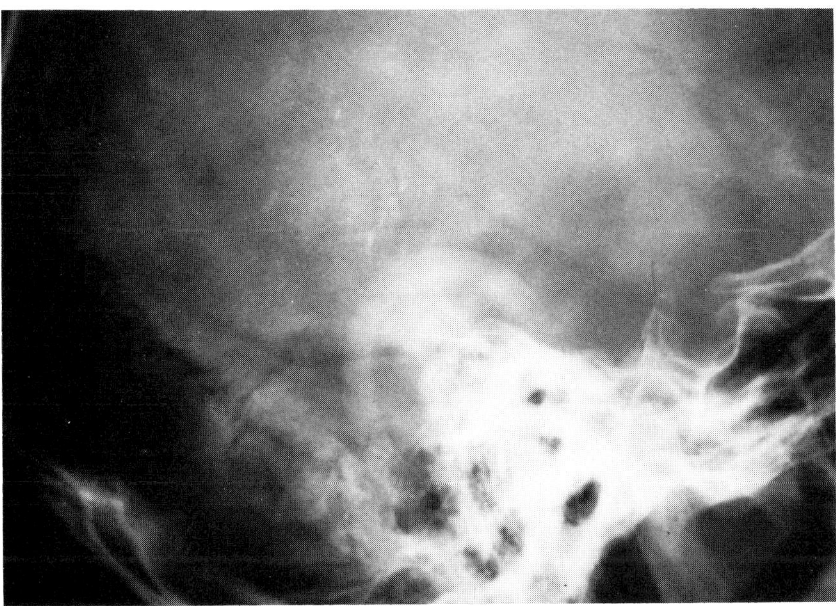

Figure 2–88. CALCIFIED ARTERIOVENOUS MALFORMATION: Multiple small speckled areas of calcifications project superior and posterior to the mastoid air cells. Curvilinear areas of arterial or venous calcification also may be seen.

Meningioma. The incidence of radiographically visible calcification has been reported to be as high as 18 per cent, but 10 per cent or less is the most commonly reported figure. As with other types of calcified brain tumors, it seems that the incidence of visible calcifications on plain skull films is lower than previously reported. This is because brain tumors in general are being diagnosed earlier and are therefore smaller in size. On the other hand, CT scans are able to detect areas of calcification not visible on the plain film examination.

The meningiomas contain psammomatous calcification, and these calcifications frequently are small stippled areas distributed homogeneously throughout the tumor. They may be distributed only peripherally or may calcify only in a portion of the tumor (see Chapter 10.

These tumors also may exhibit reactive bone formation.

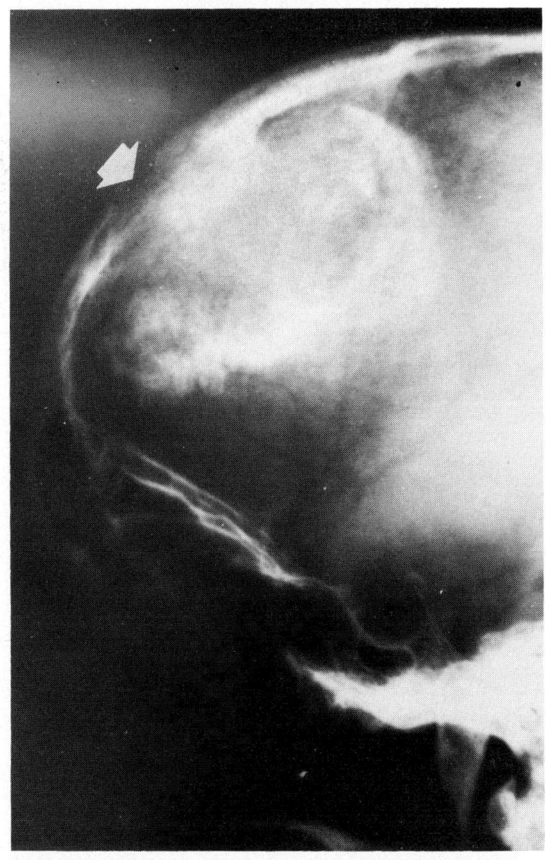

Figure 2–89. CALCIFIED MENINGIOMA WITH INVASION OF THE CALVARIA: There is invasion of the frontal bone at the point of attachment of the meningioma, without evidence of reactive bone formation. This bony invasion occurs in a small per cent of cases. (Case courtesy of Drs. O. Sugar and G. Dobben.)

Oligodendroglioma. These tumors exhibit calcification in most cases, but are uncommon. Over one half of these tumors calcify. The calcification may be amorphous and/or speckled; however, the author has frequently seen "boomerang shaped" areas of calcification in these oligodendrogliomas; this is exhibited in the present example (Fig. 2–90).

The calcification is readily demonstrated on the CT scan, even when it is only faintly visible on the plain skull examination. In this case the abnormal area is much more readily identified on the CT scan than on the plain skull examination.

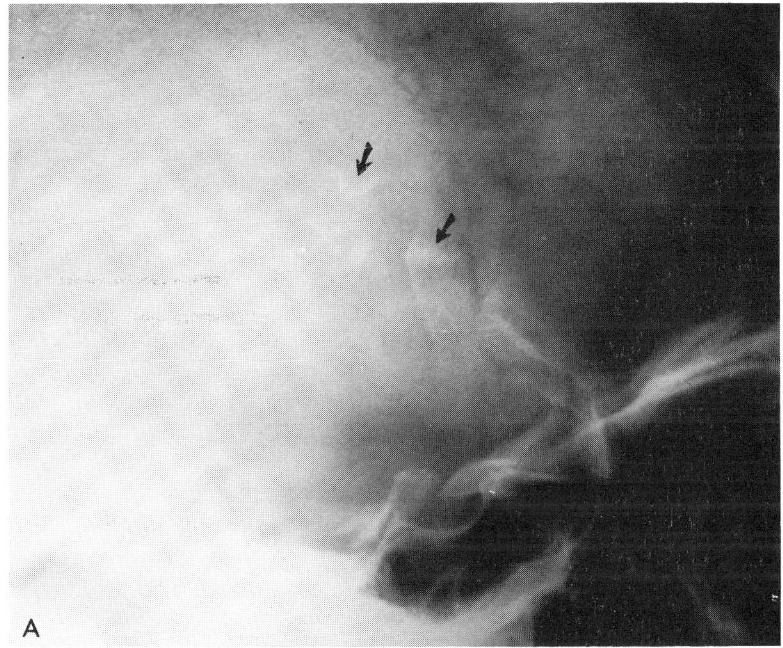

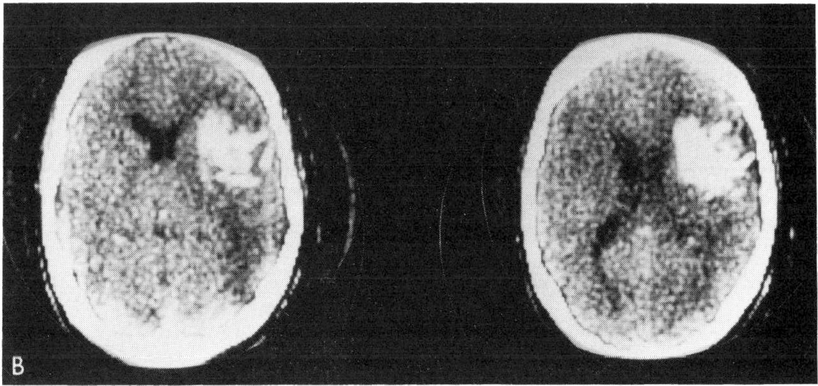

Figure 2–90. *A*, The plain skull film shows multiple curvilinear areas of calcification (*arrows*); a 3-mm shift of the pineal gland to the contralateral side also was present. The CT scan (*B*) demonstrates extensive areas of apparent dense calcification deep in the right hemisphere, associated with moderate compression of the frontal horn of the right lateral ventricle. A postinfusion scan was not performed. This is a surgically proved oligodendroglioma. (Skull film courtesy of the Carle Clinic Radiology Group.)

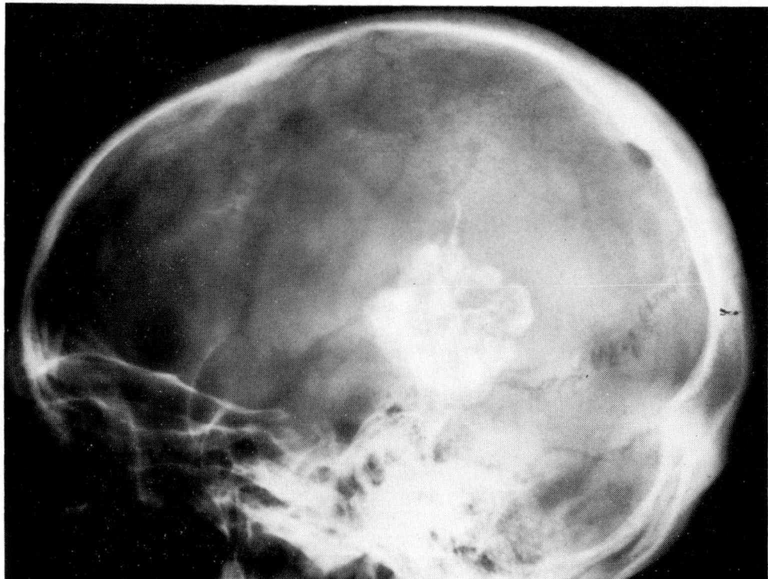

Figure 2–91. OLIGODENDROGLIOMA: The plain skull demonstrates a large, densely calcified lobulated mass. This is a spectacular case of a calcified oligodendroglioma. The pneumoencephalogram also demonstrated a cystic component to the tumor. This case was studied before the discovery of CT scanning; however, the CT scan would have beautifully demonstrated both the calcified and cystic components of the tumor.

GLIOMAS

As a group, the gliomas represent approximately 50 per cent of all the primary brain tumors. They demonstrated microscopic calcification in one third of the cases when reported in 1914. However, at the present time it appears that the incidence of calcification is far less than that previously reported. This is presumably because computed tomography and other diagnostic techniques have made possible diagnosis much earlier in the course of the disease. The calcification is due to the focal areas of necrosis that result as the tumor outgrows its normal blood supply. The calcification is amorphous and may proceed asymmetrically within the tumor mass. There may be solitary areas of calcification or large clusters.

These areas of calcification are readily detected by CT scanning, even if not visible on plain skull radiographs.

Astrocytoma – Grades I and II. Calcifications are detectable in approximately one fifth of cases. These tumors frequently have a cystic component, and calcifications also may occur in the walls of the cyst.

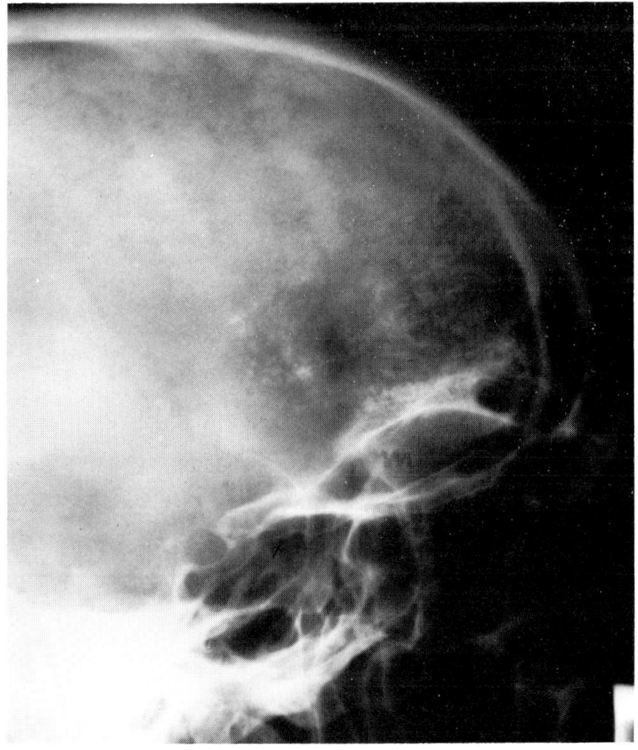

Figure 2–92. ASTROCYTOMA: Small, speckled calcifications outline a large frontal lobe astrocytoma. It has been stated that as many as 20 per cent of astrocytomas demonstrate calcifications that are visible on plain skull films. However, since the development of new diagnostic techniques, it appears that only a very small percentage of astrocytomas contain radiographically visible calcification. Indeed, we only occasionally see a calcified astrocytoma on CT scans.

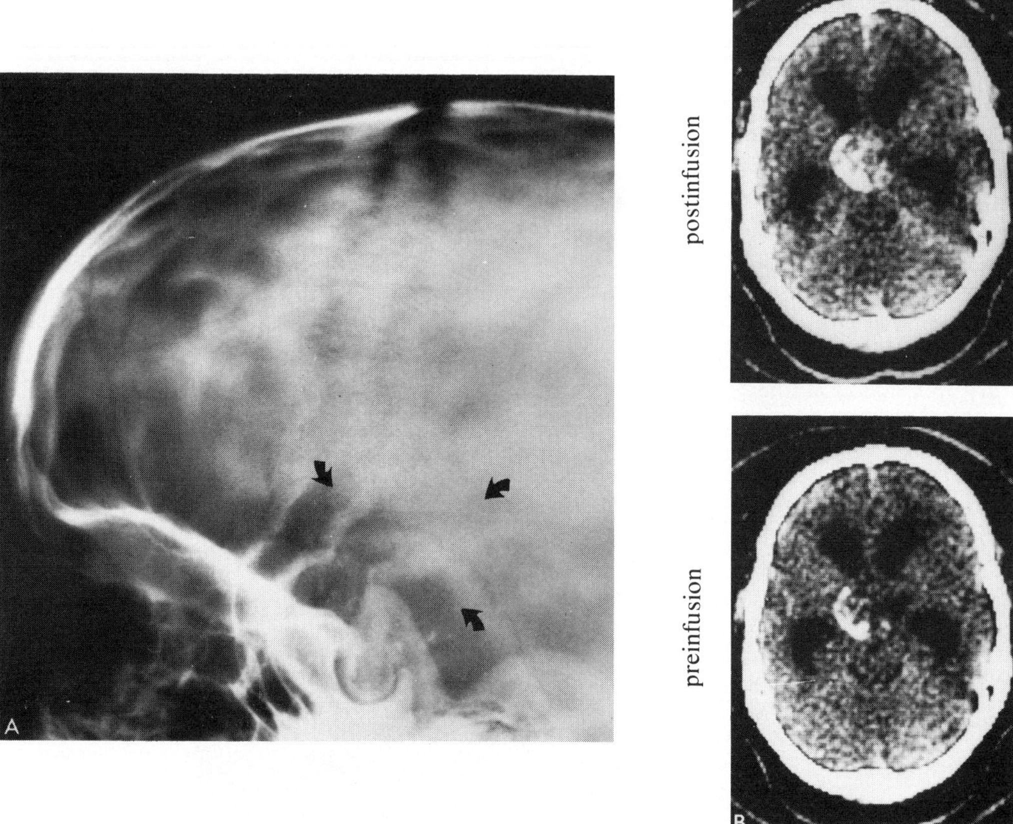

Figure 2–93. CRANIOPHARYNGIOMA: Craniopharyngiomas arise in the suprasellar area from remnants of Rathke's pouch, producing an enlargement of the sella with their intrasellar extension. There are two age group peaks for craniopharyngiomas. The lower age group ranges through the first three decades; the second is patients over the age of 50. In the younger group, approximately 60 per cent of the tumors are calcified; in the older group, only 20 per cent are calcified. These tumors are often cystic, calcifying around the periphery of the tumor (*A*). The calcification may not outline the entire tumor mass. These calcifications are often apparent on plain skull examination, but are much more readily apparent on the CT scan. They may be scattered and punctate or curvilinear in configuration.

In the case shown, the full extent of the suprasellar calcification cannot be appreciated, but the process extends into the suprasellar cistern. The pituitary gland demonstrates extensive peripheral calcifications.

Hypervascularity of the tumor may not be apparent on the arteriogram, but will be readily visualized on the CT scan (*B*) as a rim of enhancement that outlines the tumor to best advantage.

The craniopharyngiomas may not calcify at all. If this is the case, there will be simply a cystic mass in the suprasellar cistern that extends into the sella. The fluid within the cyst is of higher density than cerebrospinal fluid, and reflects the fluid that has been described as "crank-case oil" when surgically removed. These craniopharyngiomas may enlarge sufficiently to produce hydrocephalus secondary to obstruction at the level of the foramen of Monro.

It should be noted that, if hydrocephalus of this type is present, it may be necessary to shunt both ventricles so that the decompression of one ventricle does not lead to herniation of the opposite ventricle under the falx cerebri secondary to the ventricle's behaving as a mass lesion.

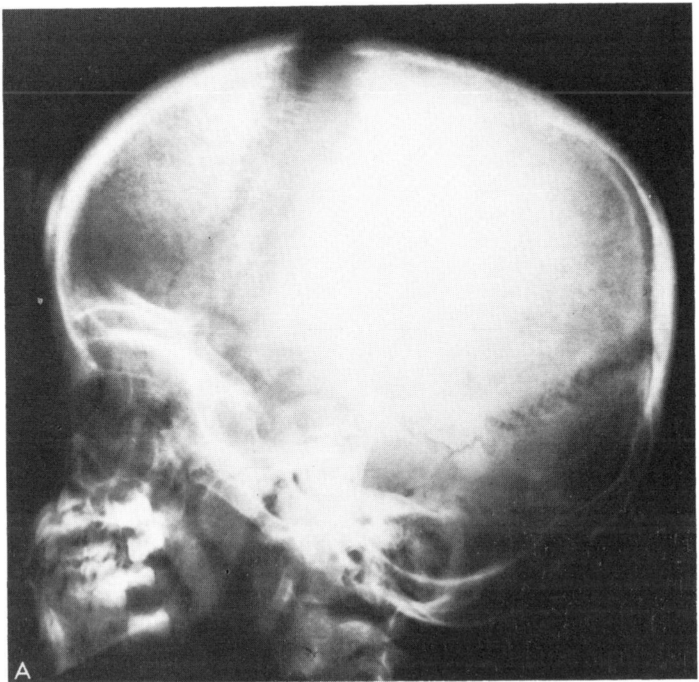

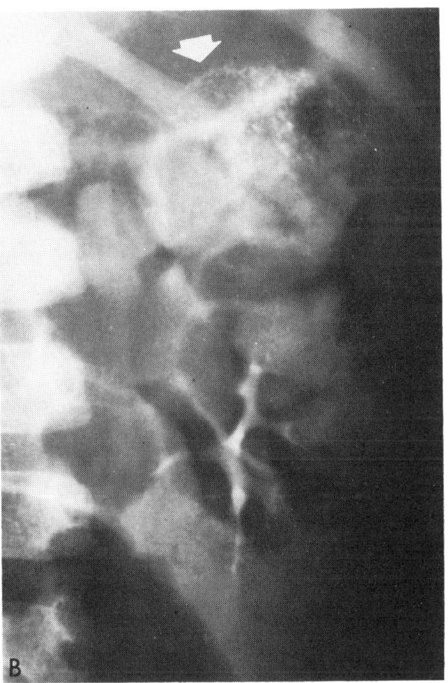

Figure 2–94. NEUROBLASTOMA: *A*, The skull film demonstrates scattered areas of lucency throughout the calvaria secondary to osteolytic metastatic deposits of neuroblastoma in the calvarial bones. In addition, there is wide separation of the coronal suture because of spread of the tumor cells into the meninges.

B, The intravenous pyelogram reveals a left suprarenal mass that is rounded and contains diffuse areas of calcification. The left kidney is displaced inferiorly. This is a primary neuroblastoma arising in the left adrenal gland. (Case courtesy of Dr. John Fennessy.)

Metastatic leukemic infiltrates may produce changes in the skull similar to those seen with neuroblastoma.

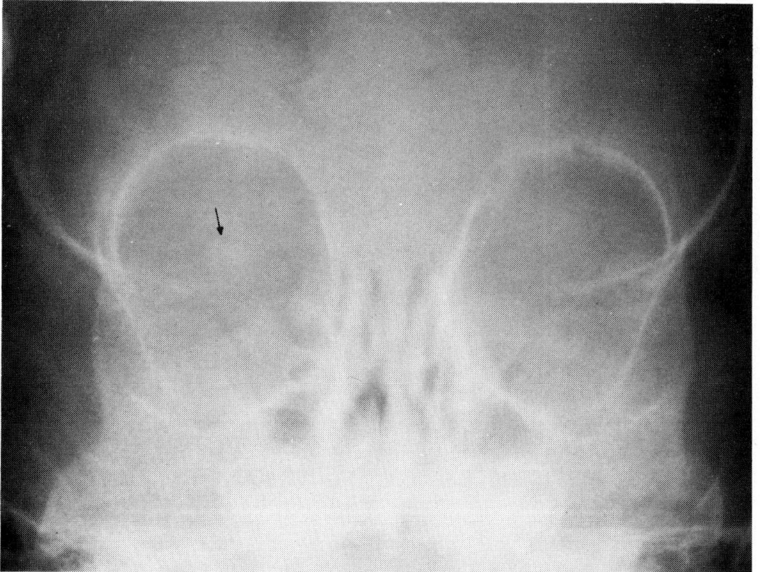

Figure 2–95. RETINOBLASTOMA: Retinoblastomas may calcify sufficiently to be visible on radiographs. The CT scan revealed similar findings. In this case, calcifications are faintly visible in the right retina (*arrow*).

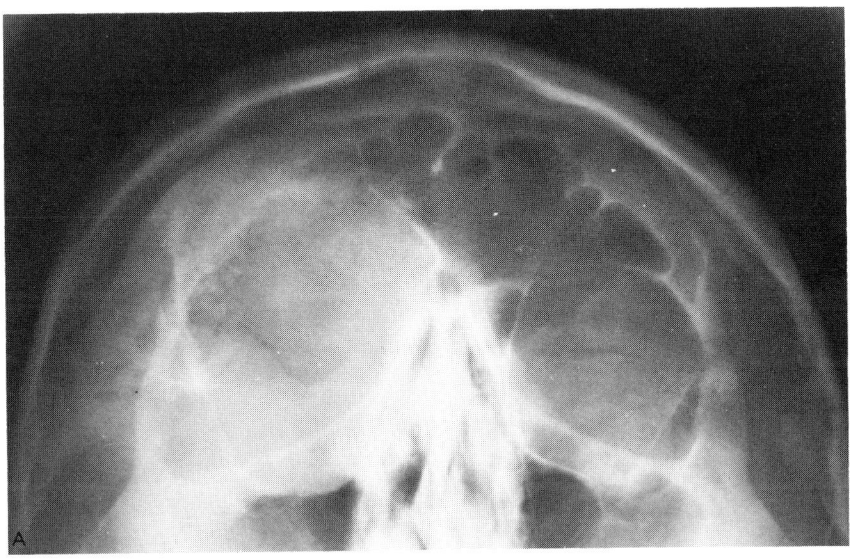

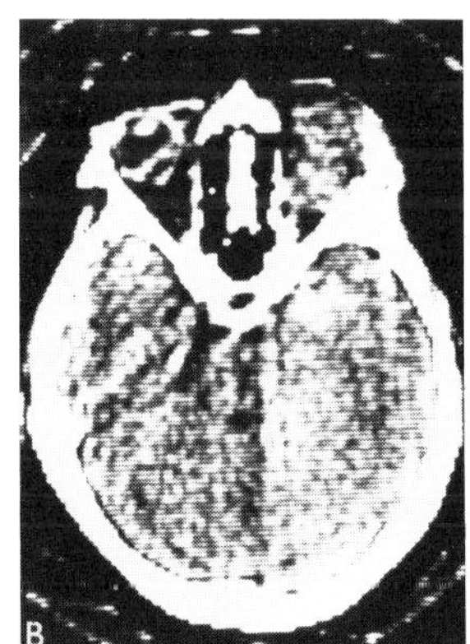

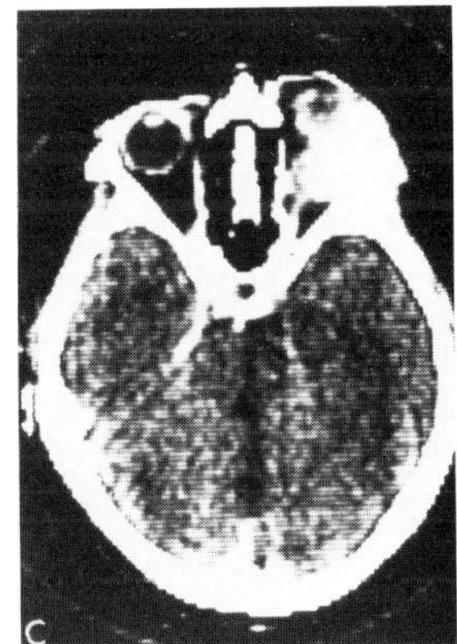

Figure 2–96. LACRIMAL GLAND CARCINOMA: The plain skull film (*A*) reveals extensive bony destructive change involving the roof of the orbit, the lateral margin of the orbit and the zygomatic process of the frontal bone. There is also soft tissue swelling. The CT scan (*B*) shows a large soft tissue mass lateral to and behind the globe on the right side. Exophthalmos is also present on the right side. The postinfusion scan (*C*) reveals homogeneous enhancement of the tumor mass. This was proved surgically to be a lacrimal gland carcinoma.

Figure 2–97. ANEURYSM: Giant aneurysms are described as those greater than 2.5 cm in size.

Aneurysm of the cavernous portion of the internal carotid artery may cause unilateral sellar enlargement if the aneurysm reaches a sufficient size. Most commonly, the changes in the sella will be unilateral and will consist of erosion of the anterior clinoid process and dorsum sellae and floor of the sella on the side of the aneurysm (*A*). In addition, there may be an associated curvilinear calcification adjacent to the sella, which substantiates the diagnosis of a vascular mass. Besides the changes in the sella, there may be erosion of the superior orbital fissure secondary to mass effect and pressure erosion of the aneurysm (*B*). Tomograms of the sella will help to confirm the configuration of the sellar erosion; in addition they may reveal areas of curvilinear calcification not apparent on the plain films.

The CT scans (*C*) of these large aneurysms have rather characteristic appearances. The preinfusion scan reveals a large area of increased density in the parasellar area. These large aneurysms may also have areas of calcification in their walls; these are readily apparent on the CT scan. After infusion of contrast material there will be enhancement of all or a portion of the aneurysm. The area of enhancement will vary with the size of the aneurysm; also, it should be noted that frequently there is only a small area of enchancement because the rest of the aneurysm is filled with clotted blood.

The increased density on the preinfusion scan is secondary to both flowing as well as clotted blood in the aneurysm. In fact, the pattern of enhancement may be somewhat unusual because of this fact. At times, one may mistakenly think of other pathologic entities, e.g., parasellar meningiomas, because of the high density on the preinfusion scan and the marked and often homogeneous enhancement. It would appear that a correct diagnosis is not always possible in these cases, but the possibility of an aneurysm should be strongly suggested—especially since the wall of the aneurysm tends to calcify, resulting in peripheral calcification rather than homogeneous calcification. Arteriography will, of course, be necessary to confirm the diagnosis and also to evaluate the full extent of the disease (see Chapters 5 and 8).

Clinically, these giant aneurysms often present as a partial or complete "cavernous sinus syndrome" with involvement of the II, III, IV, V and VI cranial nerves. Patients will complain of the gradual progression of blindness and varying degrees of extraocular muscle paralysis. There may also be retro-orbital pain with these large aneurysms. (Case courtesy of Dr. John Fennessy.)

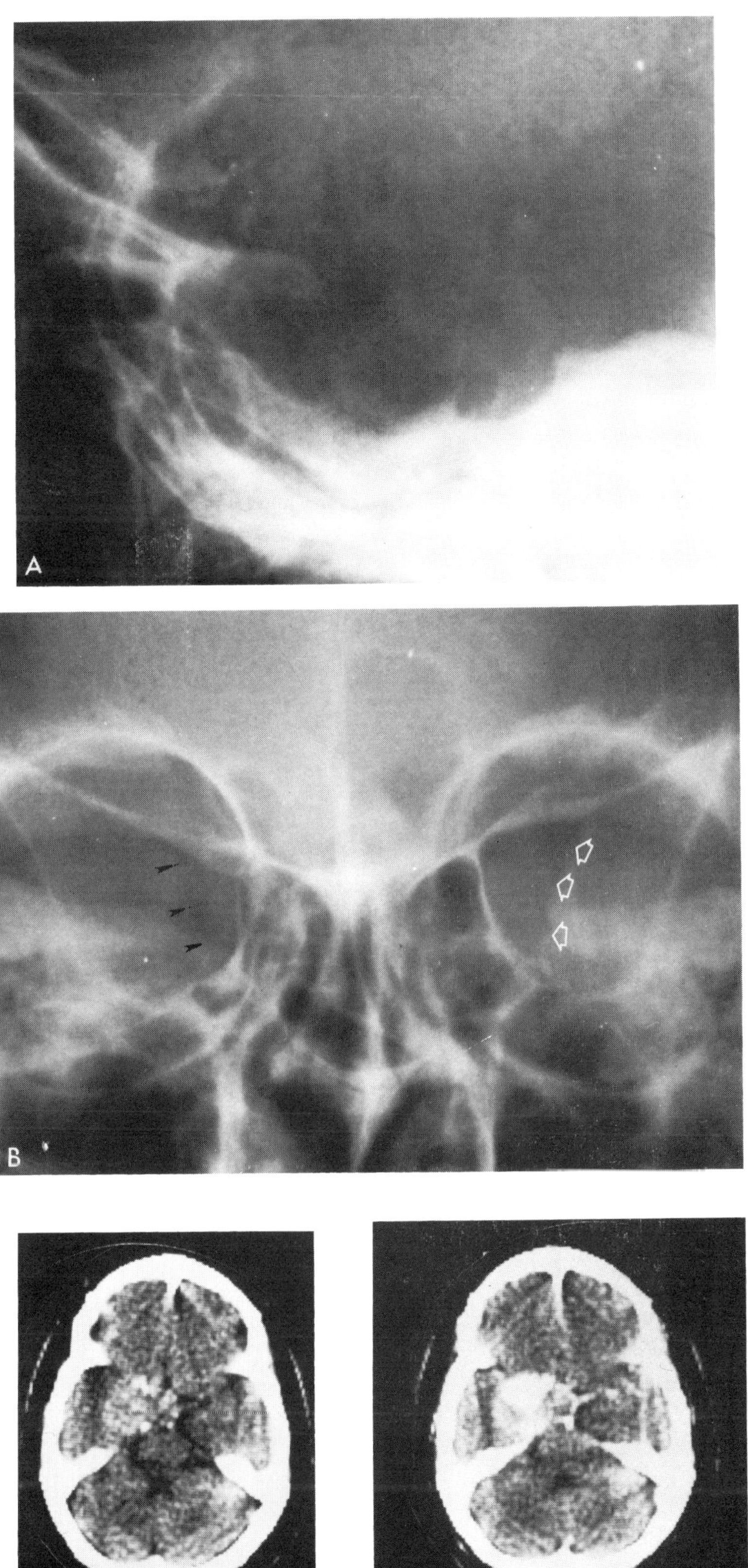

Figure 2–97. *See legend on the opposite page.*

METASTASES

Although osteoblastic metastatic deposits may be seen with prostatic carcinoma, treated osteolytic lesions (in the healing phase) or in healing hyperparathyroidism, most metastatic deposits in the cranial vault are osteolytic. The lesions frequently are of varying size, with poorly defined irregular margins. Differentiation from multiple venous lakes may be difficult.

Any tumor known to metastasize may spread to the bony calvaria; however, metastatic breast carcinoma is seen most commonly in daily practice. These lesions may be demonstrated on the CT scan of the calvaria; however, the routine skull series is a more efficient and reliable examination for the diagnosis of metastatic disease.

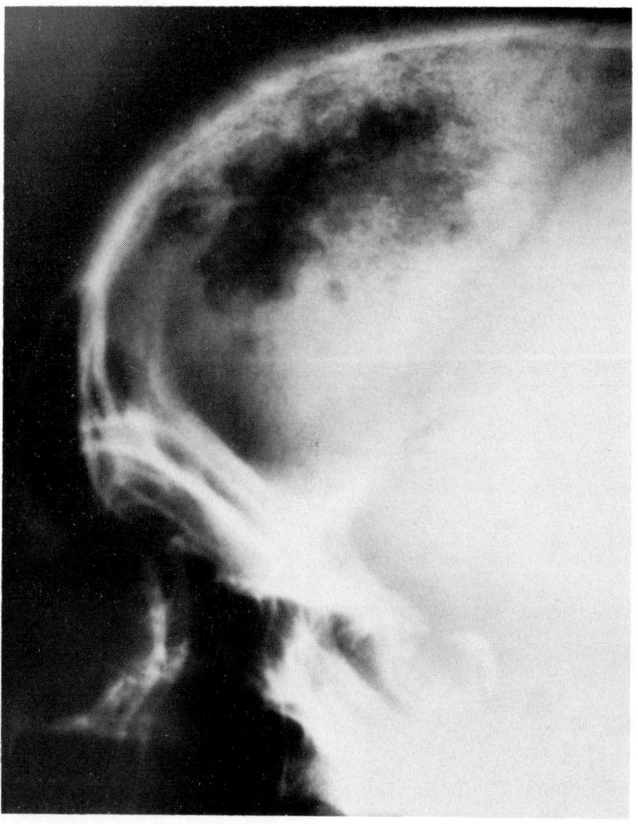

Figure 2–98. This patient demonstrates a large, poorly marginated osteolytic metastatic deposit in the frontal bone. The patient has known breast cancer.

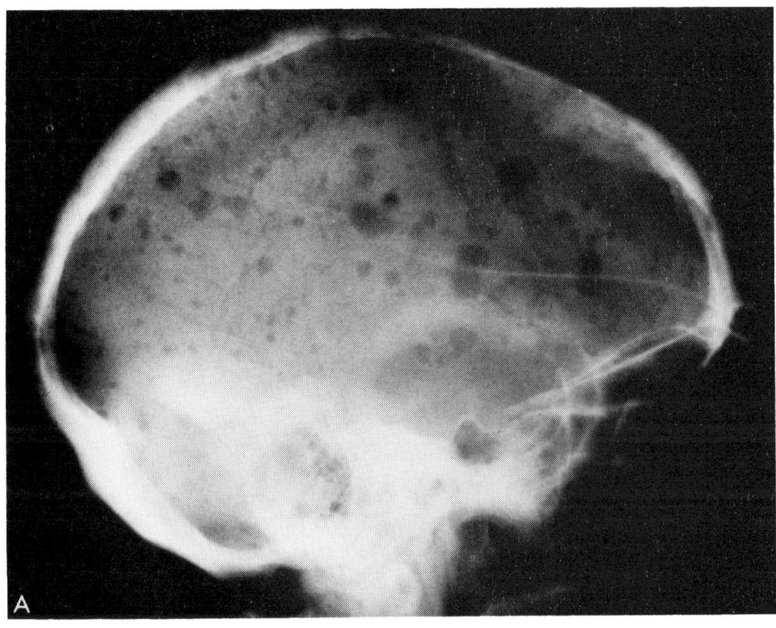

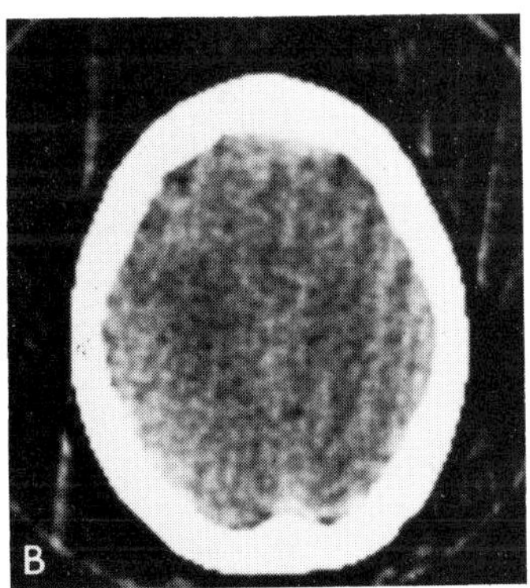

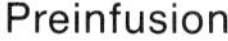
Preinfusion

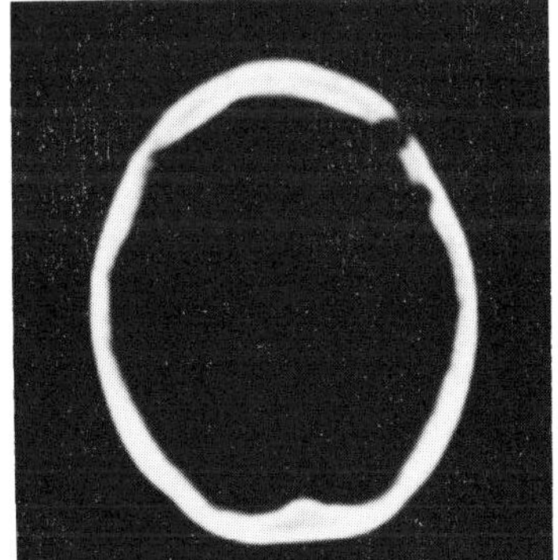

Preinfusion

Figure 2–99. MULTIPLE MYELOMA: The skull lesions seen with multiple myeloma (*A*) are scattered radiolucent areas with poorly defined margins that give the appearance of "droplets of oil on brown paper." Absolute differentiation from multiple metastases is impossible, and diagnosis rests on results of laboratory data.

Multiple myeloma may involve the mandible, whereas other types of metastases rarely do. This finding may help in differential diagnosis.

CT scans of the head (*B*) reveal that the bony calvaria appears to be normal at standard window widths and window levels, whereas on higher window widths and levels the metastatic lesions can readily be identified in the diploë of the skull. It is important to view the CT scan of the skull on high window width and window levels whenever bony metastases are suspected.

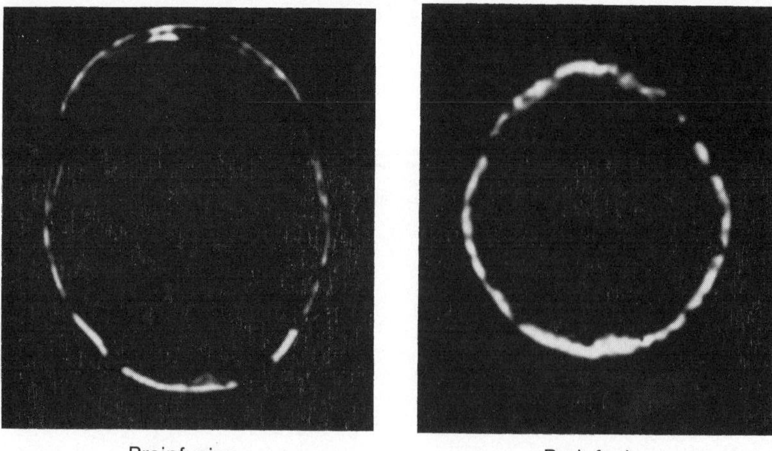

Preinfusion Preinfusion

Figure 2–100. CT SCAN OF MULTIPLE MYELOMA: The CT scan of the bony calvaria, using high window widths and window levels, reveals innumerable osteolytic metastatic deposits throughout the calvaria secondary to multiple myeloma.

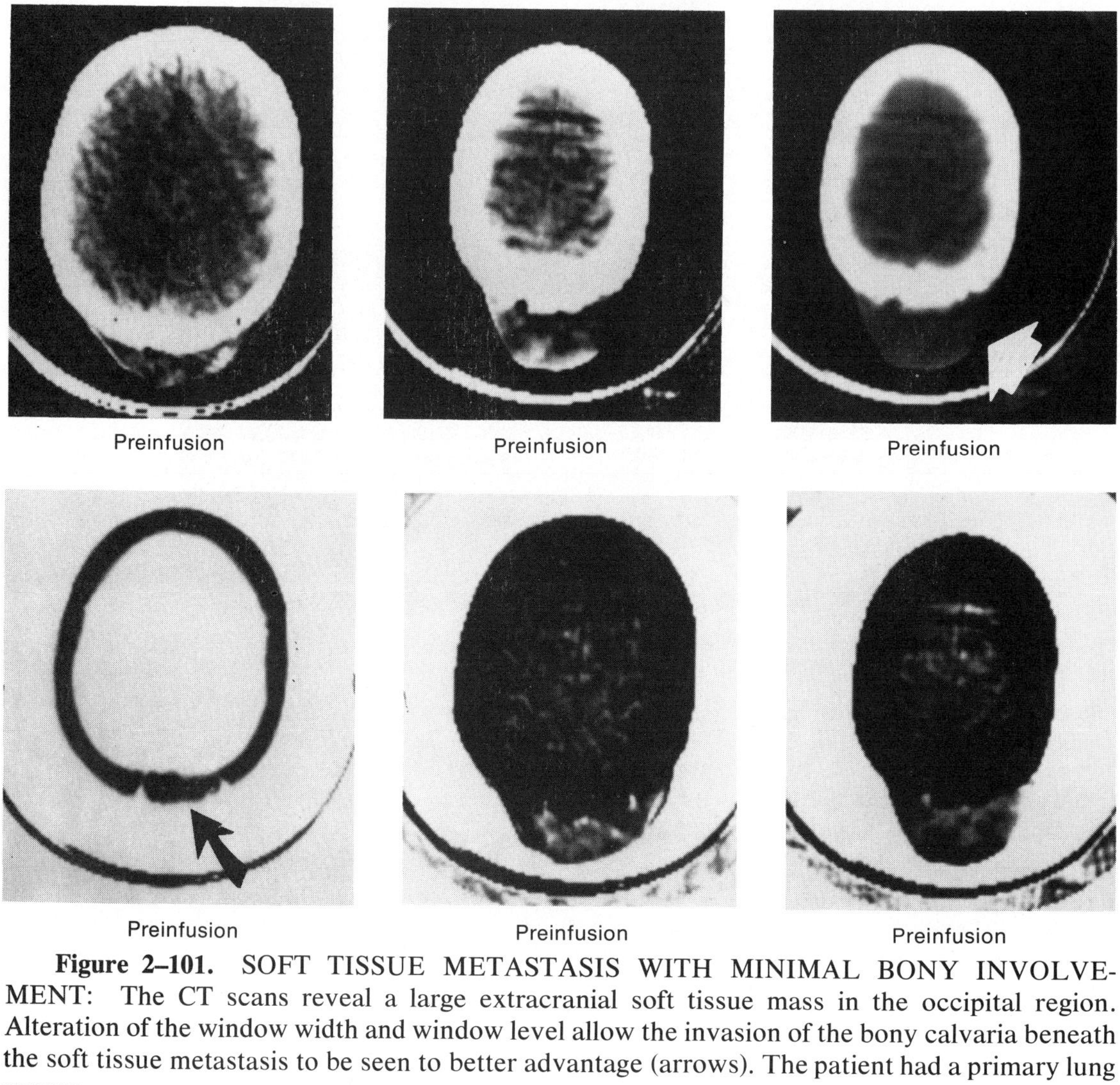

Preinfusion Preinfusion Preinfusion

Preinfusion Preinfusion Preinfusion

Figure 2–101. SOFT TISSUE METASTASIS WITH MINIMAL BONY INVOLVEMENT: The CT scans reveal a large extracranial soft tissue mass in the occipital region. Alteration of the window width and window level allow the invasion of the bony calvaria beneath the soft tissue metastasis to be seen to better advantage (arrows). The patient had a primary lung cancer.

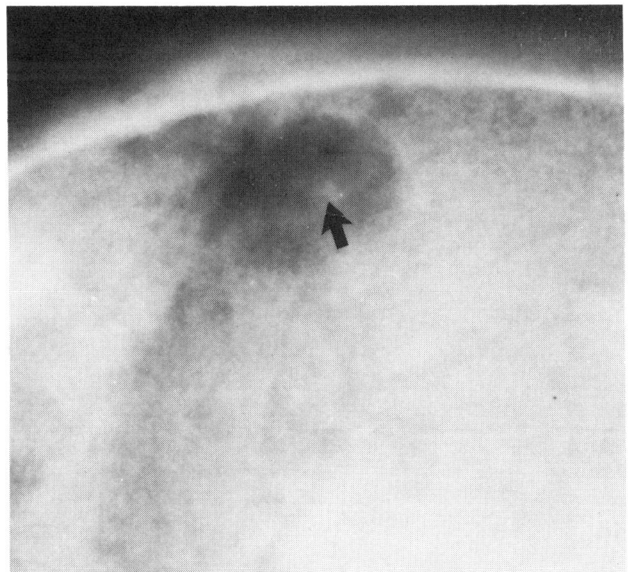

Figure 2–102. TARGET LESION, METASTATIC BREAST CARCINOMA: In the center of this osteolytic metastatic disease process there is an area of increased bony density (*arrow*). The appearance is that of a target — hence the name "target lesions" of the skull. This appearance is most common with metastatic breast carcinoma that has been treated and is in the healing phase. A similar phenomenon can be seen with healing eosinophilic granuloma and other less common disease processes.

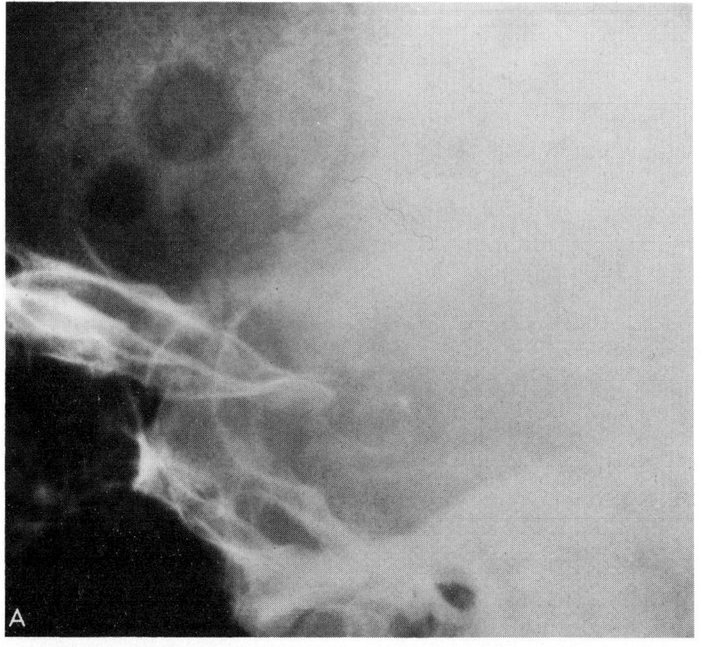

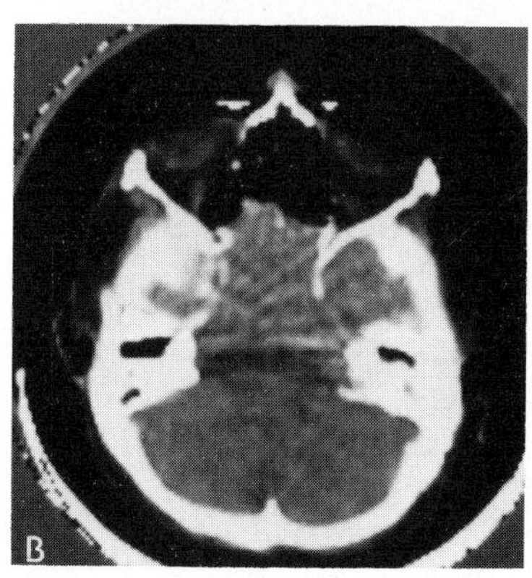

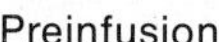

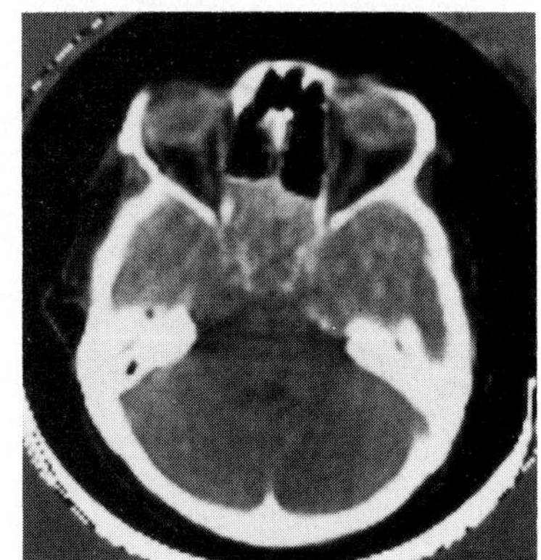

Figure 2–103. OSTEOLYTIC METASTASES INVOLVING THE BONY CALVARIA AND THE SELLA TURCICA: *A,* The lateral radiograph of the skull reveals several rounded metastatic deposits in the frontal area of the bony calvaria. In addition, there is massive bone destruction involving the entire base of the skull surrounding the sella turcica. *B,* The two low cuts of the CT scan through the region of the sella turcica reveal a large area of bone destruction. The entire sphenoid sinus is destroyed by the metastatic tumor, and there is encroachment on the ethmoid sinuses, the anterior clinoid processes and the clivus and petrous apices, both of which are amputated. The CT scan demonstrates beautifully the exact extent of involvement of the bony structures. (Case courtesy of Dr. David Neer.)

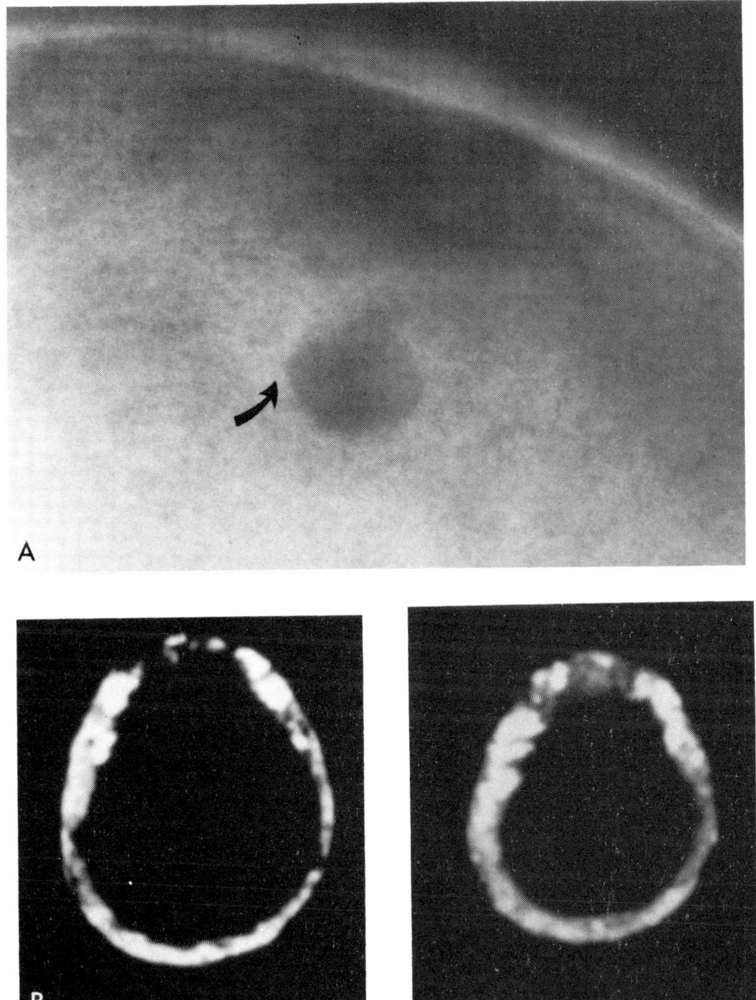

Figure 2–104. MIXED OSTEOLYTIC AND OSTEOBLASTIC METASTASES: The lateral skull film (*A*) demonstrates multiple scattered lucent skull defects as well as multiple osteoblastic lesions (*arrow*). This reflects an element of reparative bone formation and is seen most commonly following treatment of the osteolytic metastatic deposits.

The CT scan of the calvaria (*B*) also demonstrates areas of bony destructive change and areas of bone formation.

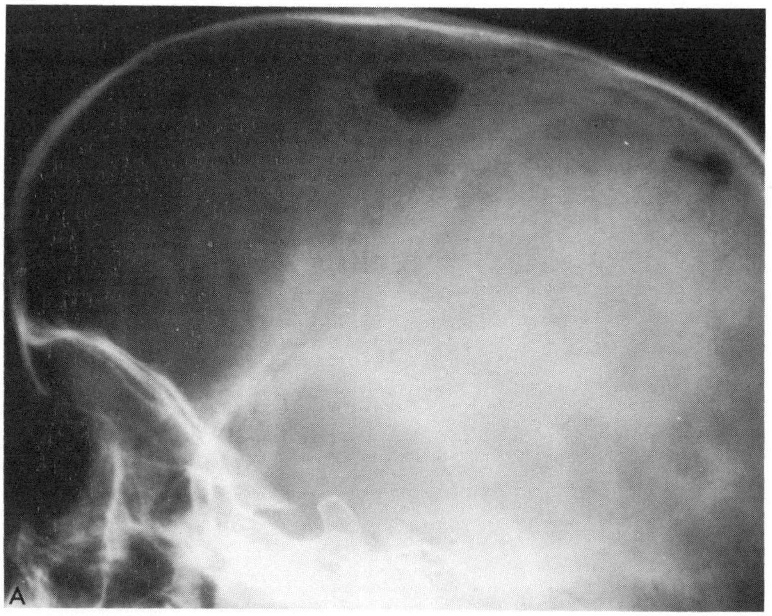

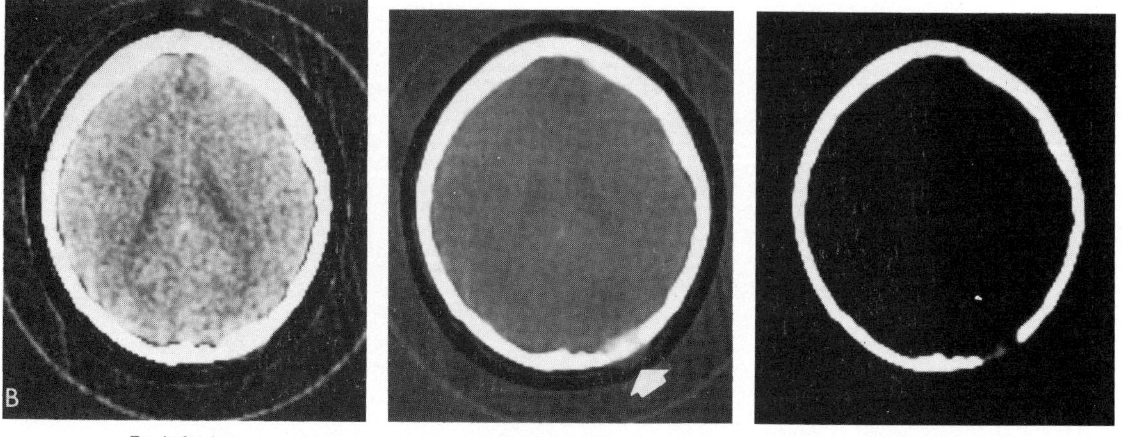

Figure 2–105. EOSINOPHILIC GRANULOMA: The skull lesion (*A*) is an area of lucent destructive change with a clear, slightly irregular border. In the healing phase, a sclerotic border may develop. The granulomas often are solitary, but may be multiple and may present as part of a syndrome of histiocytosis. These lesions may be seen in adults, but are more common in young individuals.

The lesions respond well to radiation therapy and may develop a "target" appearance.

B, CT scans of another patient reveal a well defined area of bony destructive change associated with a small soft tissue component (*arrowhead*). Note that on the standard viewing levels the bony involvement cannot be readily appreciated. It could have been overlooked if views at higher window widths and levels had not also been obtained.

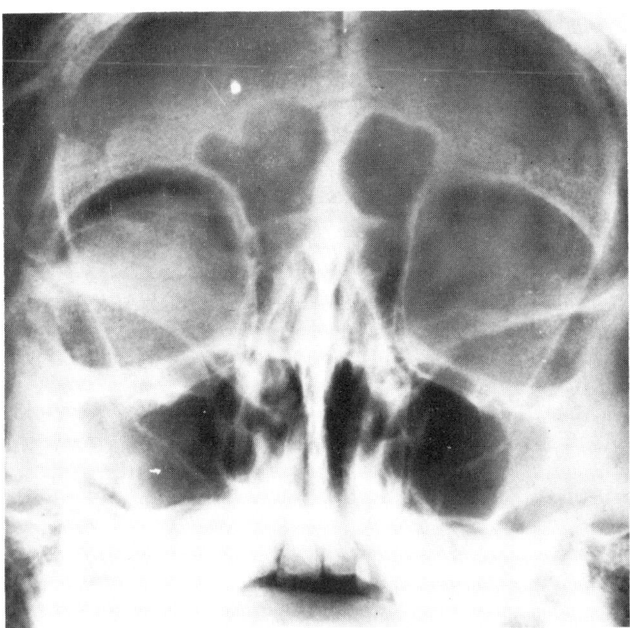

Figure 2–106. TRAUMATIC ORBITAL EMPHYSEMA: The bony defect in the lamina papyracea cannot be seen with this medial wall blow-out fracture; however, its presence can be suspected when the air is identified around the globe of the right eye.

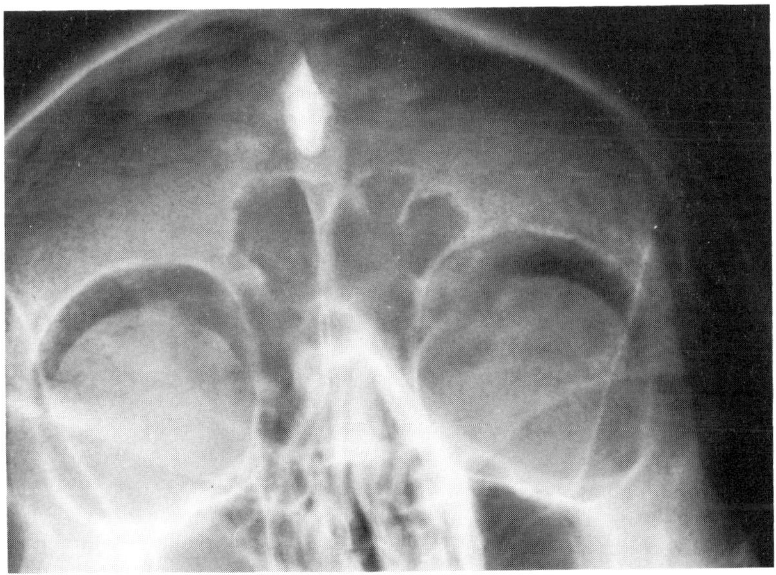

Figure 2–107. AIR UNDER EYELIDS: In patients with deep-set globes, air may be trapped over the lid, giving a false impression of orbital emphysema. This change is usually bilateral, which aids in differentiation from orbital emphysema, which usually is unilateral.

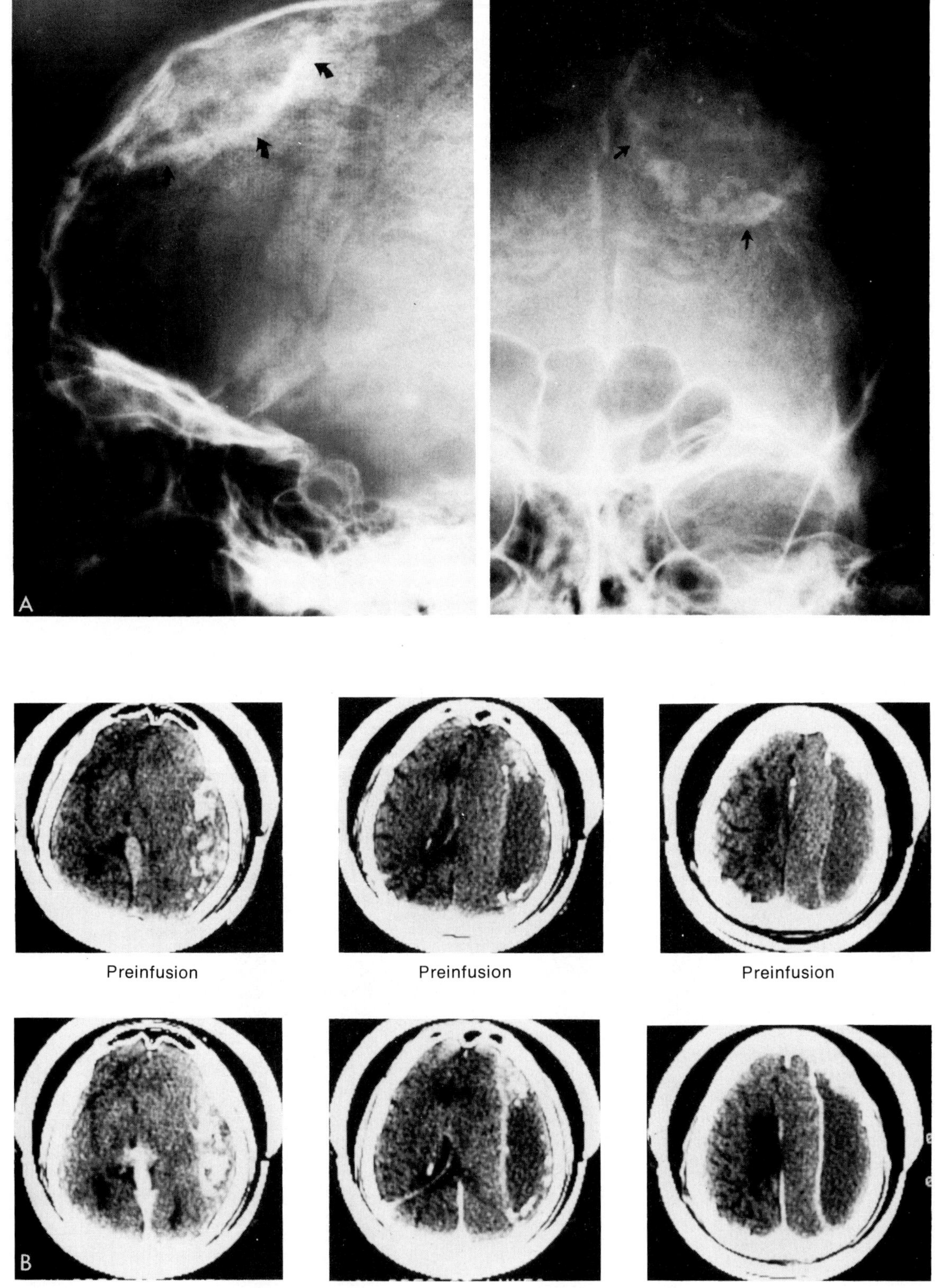

Figure 2–108. *See legend on the opposite page.*

Figure 2–108. CALCIFIED SUBDURAL HEMATOMA: A chronic subdural hematoma may be suspected when plain film radiography demonstrates a shift of the pineal gland. An appropriate history may or may not be available in these patients.

These extracerebral accumulations of blood may very rarely calcify. At times, differentiation by plain skull examination from the reactive bone formation secondary to meningioma may be difficult.

A, The plain skull films in this patient demonstrate a well defined calcified lentiform mass adjacent to the inner table in the left frontal region (*arrows*). This was proved surgically to be a chronic subdural hematoma that had calcified.

B, The CT scans demonstrate a large, chronic calcified subdural hematoma in the right temporal and parietal areas. The preinfusion scan reveals a low density lentiform accumulation with central and peripheral calcification. There is marked shift of the midline from right to left. An engorged straight sinus and vein of Galen appears posteriorly on the lowest cut, and this can be seen to enhance on the postinfusion scan. The patient developed the subdural accumulation following the placement of a shunt tubing device in the left lateral ventricle. There is also marked enhancement of the membrane of the subdural on the postinfusion scan.

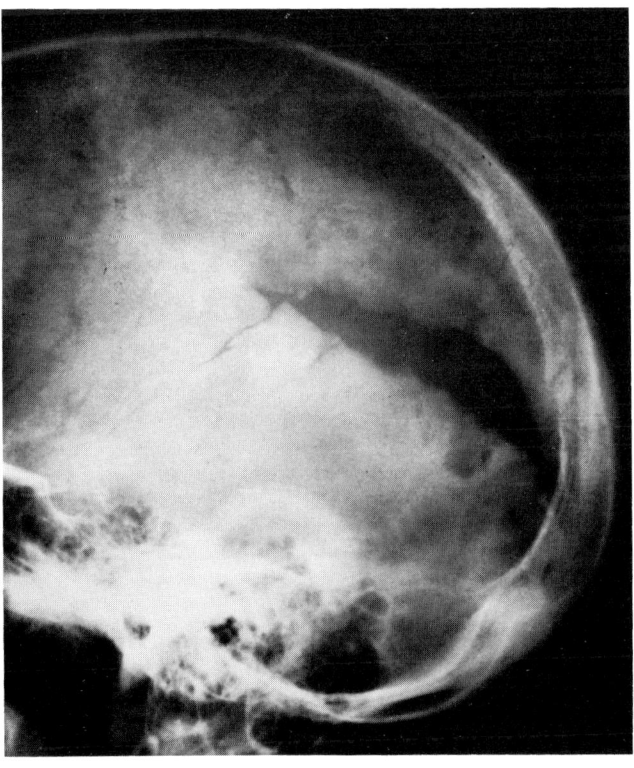

Figure 2–109. LEPTOMENINGEAL CYST: Leptomeningeal cysts may occur following a linear skull fracture. If the leptomeninges protrude through an associated tear in the dura and are trapped in the linear skull fracture, the continued transmitted pulsations of heart beat and respiration may result in gradual smoothing and expansion of the fracture line — a leptomeningeal cyst. This cyst may be associated with a palpable soft tissue mass (see Chapter 14). Underlying brain damage may also be present in these cases.

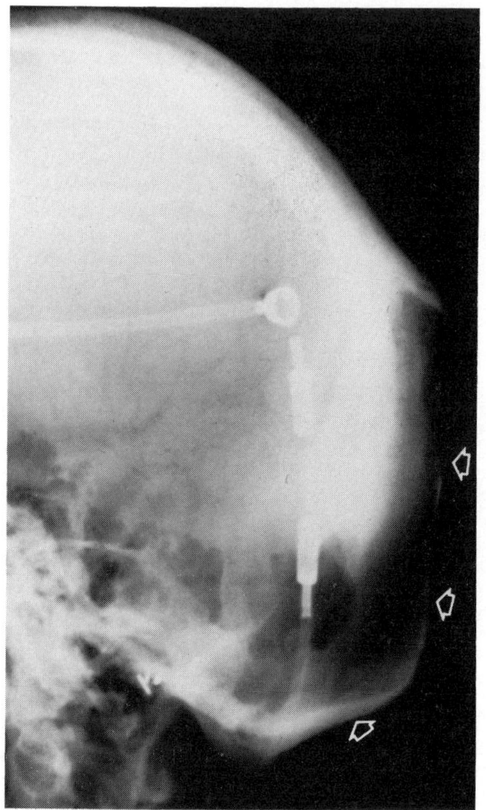

Figure 2–110. INTRADIPLOIC ARACHNOID CYST — POSTOPERATIVE: Following an operation on the posterior fossa, this patient developed an area of expansion of the skull between the inner and outer tables in the posterior fossa (*arrows*). The expansion was due to an arachnoid cyst between the tables. Note also the acquired basilar impression. (Case courtesy of Drs. Oscar Sugar and Glen Dobben.)

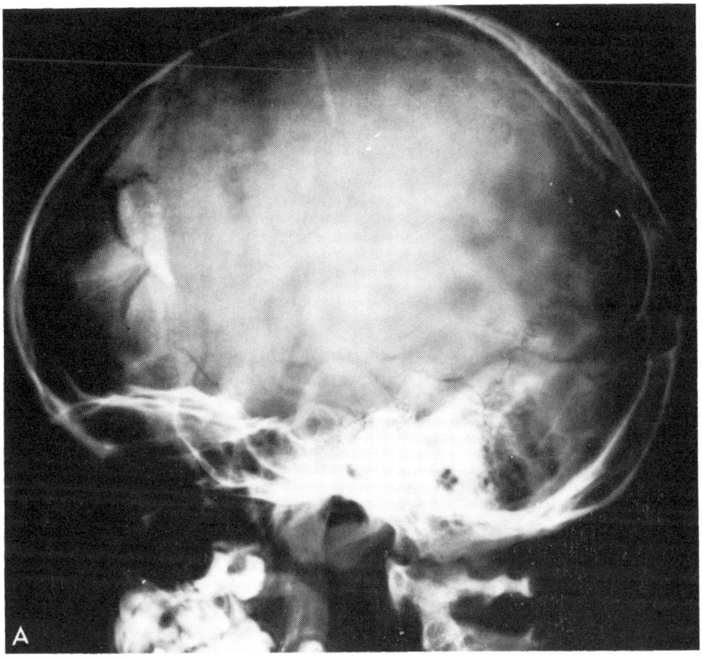

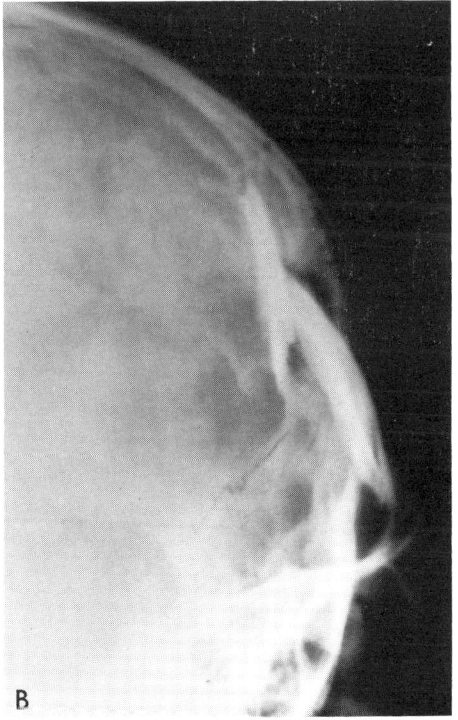

Figure 2–111. DEPRESSED SKULL FRACTURE: Following a direct blow to the frontal region, this patient developed a depressed comminuted fracture of the skull. The amount of depression is best demonstrated on the tangential view (*B*) (see also Chapter 13). These depressed skull fractures are readily demonstrated on CT scans.

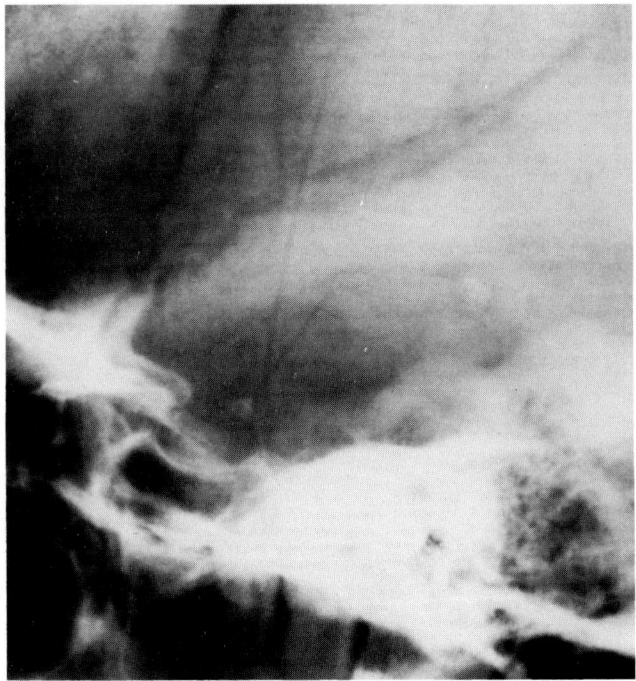

Figure 2–112. MIDDLE MENINGEAL ARTERY GROOVE SIMULATING A FRACTURE: This meningeal artery groove has been called the "resident's" skull fracture. It can be differentiated from a true fracture by the area of bony sclerosis adjacent to the lucency and by the fact that there is a similar groove on the other side (which in this case is not as long). Vascular grooves, since they involve only one table of the skull, are less lucent than true fractures, which involve both tables of the skull.

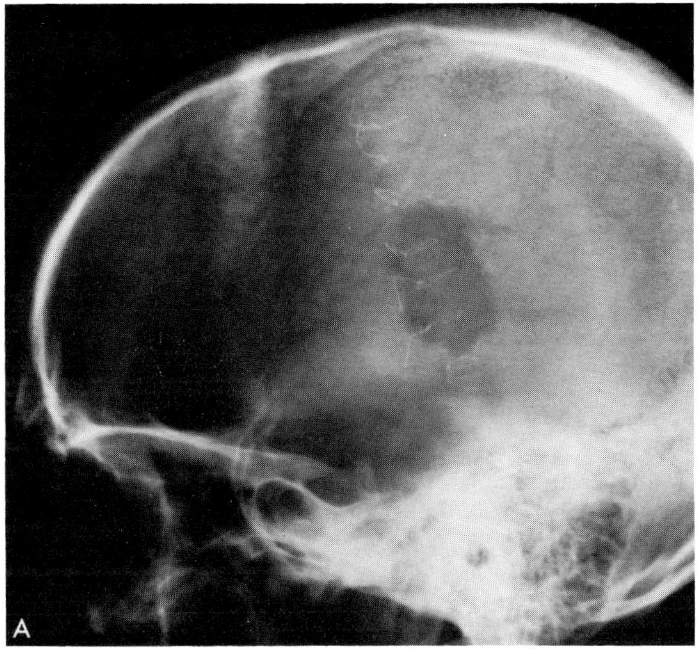

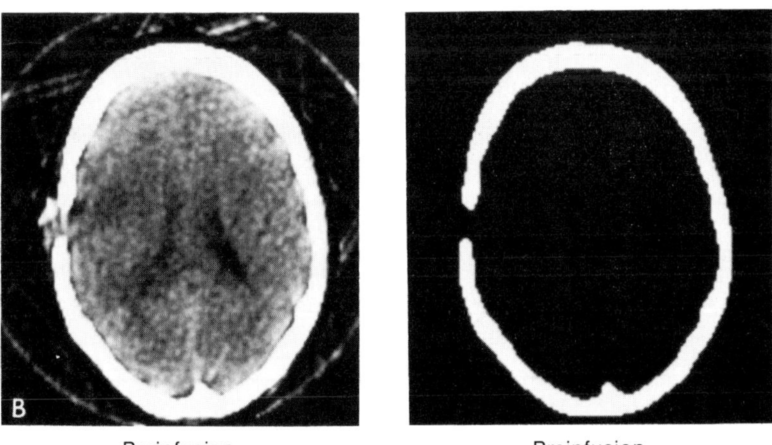

Figure 2–113. POSTOPERATIVE CHANGES: *A*, A small portion of the bony calvaria has been removed to evacuate a subdural hematoma. Metallic sutures project over the craniectomy site. *B*, The CT scan also reveals where the bone has been removed, as well as a small area of lucency under the operative site, probably an infarct. At times "bur" holes may have this appearance, but usually they are more subtle and must be looked for by manipulating the window width and window level.

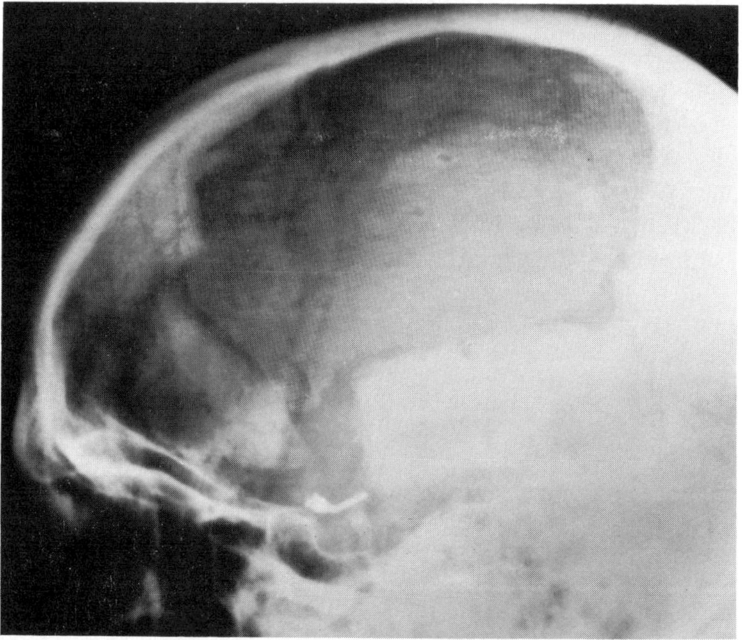

Figure 2–114. CRANIECTOMY DEFECT WITH TANTALUM WIRE IN PLACE: Because of osteomyelitis involving the bony flap, the entire flap was removed and replaced with a tantalum wire mech. This wire has a cross-hatch appearance similar to wire used for commercial purposes. The aneurysm clip is in place. Because these metallic devices interfere with CT scans they are rarely used today, and their use is strongly discouraged. Insertion of solid metallic plates is also discouraged.

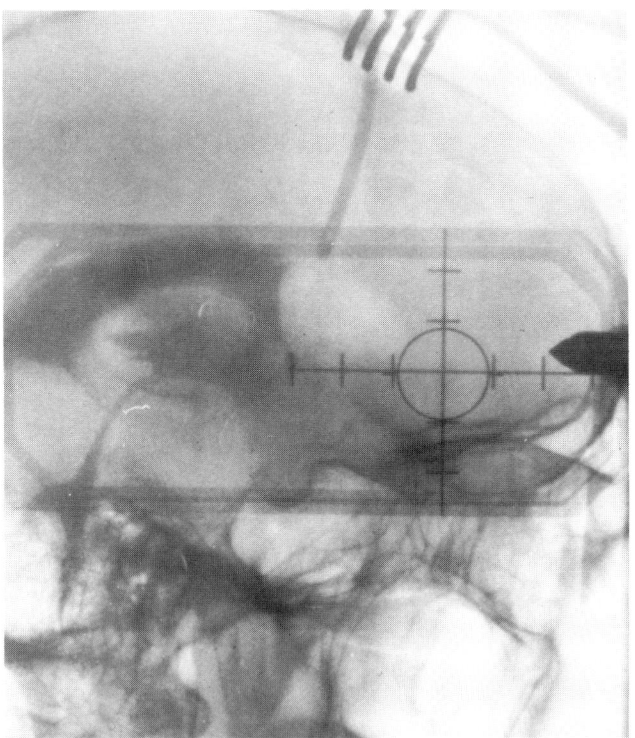

Figure 2–115. STEREOTACTIC BIOPSY USING X-RAY CONTROL: A metallic device holds the patient immobile. After an air and Conray ventriculogram, the biopsy is identified in two planes, and a small needle biopsy is made. The localizing device is projected over the frontal region on this view.

DEFINITIONS

Bur hole: A small (approximately 1.5 cm) opening made with a metal "bur" for trephination of the skull. It is used to drain chronic subdural hematomas, for ventriculogram studies and for placement of shunt tubes.

Craniotomy: The opening of the bony calvaria — usually by connecting strategically placed bur holes. Following the operative procedure, the bony flap is replaced in its original position.

Craniectomy: Following a craniotomy the bony calvaria is not replaced — a craniectomy. This is frequently seen following operative procedures on the posterior fossa.

Post-op changes: The appearance of the skull following a surgical procedure will depend upon the type of surgery performed.

CHAPTER 3

COMPUTED TOMOGRAPHY

Introduction and Normal Anatomy

The technique of computed tomography (CT) was the concept of Mr. Godfrey Hounsfield, scientist, EMI Ltd., Middlesex, England. The technique was introduced into clinical practice in England in 1972, but its use has expanded rapidly since then. The CT scan is not a direct x-ray of the brain, but rather a mathematical reconstruction of the tissue densities of the brain. The method requires the use of a computer as well as sophisticated scanning equipment.

Since the development of the original instruments there have been real advances in the field of CT scanners. The translate/rotate scanners have been modified so that scans can now be performed more rapidly, with a slice scanning time of less than 20 seconds. This, of course, has greatly enhanced our ability to obtain accurate scans, and now the scan can be done with less risk of patient-motion artifact. Further, the ability to scan faster has made it possible to examine a larger number of patients in the same amount of time.

The first scanners used a water bag that surrounded the patient's head and a thin x-ray beam with a single detector for each slice. Simply stated, in the first generation scanner, the x-ray tube traversed back and forth on a rail at the side of the patient's head. Two hundred and forty density measurements were made during each traverse of the tube by detectors placed at the side of the patient's head opposite the x-ray tube. In the example shown in Figure 3–1, a "mass lesion" has been placed in the left hemisphere. Two sodium iodide crystal detectors, which are closely aligned with the x-ray tube, simultaneously record the finely collimated beam, resulting in two cuts per scan, with a thickness of 1.3 cm per cut. After each traverse the scanning device rotates 1° until the unit has rotated 180°; at the completion of 180° of rotation the unit pauses, and in 30 seconds the computer simultaneously solves 43,200 equations of the tissue density measurements. The scan itself takes 4½ minutes. The result is a 160 × 160 dot matrix of tissue absorption density measurements of the brain, the skull and the surrounding water bag. The A and B cuts of each level are obtained simultaneously with each 180° rotation of the unit. The dot matrix is made up of 25,600 points, each of which represents a column of tissue 13 mm tall and 1.5 × 1.5 mm square. The information is presented in three different ways — on the cathode x-ray tube, where density measure-

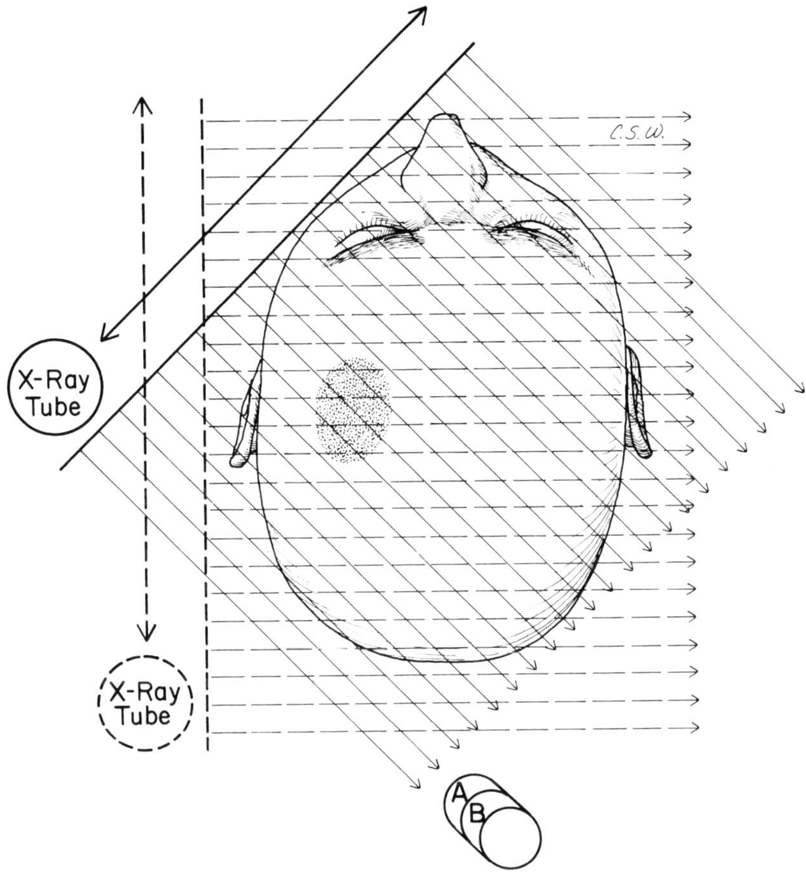

Figure 3–1

ments can be made; on the Polaroid picture, which can be used for permanent reference; and on the number print-out sheet.

Second generation scanners are based on the same principle as the original water-bag scanners, but eliminate the water-bag and replace it with a bolus that surrounds the patient's head with a material that approximates more closely the density of the intracranial contents. These scanners also use a fan beam x-ray source and multiple detectors.

Third generation scanners are based on the rotation of both the tube and the detector or detectors around the patient's head. These scanners are exceptionally fast — some requiring less than 5 seconds of actual scanning time. Fourth generation scanners use a moving source but multiple stationary detectors.

The matrix size (Fig. 3–2) varies from manufacturer to manufacturer, the initial 80 × 80 dot matrix has now increased to a matrix as large as 320 × 320 dots. There is a trade-off with increasing matrix size because more time is necessary to present the larger computed density matrix for viewing. The number print-out (Fig. 3–2) is well suited to research; however, diagnosis is usually performed by using the Polaroid picture or some other photographic method.

In Figure 3–3 the lateral ventricles are outlined by a thin black line; they exhibit the low density numbers typical of cerebrospinal fluid. The dark black line outlines a high density area which subsequently proved to be a tentorial meningioma. The small low density area posterior to the heavy black line is the superior cerebellar cistern. The number density range is stated in Hounsfield units (EMI) and extends from +1000 for bone to −1000 for air (Fig. 3–3). Water has a density of 0, and the scale is arbitrarily based on this figure (see Chart 3–1). Note that because the printed

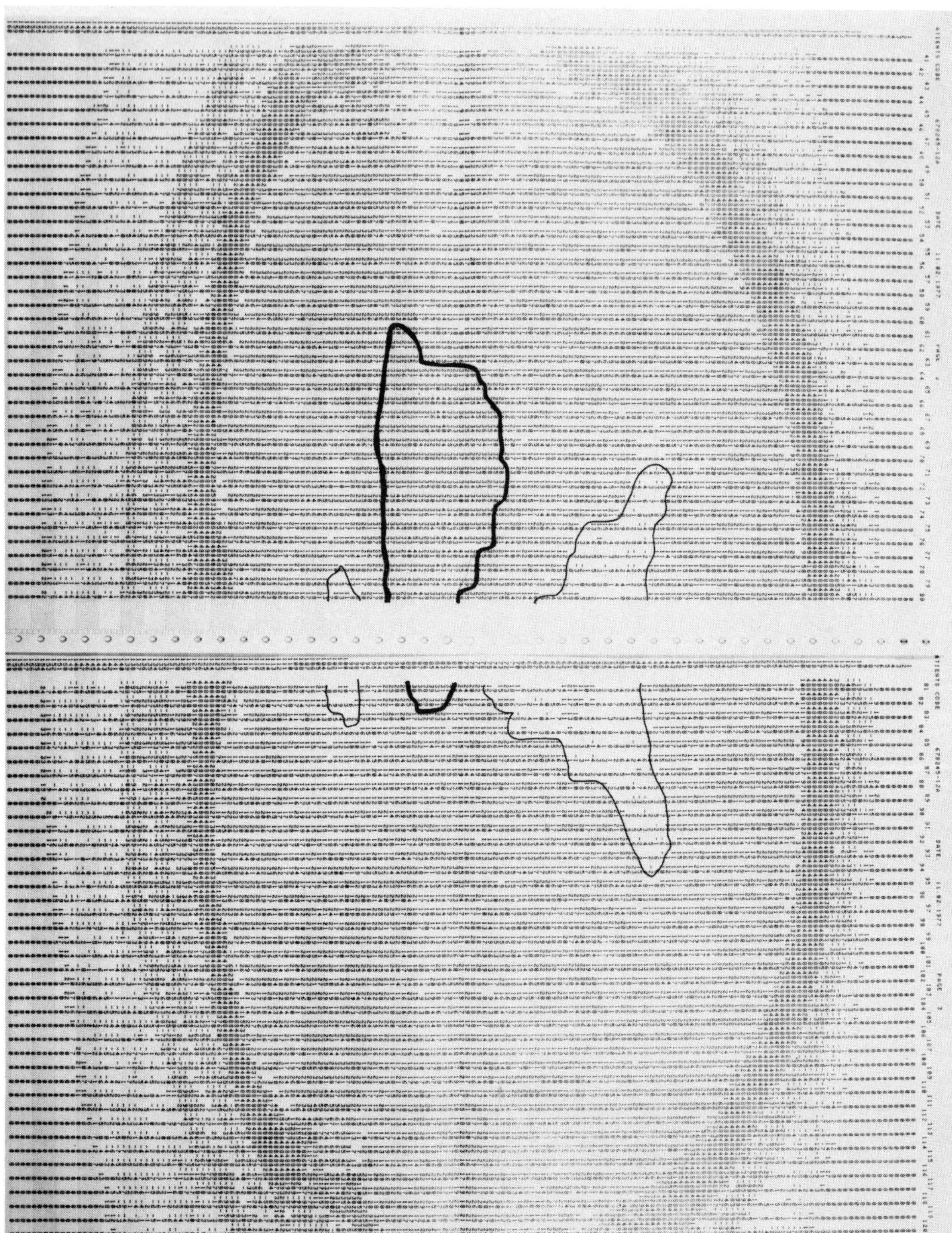

Figure 3–2

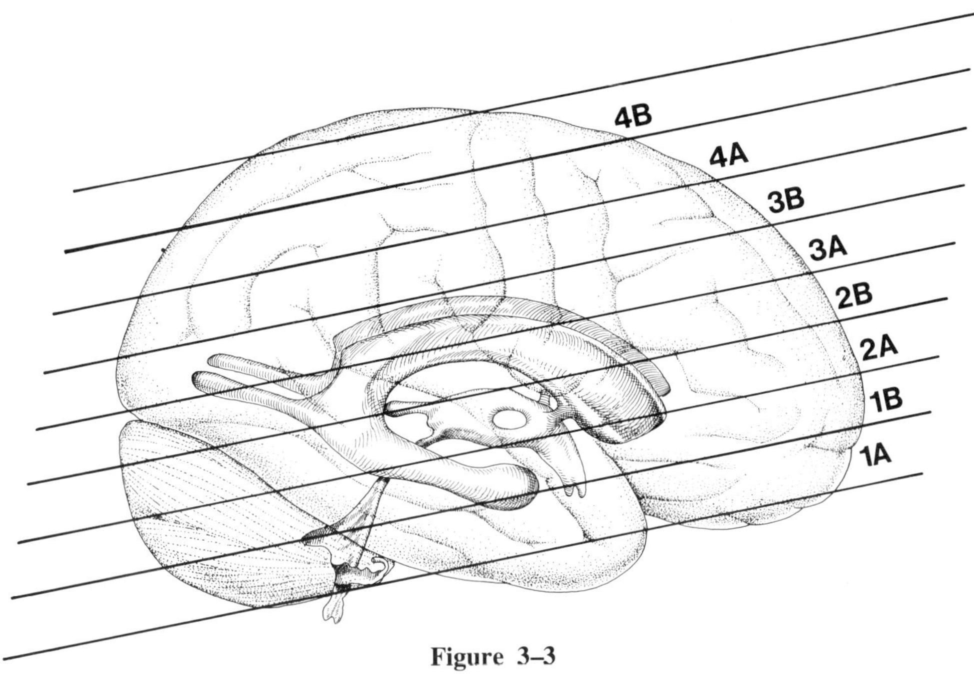

Figure 3–3

EMI COEFFICIENTS OF ABSORPTION IN HOUNSFIELD UNITS

AIR -1000 | FAT -100 | -32 | -10 | H_2O 0 | 10 | 20 | 30 | 40 | 50 | 60 | 70 | 80 | 90 | 100 | 110 | 120 | 200 | 400 | 600 | 800 | BONE +1000

CSF

EDEMA

WHITE MATTER

GRAY MATTER

FLOWING BLOOD

CLOTTED BLOOD

UNCALCIFIED MENINGIOMAS

CALCIFIED MENINGIOMAS

UNCALCIFIED GLIOMAS

HEMORRHAGIC & CALCIFIED GLIOMAS

CALCIFICATION

Chart 3–1

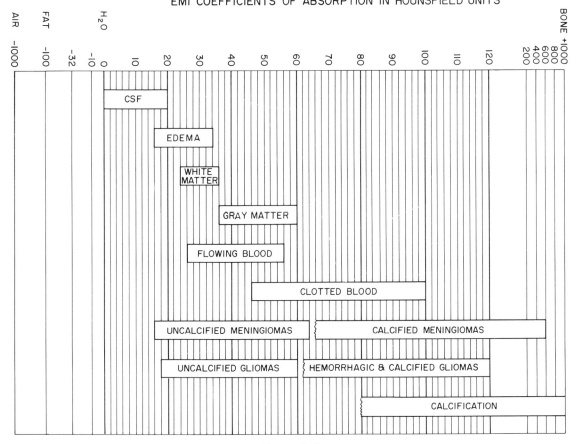

numerical densities require a certain amount of space the bony calvaria is distorted so that it appears to be short and wide rather than long and narrow.

Computed tomography of the brain has revolutionized our approach to the diagnosis of intracranial abnormalities. The CT scan demonstrates such abnormalities with an exactness and precision that never before had been possible. The technique is noninvasive, provides better definition of the extent of intracranial lesions than other methods and is especially useful in defining midline lesions and abnormalities of the posterior fossa. With proper training, the CT scan is easily performed, with essentially no discomfort to the patient, and may be done on either an outpatient or inpatient basis.

The newer rapid speed scanners allow an entire examination — including both the pre- and postinfusion portions — to be done in less than 45 minutes in the cooperative patient. Furthermore, the newer scanners also allow for alterations in the standard positioning of the head, making it possible to obtain views in the coronal and other projections.

The author recommends a standard patient positioning for every new case, regardless of the clinical presentation, because the physical signs and the patient's symptoms frequently do not actually reflect the position of the intracranial pathology. Furthermore, when the patient returns for a follow-up examination, the study can be repeated and the views compared without a great deal of difficulty. If a suspicious area is seen but the standard views are not satisfactory, or if an additional view is desired, the position of the patient's head can be changed and additional cuts can be obtained.

The patients are scanned at an angle of approximately 20 to 25° (a line from the base of the skull). Twelve to 14 cuts of 8 mm each are obtained in each patient. The number of cuts obtained necessarily varies with the patient's head size. The lowest cut is positioned so that the lowest portion of the cerebellum or even the foramen magnum is visible; with the angle of the cut, the roof of the orbit, or even the orbit itself should be visible. The cuts are then positioned so that each is above the next until the entire cranial contents up to and including the high convexities are included on each scan. The angle of the cuts is such that the higher cuts demonstrate the parietal rather than the frontal lobes — a source of confusion to those who are being initiated into the technique. This is particularly important to remember when a surgical approach is being planned.

Figures 3–4 through 3–10 demonstrate normal anatomic sections of the brain correlated with the appropriate CT scans. Anatomic structures are labeled both on the specimen and the CT scan slice. Note that there is some variation in the CT scan appearance from patient to patient. As in any biologic study, there is a good deal of variation even among normal patients, and no two scans are identical. In addition there is always some variation when the patient is positioned in the scanning unit, even though the view of a particular area of interest or the position of the patient can be altered to allow better visualization of any area under scrutiny. The sella turcica is sometimes best studied with cuts obtained parallel to the base of the skull in the region of the sella.

All the head scans presented in this text were performed on EMI model 1010 units. With each rotation of the scanner two slices are obtained, an A slice and a B slice. The slice thickness is 8 mm and the matrix dot size is 1.5 mm × 1.5 mm. Each scanning unit has a "minification" factor; to determine the true size from a measurement on the Polaroid photograph one need only scan an item of known size and relate the size on the Polaroid to the true size of the item.

After the completion of each standard preinfusion scan a repeat scan may be performed following the intravenous administration of contrast material. For adults, I use 300 cc of Conray 30 per cent in an infusion set; the first 150 cc is infused before beginning the scan; the remainder is infused slowly throughout the duration of the scan. For pediatric patients we use 4.4 cc/kg (2 cc/lb). It would appear that the type of contrast medium used is not critical, but that the amount of iodine necessary is 40 gm in the adult to insure an adequate load of contrast material. There is a

Text continued on page 136.

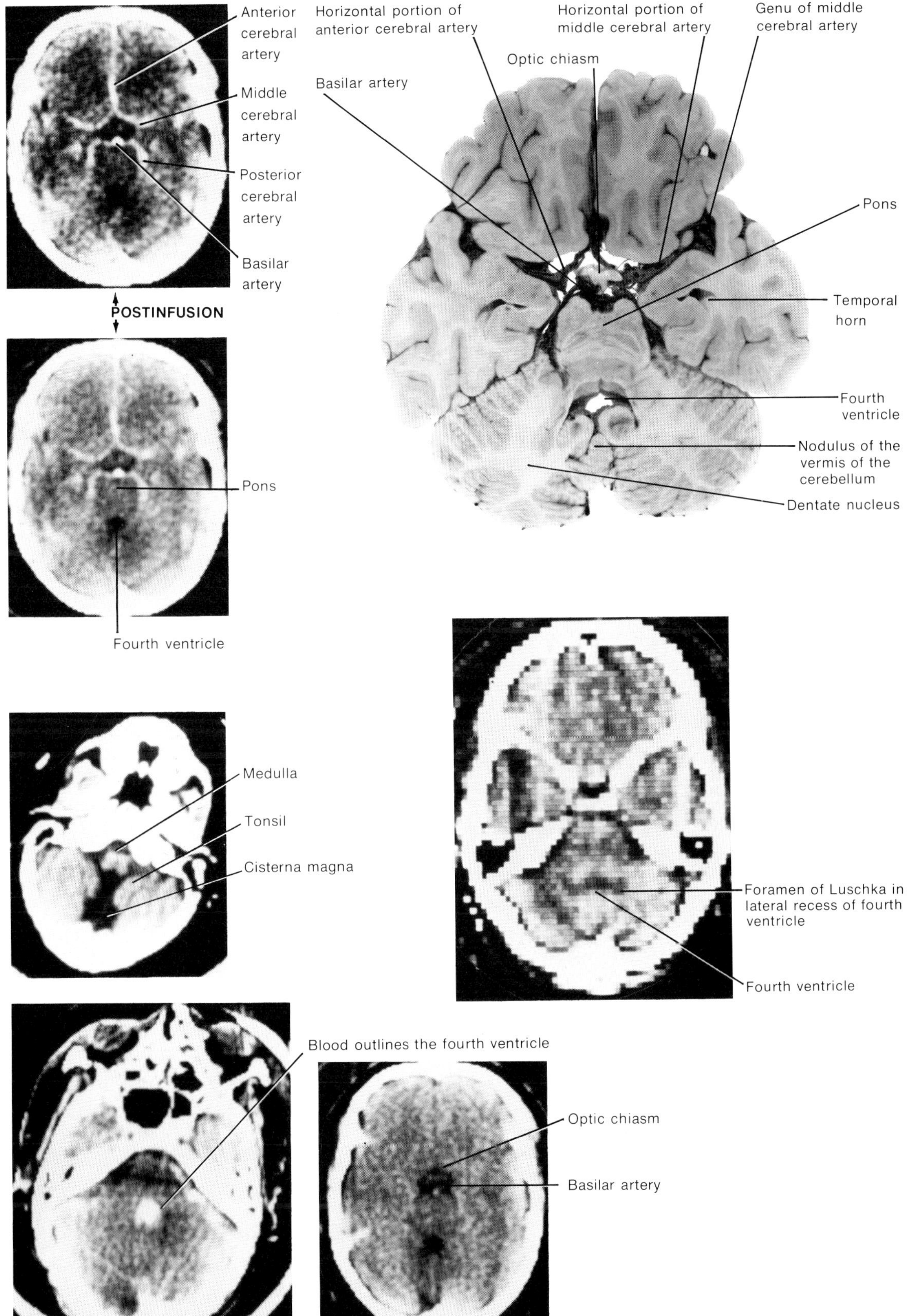
Anterior cerebral artery
Middle cerebral artery
Posterior cerebral artery
Basilar artery
POSTINFUSION
Pons
Fourth ventricle
Horizontal portion of anterior cerebral artery
Basilar artery
Optic chiasm
Horizontal portion of middle cerebral artery
Genu of middle cerebral artery
Pons
Temporal horn
Fourth ventricle
Nodulus of the vermis of the cerebellum
Dentate nucleus
Medulla
Tonsil
Cisterna magna
Foramen of Luschka in lateral recess of fourth ventricle
Fourth ventricle
Blood outlines the fourth ventricle
Optic chiasm
Basilar artery

Figure 3–4

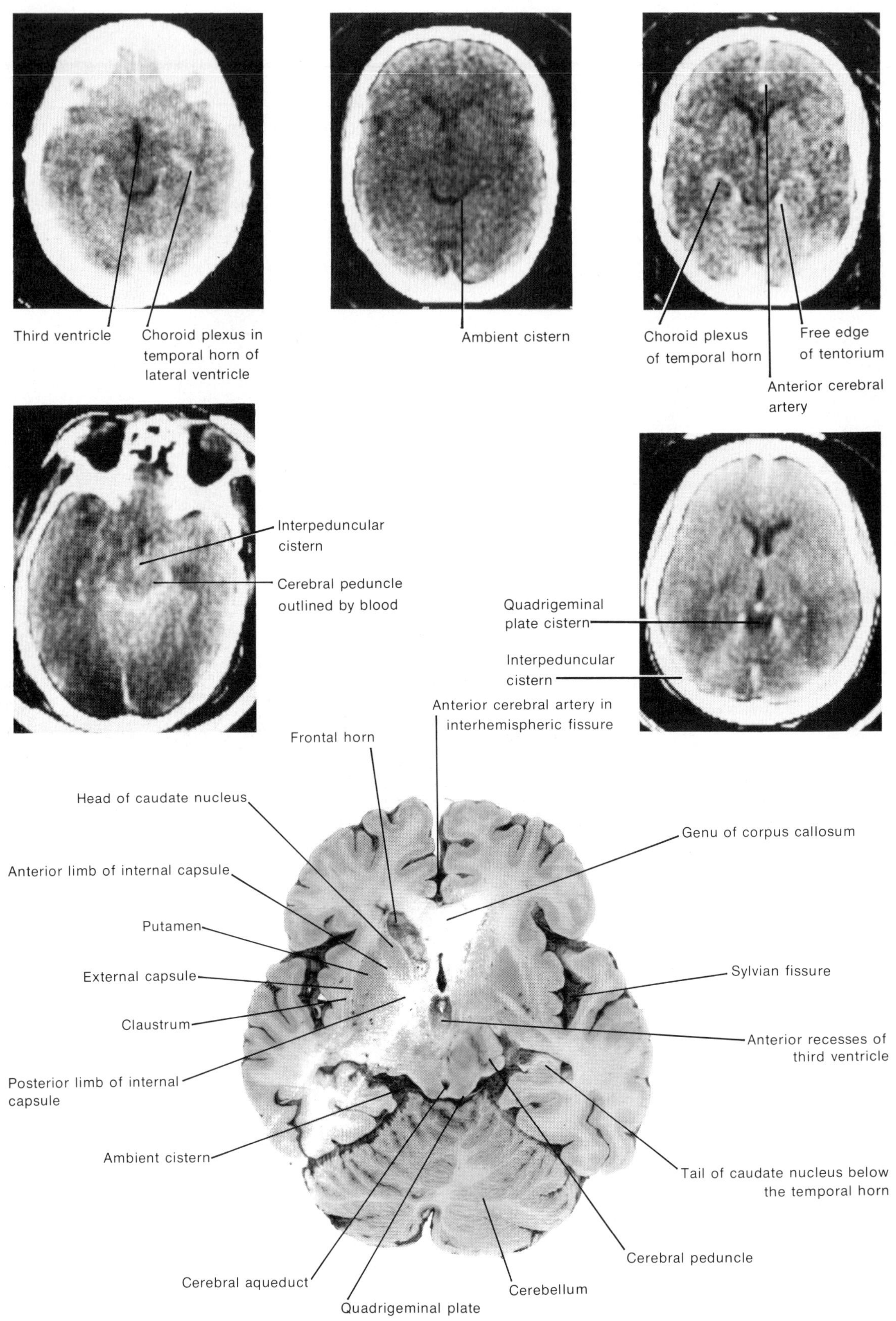
Third ventricle
Choroid plexus in temporal horn of lateral ventricle
Ambient cistern
Choroid plexus of temporal horn
Free edge of tentorium
Anterior cerebral artery
Interpeduncular cistern
Cerebral peduncle outlined by blood
Quadrigeminal plate cistern
Interpeduncular cistern
Anterior cerebral artery in interhemispheric fissure
Frontal horn
Head of caudate nucleus
Genu of corpus callosum
Anterior limb of internal capsule
Putamen
External capsule
Sylvian fissure
Claustrum
Anterior recesses of third ventricle
Posterior limb of internal capsule
Ambient cistern
Tail of caudate nucleus below the temporal horn
Cerebral peduncle
Cerebral aqueduct
Cerebellum
Quadrigeminal plate

Figure 3–5

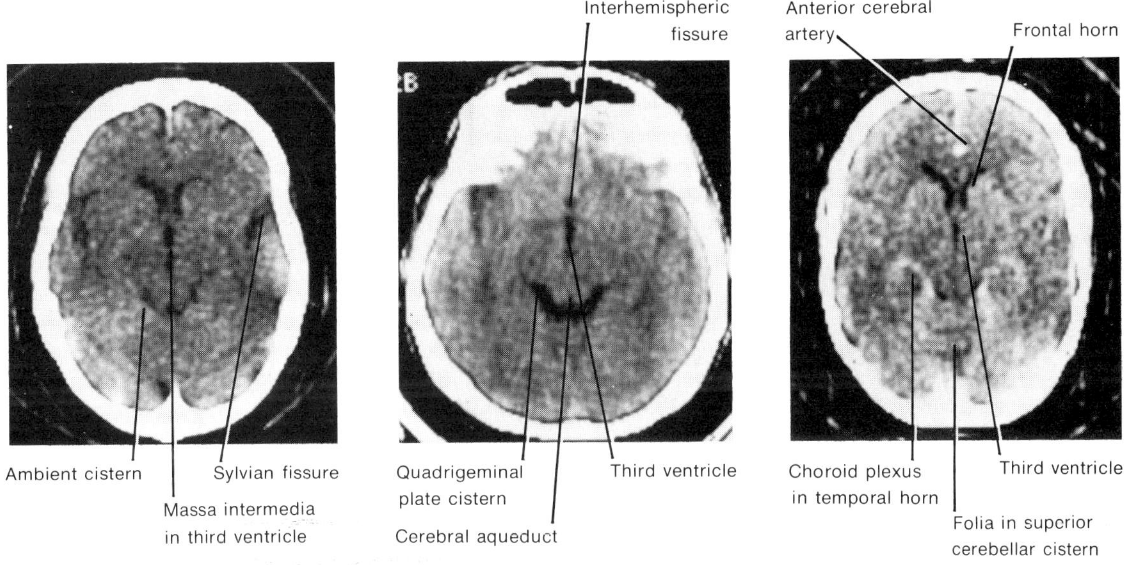
Interhemispheric fissure
Anterior cerebral artery
Frontal horn
Ambient cistern
Sylvian fissure
Massa intermedia in third ventricle
Quadrigeminal plate cistern
Third ventricle
Cerebral aqueduct
Choroid plexus in temporal horn
Third ventricle
Folia in superior cerebellar cistern

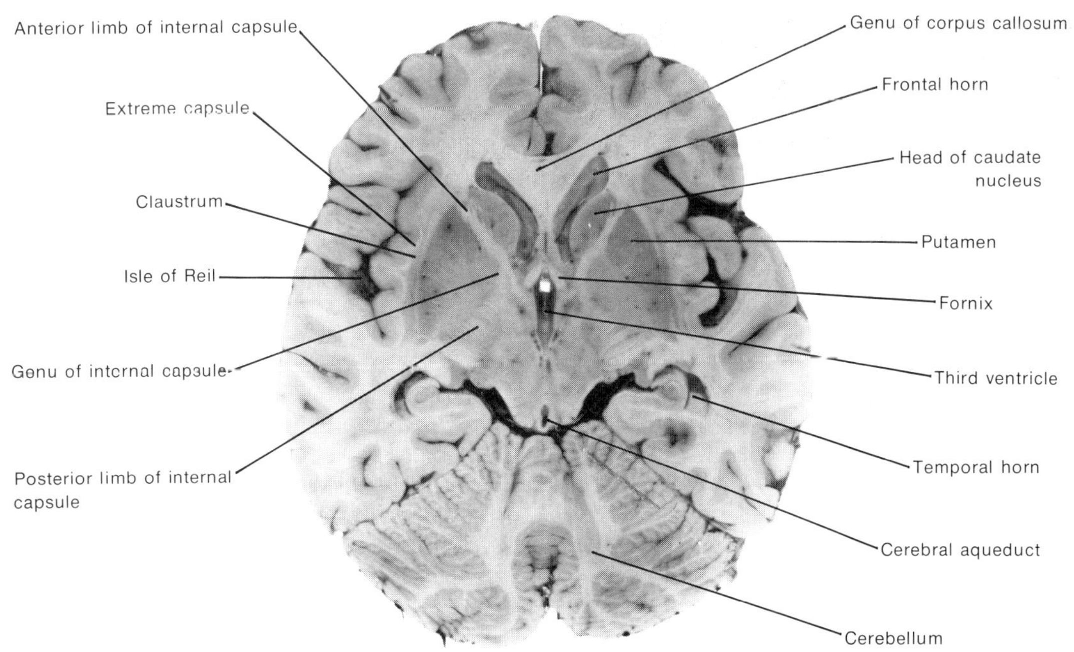
Anterior limb of internal capsule
Extreme capsule
Claustrum
Isle of Reil
Genu of internal capsule
Posterior limb of internal capsule
Genu of corpus callosum
Frontal horn
Head of caudate nucleus
Putamen
Fornix
Third ventricle
Temporal horn
Cerebral aqueduct
Cerebellum

Figure 3–6

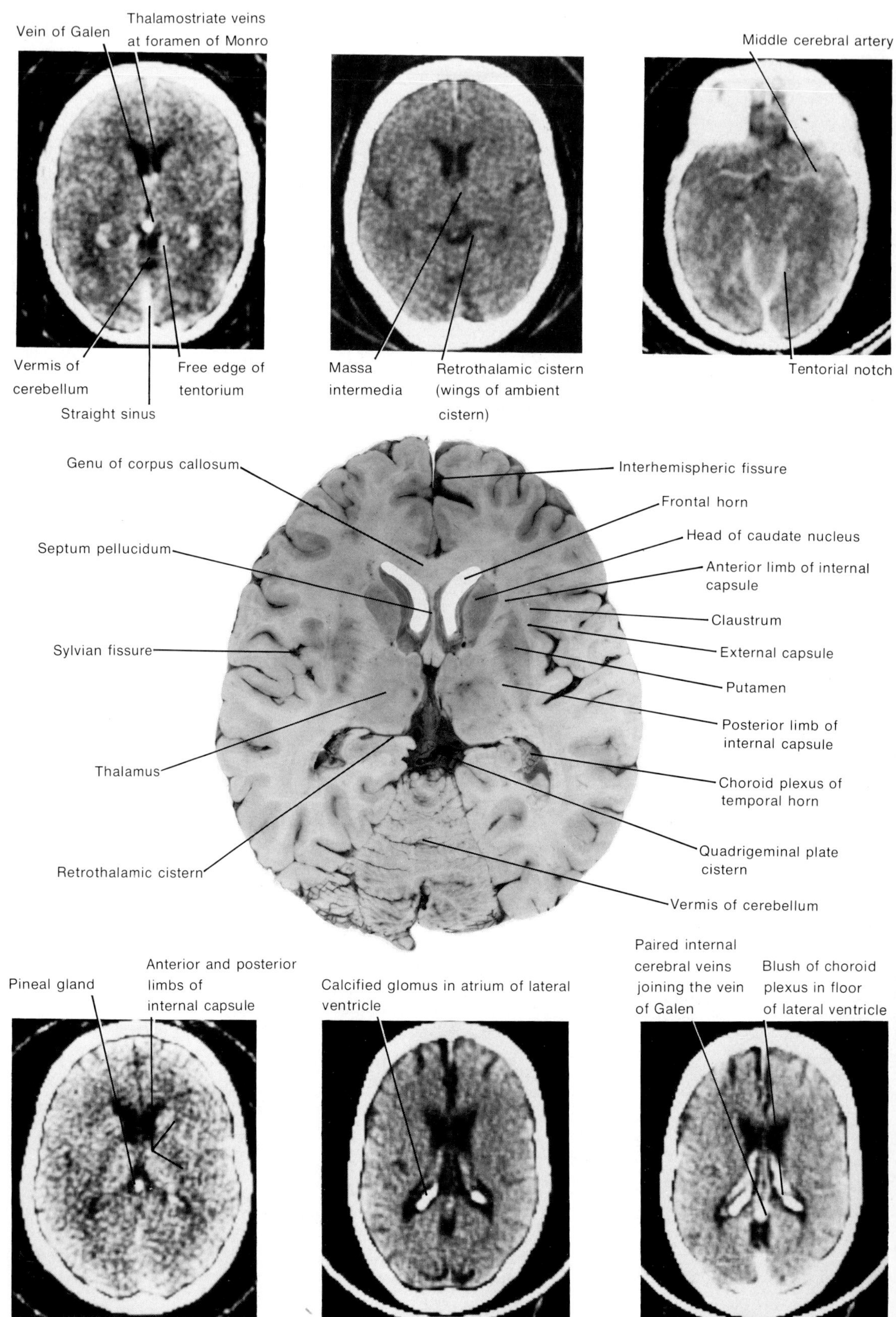
Vein of Galen
Thalamostriate veins at foramen of Monro
Vermis of cerebellum
Straight sinus
Free edge of tentorium
Massa intermedia
Retrothalamic cistern (wings of ambient cistern)
Middle cerebral artery
Tentorial notch
Genu of corpus callosum
Septum pellucidum
Sylvian fissure
Thalamus
Retrothalamic cistern
Interhemispheric fissure
Frontal horn
Head of caudate nucleus
Anterior limb of internal capsule
Claustrum
External capsule
Putamen
Posterior limb of internal capsule
Choroid plexus of temporal horn
Quadrigeminal plate cistern
Vermis of cerebellum
Pineal gland
Anterior and posterior limbs of internal capsule
Calcified glomus in atrium of lateral ventricle
Paired internal cerebral veins joining the vein of Galen
Blush of choroid plexus in floor of lateral ventricle

Figure 3–7

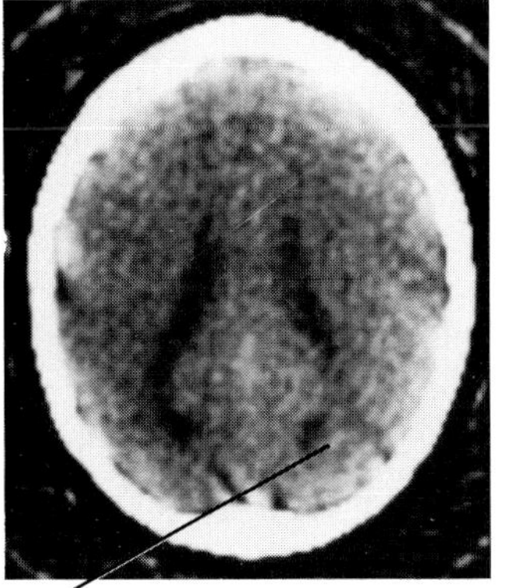
Posterior extent of occipital horn
of lateral ventricle

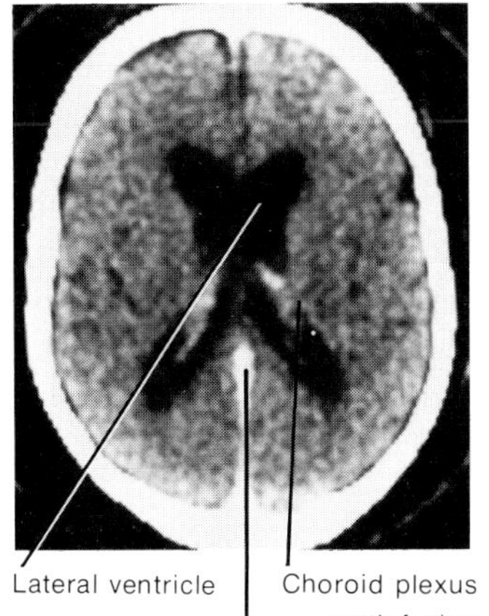
Lateral ventricle
Choroid plexus
postinfusion
Straight sinus

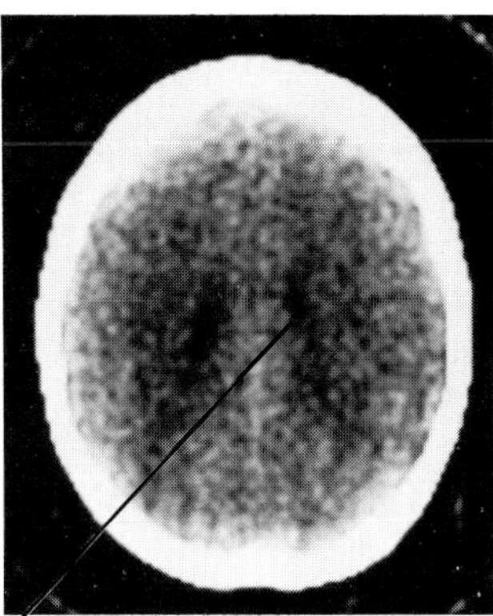
Body of lateral ventricle

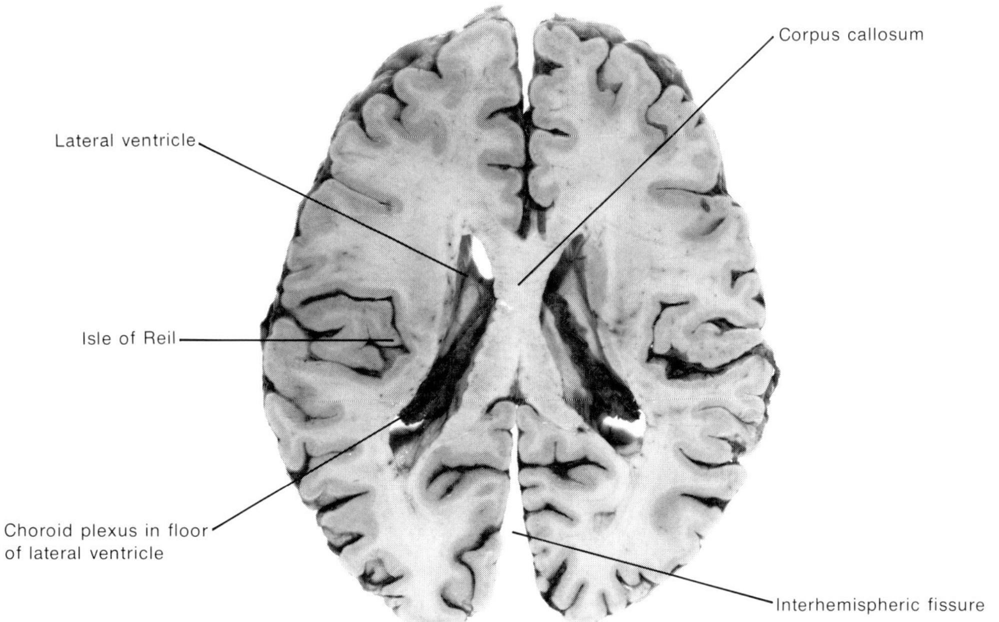
Corpus callosum
Lateral ventricle
Isle of Reil
Choroid plexus in floor
of lateral ventricle
Interhemispheric fissure

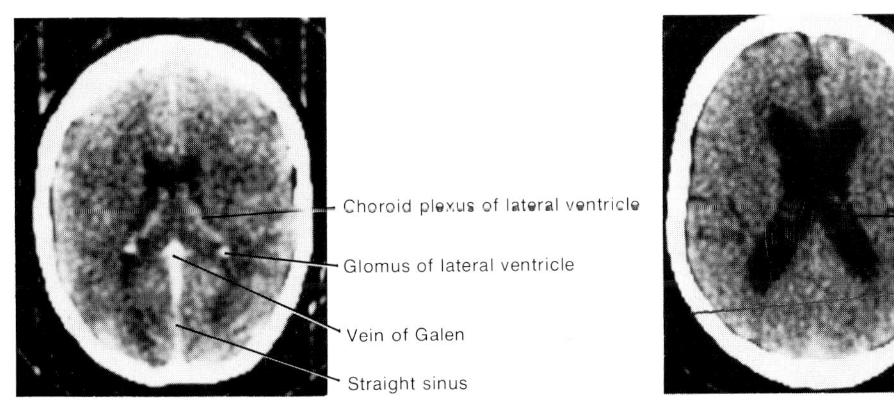
Choroid plexus of lateral ventricle
Glomus of lateral ventricle
Vein of Galen
Straight sinus
Lateral ventricle

Figure 3–8

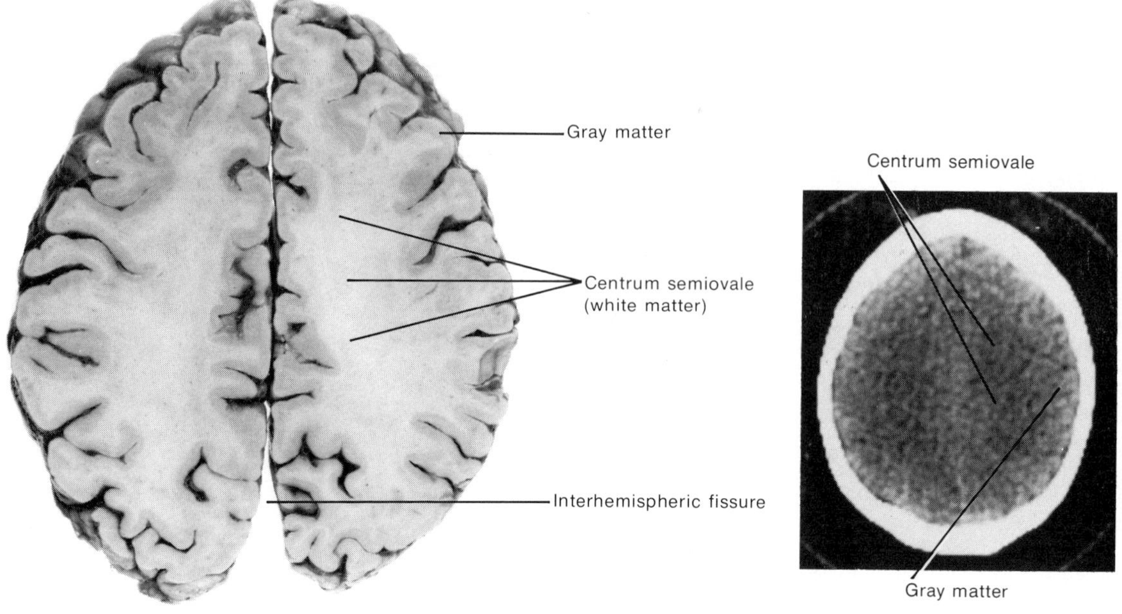

Figure 3–9

very real possibility of an anaphylactic reaction to the contrast medium as well as emesis with aspiration of gastric contents. For these reasons the use of contrast infusion should not be undertaken without some consideration.

All the scans throughout this volume are labeled so that the right hand side of the picture represents the right hemisphere — i.e., as if one is looking *down* on the patient's head. All preinfusion scans are numbered with single digit numbers; the postinfusion scans are labeled with double digit numbers. Some are simply labeled as pre- and postinfusion scans without numbers.

Although some examiners favor a postinfusion scan on each individual, the potential danger of an adverse affect on the kidneys — even including renal shut-down—precludes this approach to computed tomography. The author recommends a cautious, rather than blanket, approach to the use of contrast infusion. Those patients who should have contrast enhancement are listed below. In addition, for an initial examination, I *STRONGLY* recommend a preinfusion scan before the study following contrast infusion. Some argue convincingly that only a postinfusion scan should be performed. However, those cases where the diagnosis is obscured — e.g., the differentiation between basal ganglia, hemorrhage and a luxury perfusion, or in those cases where an infarct is obscured by the infusion — make this method less desirable than the conservative approach of a preinfusion scan followed by a postinfusion study. Perhaps the use of "postinfusion only" scans should be limited to patients with a tumor diagnosis who are returning for follow-up. There is no doubt that additional information not appreciable on the preinfusion scan is gained on the postinfusion scan. Those patients who should have a postinfusion study in addition to the preinfusion are:

1. All patients with suspected metastases.
2. All patients with evidence of a space-occupying lesion on the preinfusion scan.
3. Postoperative brain tumor patients.
4. Suspected arteriovenous malformations.
5. Individuals with demyelinating diseases or seizure disorders who are being worked-up for the first time.
6. Suspect chronic bilateral isodense subdural hematomas.
7. Initial work-up of hydrocephalus.

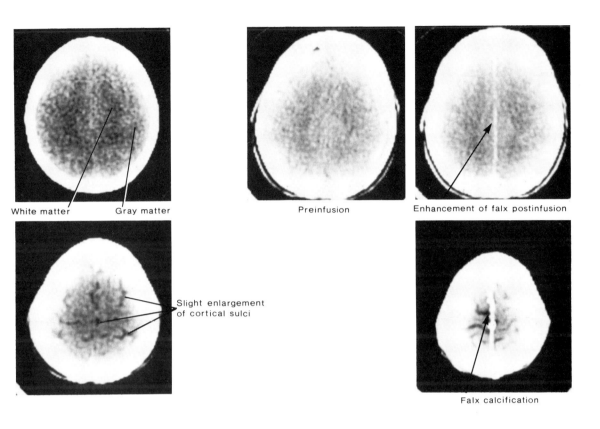

White matter Gray matter

Preinfusion

Enhancement of falx postinfusion

Slight enlargement of cortical sulci

Falx calcification

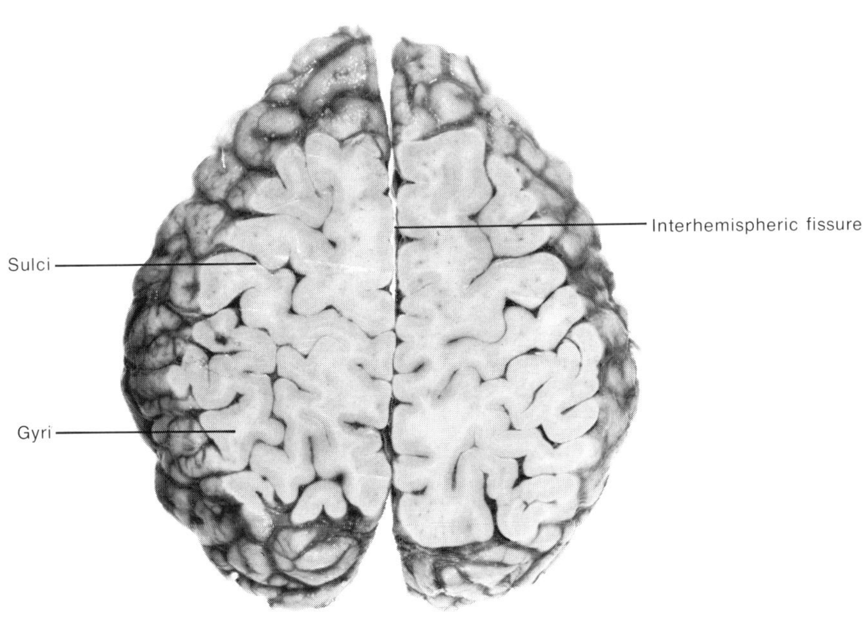

Figure 3–10

Those patients who need a routine preinfusion CT scan only:

1. Dementia.
2. Acute head trauma.
3. Follow-up of change in size of lateral ventricles post-shunting.
4. Follow-up following evacuation of a subdural hematoma.

ORBITAL TOMOGRAPHY

If the orbits are the area of interest, the patient is scanned through the orbits by positioning the head in the scanner so that the cuts are parallel to Reid's base line. Care should be taken that the entire orbit is included on the scan. Cuts are obtained both pre- and postinfusion.

POSTERIOR FOSSA

Some examiners recommend multiple overlapping cuts through the posterior fossa for evaluation of the posterior fossa. I have not found this technique necessary for diagnosis; however, it is conceivable that it may be helpful — especially for small lesions. In fact, *very* thin section tomography — 1 mm — is being suggested for diagnosis of small pituitary lesions and small tumors of the internal auditory canal.

The quality of the image depends on the patient's remaining relatively immobile throughout the scan. This can prove particularly troublesome in children, and the author recommends adequate sedation before the scan. The standard dosage schedule for pediatric neuroradiologic procedures is recommended, with the amount of sedation used on the low end of the schedule. The sedative is administered intramuscularly 45 to 60 minutes before the procedure. These patients must be observed closely for any depression of vital signs. In some patients, both children and adults, it will be necessary to perform the scan under general anesthesia.

WINDOW WIDTH AND WINDOW LEVEL

Although it has been found that certain types of intracranial abnormalities measure a specific density on the CT scan, there is a good deal of "overlap" between the lesions (see Chart 3–1). The various scanning units are equipped with devices that measure the density of the structures visualized. These numerical measurements may be helpful to determine the histologic nature of the abnormality being viewed. During the course of reviewing intracranial findings, the bony calvaria is often examined in only a cursory fashion. It may become apparent after manipulation of the "measuring" device that more information can be gained only if a more thorough examination of the cranial contents and the bony calvaria is performed.

A description of the method of examination of the bony calvaria will serve as a basis for discussion of these methods of measurement. These methods require a review of some very basic radiologic concepts, including the topics of *window width* and *window level.* The measuring devices on EMI CT scanners employ an arbitrary numerical scale that places the density of water at 0, the density of bone at +1000 and the density of air at −1000. These density units are called "Hounsfield units" after Mr. Godfrey Hounsfield, the developer of the CT scanner.

Contrast. Radiographic contrast may be considered as the difference between the blackest black and the whitest white. *High* contrast means that there is a large difference between the shades of gray, black and white. With maximum contrast, the densities on the radiograph are either black or white, and there are no shades of gray. On the EMI scanners this contrast level is obtained by placing the unit in the "measure mode." On the measure mode the image is either black or white at a given window density level (L) expressed in Hounsfield units (u). The level can be moved up or down to obtain the density range of an abnormal area. Certain abnormalities tend to fall within a certain density range, and at times a diagnosis can be made with a fair degree of certainty. This is especially true when there is clotted blood secondary to an intra- or extracerebral hematoma.

The latitude, on the other hand, is the number of shades of gray that may be seen on the photograph or radiograph. When there is a wide latitude, large numbers of shades of gray can be seen. When using the scanner, latitude can be altered by changing the *window width*. The viewing system can readily be changed from a very high contrast system to a very low contrast system in which the difference between densities becomes less in the shades between black and white.

The significance of these alterations becomes of practical importance when certain intracranial and calvarial changes can be appreciated only by altering the window width and window level. This is especially true of bony lesions, where abnormalities become apparent only after thorough inspection on the oscilloscope screen, examining each slice at varying window widths and window levels. For comparison purposes, an identical window width and window level should be used from time to time and from case to case.

The abnormalities of the bony calvaria usually are more readily apparent on the plain skull examination; however, the skull radiographs are not always available for examination at the time of the CT study. Conversely, it has been stated that after a CT scan there is no need for a routine skull series. As discussed in Chapter 2, neither view is entirely correct. In most cases, skull radiographs provide information not available from the CT scan or that is more readily apparent on the skull film than on the scan. However, when skull radiographs are not available, examination of the bony calvaria by CT scan is very helpful.

Throughout this text are examples that demonstrate the changes that become apparent when one examines the brain or calvaria by other than standard measurements. On a daily basis, our hand copy, permanent record, is printed at a window width of 100 and a window level of 36 u on a 10 × 12 x-ray film photograph taken from the oscilloscope screen of the EMI scanner.

RECONSTRUCTION TOMOGRAPHY

By utilizing advanced computer techniques, a CT image can be manipulated to provide a view in a plane other than the initial scanning plane. This is accomplished by first performing multiple overlapping cuts in a single plane and then "feeding" the density readings in the overlapping sections into a computer, which "rearranges" the data so that a scan originally performed in the axial projection can be viewed in the sagittal plane.

This can be done for any plane desired. To be successful, the method does require a cooperative, immobile patient. The overlapping cuts also result in a significant increase in radiation dose to the patient.

The method is especially useful for studies of the sella and is also helpful in diagnosing lesions of the lumbar spine.

ARTIFACTS

A variety of artifacts or false images may be produced by the CT scanners. They are generated by many different phenomena. All artifacts degrade or alter the CT image; therefore, it is helpful to understand their origins. If the origin can be determined, artifacts can at times be altered or eliminated.

The various scanners available have different scanning speeds. With the older models and with slower scanning speeds, there is a greater change of artifact secondary to patient motion. Such motion can degrade the image to such a great extent that the study becomes uninterpretable.

Metallic surgical clips are also a significant cause of artifacts, and their use should be discouraged.

Metallic plates interfere with scanning so greatly that CT examinations usually cannot be performed in such patients. The metal connecting portions of shunt tube devices also degrade scan images. This degradation usually occurs only on the scan slice at the level of the metallic device and so may not interfere with interpretation.

Various other electrical and mechanical problems also may alter the images — e.g., weak or defective photo multiplier tubes, alteration of the kilovoltage during scanning or mechanical interference with the scanner motion.

Air in the lateral ventricles causes a specific artifact. The scan will demonstrate a white line surrounding the peripheral margin of the retained air. This artifact is computer generated because of the very great density change between the air in the ventricle and the surrounding brain tissue.

Pantopaque in large quantities also can degrade the image.

A standard artifact can be found on routine CT scans with EMI head scanners. All the scans demonstrate a thin black line between the cerebrum and the inner table of the skull. This artifact is also generated by the computer. Shadowing and shading artifacts also occur and can be a relatively constant artifact on some scanners. Shading artifacts can also be seen because of the head cradle used with the scanners. Air bubbles retained in the water bags of certain scanners also produce a characteristic curvilinear artifact.

The following illustrations provide examples of the several types of artifacts seen on CT scans. It is hoped that they will aid the reader in differentiating artifacts from true abnormalities.

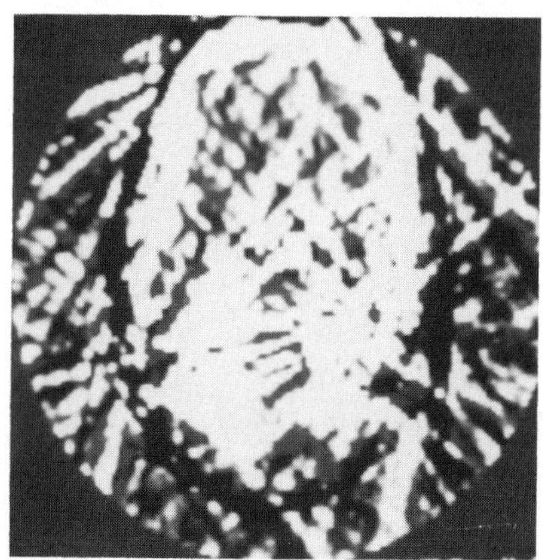

Preinfusion

Figure 3–11. Motion artifact.

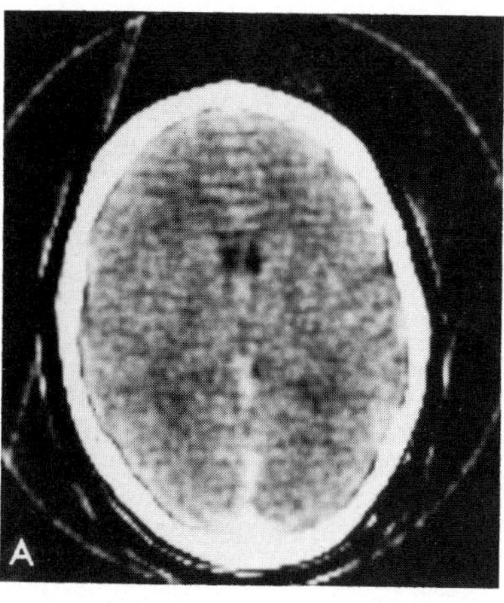

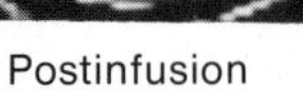

Postinfusion

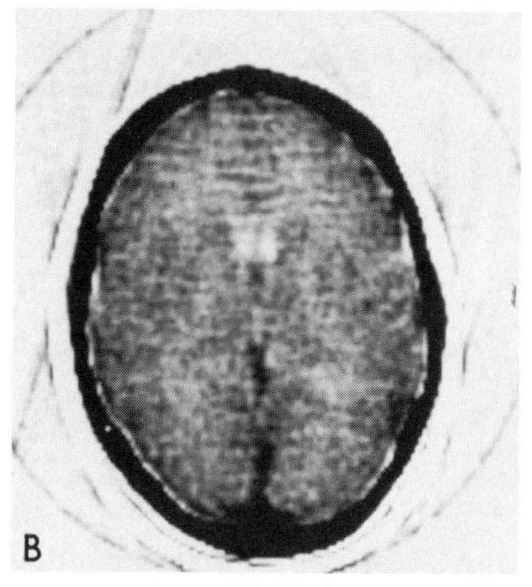

Postinfusion

Figure 3–12. *A* and *B*, Reduced tube output (caused by poor beam quality) leads to a "noisy" picture.

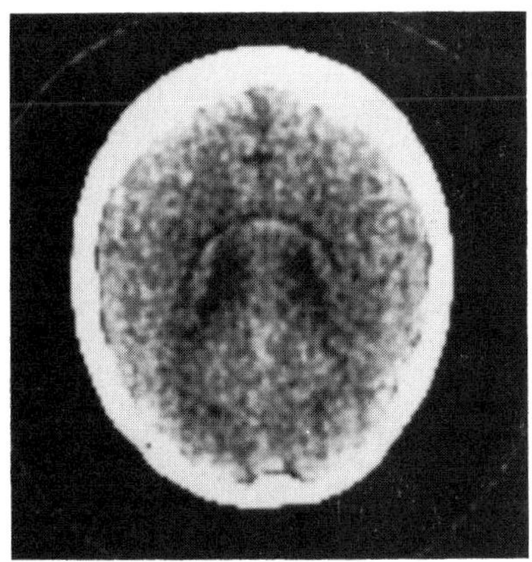

Figure 3–13. Curvilinear artifact secondary to an air bubble in the water bag.

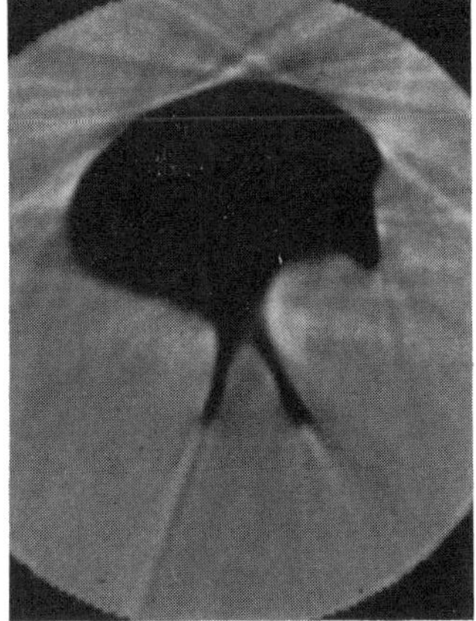

Figure 3–14. Scan of water bag.

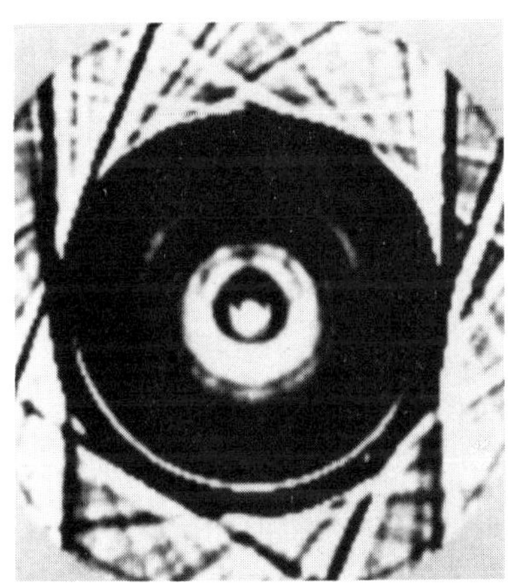

Figure 3–15. Scanning without indexing.

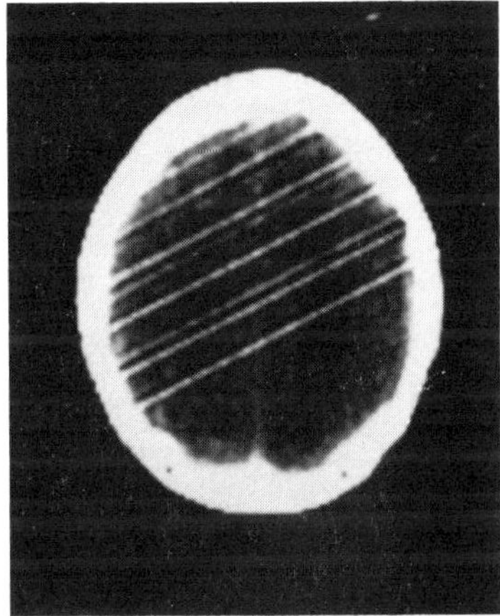

Figure 3–16. Changing detector sensitivity during scan.

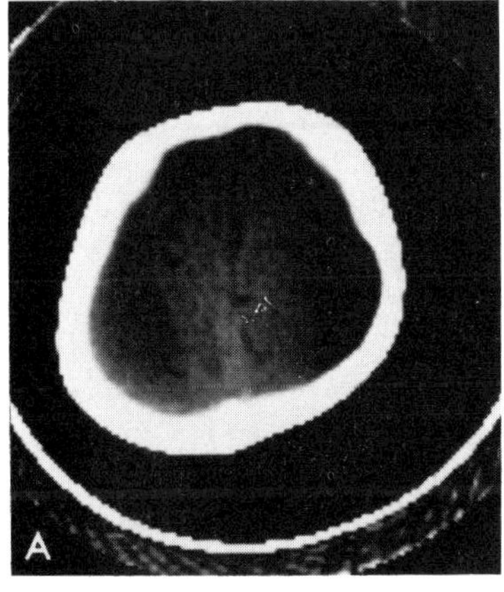

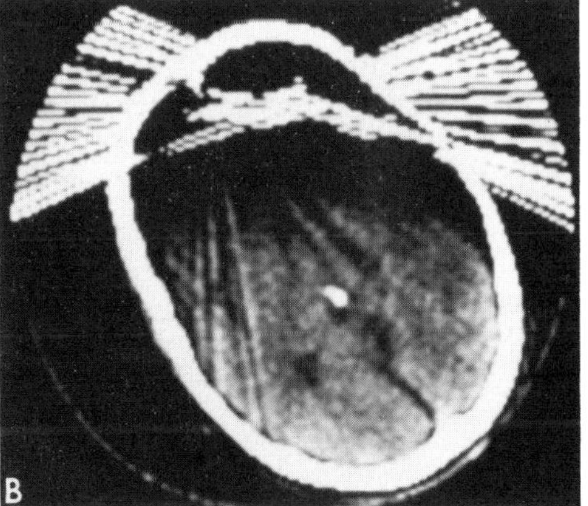

Figure 3–17. *A* and *B*, Shading artifact secondary to saturation of detectors.

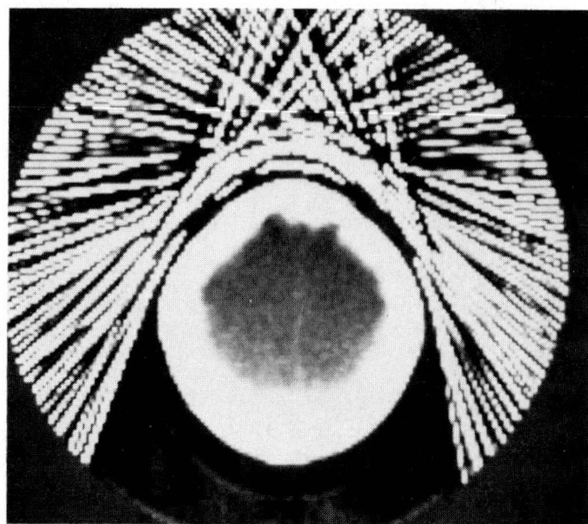

Figure 3–18. Artifact secondary to air around calvaria. This can be seen in patients with bouffant or Afro hair-styles.

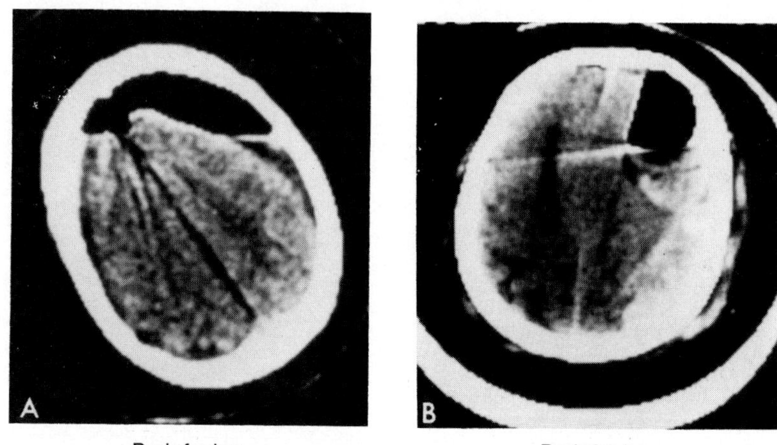

Figure 3–19. *A* and *B,* A white line computer overswing artifact caused by air within the calvaria.

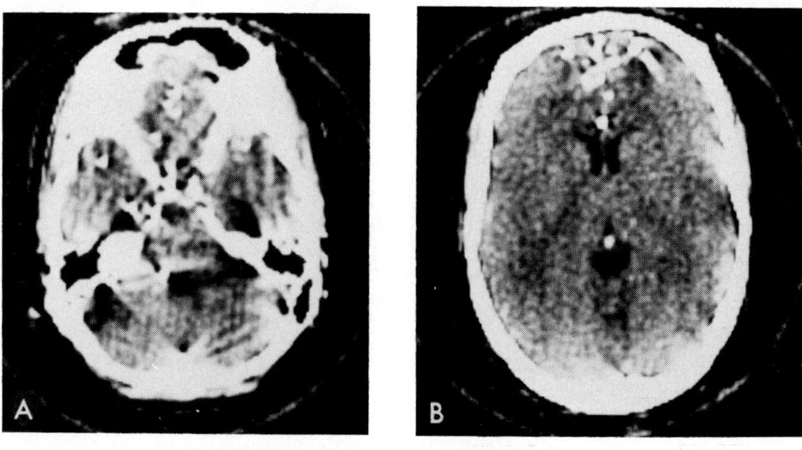

Figure 3–20. *A* and *B,* Pantopaque droplets.

CHAPTER 4

ANGIOGRAPHIC TECHNIQUE AND APPLIED CEREBROVASCULAR EMBRYOLOGY AND NORMAL ANATOMY

Angiographic Technique

SPECIAL PROCEDURE ROOM

Few hospitals have the luxury of a special procedure room devoted solely to neuroradiologic studies. More commonly, the special procedure room is used for GI studies in the morning and for the arteriographic studies in the afternoon, and often these facilities must be shared with others performing arteriography of the abdomen and lower extremities. Not uncommonly these rooms are not designed for biplane arteriography, making it necessary to use two separate injections to obtain a biplane study. This is suboptimal, but can be made to work if necessary.

Under ideal circumstances, a neuroradiologic suite should be set up such that it is equipped for biplane arteriography, including an image intensifier, so that both fluoroscopy and biplane arteriography can be performed without difficulty. The biplane technique can be either simultaneous or — if possible, and preferably — using alternating exposure technique. The table should have a free floating top and be movable in the up-down direction. A sliding top above a fixed top is helpful for patient positioning (Figs. 4–1, 4–2). The focal spot size should be 1.3 mm or less, and a small focal spot (0.3 mm or less) should also be available for selection so that magnification technique can be utilized conveniently. A high quality image intensifier should be situated so that catheter placement is possible with a minimum of patient movement and that filming can proceed with a minimum of patient motion after the catheter is in place.

A large, esthetically pleasing room away from main traffic areas is ideal and should allow access only to those involved in the procedures. The room should be quiet and set up so that the surroundings do not frighten the patient. Excess "clutter" should be eliminat-

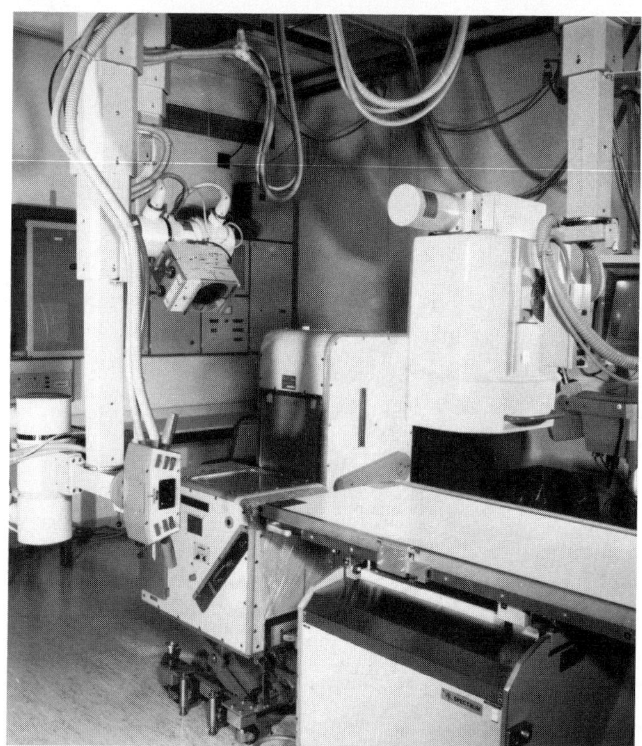

Figure 4–1. ANGIOGRAPHY EQUIPMENT: The AP and lateral tubes are in place and are aligned with the film changing units. The floating top table rests against the film changing device. The image intensifying unit rests above the table, and can be seen in the right of the picture. The room is large and well lighted.

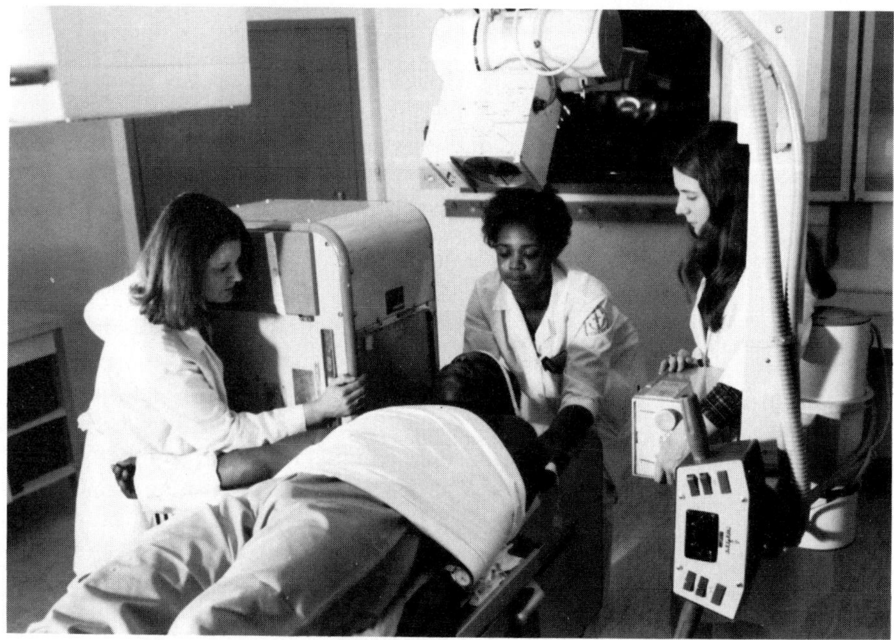

Figure 4–2. BIPLANE FILMING: The patient is being positioned for simultaneous filming in the AP and lateral projections. Note that the patient is positioned as close to the lateral film changes as possible. This is done to eliminate magnification. The AP grid is a focused grid and is "off-centered" to one side of the 14 × 14 grid. This grid is rotated, and the film changer is switched, depending on which side of the patient is being studied, so that the lateral film changer is always closest to the side injected.

ed, and the room should be well lighted and quiet. Large leaded windows should be available for patient monitoring, and remote monitors also may facilitate examination. The theory and practice of a "place for everything and everything in its place" should certainly be practiced in this setting. This is particularly true in those rare emergency conditions when equipment should be available quickly and conveniently.

An emergency cart with the necessary equipment for possible emergency and resuscitative procedures also should be readily available to be pushed to the bedside should the need arise. This emergency cart is stocked with all emergency drugs that might be needed. Any drugs used should be replaced immediately.

X-RAY EQUIPMENT

In general, the type of equipment is a matter of personal choice. Many manufacturers have equipment available for purchase that will produce a satisfactory series of radiographs. It is the author's opinion that a 1,000MA generator with three-phase equipment is preferable because it allows a wider range of technique choices and results in films with better contrast. In addition, it is helpful to have the capability of simultaneous biplane filming for adequate study of intracranial abnormalities. Magnification techniques are also necessary if an optimal study is to be performed. In general, the large focal spot for routine filming should be 1.3 to 1.2 mm in size. The small focal spot is then 0.2 to 0.3 mm in size.

INJECTORS

Manual Injections. Contrast material can be injected by hand when small amounts of contrast material are to be injected, when the vessel to be injected is very small or when it is desirable to remove the catheter from the vessel as soon as the injection is completed. On the other hand, this procedure results in excessive radiation exposure to the operating physician. In the author's opinion, injection by hand is undesirable except in unusual circumstances. The modern automatic injectors allow the injection of even small amounts of contrast material and — again in my opinion — all injections, with rare exceptions, should be made with the automatic injector.

Automatic Injectors. Injectors are available that can inject a bolus of contrast material at a pre-set pressure or at a rate of a pre-set volume per unit time. The pressure injectors reflect the pressure of the fluid at the hub of the catheter — not at its tip — making their desirability questionable. Volume injectors deliver a pre-set volume of contrast material in a predetermined period of time. For example, the volume injector can be set to deliver 10 cc per second for 2 seconds: a total dose of 20 cc. The settings of amount and time of delivery can be made at the time of injection.

The author has had many years of excellent and dependable service from the Viamonte-Hobbs injector. This unit has a built-in voltage ground to safeguard against an electric current passing through the patient. The Viamonte-Hobbs injector operates on the principle of a metered delivery rate; this can be set accurately and conveniently at the tableside just before injection. One dial is used to select the duration of the injection (variable from 1 to 4 seconds); a second dial is used to set the delivery rate (variable from 2 to 60 cc per second). There is also a back-up device, set before each injection, that prevents the delivery of more contrast material than desired. This is a mechanical stop device that also can be used to control the amount of contrast material injected. It can be set if the injection is to continue longer than 4 seconds — and maximum setting of the dial. Thus, if one would like to inject 6 cc per second for 8 seconds, the injector timer button is switched to "off." The volume per second is set on one dial and the total volume is set by using the back-up device. When the predetermined volume has been delivered, the mechanical device will stop the injector.

The Viamonte–Hobbs injector also has a dial that can be set to delay either the injector or the filming if desired. This is helpful when one needs a "blank" film at the beginning of the run to use for subtraction techniques. In this case, the unit is placed on an "injector delay" of one tenth of one second; i.e., the injection of contrast material occurs one tenth of one second after radiographic filming begins. This produces one exposed film without contrast before contrast material arrives at the area of interest. The unit also can be set for "x-ray delay" if that is desired.

FILM CHANGERS

Hand-Pulled Cassettes. After the injection of contrast material, the exposures are made, and each individual cassette is pulled out of the line of x-rays. This was the original method of filming, and it is still used today by some institutions. The films obtained with this technique are of good quality because the film screen contact is excellent. and a relatively rapid sequence of films can be obtained. The method is undesirable, however, because the firing rates are slow and inaccurate and because the scatter of radiation to the personnel increases individual exposure. Separate injections also must be made for biplane filming.

Automatic Cassette Changers. The Sanchez-Perez film changing unit uses automatically advanced cassettes and produces films of excellent quality. However, the units are noisy and are cumbersome because of the weight of the cassettes. They also are limited to the number of films that can be obtained.

Cut Film Changers. The Elema-Schonander film changing unit is the most popular of the cut film changers. The AOT changers are available for use with two film sizes — 14 × 14 inch (35 × 35 cm) and 10 × 12 inch. The 14 × 14 inch size is more desirable because it has wider uses than do the smaller film sizes, which are limited for the most part to use in studies of intracranial pathology. Departments that perform only studies of intracranial pathology also may find the small size a limitation, because it is difficult to visualize the extracranial vessels and nearly impossible to perform an arch angiogram without multiple injections. It is the rare institution that has the luxury of a room used solely for intracranial pathology studies. The 14 × 14 film changer also can be used for abdominal arteriography, and it seems wise to have a capability for both. The Schonander-AOT cut film changers are dependable, versatile and withstand years of hard use and abuse without malfunction. The receivers can easily be transported to the dark room for film processing.

The film carriers are heavy and awkward to load, but do allow easy filming in both single and series films. There is minimal film wastage if the equipment is used properly, and unexposed films can be reloaded and used. The film carriers can be loaded with up to 30 films, and filming can be performed at a rate of up to 6 films per second. The filming program can be pre-selected so that most any series can be obtained. Films can be exposed simultaneously in biplane projection; to prevent cross-fogging, the films can be loaded in the carriers alternately for single plane filming. At our institution we have an electronic system that allows for alternating filming without cross-fogging and without alternating film loading. This has resulted in increased film quality.

Puck. Elema-Schonander manufactures a lightweight movable unit that also uses 14 × 14 inch cut films. Films are limited to two per second, and the carrier is limited to 20 films. This is inadequate for use in a neuroradiology section where more rapid filming is desired. Computer cards are used to program the units, but this method does not seem advantageous. Motion artifacts may occur with these lightweight units.

Roll Film Changers. *Franklin Changer.* This is the best known of the roll film units. It can be used with the biplane technique, and the dimensions of the units allow for an area 11 × 14 inches.

Alternating exposures results in single plane filming — but also in a waste of film. Films may be exposed at a rate of up to 6 per second.

Roll film changers waste more film than do cut film changers. A single test film requires one exposure on a large sheet of film. The last length of film often is too short for a full run, resulting in excessive wastage.

SUMMARY

Although each injector and film changer has its advantages and disadvantages, the author has found the Elema-Shonander 14 × 14

AOT changers and the Viamonte-Hobbs injector to be safe, versatile, dependable and efficient for use in our neuroradiology procedures.

TECHNICAL COMPLICATIONS

It is clear that the inexperienced operator will have greater difficulty performing angiographic procedures, leading to a greater complication rate. It is imperative that the angiographer be given a basic introduction to standard angiographic methods and techniques — preferably an introduction to angiography using the Seldinger technique for the femoral approach. A sound knowledge of the fundamentals will facilitate the technique of angiography. For neurosurgery residents, who must, by necessity, learn cerebral angiography without the benefit of prior angiography experience, close monitoring of these procedures — preferably by a neuroradiologist — is necessary. The neuroradiologist is versed in film technique and the proper use of equipment as well as in angiographic techniques.

The first introduction to cerebral angiography following thorough verbal instructions should be observation of an experienced operator. There are some basic techniques that should be followed and certain precautions always to be taken; however, each operator soon develops his or her own techniques. These include minor personal variations on the basic technique.

PREMEDICATION

For adults the author recommends 100 mg Nembutal and 0.4 mg of atropine IM before angiography. For children, I recommend the dosage originally suggested by Taveras:

Age (yrs)	*Secobarbital (mg/kg)*	*Meperidine (mg/kg)*	*Atropine, Total Dose (mg)*	*Chlorpromazine (mg/kg)*
1–4	8–10	1–1.5	0.1–0.2	1.5
5–8	5–7	1–1.5	0.3	1.0
9–12	3–4	1.0	0.4	0.75

ARTERIOGRAPHY

Definition. *Arteriography* is the visualization of an artery or arteries by x-ray after injection of a radiopaque contrast material. *Angiography* is the radiography of vessels after the injection of a radiopaque material.

HISTORY

Cerebral arteriography was first introduced by Egazs Moniz in 1927. The procedure at first employed Thorotrast as a contrast material. It was found later that Thorotrast, because of its properties as both a B^- emitter and an alpha particle emitter, and because it was taken up by the reticuloendothelial system and not excreted, caused the development of certain types of tumors. The alpha particles are especially implicated because of their short tissue penetration and the great ionization of the tissues through which they pass. Therefore, Thorotrast is no longer used as a contrast material. Through the years many materials have been developed that provide excellent visualization and have only slight toxicity. At the present time, Conray 60 per cent is used most commonly for study of the intracranial vessels. It appears that the meglumine salt of Conray is less toxic to the nervous system than is the sodium salt of other contrast materials. However, many other contrast materials have been and continue to be used for cerebral angiography.

INFORMED CONSENT

Before angiography, it is wise for the individual who will be performing the examination to discuss the procedure with the patient, explaining in some detail what will be done. Without going into excessive detail, one must explain both the procedure itself and the possible complications in such a fashion that the patient will readily understand. At the present time the public is well aware of the "informed consent"; because of this, the patient should be told of possible complications, including the possibility of a "stroke." In order to avoid frightening the patient away from a needed procedure, it is wise to use a good deal of discretion when explaining such possibilities to the individual or the family. Such possible difficulties as soreness of the neck, arm or leg for several days following the procedure and "black and blue" marks at the puncture sites will be readily accepted as normal consequences if the patient is told about them well in advance. Fear of the unknown often frightens the patient most, and any information about the procedure that will alleviate such fears not only will help the patient, but will most certainly be to the operator's advantage.

ANESTHESIA

As a general rule, all our angiograms are done with the patients awake. General anesthesia can be used, and may be necessary in certain cases. It is often used in the pediatric age group.

FILMING TECHNIQUE

Routine filming technique for carotid angiograms is 2 films per second for 3 seconds, and 1 film per second for 6 seconds. We inject 10 cc for a routine common carotid arteriogram, 7 cc for an internal carotid arteriogram and 3 to 7 cc for an external carotid angiogram, depending on the size of the external carotid or branch vessel being studied. By knowing the filming sequence, one can evaluate the circulation time in the intracranial system.

ARTERIOVENOUS CIRCULATION TIME

The period from the greatest beginning concentration of contrast material in the carotid siphon to the maximum concentration in the parietal veins is called the "arteriovenous circulation time." According to various authors, the average time is 4.13 seconds to 4.37 seconds. The circulation time is normally faster in children, and a circulation time greater than 6 seconds is definitely prolonged.

The time can be determined by knowing the timing of the filming sequence, i.e., 2 films per second for 3 seconds and then 1 film per second for 6 seconds. Therefore, one can determine the various circulation times simply by counting the number of films.

TABLE 4–1 FILMING TECHNIQUE AND CONTRAST AMOUNTS—CONRAY 60 PER CENT

Procedure	*Contrast Material Amounts*	*Total*
Common carotid arteriogram	10 cc/sec for 1 sec	10 cc
Internal carotid arteriogram	10 cc/sec for 0.7 sec	7 cc
External carotid arteriogram	10 cc/sec for 0.3 to 0.7 sec	3–7 cc
	or	
	0.3 to 0.7 cc/sec for 1 sec	3–7 cc
Brachial arteriogram	25 cc/sec for 1.8 sec	45 cc
Arch arteriogram	25 cc/sec for 2 sec (Renografin-76)	50 cc
Innominate or subclavian arteriogram for visualization of vertebral when selective catheterization cannot be performed	10 to 14 cc/sec for 2 to 3 sec	20–40 cc
Vertebral arteriogram	10 cc/sec for 0.3–0.7 sec	3–7 cc
	or	
	0.3 to 0.7 cc/sec for 1 sec	

In brain death the circulation time is markedly prolonged, and the contrast material does not proceed above the supraclinoid portion of the internal carotid artery. Other causes of a prolonged circulation time are marked increased intracranial pressure, arterial thromboses, diffuse arteriosclerosis and arterial spasm.

A shortened circulation time is seen with arteriovenous malformations and arteriovenous fistula; it also may be seen with any process that results in early venous drainage, such as infarcts, glioblastoma multiforme, metastases and brain abscesses.

The author recommends that more than 7 or 8 cc should never be injected into the vertebral artery, except in the presence of an arteriovenous malformation or a very vascular tumor, where a higher volume injection is necessary for visualization of the abnormality.

PUNCTURE NEEDLES

A variety of different needles may be used for cerebral angiography. Figures 4–3 — 4–5 illustrate the various needles and guidewires that the author has found satisfactory in daily use.

Cournand-Potts Needle. This needle has a beveled tip and a matching beveled needle hub. In Figure 4–4 it is shown locked into position on the Davis rake. The needle is correctly positioned with the bevel down. The metallic needle extends out beyond the hub of the needle to eliminate "dead space" and to avoid the risk of clot formation within the lumen. The Luer-Lok fitting fastens tightly over the needle hub.

The Davis rake helps to immobilize the needle while it is in the vessel.

Davis Needle. The Davis needle is a long, firm plastic needle with a slight curve at its distal end. The needle has a blunt plastic cannula that occludes the needle between injections. The needle–catheter is placed into the carotid artery using the Seldinger technique. Under fluoroscopic control, the catheter can be manipulated selectively into the internal and external carotid arteries by taking advantage of the distal curve and using the guidewire if necessary.

BRACHIAL ANGIOGRAPHY

The brachial angiogram is one of our safest and most frequently performed procedures, and usually can be done rapidly and with minimal patient morbidity. As with carotid angiography, the procedure should be discussed at length with the patient. It should be stated that the needle puncture will be in the arm — right or left — and that the injection itself will be quite painful, causing a stinging and burning sensation that will last approximately 10 to 15 seconds. If the injection is into the right arm, pain will be felt in the right elbow, the right shoulder, the right side of the face and neck, in the teeth and behind the eye. If the right brachial injection fills the left carotid these sensations also will be felt in the left carotid distribution. In addition, a less strong sensation will be felt in the rectum and lower extremities caused by the contrast material that enters the arch of the aorta and the descending aorta. The injector and the film changer will create a certain amount of noise while the film series is generated. All these things ideally should be explained to the patient before the examination, and a brief description of the events that will occur during the study should help greatly in allaying the patient's fears.

Technique

The patient should be positioned on the table as comfortably as possible so that the area of interest can be filmed without moving the patient after the needle is in place. The arm is then placed palm up in a 30 to 45° abducted position on a firm arm board. A blood pressure cuff is positioned on the lower portion of the forearm (see Figure 4–6). A rolled towel is placed below the distal humerus just above the elbow. This serves to hyperextend the arm and allows for easier puncture of the brachial artery by making the pulse more readily palpable. The arm is then fixed to the armboard by two strips of adhe-

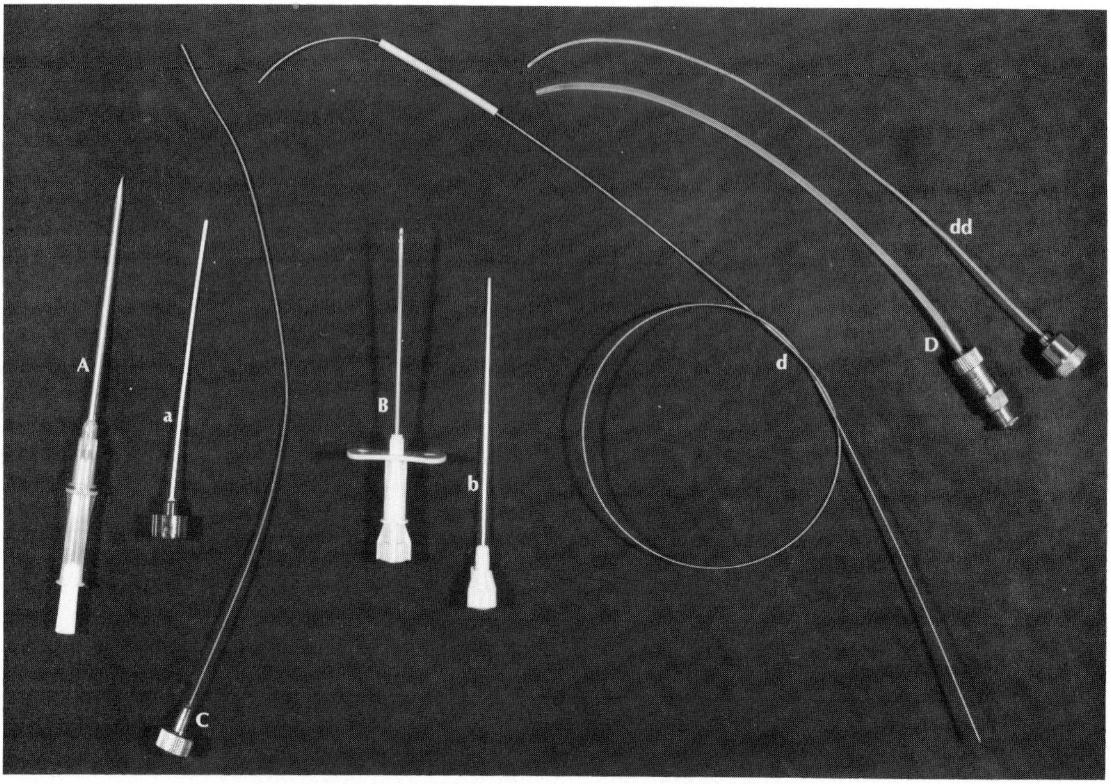

Figure 4–3 *See legend on the opposite page.*

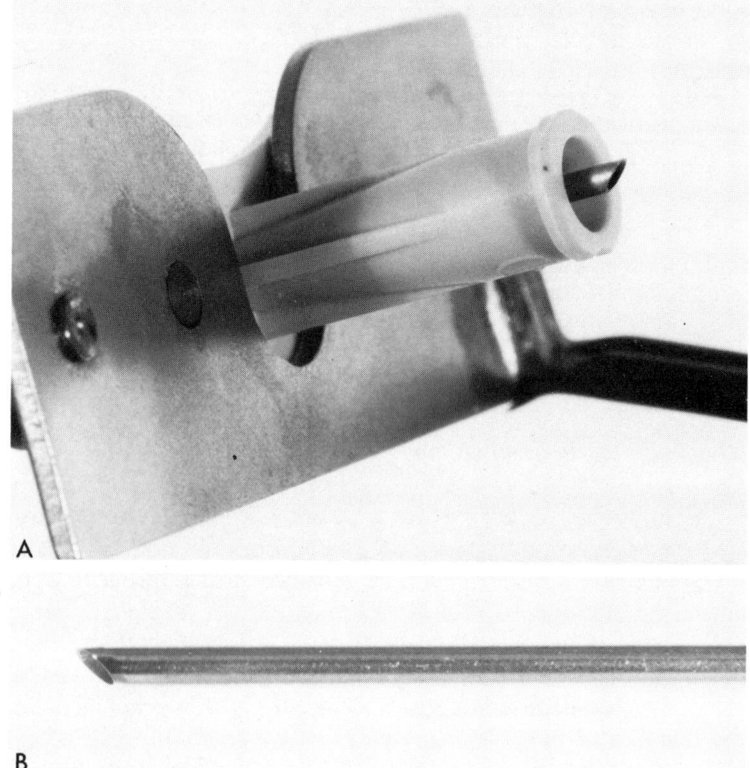

Figure 4–4 *See legend on the opposite page.*

Figure 4–3. TYPICAL ANGIOGRAM NEEDLES: *A*, Brachial angiogram needle. The needle is metal and has an outer plastic sheath. The solid plastic obturator *(a)* occludes the needle between injections.

B, Cournand-Potts needle. This metal needle is used for carotid angiography and has a beveled tip and a hub with a matching bevel. The metallic obturator *(b)* occludes the needle between injections.

C, The soft-tipped metal guidewire is used to position both the brachial and carotid needles.

D, Davis needle. This short catheter needle can be used for selective internal and external carotid angiography. The short guidewire *(d)* is passed through the puncture; then, using the Seldinger technique, the Davis needle is advanced over the guidewire and into the carotid artery. The plastic obturator *(dd)* occludes the needle between injections. The Davis needle also can be used for jugular venography.

Figure 4–4. *A*, COURNAND-POTTS NEEDLE: The needle is held immobile by the Davis rake. The inner core of the needle extends beyond the hub of the needle so that, when connected to the tubing for contrast injection with a Luer-Lock fitting, all dead space is eliminated.

B, The bevel of the needle faces down and corresponds to the bevel at the tip of the needle.

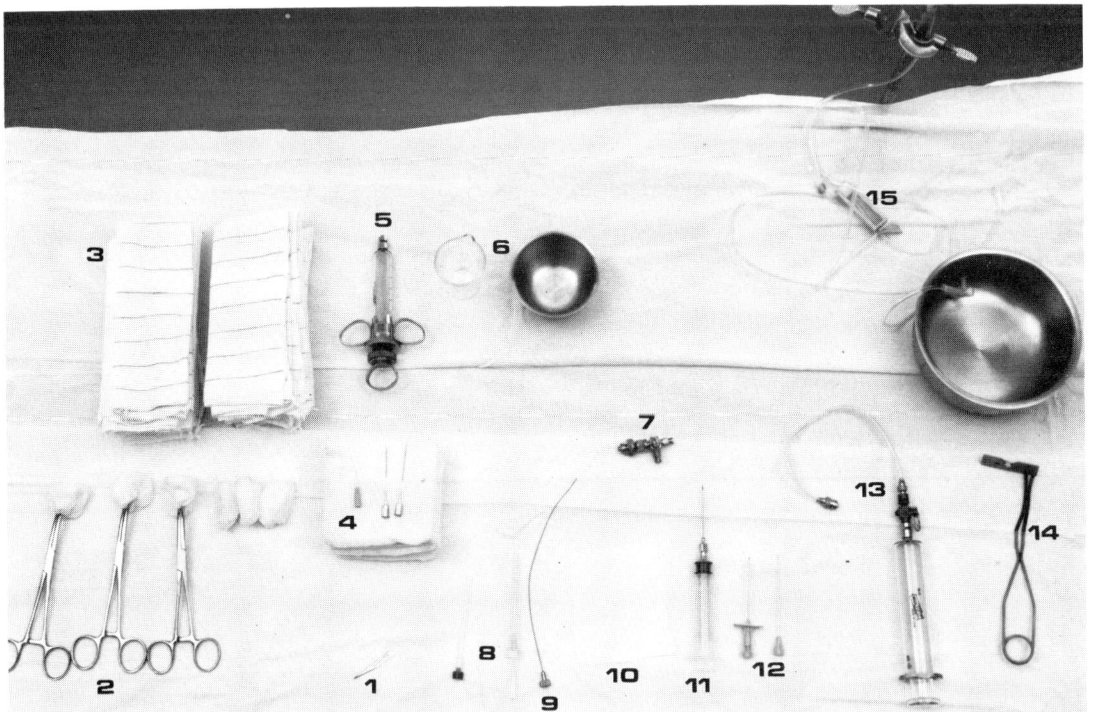

Figure 4–5. TYPICAL ANGIOGRAM TABLE SET-UP: 1. Scalpel blade; 2. clamps and sponges; 3. towels; 4. needles for local anesthesia; 5. syringe; 6. containers for contrast material; 7. high pressure stopcock; 8. brachial angiogram needle and obturator, 16 gauge; 9. guidewire; 10. sterile tape to hold brachial needle in place; 11. syringe for local anesthetic; 12. Cournand-Potts needle, 18 gauge; 13. syringe with stopcock and low pressure tubing for carotid angiograms; 14. Davis rake; 15. IV set-up for flushing solution.

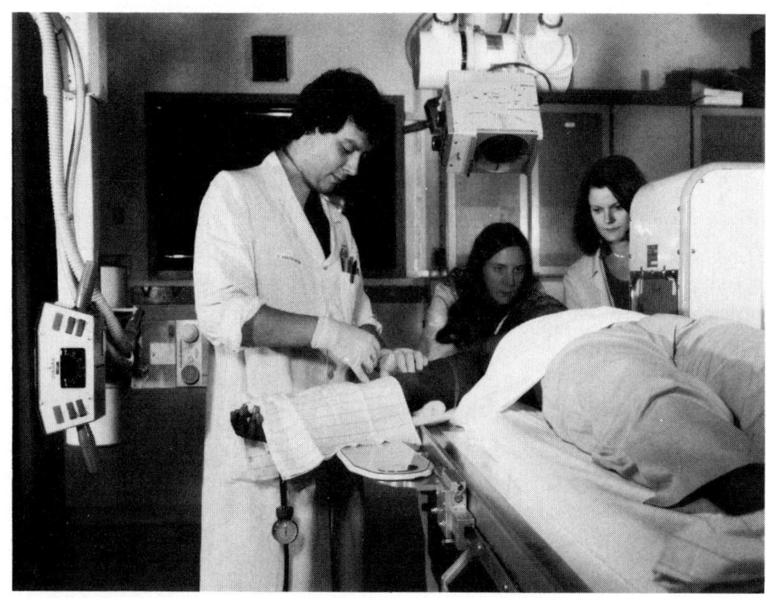

Figure 4–6. BRACHIAL ARTERIOGRAPHY: The patient is in position for filming after the needle is inserted into the right brachial artery. The arm to be punctured (either right or left) is placed on an armboard in the anatomic position — with the palm facing toward the ceiling. The arm is hyperextended at the elbow by placing a rolled towel under the distal end of the humerus just above the elbow. A blood pressure cuff is wrapped around the patient's wrist, and the patient's arm is then taped to the armboard so that it cannot be bent. The arm is then prepped, the brachial pulse palpated, and the artery punctured just above the crease in the elbow.

sive tape that circle the arm and attach to the armboard in the upper humeral region and at the level of the wrist.

The brachial artery is palpated and an antiseptic solution applied to the area surrounding the puncture site. A bleb of local anesthetic is then introduced into the skin just over the brachial artery. The artery should be punctured just above the elbow skin crease, where it is most readily palable. A tiny nick is then made in the anesthetized skin over the brachial artery. The skin nick is made with a surgical blade and prevents dulling of the needle tip by the strong layer of skin. The puncture is then made by piercing the brachial artery. The author prefers a through-and-through puncture of the vessel followed by slow withdrawal of the needle after the inner cannula has been removed. As the needle enters the lumen of the vessel there will be free flow of pulsating blood from the hub of the needle. A flexible guidewire is then introduced and the needle is advanced over the guidewire until it is positioned well in the vessel.

I strongly recommend the use of a 16-gauge disposable needle that has a metal inner core with a needle tip and an outer plastic sheath with a blunt tip (see Figure 4–3,*A*). This needle is also supplied with a firm plastic inner stylet to occlude the needle between injections, obviating the need for continuous flushing of the system. The puncture also may be performed with a Cournand-Potts needle, but this is less satisfactory.

At times the brachial vein will be entered and only venous blood will exit from the hub of the needle. The needle puncture should then be made slightly more laterally, as the brachial artery is lateral to the vein with the patient in the anatomic position.

Steps in Needle Puncture

1. The pulse is palpated by the free hand, and the needle is then passed through the skin nick and soft tissues until its tip rests on the brachial artery and a transmitted pulse can be felt through the needle.

2. The brachial artery is then punctured just above the elbow crease with a sharp forward thrust.

3. The needle should pass through-and-through the vessel; the inner metal cannula is then removed and the plastic sheath slowly withdrawn until there is free flow of pulsating arterial blood.

4. The soft-tipped guidewire is then advanced through the plastic sheath until the tip of the guidewire extends beyond the tip of the needle. The plastic needle is then advanced over the guidewire to the hub of the needle so that its entire length rests in the vessel.

5. The guidewire is then removed and the plastic needle is occluded with the obturator.

6. If there is difficulty advancing the needle — because of an area of narrowing from arteriosclerosis or previous arterial cutdown — the vessel may then be punctured at a more proximal point. If the puncture is performed at a higher than usual level, great care must be taken to be certain that the vessel is firmly compressed at the puncture site when the needle is removed.

7. At the termination of the procedure, the needle is removed. Firm pressure is applied at the puncture site for 10 minutes.

Occasionally both the brachial artery and vein will be entered simultaneously. Initially one obtains venous blood, followed by pulsating arterial blood. If this is the case, after the needle has been advanced into the artery, pressure should be applied to the puncture site for several minutes to prevent the occurrence of a hematoma.

Volume of Injection

The injections are made using a volume injector. The injector is connected to the needle with a high-pressure clear plastic tubing with an intervening stopcock that allows removal of air bubbles without disconnecting the tubing device. *45 cc of Conray 60 per cent is injected at a rate of 25 cc/second for 1.8 seconds.*

Technique of Filming

If examination of the vessels of the neck is desired, 0.5 second of x-ray delay is recommended, and films are obtained at a rate of 4 films per second for 2 seconds. For the intracranial series, a similar injection is made with 0.7 to 1.0 second of x-ray delay, and filming is done at a standard rate of 2 films per second for the first 3 seconds and 1 film per second for the next 6 seconds. At the time of the injections, the cuff is inflated at the wrist to promote retrograde flow of the contrast material and to prevent antegrade flow of the contrast down to the hand, which is quite painful. All filming is done using a biplane technique.

Some operators perform a single test radiograph of the brachial artery at the puncture site, using a small amount of contrast material. Using our present needle puncture technique, we have found this unnecessary, except in rare cases (Fig. 4–7).

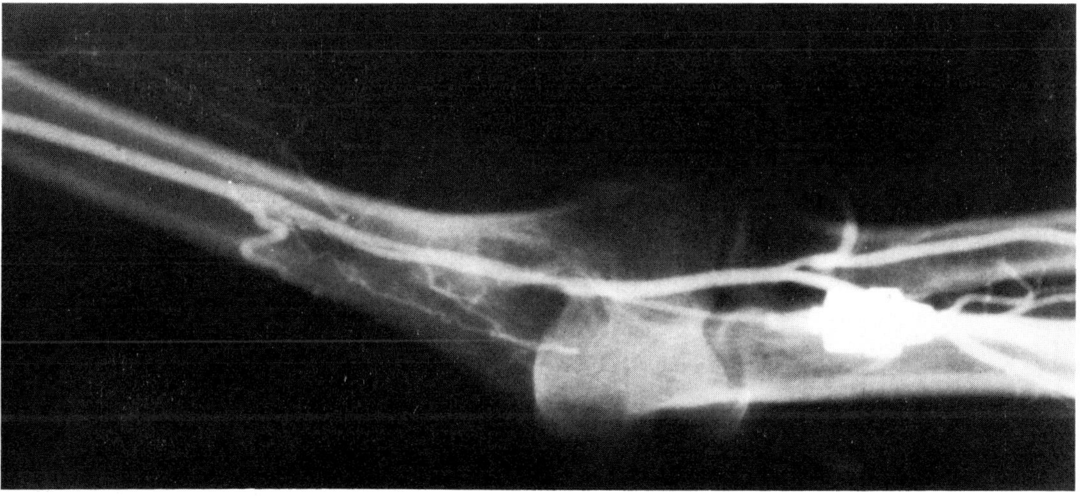

Figure 4–7. RIGHT BRACHIAL ARTERIOGRAM: The needle is in place in the brachial artery, and contrast material has been injected to confirm the correct position of the needle.

Following the injection, the cuff is deflated at the wrist and the obturator is replaced in the needle. For more exact timing on the intracranial series, the operator should inspect the films to determine how many seconds or what fraction of a second will be required in order to set an appropriate "x-ray delay." Thus, there will be one blank film followed by films with contrast material in the intracranial circulation.

This method of filming allows for adequate visualization of the intracranial circulation in nearly all cases. Slower and more prolonged filming may be needed when there is slow circulation of contrast material owing to elevated intracranial pressure.

Complications

Occasionally contrast material will extravasate from the vessel into the muscle of the arm. This is very painful for the patient, and a film will reveal the radiodense contrast in the soft tissues (Fig. 4–8). When this occurs the needle should be removed and compression applied. No further puncture attempt should be made until 48 hours have passed.

A subintimal injection also may occur that dissects the vessel over a variable length. Figure 4–9 demonstrates the intimal flap.

Because of the force of the injection, the needle rarely may be pushed backward out of the vessel; for this reason, precautions should be taken that the needle is secured in place before injection.

Anatomic Variations

In approximately 1 per cent of patients one will encounter an aberrant right subclavian artery. In such a case, only the vertebral artery will fill from the brachial injection, and right carotid arteriography will have to be performed. In 20 to 25 per cent of cases, the left carotid artery arises as a common trunk with the right innominate vessel. This normal anatomic variation may or may not be of help. If one does not wish to fill the left carotid circulation, the left carotid vessel can be compressed during the time of the injection and into the early venous phase. This will prevent contrast from entering the left carotid artery, allowing visualization of only the right carotid artery and the right carotid and right vertebral circulation. Obviously, a second injection without left carotid compression will allow

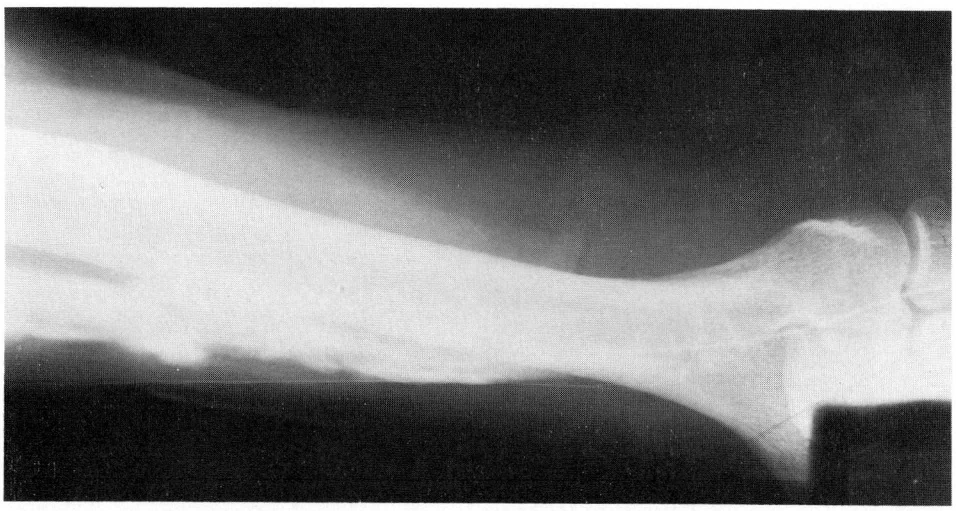

Figure 4–8. EXTRAVASATION OF CONTRAST MATERIAL: The brachial catheter has dislodged from the lumen of the vessel, and the injection has resulted in the accumulation of contrast material in the muscles and soft tissue of the arm. This is very painful for the patient, and may result in occlusion of the brachial artery.

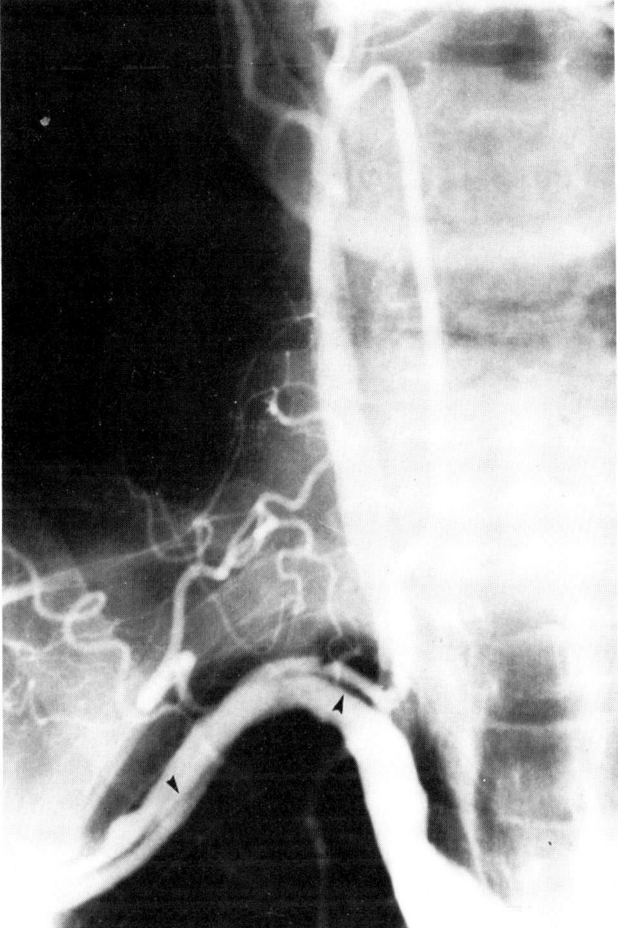

Figure 4–9. SUBINTIMAL INJECTION: A large subintimal flap has been raised in this patient secondary to the brachial arteriogram. The arrows mark the flap of the intima, which extends to the level of the origin of the vertebral artery.

comparison between the two sides (see Figure 4 28). On the other hand, compression of the left carotid artery may cause the contrast material to cross over to the left side via the anterior communicating artery — again filling the left internal carotid system.

The left vertebral artery arises as a separate trunk from the aortic arch in approximately 5 per cent of cases. In the vast majority of patients, the left vertebral circulation will be visualized by left brachial injection. In the majority of cases the left vertebral artery is the dominant supplying vessel to the vertebral–basilar system. It should be noted that, in 5 per cent of cases, the vertebral artery will end in the posterior inferior cerebellar artery, and there will be no visualization of the remainder of the posterior fossa. In such instances, contralateral brachial arteriography will be needed.

PERCUTANEOUS CAROTID ARTERIOGRAM

This procedure should be discussed with the patient before it is undertaken. It is important that both the procedure itself and its risks should be discussed at sufficient length to ensure informed consent. The more a patient knows about the procedure, the better. The fear element is reduced, and, in general, the patient is able to co-operate better. The physician who is to perform the procedure should visit the patient in the hospital room. I recommend a step-by-step explanation, telling the patient what vessel is to be studied. The following are some of the things that may be discussed during this meeting.

1. You will be brought to the radiology department on a cart.

2. I will meet you there, and any additional questions you may have will be answered.

3. You will be placed on the angiogram table and made as comfortable as possible.

4. An intravenous infusion may be started if necessary; also, a cardiac monitor may be started.

5. Your neck will be extended by elevating the table and allowing your head to fall back over the end of the table. (Your shoulders may be elevated by an inflatable balloon.) Your head will be positioned over the film changer so that only minimal movement will be necessary after the needle is in place before filming.

6. Your neck will be prepared with three washes of antiseptic solution, the last being alcohol. After injection of a local anesthetic, the needle will be placed in the vessel.

7. Enough injections will be made to outline any abnormalities.

8. The needle will then be removed and firm pressure applied at the puncture site for 10 minutes or until bleeding stops.

Puncture Technique

Individual angiographers soon develop a personal technique that is satisfactory and comfortable for them. However, while learning the methods, the beginning angiographer will be assisted by these guidelines for puncture technique:

1. Extend the neck by elevating the table and allowing the head to fall over the end of the table or by inflating a balloon under the patient's shoulders. These steps result in extension of the neck.

2. The area is then cleaned widely with three washes of antiseptic solution, the last an application of alcohol.

3. The carotid artery is then palpated in the neck with the hand that will not hold the puncture needle.

4. When the pulse is well localized, a local anesthetic is injected into the skin at the anticipated point of puncture. The author recommends puncturing the vessel two fingerbreadths above the clavicle. This way, the puncture should always be well below the bifurcation. A second injection of local anesthetic is then introduced between the trachea and carotid artery and beneath the carotid artery. This second bolus should be approximately 5 to 6 cc and it serves several purposes.

(a) It anesthetizes the local area in the neck where the puncture needle will be thrust when the puncture attempts are made.

(b) The bolus serves to immobilize the vessel, therefore allowing an easier puncture.

(c) If the carotid artery is situated too far medially and under the trachea, this bolus of local anesthetic will move the vessel laterally and forward into a more accessible position. This bolus of anesthetic should be injected deep enough so that it is *below* the vessel. Putting the local anesthetic in the tissues between the skin and the vessel only serves to obscure the pulse and make the puncture more difficult.

5. A small nick is then made in the skin with a scalpel blade so that the tip of the puncture needle is not dulled while entering through the skin.

6. The vessel is then palpated and immobilized by the free hand. This can be done by reaching lateral to the vessel with the fingertips and pulling the vessel medially, thus trapping the vessel between the fingers and the bolus of local anesthetic. Or the vessel can be immobilized by trapping it between the tips of the index and middle finger — one finger on either side of the vessel.

7. The puncture needle is then advanced through the skin nick and soft tissues until the tip of the needle rests directly on the carotid artery and the pulsations transmitted from the vessel can be felt in the needle.

8. The vessel is then impaled by a single forward thrust of the needle or by multiple short forward thrusts.

9. If a Potts-Cournand needle (see Figure 4–4) is used, the needle puncture is performed with the bevel up.

10. I recommend through-and-through puncture of the vessel, although some operators prefer to puncture only the anterior wall.

11. The needle is then rotated 180° so that the bevel is down and is slowly withdrawn, holding the hub close to the patient's neck and chest, until bright red pulsating blood appears from the hub of the needle.

12. The soft-tipped guidewire is then advanced through the needle until the tip of the wire is well beyond the tip of the needle. The needle is then advanced over the guidewire approximately 1 cm. The guidewire is then withdrawn, the obturator is placed in the needle, and the needle is immobilized with a Davis rake (see Figs. 4–3 and 4–10).

13. The patient is then placed in position for filming. If desired a short run of films or even a single film may be exposed following the injection of contrast material to rule out the presence of a subintimal injection.

There should be free flow of blood from the needle at all times and easy flushing of the vessel with nonheparinized saline throughout the procedure. The absence of a free flow of blood or easy flushing may mean that the needle tip is subintimal or has become dislodged from the vessel lumen. *NEVER* inject contrast if these criteria are not met. The injection of contrast under less than optimal conditions presents significant danger to the patient. Complete occlusion of a vessel could prevent flow to the hemisphere, possibly resulting in a stroke or even death.

The author recommends the use of the obturator between injections rather than continuous or intermittent flushing. At the time of injection, a short, flexible connecting tube is attached to a syringe filled with saline. A stopcock is placed between the saline-filled tube and the syringe. The tubing is connected to the hub of the needle after the obturator is removed; then the closed stopcock is opened, and blood is allowed to fill the clear plastic tubing. If no bubbles of air are present, the tube is flushed with saline. Then the patient may be asked whether there is a cold, salty taste in his mouth from the flushing solution (confirming injection into the carotid system) or whether he feels pain in his neck (possibly implying a subintimal or extravascular injection). If all is well, the syringe is disconnected, the tubing is connected to the tubing on the injector, and the study is performed. I recommend the use of a volume injector and a dose of 10 cc/second over a 1 second period. The injection can be made by hand, but this is less readily reproducible and results in needless radiation exposure to the operator. There is no advantage to hand injection of contrast, and I do *not* recommend it.

Film exposure should begin with the contrast injection. This will ensure a blank film followed by films showing contrast material in the circulation.

The normal carotid bifurcation is at the level of C_4. At the time of intravascular injection, the contrast material will be seen as a "jet stream" (Fig. 4–10); later films demonstrate the normal carotid bifurcation. A slight dilatation of the proximal internal carotid artery is normal; this is the carotid sinus.

The location of the bifurcation can vary, and it may be seen either above (Fig. 4–11) or below (Fig. 4–12) the C_4 level.

Occasionally an enlarged superior thyroid artery will be punctured in the mistaken belief that it is the carotid artery (Fig. 4–13). A successful examination is unlikely if this occurs.

If a clamp has been placed on the common carotid artery that partially occludes the vessel (Fig. 4–14), puncture can be performed above the clamp.

The carotid artery occasionally may exhibit a "buckle" along its course. This may vary in size or position (Fig. 4–15).

Complications

If there is a *subintimal injection* demonstrated on the neck series, or if there is some other technical difficulty with the procedure, the needle should be removed and 10 minutes of compression applied to the puncture site. It should be remembered that, even with a subintimal injection, there may be excellent flow from the needle — apparently because the intimal flap "holds" the cephalad flow of blood and actually directs the blood to the tip of the

Text continued on page 162

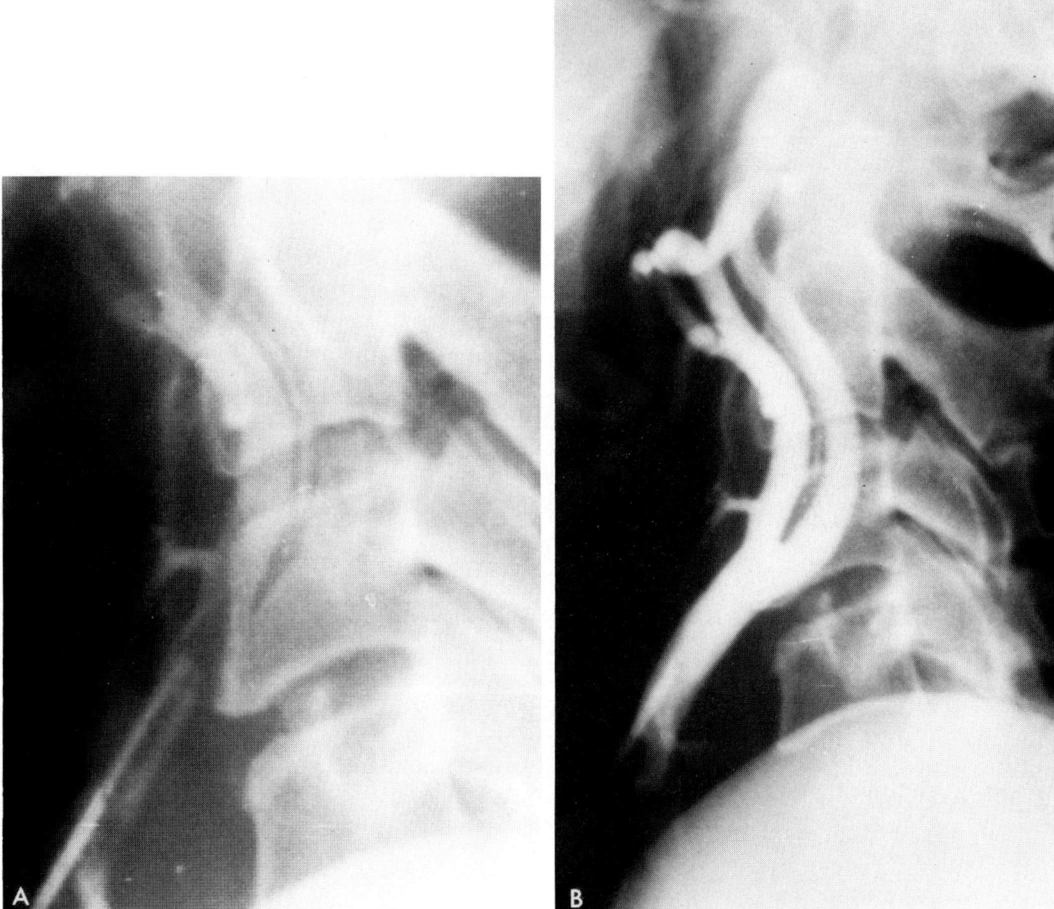

Figure 4–10. NORMAL CAROTID BIFURCATION: *A*, The needle is in place in the carotid artery, and the bevel of the needle is directed downward. A jet stream of contrast material is visible exiting from the tip of the needle.

B, The carotid bifurcation is visualized and is normal. The internal carotid artery is posterior to the external carotid artery, and the slight dilatation of the internal carotid artery is the carotid sinus.

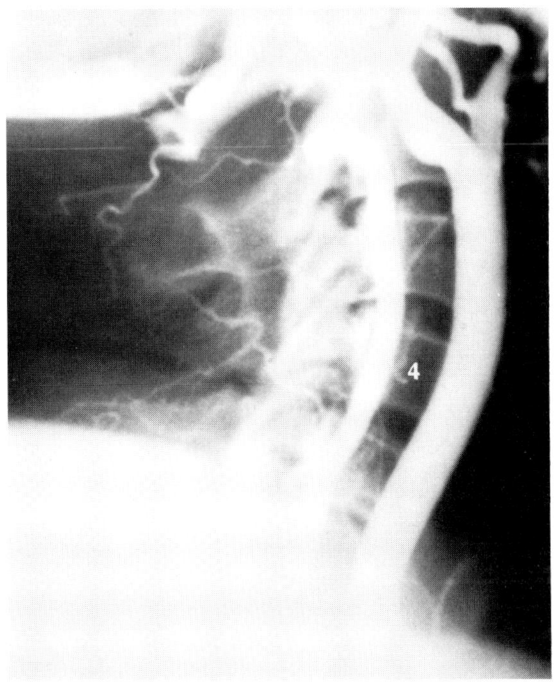

Figure 4–11. HIGH CAROTID BIFURCATION: The carotid bifurcation is at the level of C_2; the normal level is C_4.

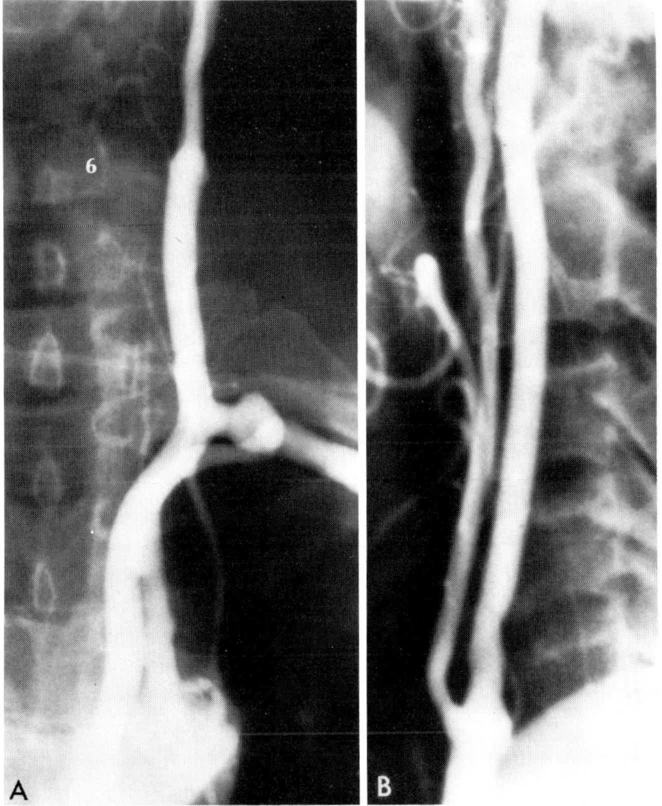

Figure 4–12. LOW CAROTID BIFURCATION: The carotid bifurcation is at the level of C_6. In this case it was visualized via a left branchial angiogram because there a surgical anastomosis had been made between the left subclavian and the left common carotid artery to prevent a "steal" down the left vertebral artery secondary to stenosis of the proximal left subclavian artery.

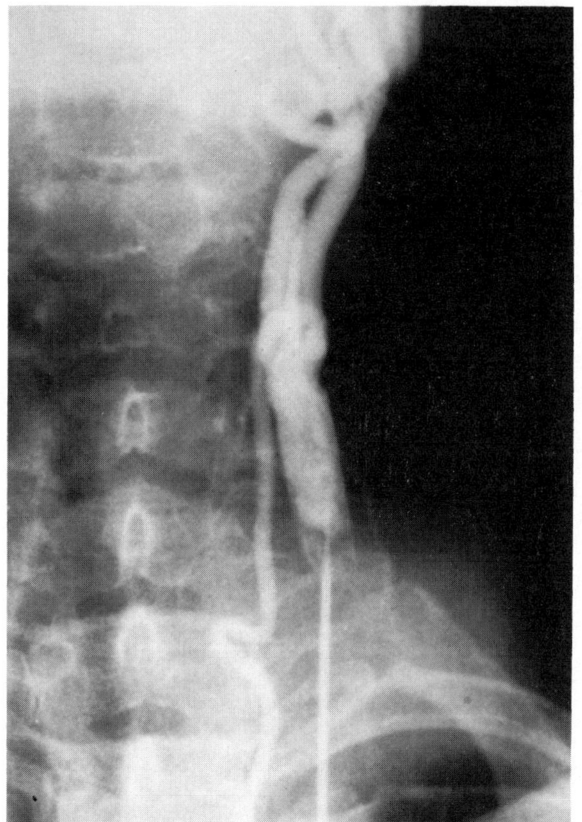

Figure 4–13. SUPERIOR THYROID ARTERY: This left common carotid angiogram demonstrates a large superior thyroid artery. At times, this vessel probably is inadvertently punctured and catheterized, resulting is local complications. Note the deviation of the trachea secondary to the local hematoma in the neck.

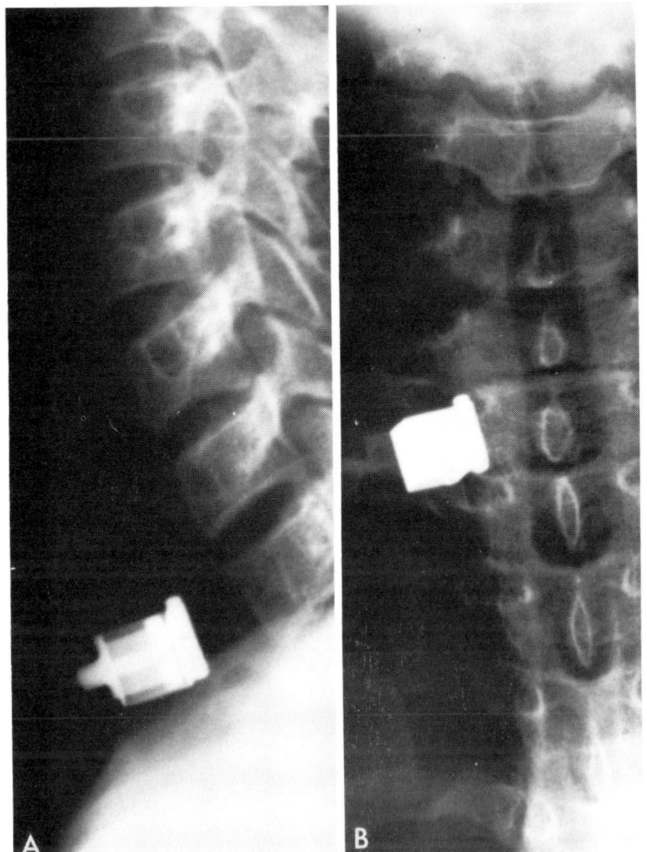

Figure 4–14. CAROTID CLAMP: A metallic clamp is in place that completely or partially occludes the common carotid artery.

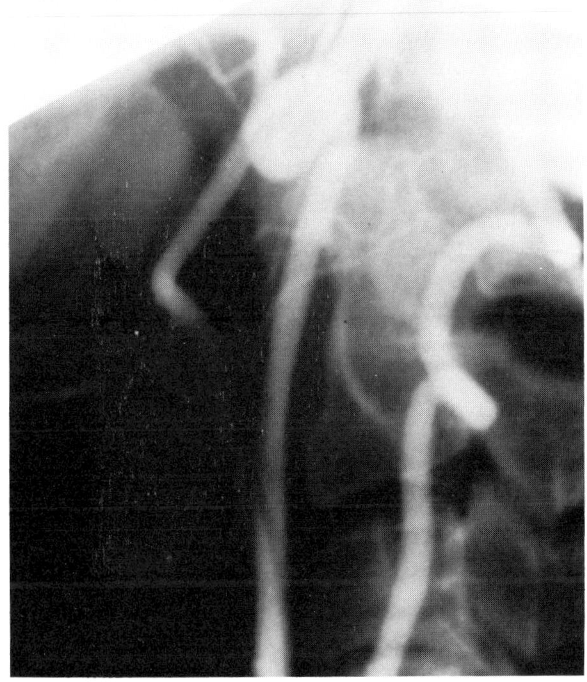

Figure 4–15. LOOP IN CAROTID ARTERY: Just below the base of the skull there is a large loop or "buckle" in the carotid artery. This is of no consequence, but may create a bruit.

needle. The author has noted that patients frequently complain of pain in the ear or in the angle of the jaw when there is a subintimal injection. This pain also occurs occasionally without a subintimal injection; thus it should not be used as a definite sign of this complication (Figs. 4–16, 4–17, 4–18).

Injection into the soft tissues of the neck is very painful for the patient and results in an amorphous collection of contrast in the patient's neck on the radiographs. If injection is subintimal or extravascular the needle should be removed and compression applied for 10 minutes. The procedure is then delayed for 48 hours (Fig. 4–19).

Occasionally a hematoma will develop in the neck during the procedure. If this occurs, pressure should be applied locally. If a hematoma develops while the needle is in place, gentle but firm pressure should be applied over the needle and the study performed and completed without further delay. In this situation, it may be necessary to remove the needle before viewing the films. It appears that these hematomas occur from bleeding from small muscular branches or from the back wall puncture site in the common carotid artery. This may occur because of a coagulopathy secondary to anticoagulation therapy or liver disease, or a hematoma may develop second-

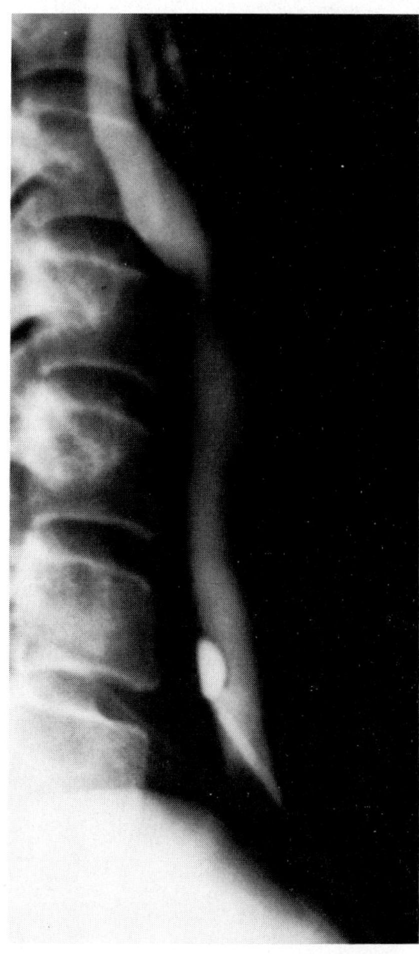

Figure 4–16. SUBINTIMAL INJECTION: The needle is in place in the vessel, and a small subintimal flap has been raised at its tip. No further injections should be made unless the tip of the needle can be manipulated beyond the subintimal flap — which often is not possible. A good antegrade flow of the contrast material demonstrates stenosis of the vessel distal to the injection site.

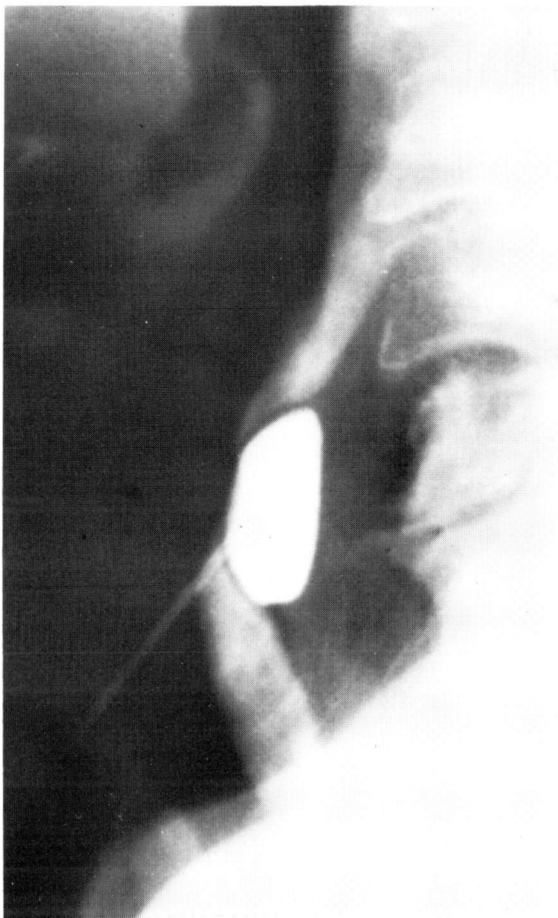

Figure 4–17. SUBINTIMAL INJECTION: A large subintimal accumulation of contrast material has almost completely blocked the antegrade flow of contrast material.

ary to bleeding from the back wall puncture site when the needle has gone through-and-through the vessel. If the hematoma becomes so large that it compromises the airway, the study should be terminated.

At the time of administration of the local anesthetic, *great* care should be taken to prevent the intra-arterial injection of xylocaine, since this leads to grand mal seizures. If this should occur, the study should be terminated and undertaken at another time.

Percutaneous vertebral artery puncture was first performed in 1940. With the use of femoral artery catheterization and selective study of the intracranial vessels, this method is no longer in popular use. The author has had no experience with this technique and does not recommend its use. The vertebral artery arises from the subclavian vessels and enters into the foramina transversaria at the level of the sixth cervical vertebra in most of the cases. There is some variation in the level of entrance into the foramina transversaria, however, and the vessel may enter at any level (Fig. 4–20). The vessel is probed and punctured as it travels in the foramina transversaria. Following the procedure, there is no way to apply adequate pressure to the puncture site, and conceivably excess bleeding could lead to a hematoma and occlusion of the vertebral artery. At the present time, vertebral angiography is performed using direct catheterization. Approximately 4 to 7 cc of contrast material is used with either percutaneous angiography or the catheterization technique.

The catheterization technique can provoke arterial spasm. An example is shown in Figure 4–21.

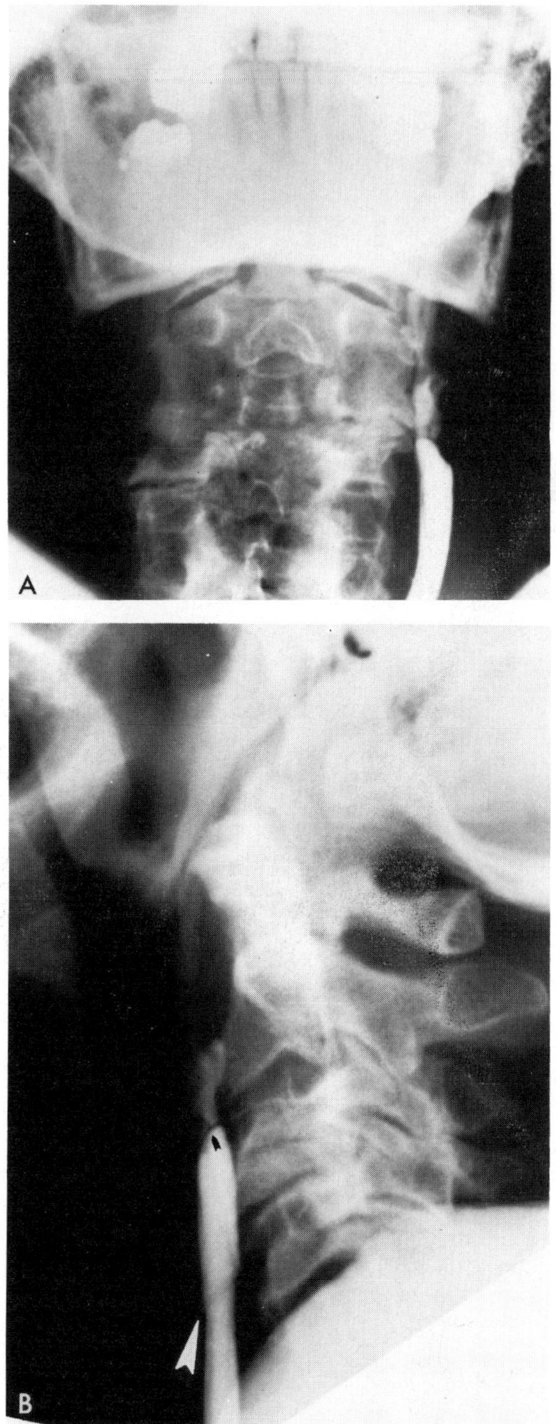

Figure 4–18. SUBINTIMAL INJECTION: *A,* The use of a soft plastic catheter has resulted in a large subintimal flap that has completely blocked the antegrade flow of contrast material through the internal carotid artery. The internal carotid artery was subsequently shown to be widely patent.

B, The small black arrow indicates the intimal flap; the white arrow shows the point of entry of the needle into the carotid artery.

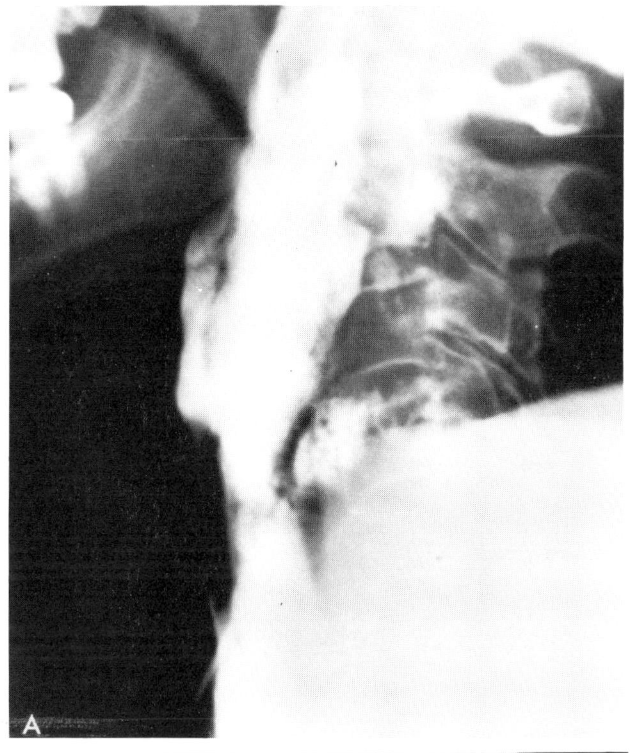

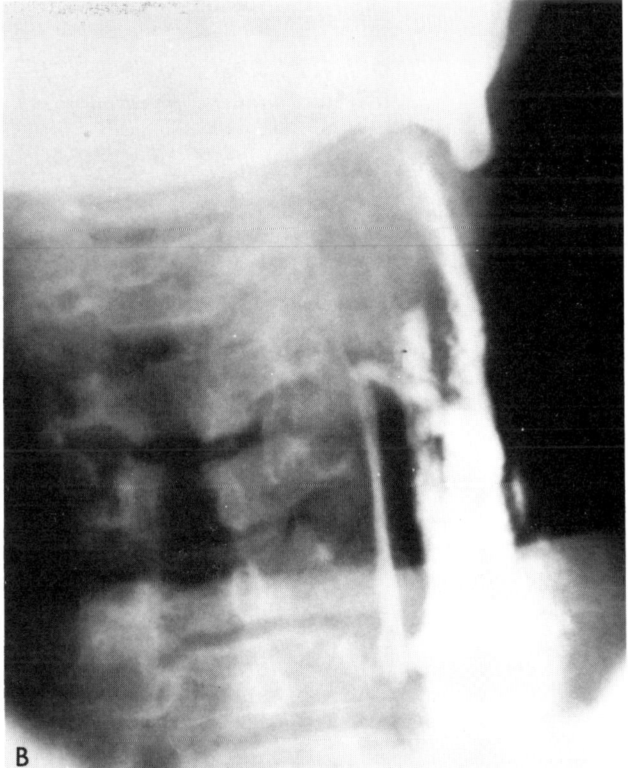

Figure 4–19. EXTRAVASATED CONTRAST MATERIAL: *A,* The tip of the needle had pulled out of the vessel before injection of the contrast material, resulting in the injection of contrast into the soft tissues of the neck.

B, The AP view reveals the extravasated contrast material; it also demonstrates the superior thyroid artery as the contrast follows the adventitia of the blood vessels. This is very painful for the patient, and may compress and occlude the vessel.

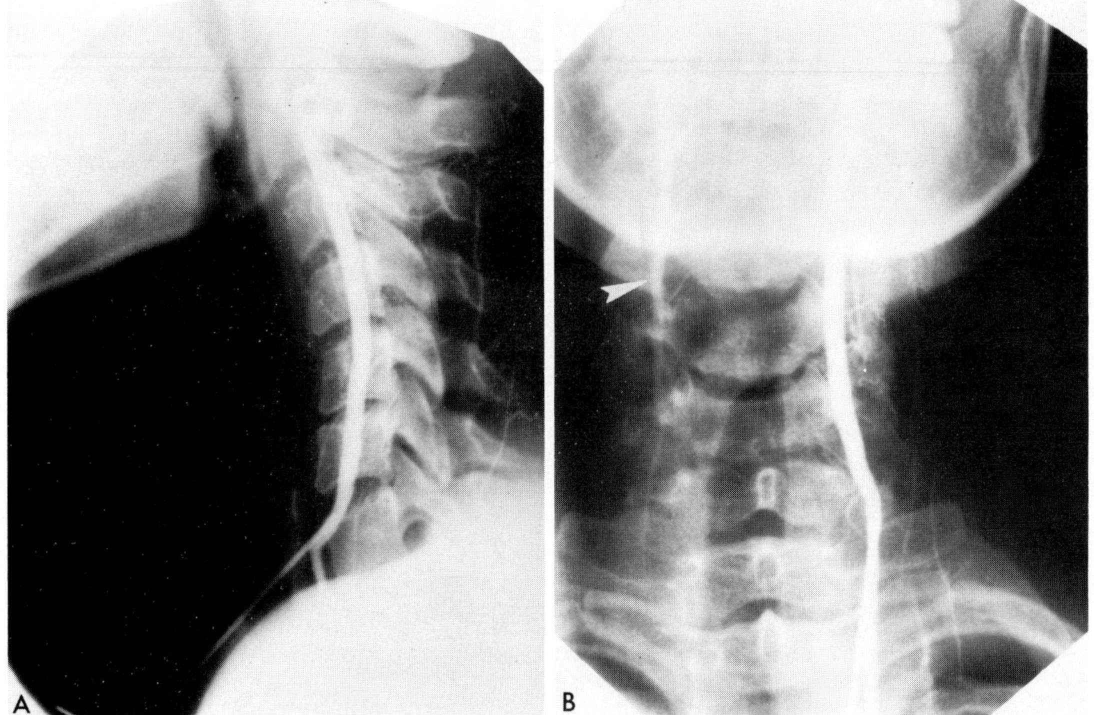

Figure 4–20. PERCUTANEOUS VERTEBRAL ARTERIOGRAM: The needle has been threaded into the vertebral artery. With the injection of contrast material the flow is also noted to go retrograde down the contralateral vertebral artery *(arrow)* because of the force of the injection.

Occasionally at the time of carotid angiography, the vertebral artery will be entered inadvertently. In this case, the puncture needle is usually found to be quite deep in the soft tissues of the neck. In addition, it will be noted that while the guidewire may thread up the vessel, the puncture needle will not follow because the vessel is within the foramina transversaria. This is particularly common when the metallic puncture needle is used; the plastic needle occasionally will thread without difficulty.

The true nature of the puncture site may not become apparent until the films are processed. Fairly commonly both the vertebral and carotid arteries will be entered simultaneously. If this is suspected, the puncture needle should be withdrawn slowly and correctly positioned when there is pulsating flow from the carotid artery after the needle has been removed from the vertebral vessel.

FEMORAL ARTERY CATHETERIZATION

History and Complications

Femoral artery catheterization and selective injection of the visceral vessels was first described by Seldinger in the 1950s. This method has increased greatly in popularity since its discovery, and is now used quite commonly in most centers. It has greatly facilitated the study of those patients requiring study of multiple vessels. With this method, multiple vessel studies can be accomplished without a great deal of difficulty or trauma to the patient. There are, of course, certain dangers.

The limitations are obvious in older patients who have significant peripheral vascular disease and interruption of the vascular supply to the legs. The placement of the femoral catheter may compromise blood flow to such a

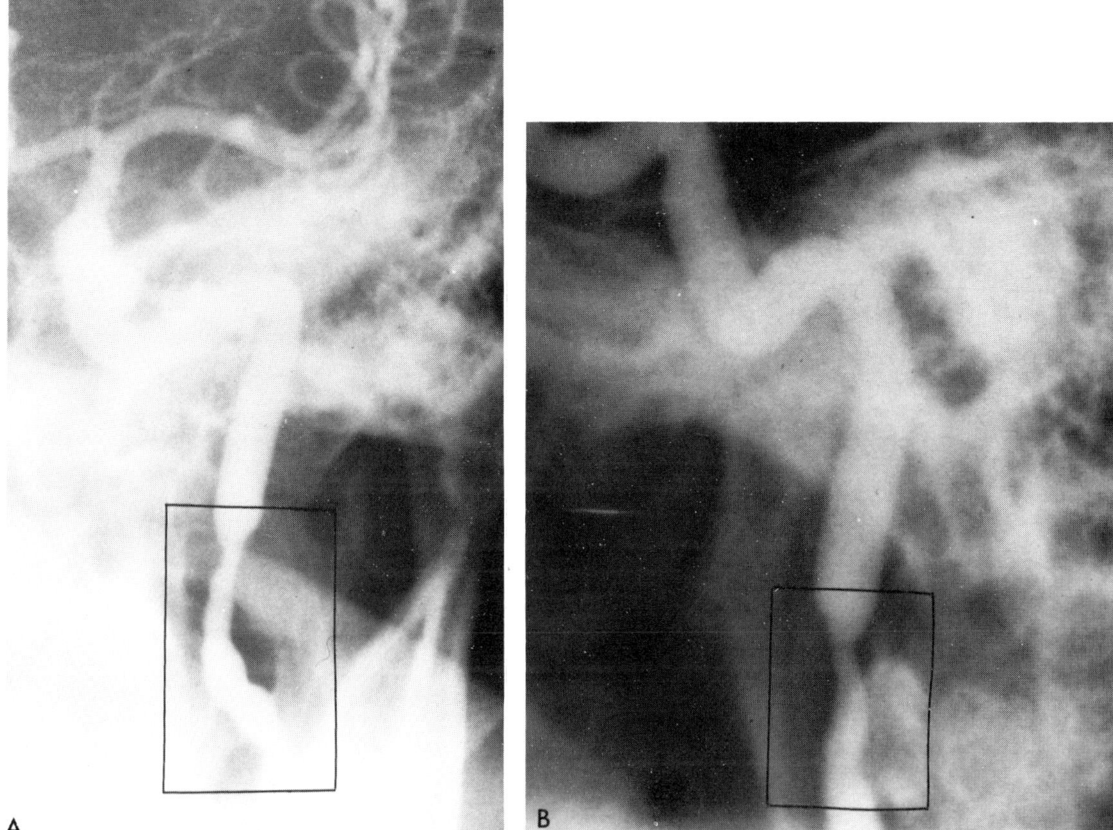

Figure 4–21. SPASM ASSOCIATED WITH A CEREBRAL CATHETER: A catheter is in place in the common carotid artery. With the injection of contrast material, the AP *(A)* and lateral *(B)* views demonstrate marked spasm of the proximal portion of the internal carotid artery. Subsequent injections showed the vessel to be normal. This spasm may be remote from the injection site and may even be seen in the cranial vault in the cerebral circulation.

degree that the leg may become cold and pulseless. If there is any possibility that this may occur, another approach should be used. In addition, in the older age groups, the femoral vessels may have become so tortuous that retrograde catheterization is impossible. In addition to the arteriosclerotic changes that occur in the lower limbs and the tortuosity of the vessels, one must also contend with similar changes in the great vessels as they arise from the arch of the aorta. It has been shown by pathologic studies that the great vessels tend to be spared from arteriosclerotic change from their point of origin at the arch to the levels of the carotid artery bifurcations. While there is little arteriosclerotic change, there is often a good deal of tortuosity, making the catheterization of the vessels impossible in some cases. The age of 50 years has been used as an arbitrary cut-off for catheterization and study from below. This, of course, is not an invariable rule, and some reports have been made of successful studies of patients in their ninth decade. The changes secondary to aging appear to become much more pronounced in hypertensive patients; therefore, in the presence of long standing hypertension one may want to consider a different approach. Since the vertebral arteries often have a stenotic origin in the older patients, when the posterior fossa is the site of suspected pathology one may have difficulty attempting catheterization. Because of the need to study many different vessels, it may be most expeditious to study all those that can be visualized by the femoral approach and then examine the remainder of the vessels using the percutaneous technique.

Catheters Available

Various types of catheters have been used (Fig. 4–22), and each has advantages in certain situations. In the very young age groups, and in the absence of anomalous vessels, a straight or gently curved catheter may be all that is necessary to selectively catheterize all the cerebral vessels. The order of study would appear to be in part arbitrary. However, if there is a particular area of interest, it would seem prudent to review the circulation in this vessel distribution first. If the study should be ended prematurely, the area of interest will be visualized. In patients in their second and third decades, the gently curved catheter may be used with a good deal of success. At some institutions an arch angiogram is performed initially to visualize the origins of the great vessels as they arise from the aorta; following this, a judgment is made as to the catheter needed to complete the study. We have found this step necessary, and proceed directly to catheterization without an arch injection. In most instances, the left carotid artery is the most difficult vessel to visualize, and, anticipating this, one would proceed directly to the catheterization of this artery. An argument can be made in favor of this approach since the catheter loses its rigidity while it remains in the body heat. In anticipation of these various vascular patterns, some operators do not use standard manufactured catheters but choose to create

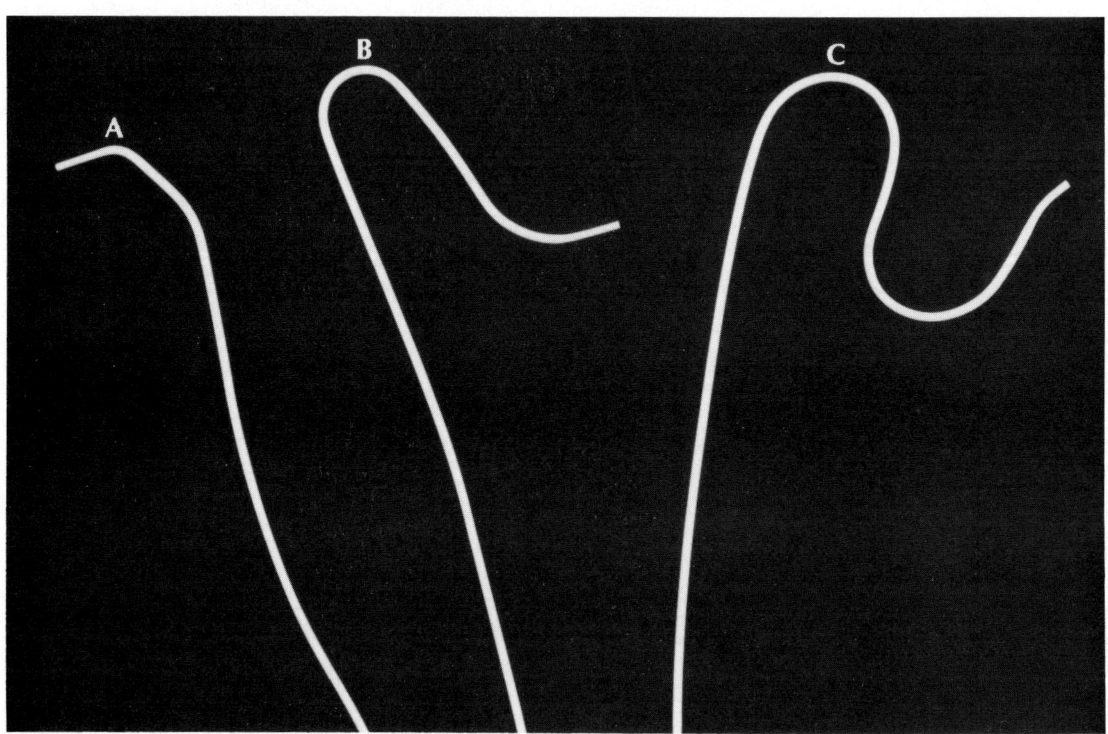

Figure 4–22. CEREBRAL CATHETERS: *(A)* Femoral-cerebral #1; frequently used in younger patients and pediatric cases. *(B)* Sidewinder #3; this catheter is frequently used in older individuals with tortuous brachiocephalic vessels. The author has had excellent success with this catheter, particularly in demonstrating the left carotid artery circulation. *(C)* Headhunter. This catheter has also been used for cerebral angiography, but has a tendency to knot and therefore should be used with great caution.

their own from basic materials. In this way the curve of the catheter can be formed to meet the needs of each case. This works well for some; however, I have found that the standard, preformed manufactured catheters have served our purposes well.

With the development of newer catheters it has become possible to perform catheterization studies in some older individuals; however, it is at times difficult to select those in whom it is possible. Patients with iliofemoral vascular occlusive disease cannot, of course, undergo femoral catheterization, and any needed studies will require percutaneous techniques.

A variety of standard-shaped catheters are now available from multiple manufacturers. The individual operator will discover, through trial and error, which catheters best suit his or her needs. A straight or pigtail multiple-end and side-hold catheter is necessary for arch angiography.

In older patients, I have found the "Sidewinder-Femoral Cerebral #III" catheter manufactured by the Cordis company to be especially satisfactory. In more difficult cases, the right carotid and either the left or right vertebral artery are catheterized with the "Femoral-Cerebral I" with the gentle curve. The catheter is then changed to the "Sidewinder" for catheterization of the left carotid artery.

This "S"-shaped catheter is unique, but, with experience, the individual angiographer can become accustomed to its use. The manufacturer recommends forming a loop with the catheter so that the large curve of the catheter rests in the ascending aorta, the distal part of the catheter curls back upon itself and the small curve is directed cephalad. The tip of the catheter is then manipulated until it rests in the origin of the vessel to be catheterized. A small amount of injected contrast ensures that the proper vessel has been catheterized. At times it is necessary to perform the study by injection from this point. If this is the case, 12 cc of Conray 60 per cent should be injected rather than the usual 10 cc. To position the catheter tip higher in the vessel, it is necessary to pull *back* on the catheter at the puncture site. This will cause the catheter to unroll and advance up into the vessel. The author has found this catheter unsatisfactory for catheterization of the vertebral arteries.

For any catheter and catheterization technique, liberal use of the guidewire is recommended to facilitate both catheter placement and advancement. At our institution the guidewires and catheters are used once and then discarded.

Injections in the common carotid artery should be 1.5 cm below the carotid bifurcation. Intermittent flushing should be done with saline containing 1 cc of 1000μ/cc of heparin/500 cc of saline.

With experience and practice each operator develops an individual technique for both puncture and catheter placement.

COMPLICATIONS OF CEREBRAL ANGIOGRAPHY

Other complications that may occur with any type of arteriographic study are:

1. hematoma
2. subintimal injection
3. hypotension or hypertension
4. allergic reaction
5. femoral embolus
6. cerebral embolus
7. angina
8. emesis
9. nausea
10. change in mentation
11. monoparesis
12. hemiparesis
13. aphasia
14. visual disturbance
15. seizure
16. vertigo
17. numb fingers
18. headache
19. global amnesia
20. death

During the course of the study, it is wise to converse with the patient so that any change in the mental status will be readily appreciated. If such a change does occur, the study should be stopped and performed at another time.

General Guidelines for Post-Angiogram Orders

POST-ANGIOGRAM ORDERS

For brachial angiogram:
1. Bed rest for 4 hours
2. Keep arm straight for 1 hour
3. Vital signs every 15 minutes for 2 hours, every 30 minutes for 2 hours, every 60 minutes for 2 hours and until stable
4. Resume previous diet and orders
5. IV orders as needed
6. Cold packs to puncture site for pain

For carotid angiogram:
1. Bed rest for 8 hours
2. Vital signs every 15 minutes for 2 hours, every 30 minutes for 2 hours, every 60 minutes for 2 hours and until stable
3. Resume previous diet and orders
4. Cold packs to puncture site for pain
5. IV orders as needed

For femoral angiogram:
1. Flat in bed for 8 hours and complete bed rest for 24 hours
2. Vital signs every 15 minutes for 2 hours, every 30 minutes for 2 hours, every 60 minutes for 2 hours and until stable
3. Check peripheral pulses and puncture site when taking vital signs
4. IV orders as needed
5. Cold packs to puncture site as needed for pain
6. Resume previous diet and orders

Knotted Catheter

It should be mentioned that certain catheters with multiple loops at the end sometimes tie in a knot (Fig. 4–23). In addition to the hazard of knot formation, the catheter may loop back upon itself and form a functional knot. Various methods have been described to remove these knots or untie them without operative intervention. If this unfortunate event should occur, *DO NOT* remove the catheter from the aortic arch, which provides sufficient room for catheter manipulation.

Most frequently, knotting occurs when the catheter is being torqued rapidly in 360° circles in an attempt to enter a vessel; with multiple-end curved catheters, however, this rapid torquing should *not* be used for just this reason. The steps described below should be followed when attempting to unknot the catheter:

1. Pass a guidewire through the catheter, using the firm end in the hope of loosening the knot.

2. Inject the maximum amount of contrast material in an attempt to open or loosen the knot and to provide space for a guidewire to open the catheter.

3. The opposite femoral artery can be punctured and a straight catheter passed through the loop in the knot. The knotted catheter is then pulled against this to open the knot.

4. If the catheter is kinked upon itself but is not knotted, firm pressure over the groin while the catheter is pulled down and removed will forcibly open the catheter as it exits from the vessel. With such traumatic removal of the catheter, the limb should be observed very carefully for compromise of the circulation.

5. If all attempts fail, the catheter will have to be removed surgically.

The long multicurved catheters should be manipulated gently and never "twirled" in an attempt to achieve placement. Indeed, because of the possibility of complications, a vascular surgeon should be available for consultation and emergency procedures if needed.

SUBTRACTION

The technique of subtraction was originally described by Ziedses des Plantes in 1935. The purpose of "subtraction" is to remove or "subtract" the image of the bony structures from the radiograph by using various photographic techniques. This allows visualization of the normal vasculature, but, more important, exposes areas of abnormal vascularity which are seen only faintly or not at all without the use of subtraction. The technique is especially helpful when studying the vessels at the base of the brain and in the study of the posterior fossa anatomy, where there are dense overlying bony structures.

We use a subtraction unit that has a timer that allows for fixed exposure times. Times can be varied from one tenth of a second through 15 seconds. This type of unit makes possible dependable reproduction and repetition of the desired exposure times. In addi-

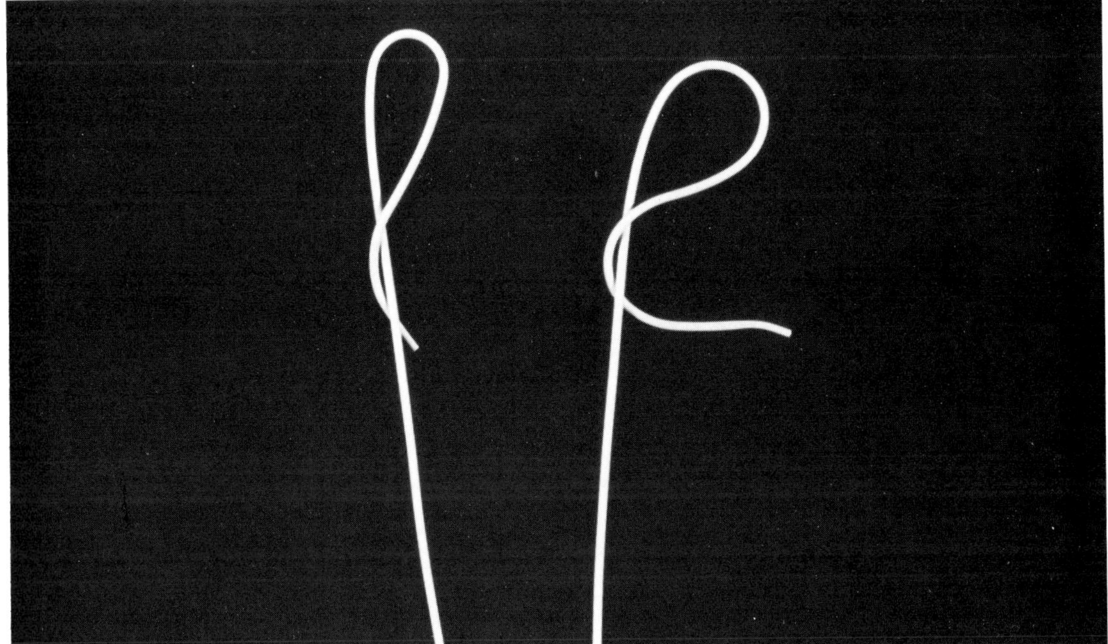

Figure 4–23. KNOTTED CATHETERS: The long curved catheters may loop back upon themselves, therefore resulting in a functional knot. At times the tip of the catheter may even pass through the loop, resulting in a true knot. Great caution should be taken to avoid this complication. These catheters should not be twirled, but should always be moved slowly and deliberately.

tion, the unit can function as a view-box for continuous viewing. There are also a variety of light bulbs of varying intensity that have independent switches for alteration of the light exposure level. The unit has the appearance of a view-box with a glass top; the lights of varying intensity are positioned below the viewing area and the exposure timer. The technique requires the use of a darkroom.

Although many different methods for performing the subtraction have been worked out using a variety of films, at our institution we use Kodak subtraction masking film and Dupont Cronex subtraction print film.

The technique requires the use of a "blank" film of a standard serial run of films plus a film taken after contrast material has been introduced into the vessels. It is important that the patient remain motionless during the serial run of films.

The first step is making of the subtraction mask film. The blank film of the run is placed in the view-box of the unit. A single sheet of Kodak subtraction masking film is placed emulsion side down over the area to be subtracted. The unit's lid is closed, and an exposure is made using a 7-watt bulb for 3 seconds. When this mask film is processed it will be a very dark reversal image of the original blank film.

The mask film is then placed on the view-box and taped in position. A film from the serial run demonstrating contrast material within the vessels is then exactly superimposed on the subtraction mask. Exact superimposition will be impossible if the patient moved during the film run. This second film is taped in place so that it too is immobile. The films are superimposed while the unit is on continuous view, and the operator will be able to see the "subtraction" of the bones and the exposure of the previously unvisualized portions of the vascular system.

A single sheet of Dupont subtraction print film is then placed over the area of interest (emulsion down), and the lid of the unit is closed so that good film contact is obtained. The final exposure is then made, using a 40-watt bulb and an exposure time of 0.5 second. When this film is processed, the final image will demonstrate the vessels without the overlying bony structures.

One may choose to subtract only one film of a series, or the entire film run can be subtracted. The technique of making the mask or final print can be varied from case to case, depending on the exposure of the films. In general, however, the method described will prove satisfactory for most cases.

Tips for Use

1. Either the arterial or venous phase may be subtracted.
2. The exposure times may be varied to obtain a more precise technique in an individual case.
3. If the patient moved during the filming, the final print film may still prove satisfactory if an attempt is made to subtract the image in a small area of interest. The remainder of the image may be blurred, but that is of no consequence.
4. If several areas must be viewed, subtractions can be made individually in the areas of interest.
5. If no blank films are obtained at the start of a serial run, the late venous phase or last film of the run sometimes can be used as the "blank."

AMIPAQUE (METRIZAMIDE) CISTERNOGRAPHY

A lumbar puncture is performed and 4 to 6 cc of 180 mg^{I}2/cc Amipaque is instilled in the lumbar subarachnoid space. The patient is then placed in the head-down position for 5 minutes and kept in the 15 head-down position until the completion of the scan. The contrast may be allowed to flow cephalad with the patient either prone or supine, and the patient may be rotated 360° several times to facilitate entry of the material into the lateral ventricles. Initially, the contrast should be kept below the puncture site; it is then allowed to flow rapidly cephalad in order to prevent leakage from the puncture site.

The CT scan is then performed either immediately or after several hours, with the contrast outlining the basilar cisterns, the fourth ventricle, the lateral ventricles and the cortical sulci. The patient should be kept in the 15° head-down position during the scan.

Mass lesions appear as areas of negative contrast bathed by the high density of the Amipaque. It would appear that the availability of this new contrast material for cisternography will further decrease or eliminate the need for pneumoencephalography.

Applied Cerebrovascular Embryology and Normal Anatomy

EMBRYOLOGY

During the course of embryologic development there are six brachial arches and clefts. A number of these disappear entirely; however, some remain to form the brachiocephalic system as we know it. Figure 4–24 demonstrates the origin of the various segments of the cleft and arches and the vessels that are present in the normal adult. These development changes need not be committed to memory, but do aid in achieving an understanding of the anatomy of the great vessels.

Aberrant Right Subclavian Artery. This anomaly is of some significance to the angiographer. The aberrant right subclavian artery arises distal to the origin of the left subclavian artery. This occurs because the stem of the right subclavian artery originates from the right dorsal arch and the seventh intersegmental artery. With shortening of the aorta between the left common carotid arte-

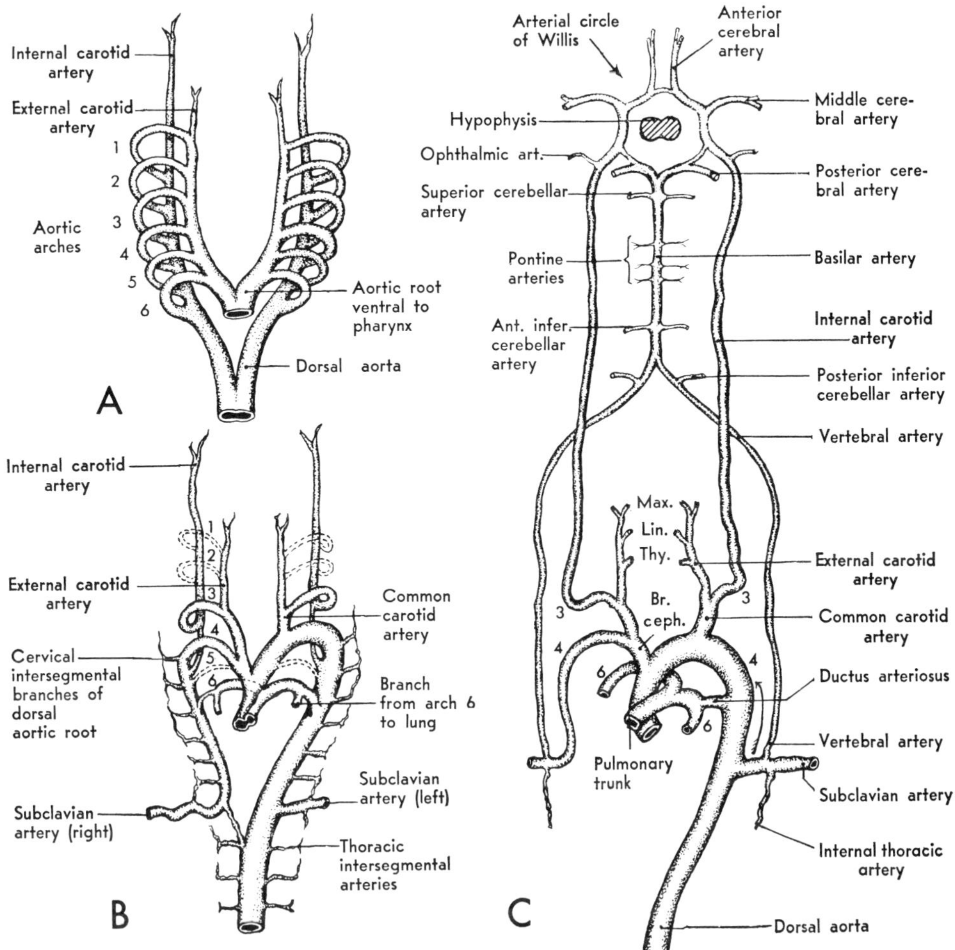

Figure 4–24. The primitive brachial arches and clefts are variously resorbed and persist to form the brachiocephalic vessels as we know them in the normal individual. These diagrams illustrate the major changes that occur in the aortic arches of mammalian embryos. *A*, Ground plan of complete set of aortic arches. *B*, Early stage in modification of arches. *C*, Adult derivatives of the aortic arches. *Abbreviations:* Br. ceph. = brachiocephalic (innominate) artery; Lin. = lingual artery; Max. = maxillary artery; Thy. = thyroid artery. The arrow in *C* indicates the change in position of origin of left subclavian artery that occurs in the later stages of development. (Reproduced, by permission, from Carlson, B. M.: Foundations of Embryology, 3d ed. New York, McGraw-Hill, 1974.)

ry and the left subclavian artery, the abnormal right subclavian artery is found below the left subclavian. Because its origin is from the right side, it must cross the midline to reach the right arm.

When this happens, the right common carotid artery arises directly from the arch as an independent branch, and only the right vertebral artery arises from the right subclavian. Therefore, a right brachial arteriogram demonstrates only the vertebral circulation; the right carotid circulation must be studied separately. Catheterization of these vessels will also need to be adapted to the anatomic variations.

ANASTOMOSES

PRIMITIVE INTERNAL CAROTID — VERTEBROBASILAR

Three main vessels connect the internal carotid with the vertebrobasilar system. They

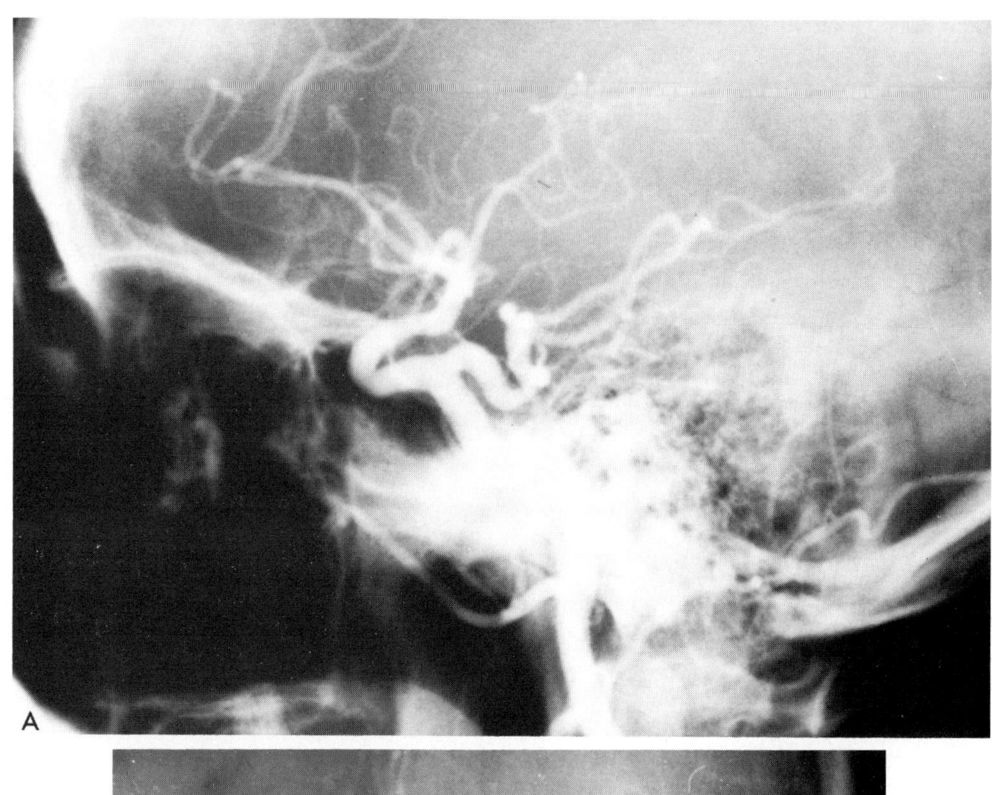

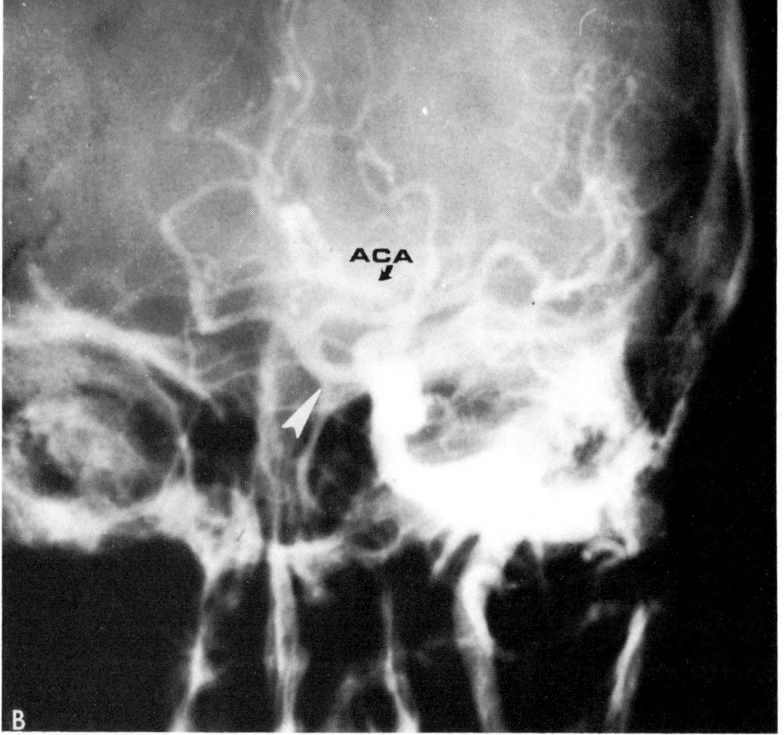

Figure 4–25. PERSISTENT TRIGEMINAL ARTERY: *A*, The lateral view demonstrates a large trigeminal artery coursing posteriorly to fill both posterior cerebral arteries.

B, The AP view demonstrates the trigeminal artery which courses posteromedially *(arrow)* to fill the posterior cerebral arteries. The anterior cerebral artery *(ACA)* projects just above the trigeminal artery.

are, in order of occurrence, the persistent trigeminal artery, the primitive acoustic artery and the primitive hypoglossal artery. The possibility of one of these persistent primitive communications should come to mind when a common carotid injection also fills in a large part of the anatomic distribution of the vertebrobasilar system. However, with advanced arteriosclerotic occlusive vascular disease there may be filling of the vertebrobasilar system via collateral circulation from the external carotid artery. In such patients, close examination is required to be certain that indeed a primitive communication is present between the internal carotid artery and the basilar artery.

Persistent Trigeminal Artery. Of the three persistent primitive communications between the internal carotid and vertebrobasilar system the persistent trigeminal artery is the most common (Fig. 4–25).

The trigeminal artery originates from the internal carotid artery just proximal to the intracavernous portion of the carotid artery and follows a tortuous curvilinear course posteriorly to join the basilar artery. Without proper attention, this vessel may be mistaken for a large posterior communicating artery; however, the point of origin is different. The posterior communicating artery arises from the supraclinoid portion of the internal carotid artery.

The persistent trigeminal artery is associated with an increased incidence of aneurysms.

Primitive Acoustic Artery. The second most common primitive communicating vessel is the acoustic artery. This vessel connects the petrous portion of the internal carotid artery with the basilar artery.

Primitive Hypoglossal Artery. This rare persistent communication (Fig. 4–26) con-

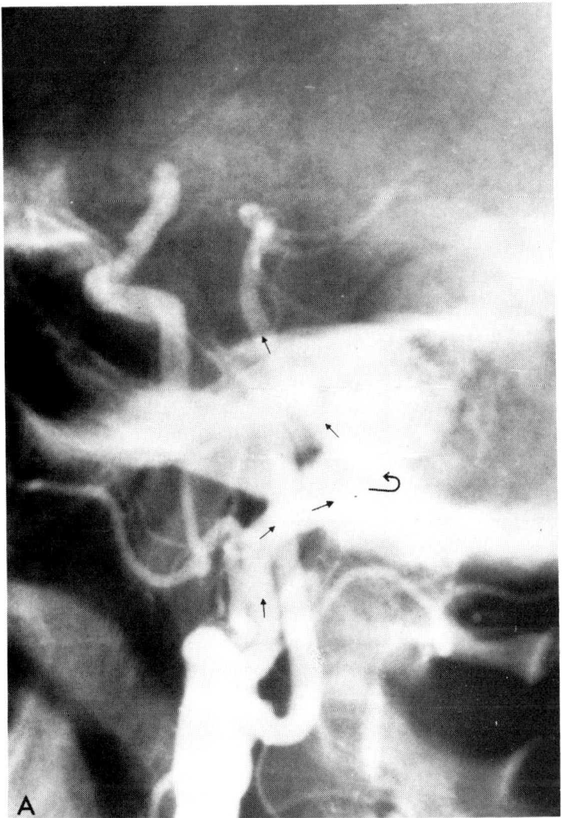

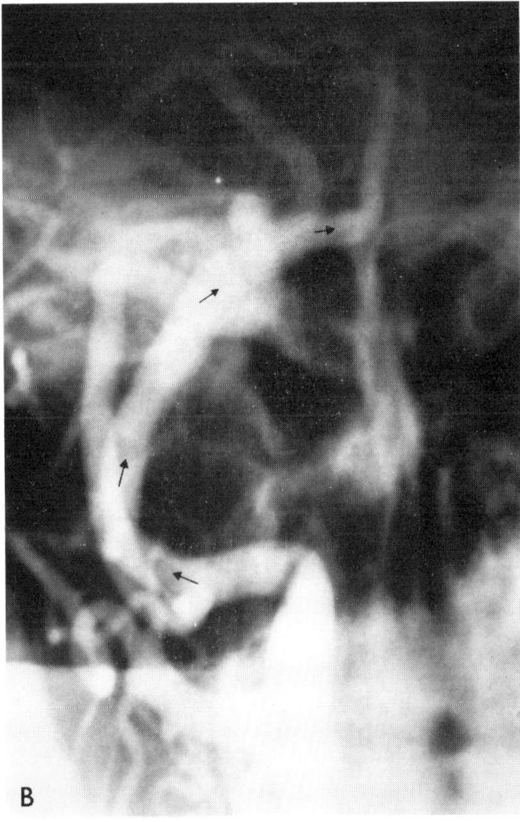

Figure 4–26. *A* and *B*, PRIMITIVE HYPOGLOSSAL ARTERY: The hypoglossal artery arises from the internal carotid artery in its cervical portion. As seen in these AP and lateral views, the vessel then courses through the hypoglossal canal to join with the basilar artery *(arrows)*. The carotid artery overlies the hypoglossal artery on the AP view.

nects the cervical portion of the internal carotid artery with the basilar artery via the hypoglossal canal.

NORMAL ANATOMY

The right carotid artery arises from the innominate artery shortly after its take-off from the arch of the aorta. The left common carotid artery arises as a separate trunk from the arch of the aorta (Figs. 4–27 — 4–32). The left subclavian artery arises just distal to the left carotid aorta.

The bifurcations of the carotid arteries into the internal and external carotid arteries occur at the level of the fourth cervical vertebra. The bifurcation level varies from individual to individual, but the bifurcations usually are at the same level on each side. At the level of the bifurcation in the neck, the internal carotid artery usually courses lateral and posterior to the external carotid artery. The artery runs in the carotid sheath, and is medial to the internal jugular vein. The vagus nerve runs posteriorly between the two vessels. The internal carotid artery then courses cephalad until it enters the carotid canal at the base of the skull. The internal carotid artery may have kinks or tortuous loops in the neck. These are normal anatomic variations (see illustration). There are four divisions of the internal carotid artery. They are: (1) cervical portion; (2) petrous portion; (3) cavernous portion and (4) supraclinoid portion or the intradural portion. There are no branches of the cervical portion of the internal carotid artery. The other three segments have various branches — only some of which are of consequence to the neuroradiologist. The petrous portion: caroticotym-

Text continued on page 180

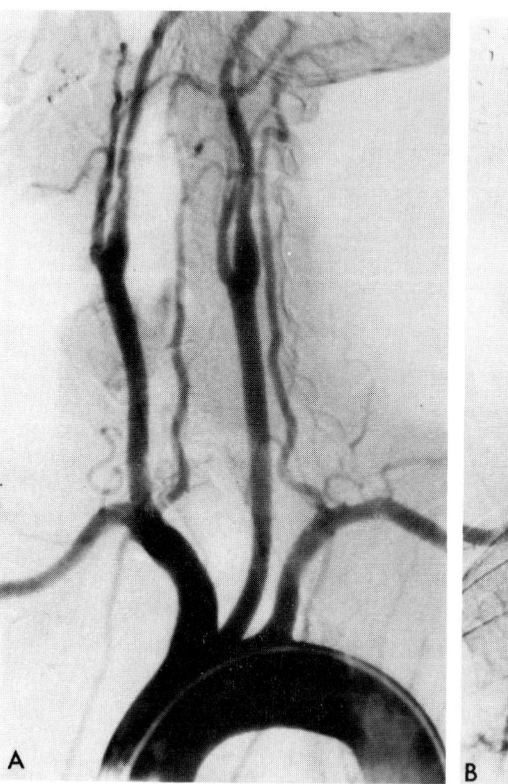

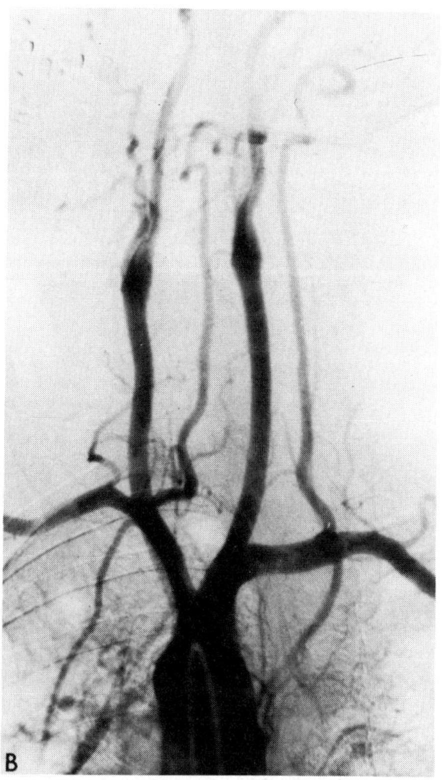

Figure 4–27. NORMAL ARCH ANGIOGRAM: The catheter is in place, with the tip of the multiple-end and side-hole catheter in the ascending aorta approximately 2 cm above the aortic valve. Films obtained in the right posterior oblique (RPO) and left posterior oblique (LPO) projections demonstrate good antegrade flow through the normal great vessels. Both carotid and both vertebral arteries are demonstrated and appear normal.

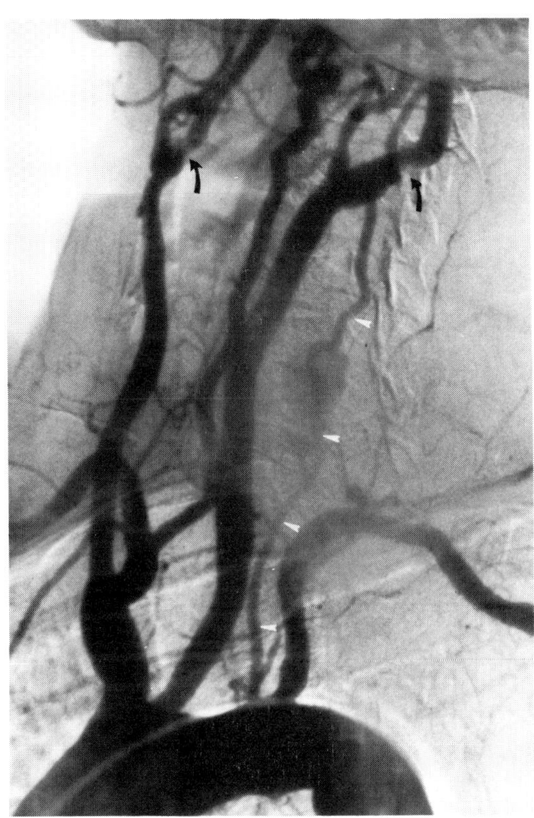

Figure 4–28

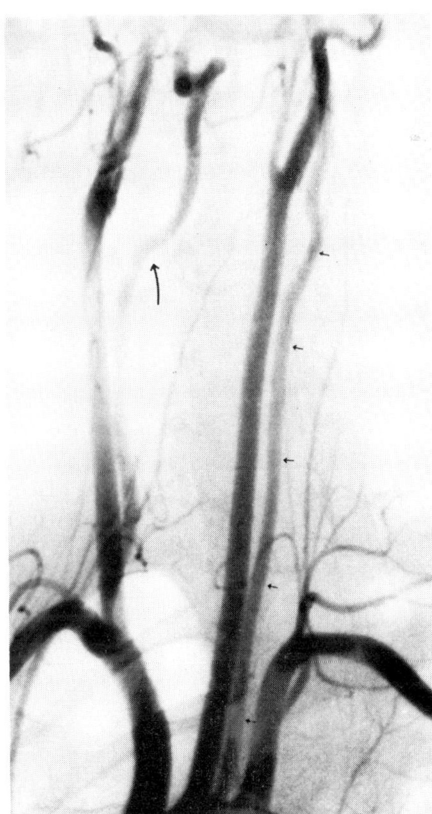

Figure 4–29

Figure 4–28. ABNORMAL ARCH ANGIOGRAM: The arch angiogram in the RPO projection demonstrates bilateral carotid stenosis *(black arrows)* and a left vertebral artery that arises directly from the arch of the aorta *(white arrows)*.

Figure 4–29. ARCH ANGIOGRAM — ANATOMIC VARIATIONS: The arch angiogram in the RPO projection demonstrates that the left vertebral artery arises directly from the arch of the aorta *(small arrows)* and that both vertebral arteries enter into the foramina transversaria of the cervical vertebrae at the C_4 level rather than the normal C_6 level. This is a normal anatomic variation, and should not be mistaken for a mass displacing the vessels. A separate origin of the left vertebral artery occurs in 5 to 6 per cent of individuals.

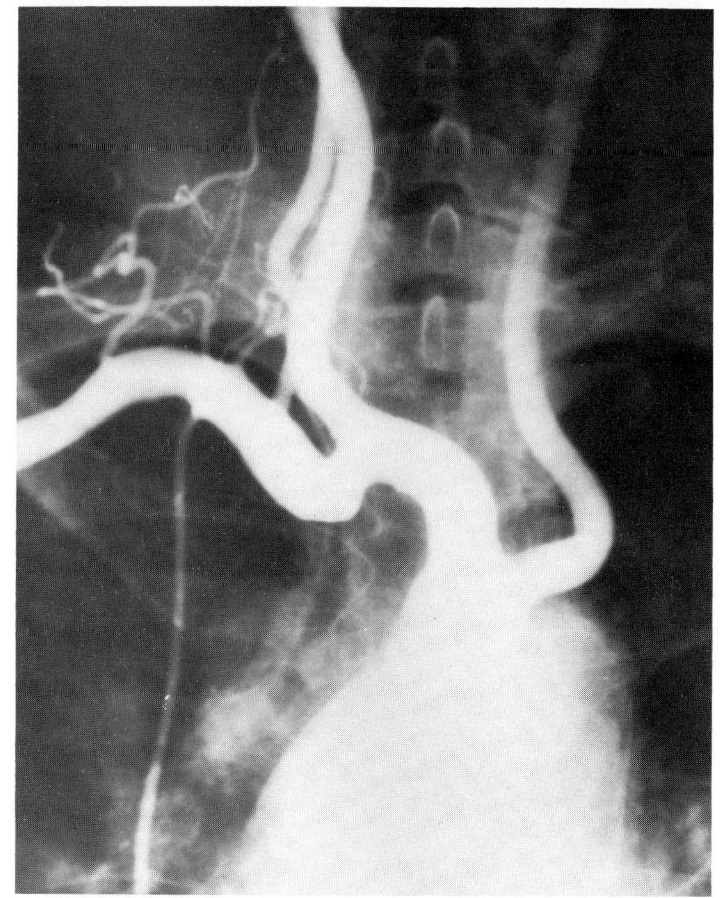

Figure 4–30 *See legend on the opposite page.*

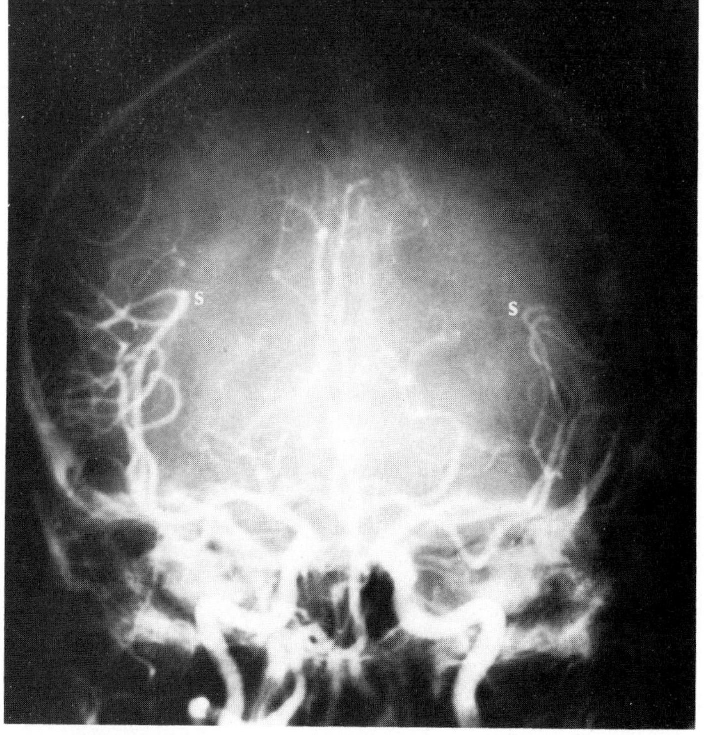

Figure 4–31 *See legend on the opposite page.*

Figure 4–30. BOVINE ARCH: The left common carotid artery arises from the innominate artery. This common origin occurs to a varying degree in 25 per cent of individuals.

Figure 4–31. BOVINE ARCH: Because the left common carotid artery arises from the innominate artery, a right brachial injection results in filling of the left internal carotid artery circulation as well as the right carotid and right vertebral artery circulations. Note that the sylvian points are symmetric *(s)*.

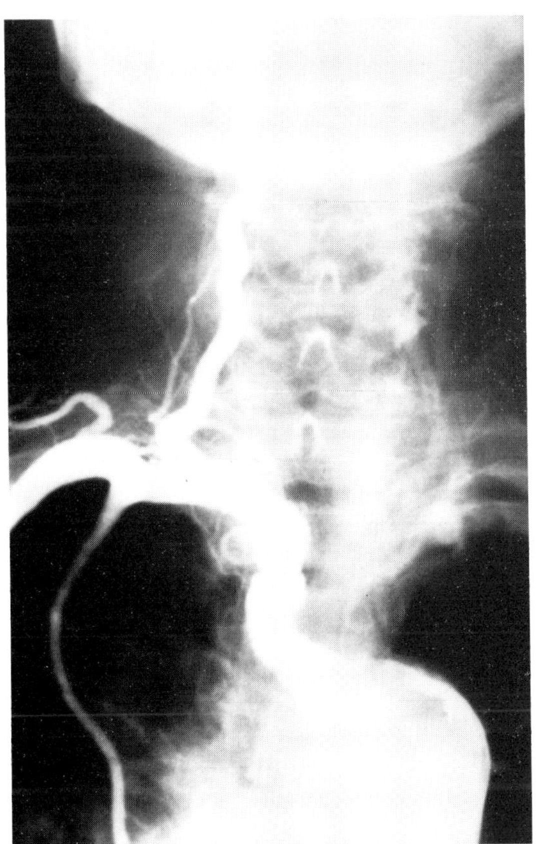

Figure 4–32. ABERRANT SUBCLAVIAN: The right subclavian artery arises distal to the left subclavian artery. In this case the right common carotid artery arises directly from the arch of the aorta; therefore, only the right vertebral artery fills from the right brachial injection.

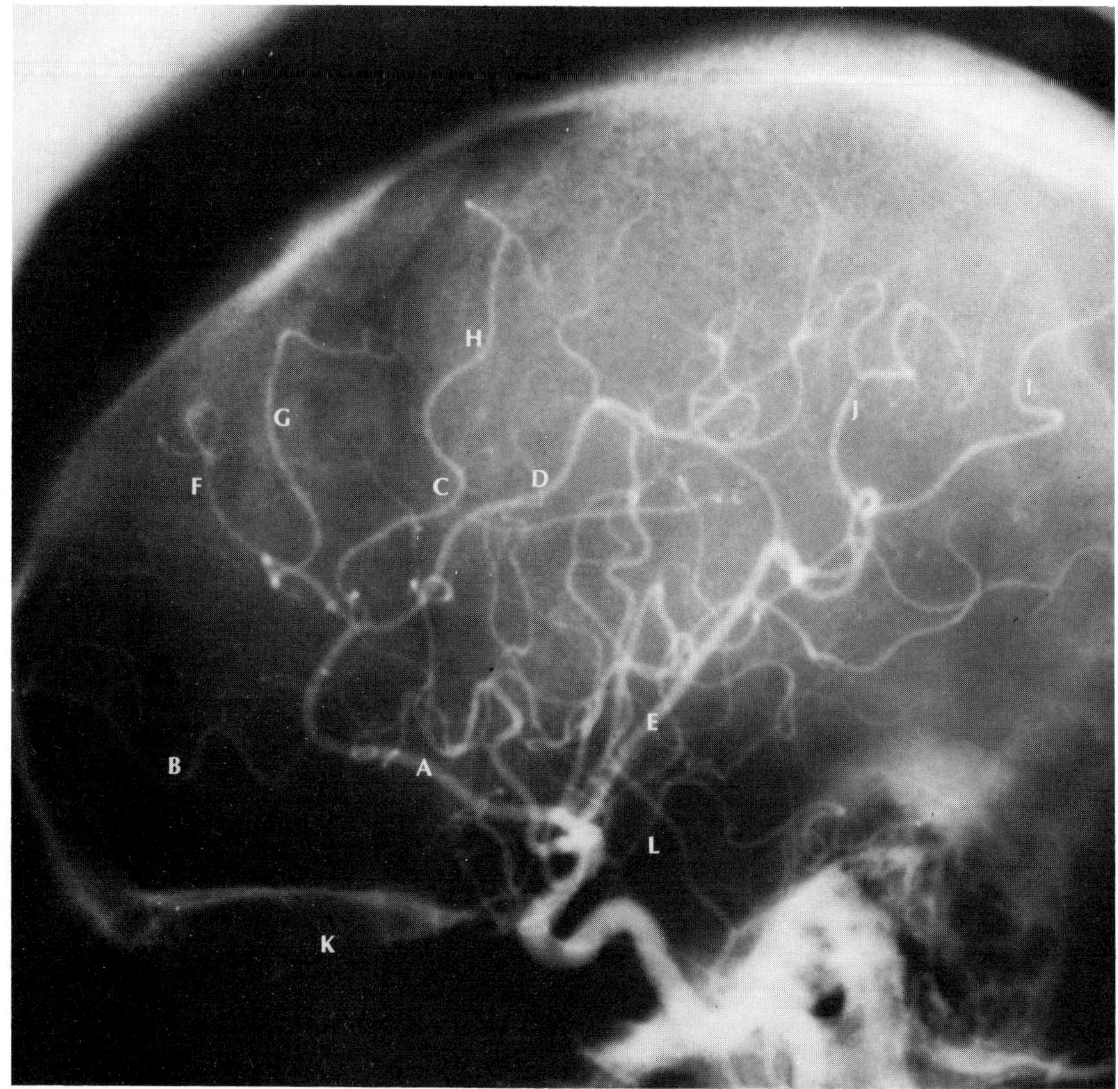

Figure 4–33. NORMAL CAROTID ANGIOGRAM: *A,* Anterior cerebral artery; *B,* Frontal polar a.; *C,* Callosal marginal a.; *D,* Pericallosal a.; *E,* Middle cerebral artery branch; *F,* Anterior internal frontal a.; *G,* Middle internal frontal a.; *H,* Posterior internal frontal a.; *I,* Angular a.; *J,* Anterior parietal a.; *K,* Ophthalmic a.; *L,* Anterior choroidal a.

panic; artery of the pterygoid canal (vidian artery). The cavernous portion: cavernous branches; hypophyseal branches; semilunar branches; meningeal branches; ophthalmic artery. The supraclinoid portion: posterior communicating artery; anterior choroidal artery; anterior cerebral artery; middle cerebral artery.

After its entrance into the carotid canal, the internal carotid artery courses anteromedially until it lies adjacent and just lateral to the sella turcica. As the internal carotid artery courses in the carotid canal it passes endocranially past the foramen lacerum. Indeed, as viewed from below, the internal carotid artery can be seen in the foramen lacerum, but the artery does not pass ''through-and-through'' the foramen lacerum. As the carotid enters into the cavernous portion of its course, it turns to course superiorly toward the posterior clinoid process; it then turns to course first anteriorly and then superiorly on the medial side of the anterior clinoid process and perforates the dura matter. In the cavernous portion, the internal carotid artery lies in close relationship to the third, fourth, sixth and ophthalmic and the maxillary branches of the fifth cranial nerves. Because of the close relationship of these nerves at the level of the cavernous sinus, a cavernous sinus thrombosis may be diagnosed clinically by pareses of these nerve branches. Beneath the anterior clinoid process the internal carotid artery turns to course first superiorly and then posteriorly. Because of this "S"-shaped course, this is called the carotid siphon. Just at the level of the exit of the internal carotid artery as it pierces the dura to become intracranial, the ophthalmic artery arises and courses anteriorly to supply the globe.

Text continued on page 186

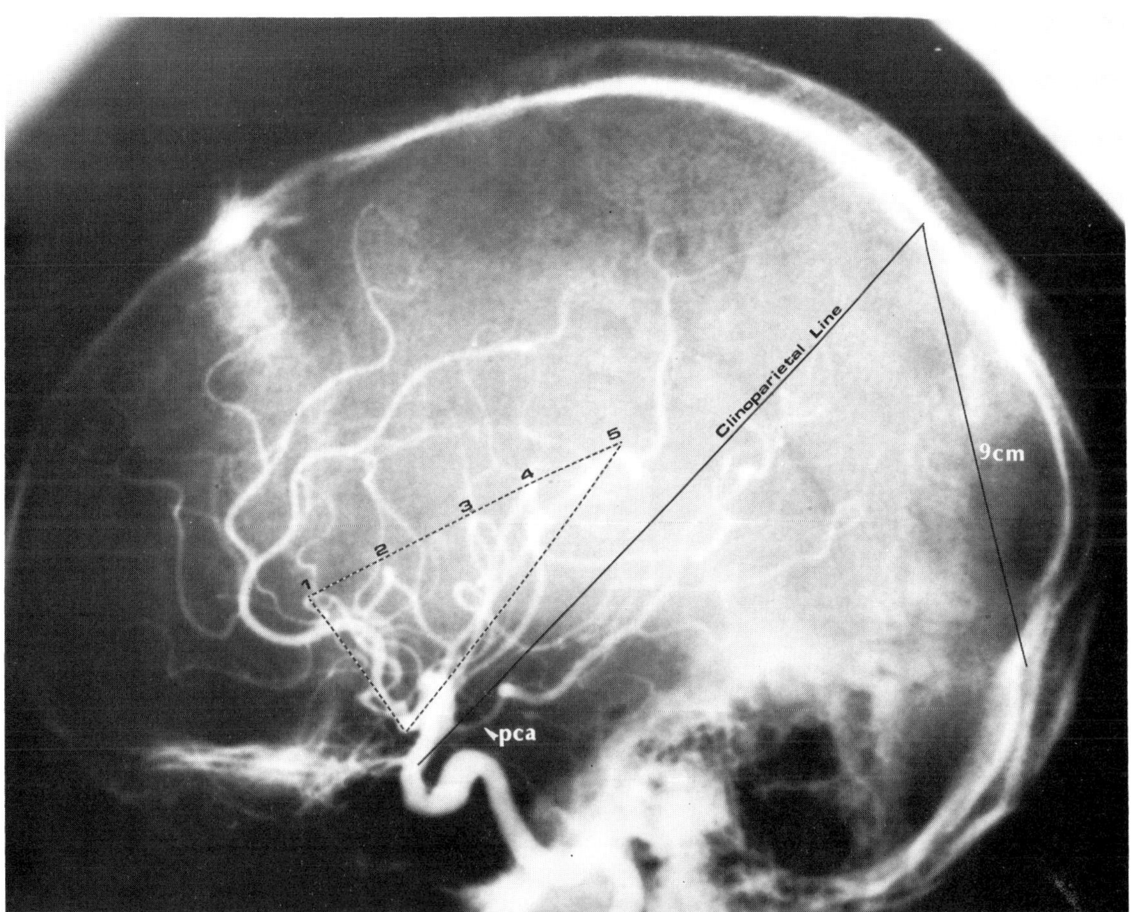

Figure 4–34. CLINOPARIETAL LINE: To determine the anticipated normal position of the sylvian triangle, a line is drawn from the internal occipital protuberance 9 cm up to the inner table of the skull in the parietal region. A line is then constructed from this point to the anterior clinoid process — the *clinoparietal line*. The main middle cerebral artery branch should fall within 1 cm above or below this line.

The dotted lines demonstrate the sylvian triangle. The tops of the loops of the middle cerebral artery branches are numbered 1 to 5 as they rise to the top of the sylvian fissure. Point 5 is the *sylvian point* — the last branch of the middle cerebral artery to exit from the sylvian fissure.

The posterior communicating artery *(pca)* and posterior cerebral artery point below the clinoparietal line. The origin of the anterior choroidal artery projects above the clinoparietal line just distal to the posterior communicating artery.

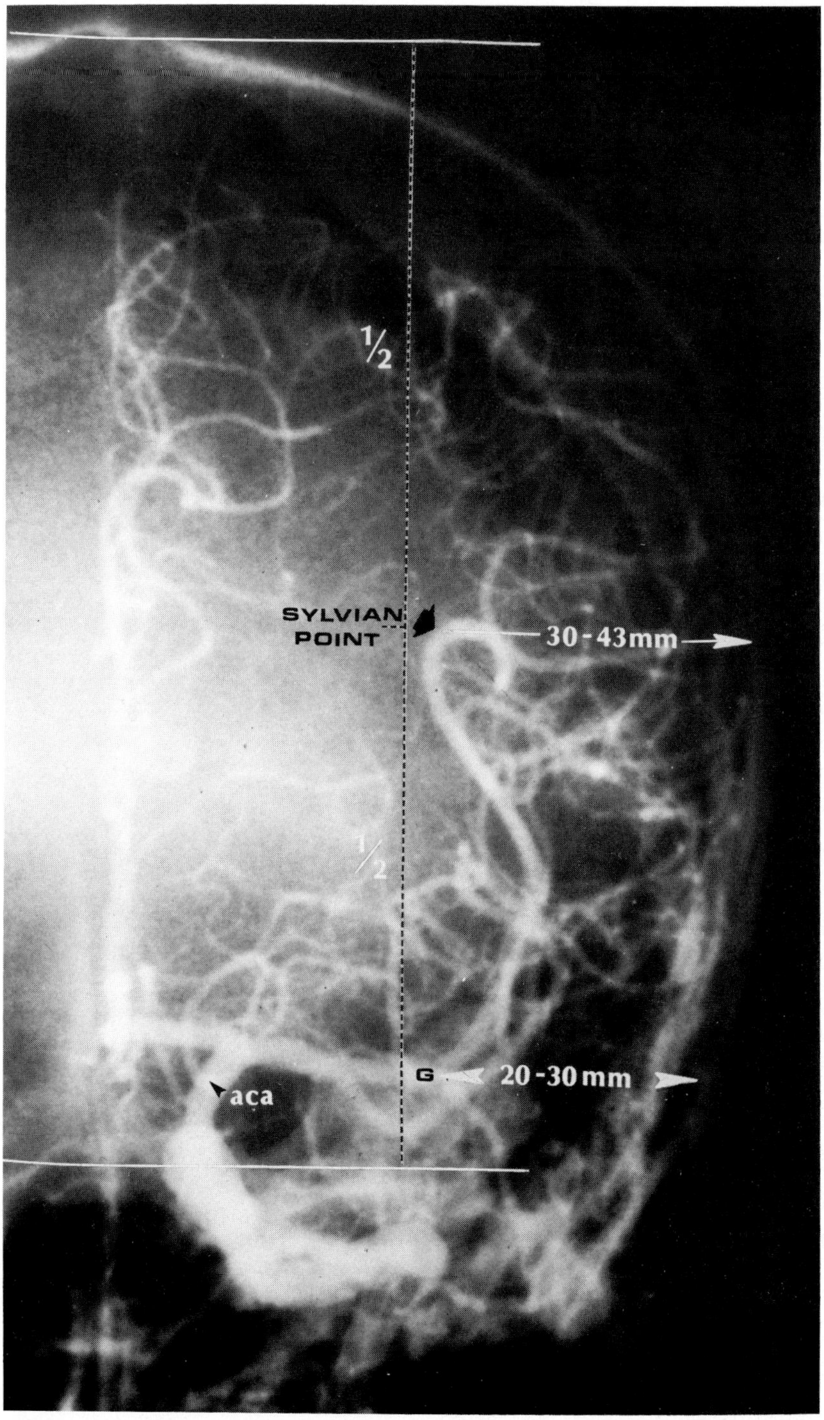

Figure 4–35. AP VIEW OF NORMAL SYLVIAN POINT: The sylvian point normally projects 30 to 43 mm from the inner table of the skull. The point normally lies half-way along a line *(dotted line)* perpendicular to a tangent to the inner table in the high convexity area and the orbital roof or the petrous pyramid, whichever is lower. There is a ±1 cm range of normal.

The genu *(G)* of the middle cerebral artery normally measures 20 to 30 mm. from the inner table of the skull.

The anterior choroidal artery *(aca)* can be seen as it arises from the internal carotid artery.

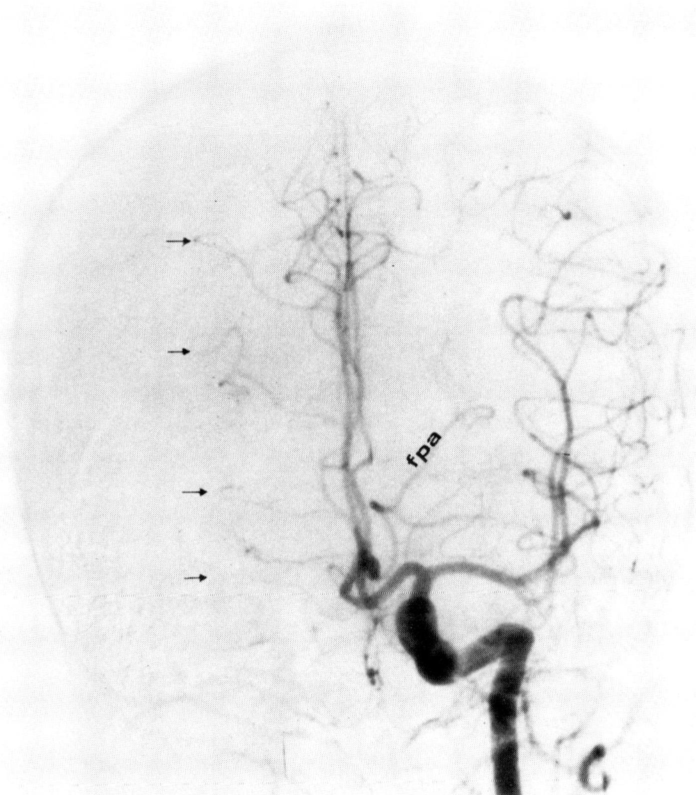

Figure 4–36. NORMAL AP VIEW OF LEFT CAROTID ARTERIOGRAM. Both pericallosal arteries fill from the left carotid artery. The normal distribution of the anterior cerebral artery and its branches as they distribute over the cerebral convexity are well demonstrated on the right side *(small arrows)*. The frontal polar artery is well seen *(fpa)*.

Figure 4–37. SUBMENTOVERTEX VIEW OF RIGHT BRACHIAL ANGIOGRAM WITH FILLING OF LEFT CAROTID ARTERY. The right brachial arteriogram *(A)* demonstrates filling also of the left common carotid circulation, providing an excellent demonstration of the anatomic structures in the circle of Willis, and throughout the normal circulation. (*A*, Common carotid artery; *B*, Vertebral artery; *C*, Carotid bifurcation; *D*, External carotid artery; *E*, Basilar artery; *F*, Anterior superior cerebellar artery; *G*, Posterior cerebral arteries; *H*, Internal carotid artery in the carotid canal; *I*, Bifurcation of internal carotid artery; *J*, Genu of middle cerebral artery; *K*, Horizontal portion of anterior cerebral artery; *L*, Anterior communicating artery; *M*, Posterior communicating artery; *N*, Anterior cerebral arteries; *O*, Middle cerebral artery branches in the isle of Reil.)

The CT scan *(B)* also demonstrates the posterior communicating arteries as they are bathed in the cerebrospinal fluid in the suprasellar cistern *(arrow)*. They are faintly seen on the preinfusion scan.

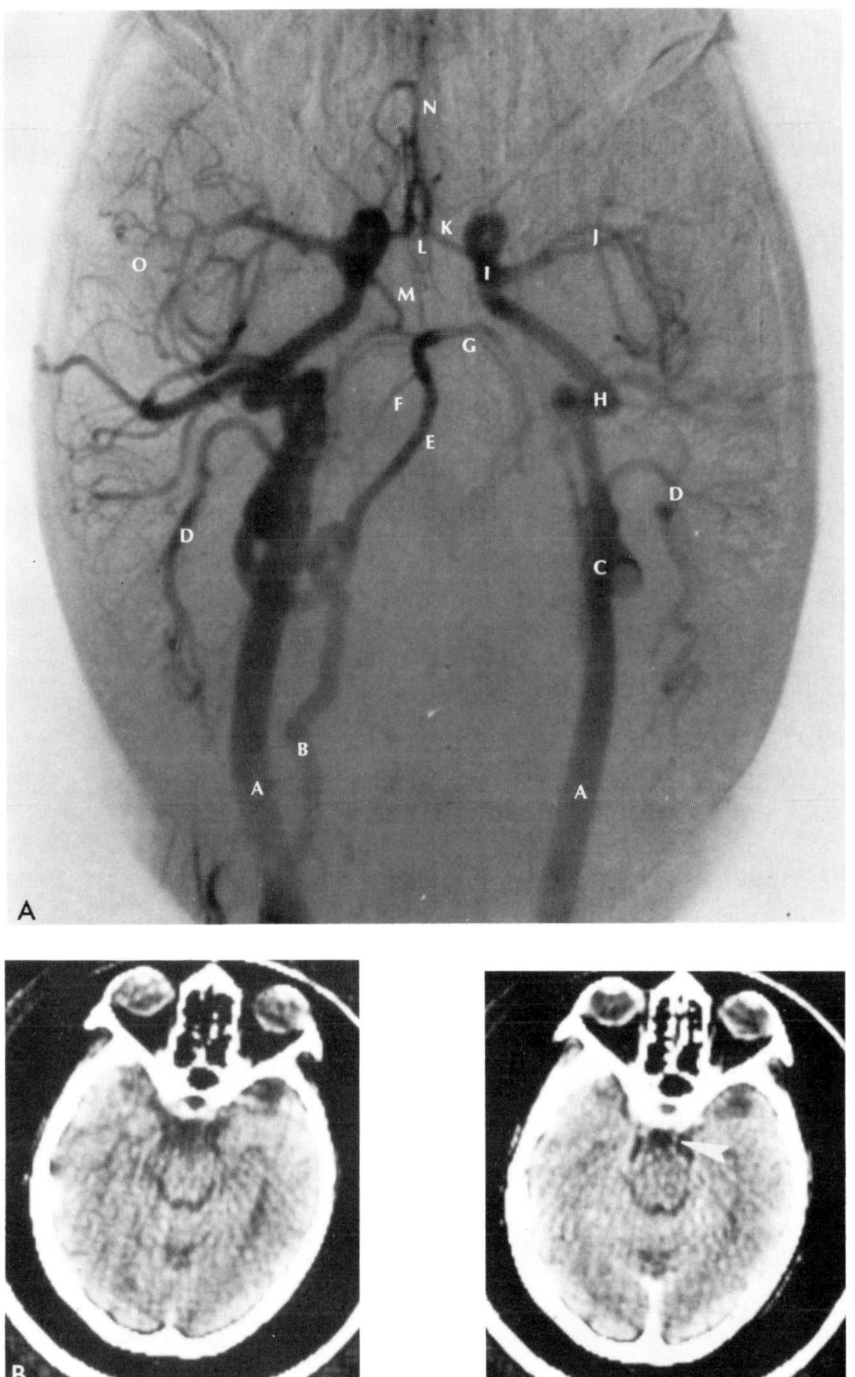

Figure 4–37 *See legend on the opposite page.*

At its origin, the ophthalmic artery lies lateral to the optic nerve. More distally, the artery will be seen to cross superiorly over the optic nerve and then to lie on the medial side of the optic nerve. The ophthalmic artery then gives off multiple retinal arteries, ethmoidal branches, and may give rise to an angiographically visible anterior meningeal artery. The terminal branches of the ophthalmic artery exit through the supraorbital foramen and distribute themselves over a small patch of skin covering the medial end of the eyebrow and forehead on each side. It is the branches of the external carotid feeding the teeth, tongue, cheek and the soft tissues of the neck and scalp that cause the stinging and burning sensations felt when contrast material is injected. By avoiding injection of contrast material into the external carotid system, one can prevent considerable discomfort to the patient. Also, in a combative patient, if an internal carotid angiogram is performed rather than a common carotid artery angiogram, there is less likely to be motion artifact on the study. This is, of course, in the absence of a tumor (e.g., a meningioma), where the external carotid feeders may supply vital information concerning vascular supply to the tumor.

As the carotid artery makes its final bend superiorly above the anterior clinoid process, the posterior communicating artery arises. The posterior communicating artery is one portion of the circle of Willis. It courses posteromedially to join with the posterior cerebral artery on the same side. This vessel does not fill on each arteriogram. Indeed, it may vary greatly in size from individual to individual, and may even be hypoplastic and nonfunctioning in some cases. There is sometimes a junctional dilatation at the level of the vessel's origin. This is called an *infundibulum*. If the junctional dilatation measures more than 3 mm, it may be considered an aneurysm. If the posterior cerebral artery arises directly

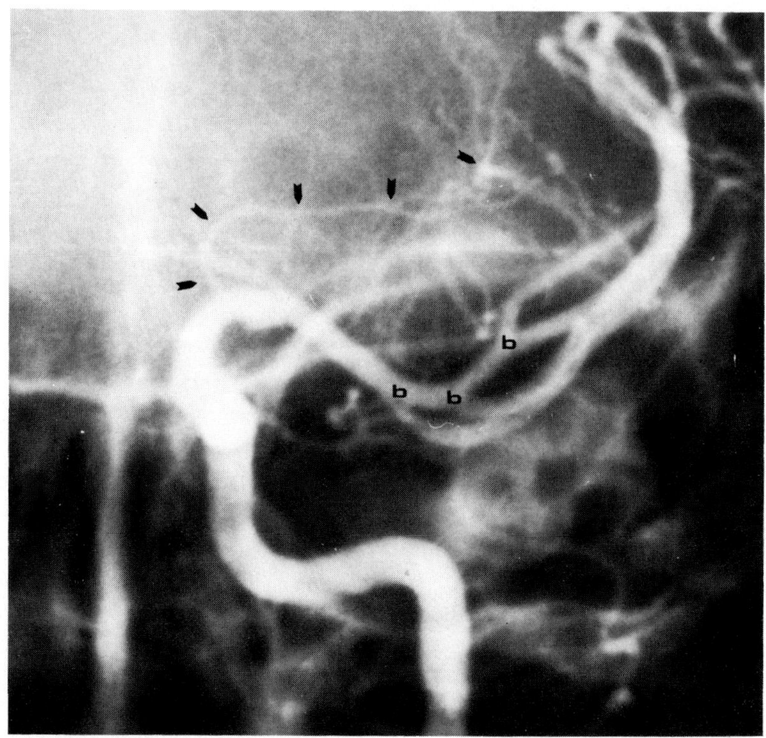

Figure 4–38. ANTERIOR CHOROIDAL ARTERY: The anterior choroidal artery arises from the carotid artery and courses posteriorly. It then curves laterally, continuing in a lateral course until the vessel enters the choroid plexus of the temporal horn of the lateral ventricle *(black arrows)*. It is said that a dime will fit beneath the first curve of the anterior choroidal artery. The multiple bifurcations (*b*) of the middle cerebral artery were well demonstrated on this examination.

from the internal carotid artery, as it does occasionally, it is considered a primitive posterior cerebral artery.

Just above the origin of the posterior communicating artey the anterior choroidal artery arises (Fig. 4–38). This vessel may also have a junctional dilatation. On the anterior view, this vessel will be seen to course laterally in a curvilinear fashion. The anterior choroidal also simultaneously courses posteriorly until it enters the anterior tip of the temporal horn, where it feeds the choroid plexus in the roof of the temporal horn. Occasionally, on the lateral view one may see the blush of the choroid plexus in the temporal horn as it feeds the very vascular capillary plexus of the choroid.

VASCULAR ALTERATIONS WITH TRANSTENTORIAL HERNIATION

One should remember that there is a choroid plexus in all of the ventricles. The choroid plexus of the lateral ventricle lies in the floor of the ventricle; it then follows around to the atrium of the lateral ventricle and then continues to the roof of the temporal horn. The hippocampal gyrus of the temporal horn runs in the floor of the temporal horn; thus, when transtentorial herniation is present, the anterior choroidal vessel will be seen to have a more medial position than normal.

The posterior cerebral artery and the basal vein of Rosenthal also follow a similar course. Therefore, with transtentorial herniation, it will be seen that these vessels are displaced medially. One must remember that the free edge of the tentorium extends forward from the level of the attachment of the falx and the straight sinus up to the posterior clinoids; its most anterior extent is up to the anterior clinoids. Through this tentorial notch extends the midbrain. The midbrain itself consists of the cerebral peduncles, the collicular plate and a portion of the cerebral aqueduct.

CORRELATION WITH MIDBRAIN ANATOMY

All the descending tracts from the cerebral hemispheres descend and coalesce at the level of the cerebral peduncles. At this level, all these tracts pass from the supratentorial to the infratentorial areas through the tentorial notch or "slit" as it is sometimes called. Because all the tracts are confined to a small area at this level, even a small lesion will produce considerable neurologic damage. For a lesion on the cerebral cortex to produce the same amount of damage, the affected area would have to be quite large.

The third cranial nerve arises along the inferior portion of the belly of the pons and also courses forward along the free edge of the tentorium. Because of this anatomic proximity, the third nerve is also affected when there is temporal lobe herniation, and the third nerve is trapped by the free edge of the tentorium as the uncus of the hippocampal gyrus is forced over and below the free edge of the tentorium. This will be reflected by physical examination as a third nerve palsy on the affected side.

ANTERIOR CEREBRAL ARTERY

Above the origin of the anterior choroidal artery, the supraclinoid internal carotid artery divides into the anterior and middle cerebral arteries. The anterior cerebral artery courses anterior and medially, lying along and supplying the medial surface of the cerebral hemisphere.

Anterior Communicating Artery

Just anterior to the lamina terminalis, the anterior cerebral arteries are very close together and are connected by the anterior communicating artery. This also is a portion of the circle of Willis. Proximal to the anterior communicating artery, the horizontal portion of the anterior cerebral artery gives rise to the medial group of lenticulostriate arteries (Fig. 4–39).

The anterior cerebral artery then gives rise to the frontopolar artery, which supplies the frontal lobe along its medial surface and laps over the anterior inferior surface to become visible on the lateral view. The anterior cerebral trunk then gives rise to the pericallosal artery, which roughly parallels the course of the callosal artery but is more superiorly

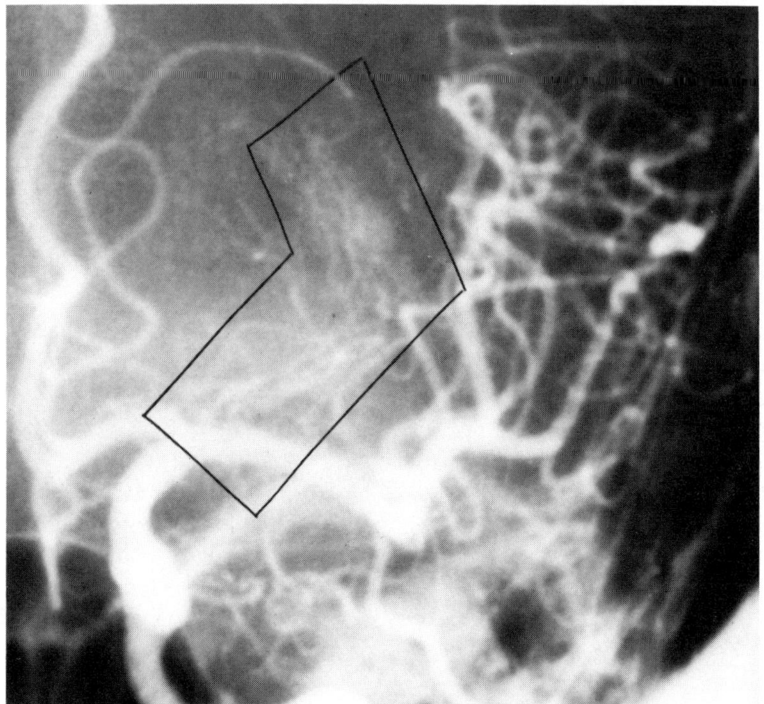

Figure 4–39. LENTICULOSTRIATE ARTERIES: The multiple small vessels that arise from the horizontal portions of the anterior and middle cerebral arteries and supply the lentiform nucleus are the lenticulostriate arteries. The medial lenticulostriate arteries arise from the anterior cerebral artery; the lateral lenticulostriate arteries arise from the middle cerebral artery.

placed. The callosal marginal artery and its branches also supply the frontal lobe; it extends up and over the medial surface of the frontal lobe to become visible on the lateral surface of the brain (see Fig. 4–36).

The pericallosal artery follows along the edge of the corpus callosum, although it is not closely applied to it in the normal state. This pericallosal artery then breaks up posteriorly into a small but vascular capillary plexus that lies on top of the corpus callosum and appears as a tiny "moustache" on the arteriogram (see Fig. 4–49). The position of the pericallosal plexus can give an important clue about the presence of a tumor or space-occupying lesion when there is a tilting of the "moustache" on the AP view. This pericallosal plexus is not readily seen on the lateral view. In addition, there are potential collateral anastomoses with the posterior pericallosal branches of the posterior cerebral artery. These anastomoses may open if there is a block of the more proximal pericallosal artery.

Recurrent Artery of Heubner

The recurrent artery of Heubner arises from the anterior cerebral artery distal to the anterior communicating artery. The artery then courses laterally behind the anterior cerebral artery. Its position is approximately horizontal to the horizontal portion of the anterior cerebral artery. The artery then enters the medial portion of the anterior perforated substance, where it supplies the anterior limits of the internal capsule, the rostral and medial aspects of the putamen and the head of the caudate nucleus. In standard angiographic projections this vessel is obscured by the horizontal portion of the anterior cerebral artery.

MIDDLE CEREBRAL ARTERY

The middle cerebral artery runs anteromedially in the sylvan fissure between the frontal lobes and the anterior tip of the temporal lobe. Along its horizontal portion, the middle cerebral artery gives rise to the orbital frontal branch, which feeds the inferior portion of the frontal lobe over the roofs of the orbits. Also along its horizontal portion, the middle cerebral artery gives rise to the lateral lenticulostriate vessels which pierce the anterior perforated substance and supply the basal ganglia. (*Stria* is another term for basal ganglia; *lentiform* nucleus means the putamen, the internal capsule and the globus pallidus.) The middle cerebral artery branches in its more lateral extent in a rapid series of bifurcation or into a single trifurcation (see Fig. 4–41). This region of the middle cerebral artery is known as the genu (or knee) of the middle cerebral artery, or, more generally, as the region of the "trifurcation" of the middle cerebral artery. The middle cerebral artery then enters the region of the isle of Reil. This island of tissue develops as the brain enlarges, and the temporal and parietal lobes grow over this area of tissue. Indeed, in the anatomic specimen, if one pulls open the sylvian fissue by pulling the parietal lobe up and the temporal lobe down, the isle of Reil is visible. The main branches of the middle cerebral artery are contained in this isle before they exit and distribute themselves over the convexities of the brain.

It is at this point that the branches of the middle cerebral artery in the isle of Reil course posteriorly and superiorly. Each branch of the middle cerebral artery courses superiorly in the sylvian fissure until it reaches the isle of Reil; the branches then turn inferiorly and then laterally along the operculum (lid) of the isle until they reach the opening of the sylvian fissure, where they exit, turn superiorly or

Text continued on page 196

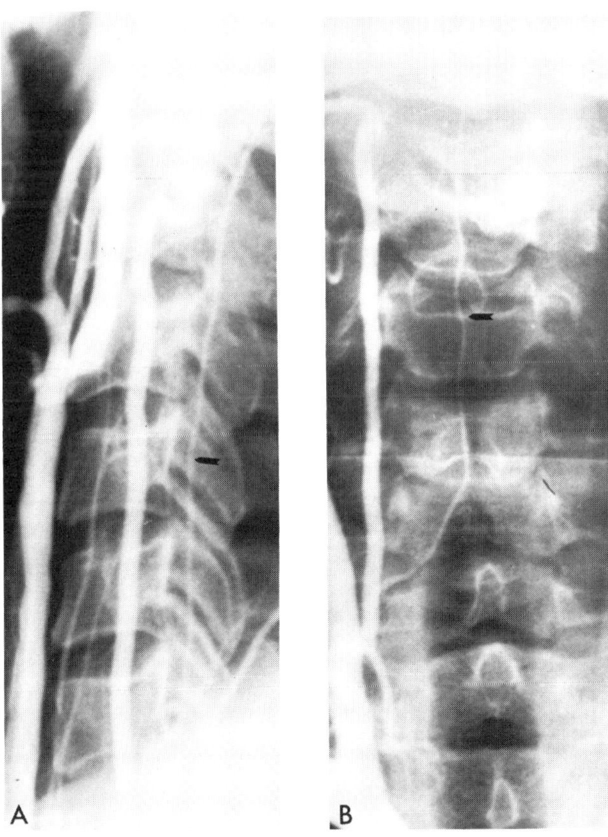

Figure 4–40. ANTERIOR SPINAL ARTERY: The anterior spinal artery is greatly enlarged in this patient because it is used as a source of collateral blood supply. Note its position in the midline along the anterior margin of the cervical spinal cord *(arrows)*.

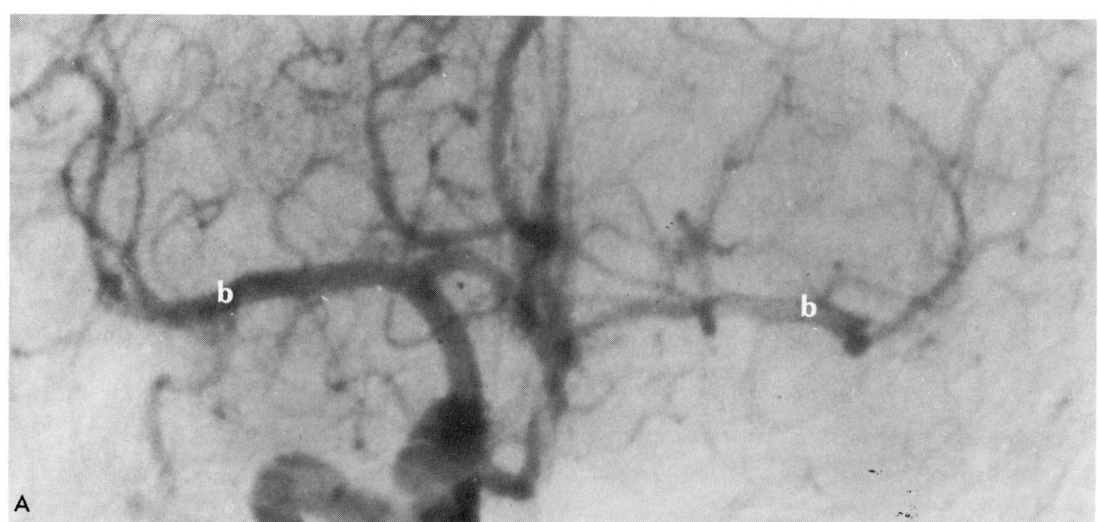

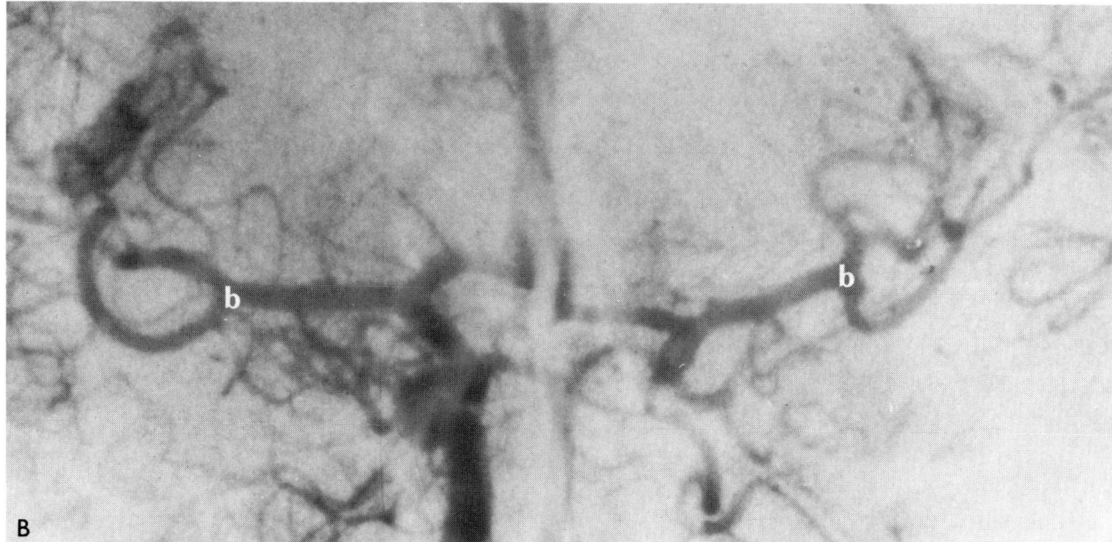

Figure 4–41. CROSS COMPRESSION: This RBA was performed with cross compression of the contralateral carotid artery in the neck. This causes the blood to cross over to the opposite hemisphere via the anterior communicating artery. The *(b)* marks the bifurcations of the middle cerebral arteries.

B, The patient is positioned with the chin elevated so that the region of the middle cerebral artery projects through the orbit, providing an excellent demonstration of the region of the middle cerebral bifurcation. This view is especially useful in patients with an aneurysm at this level.

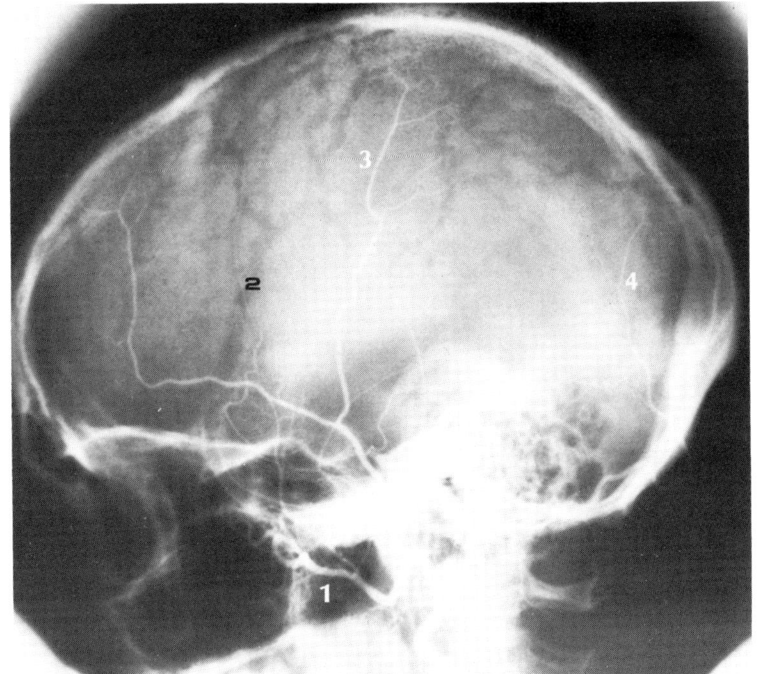

Figure 4–42. EXTERNAL CAROTID ARTERIOGRAM: This normal external carotid arteriogram demonstrates: (*1*) the internal maxillary branch; (*2*) the middle meningeal artery, which arises from the internal maxillary artery; (*3*) the superficial temporal artery and (*4*) the occipital branch of the external carotid artery.

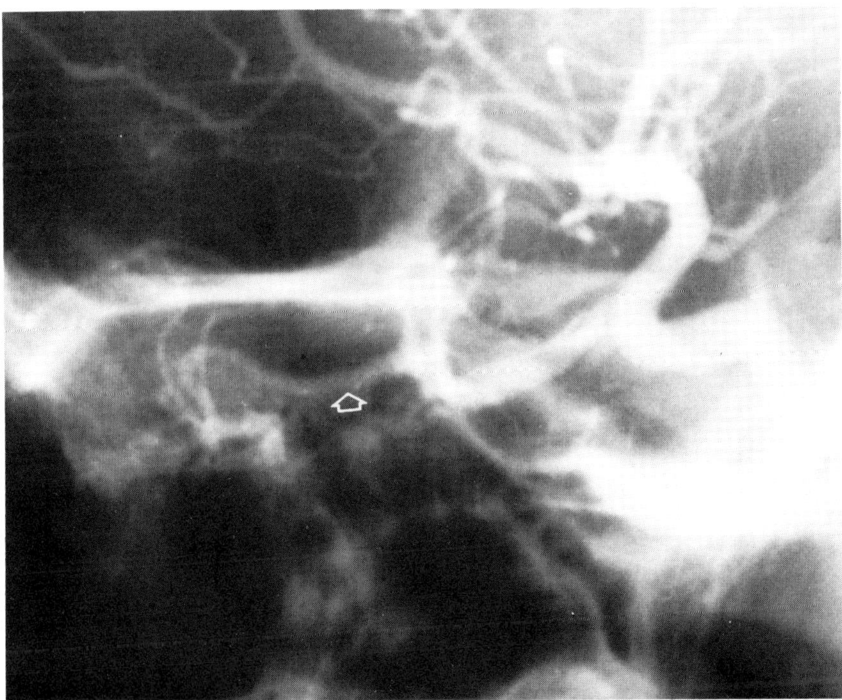

Figure 4–43. OPHTHALMIC ARTERY: The ophthalmic artery arises from the internal carotid artery, and then passes through the optic canal lateral to the optic nerve. The artery then courses superiorly and medially, up and over the optic nerve, and then anteriorly, when it gives rise to the retinal branches, the ethmoidal branches and the supraorbital artery. The vessel is greatly enlarged in this case because the terminal branches supplied a hemangioma of the face.

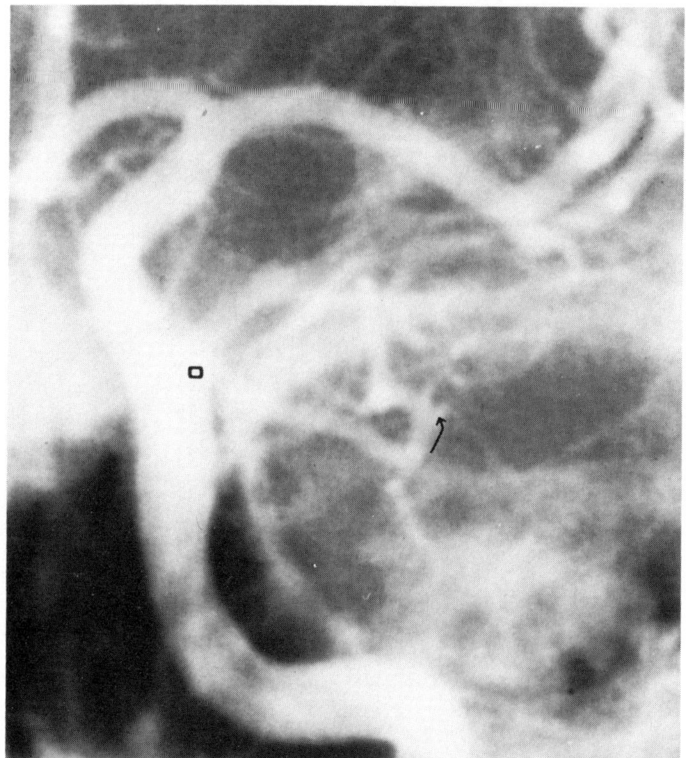

Figure 4–44. AP VIEW OF THE OPHTHALMIC ARTERY: The artery can be seen from its point of origin from the internal carotid artery (□). It then courses anterolaterally, following the lateral aspect of the optic nerve. The vessel then crosses superomedially to rest medial to the optic nerve (*curved arrow*) and then anteriorly to give its terminal branches.

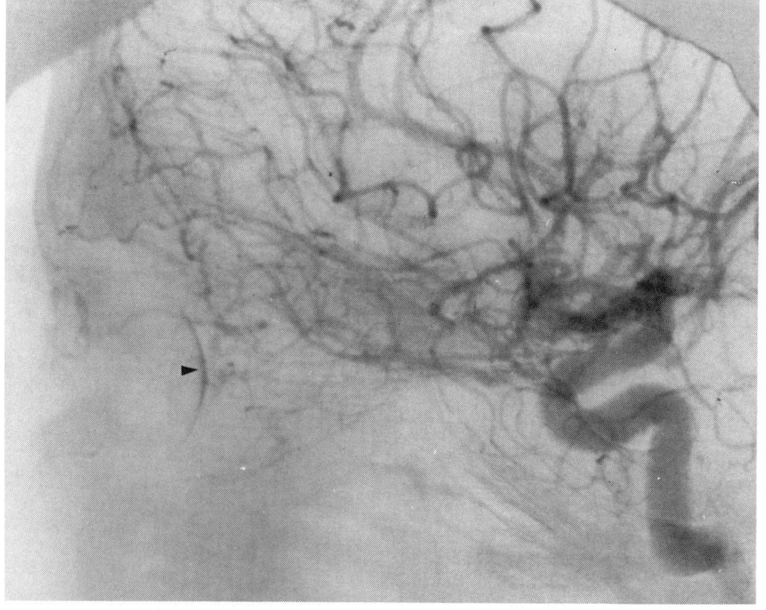

Figure 4–45. CHOROIDAL BLUSH OF THE RETINA: The blush of the retina can be seen in most cases. It is best demonstrated with subtraction techniques *(arrow)*, as in this case. It is a curved line that follows the posterior margin of the globe of the eye.

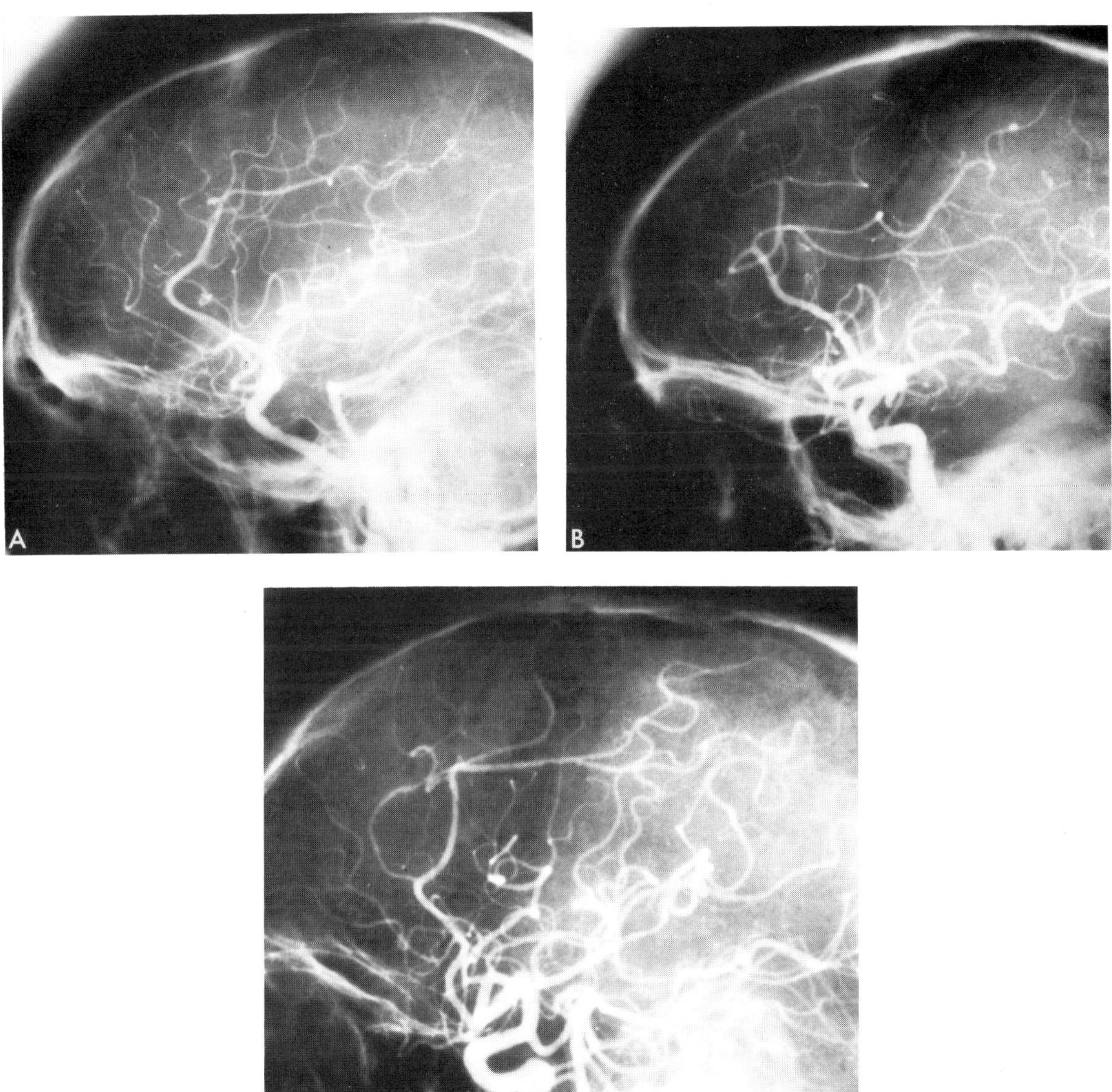

Figure 4–46. NORMAL ANATOMIC VARIATIONS OF THE PERICALLOSAL ARTERY: *A—C,* The normal course of the pericallosal artery can vary greatly and should not be mistaken for displacement secondary to a mass lesion.

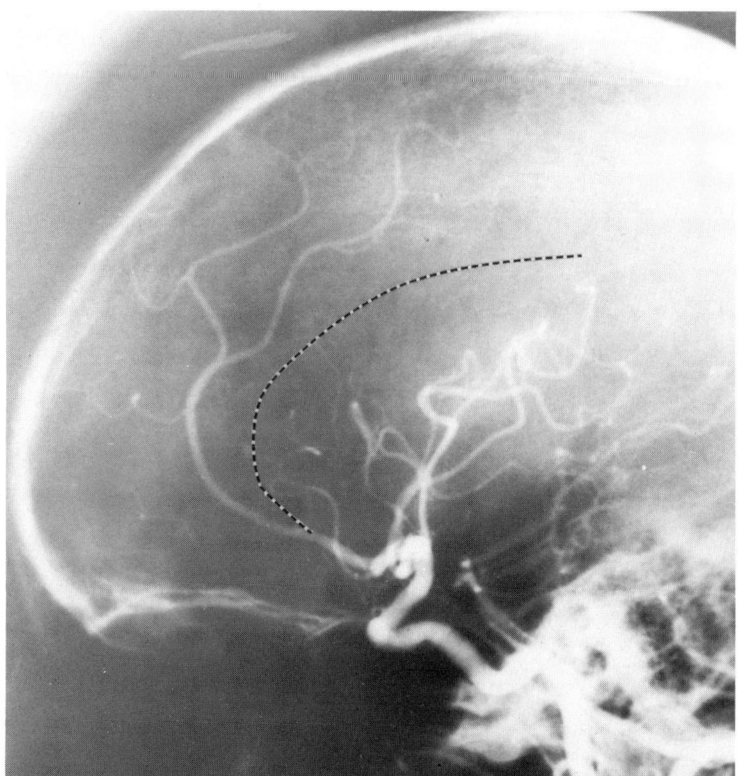

Figure 4–47. NORMAL VARIATION: In this example the pericallosal artery is not filled, and only the callosal marginal artery is seen. The pericallosal artery was demonstrated to fill from the other side. In this case a mistaken diagnosis of hydrocephalus might be made. The dotted line indicates the anticipated position of the pericallosal artery.

Figure 4–48. ABSENT FILLING OF THE ANTERIOR CEREBRAL ARTERY: *A*, The internal carotid injection in this case demonstrates filling only of the middle and posterior cerebral arteries. *B*, The posterior cerebral artery is readily demonstrated on the lateral view *(pc)*. This appearance should not be mistaken for a shift of the anterior cerebral artery on the AP view. The anterior cerebral artery filled when an injection was made on the opposite side.

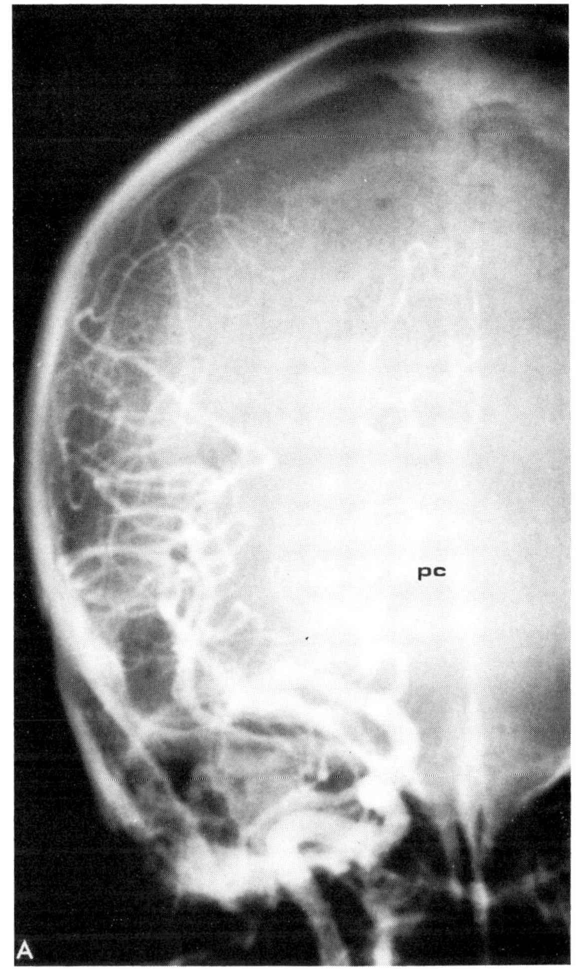

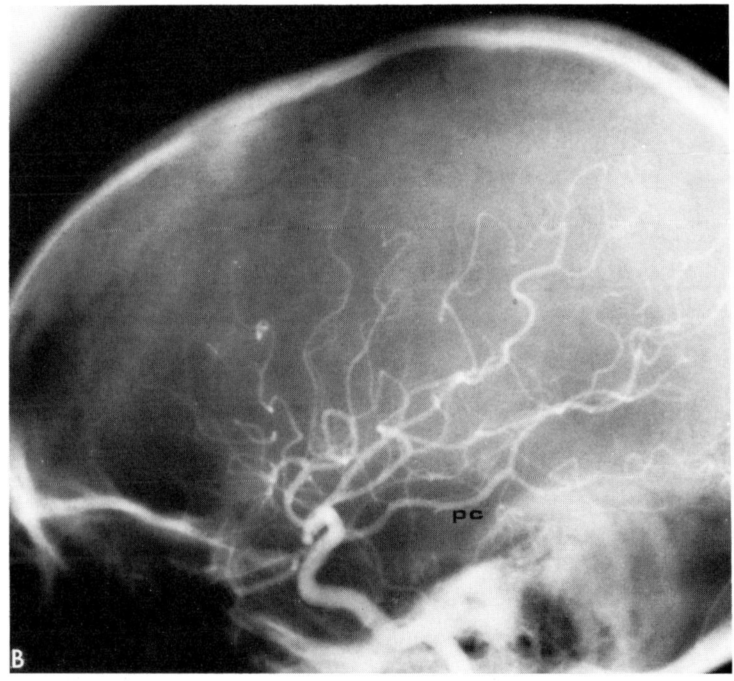

Figure 4–48 *See legend on the opposite page.*

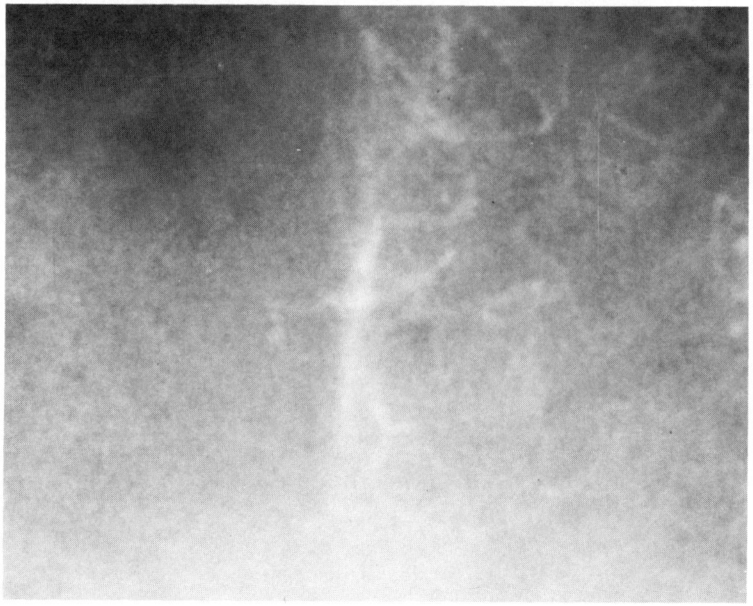

Figure 4–49. PERICALLOSAL PLEXUS: The pericallosal artery breaks up into a capillary plexus — the pericallosal plexus — that has the appearance of a "moustache." On the right the pericallosal plexus is normal in position, but on the left it is tilted upward. This "tilting" of the pericallosal plexus may be either upward or downward when a mass lesion is present. This sign may help to delineate the position of the mass.

inferiorly, and then distribute themselves over the cerebral convexities.

As a rule, each of these branches is named after the area it supplies: e.g., the frontoparietal opercular branches, the parieto-opercular branches, etc. Meticulous anatomic studies have been performed to provide individual labels for each of the branches of the middle cerebral artery, but such detail is beyond the scope of this book. The branches that supply the temporal lobe course inferiorly and are named the temporal opercular branches.

It can be seen that the isle of Reil is triangular, with one limb along the upper portion of this area of tissue. This part is known as the roof of the sylvian triangle. A line can be drawn along the tops of the middle cerebral branches as they rise to the top of the isle of Reil and then turn down and laterally to exit. This line connecting the upper portions of the loops of the middle cerebral artery, from the most anterior to the most posterior branch, forms the angiographic roof of the sylvian triangle. Normally, four to six loops form the roof of the triangle. The other two sides of the sylvian triangle are established by connecting a point placed at the level of the genu of the middle cerebral artery (as seen on the lateral view) with the most anterior and most posterior points of the roof (see Fig. 4–33).

THE SYLVIAN TRIANGLE

The sylvian triangle is one of our most useful angiographic landmarks. Each time an angiogram is reviewed, the sylvian triangle should be identified and its position checked relative to the anticipated normal. The beginning angiographer should *measure* the position of the triangle after identifying it. According to Taveras, in the normal individual the sylvian point — which is the last branch to exit from the sylvian triangle — should be 30 to 43 mm from the inner table of the skull in its side-to-side position, as measured on the AP film. The sylvian point should lie approximately midway, ± 1 cm, between a line drawn tangent to the inner table of the skull and the top of the petrous bone or the orbital roof, whichever is lower. Any displacement from this anticipated normal position should be noted (Fig. 4–35).

On the lateral view, the top of the sylvian triangle is identified by drawing a line connecting the tops of the 4 to 6 loops of the middle cerebral artery branches as they rise to the upper limit of the isle of Reil (Fig. 4–34). As previously noted, this line represents the "roof" of the sylvian triangle, and normally should be straight — although one of the loops may be displaced above or below the line without definitely suggesting the presence of pathology. The anterior inferior limit of the sylvian triangle is the genu of the middle cerebral artery, and the floor of the triangle is determined by connecting the genu of the middle cerebral artery to the sylvian point. The anterior limb is a line connecting the anterior loop to the genu of the middle cerebral artery. These three lines thus make the sylvian triangle. Normally, the position of the triangle is such that the main middle cerebral artery branch along the floor of the triangle lies above the clinoparietal line (Fig. 4–34). The position of this line is determined by drawing a line 9 cm up from the internal occipital protuberance to the inner table of the skull in the parietal region. A line is then drawn from this point on the parietal bone to the anterior clinoid process — hence the *clinoparietal* line. The main middle cerebral artery branch should be within 1 cm above or below this line. In the normal individual, the middle cerebral artery branch generally is above this line. In children, the middle cerebral artery branches ride even higher than in the adult. Any deviation from this anticipated normal position should be noted.

The author has also found that the horizontal portions of the anterior and middle cerebral arteries usually are superimposed upon each other in the normal individual. Although there can be normal variations in position of the initial segments of these vessels, if they are readily visible as separate vessels on the lateral view one should anticipate that there *may* be displacement of these vessels from their normal position.

Similarly, in the normal individual only the first or possibly the first two branches of the middle cerebral artery should project anterior to a line drawn superiorly from the internal carotid artery at the level of its bifurcation into the anterior and middle cerebral arteries. If more branches are anterior to the internal carotid artery bifurcation, one should consider the possibility of forward displacement of the sylvian triangle. Conversely, if no loops are anterior to the internal carotid artery bifurcation, there may be posterior displacement of the sylvian triangle. In addition, one may see a telescoping together of the various branches of the middle cerebral artery when a mass lesion is present. The telescoping may be either anterior or posterior in direction, depending on the position of the mass lesion. There may also be superior or inferior displacement of the sylvian triangle — or any combination of these changes — depending on the position of the mass or whether multiple lesions are present.

Because of the standard angiographic projection, which is 12° toward the feet in the AP projection, a forward displacement of the sylvian triangle may give the impression that the sylvian point is being displaced inferiorly. On the other hand, a posterior displacement of the sylvian point may translate to a superior displacement of the sylvian triangle on the AP view. These changes should be kept in mind when reviewing an angiogram. No final opinion should be made on an angiogram without thorough examination of both the AP and lateral views.

It is sometimes difficult for the beginning angiographer to identify the sylvian triangle. If there is such difficulty, the very early films should be reviewed in the lateral projection, where the early filling of the middle cerebral artery branches in the sylvian triangle are not obscured by the contrast-filled opercular branches of these vessels. The sylvian triangle can then be identified and any changes in the anticipated normal position of the vessels noted.

On some occasions, a very large mass lesion of the temporal lobe will cause such marked elevation of the sylvian triangle that, on the lateral view, it takes on the anatomic appearance of the anterior cerebral artery. Only comparison with the AP view will reveal the true nature of the angiographic changes. On the other hand, occlusion of the middle cerebral artery may be mistaken for gross distortion of this vessel. Again, comparison with the AP view will reveal the true nature of the abnormality.

The triangle is of great angiographic significance because it lies roughly in the midportion of the brain, deep in the cerebral hemisphere. It is therefore affected by most mass lesions. In fact, many lesions are named by their position relative to the triangle, e.g., presylvian, suprasylvian, infrasylvian or retrosylvian. When interpreting arteriograms it is important to attempt to visualize the triangle *in each instance* because of its critical anatomic position. The branches of the middle cerebral artery form a "candelabra" appearance on the lateral view.

Each vessel is a named branch, but as noted earlier they are grouped according to the anatomic area they supply. The last branch out of the triangle is called the angular branch. This last branch courses posteriorly, and is the middle cerebral artery's contribution to the visual cortex, supplying the area of macular vision. The remainder of the visual cortex is supplied by the calcarine branch of the posterior cerebral artery.

Inspection of the cerebral cortex from the lateral view reveals that the middle cerebral artery and its branches supply the bulk of the visible cerebral cortex. The anterior cerebral artery extends up and over from the medial side to supply a small peripheral area of the cortex; the posterior cerebral artery supplies a similar territory posteriorly.

Anatomic/Neurologic Correlation

Thinking back to basic neurology, one remembers that the homunculus is placed over the cerebral cortex so that its foot is at the high convexity while the trunk, chest, arm and face are placed low over the convexity — the homunculus being upside down on the cerebral convexity. In addition, one will remember that the tongue and fingers are disproportionately enlarged, with the thumb even more so to reflect its large representation on the cerebral cortex.

These relative sizes and positions are important in the presence of occlusive cerebrovascular disease. When the middle cerebral artery is occluded, the face and arm will be affected much more than the leg because of the blood supply to the cortex. Conversely, in the presence of a high-convexity meningioma, the foot and leg will be much more affected — not only because of the blood supply, but because of the pressure on the cerebral cortex represented by the foot and leg in the high-convexity region.

In addition to major vascular occlusions, one can also see branch occlusions in any vascular distribution. In many cases, retrograde collateral flow from other vessels will attempt to fill these branches. Without adequate collateral flow, occlusion of these vessels usually results in permanent neurologic damage.

POSTERIOR CEREBRAL ARTERY

The basilar artery is formed by the joining of the two vertebral arteries. It courses up in the prepontine cistern just posterior to the clivus until it reaches the interpeduncular fossa. Here the terminal bifurcation of the basilar artery becomes the posterior cerebral arteries. From their bifurcation in the interpeduncular cistern, the posterior cerebral arteries must course first laterally, under the cerebral peduncles, and then posterosuperiorly to the level of the quadrigeminal plate. On the AP view this course is readily apparent (see Chapter 14); indeed, they often outline the cerebral peduncles very well. On the lateral view, however, the horizontal portion of the posterior cerebral arteries is not appreciated because we are seeing the vessels "end-on." This results in a telescoping of the vessels and a failure to appreciate their initial lateral course.

The posterior cerebral arteries then course around the brain stem in the perimesencephalic cistern, which makes up only a small portion of the ambient cistern. More posteriorly and superiorly, the perimesencephalic cistern and the quadrigeminal plate cistern converge. At the quadrigeminal plate cistern, the posterior cerebral arteries nearly meet at the midline. In the region of the quadrigeminal plate, the posterior cerebral arteries are closely related to the pineal gland and the vein of Galen. The superior cerebellar arteries arise just inferior to the posterior cerebral arteries — also in the interpeduncular cistern. The posterior cerebral and superior cerebellar arteries are separated from each other by the tentorium, which extends forward at this point and divides the supratentorial compartment from the infratentorial compartment. In the presence of a tentorial meningioma that arises along the free edge of the tentorium, the posterior cerebral and superior cerebellar arteries will be splayed apart from each other by the tumor mass.

The posterior communicating artery arises from the horizontal portion of the posterior cerebral artery, a short distance from the midline (see Chapter 14). The posterior communicating artery then courses anteriorly and slightly laterally to join with the internal carotid artery in its supraclinoid portion. One may see this posterior communication artery fill retrograde when contrast material is injected into the vertebral artery. On the other hand, if the posterior communicating vessel does not fill retrograde, one may see a filling "defect" in the posterior cerebral artery from "washout" of unopacified blood from the posterior communicating artery, which fills from the carotid artery system. This area of "washout" should not be mistaken for an area of vascular spasm or arteriosclerotic narrowing.

In some cases, the posterior cerebral artery does not fill from the vertebrobasilar system, but arises directly from the internal carotid artery — a variation known as a "primitive posterior cerebral artery" (see Fig. 4–48). The significance of this anatomic finding becomes most apparent when one wishes to examine the left posterior cerebral artery distribution and finds that neither right nor left brachial arteriography is helpful. Percutaneous left carotid arteriography will then be required. If catheterization is performed, an additional injection will be needed.

The anterior and posterior thalamoperforating arteries arise from the posterior communicating artery and the proximal portions of the posterior cerebral arteries, respectively. The posterior pericallosal artery then arises, followed by the medial and lateral posterior choroidal arteries (see Chapter 14). These later branches are not well seen in the AP view. The posterior pericallosal artery supplies the posterior portion of the corpus callosum and has the potential to provide collateral flow to the distribution of the pericallosal artery. The medial posterior choroidal arteries project anteriorly on the lateral view, have a "reverse three" configuration in many cases, and supply the choroid plexus of the third ventricle as it runs in the roof of the third ventricle. The lateral posterior choroidal vessels project more posteriorly on the lateral view; they supply the choroid plexus of the lateral ventricles in the region of the atrium of the lateral ventricle. The posterior cerebral artery then gives rise to the posterior temporal branch, which supplies all of the medial and undersurface of the temporal lobe, with a small portion of its distribution over the convexities of the temporal lobe. Coursing further posteriorly, the posterior cerebral then becomes the internal occipital artery; this branches into the calcarine artery, which supplies the visual cortex, in the region of the calcarine fissure along the medial surface of the occipital lobe. The other branch is the parieto-occipital artery, which supplies the bulk of the occipital lobe and a portion of the posterior aspect of the parietal lobe.

The branches of the posterior cerebral artery are:

1. Posterior communicating a.
2. Thalamoperforating a.
3. Posterior pericallosal a.
4. Medial posterior choroidal a.
5. Lateral posterior choroidal a.
6. Posterior temporal a.
7. Internal occipital a.
   a. parieto-occipital a.
   b. calcarine a.

EXTERNAL CAROTID ARTERY

The external carotid artery (Fig. 4–42) is the smaller of the two vessels at the level of the bifurcation of the common carotid artery in the neck. External carotid angiography is of particular importance in the study of a meningioma because these tumors obtain the bulk of their blood supply from the external carotid system via the internal maxillary artery, which gives rise to the middle meningeal artery. At the level of the carotid bifurcation in the neck, in most cases, the external carotid artery courses medial and anterior relative to the internal carotid artery. The external carotid artery then gives rise to eight main branches:

1. Superior thyroid artery; supplies the thyroid gland.
2. Lingual artery; supplies the tongue.
3. Facial artery (often arises in common with the lingual artery); supplies the face.
4. Occipital artery; supplies the muscles of the neck and the scalp over the occipital portion of the skull.
5. Posterior auricular artery; supplies the ear and the scalp above and behind the ear.
6. Ascending pharyngeal artery; may give rise to various inconstant branches, including pharyngeal and meningeal branches.
7. Superficial temporal artery; supplies mainly the scalp over the parietal region.
8. Internal maxillary artery.

Of all the branches, the internal maxillary artery gives rise to the artery that most concerns us from an arteriographic and diagnostic point of view, for it gives rise to the middle meningeal. When a meningioma is present, the internal maxillary artery may be greatly enlarged, and the middle meningeal branch may be very apparent on the arteriogram. Indeed, if one suspects a meningioma, one should be particularly careful to puncture the common carotid artery *well below* the level of the bifurcation so as not to miss the external carotid vessel. If catheterization is performed, the tip of the catheter should be positioned *below* the bifurcation.

Examination of the external carotid distribution will reveal that the middle meningeal artery is visualized in almost all cases as a small vessel that originates from the internal maxillary artery and courses superiorly and medially. This middle meningeal vessel enters the bony calvaria via the foramen spinosum and supplies the meningeal coverings of the brain. The vessel will be seen to travel in the meningeal artery groove in the inner table of the skull in the adult. The foramen spinosum will be enlarged in some cases of meningioma, as will the meningeal artery groove. However, normal variations occur in the size of both the foramen spinosum and the meningeal artery groove, and so this finding is certainly not pathognomonic. It merely serves to substantiate other findings (see Chapter 9).

External Carotid Angiography. In the presence of such meningeal supply to a brain tumor, selective catheterization of the external carotid artery can be performed, and a selective external carotid artery angiogram performed (Fig. 4–42). Depending on the size of the vessel, one may inject from 3 to 8 cc of contrast material. If superselective catheterization of the vessel of interest is possible, this is also advantageous. By test injections under fluoroscopic control, the size of the vessel can be determined so that an appropriate amount of contrast material can be injected. This must be balanced against the amount of contrast material that may represent excessive filling, consequently resulting in overfilling of the external carotid system and retrograde flow into the external carotid system. In addition to the mechanical and technical difficulties of this type of injection, the patient will feel considerable discomfort from injection into the external carotid system. The patient should be forewarned against this. Both the presence of the catheter in the vessel and the injection of contrast material into the vessel irritate to the vessel wall. This may result in spasm of the vessel, which will also promote retrograde flow into the internal carotid system. This spasm of the external carotid artery often will be visible fluoroscopically at the time the catheter is placed. The author has seen one case of this type of vascular spasm that resulted in a remote spasm involving one major branch of the middle cerebral artery group.

ANATOMIC DISSECTION AND CORRELATION

During the course of each resident group rotation on the neuroradiology service, we dissect a preserved brain in order to gain a greater appreciation of the intracerebral structures in their three-dimensional positions. This anatomic dissection is carried out by very loosely structured groups of three to five residents. Axial sections are dissected to establish correlation with the CT scan findings. The standard coronal sections are also done. A single brain cut in two through the corpus callosum will serve both purposes. Initially, a superficial inspection of the brain is made, noting the positions of the falx cerebri and the tentorium cerebelli, and making particular note of the free edge of the tentorium and the dural sinuses and arachnoid villi. Following this, the parietal and temporal lobes are opened, and the isle of Reil or insula is inspected. Thus, the course of the cerebral arteries can be visualized: the pattern of rising to the highest portion of the isle of Reil by the middle cerebral artery branches, followed by the descent of each branch until it reaches the operculum of the isle of Reil and then turns either superiorly to course over the frontal and parietal lobes or inferiorly to distribute over the temporal bone. This visual reinforcement of understanding the distribution of the middle cerebral vessels serves to crystalize in the student's mind the anatomic course and position of these branches in the isle of Reil. Further dissection of the brain can proceed in a random fashion at the discretion of the neuroanatomy students or the instructor. Often, following the course of individual vessels is quite helpful. Certainly the position of the ventricles relative to the other structures of the brain should be noted. The identification of as many landmarks as possible is very useful for review and helps the uninitiated student to learn more about the normal anatomy. The quadrigeminal plate cistern with the pineal, internal cerebral veins, vein of Galen and posterior continuation into the superior cerebellar cistern certainly should be pointed out. The close relationship to the splenium of the corpus callosum, and the pulvinar of the thalamus (most posterior nucleus of the thalamus) also should be noted.

In many cases, the veil-like membrane of the cisternae magna will be seen as it extends posteriorly from the lobes of the cerebellum as a fold of the arachnoid membrane of the leptomeninges. Close inspection of this area will also reveal the normal pathways of the posterior inferior cerebellar artery (PICA) and anterior inferior cerebellar artery (AICA) as well as the vertebrobasilar system itself. It also will show the multiple small pontine perforating vessels, which are not seen on angiograms. In addition, of course, with review of a large number of specimens, one begins to get a feel for the many normal anatomic variations that may be seen. This is particularly noteworthy when one compares the various sizes of the cisternae magna and the inverse relationship between the size of the PICA and the size of the AICA.

JUGULAR VENOGRAPHY

Indications. Jugular venography may be used to outline the cavernous sinus — for example, to determine the lateral extension of a pituitary tumor. It also may be used to demonstrate invasion of the internal jugular vein by a glomus jugulare tumor.

Technique. The internal jugular vein lies lateral to the internal carotid artery in the carotid sheath. The neck is prepared and draped in a fashion similar to the procedure followed for carotid puncture. A local anesthetic should be injected around the puncture site. Since the internal jugular vein is lateral to the carotid in the neck, the needle should be directed lateral to the carotid artery for the puncture. Suction should be applied to the hub of the needle as it is being withdrawn. When free flow of venous blood is obtained, a guidewire is threaded through the needle and a polyethylene catheter or Davis needle is placed into the internal jugular vein, using the Seldinger technique. The needle is advanced until its tip is at the jugular bulb. Contrast material is injected at a rate of 8 cc per second for 2 to 2.5 seconds to visualize the jugular vein. To visualize the cavernous sinus, pressure should be applied at the time of injection to the jugular vein below the injection site; it may be necessary to compress both internal jugular veins during injection.

EMBOLIZATION

With advances in techniques, invasive radiology has become a part of many neuroradiologic practices. Catheters are used to introduce small spheres or particles of occlusive materials in order to decrease the blood supply to arteriovenous malformations and certain types of vascular tumors. This method may be the definitive treatment for arterioven-

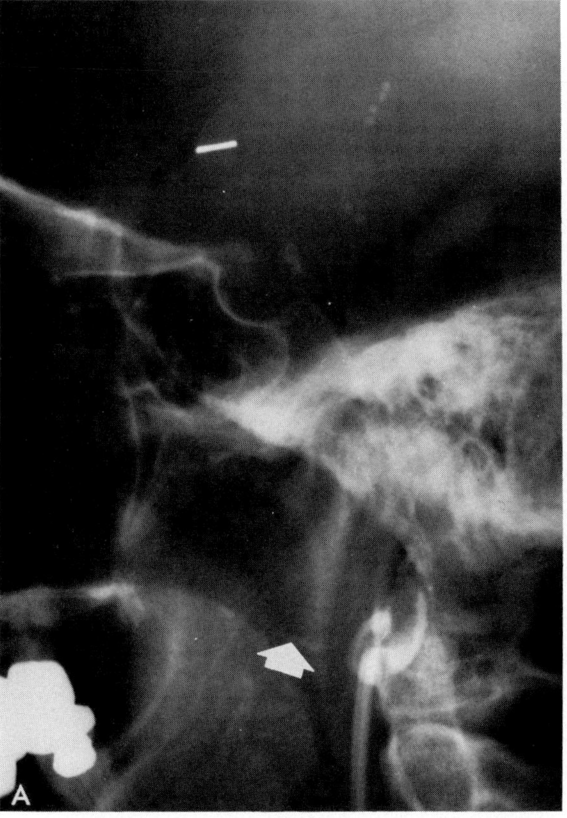

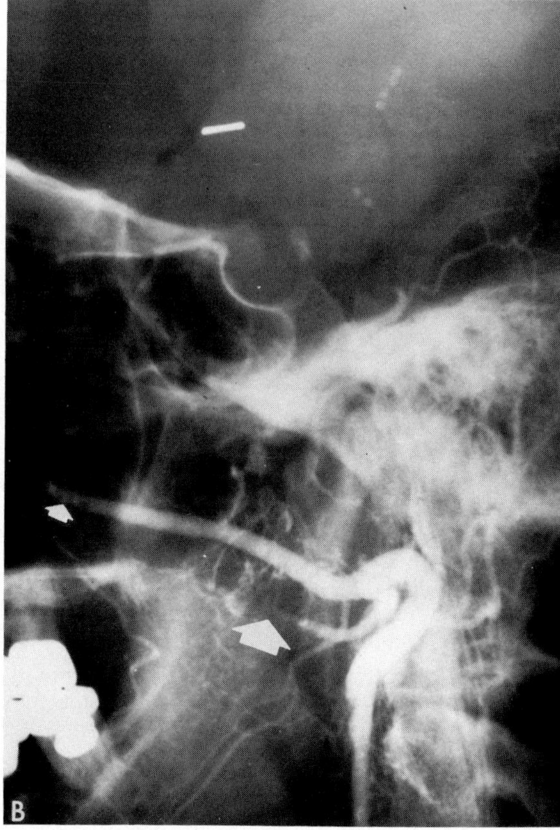

Figure 4–50. EMBOLIZATION: The preliminary film *(A)* demonstrates multiple small Silastic balls in the terminal branches of the external carotid artery. Some are in the superficial temporal artery over the bony calvaria; others are in branches of the internal maxillary artery *(arrow)*. Following the injection of contrast material *(B)*, there is interruption of the flow of the contrast material through these branches because of the mechanical obstruction.

ous malformations; it also decreases the vascularity of tumors, making them more readily amenable to surgical removal. Meningiomas and glomus jugulare tumors in particular may benefit from embolization.

The technique of embolization is beyond the scope of this book. It is enough to say that great care is needed to prevent the embolic materials from entering the internal carotid system and causing a stroke (Fig. 4–50).

NORMAL VENOUS ANATOMY

FALX CEREBRI AND TENTORIUM CEREBELLI

For a full understanding of the venous drainage of the cerebrum, one must know the structure of the falx cerebri and the tentorium cerebelli.

The brain is enclosed in three meningeal layers:

The *pia mater* is a thin, delicate connective tissue closely applied to the brain and spinal cord that carries the rich network of blood vessels that supply the brain and cord. The pia dips into each fissure and sulcus and forms the choroid plexuses of the lateral, third and fourth ventricles.

The *arachnoid layer* is a delicate, avascular membrane lying between the dura mater and the pia mater. The subarachnoid space contains the arteries, the veins, and the cerebrospinal fluid.

The *dura mater* is a dual-layered membrane that is composed of dense fibrous connective tissue and collagen. The outer periosteal layer forms the periosteum of the inner table of the skull. The inner meningeal layer is smooth and forms the various partitions of the brain. The falx cerebri is a thin dural reflection of the *meningeal* layer, which extends down between the cerebral hemispheres. This inner layer also forms the tentorium cerebelli and the falx cerebelli, which separates the two cerebellar hemispheres.

The falx cerebri is attached anteriorly at the crista galli. At its anterior extent, the falx is not very wide, but it widens progressively as it extends from front to back. The straight sinus is the posterior point of attachment of the falx, and the length of the straight sinus reflects the width of the falx posteriorly. The superior sagittal sinus is formed by the dural reflection; it is triangular in shape. The inferior sagittal sinus runs along the inferior margin of the falx cerebri to enter the straight sinus at the level of the vein of Galen posteriorly. The straight sinus then courses posteroinferiorly to the level of the torcular Herophili or confluence of sinuses. This confluence of sinuses is at the level of the internal occipital protuberance, which is opposite the external occipital protuberance. Extending laterally from the confluence of sinuses are the right and left transverse or lateral sinuses. The transverse sinuses drain into the sigmoid sinuses just posterior to the petrous bones bilaterally and from there into the internal jugular veins bilaterally. In most cases, the right transverse sinus is larger than the left. It has been shown that most of the blood from the superior sagittal sinus drains into the right transverse sinus, whereas most of the blood from the inferior sagittal sinus drains into the left transverse sinus. There is a great deal of anatomic variation in the position of the superior sagittal sinus as it drains into the transverse sinus; in some cases, the superior sagittal sinus may enter the transverse sinus far lateral to the midline (see Fig. 4–56).

The transverse sinuses follow the tentorium at the level of its attachment to the occipital bone. The transverse sinuses also are triangular, and they lie just below the tentorium. The straight sinus, at the level of its junction with the inferior sagittal sinus and the vein of Galen, is superior to the transverse sinuses. The middle of the tentorium is then also in a higher position than the lateral portions of the tentorium; indeed, from the level of the straight sinus, the tentorium slants downward and forward to cover the cerebellum. The tentorium is attached bilaterally to the petrous bones along their upper margins; the free edge of the tentorium slants forward from the tentorial notch around the midbrain and extends anteriorly to attach as far forward as the anterior clinoid processes bilaterally. The tentorium is then "tent-shaped," as its name would suggest. The top peak is at the level of the junction with the inferior sagittal sinus and the vein of Galen. The straight sinus then forms the roof, and the remainder of the tentorium slants downward and forward to cover the posterior fossa structures (see Fig. 4–58). Because the dural structures are enhanced by contrast infusion, they are visualized readily on the postinfusion scan. The superior sagittal sinus, the inferior sagittal sinus and the falx are readily visualized on the CT scan (see Chapter 3).

Because it is in the same plane, or nearly the same plane as the standard CT scan cut, the tentorium may be seen as a sheet like area of enhancement rather than a linear structure. Depending on the angle of the cut, one may visualize much or little of the tentorium on a single scan slice.

The tentorial notch is formed by the anteriorly sloping free edges of the tentorium as they slope down and forward from the straight sinus. This notch appears as a "V"-shaped area on the postinfusion scan. In addition to the notch, one sees a contiguous portion of the straight sinus posterior to the notch as the straight sinus drains toward the torcular Herophili or confluence of sinuses. The visualization of this notch and the blush of the tentorium are helpful when one is attempting to decide whether a lesion is above or below the tentorium. Obviously, the vermis and midportion of the cerebellum extend higher than the rest of the cerebellar structures; therefore, on an individual CT scan cut, a more medially placed lesion is likely to be in the vermis of the cerebellum, whereas a more laterally placed lesion is more likely to be in the occipital lobes. If there is any question about the position of the mass — whether it be in the supratentorial or infratentorial compartment — arteriography may be needed. In addition, one may perform tomographic cuts in the coronal projection by hyperextending the patient's head. This will make the position of the lesion graphically clear. Reconstruction tomography

Text continued on page 213

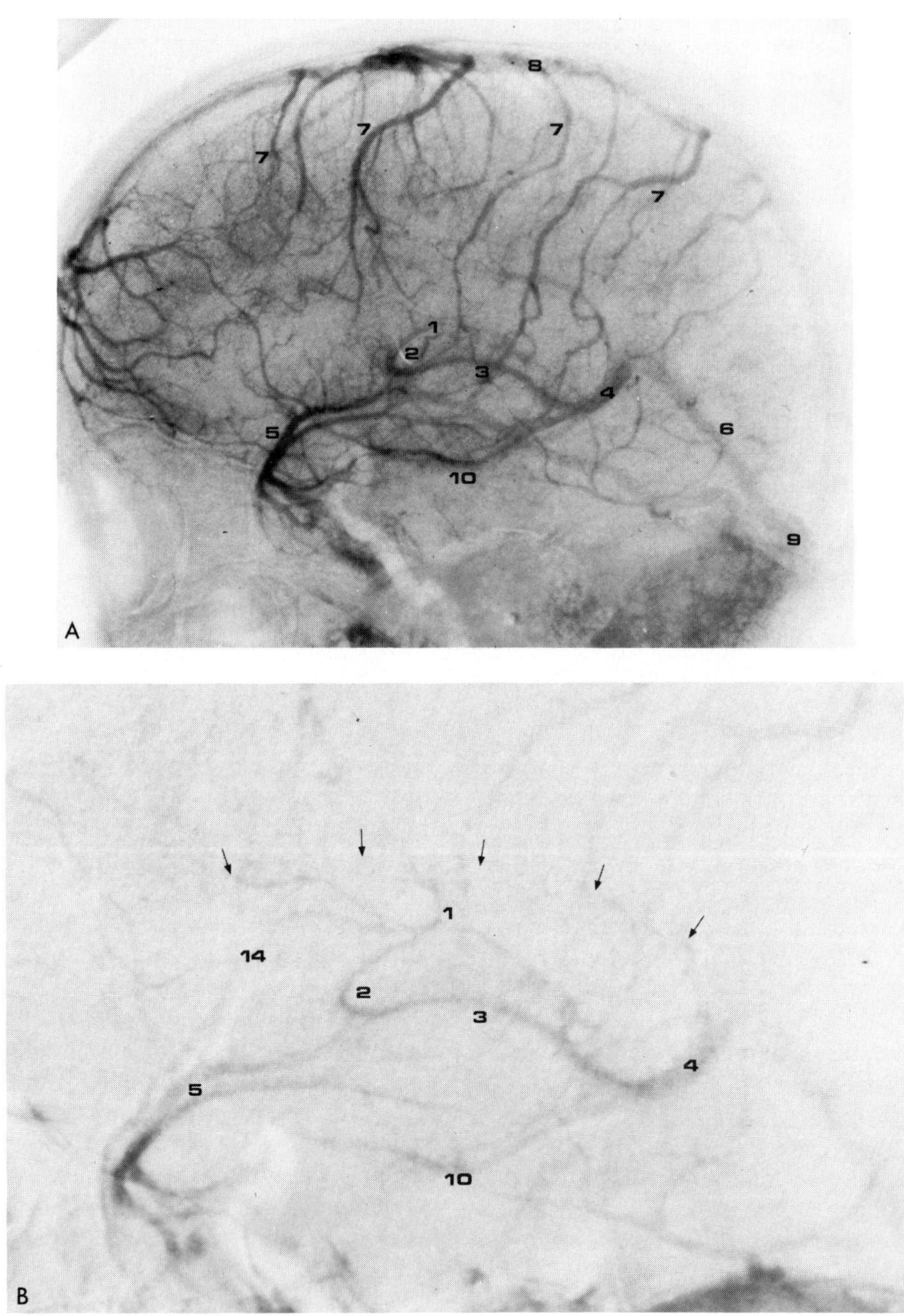

Figure 4–51 *See legend on the opposite page.*

Figure 4–51. NORMAL VENOUS ANATOMY: The deep and superficial venous structures are readily identified in most cases.

1. Thalamostriate vein.
2. Venous angle.
3. Internal cerebral vein.
4. Vein of Galen.
5. Middle cerebral vein.
6. Straight sinus.
7. Superficial cortical veins.
8. Superior sagittal sinus.
9. Torcular Herophili.
10. Basal vein of Rosenthal.

In *(B)* the small arrows demonstrate the subependymal course of the veins. A linear measurement made from one of the small veins to the internal cerebral vein reflects the height of the lateral ventricle. (14) is an anomalous course of the septal vein.

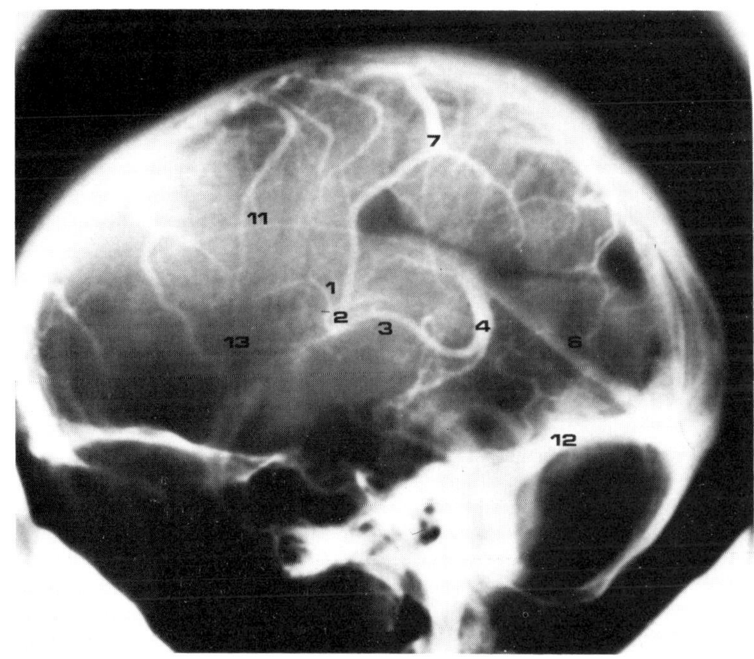

Figure 4–52. NORMAL SUPERFICIAL AND DEEP VENOUS ANATOMY:

1. Thalamostriate vein.
2. Venous angle.
3. Internal cerebral vein.
4. Vein of Galen.
5. Middle cerebral vein.
6. Straight sinus.
7. Vein of Trolard.
8. Superior sagittal sinus.
9. Torcular Herophili.
10. Basal vein of Rosenthal.
11. Inferior sagittal sinus.
12. Transverse sinus.
13. Septal vein.

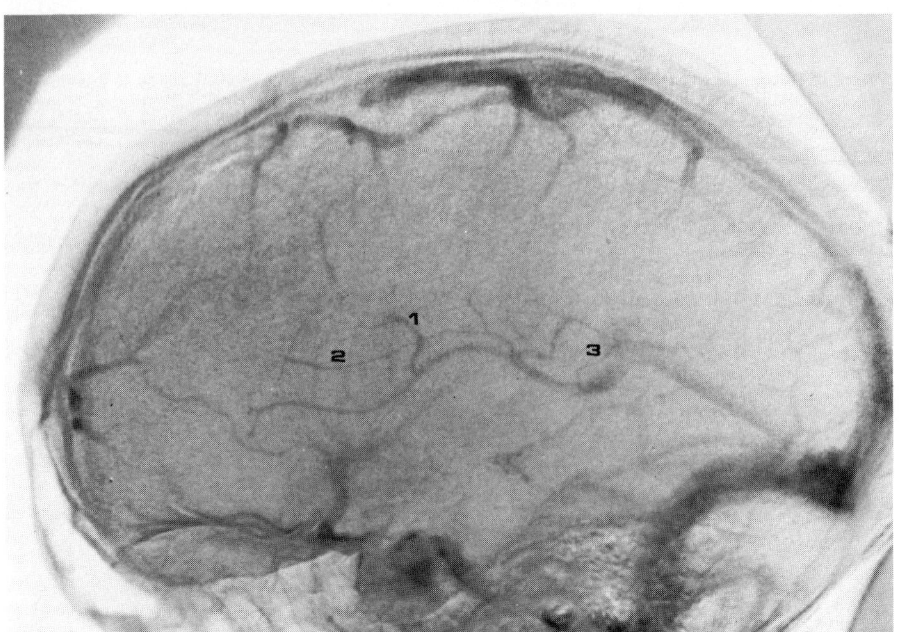

Figure 4–53. NORMAL DEEP VENOUS ANATOMY:
1. Thalamostriate vein.
2. Middle terminal vein.
3. Common atrial veins.

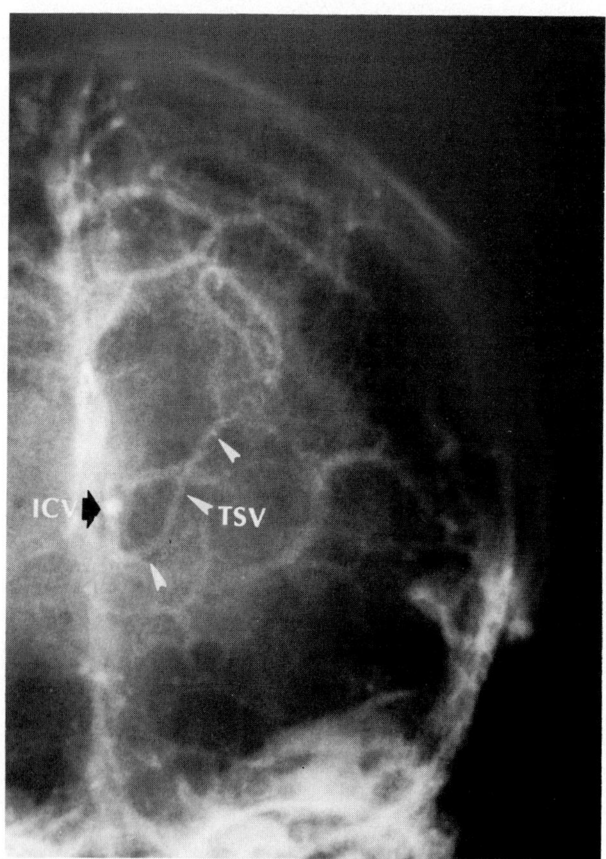

Figure 4–54. Normal AP view of the deep venous system, showing the internal cerebral vein *(ICU)* and the thalamostriate vein *(TSV)*.

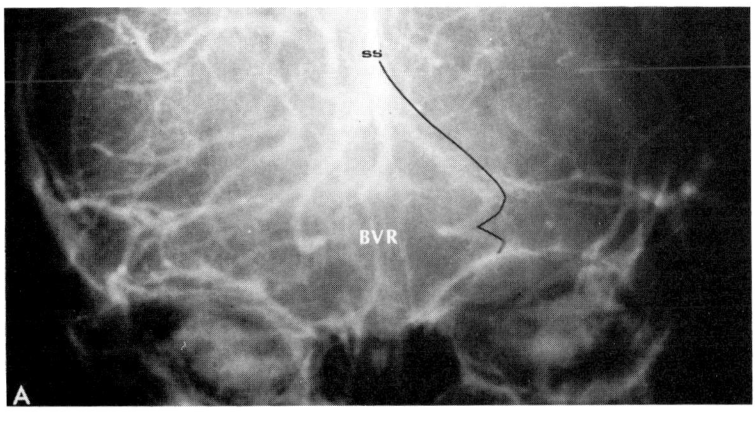

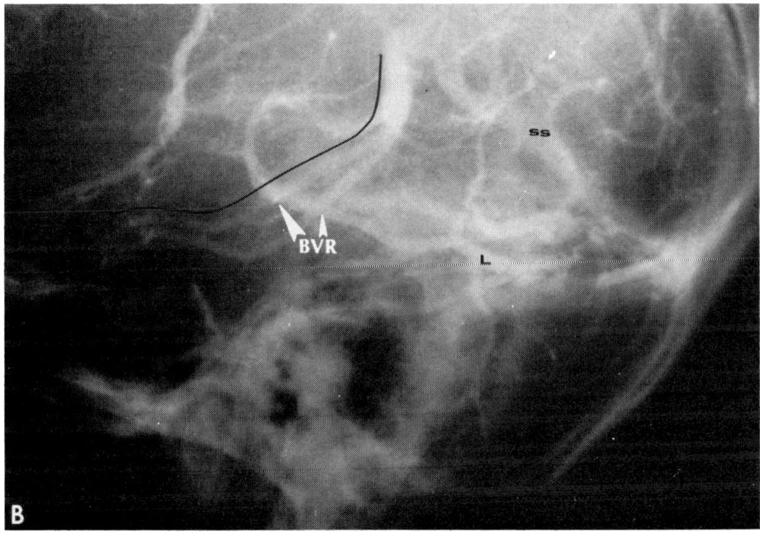

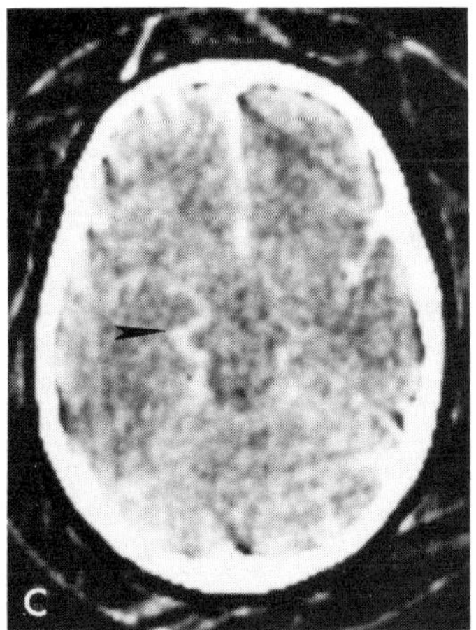

Figure 4–55. BASAL VEIN OF ROSENTHAL: The basal vein of Rosenthal can be followed from its origin at the anterior perforated substance posteriorly and around the brain stem, where it joins with the vein of Galen and then drains into the straight sinus *(SS)*. The course of this vein is demonstrated on one side in both the AP *(A)* and the lateral *(B)* views *(black line)*. In *B*, *L* is the vein of Labbé which drains into the transverse sinus.

C, The CT scan also demonstrates the course of the basal vein in the axial projection.

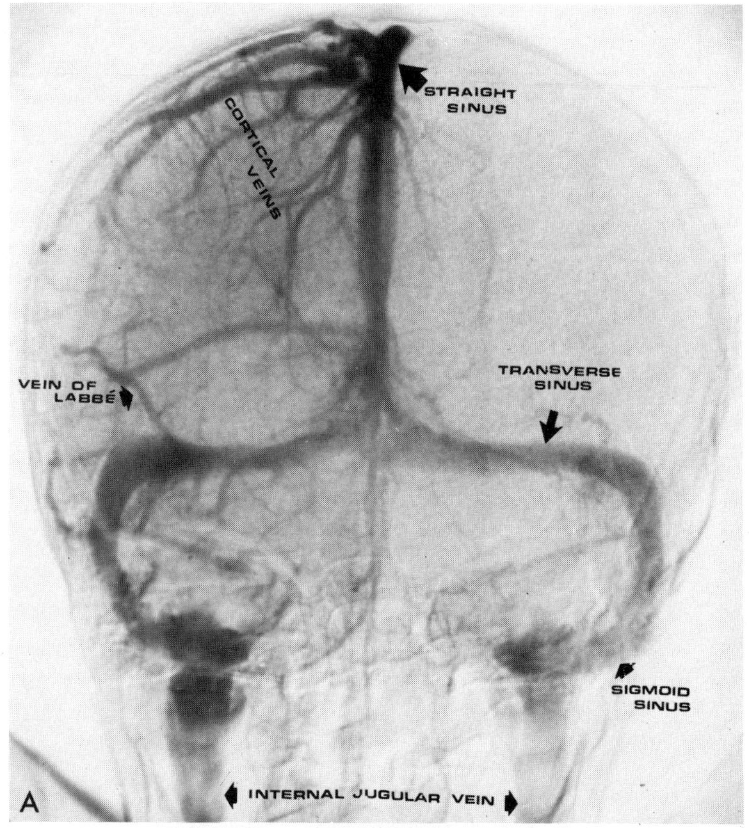

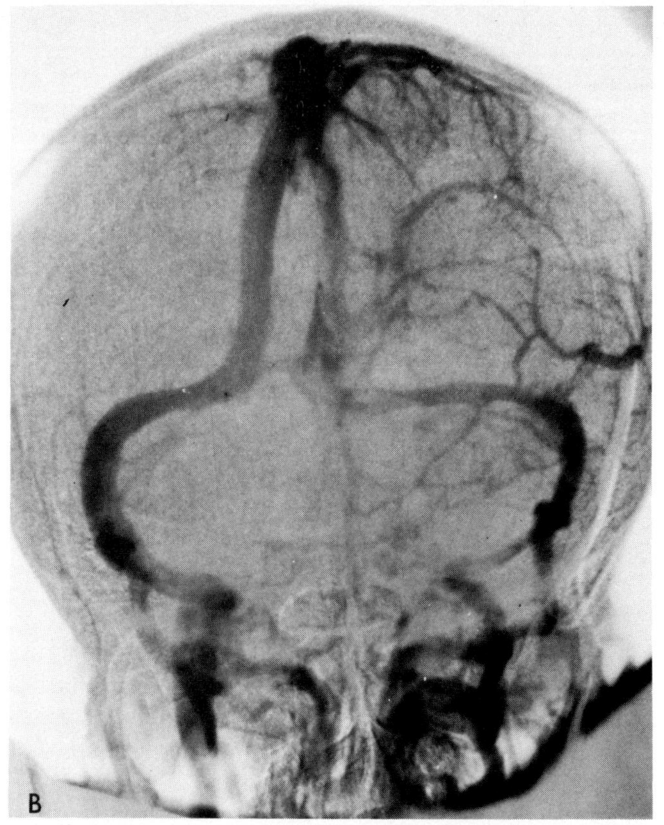

Figure 4–56 *See legend on the opposite page.*

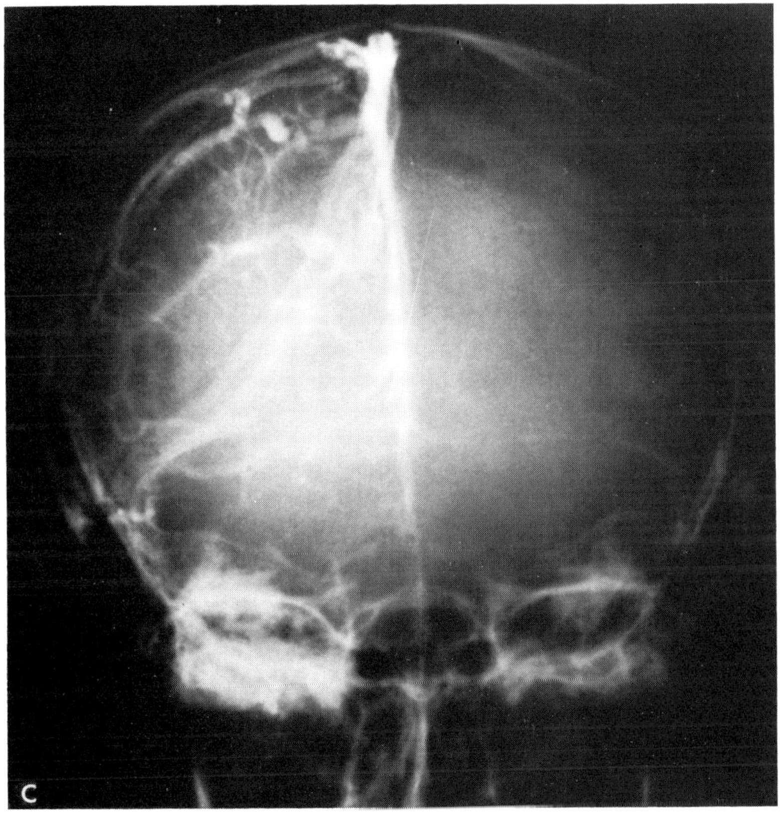

Figure 4–56. *A, B, C,* SUPERIOR SAGITTAL SINUS: The superior sagittal sinus normally lies at the midline, but can drain in an off-centered manner and still be considered entirely normal. The sinus may be placed to the right or the left of the midline.

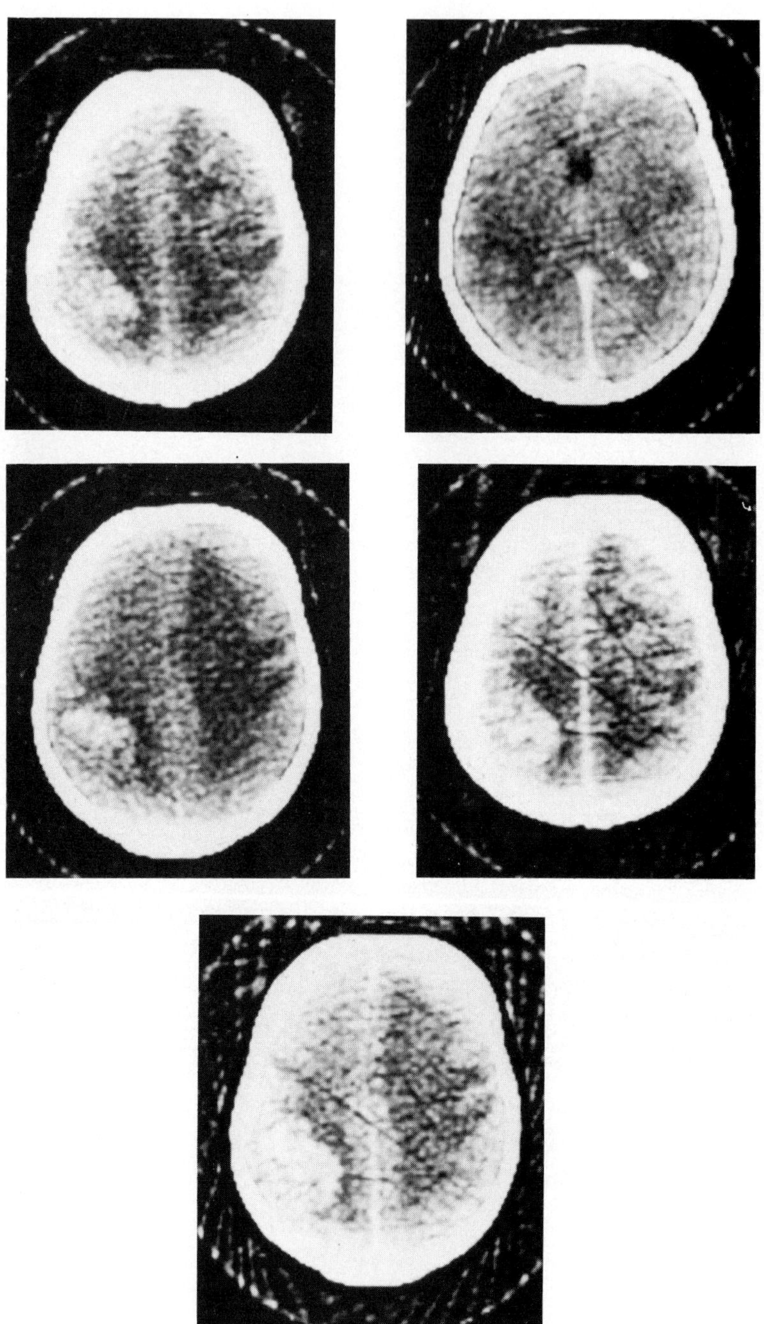

Figure 4–57. SUPERIOR SAGITTAL SINUS THROMBOSIS: With occlusion of the superior sagittal sinus by clot, there are infarcts in the areas of distribution of the superficial cortical veins. In many cases, hemorrhagic infarcts may develop, as are present in this case.

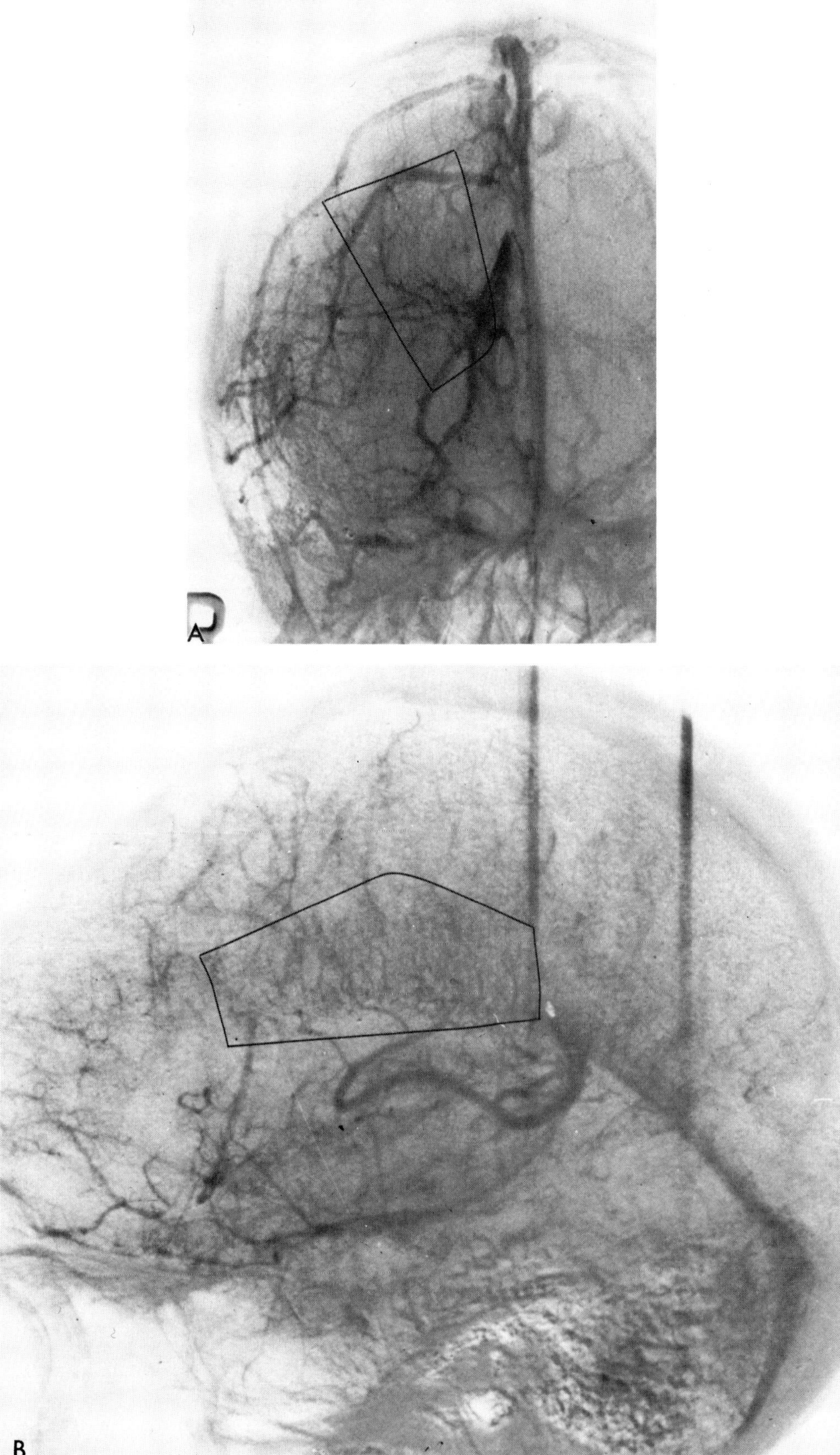

Figure 4–58. MEDULLARY VEINS: These veins have developed secondary to an infarct deep in the cerebral hemisphere. The veins are longer than 1.5 cm, and can be seen draining into the deep venous system on both the AP *(A)* and lateral *(B)* views.

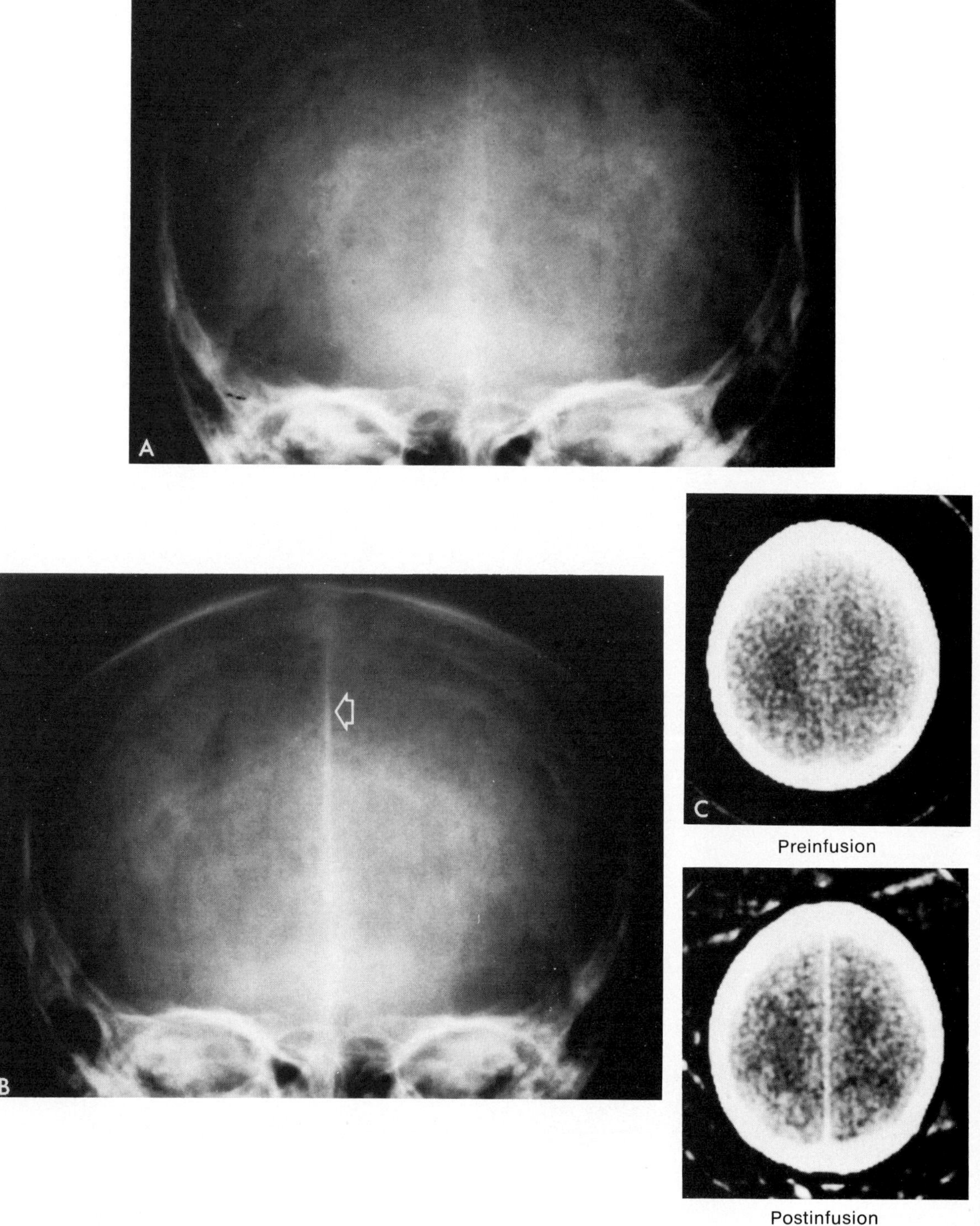

Figure 4–59. BLUSH OF THE FALX: The falx cerebri normally concentrates the contrast material. This is demonstrated on this patient, where the falx is seen on the postinjection film *(arrowhead)*. This phenomenon is also seen on the CT scans.

may also be used for better delineation of the position of such lesions. Of course, in many cases the clinical presentation may supply the answer to the question of where the abnormality is situated.

The main diagnostic difficulty is the question of an occipital pole versus a cerebellar lesion. If one remembers basic neurology, it will be recalled that a *left* homonymous hemianopsia is consistent with a *right* occipital pole lesion and that a *right* homonymous hemianopsia is consistent with a *left* occipital pole lesion. The presence of a visual field defect therefore is quite suggestive of an occipital pole lesion. Ataxia is more suggestive of a cerebellar mass lesion, particularly in the presence of obstructive hydrocephalus or displacement of the fourth ventricle.

SUPRATENTORIAL VENOUS SYSTEM

The venous drainage of the supratentorial system can be roughly divided into superficial and deep venous systems. The deep venous system is of the greatest clinical importance because of the displacements that are caused by mass lesions in various positions in the brain. On the other hand, there are a good many superficial veins that can be of some assistance in diagnosing abnormalities within the cranial vault.

Superficial Veins

Close inspection of any angiogram will show that the superficial cortical veins drain upward for the most part and enter the superior sagittal sinus. In addition to draining in an upward direction, the veins will be seen to enter the superior sagittal sinus in such a fashion that the flow will be against the normal front-to-back flow in the sinus. This pattern of venous drainage occurs because the normal growth and development of the cerebral cortex draws the veins forward. Only two of the superficial veins are of any real consequence: (1) The vein of Trolard is a large superficial cortical vein in the parietal region. It will be seen to drain upward and then forward into the superior sagittal sinus. (2) The vein of Labbé is a superficial cortical vein that drains from the parietal region inferiorly and posteriorly to enter the transverse sinus. To commit the two to memory, one must only recall that "Trolard" begins with a "T," and the vein drains to the *Top*; whereas Labbé begins with "L," and the vein drains to the *L*ateral sinus (transverse sinus) over the *L*ateral aspect of the brain and is *L*ower over the cortex.

The middle cerebral vein, as its name suggests, is formed by a group of superficial tributary veins that drain the middle cerebral artery distribution and course anteriorly and inferiorly to enter the cavernous sinus. Gross vascular displacements are unusual in the superficial venous system, and so these veins do not often provide significant diagnostic value. On the other hand, the neurosurgeon uses these cortical veins as a guide to the position of an underlying mass lesion. These cortical veins provide landmarks for the neurosurgical approach to the area of abnormality.

It will be noted also that the normal sequence of filling of the cortical veins is from the frontal region initially, then progressing posteriorly. When reviewing a serial run of films, this does not mean that the frontal veins will be filled on the first film, the parietal veins on the second film, and so on — but it does mean that the occipital veins should not be filled before filling of the frontal veins. Review of the serial film run may reveal that the cortical veins fill simultaneously. This finding may be normal, or it may imply some slowing of filling in the frontal region. Slow filling of the cortical venous system is a reflection of a localized increase in intracranial pressure that prevents blood from entering the cortical veins. With some mass lesions there will be a total absence of filling of the veins. Such absence of venous filling provides further confirmatory evidence of the presence of a mass lesion.

If the anterior cerebral artery on the side of the injection is occluded, or, more commonly, if an anterior cerebral artery fills from the contralateral carotid artery as a normal variation, there will be poor arterial flow to the frontal region. This poor flow will appear as slow or even absent venous filling in the frontal region. If this is the case, the condition should not be mistaken for evidence of a frontal mass lesion. Because of poor arterial opacification of the frontal region, there will be poor venous opacification — even in the absence of a mass lesion. In these cases, there generally are other signs, such as the presence or absence of a midline shift, that will help one decide whether a mass lesion is present or absent.

Deep Veins

Not many of the deep veins are of major significance in the diagnosis of mass lesions. The internal cerebral veins are of major importance and command our greatest attention. These veins are paired and lie just on either side of the midline. They begin anteriorly at the level of the foramen of Monro and travel in the roof of the third ventricle posteriorly until they terminate in the vein of Galen. The internal cerebral veins are enclosed in the velum interpositum. This is a thin, veil-like membrane that envelops the veins and is of no real significance except that air may sometimes enter between the leaves of the velum interpositum and form what is called a "cavum velum interpositum." On the lateral view it will be seen that the internal cerebral veins will form a gentle hump in the midportion of its course (see Fig. 4–54). Anteriorly, the internal cerebral vein is joined at the level of the foramen of Monro by the thalamostriate vein and the septal vein.

The angiographically visible portion of the thalamostriate vein runs in the floor of the lateral ventricle, and courses gently forward to join the internal cerebral vein at the level of the foramen of Monro. On the anteroposterior view, the thalamostriate vein will be seen to form a curvilinear outline of the body of the lateral ventricle as it curves inferiorly to join the internal cerebral vein. In fact, when one compares the normal brow-up view of a pneumoencephalogram with the anteroposterior view of the angiogram, the correlation between the two is easy to appreciate. The body of the lateral ventricle as it is outlined by air will be seen to correspond with the position of the thalmostriate vein — thus providing the arteriographic and pneumoencephalographic correlation (see Chapter 16).

Also joining the internal cerebral vein at the level of the foramen of Monro is the septal vein. This vein originates in the septum pellucidum and follows a curvilinear course posteriorly to enter the internal cerebral vein. At the level of the junction between the internal cerebral vein and the thalamostriate vein is the anatomic position of the foramen of Monro. This junction and the angle that is formed are known as the "venous angle" (see Fig. 4–52). If the thalmostriate vein enters the internal cerebral vein posterior to the foramen of Monro so that the internal cerebral vein is divided into two segments, making the upward hump smaller than the descending hump, one has a "false venous angle." The significance of the false venous angle is that it no longer marks the foramen of Monro; additionally, the evaluation of hydrocephalus on the anteroposterior venous angiogram can no longer be made. In other words, when judging the presence of hydrocephalus, one must first rule out the presence of a false venous angle.

The paired internal cerebral veins course posteriorly until they join the vein of Galen at the level of the quadrigeminal plate cistern. The unpaired vein of Galen then enters into the straight sinus in the tentorium of the cerebellum at the level of its attachment with the falx cerebri. The straight sinus is also joined by the inferior sagittal sinus at the level of the junction with the vein of Galen.

The internal cerebral vein may be up to 2 mm in diameter. Therefore, when the internal cerebral vein is measured to determine whether there is or is not a shift, the point of measurement should be to the medial side of the vein. The medial side theoretically should lie just lateral to the midline. Up to 2 mm of shift of the internal cerebral vein are accepted as within normal limits.

In addition to the thalamostriate vein, multiple small veins also lie in the floor of the lateral ventricle at different levels. These veins run in the subependymal layer and will, on close inspection, reveal a "Y" shape at their superior margin as they follow the roof of the lateral ventricle. By measuring the height of these subependymal veins as they form the "Y" shape at the top of the ventricle down to the level of the internal cerebral veins, one can obtain an accurate measurement of the size of the lateral ventricle (see Fig. 4–00). The normal ventricular size appears to increase with age. By comparing the anticipated normal size and the measured size one can evaluate the presence of abnormal ventricular enlargement. The lateral vein of the atrium drains the lateral ventricle and enters the internal cerebral vein at the level of the vein of Galen. Since the development of CT scanning these measurements have been de-emphasized, and the reader is referred elsewhere for precise measurements.

The basal vein of Rosenthal (Fig. 4–55) drains the posterior portion of the frontal lobe and the anterior tip of the temporal lobe. The basal vein of Rosenthal is seen arteriographically in both the anteroposterior and lateral projections. The basal vein of Rosenthal is seen to begin deep in the hemisphere at the anatomic level of the anterior perforated substance. This is the same point where the lenticulostriate arteries perforate into the region of the basal ganglia. The vein then courses posteriorly along the medial edge of the hippocampal gyrus of the temporal lobe, where it then follows the free edge of the tentorium and curves around the midbrain in the perimesencephalic (ambient) cistern to enter the vein of Galen. Most of its course is similar to that followed by the posterior cerebral artery; thus, changes in the position of thc posterior cerebral artery are also reflected in changes in the position of the basal vein of Rosenthal. It should also be noted that the third nerve, which arises from the pons and passes forward between the posterior cerebral arteries and the superior cerebellar arteries, follows a similar course. It also is affected in the presence of other mass lesions which affect the adjacent artery and vein. The basal vein lies medial to the temporal horns of the lateral ventricles.

The veins just described represent the major veins that concern us. The deep veins — particularly the midline veins — are of great importance in the diagnosis of mass lesions in the supratentorial region.

Medullary Veins

Medullary veins normally are present but usually are not seen on the normal angiogram except by magnification techniques. They are abnormal if greater than 1.5 cm in length. They are seen with glioblastomas, arteriovenous malformations and infarcts (Fig. 4–58).

CHAPTER 5

THE ABNORMAL ANGIOGRAM

VASCULAR DISPLACEMENTS SECONDARY TO MASS LESIONS

Intracranial mass lesions can cause a variety of abnormal angiographic appearances. In some instances, particularly that of meningiomas, the pattern is quite typical, and the diagnosis can be made with a high degree of certainty from the angiographic appearance alone. For this reason, Chapter 9 has been devoted entirely to meningiomas. Some other tumors also have a relatively characteristic angiographic appearance — particularly the malignant glioblastoma multiforme, which presents with a host of abnormal vessels, early draining veins and marked mass effect. Rarely, however, is it possible to make an unequivocal statement about the histology of a specific mass from the angiogram alone. The development of computed tomography has added greatly to our ability to diagnose the nature of a mass; in certain entities the CT scan has decreased or eliminated the need for angiography. This is especially true in patients who have had cerebral trauma or have suffered an intracerebral hemorrhage. In these, the need for angiography has been nearly eliminated. On the other hand, in other disease entities angiography and computed tomography are complementary techniques.

The present chapter on the abnormal angiogram first offers a general overview of the various disease processes and their anticipated histologic, plain skull, angiographic and computed tomographic findings. Then, illustrations are provided to demonstrate the variety of vascular displacement patterns seen with mass lesions in several supratentorial anatomic locations. Mass lesions in these various locations tend to provoke typical patterns of shift of arterial and venous structures. The author has attempted to correlate the angiograms with corresponding CT scans whenever possible. The CT scans follow the angiograms in most cases so that the reader can "test" his or her diagnostic acumen before correlation with the CT scan. Because a variety of lesions can be seen in a given anatomic site, these cases have been grouped by location rather than by disease process.

Typical or classic cases have been chosen whenever possible. The angiogram and CT scan are from the same patient when possible, and from a very similar patient when corresponding studies were not available.

GLIOBLASTOMA MULTIFORME

Glioblastomas are malignant tumors of astrocytic origin. The tumors usually have a rapidly progressive course, leading to death. They are encountered in all age groups, but their incidence decreases after the age of 40. After surgical removal, glioblastomas recur in the bed of the surgical site, and have rapid local extension. These tumors may rarely metastasize outside the central nervous system.

Not infrequently the patients present with the adult onset of a seizure disorder; a progressive hemiparesis is fairly common. If located in a relatively "silent" area, such as the frontal lobes, the tumor may become quite large before there is any apparent problem. In point of fact, however, it seems that glioblastomas commonly are quite large at the time of initial presentation.

Pathology. These tumors are highly pleomorphic. There are polygonal cells with mitotic figures, some with multinucleated giant cells, fusiform cells with pseudopalisades and areas of necrosis, astroblasts in perivascular pseudorosettes and a variety of astrocytes. The tumors invade the corpus callosum and grow across the midline to the opposite side, demonstrating a "butterfly" pattern of growth. Areas of necrosis are also commonly seen in these tumors as their rapid growth exceeds the blood supply.

Plain Skull. There may be a shift of the pineal gland to the contralateral side. Usually the growth of the tumor is so fast that the patient becomes clinically symptomatic before the secondary changes of increased intracranial pressure can develop. Rarely, areas of calcification may be seen.

Computed Tomography. The preinfusion scan usually demonstrates a poorly defined low density area of varying size associated with shift of the midline to the contralateral side. There may rarely be scattered areas of calcification and/or hemorrhage. The area of involvement often is surprisingly large, even in a patient with minimal symptomatology. On the other hand, it is not uncommon to have a patient who is symptomatic demonstrate a normal CT scan initially — only to return in 6 weeks to 6 months with a spectacularly abnormal scan.

After the infusion of contrast material there is commonly an irregular ring of enhancement with a lucent center — apparently secondary to tumor necrosis in some cases — and a varying amount of surrounding edema. Less commonly, there is homogeneous enhancement of the tumor mass, also with varying degrees of surrounding edema. Rarely there will be no demonstrable areas of enhancement on the postinfusion scan.

Angiography. These tumors usually are supplied by branches of the internal carotid artery. Rarely they may demonstrate blood supply from the external carotid system. They may present as avascular masses or very vascular tumors with large feeding arteries and early draining veins. The presence of neovascularity and early draining veins, particularly with drainage into the deep venous system, usually correlates with a high degree of malignancy. Frequently the size of the tumor mass as reflected by the abnormal vessels is much smaller than the mass effect, reflecting a large amount of surrounding edema.

If there is no neovascularity to demonstrate the true position of the tumor, one of the great benefits of the CT scan is that it can show the true anatomic location of the tumor relative to the surrounding edema, which not uncommonly is asymmetric in its distribution around the tumor. In demonstrating the anatomic location more accurately, the CT scan aids in treatment planning, whether it be surgery or radiation therapy.

OLIGODENDROGLIOMA

These tumors are rare, usually occur in adults and, of all brain tumor types, are reported to be calcified in the highest percentage of cases. Oligodendrogliomas not uncommonly contain areas of calcification which can be seen by plain skull radiography and are readily demonstrated by CT scanning. In addition, oligodendrogliomas may also contain areas of hemorrhage — again readily demonstrable by CT scan.

ASTROCYTOMAS

These are tumors of astrocytes — the supporting cells of the brain. They are seen at all ages but are less common after 40. Astrocytomas are relatively benign brain tumors and are found in all parts of the central nervous system. They can rarely be removed entirely at surgery and frequently undergo malignant transformation.

Histology. These tumors are made up of astrocytes; frequently they demonstrate either gross or microscopic evidence of cyst formation. There may also be perivascular cuffs of lymphocytes. It is important to remember that astrocytomas lack: (1) areas of necrosis and hemorrhage; (2) capillary endothelial proliferation; (3) cellular pleomorphism; (4) mitotic figures. Evidence of any of these four characteristics may signify the presence of a glioblastoma. Therefore, a limited surgical biopsy might not include a more abnormal area and would not reflect the true nature of the tumor.

Computed Tomography. These tumors may demonstrate areas of calcification and not uncommonly are cystic. Areas of either central or peripheral calcification may be seen.

Astrocytomas of the cerebellum are discussed in Chapter 14. Brain stem gliomas are also included in that chapter.

EPENDYMOMAS

These tumors arise from ependymal cells and may occur in any part of the ventricular system. They also sometimes develop from the ependymal lining of the central canal of the spinal cord. They may contain areas of calcification.

CHOROID PLEXUS PAPILLOMAS

These tumors, which arise from the normal choroid plexus, are very similar in histologic appearance to normal tissue. They are rare and usually are found in children. Positional headaches may be the presenting complaint if a tumor blocks the foramen of Monro and causes obstructive hydrocephalus when the head is in a certain position. They may be associated with an excessive production of cerebrospinal fluid.

COLLOID CYSTS

These cystic tumors arise from the anterior part of the third ventricle and frequently cause obstructive hydrocephalus because of obstruction of the foramen of Monro. They are rounded and isodense or demonstrate increased density on the preinfusion CT scan. However, they enhance homogeneously on the postinfusion scan.

METASTASES

Patients of any age group may present with cerebral metastases. The finding of multiple lesions support the diagnosis of metastases, although it is not uncommon to see a solitary metastatic lesion. On the other hand some primary brain tumors such as the microglioma may develop from multiple sites. In an active clinical practice there is rarely a day that passes that one does not see an example of multiple brain metastases. This is the most common type of brain tumor that is seen (see section on Metastases).

Plain Skull. The routine skull series usually is normal. There may be a shift of the pineal gland, but, if the metastases are multiple and "balancing," there will be no shift of the midline structures. Multiple metastatic deposits also may be found in the bony calvaria.

Computed Tomography. The CT scan with infusion is the most efficient and accurate method of demonstrating the presence of metastatic lesions. The CT scan should be performed both with and without the infusion of contrast material, although after the diagnosis is established the patient's response to treatment may be followed with a postinfusion scan only. Lesions may be seen on the postinfusion scan that cannot be identified on the preinfusion scan. In such patients the preinfusion scan may be normal or there may be an increased number of metastatic lesions demonstrated on the postinfusion scan. This finding may alter the approach to treatment.

Metastatic nodules may be isodense, lucent or of greater density than the normal brain. They may even present a combination of these findings. Metastatic squamous cell carcinoma tends to be of lower than normal brain density, whereas metastatic adenocarcinoma shows higher than normal density. These lesions may or may not be space-occupying; there may be no edema or spectacular surrounding edema. They usually are distributed homogeneously, but may be of a "ring" type. At times differentiation from a primary brain tumor is impossible — especially when only a solitary metastatic deposit is present.

The bony calvaria may be evaluated for metastases by reviewing the standard cuts at high window width and window level. The skull film is more accurate for diagnosis of metastases.

Angiography. Multiple lesions may be demonstrated angiographically, but far less accurately than by CT scan. The lesions may be avascular, or they may demonstrate abnormal vascularity with early draining views. Generally speaking, if multiple lesions consistent with metastases are demonstrated by other means, angiography is not performed as part of the work-up. However, with a solitary lesion, or when the diagnosis is in doubt, angiography may be performed to aid in diagnosis. The mass or masses may be avascular, demonstrating only vessel displacement and a shift to the contralateral side. On the other hand, metastatic lesions may demonstrate neovascularity, with an abnormal accumulation of vessels and early draining veins. At times, differentiation from a glioma may be difficult — especially with a solitary mass — regardless of whether it is avascular or demonstrates abnormal vessels. With balancing lesions, there may be little or no shift of the midline structures.

ABSCESS

Abscesses usually are caused by pyogenic bacteria, which may spread from middle ear infections, sinusitis, mastoiditis or from hematogenous spread. The latter occurs most often with endocarditis or intravenous drug abuse. A history of recent dental manipulation is not uncommon. Brain abscesses may act as a mass lesion in the same way as any other mass. Rupture into the ventricular system may cause death. Multiple abscesses are occasionally seen — especially in association with subacute bacterial endocarditis.

Plain Skull. The plain skull examination usually is normal, but it may show a shift of the pineal gland if there is sufficient mass effect. The source of infection, e.g., sinus or ear, may be visible by plain film examination.

Actually, it is impossible to differentiate with absolute certainty between an abscess or a glioblastoma in most cases. A high index of suspicion is helpful in diagnosis.

Arteriography. Most commonly there is an avascular mass; however, a capsular stain may be seen, and rarely a thick-walled, prolonged capsular stain may be visualized that persists into the venous phase. With multiple abscesses the arteriogram will reflect this finding, showing stretching of vessels in separate areas and scattered areas of capsular stain —a sign typical of abscess formation. Early draining veins also may be seen.

Computed Tomography. Typically, there is a large irregular area of radiolucency associated with a shift of the ventricular system to the contralateral side. In the rare case of multiple abscesses, scattered low-density areas are seen. The areas of lucency have irregular margins; rarely, the higher density rim of the actual abscess may be visible within the area of radiolucency, even on the preinfusion scan. Postinfusion, there is enhancement in a ring pattern that usually demonstrates a thick-walled rim of enhancement surrounded by edema. Occasionally, there is a multilobulated pattern of enhancement in one area or multiple separate rings of enhancement.

If there is a cerebritis without actual abscess formation, there may not be any evidence of enhancement — only an area of radiolucency that may or may not demonstrate mass effect.

MEDULLARY VEINS

These veins, which drain the white matter, are normally present but usually are not visible at arteriography. With magnification and subtraction techniques, it is sometimes possible to demonstrate the medullary veins, even in the normal individual. In the normal state, these very numerous veins are less than 1.5 cm long and are very fine vascular structures that run parallel to each other. They drain into the deep veins around the walls of the lateral ventricles. At times, these veins will outline the position of the lateral ventricle.

The medullary veins become enlarged in the presence of arteriovenous malformations, glioblastoma multiforme or infarction. Abnormal medullary veins can be seen on routine arteriography because they are enlarged and longer than 1.5 cm.

THE ABNORMAL ANGIOGRAM

Each mass lesion in the various lobes of the brain and in the region of the basal ganglia, the pituitary and the midline structures demonstrates a relatively typical pattern of vascular displacement. The following pages offer discussions and summaries of the types of arterial and venous displacement that may be seen with a space-occupying lesion in these various positions. The reader must remember that it is not uncommon for a mass to cross over these boundaries; thus, each angiographic appearance usually cannot be absolutely categorized into an individual lobar position. However, an attempt has been made in the following illustrations to categorize these lesions by anatomic location and to demonstrate the "classic" vascular dislocations that occur. The section on mass lesions has been divided into anatomic locations without regard to histologic type. Whenever possible, each case is correlated with the corresponding CT scan or with a scan from a similar patient.

If the reader commits to memory the anticipated vascular dislocations caused by the various space-occupying lesions, an individual angiogram can be evaluated and interpreted without a great deal of difficulty. One must keep in mind that it is a rare lesion that can be diagnosed with certainty by its angiographic appearance alone. The differential diagnosis should be an important part of the interpretation of each angiogram, even when a CT scan is also available.

FRONTAL LOBE MASS LESIONS

When a mass is present in the frontal lobe there is displacement of the anterior cerebral artery to the contralateral side. Because the mass is anteriorly placed, most of the effect on the anterior cerebral artery will be on its proximal portion. This results in a rounded appearance of the vessel as it is displaced across the midline on the AP arteriographic views. This has been called a "round shift of the anterior cerebral artery," but could also be called a "proximal shift" of the artery. Before the vessel returns to the ipsilateral side of the falx, the pericallosal artery returns to a more normal position, so that there is not an abrupt shift under the falx. An anteriorly placed mass lesion also creates little or no displacement of the internal cerebral vein because it is remote from the anatomic position of the vein. If there is any shift of the internal cerebral vein, it will certainly be less than the shift of the anterior cerebral artery.

By using this approach to diagnosis of the

Text continued on page 231

Figure 5–1. FRONTAL LOBE ABSCESS: *A*, The AP view demonstrates a greater shift of the proximal than the distal portion of the anterior cerebral artery. Note that the falx cerebri is displaced to the contralateral side. The anticipated normal position is marked by the dotted line.

B, The early arterial lateral view shows posterior displacement of the anterior cerebral artery *(arrows)*, which also demonstrates some areas of narrowing. There is an avascular area in the frontal region. The anterior meningeal artery as it arises from the ophthalmic artery is also enlarged *(white arrows)*.

C, The capillary phase of the angiogram demonstrates a capsular blush *(arrowheads)* with a lucent center.

D, CT scans from a different patient demonstrate a thick-walled, rounded mass in the frontal region that has a radiolucent center and is surrounded by edema. The edema is quite marked and has an irregular distribution. There is marked shift to the contralateral side. There is distortion of the right frontal horn and dilatation of the left lateral ventricle. The postinfusion scan demonstrates marked enhancement of the thick rim of the abscess.

Differential diagnosis includes primary glioma and metastatic tumor.

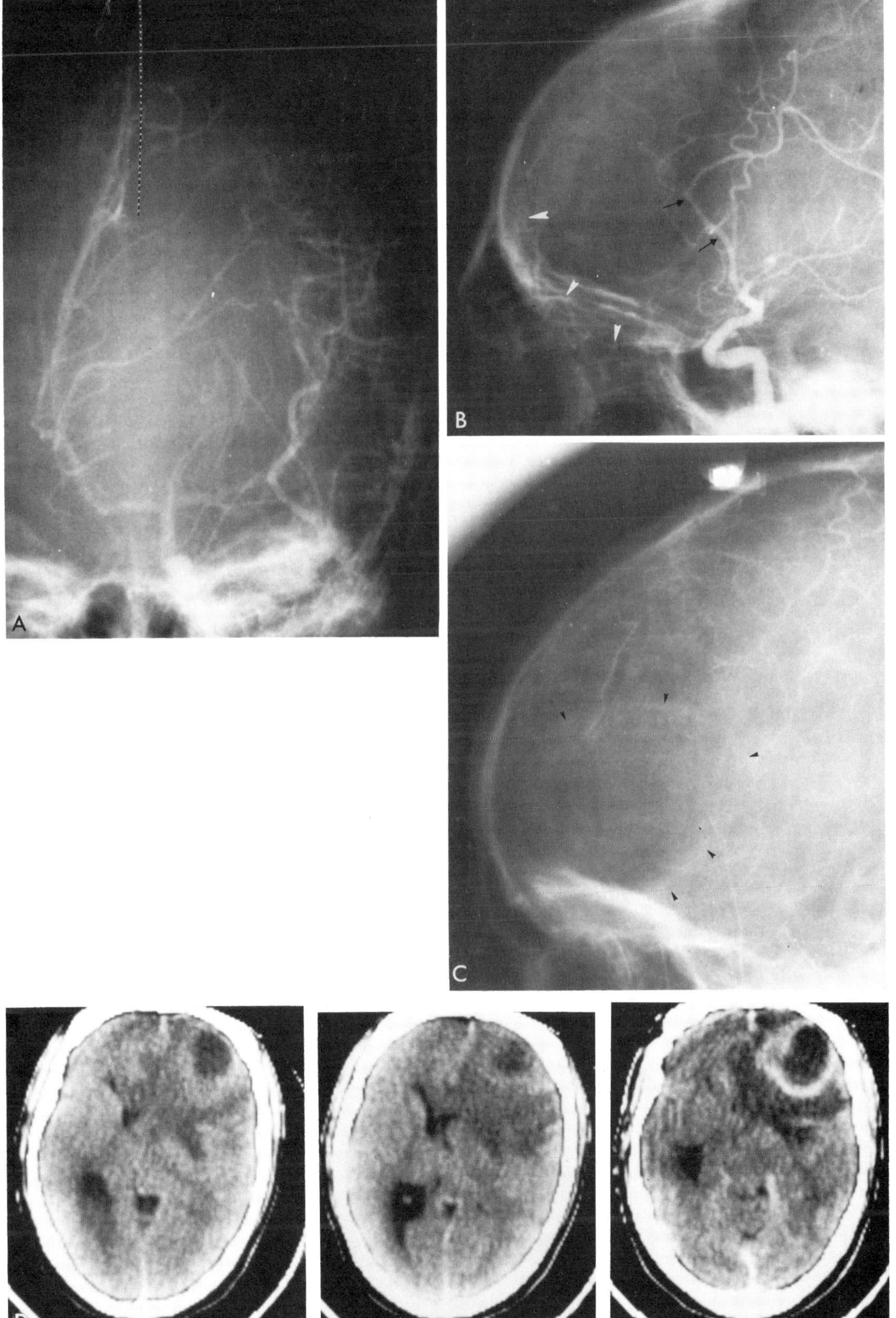

Figure 5–1. *See legend on the opposite page.*

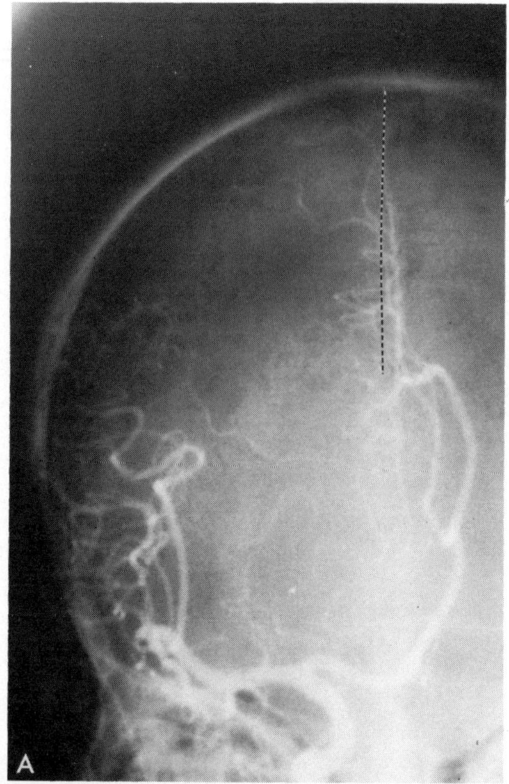

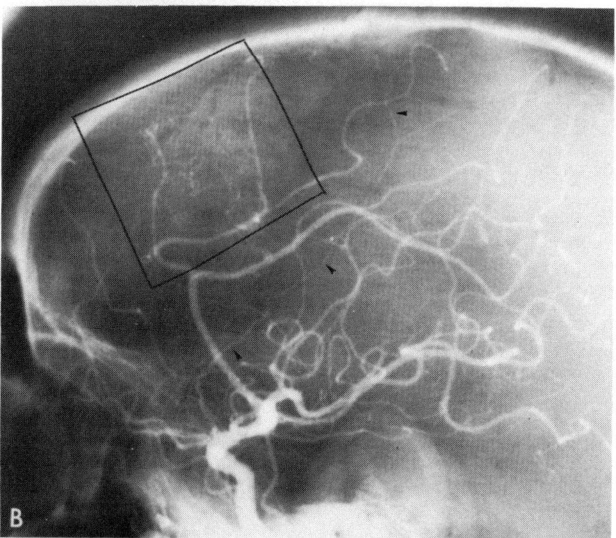

Figure 5–2. FRONTAL GLIOBLASTOMA MULTIFORME: *A*, In the AP view a shift of the pericallosal artery is more marked distally than in its proximal portion. The pericallosal artery demonstrates a sharp angulation under the falx *(dotted line)*, which is displaced to the left of the midline.

B, The lateral view reveals an area of neovascularity *(black lines)* with inferior displacement of the pericallosal artery and sylvian triangle. There is posterior displacement of the sylvian triangle. The middle meningeal artery is prominent *(small black arrows)* because of increased flow into the external carotid system due to increased intracranial pressure.

In addition to glioblastoma, the differential diagnosis includes metastasis.

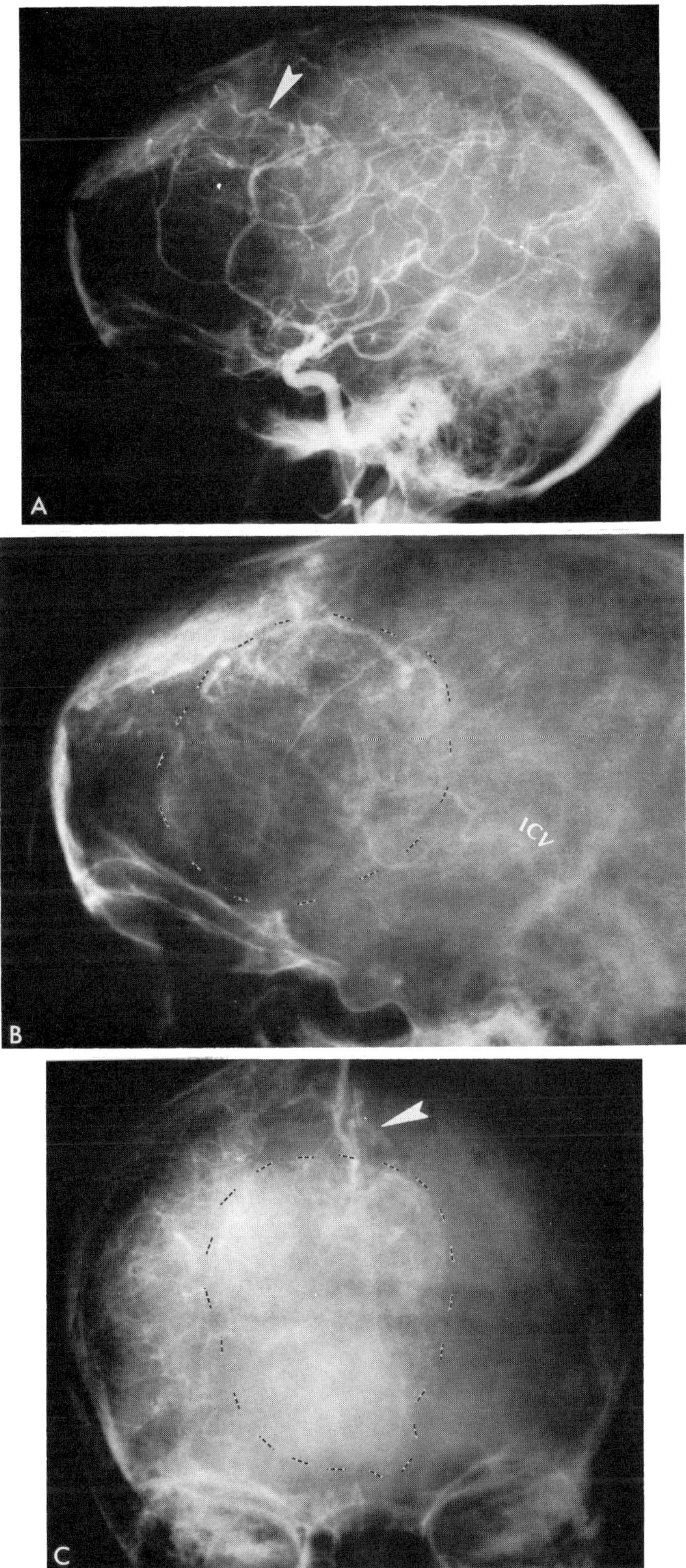

Figure 5–3. *See legend on the following page*

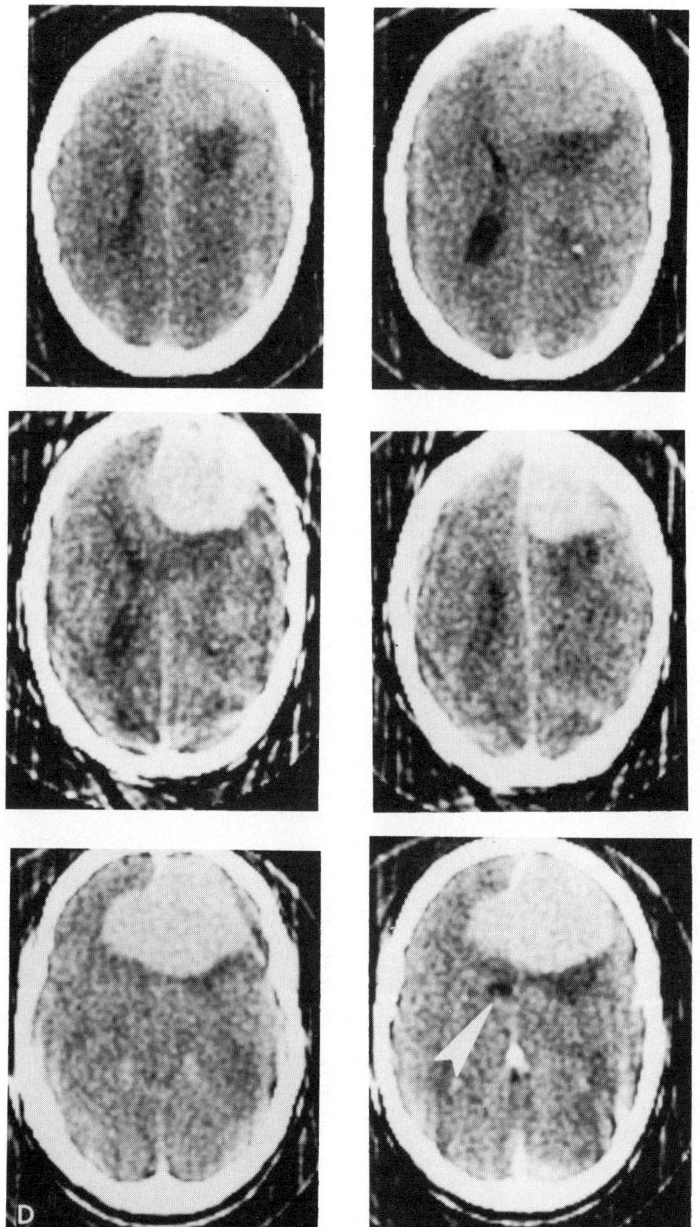

Figure 5–3. GLIOBLASTOMA MULTIFORME WITH EXTENSION VIA THE CORPUS CALLOSUM: *A*, In the lateral arteriogram there is evidence of neovascularity in the midfrontal region. Irregularity of the branches of the callosal marginal and pericallosal arteries also is evident in this region. There is downward displacement of the pericallosal artery. An early draining vein is seen in the high parasagittal region *(white arrow)*.

B, The late capillary phase demonstrates a large tumor mass with a diffuse tumor stain *(dotted lines)* and multiple draining veins. The internal cerebral vein is displaced and buckled posteriorly *(ICV)*.

C, The AP view demonstrates the deep blush *(dotted lines)* and the early draining vein in the high parasagittal region *(white arrow)*. Note that the tumor extends contralaterally across the midline.

Legend continued on the opposite page

Figure 5–3. *Continued*

D, CT scans reveal a large tumor of slightly higher density than normal brain tissue in the right frontal region. The mass extends across the midline. An area of edema extends around the tumor posteriorly. There is compression of the body of the right lateral ventricle and distortion of the frontal horns of the ventricular system. The postinfusion scan shows marked homogeneous enhancement of the tumor mass, which can be seen to extend across the midline. The frontal horns are displaced far posteriorly *(white arrowhead)*. The true extent of the tumor and its extension across the midline via the corpus callosum can be readily demonstrated on the CT scan.

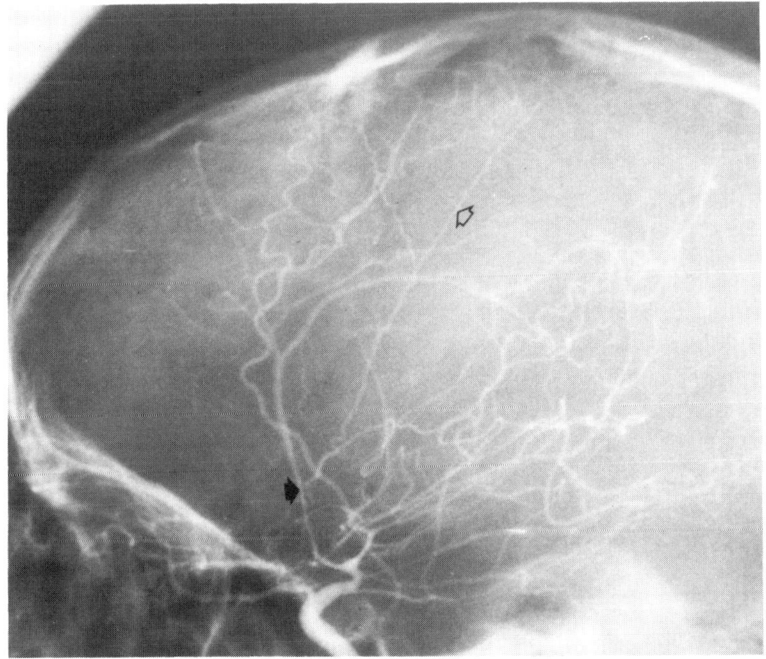

Figure 5–4. BIFRONTAL INTRACEREBRAL HEMATOMA: This angiogram demonstrates both straightening and posterior displacement of the pericallosal artery, as well as spasm of the proximal position of the vessel *(closed arrowhead)*. There is a large avascular area in the frontal region. The sylvian triangle is telescoped posteriorly. The spasm of the vessel is caused by blood in the subarachnoid space, which may be secondary to the intracerebral hematoma or may occur independently. Note also the excessive filling of the middle meningeal artery *(open arrowhead)* and the superficial temporal branch of the external carotid artery. This filling is secondary to the increased intracranial pressure, which does not allow filling of the internal carotid circulation. The AP view (not shown) demonstrated no shift of the midline because the hematoma is bilateral and symmetrical.

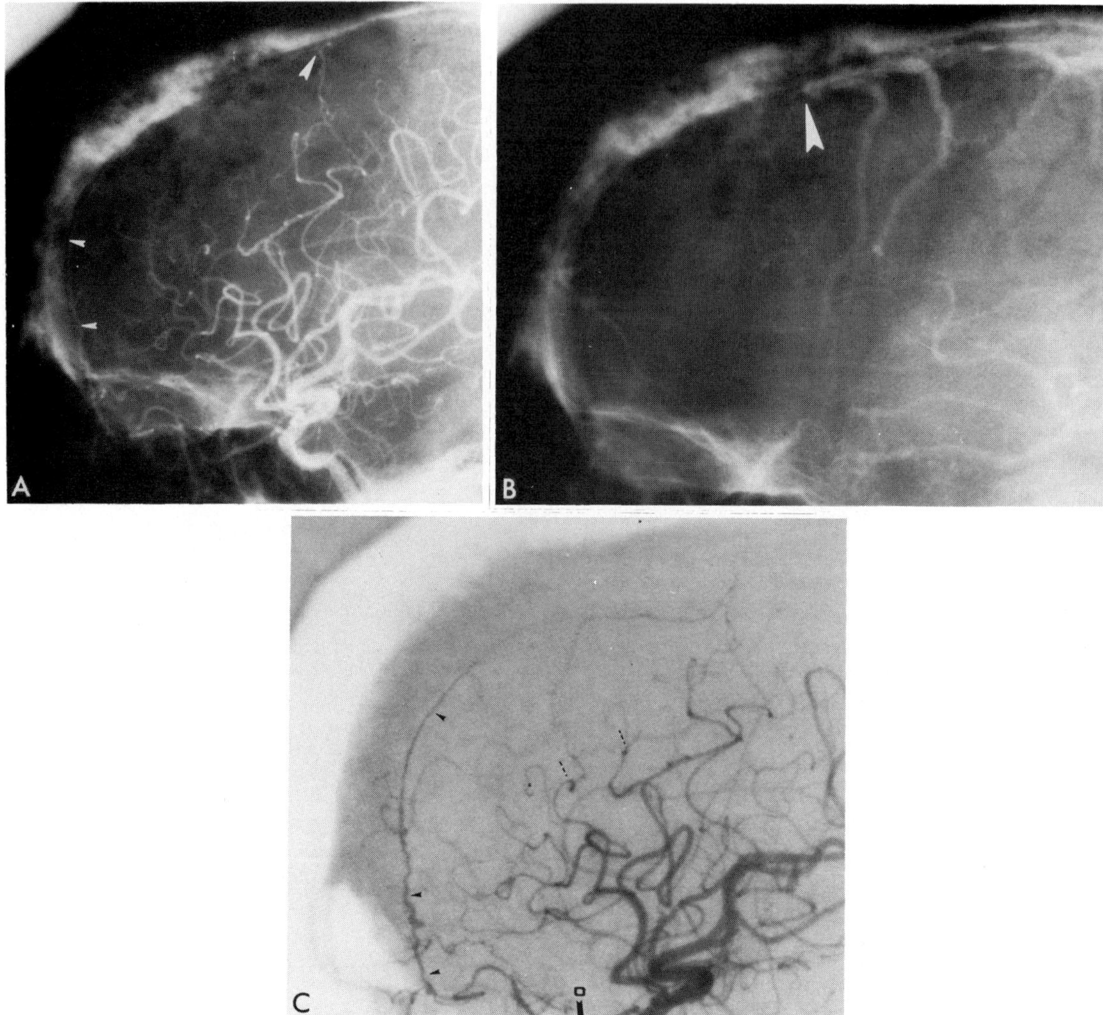

Figure 5–5. METASTASES TO THE CALVARIA AND FRONTAL REGION: An irregular lytic and blastic metastatic process involves the frontal bone of this skull. *A,* The angiogram demonstrates both an enlarged middle meningeal artery *(large arrow)* and enlarged anterior meningeal artery, which arises from the ophthalmic artery *(small arrows).* These vessels supply the tumor, which involves the meninges in the frontal region.

B, The venous phase demonstrates invasion of the superior sagittal sinus *(arrow)* and a large avascular area, both in the frontal region. The pericallosal artery fills from the opposite carotid artery.

C, The subtraction view better demonstrates the enlarged anterior meningeal artery *(black arrows),* which is dilated and tortuous and arises from the ophthalmic artery *(O).* The frontal opercular branches of the middle cerebral artery are attenuated and displaced inferiorly by the tumor in the frontal region *(dashed lines).*

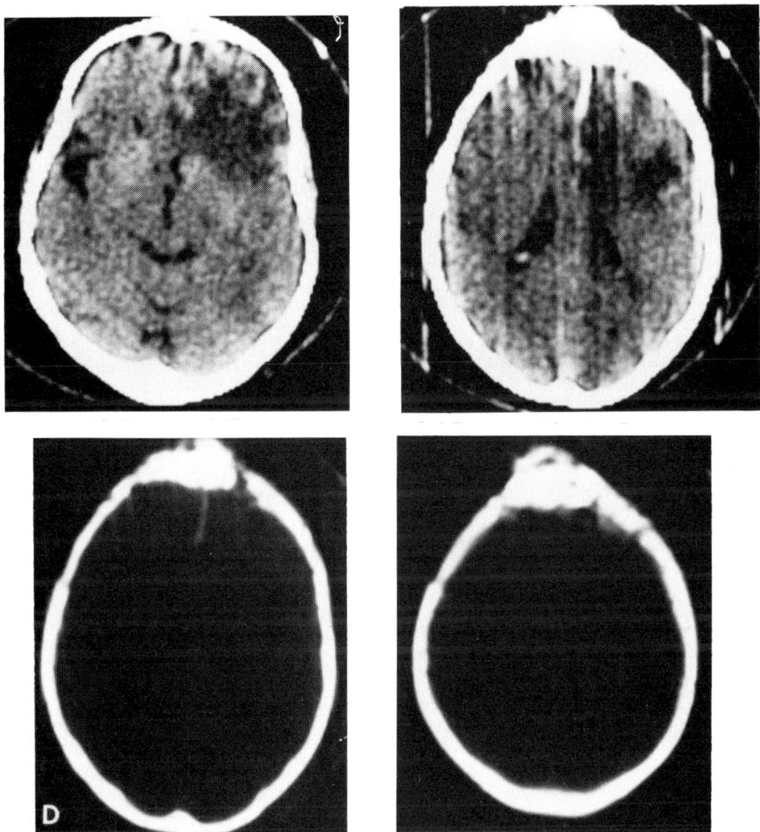

Figure 5–5. *Continued*

D, The CT scans reveal the irregular metastatic deposit involving the frontal bone bilaterally. They also demonstrate the edema in the frontal region, mainly on the right side, which is secondary to intracranial tumor extension. There is posterior displacement of the right frontal horn, compression of the body of the right lateral ventricle and minimal shift of the midline to the contralateral side.

The CT scan at high window widths and window levels demonstrates the involvement by the metastatic tumor, which is both osteoblastic and osteolytic.

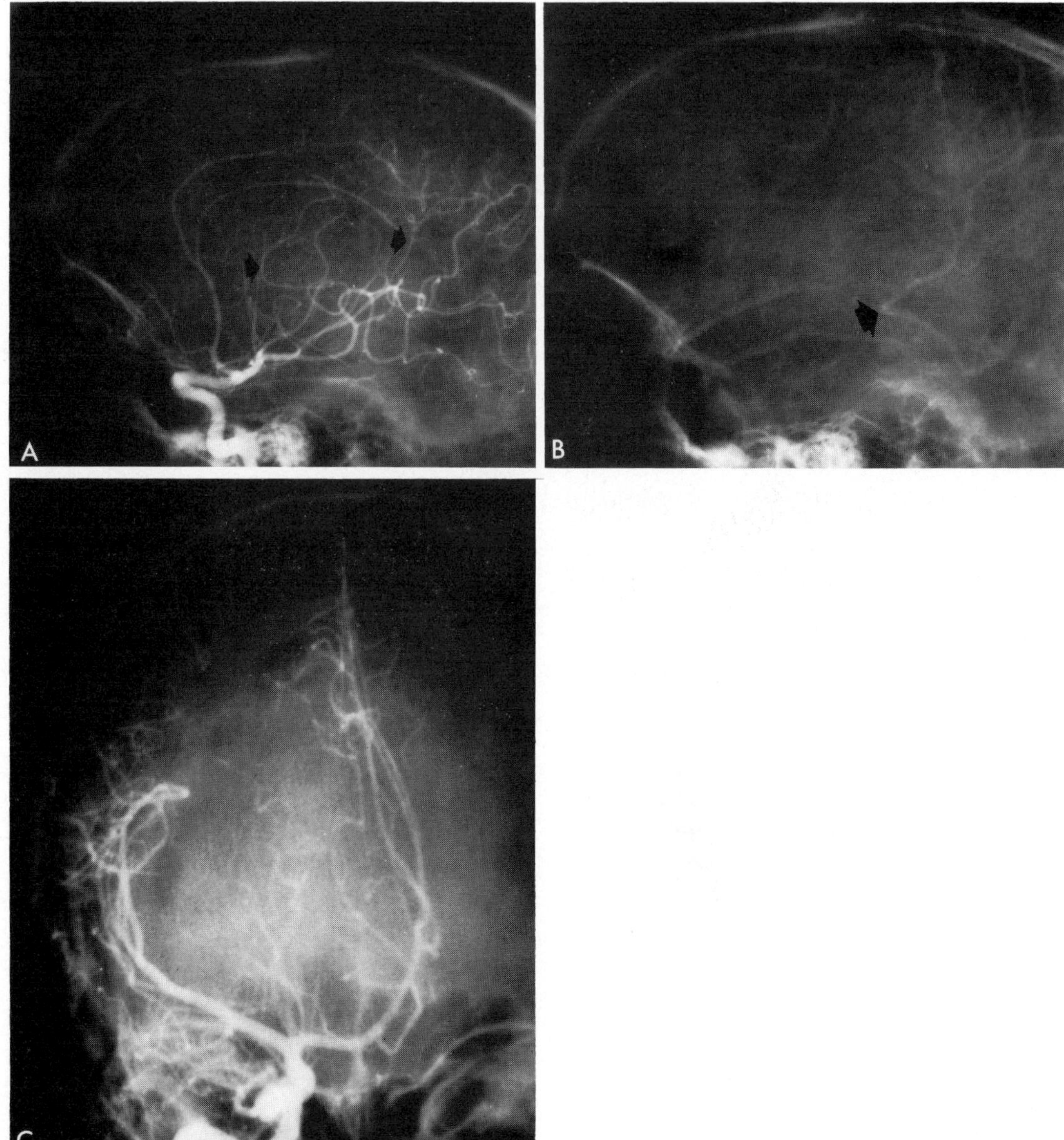

Figure 5–6. *See legend on the opposite page*

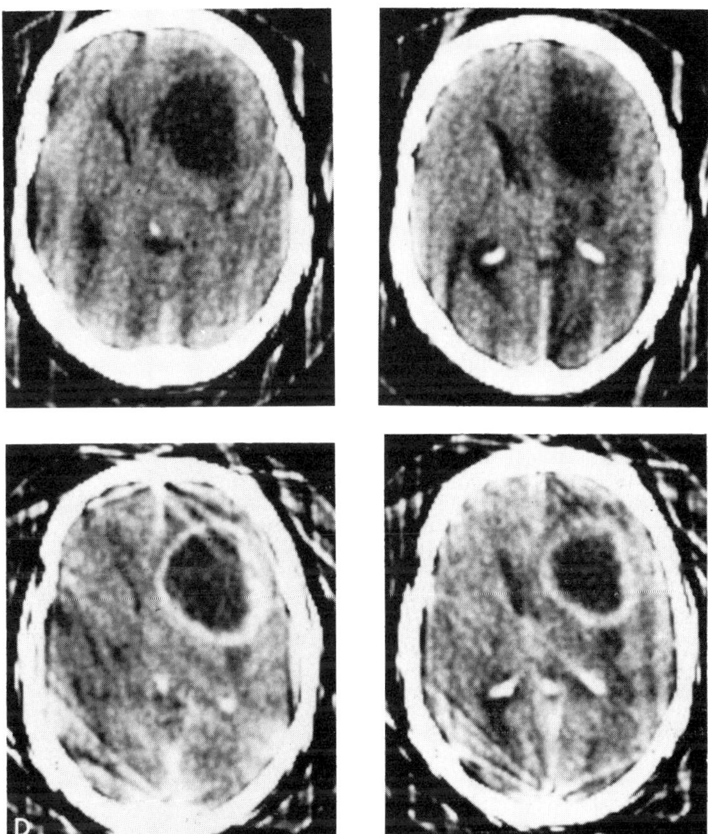

Figure 5–6. RIGHT FRONTAL PARIETAL METASTASIS: *A*, The late arterial phase of the angiogram demonstrates posterior telescoping of the sylvian triangle and stretching of all the vessels in the frontal and parietal opercular regions *(arrows)*. The sylvian triangle is displaced inferiorly.

B, The venous phase shows a closed venous angle *(arrow)* that is displaced posteriorly. There is a large avascular area in the frontal region.

C, The AP view discloses a proximal and distal shift of the pericallosal artery under the falx cerebri.

D, The AP venous phase demonstrates that the thalamostriate vein is displaced to the contralateral side *(small arrows)*, as is the venous angle *(large arrow)*. The internal cerebral vein courses superiorly and then inferiorly, returning to the midline at the junction with the vein of Galen *(dashed line)*.

E, CT scans show a large, well defined low density lesion in the right frontal region with marked shift to the contralateral side. The density of the fluid within the mass is higher than that of the cerebrospinal fluid. The postinfusion scan demonstrates a thick, slightly irregular rim of enhancement around the periphery of the mass. At surgery this proved to be a metastatic lesion with central necrosis.

The differential diagnosis includes glioblastoma and abscess.

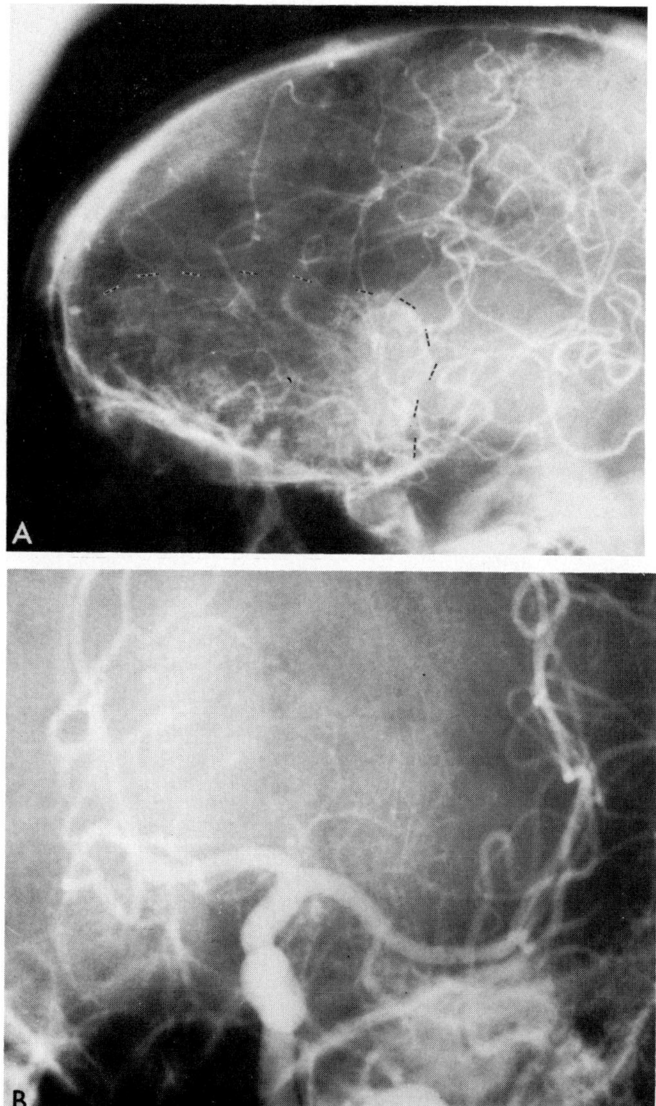

Figure 5–7. FRONTAL GLIOBLASTOMA: *A,* The lateral view reveals a large tumor stain above the roof of the orbit that extends from the frontal region to the level of the sella turcica *(dotted lines).* There are myriad small vessels, and the appearance is not unlike that of an orbital roof meningioma. There is posterior telescoping of the sylvian triangle.

B, The AP view demonstrates a proximal shift of the anterior cerebral artery and its branches; it also shows the multiple small vessels that project over the horizontal portion of the middle cerebral artery.

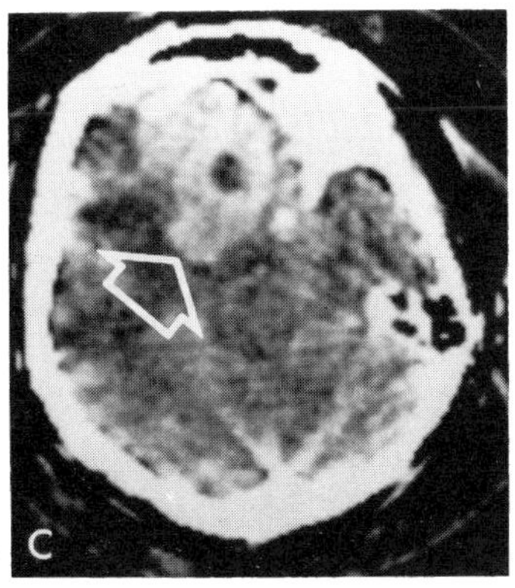

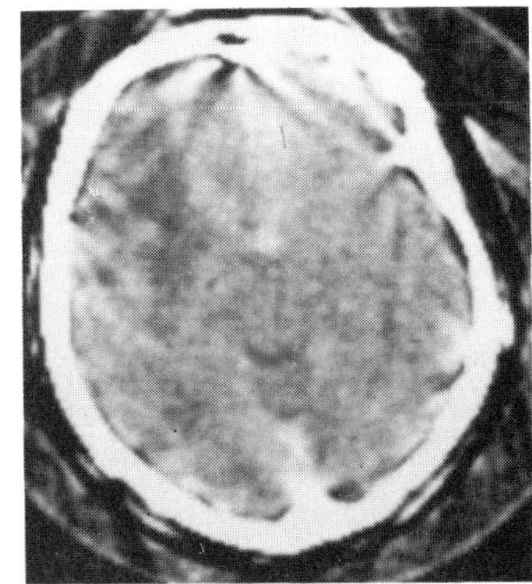

Figure 5–7. *Continued*

C, The CT scans (postinfusion only is available) demonstrate a large area of enhancement in the left low frontal region *(arrow)* which has a small central lucency of unknown etiology. The higher cut shows the abnormality more faintly and reveals some surrounding edema along the left side of the mass. The scan is greatly degraded by patient motion artifact.

The differential diagnosis includes metastasis with a necrotic center.

position of the mass, the observer should be able to determine the position of the mass before proceeding to the lateral view. In other words, if the pericallosal artery is shifted more than the internal cerebral vein, the mass is anterior in position.

The lateral view will not reveal the normal undulations of the anterior cerebral artery because the vessel is stretched as it is displaced from its normal plane toward the contralateral side. Depending on the intrinsic vascularity of the mass, one will find an avascular area in the frontal lobe region with stretching of the vessels in the frontal region together with evidence of poor or delayed venous filling secondary to localized increased intracranial pressure. Depending on the size of the mass, there may or may not be posterior displacement of the branches of the middle cerebral artery group. Most frequently, if there is any change it will be seen at the anterior portion of the sylvian triangle, leading to posterior displacement and posterior telescoping of the triangle.

The venous phase of the lateral view reveals that there is closing of the venous angle — i.e., the thalamostriate vein is displaced posteriorly and downward closer to the internal cerebral vein, making a more acute or "closed" venous angle. There is also posterior displacement of the venous angle and poor venous filling in the frontal region.

In summary, the angiographic findings with a frontal lobe mass lesion are:

AP View.

1. Proximal shift of the anterior cerebral artery.
2. Less shift of the internal cerebral vein.

Lateral View.

3. Disruption of the anterior portion of the sylvian triangle.
4. Posterior displacement of the sylvian point and posterior telescoping of the sylvian triangle.
5. Posterior displacement of the venous angle and a closed venous angle.
6. An area of avascularity in the frontal region.
7. Delayed filling of the frontal veins.

Subfrontal mass lesions and their pattern of vascular displacement are discussed in Chapter 9.

Text continued on page 244

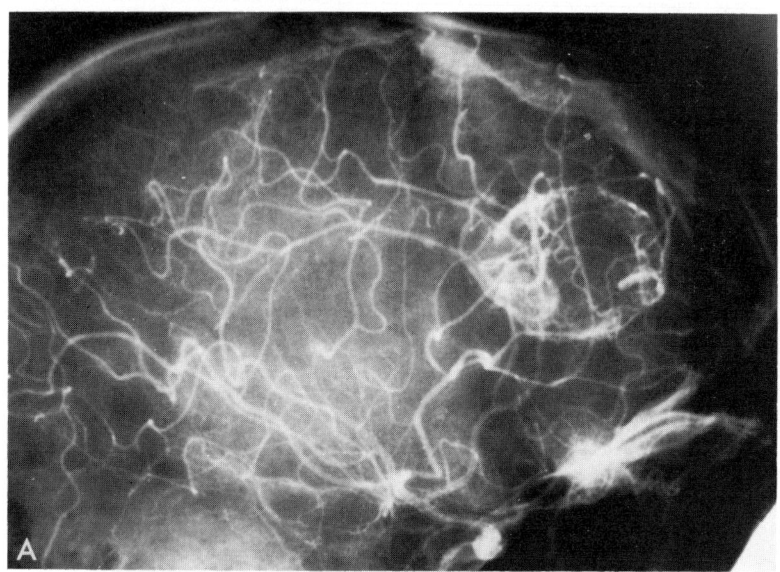

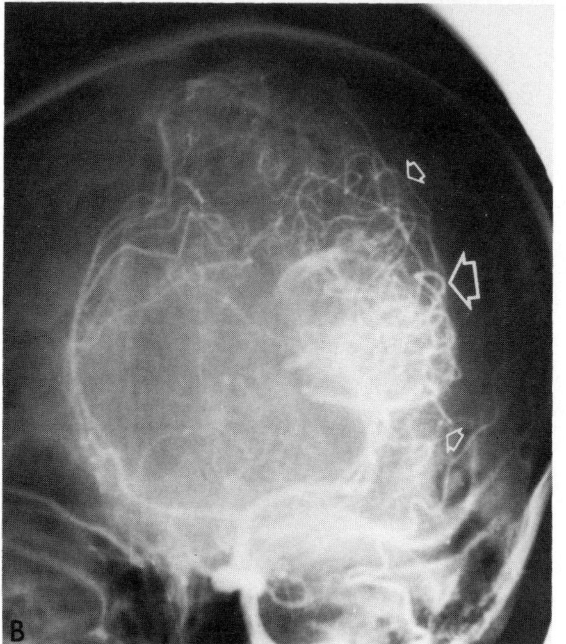

Figure 5–8. METASTASES AND CHRONIC SUBDURAL HEMATOMA: *A,* The lateral angiographic view reveals a large vascular mass lesion of the frontal region. There is stretching of all the vessels in the frontal region and stretching of the vessels of the middle cerebral artery as well. Marked inferior and posterior displacement of the sylvian triangle is evident. *B,* The AP view demonstrates the large vascular mass and also reveals the presence of a large avascular area (*arrows*) over the cerebral hemisphere, where the branches of the middle cerebral artery fail to meet the inner table of the skull. There is marked proximal and distal shift of the pericallosal artery to the contralateral side.

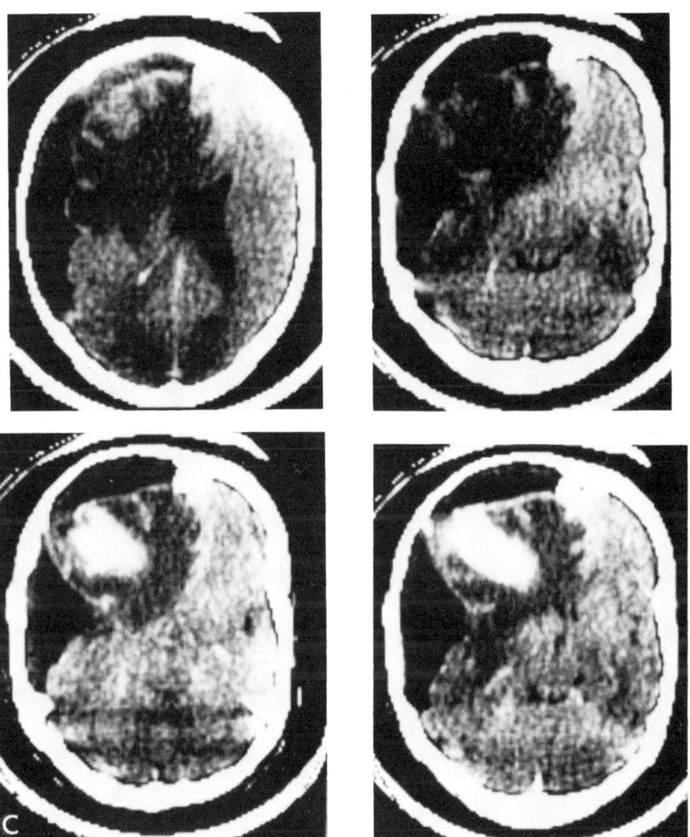

Figure 5–8. *Continued*

C, The CT scans demonstrate a large irregular area of lucency on the left frontal lobe associated with marked shift of the midline to the contralateral side. In addition, there is a large low density accumulation of fluid over the left cerebral hemisphere in both the frontal and parietal regions that appears to be lobulated. The postinfusion scan shows pronounced homogeneous enhancement of the metastatic lesion in the left frontal region with marked surrounding edema; it also reveals a thin-walled membrane around the chronic, lobulated subdural hematoma. (Case courtesy of Dr. David Neer.)

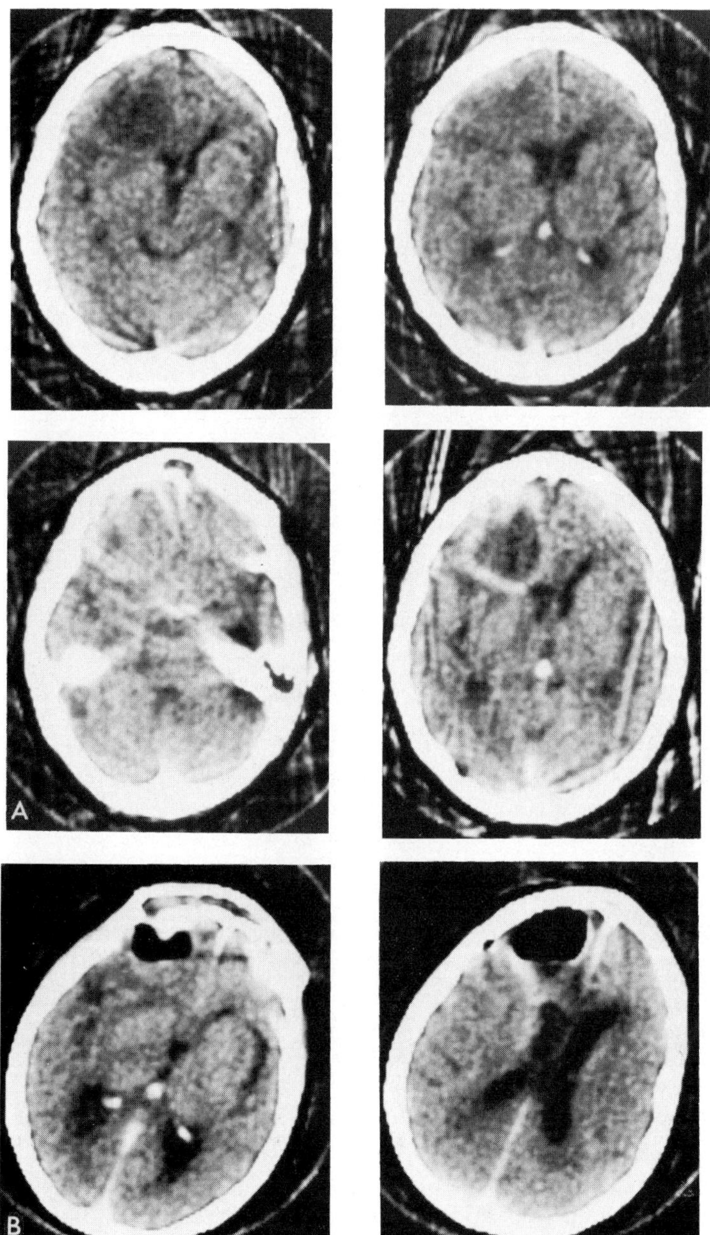

Figure 5–9. ABSCESS: *A,* The preinfusion scan revealed a large low density lesion in the left frontal region associated with posterior displacement of the frontal horn of the left lateral ventricle and a contralateral shift of the midline. *B,* Postinfusion, a thick-walled rim of enhancement was seen around the low density area.

Differential diagnosis includes a primary or secondary brain tumor.

C, The postoperative scans demonstrate that the abscess has been removed. There is now a moderate amount of air in the bed of the abscess. The lateral ventricles have increased in size compared to preoperative scans. There is a small amount of surrounding edema, and there continues to be mild distortion of the anterior portion of the left lateral ventricle.

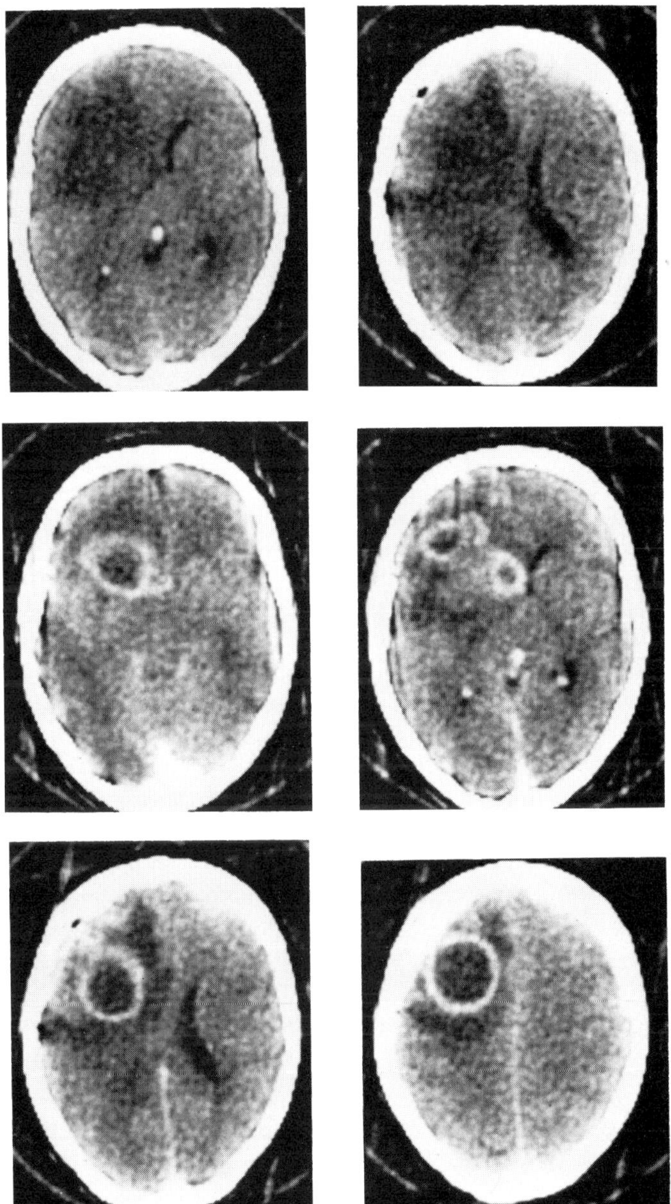

Figure 5–10. MULTILOBULATED ABSCESS. The preinfusion scan demonstrates a large lucent lesion in the left frontal and parietal region. Compression of the body of the left lateral ventricle and shift of the midline to the contralateral side are seen. There is posterior displacement of the choroid plexus calcification of the left lateral ventricle as compared to the right. The postinfusion scan shows a multilobulated area of enhancement involving the left frontal and parietal regions with irregular rims of enhancement and surrounding edema. The lesions are multiple abscesses. The differential diagnosis includes multiple metastases.

Figure 5–11. FRONTAL ABSCESS AND PARIETAL ABSCESS: *A*, The arterial phase of the angiogram demonstrates stretching of the vessels in the frontal region and curvilinear displacement of the distal branches of the middle cerebral artery in the posterior parietal region *(white arrows)*. Note the improper needle placement *(open arrow)* with the tip of the needle high in the internal carotid artery just below the base of the vault.

B, The venous phase reveals a faint rim of enhancement around the frontal abscess. This patient has cyanotic congenital heart disease and has developed two train abscesses (*black lines*).

C, CT scans from a different patient with a similar history show a large low density lesion in the right frontal region, which also has surrounding edema. A thick wall of enhancement is seen on the postinfusion scan. The lesion continues to have a lucent center.

In a different clinical setting the presence of multiple lesions should suggest the possibility of multiple metastases.

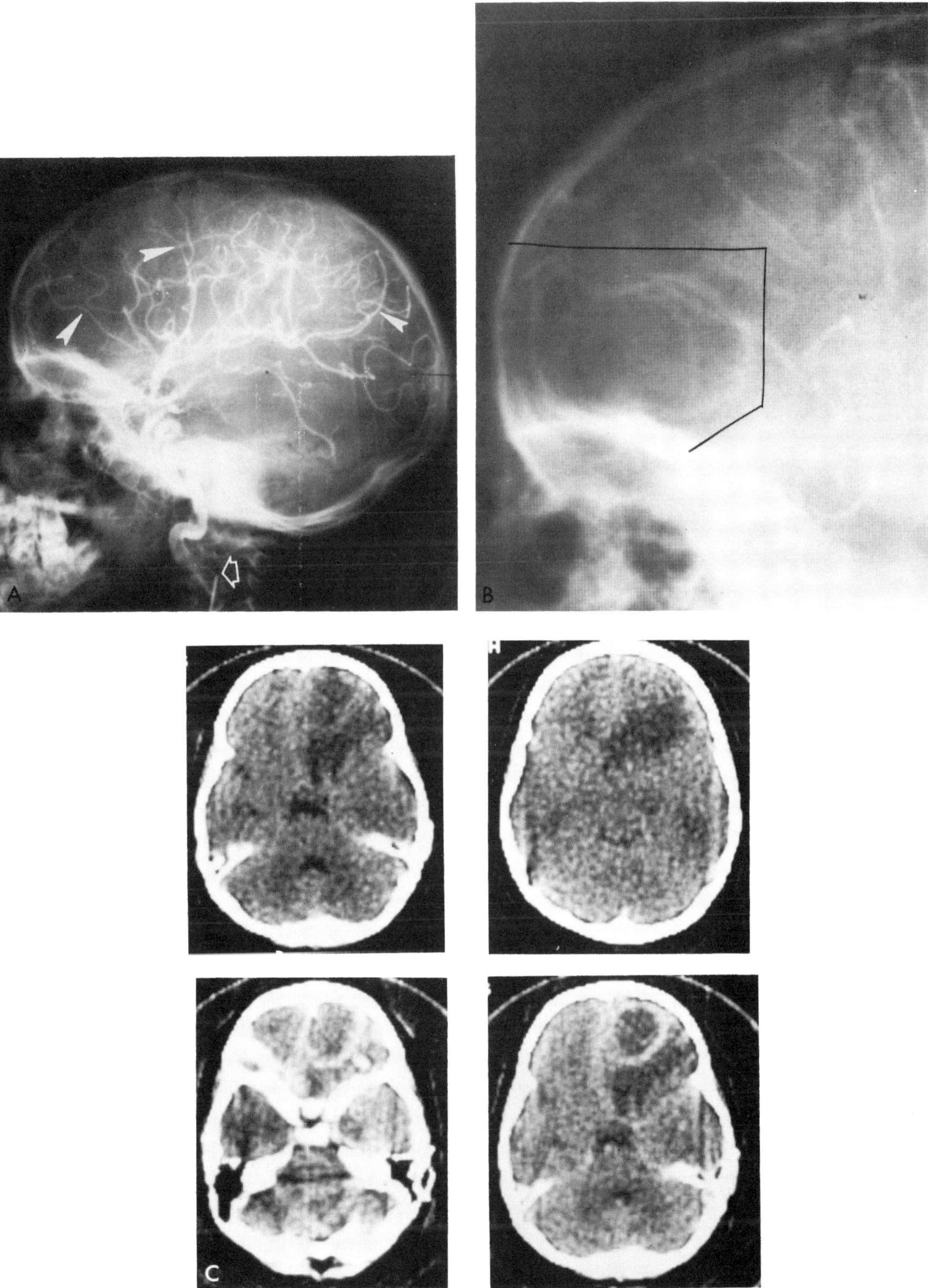

Figure 5–11. *See legend on the opposite page*

Figure 5–12. INTRACEREBRAL HEMATOMA: The left carotid arteriogram *(A)* is entirely within normal limits. However, the CT scans *(B)* demonstrate a left frontal and right anterior temporal hematoma *(small arrow). C,* There is no change on the postinfusion scan. There is mild dilatation of the lateral ventricles of unknown etiology and slight distortion of the frontal horn of the left lateral ventricle secondary to the mass.

Biopsy demonstrated evidence of hemorrhage but no tumor. However, differential diagnosis would include multiple metastases from a metastatic melanoma or some other hemorrhagic or vascular tumor.

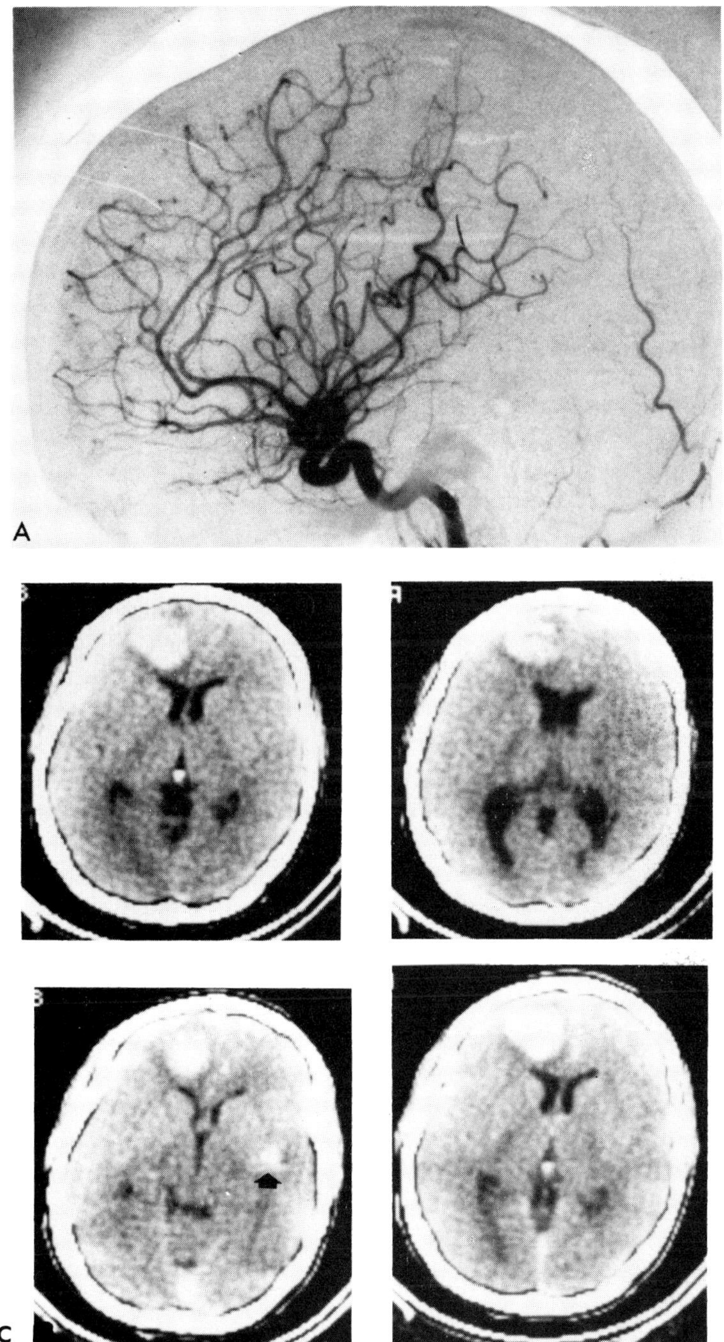

Figure 5–12. *See legend on the opposite page*

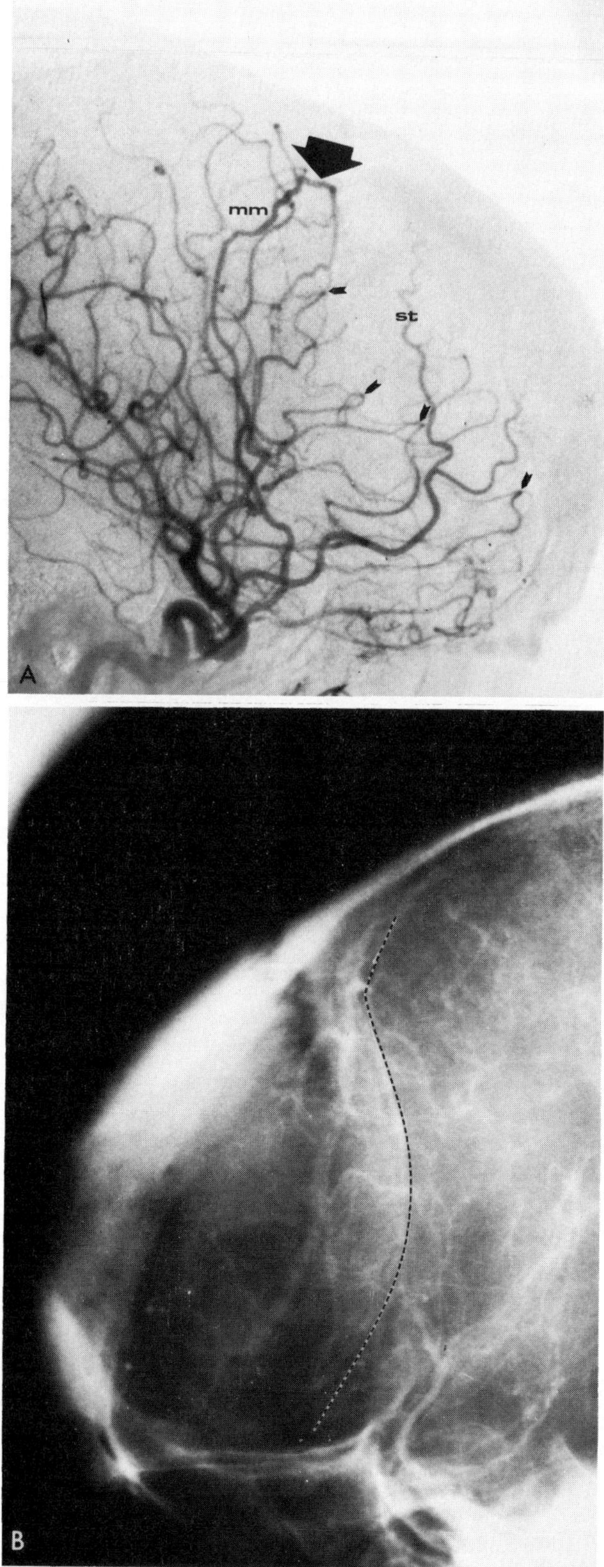

Figure 5–13. *See legend on the opposite page*

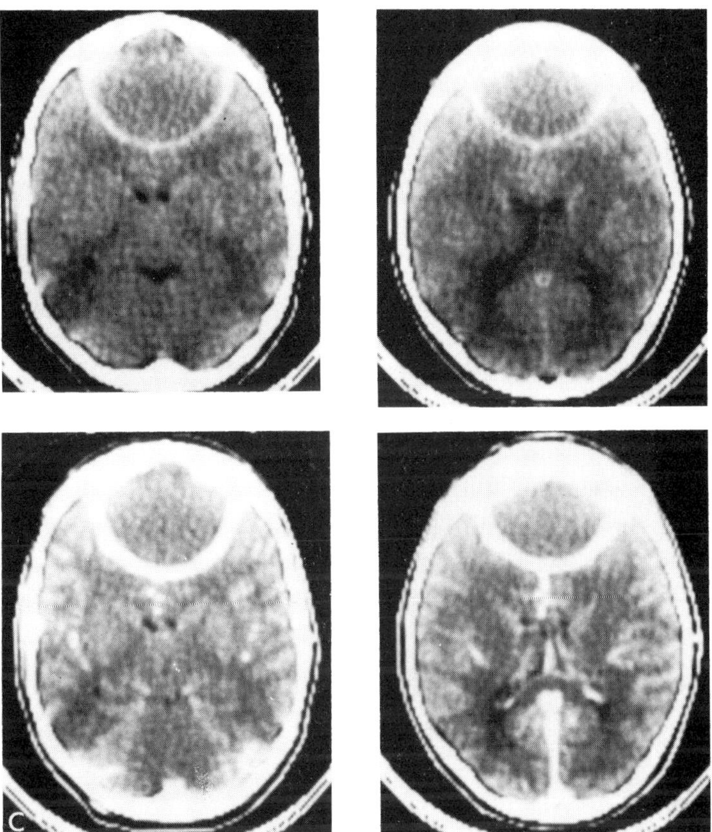

Figure 5–13. BIFRONTAL CHRONIC EPIDURAL EMPYEMA: *A*, The left lateral arteriographic view of the left carotid shows that all the distal branches of the middle cerebral artery are displaced posteriorly and inferiorly *(arrowheads)* and that there is a large avascular area in the frontal region. The middle meningeal artery *(mm)* is greatly enlarged to supply the inflamed and thickened meninges. The superficial temporal artery *(st)* also is very prominent.

B, The lateral view of the venous phase of the right carotid angiogram demonstrates that the superior sagittal sinus is displaced posteriorly away from the inner table of the skull by the large epidural collection *(dotted line)*. The cortical veins that are more laterally positioned reach more anteriorly, but never approximate the inner table of the skull. Note that the skull is thickened and sclerotic but that there is an area of thinning in the low frontal region. These findings are consistent with a chronic osteomyelitis.

C, The CT scans are spectacularly abnormal. There is a large rounded mass in the frontal region bilaterally, causing massive posterior displacement of the frontal horns of the lateral ventricles. The contents of the mass are isodense with the normal brain, but its wall is dense and well defined. The postinfusion scan provides marked enhancement of the wall of the mass as well as marked vascular prominence of the remainder of the cerebral vessels.

At surgery the lesion proved to be a large epidural abscess secondary to chronic frontal sinusitis and associated with chronic osteomyelitis of the frontal bone.

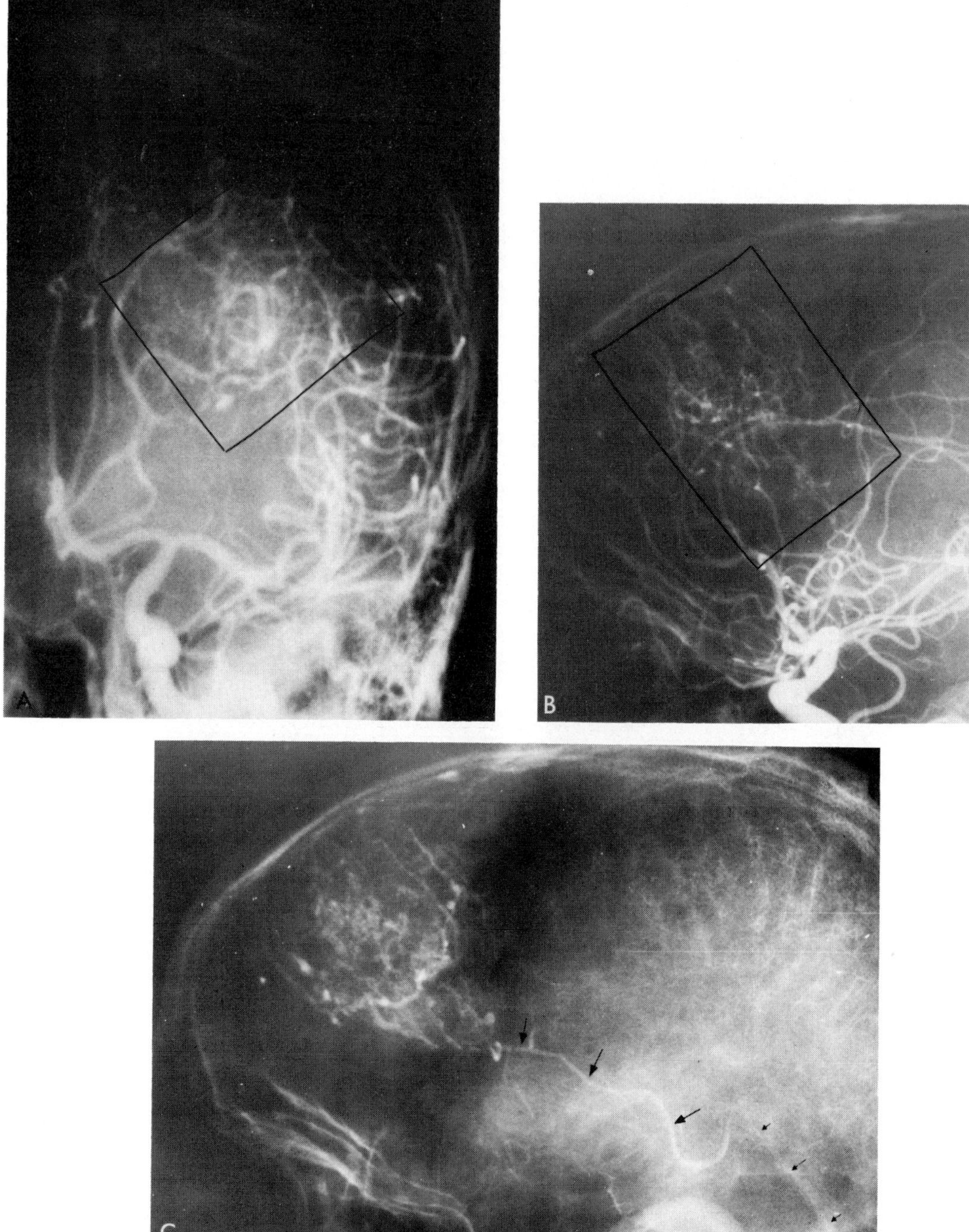

Figure 5–14. *See legend on the opposite page*

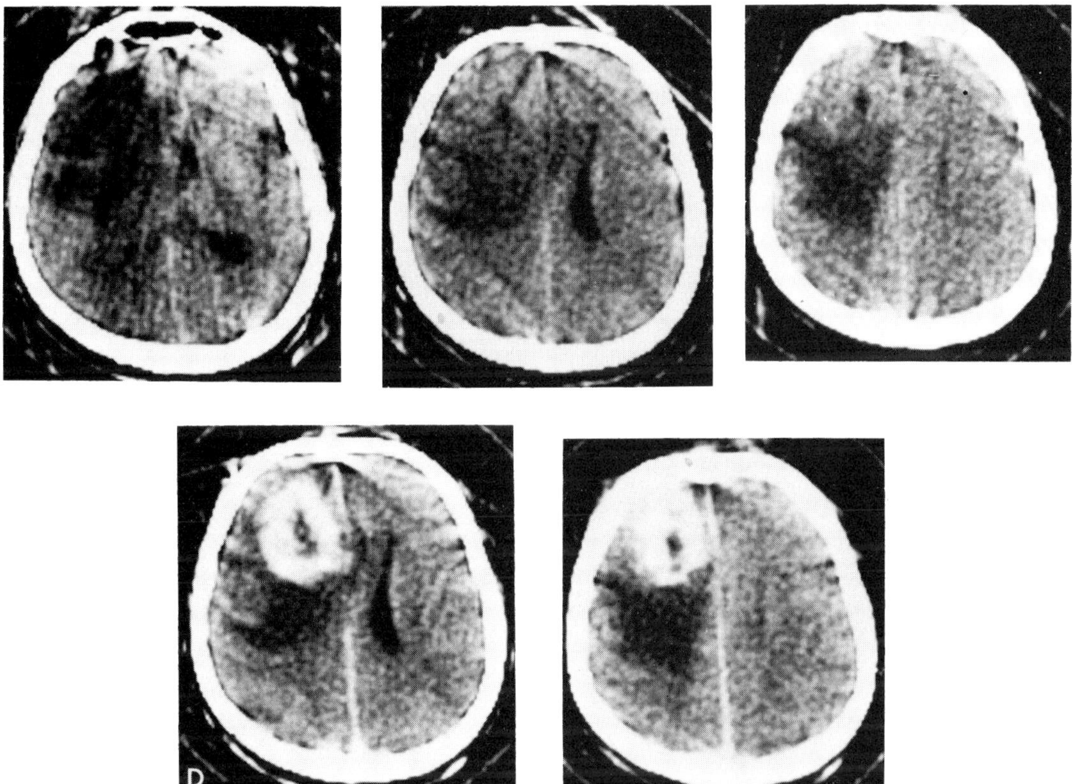

Figure 5–14. FRONTAL GLIOBLASTOMA: *A,* The AP view shows a large vascular mass *(black lines)* that is supplied by branches of both the anterior and middle cerebral arteries. There are myriad small vessels within the tumor; a marked shift of the anterior cerebral artery in both its proximal and distal portions also is seen. In the lateral view *(B),* the lesion is seen in the mid- and posterior frontal regions. There is inferior displacement of the sylvian triangle and stretching of multiple branches of the middle cerebral artery, even in the parietal region. The remote effect of the tumor outside the area of neovascularity is secondary to the surrounding edema.

C, The capillary phase reveals a large area of tumor stain with multiple capsular draining vessels and a large draining vein that feeds directly into the septal vein and then into the internal cerebral vein *(large arrows),* and then into the straight sinus *(small arrows).*

D, CT scans demonstrate a large irregular area of lucency in the left hemisphere associated with marked shift of the midline structures to the contralateral side. The tumor itself is well visualized on the postinfusion scan, but appears isodense with the normal brain on the preinfusion scan. It really is demonstrated with certainty only after the infusion of contrast material. The tumor has a thick wall of enhancement and a small lucent center that is somewhat irregular in appearance.

Differential diagnosis includes a brain tumor, either primary or secondary.

PARIETAL LOBE MASS LESIONS

Mass lesions in the parietal lobe cause a distal shift of the anterior cerebral artery to the contralateral side. Because the mass is situated adjacent to the more distal portion of the vessel, there is a rather abrupt return of the pericallosal artery to its own side of the falx. This results in a rather sharp angle of the pericallosal artery just at its point of return under the falx. This point of shift under the falx is readily identifiable on the AP view; it often can be identified on the lateral view as well. There is inferior displacement of the sylvian point. If the mass is in a parasagittal position, there will be lateral displacement of the sylvian point; if the mass is low over the convexity, there will be medial displacement of the sylvian point.

The internal cerebral vein will be shifted to the contralateral side. The degree of shift is approximately equal to the shift of the pericallosal artery.

The lateral view reveals downward displacement of the sylvian triangle and stretching of the anterior and middle cerebral artery branches around the mass lesion. Depending on the intrinsic vascularity of the mass, there is an area of avascularity. There may be delayed venous filling. The sylvian point will be inferiorly displaced.

The venous phase of the lateral view will reveal that there is an "open" venous angle, and downward displacement of the internal cerebral vein may be seen.

In summary, the angiographic findings with a parietal lobe mass lesion are:

AP View.

1. Distal shift of the pericallosal artery.
2. An approximately equal shift of the internal cerebral vein.

AP and Lateral View.

3. Downward displacement of the sylvian triangle.
4. Downward displacement of the sylvian point.

Lateral View.

5. Stretched vessels in the parietal region, arterial phase.
6. An "open" venous angle.
7. An area of avascularity or neovascularity in the parietal region.

Text continued on page 268

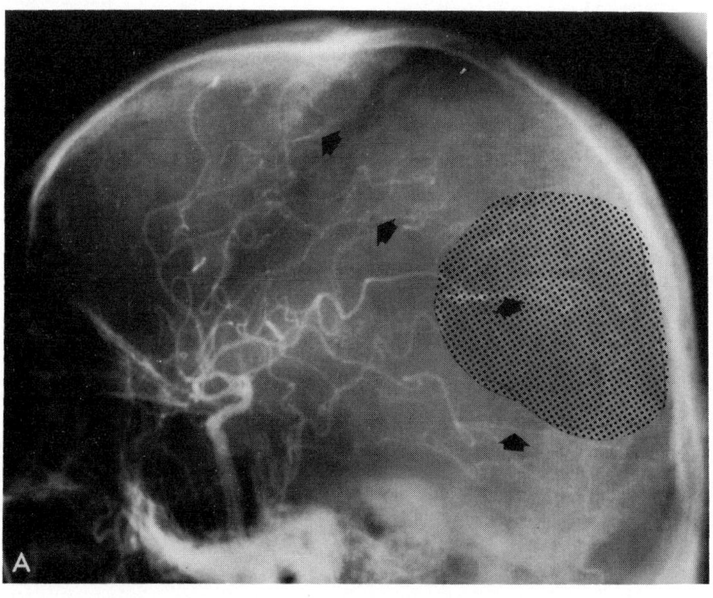

Figure 5–15. *See legend on page 246*

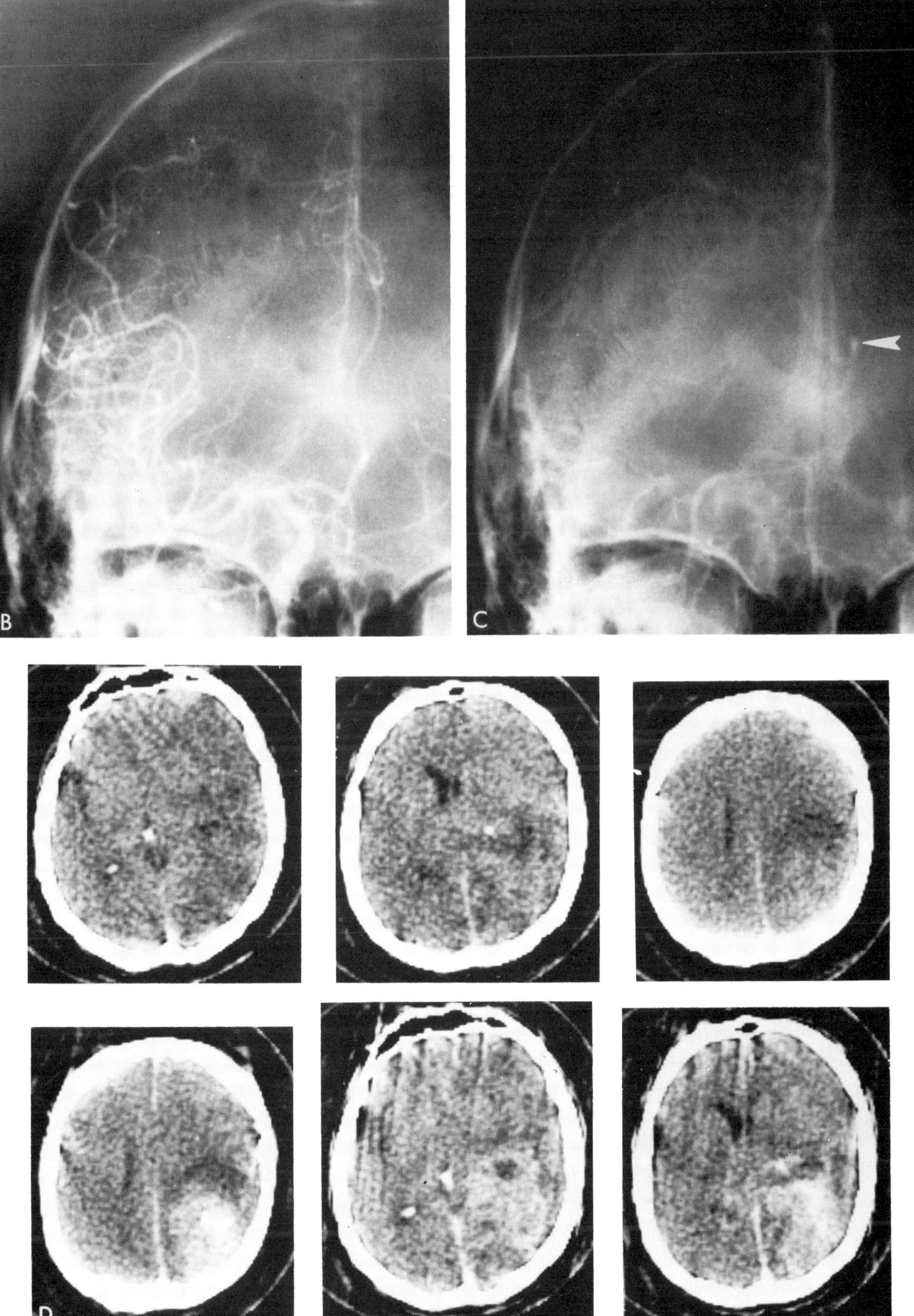

Figure 5–15. *(Continued) See legend on the following page*

Figure 5–15. PARIETO-OCCIPITAL GLIOBLASTOMA: *A,* The lateral view demonstrates marked forward telescoping of the entire sylvian triangle. At least half the loops of the middle cerebral artery vessels *(arrows)* are anterior to the level of the internal carotid artery bifurcation. There is stretching of all the branches of the middle cerebral artery, even in the posterior frontal region. The most marked stretching of the vessels occurs in the posterior parietal region, where the approximate location of the mass is marked by the dotted area.

B, The AP view of the arterial phase reveals a greater shift of the distal portion of the pericallosal artery than of the proximal portion. There is a relatively sharp angular deformity as the vessel crosses beneath the falx cerebri. Because of the angle of the projection used for the angiogram, the sylvian point appears to be displaced downward.

C, There is a greater shift of the internal cerebral vein than of the artery, indicating a more posteriorly placed mass *(arrow).*

D, The CT scans disclose a poorly defined lesion in the right hemisphere with areas of increased and decreased density. The abnormal area involves the right temporal, parietal and occipital lobes. There is shift of the frontal horns to the contralateral side and compression of the body of the right lateral ventricle. The postinfusion scan demonstrates an irregular pattern of enhancement in the tumor bed and a small amount of edema anterior to the tumor itself. On the highest cut there is evidence of extension of the tumor through the corpus callosum to involve the opposite hemisphere.

Differential diagnosis includes a primary or secondary brain tumor.

See illustrations on pages 244 and 245

Figure 5–16. PARIETAL GLIOBLASTOMA: *A,* The lateral view demonstrates forward telescoping of the sylvian triangle *(long arrow)* and stretching of all the vessels in the frontal, parietal and occipital regions *(small arrows).*

B, The late arterial view (using magnification technique) reveals multiple small irregular "tumor" vessels in the midparietal and posterior temporal regions *(black lines).* The surrounding vessels are displaced around the tumor mass.

C, The AP view shows that the very proximal portion of the anterior cerebral artery meanders across the midline but then returns to the midline and remains there for the rest of its course. The sylvian point *(SP)* is displaced both inferiorly and medially by the convex tumor. There was a mild to moderate shift of the internal cerebral vein (not shown).

The CT scans originally obtained seven months before angiography were within normal limits — even in retrospect. The present CT scans *(D)*, obtained at the same time as the angiogram, demonstrate an abnormal area of mixed high and low density in the left parietal convexity region. The higher density portion of the tumor seems to be central and surrounded by an area of edema. There is compression of the left frontal horn, but no real evidence of shift of the frontal horns — confirming the angiographic findings. There is a slight shift of the third ventricle that correlates with the shift of the internal cerebral vein.

Because of the rather superficial location, differential diagnosis includes meningioma as well as glioma and/or metastatic tumor.

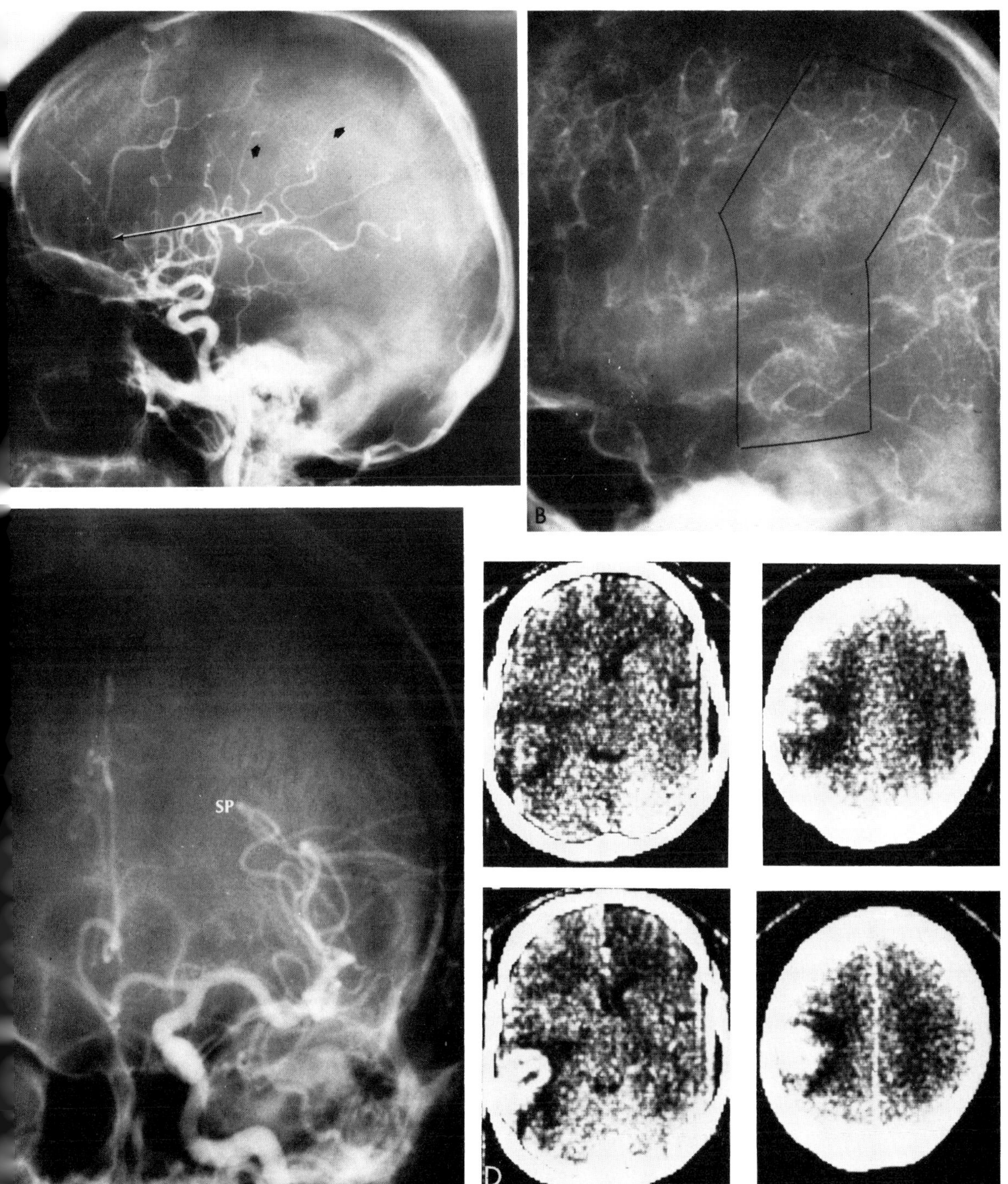

Figure 5–16. *See legend on the opposite page*

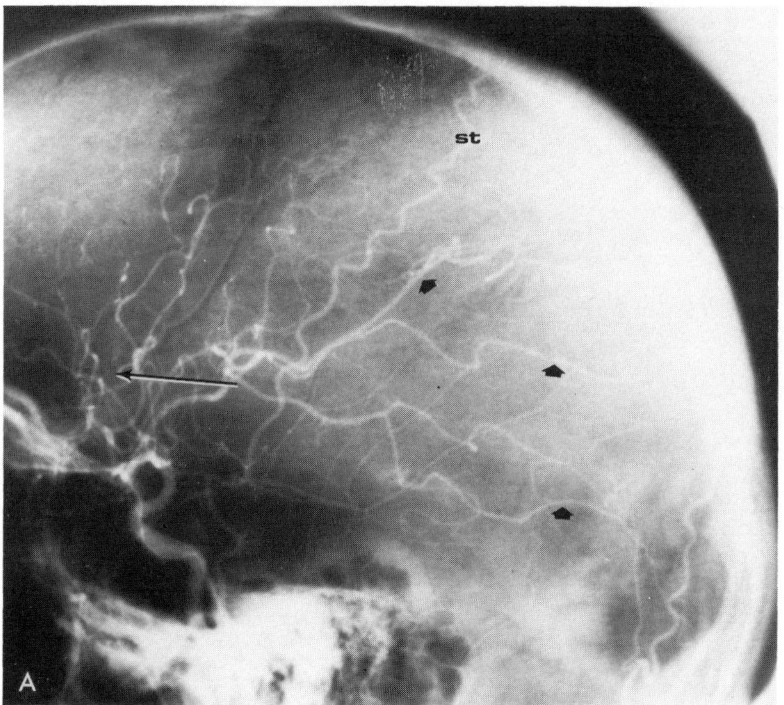

Figure 5–17. PARIETAL GLIOBLASTOMA: *A*, The angiogram reveals forward telescoping of the sylvian triangle and marked stretching of the vessels in the parietal and occipital regions *(arrowheads)*. There is no evidence of neovascularity. There is increased filling of the superficial temporal artery *(st)* because of the increased intracranial pressure.

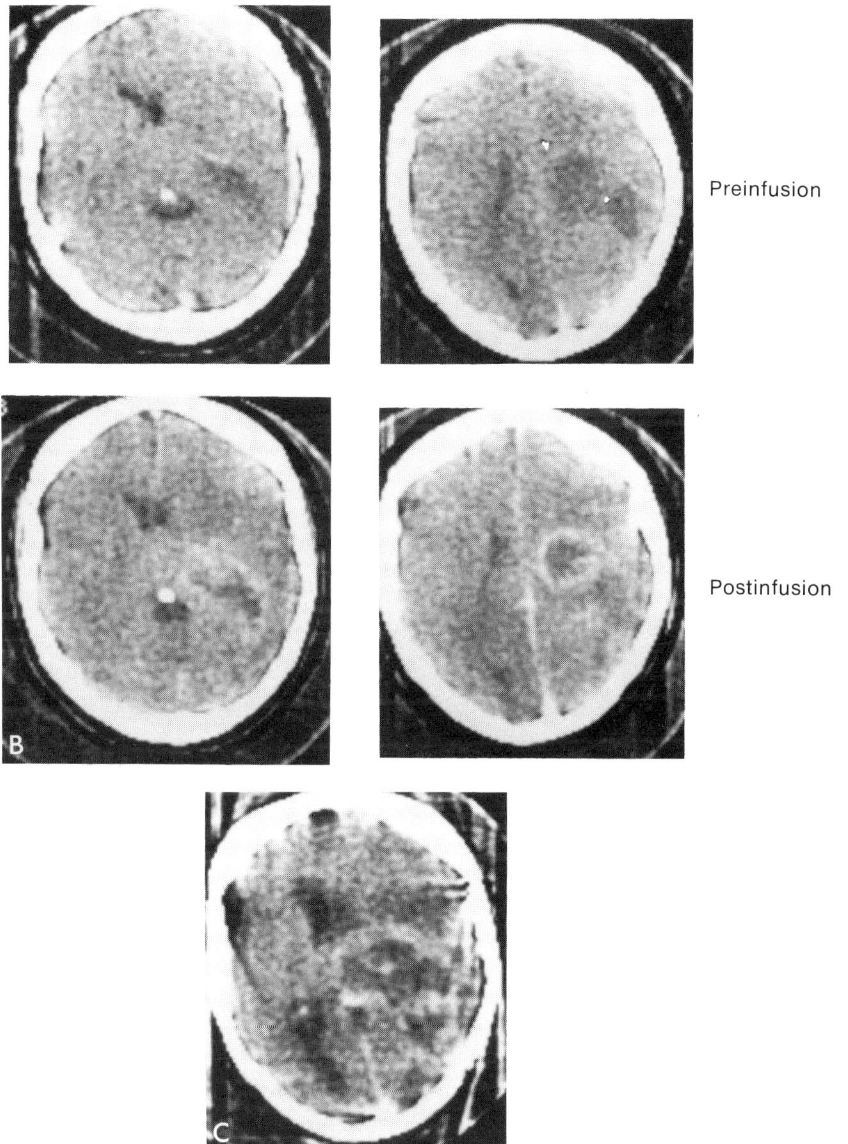

Figure 5–17. *Continued*

B, The initial CT scans demonstrate an area of radiolucency in the right parietal region that extends deep into the hemisphere in the region of the centrum ovale. There is shift of the midline to the contralateral side and compression of the body of the right lateral ventricle. The postinfusion scan demonstrates an irregular lobulated area of enhancement around the periphery of the radiolucent area.

Differential diagnosis includes abscess formation as well as glioma and/or metastatic brain tumor.

C, A follow-up scan following both surgical and radiation treatment demonstrates that the area of radiolucency and enhancement has enlarged over a three-month period. This follow-up scan was degraded by patient motion artifact.

Figure 5–18. SOLITARY METASTASIS: *A,* The CT scan demonstrates a single enhancing lesion deep in the left hemisphere surrounded by a marked amount of symmetrical edema. There is only slight compression of the body of the left lateral ventricle.

B, The postmortem pathologic specimen demonstrates the solitary metastatic lesion deep in the left hemisphere *(arrow)* which is surrounded by marked swelling of the cerebral tissues.

A solitary metastatic nodule is the most likely diagnosis, although a small early primary brain tumor is a possibility.

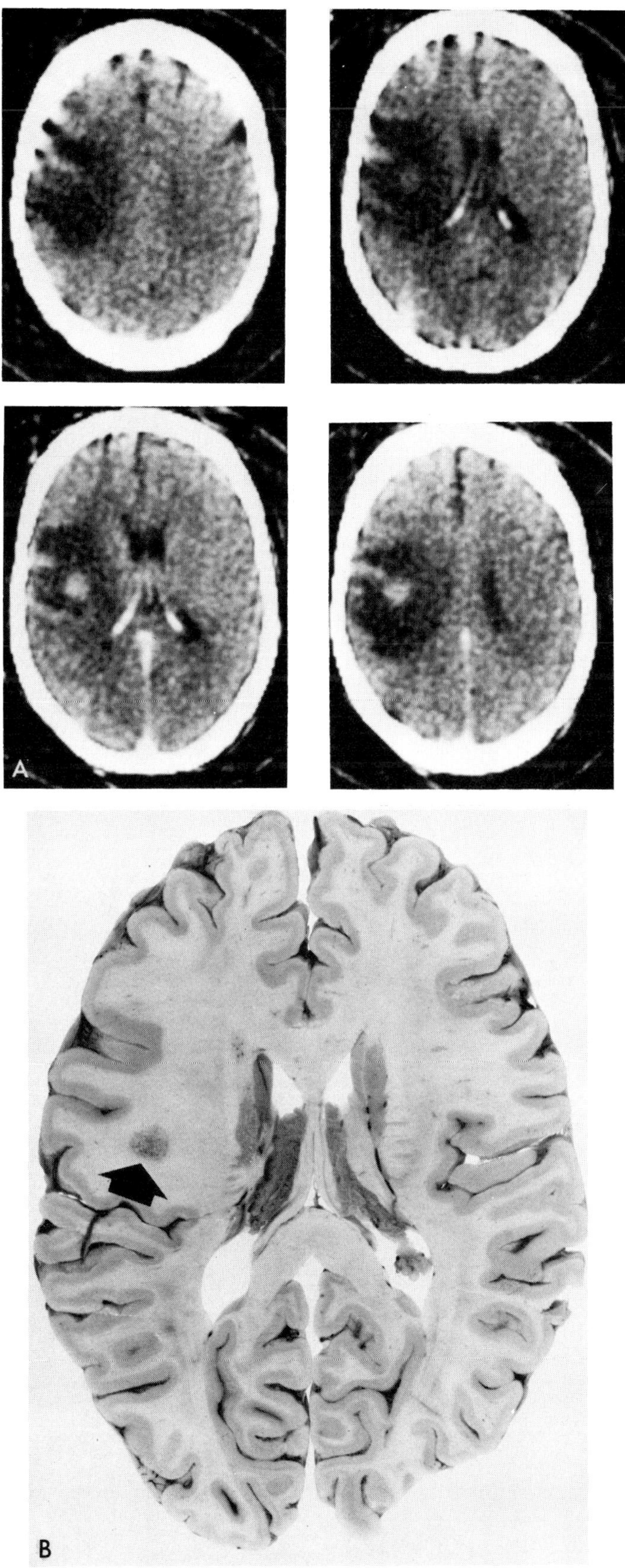

Figure 5–18. *See legend on the opposite page*

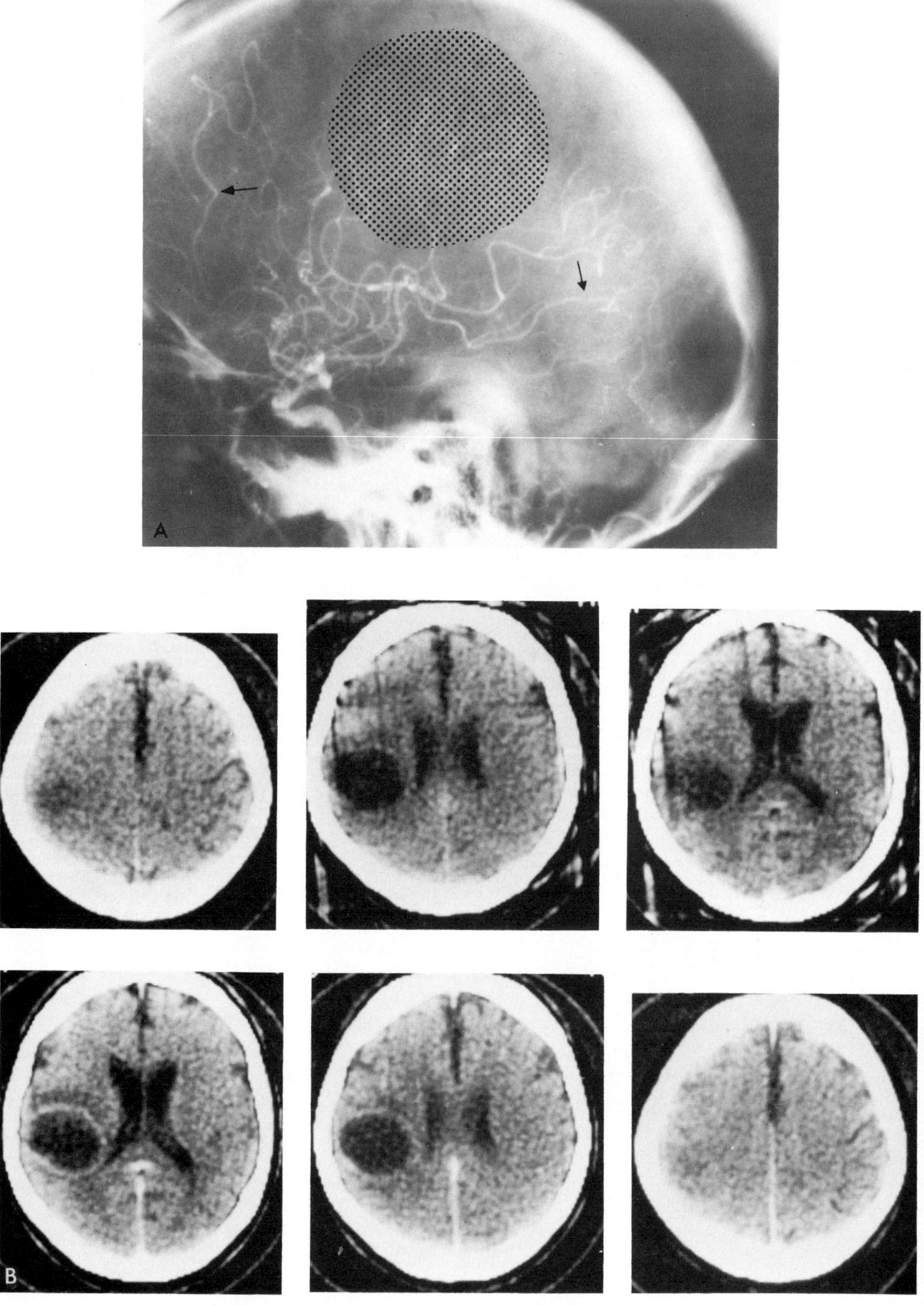

Figure 5–19. *See legend on the opposite page*

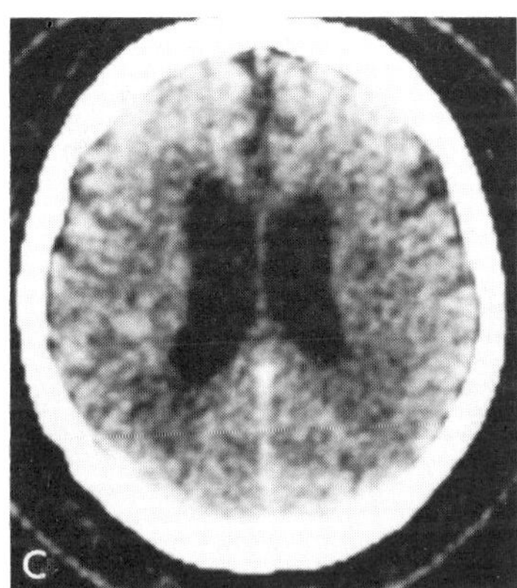

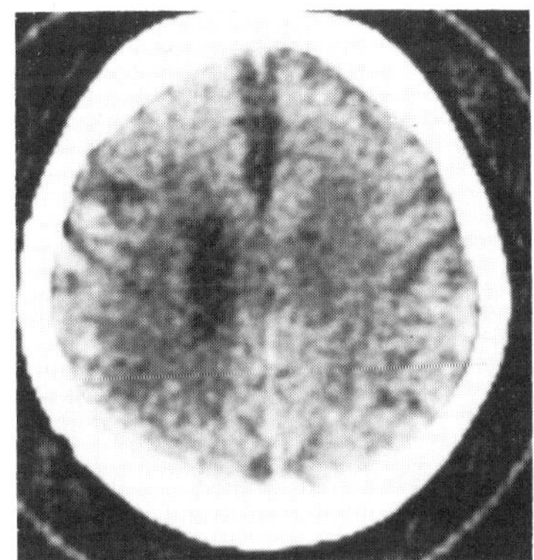

Figure 5–19. SOLITARY METASTASIS: *A,* The angiogram shows mild inferior displacement of the sylvian triangle with stretching of the vessels of the middle cerebral branches and anterior displacement of the pericallosal artery *(anterior arrow)*. The shaded area demonstrates the approximate position of the tumor. The mass demonstrated no evidence of neovascularity. There was no shift of the midline structures on the AP view.

B, The CT scan demonstrates a well defined radiolucent lesion in the left parietal region with a rim of high density that is enhanced on the postinfusion scan. Although there is no shift of the midline structures, there is very slight compression of the body of the left lateral ventricle. The fluid within the mass measured of higher density than CSF. On the higher cuts there is obliteration of the cortical sulci on the side of the mass secondary to some mass effect.

C, A follow-up scan after surgery demonstrates that there has been complete removal of the mass, and the left lateral ventricle appears slightly larger than the right.

Differential diagnosis includes a cystic glioblastoma and abscess in addition to metastasis.

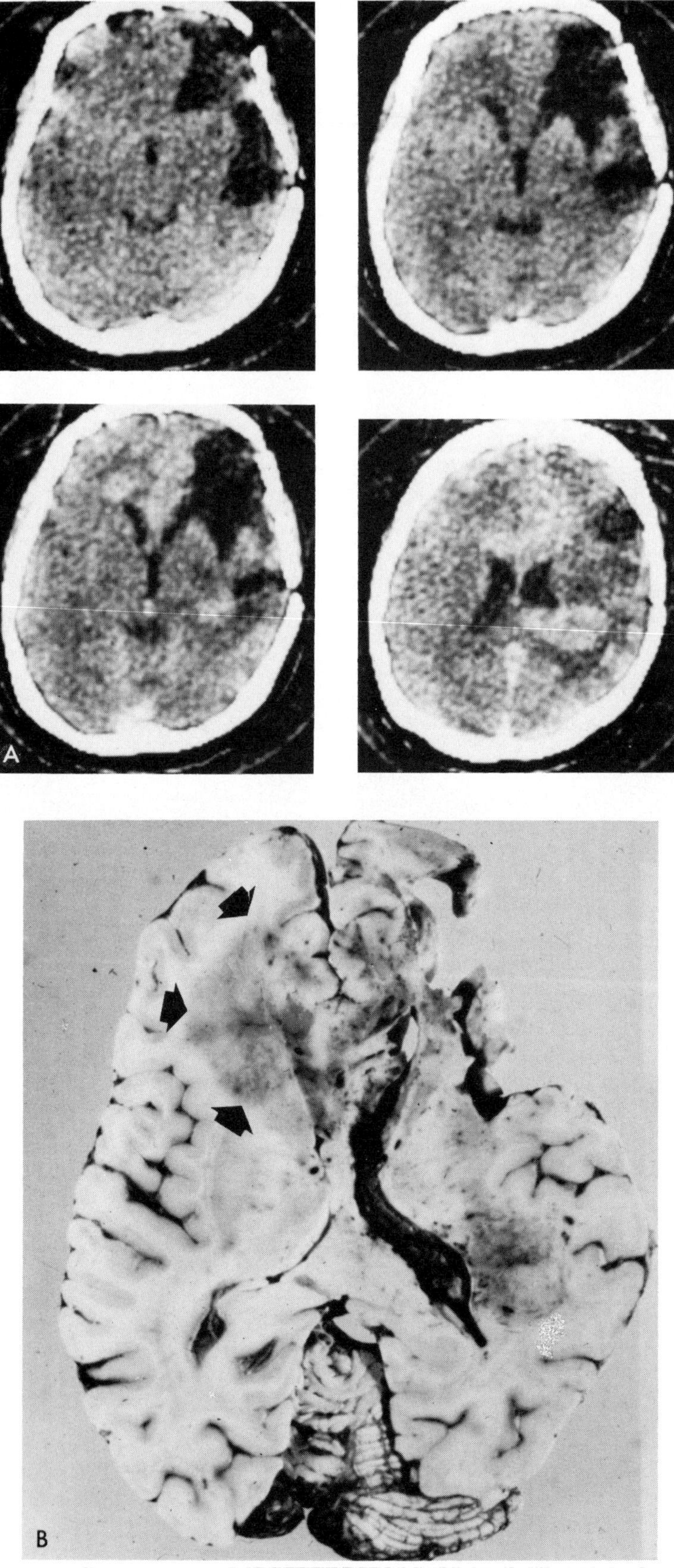

Figure 5–20. *See legend on the opposite page*

Figure 5–20. FRONTOPARIETAL TUMOR WITH EXTENSION ACROSS THE CORPUS CALLOSUM: *A*, The preinfusion CT scans reveal postoperative changes in the right frontal and parietal regions with large irregular areas of radiolucency in the obvious bony defects. There is no shift of the midline structures. The postinfusion scans demonstrate poorly visualized areas of enhancing tumor deep in the frontal region that extend across the midline in the region of the genu of the corpus callosum. The frontal horns of the lateral ventricles are splayed apart by the tumor. In addition, there is evidence of enhancing tumor in the right hemisphere posterior to the area of surgery and deep in the right hemisphere. On the highest cut the tumor extends almost to the splenium of the corpus callosum.

B, The pathologic specimen shows that the growth of the tumor to the contralateral side *(arrows)* has progressed beyond that demonstrated on the CT scan. The postsurgical change is present in the right frontal region. The tumor growth has a "butterfly" distribution typical of glioblastoma.

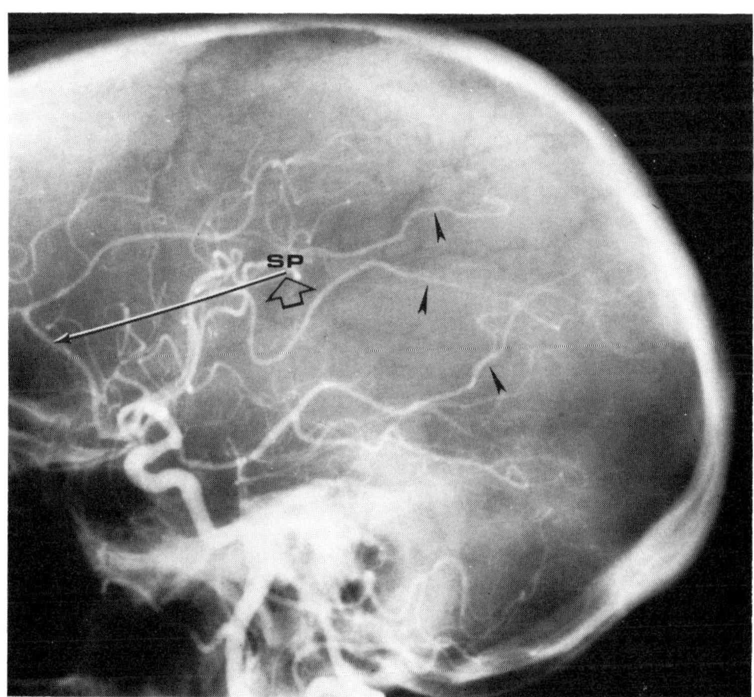

Figure 5–21. PARIETAL AND OCCIPITAL INTRACEREBRAL HEMATOMA: The angiogram demonstrates elevation and anterior telescoping of the sylvian triangle *(long arrow)* and superior displacement of the sylvian point *(open arrow)*. There is stretching of all the vessels in the posterior parietal and occipital areas. The mass is avascular.

Surgery revealed an intracerebral hematoma. Differential diagnosis includes glioblastoma or metastasis.

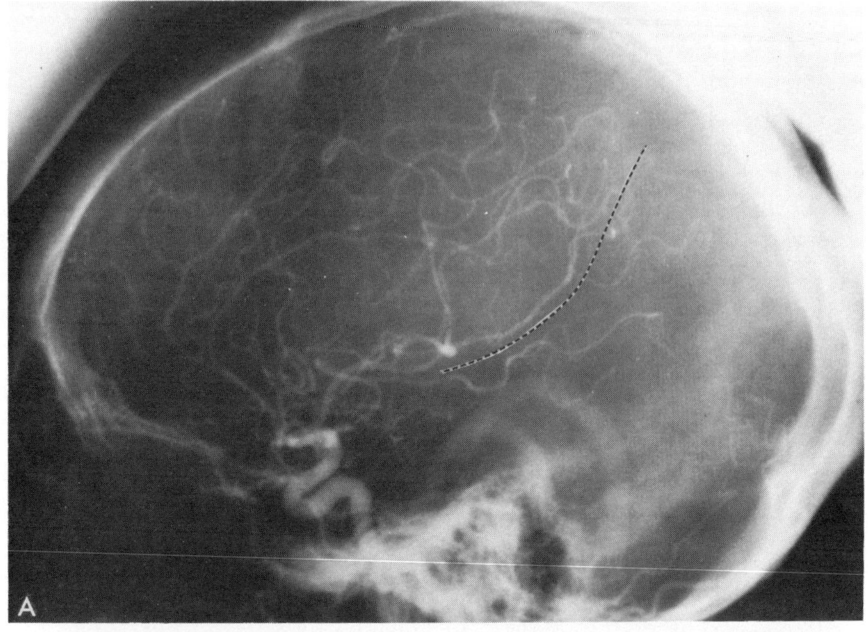

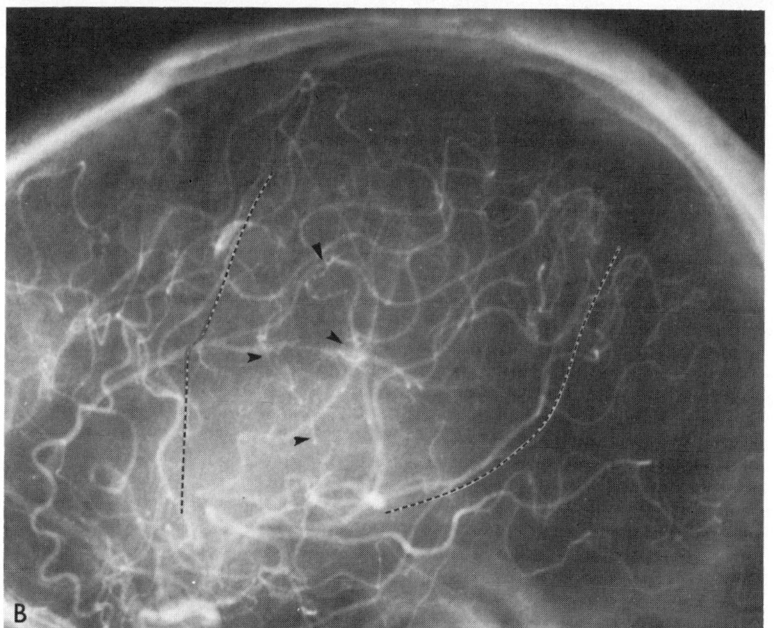

Figure 5–22. PARIETAL GLIOBLASTOMA: *A*, The lateral angiographic view reveals downward displacement and some forward telescoping of the sylvian triangle. The posterior branches of the middle cerebral artery are displaced in a curvilinear fashion around the mass *(dashed line)*.

B, A magnified view of the same area demonstrates multiple, small abnormal "tumor" vessels in the parietal region that could not be visualized in the standard angiogram *(small arrows)*. The curvilinear displacement of the vessels around the abnormal area is again demonstrated *(dashed line)*.

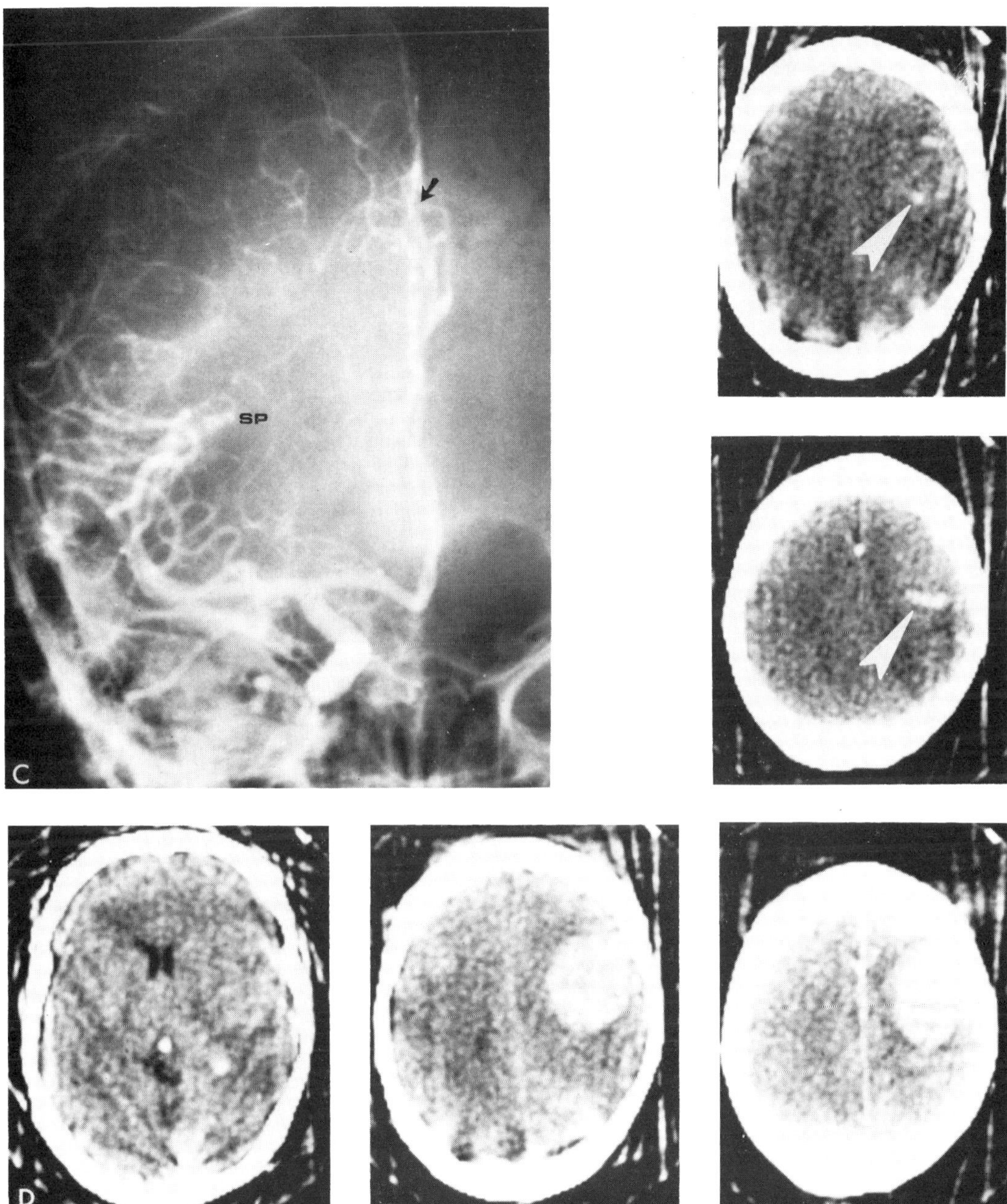

Figure 5–22. *Continued*

C, The AP view shows a distal shift of the pericallosal artery with a right-angle turn at the point of shift under the falx cerebri *(arrow).* The sylvian point *(SP)* is displaced inferiorly and medially.

D, CT scans demonstrated a calcified mass high in the right parietal convexity region *(arrows).* The mass is of higher density than normal brain tissue and contains multiple small areas of curvilinear calcification. On the postinfusion scan there is marked homogeneous enhancement of the tumor.

Surgically, this proved to be a glioblastoma, although differential diagnosis includes meningioma, oligodendroglioma and astrocytoma.

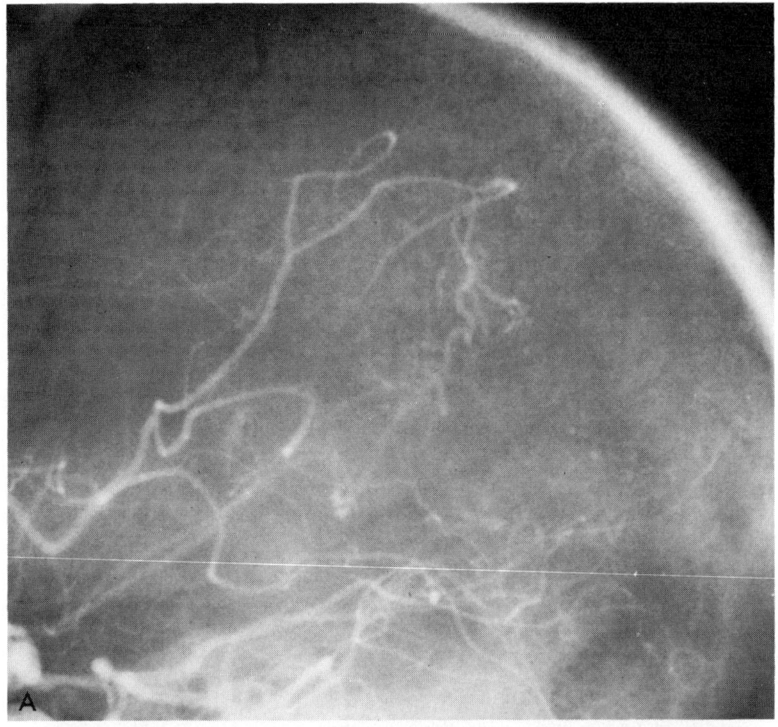

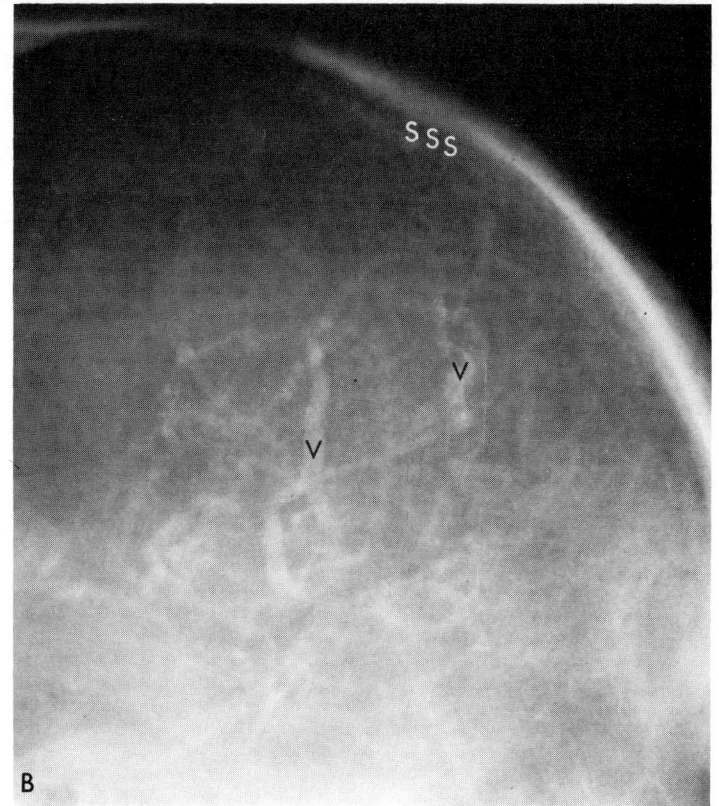

Figure 5–23. *See legend on the opposite page*

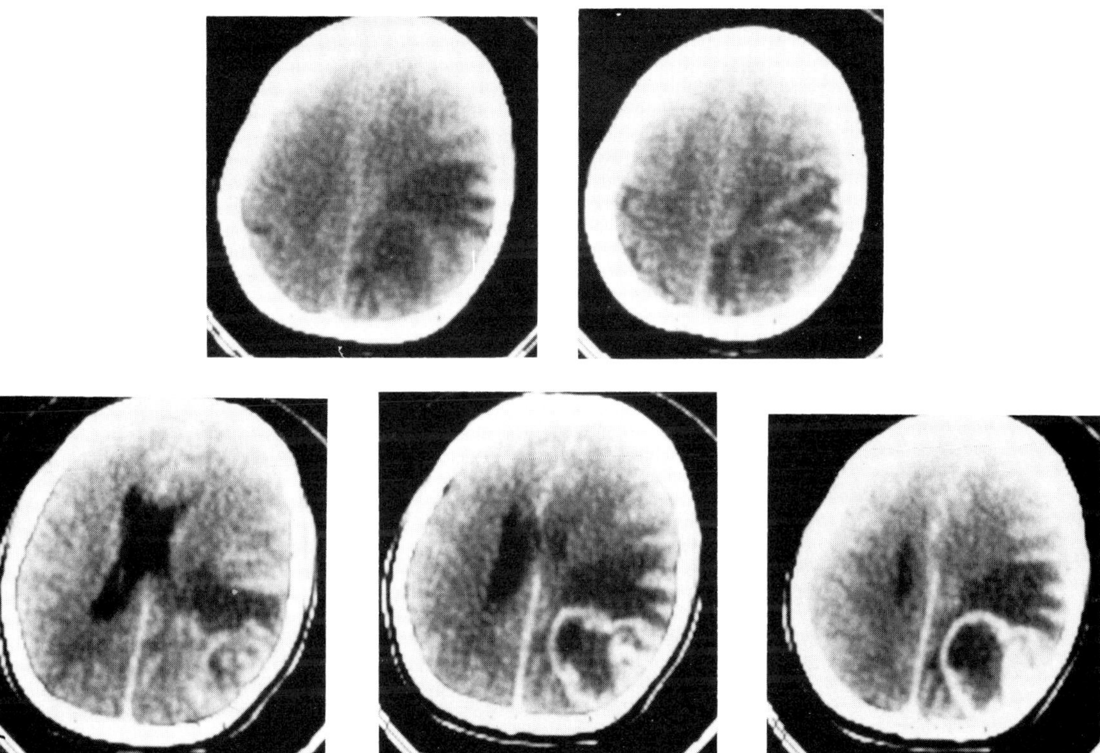

Figure 5–23. PARIETAL GLIOBLASTOMA: *A*, The angiogram reveals a large area of neovascularity in the parietal region that is supplied by enlarged branches of the middle cerebral artery. The supplying branches also demonstrate curvilinear displacement around the area of neovascularity. *B*, The capillary phase shows a large area of stain with multiple early draining veins *(V)* that drain to the superior sagittal sinus *(SSS)*.

C, CT scans from a different patient with a similar tumor demonstrate a large irregular area of radiolucency in the right parietal region. There is a surrounding area of scalloped edema. On the postinfusion scan, an irregular ring of enhancement is seen — also a solid portion of the tumor that is positioned posteriorly and is superficial. There is compression of the body of the right lateral ventricle.

This appearance is quite typical of glioblastoma, although a metastatic tumor could look this way.

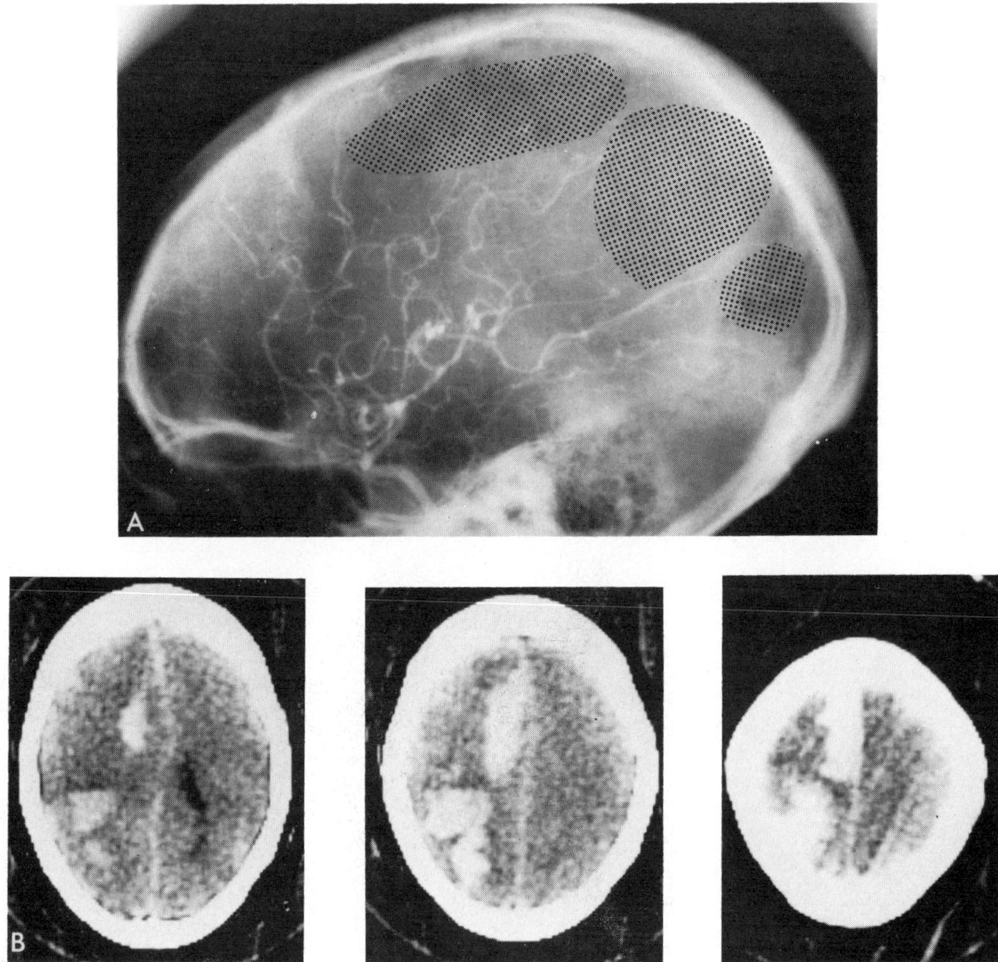

Figure 5–24. MULTIPLE INTRACEREBRAL HEMATOMAS: *A,* The angiogram is diffusely abnormal. There are three avascular areas, indicated here by shading. There is inferior and anterior displacement of the sylvian triangle.

B, The CT scans demonstrate the true nature of the abnormality by revealing multiple scattered areas of intracerebral hematoma. There is compression of the body of the left lateral ventricle. The falx is shifted in a curvilinear fashion to the contralateral side. The falx also appears thickened and of increased density because there is blood on either side of the falx secondary to an element of subarachnoid hemorrhage, which has occurred along with the intracerebral hematomas.

The etiology of these hemorrhages in this young, postpartum patient remains obscure

Figure 5–25. SOLITARY METASTASIS: *A,* The lateral view reveals a large vascular tumor that exhibits evidence of neovascularity *(black lines)* as well as a larger area of mass effect with stretching of the vessels secondary to surrounding edema. There is forward telescoping of the entire sylvian triangle.

B, The AP view demonstrates that the area of neovascularity lies just adjacent to the falx cerebri *(arrows)*. There is a distal shift of the anterior cerebral artery under the falx. The sylvian point appears to be displaced inferiorly.

At surgery this proved to be a solitary metastatic deposit from primary renal carcinoma. Differential diagnosis includes glioblastoma multiforme.

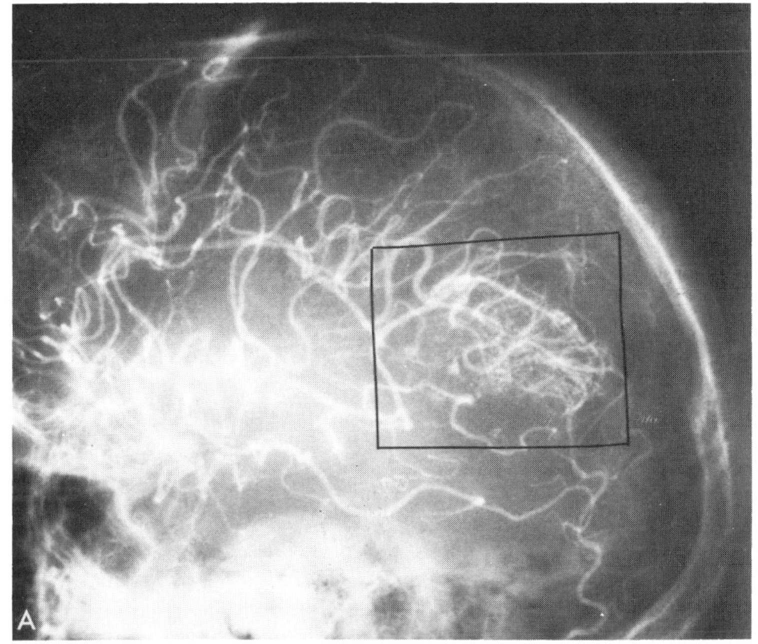

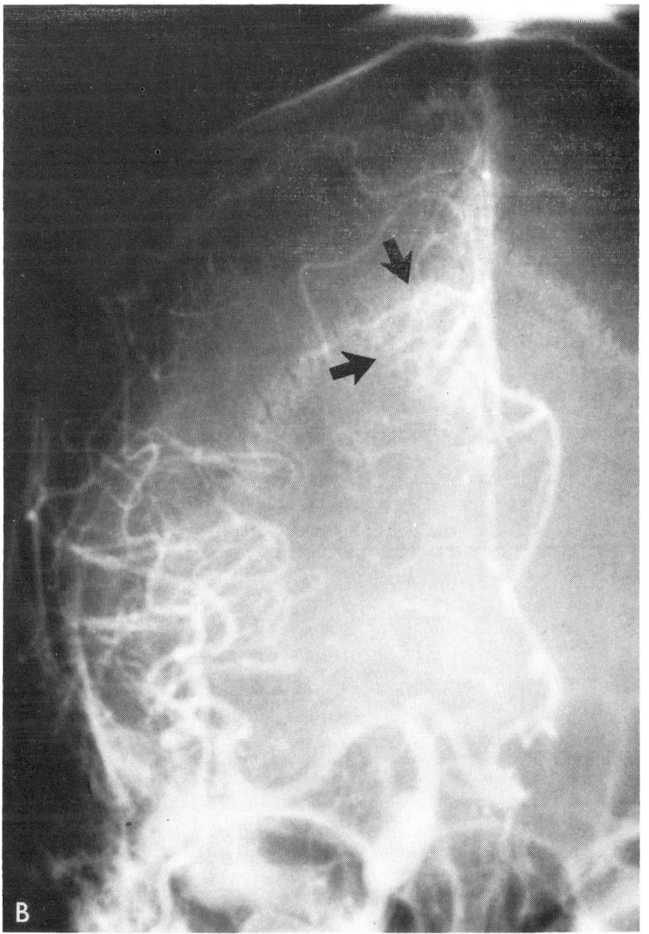

Figure 5–25. *See legend on the opposite page*

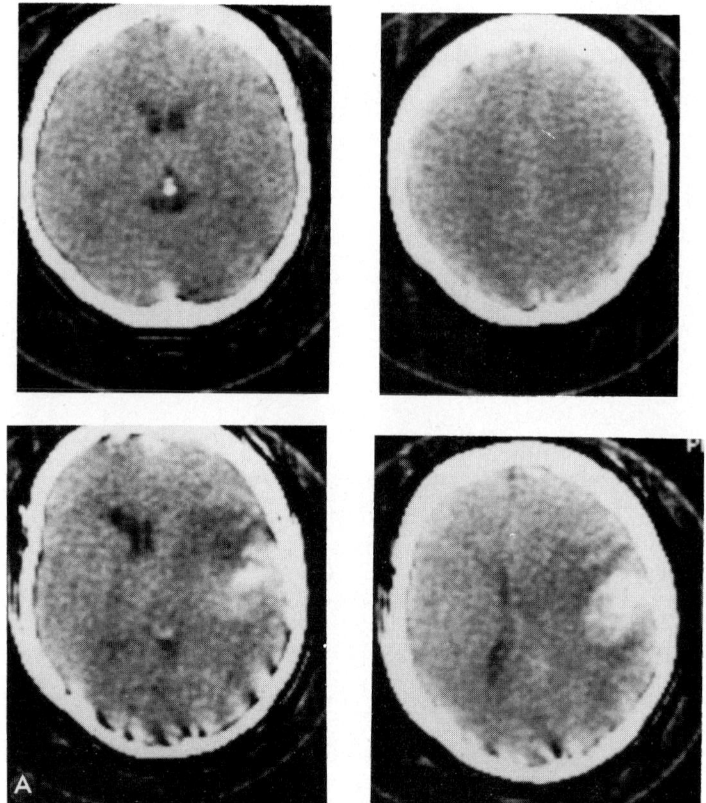

Figure 5–26. SPONTANEOUS INTRACEREBRAL HEMATOMA: *A*, The initial scans were within normal limits. Two years later the patient presented with acute onset of left hemiparesis. CT scans made then demonstrate an irregular intracerebral hematoma in the right hemisphere. Moderate surrounding edema is present, primarily anterior to the hematoma. There is compression of the lateral ventricle and shift of the midline to the contralateral side.

B, The lateral angiographic view shows marked inferior displacement of the sylvian triangle and forward telescoping of the branches of the middle cerebral artery group *(arrows)*. The mass is avascular. The anterior cerebral artery fills from the opposite side.

C, The distal branches of the middle cerebral artery are seen as they course around the large intracerebral mass *(arrows)*. There is marked inferior and medial displacement of the sylvian point *(SP)*. The posterior cerebral artery is displaced medially because of early transtentorial herniation.

At surgery this proved to be an intracerebral hematoma. The etiology is unknown.

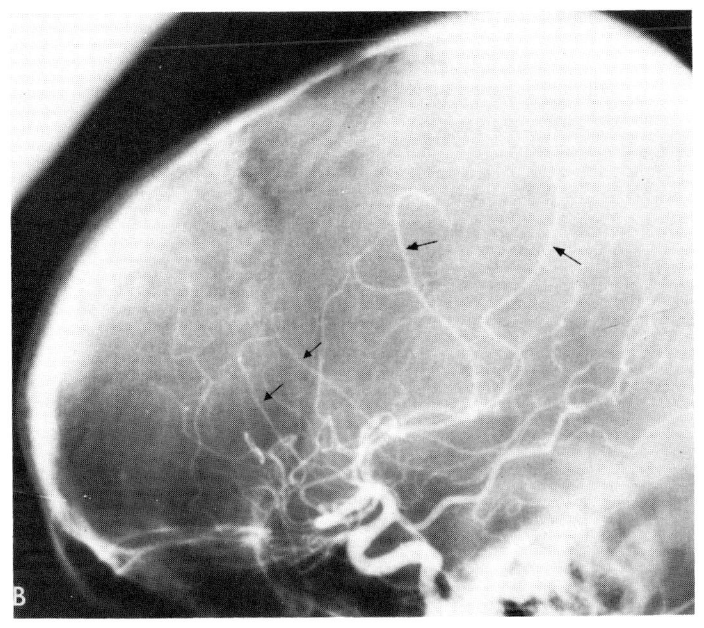

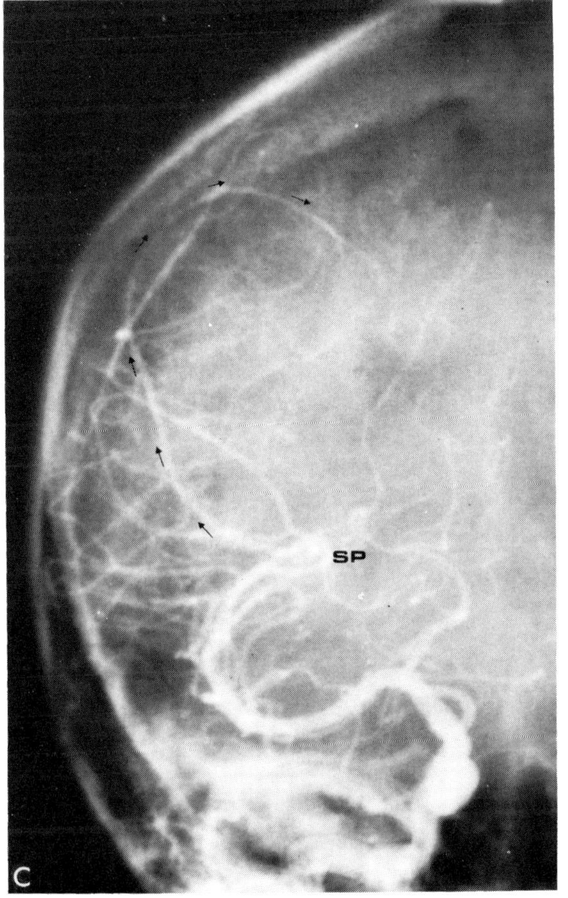

Figure 5–26. (*Continued*) *See legend on the opposite page*

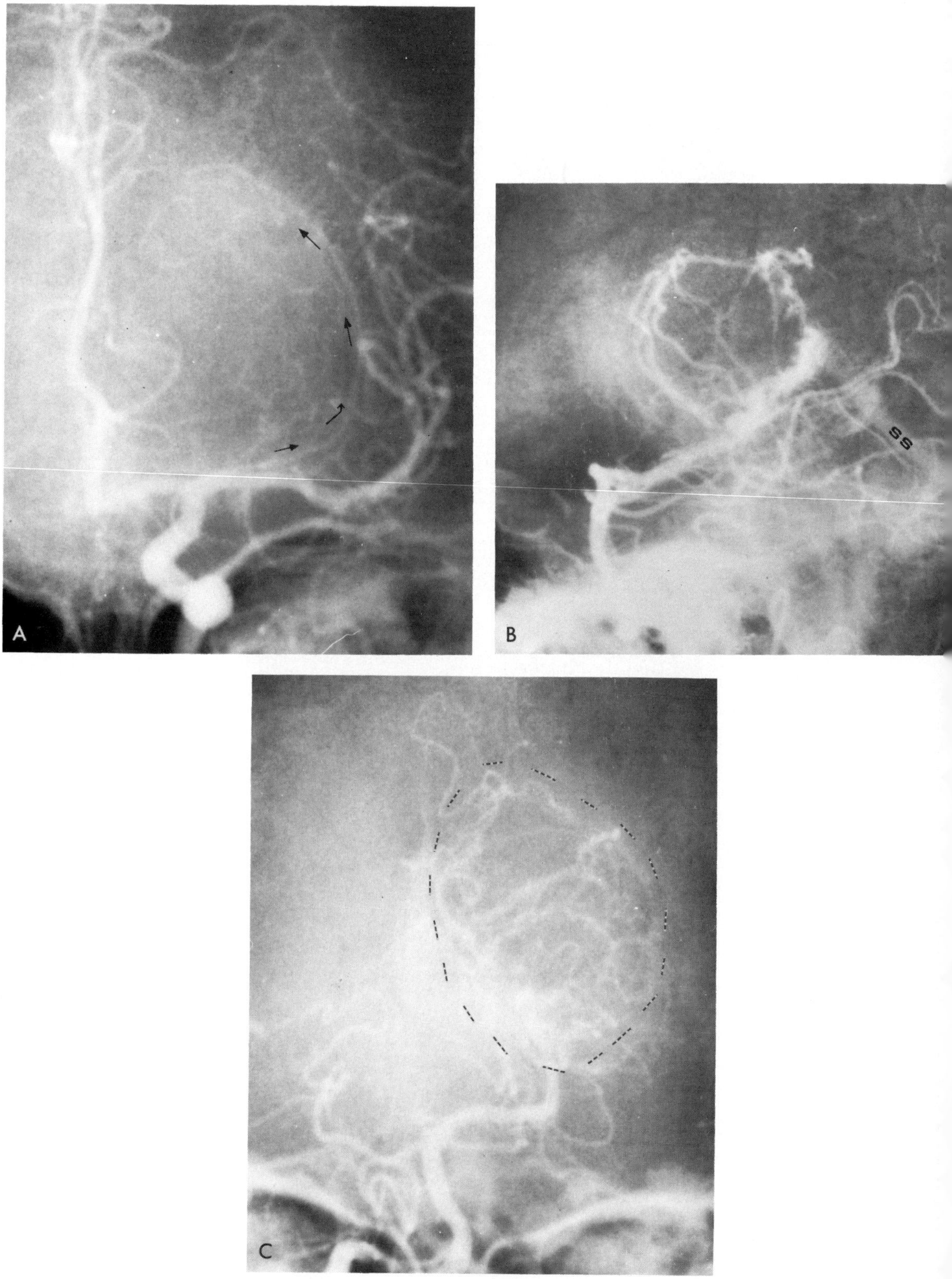

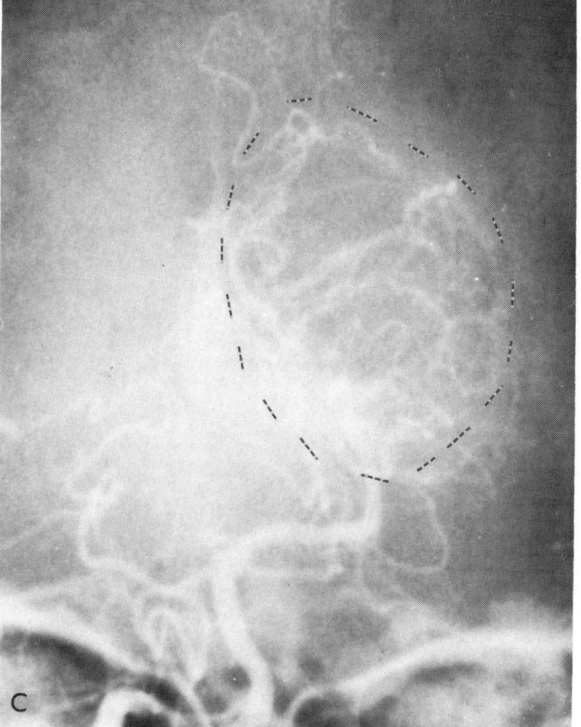

Figure 5–27. *See legend on the opposite page*

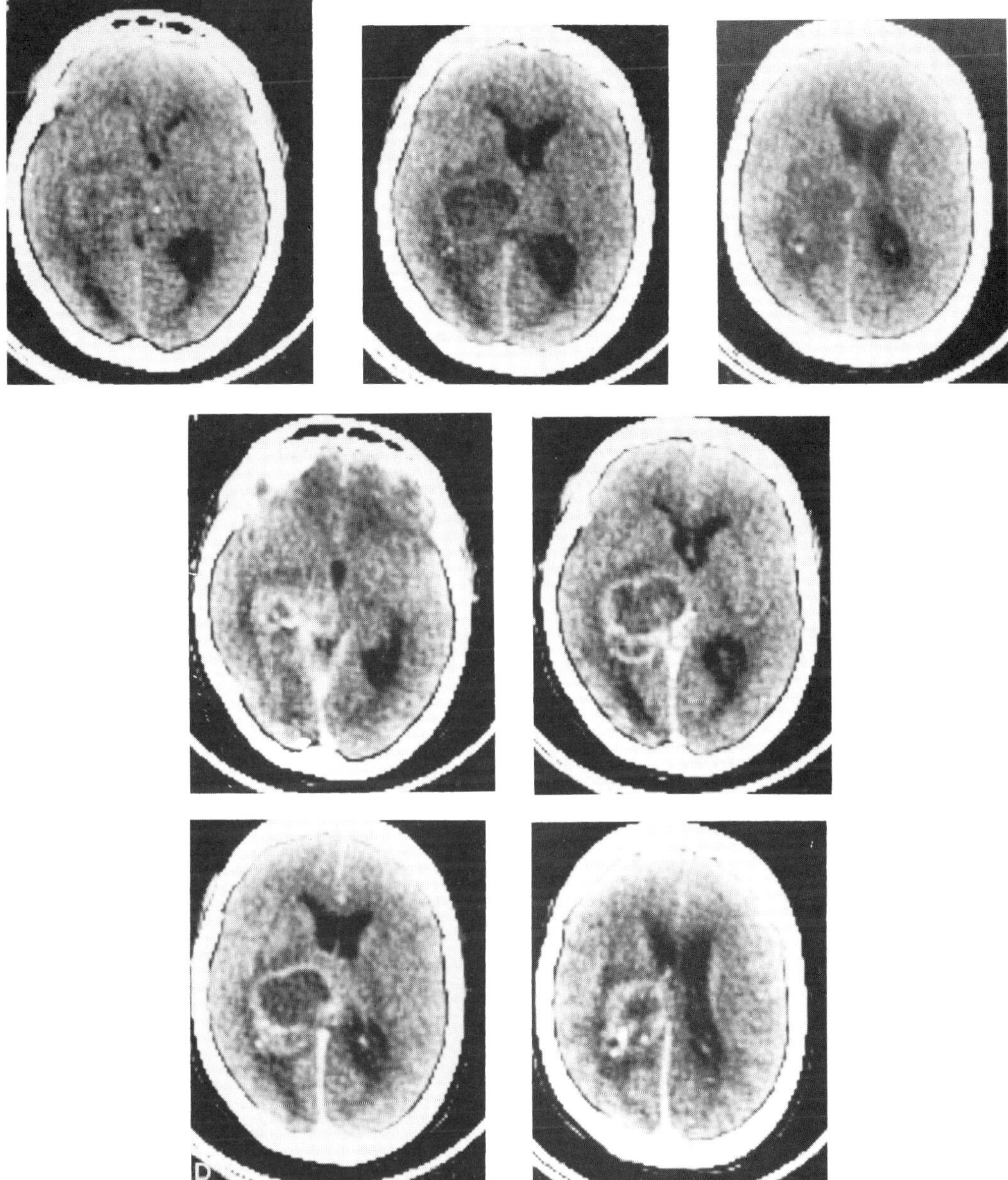

Figure 5–27. DEEP PARIETAL GLIOMA: *A*, The AP view of the carotid angiogram reveals enlargement of the anterior choroidal artery *(arrows)*, which courses posteriorly and then medially to supply a large, deep-seated tumor in the left hemisphere. There is lateral displacement of the middle cerebral vessels secondary to the mass.

B, The lateral view of the vertebral angiogram shows marked hypertrophy of the medial and lateral posterior choroidal arteries that supply the tumor. There are also anomalous vessels that arise from the posterior cerebral artery to supply the area of neovascularity. There is evidence of early venous drainage with filling of the straight sinus *(SS)* on this early arterial film. On the AP view of the vertebral angiogram *(C)*, the large area of neovascularity is seen deep in the left hemisphere *(dashed lines)*.

D, The preinfusion CT scans demonstrate a large radiolucent area deep in the left hemisphere with an irregular ring of higher density that enhances markedly on the postinfusion scan. There is also a moderate amount of irregular surrounding edema. There is distortion of the left lateral ventricle and shift of the midline to the contralateral side.

Surgically proved glioblastoma multiforme.

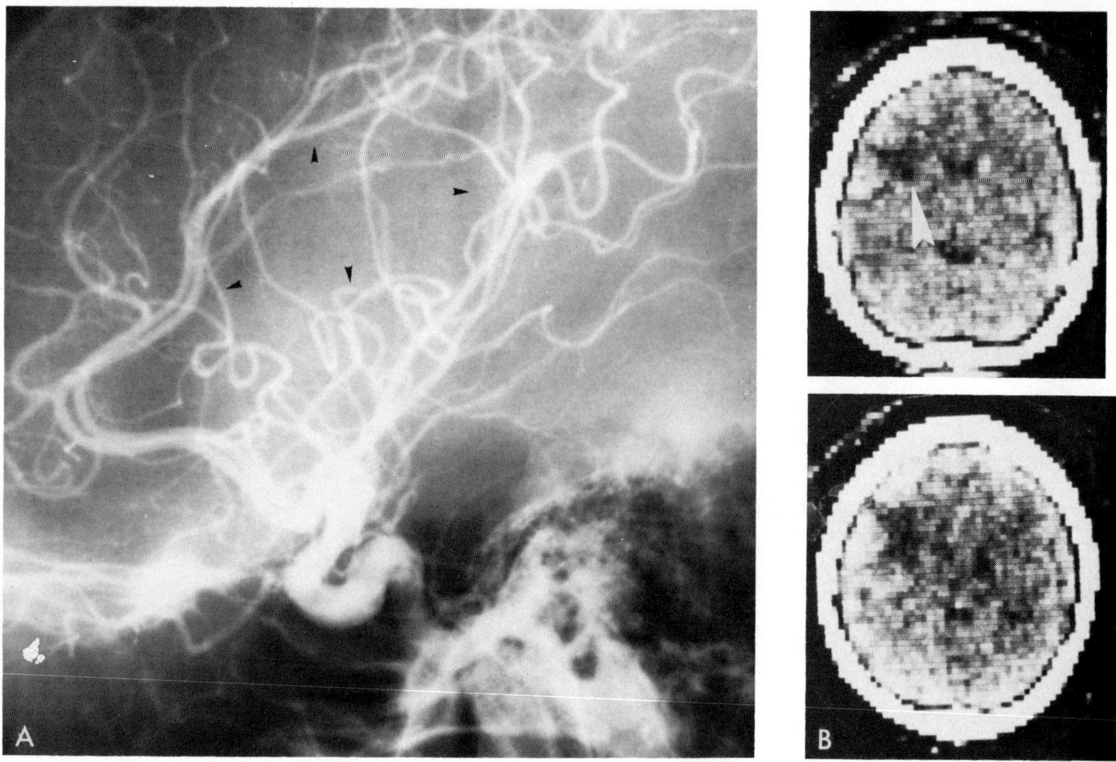

Figure 5–28. THROMBOSED ARTERIOVENOUS MALFORMATION: *A*, The angiogram demonstrates only stretching of the opercular branches of the middle cerebral artery just above the sylvian triangle *(arrows)*. The area is avascular.

B, The CT scan shows a moderate sized area of radiolucency deep in the hemisphere in the anterior parietal region *(arrow)*. There is slight distortion of the frontal horn of the left lateral ventricle.

Surgically proved old thrombosed arteriovenous malformation.

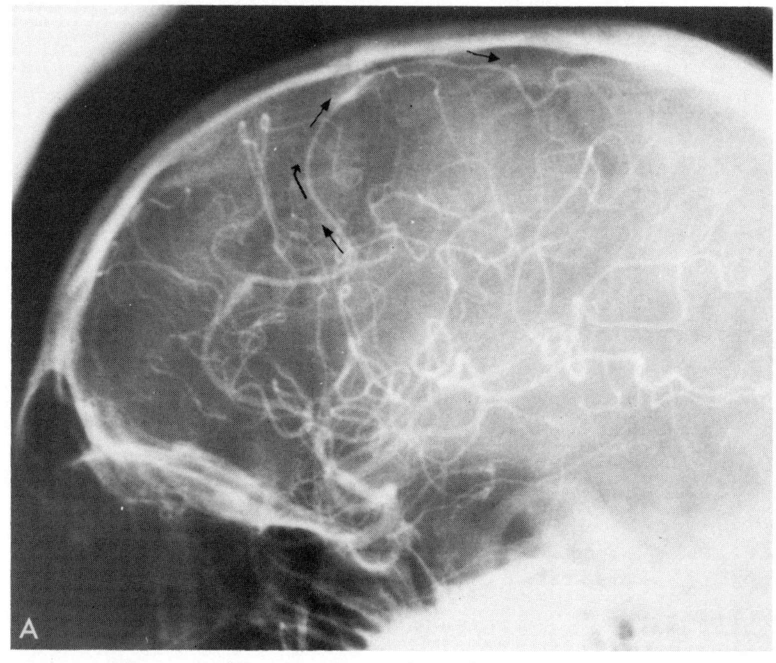

Figure 5–29. *See legend on the opposite page*

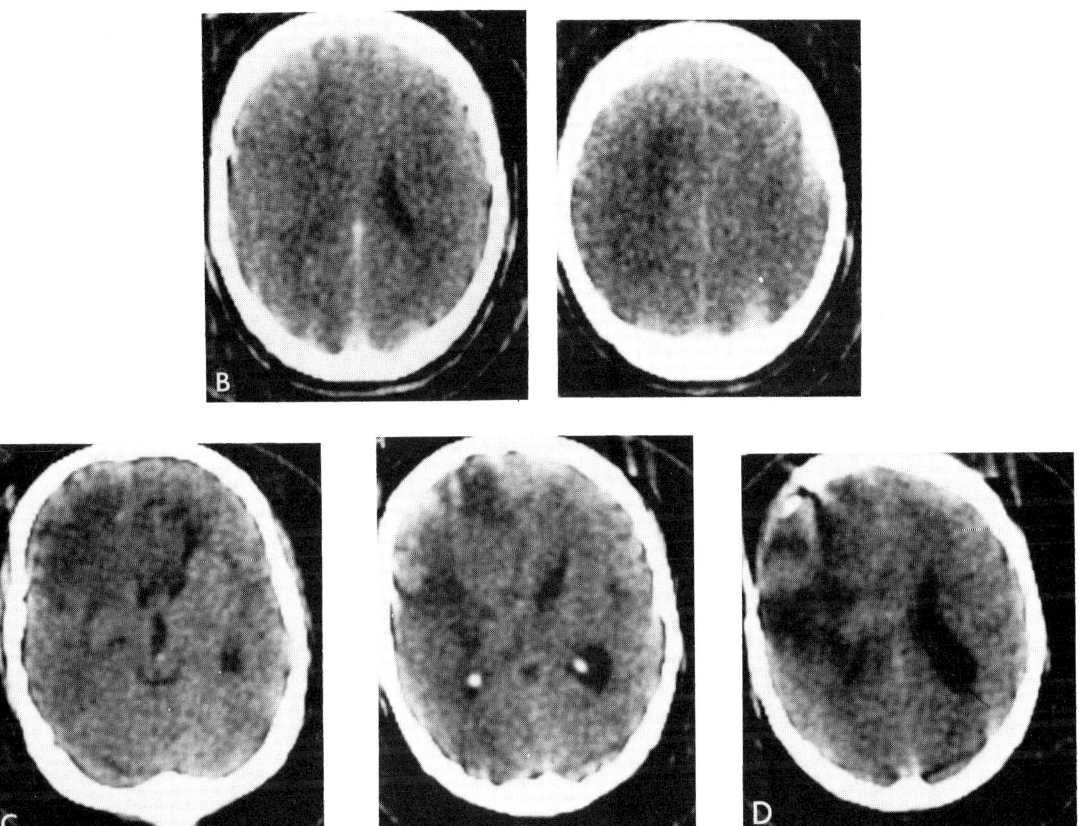

Figure 5–29. ANTERIOR PARIETAL GLIOBLASTOMA: *A*, The angiogram reveals a curvilinear displacement of one of the distal branches of the anterior cerebral artery around an avascular mass in the posterior frontal–anterior parietal region *(arrows)*. There is inferior displacement of the pericallosal artery below the tumor.

B, CT scans done 15 months before the angiogram demonstrated a poorly defined area of radiolucency deep in the left hemisphere and some compression of the body of the left lateral ventricle.

C, CT scans made at the time of the angiogram show a large irregular area of radiolucency in the left frontal and parietal regions that extends across the midline, distorting the frontal horns of the lateral ventricles and splaying the frontal horns. There is also posterior displacement of the anterior portions of the ventricular system. A postinfusion scan is not available.

D, A postoperative scan demonstrates postsurgical changes in the frontal region and a large craniotomy defect.

Surgically proved glioblastoma multiforme.

OCCIPITAL LOBE MASS LESIONS

Mass lesions in the occipital lobe may or may not produce a shift of the anterior cerebral artery. If a shift is detected, there will be slight posterior shift of the pericallosal artery under the falx cerebri. In rare instances there may be a shift of the more proximal anterior cerebral artery (see Figures 5–32 and 5–34). There is a greater shift of the internal cerebral vein; indeed, this may be the only arteriographic finding in some cases. The sylvian point may be displaced anteriorly; because of the angiographic projection, this will give the appearance of superior displacement on the AP view. Superior and anterior displacement also may occur.

The lateral view may appear to be within normal limits. A relatively normal appearance is seen, especially when the posterior cerebral artery does not fill from the internal carotid. Then one normally can anticipate an area of relative avascularity in the occipital region on the lateral view. If the mass is sufficiently large, there is stretching of the vessels in the parietal as well as the occipital region. Depending on the intrinsic vascularity of the mass, an area of avascularity associated with delayed venous filling may be noted.

The lateral view of the venous phase reveals an open venous angle.

The sylvian triangle will be displaced anteriorly, with telescoping of the branches of the middle cerebral artery group. The sylvian point will be displaced anteriorly and, on occasion, superiorly.

In summary the angiographic findings with an occipital lobe mass lesion are:

AP View.

1. Slight or no distal shift of the anterior cerebral artery.
2. A greater shift of the internal cerebral vein.

Lateral View.

3. Anterior telescoping of the sylvian triangle.
4. There may be superior and/or anterior displacement of the sylvian point.
5. An "open" venous angle.
6. An area of avascularity or neovascularity in the occipital region.

Text continued on page 281

Figure 5–30. OCCIPITAL LOBE ABSCESS: *A*, The lateral angiographic view reveals forward telescoping of the sylvian triangle *(large arrow)* and stretching of the distal branches of the middle cerebral artery group in the posterior parietal and occipital regions *(open arrows)*. The mass is avascular.

B, The AP arterial view demonstrates downward and medial displacement of the sylvian point *(arrow)* and a distal shift of the pericallosal artery under the falx cerebri.

C, The venous phase shows a shift of the internal cerebral vein that is equal to or slightly greater than the arterial shift *(arrow)*.

This was proved surgically to be an occipital abscess.

Differential diagnosis includes a primary or secondary brain tumor, an intracerebral hematoma or even a porencephalic cyst.

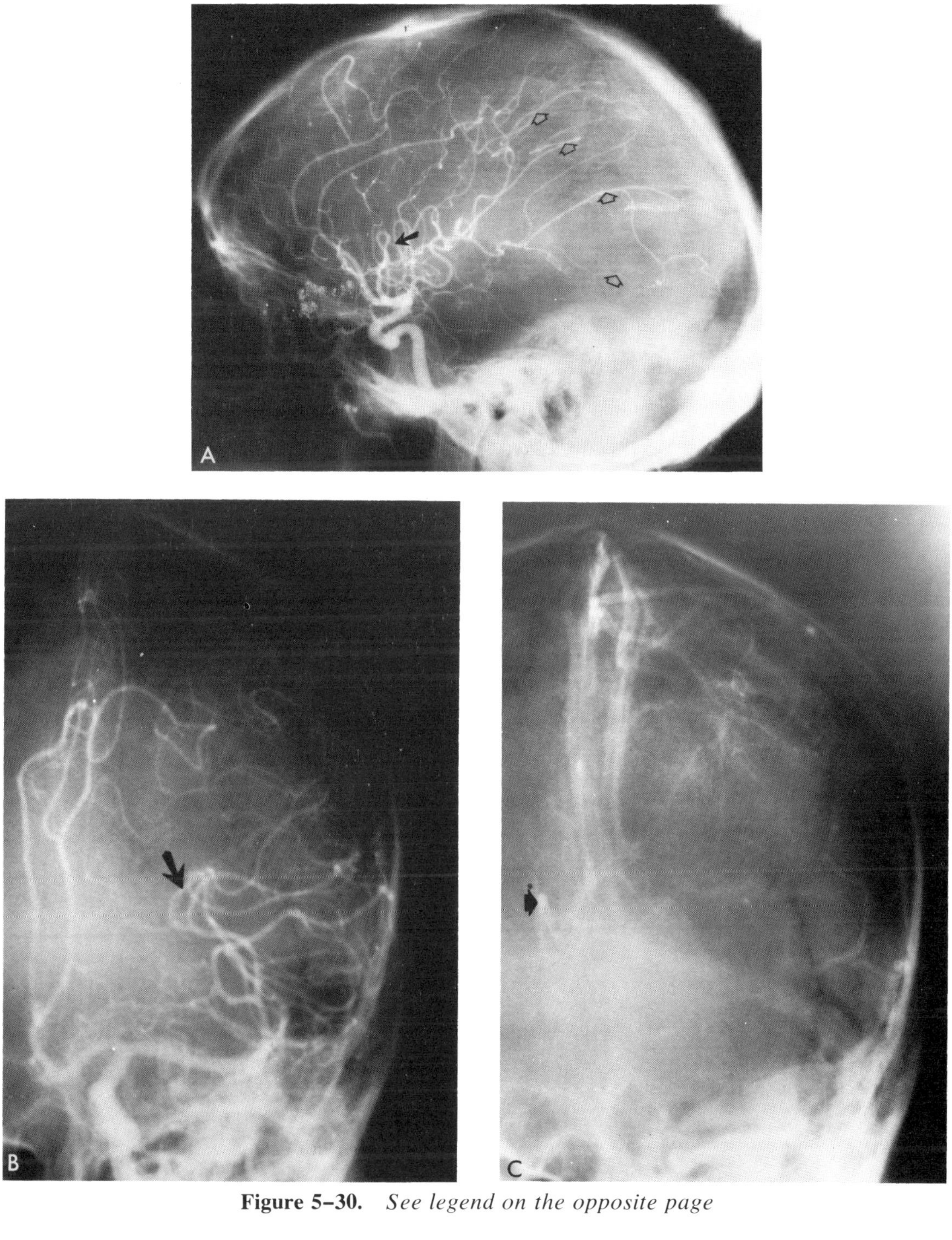

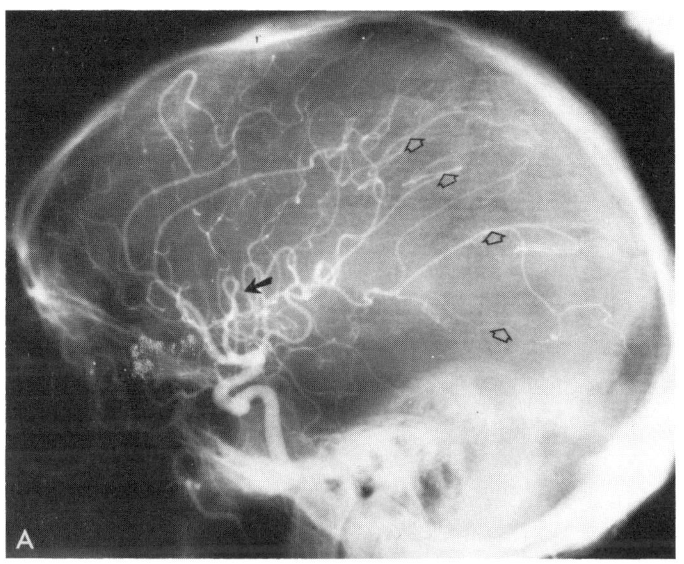

Figure 5–30. *See legend on the opposite page*

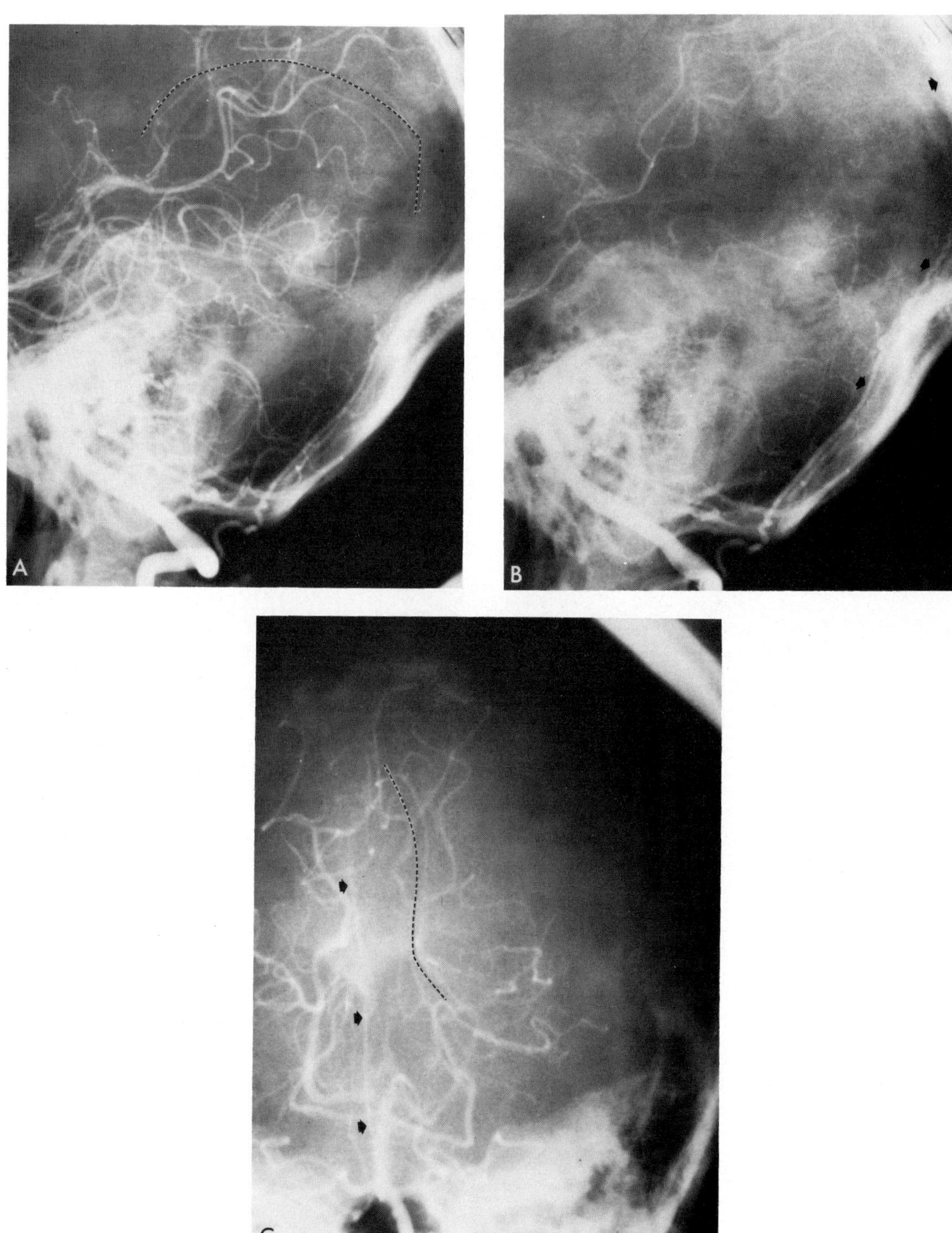

Figure 5–31. *See legend on the opposite page*

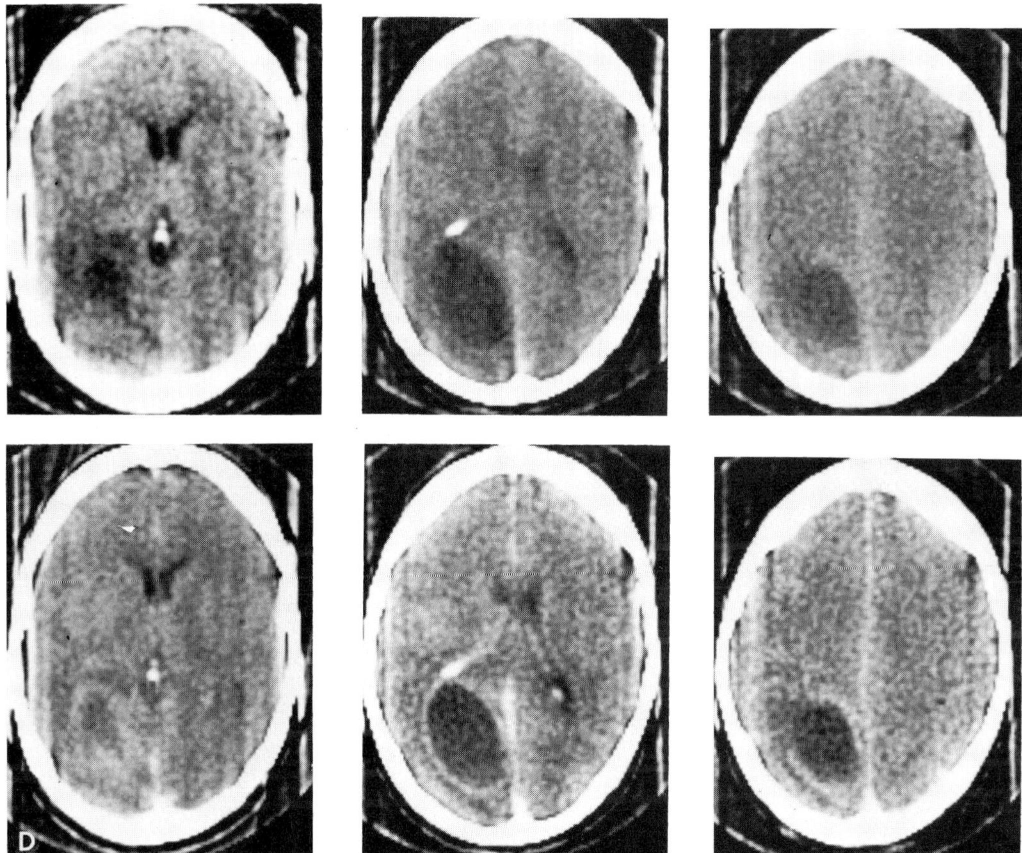

Figure 5–31. CYSTIC GLIOMA, OCCIPITAL LOBE: *A,* The lateral view of the vertebral angiogram reveals curvilinear displacement of the parieto-occipital branch of the posterior cerebral artery *(dashed line).* There is also a very large posterior meningeal artery, which arises from the vertebral artery and is best seen on *(B) (arrows).*

B, The vessel *(arrows)* remains generous in size throughout its course and becomes more tortuous distally — a finding that makes one think of a meningioma. There is no tumor blush, however. The late arterial phase reveals a relatively avascular area in the occipital pole.

The AP view *(C)* also demonstrates the large posterior meningeal artery (*arrows*) and curvilinear displacement of the branch of the posterior cerebral artery *(dashed line)* around the mass in the occipital pole.

D, CT scans reveal a well defined radiolucent lesion in the occipital lobe on the left side. There is anterior displacement of the choroid plexus calcification of the lateral ventricle. There is slight shift of the frontal horns, even though the pineal gland does not appear to have shifted. The fluid within the cyst is of higher density than CSF. There is a rim of enhancement on the postinfusion scan. This was a surgically proved cystic glioblastoma multiforme. Differential diagnosis includes abscess or cystic metastases.

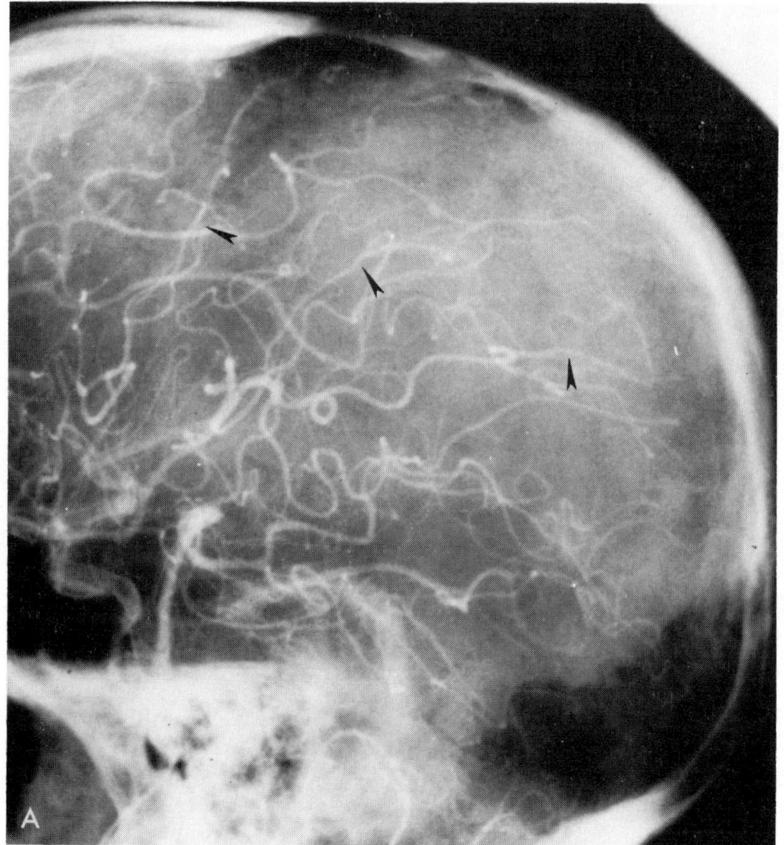

Figure 5–32. OCCIPITAL LOBE ABSCESS: *A*, The lateral angiographic view reveals stretching of all the vessels in the posterior parietal and occipital lobes *(arrows)*. There is no evidence of neovascularity or of a capsular stain. The patient had had a lung abscess removed approximately $1\frac{1}{2}$ months before this admission, and now presented with a left homonymous hemianopia.

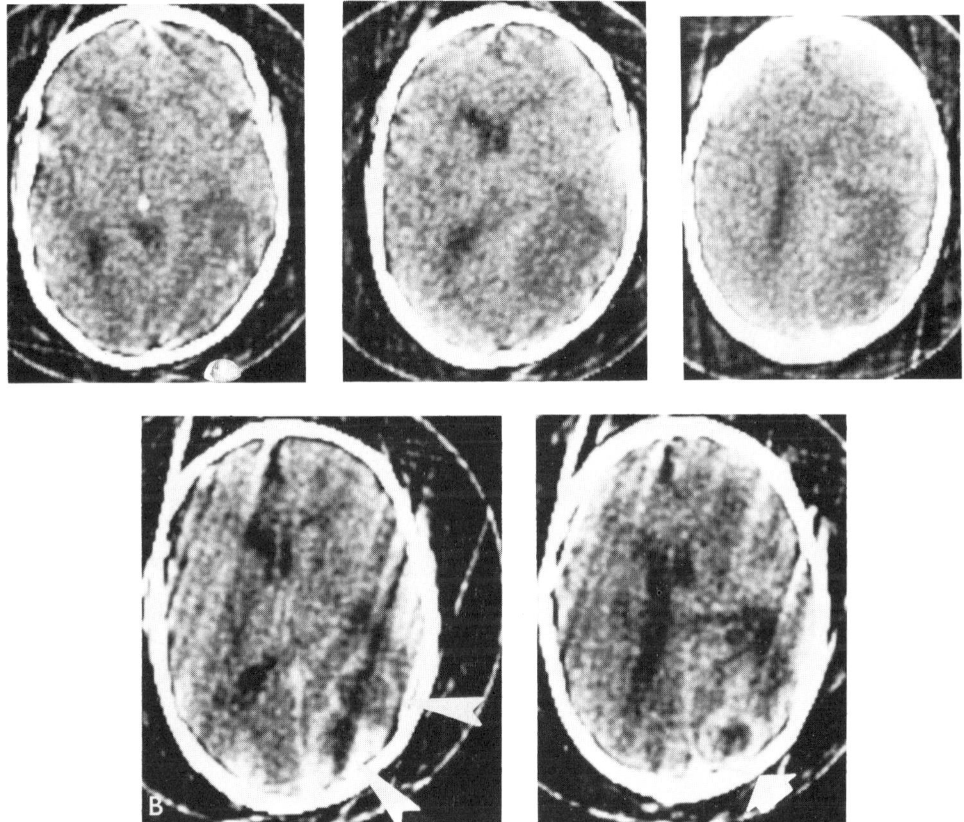

Figure 5–32. *Continued*

B, The CT scans reveal an irregular, poorly defined area of radiolucency in the right occipital lobe, which had a multilobulated appearance on the postinfusion scan. Several separate ring-shaped areas of enhancement can be identified, even though the scan is somewhat degraded by patient motion artifact *(arrows)*. There is also shift of the midline structures and compression of the body of the right lateral ventricle.

An abscess was removed at the time of surgery. Considering the patient's history, abscess seems the most likely diagnosis.

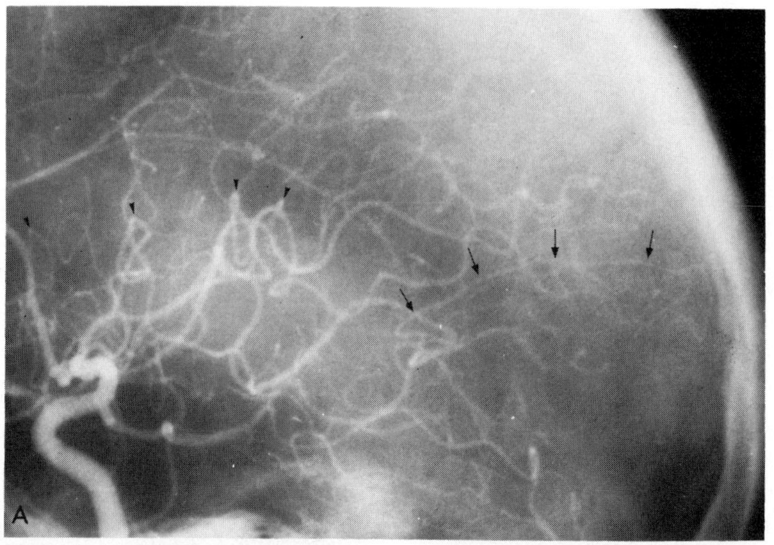

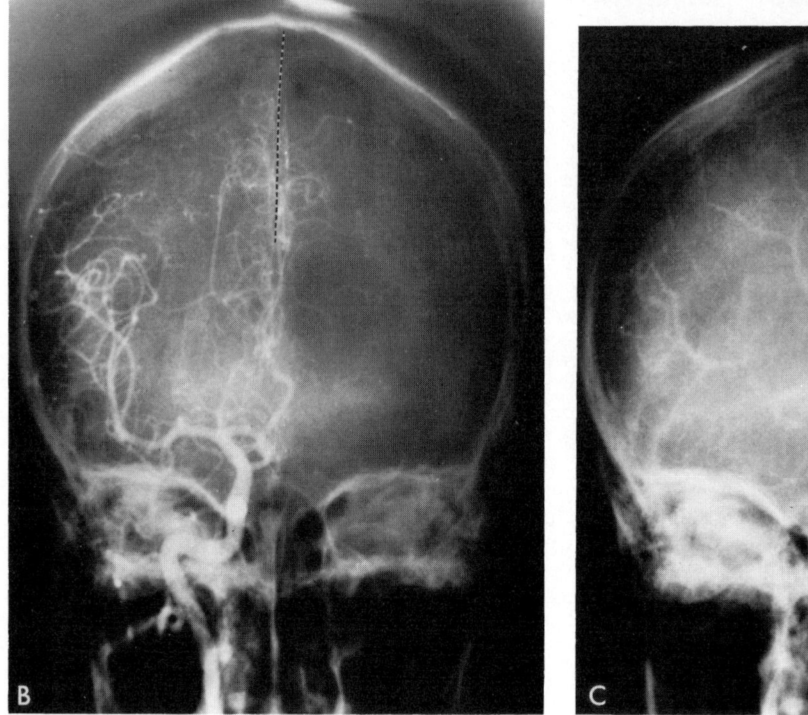

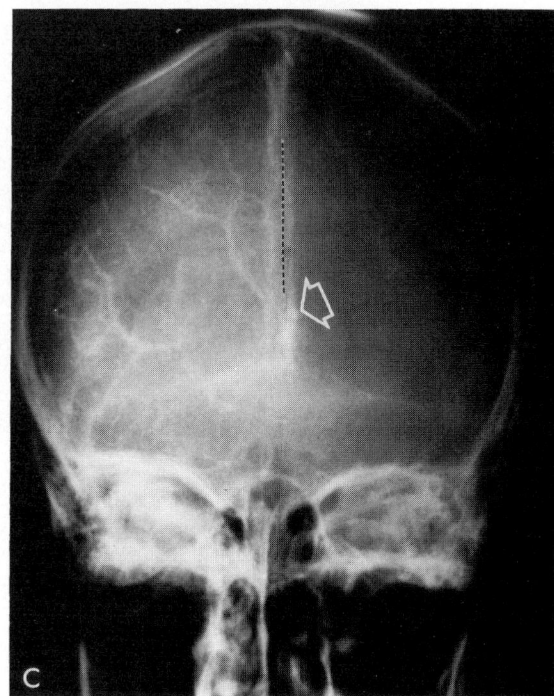

Figure 5–33. OCCIPITAL GLIOBLASTOMA: *A,* The lateral angiographic view shows stretching of a single branch of the posterior cerebral artery in the occipital region *(long arrows).* The sylvian triangle *(arrowheads)* is in normal position. There is no evidence of either neovascularity or a capsular stain.

B and *C,* The AP arterial phase is entirely within normal limits (the dotted line indicates the falx), and there is only a very slight shift of the internal cerebral vein *(arrow),* which still measures within normal limits.

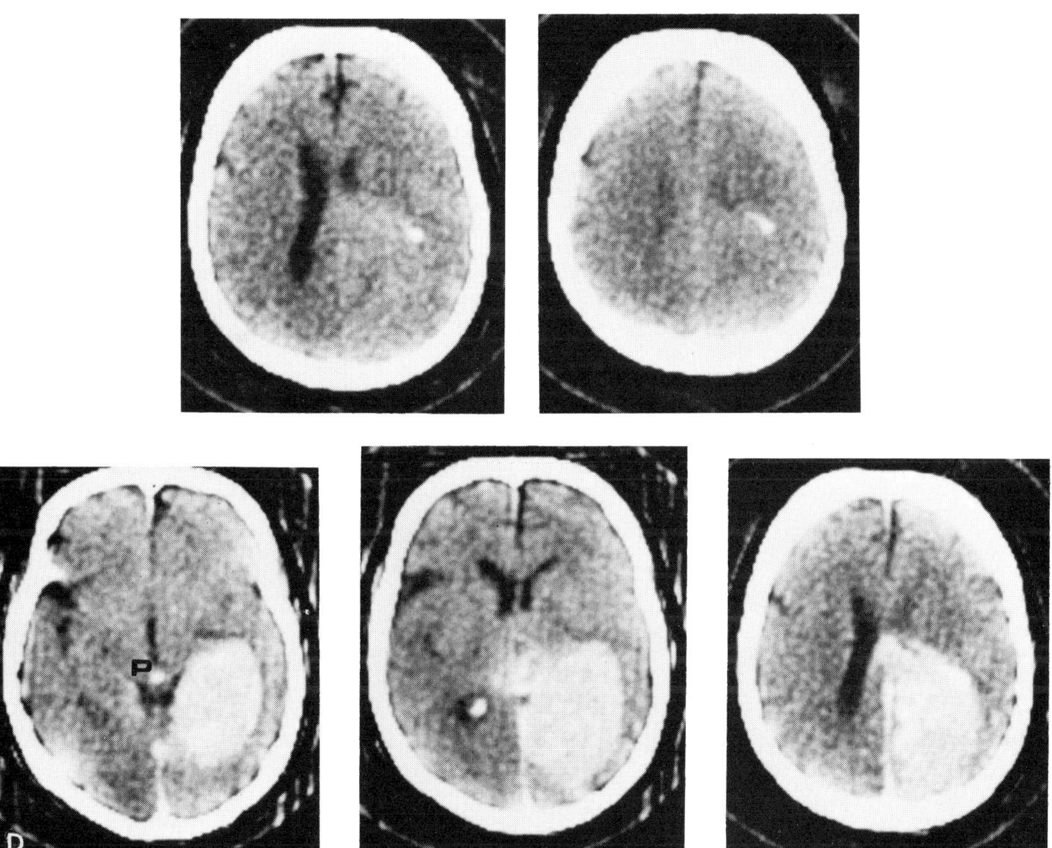

Figure 5–33. *Continued*

D, Ct scans from another patient reveal a slight increase in the density of the brain tissue in the right occipital region on the preinfusion scan with anterior displacement of the choroid plexus calcification in the atrium of the lateral ventricle. Forward displacement of the body of the right lateral ventricle is also seen. The postinfusion scan reveals homogeneous enhancement of a large mass in the right parietal and occipital regions that extends into the posterior aspect of the corpus callosum. The pineal *(P)* is in the midline.

This was proved surgically to be a glioblastoma.

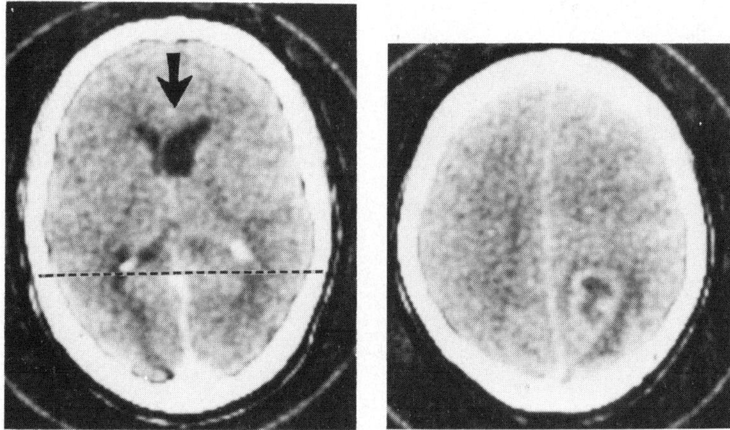

Figure 5–34. OCCIPITAL GLIOBLASTOMA: The postinfusion scan reveals a bilobed area of enhancement in the right occipital region secondary to a glioblastoma. There is forward displacement of the choroid plexus calcification (dotted line marks normal position) and a shift of the frontal horns (arrow marks midline) of the lateral ventricle; the pineal gland has not shifted. This finding sometimes is seen with occipital lobe lesions.

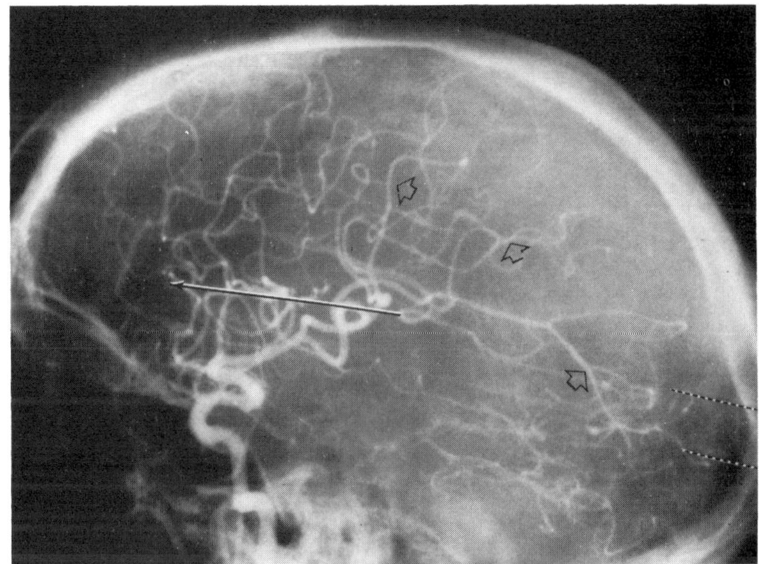

Figure 5–35. OCCIPITAL HEMATOMA: The angiogram reveals marked anterior telescoping of the sylvian triangle *(long arrow)* and stretching of the branches of the middle cerebral artery in the entire parietal lobe and in the occipital lobe *(open arrowheads)*. There is a large avascular area in the occipital lobe, and there is no evidence of neovascularity. The dashed lines follow several straight lines that extend across the head; these are secondary to the adhesive tape used to immobilize the patient.

Surgically proved intracerebral hematoma.

Differential diagnosis includes a primary or secondary brain tumor, an abscess or contusion.

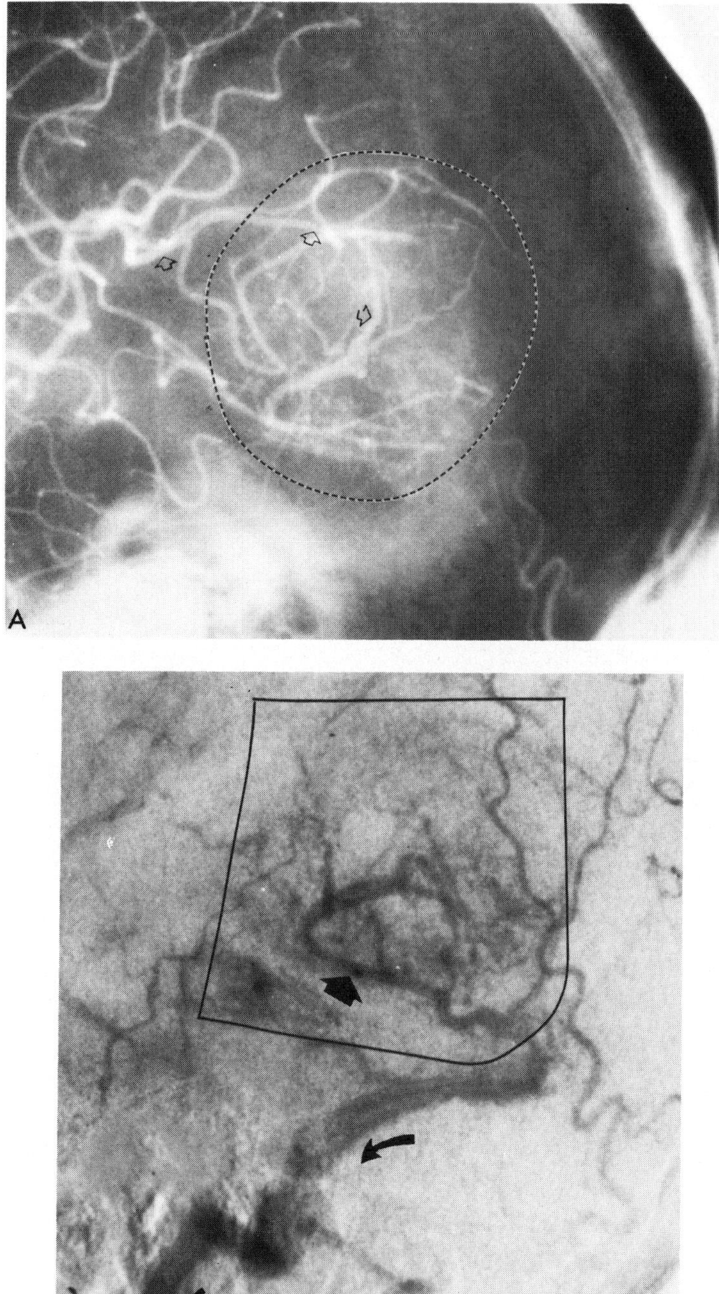

Figure 5–36. OCCIPITAL LOBE GLIOBLASTOMA: *A,* The lateral magnification view of the occipital region shows multiple branches of the middle cerebral artery; these follow an abnormal and tortuous course *(arrows)* and supply a large area of neovascularity *(dotted lines).* The capillary phase *(B)* demonstrates the large abnormal stain *(black lines)* and a large early draining vein, which drains directly into the lateral sinus and then into the sigmoid sinus and the internal jugular vein.

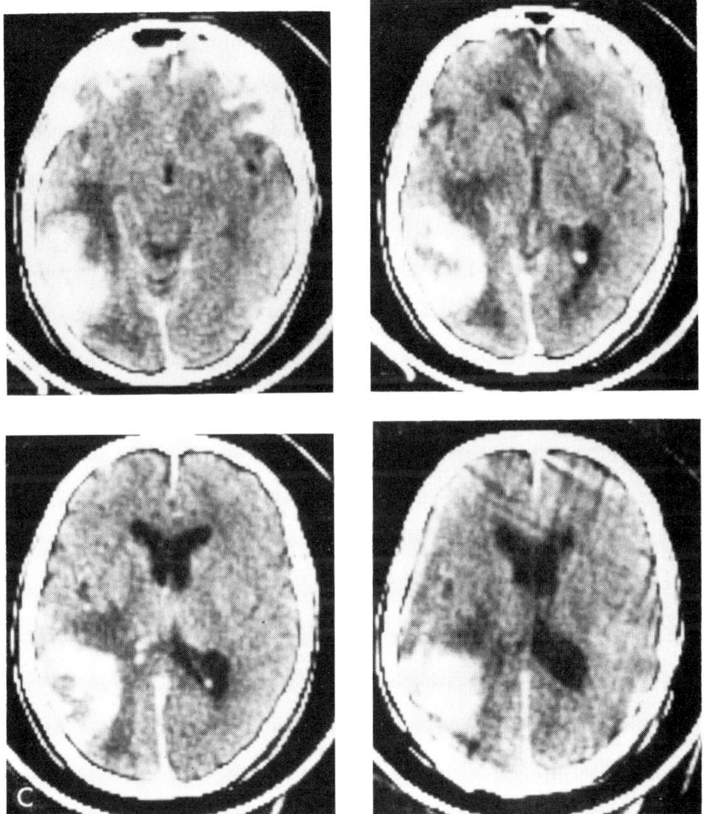

Figure 5–36. *Continued*

C, The CT scans (postinfusion only) reveal a large, thick-rimmed enhancing lesion with a radiolucent center in the left occipital lobe. The lesion has poorly defined outer margins and exhibits an irregular area of surrounding edema. There is minimal mass effect with little shift of the midline.

Surgically proved glioblastoma. Differential diagnosis also includes a vascular metastasis.

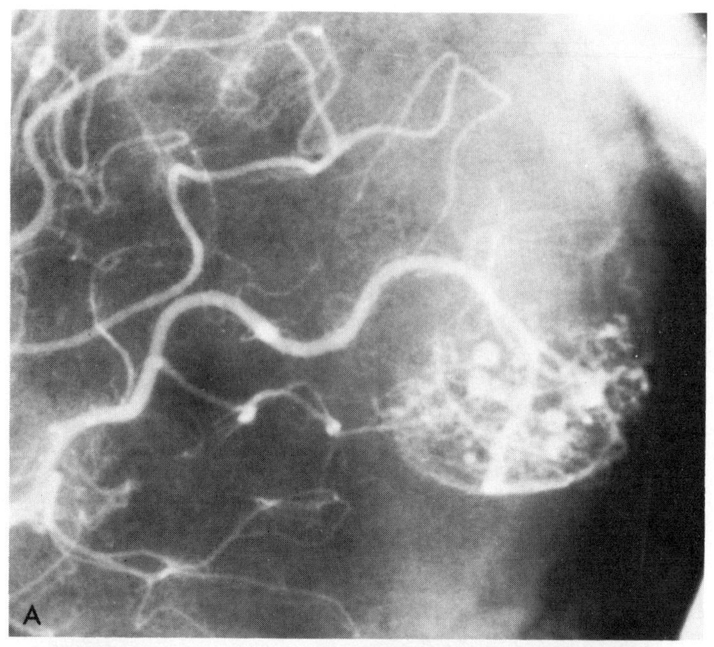

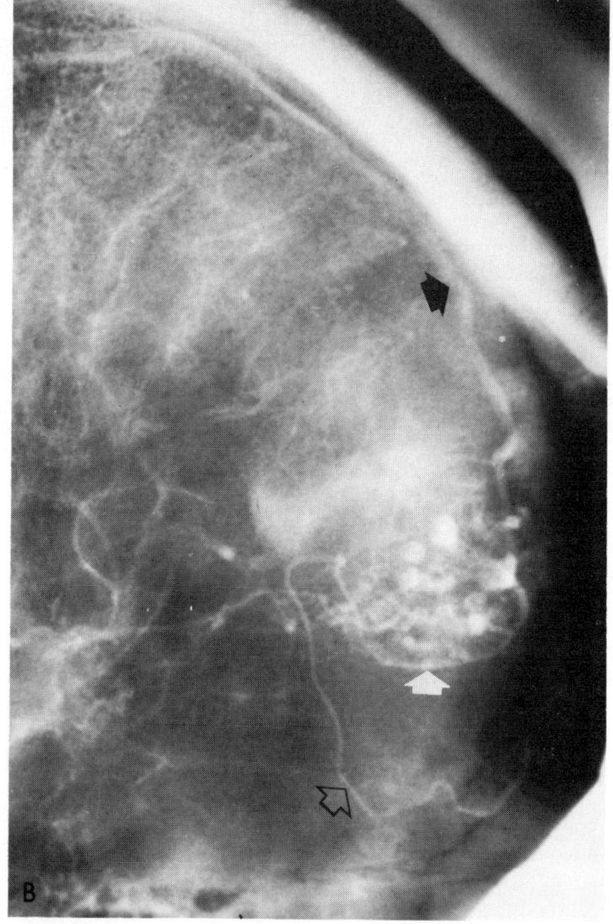

Figure 5–37. *See legend on the opposite page*

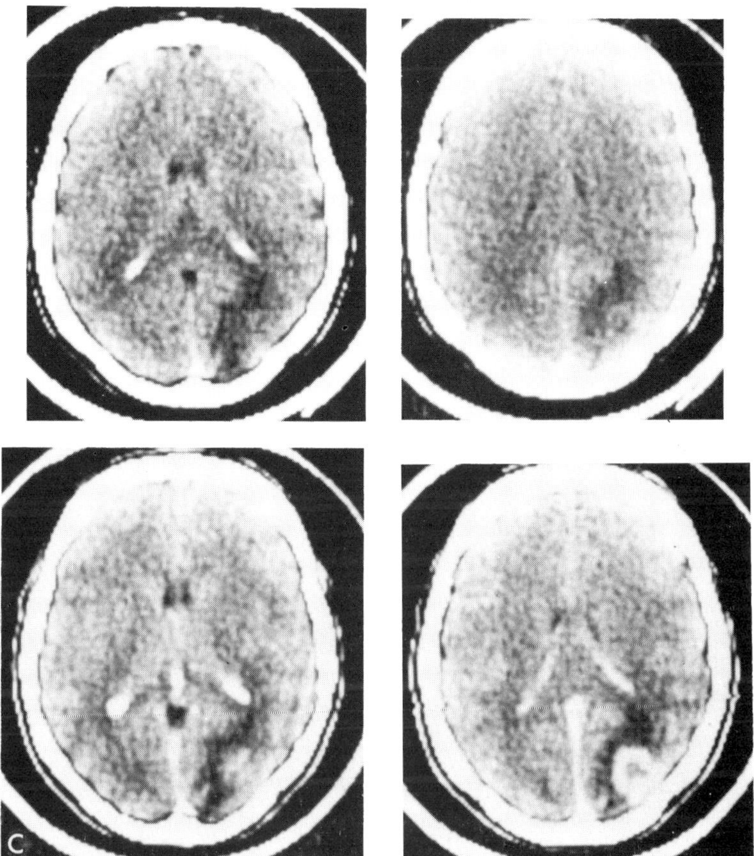

Figure 5–37. OCCIPITAL GLIOBLASTOMA: *A,* The lateral view of the selective internal carotid angiogram demonstrates an enlarged branch of the middle cerebral artery, which courses posteriorly to supply an area of abnormal vascularity in the occipital region. There are multiple abnormal vessels and puddling of the contrast material in multiple scattered abnormal accumulations. There is a surrounding area of avascularity secondary to the surrounding edema.

B, The capillary phase shows the abnormal area *(white arrow)* with a tumor stain and multiple early draining veins — one that drains inferiorly *(open arrow)* and another that drains superiorly into the superior sagittal sinus *(black arrow).*

C, CT scans reveal an area of radiolucency in the occipital region that surrounds an enhancing lesion with a lucent center in the right occipital pole. There is slight anterior displacement of the choroid plexus of the right lateral ventricle.

Surgically proved glioblastoma multiforme.

TEMPORAL LOBE MASS LESIONS

Large temporal lobe mass lesions cause both superior and medial displacement of the sylvian point. The branches of the middle cerebral artery will be displaced medially, and the genu of the middle cerebral artery, which normally is 20 to 30 mm from the inner table of the skull, also will be displaced medially. (This latter measurement is one of the least reliable of the angiographic measurements.) The anterior cerebral artery usually demonstrates an equal proximal and distal shift under the falx cerebri. There is a greater shift of the internal cerebral vein. The thalamostriate vein is medially displaced. The lenticulostriate vessels are medially displaced, as is the anterior choroidal artery.

The lateral view reveals superior displacement of the sylvian point and the entire sylvian triangle. If the mass is sufficiently large, the main branch of the middle cerebral artery will simulate the normal anatomy of the anterior cerebral artery; on the lateral view this may be mistaken for occlusion of the middle cerebral artery rather than the marked distortion that is really present. The temporal opercular branches will be markedly stretched.

If the mass is intrinsic within the temporal lobe, the branches of the middle cerebral artery will be "draped" over the mass. This draping sign is helpful when there is difficulty differentiating an intrinsic from an extrinsic mass of the temporal lobe. An extrinsic mass, such as a sphenoid wing meningioma, may have a similar pattern of vessel dislocation but will not demonstrate the draped appearance of the temporal opercular branches.

Depending on the intrinsic vascularity of the mass, there may be an avascular region in the temporal lobe.

In summary, the angiographic findings with a temporal lobe mass lesion are:

AP View.

1. Varying shift of the pericallosal artery, which may be equal proximally and distally or have only distal shift.
2. A greater shift of the internal cerebral vein.
3. Superior displacement of the sylvian point and medial displacement of the middle cerebral vessels.

Lateral View.

4. Superior displacement of the sylvian point and the sylvian triangle.
5. Stretching of the vessels in the temporal lobe region.

Text continued on page 308

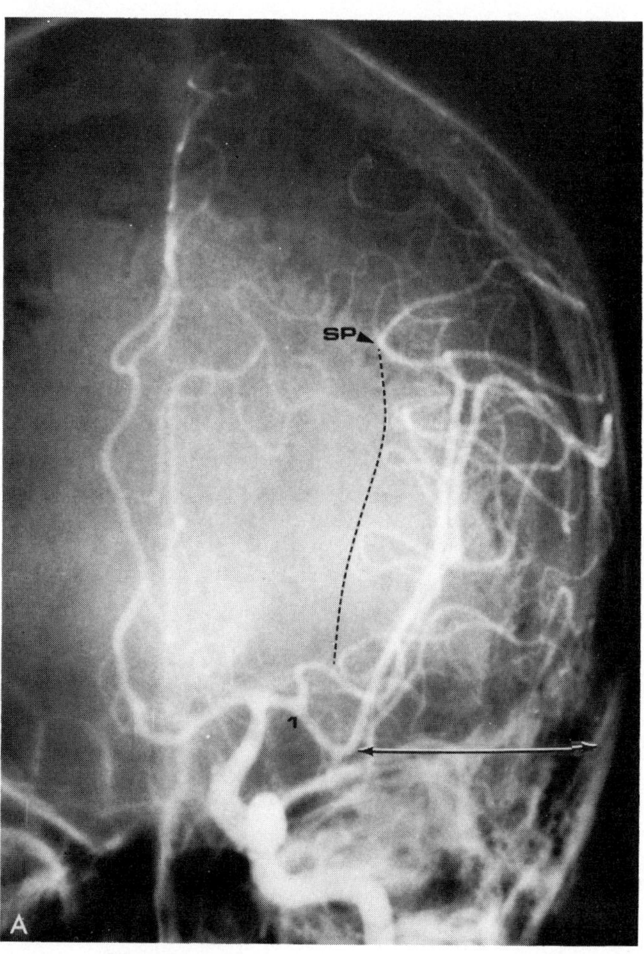

Figure 5–38. *See legend on page 284*

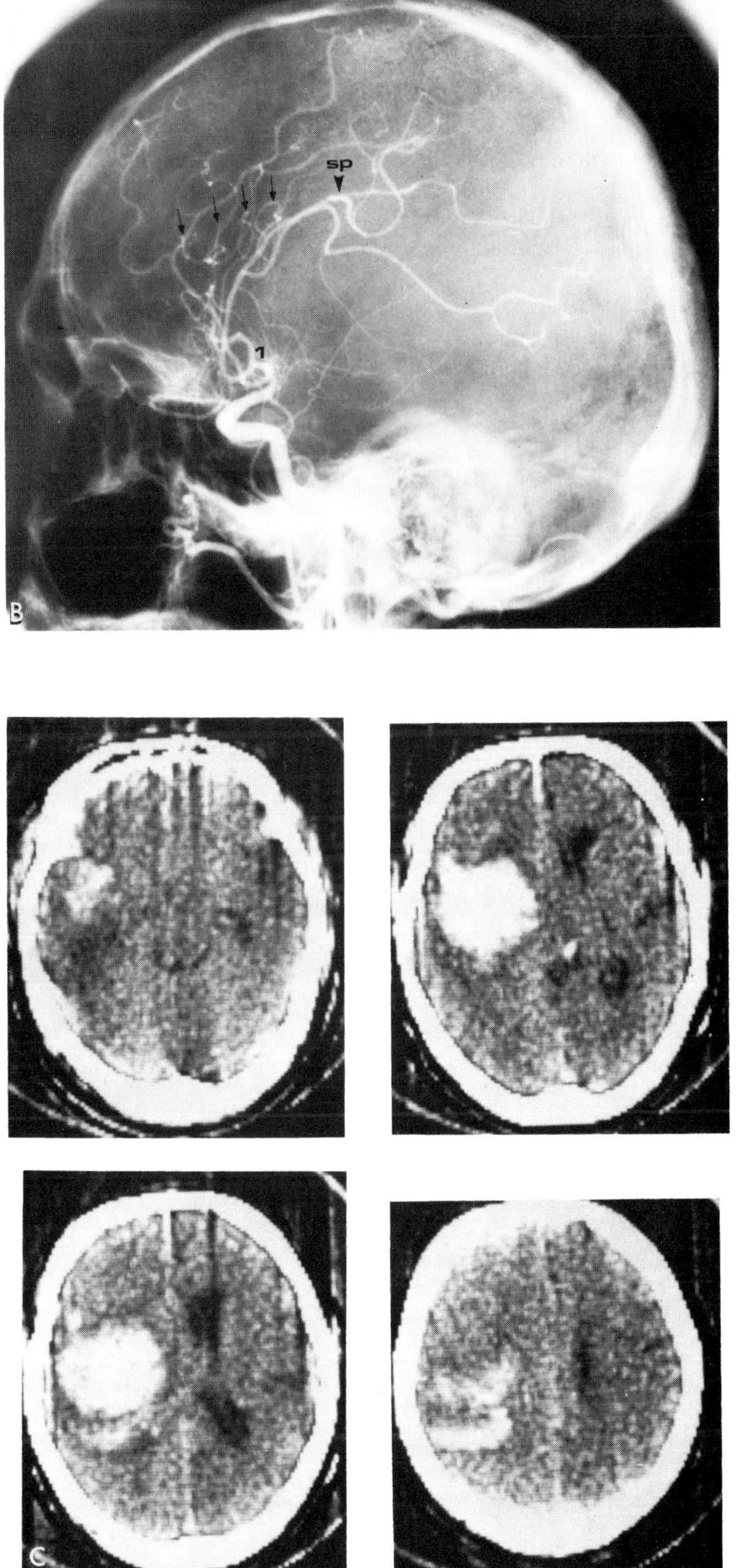

Figure 5–38. *(Continued) See legend on the following page*

Figure 5–38. TEMPORAL LOBE HEMATOMA: *A,* The AP angiographic view shows superior displacement of the sylvian point *(SP)* and medial displacement of all the branches of the middle cerebral artery. The genu of the middle cerebral artery is displaced medially *(double-headed arrow).* The middle cerebral artery bifurcation is well demonstrated *(1).* There is proximal and distal shift of the anterior cerebral artery.

B, The lateral view demonstrates that there is marked superior displacement of the entire sylvian triangle and the sylvian point (*arrows* and *sp*). In fact, the sylvian triangle is so elevated that the main branches of the middle cerebral artery appear to follow the course of the anterior cerebral artery. The bifurcation of the middle cerebral artery is well seen *(1)* because of the distortion of the middle cerebral artery group.

C, The CT scans reveal a large intracerebral hematoma in the left temporal lobe. There is marked shift to the contralateral side. There is an area of radiolucency posterior to the hematoma in the low temporal region; there is also obliteration of the cortical sulci on the side of the hematoma.

IMP: Giant temporal lobe hematoma.

See illustrations on pages 282 and 283

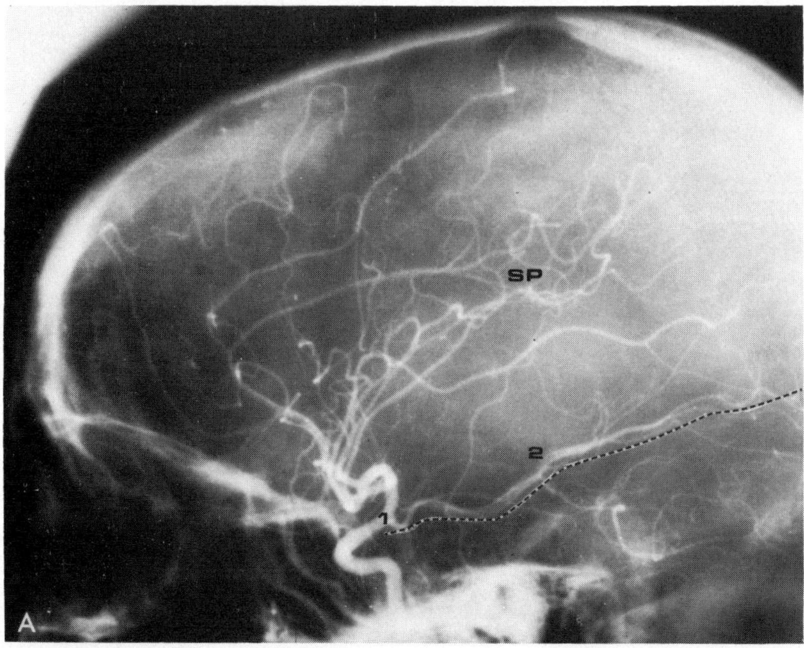

Figure 5–39. TEMPORAL LOBE HEMATOMA: *A,* The lateral angiographic view reveals superior displacement of the sylvian point *(SP)* and the entire sylvian triangle. The posterior cerebral artery arises directly from the internal carotid artery *(1)* on the AP *(B)* and lateral views and is displaced inferiorly and medially. This displacement occurs because the hematoma is pushing the hippocampal gyrus of the temporal lobe (and therefore the adjacent posterior cerebral artery) downward through the tentorial notch — *transtentorial herniation* — and at the point where the vessel returns to the supratentorial position there is a "step upward" of the artery over the free edge of the tentorium *(2).* Dotted line indicates posterior cerebral artery.

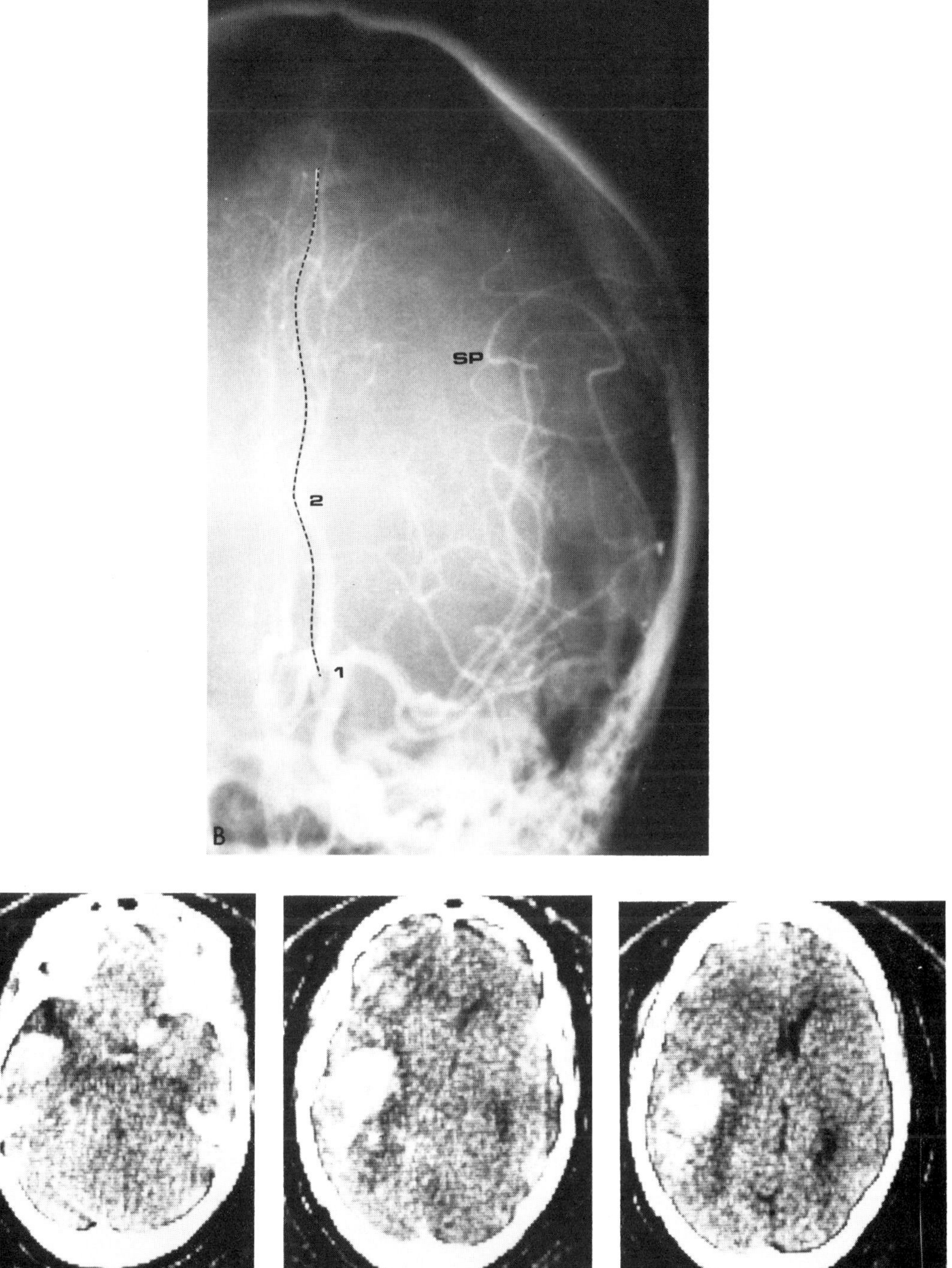

Figure 5–39. *Continued*

The AP view *(B)* reveals marked medial displacement of the posterior cerebral artery because of the herniation. The sylvian point *(SP)* is displaced superiorly, as are the rest of the vessels of the middle cerebral artery.

There is an avascular mass involving the entire temporal lobe — a "holotemporal" mass lesion.

C, CT scans demonstrate a large left temporal lobe hematoma associated with an area of surrounding edema and shift to the contralateral side. Also present is an intracerebral hematoma in the left frontal region, which was not previously suspected and is best seen on the middle cut.

IMP: Left posterior frontal and temporal hematoma.

Figure 5–40. TEMPORAL HEMATOMA SECONDARY TO ARTERIOVENOUS MALFORMATION: *A,* The lateral view demonstrates very marked elevation of the middle cerebral artery branches *(dashed line)* and a large avascular area in the temporal lobe region. The anterior choroidal artery *(ant ch)* is displaced inferiorly by the mass, but is seen to be enlarged in its distal portion and to supply an abnormal collection of vessels in the posterior temporal region.

B, The later arterial phase reveals that the branches of the middle cerebral artery are "draped" in a curvilinear fashion over the mass within the temporal lobe *(open arrowheads).* The small abnormal collection of vessels of an arteriovenous malformation are again seen *(large curved arrow),* and there is early filling of the straight sinus with contrast material *(black arrow heads).*

IMP: Large temporal hematoma secondary to hemorrhage from an arteriovenous malformation.

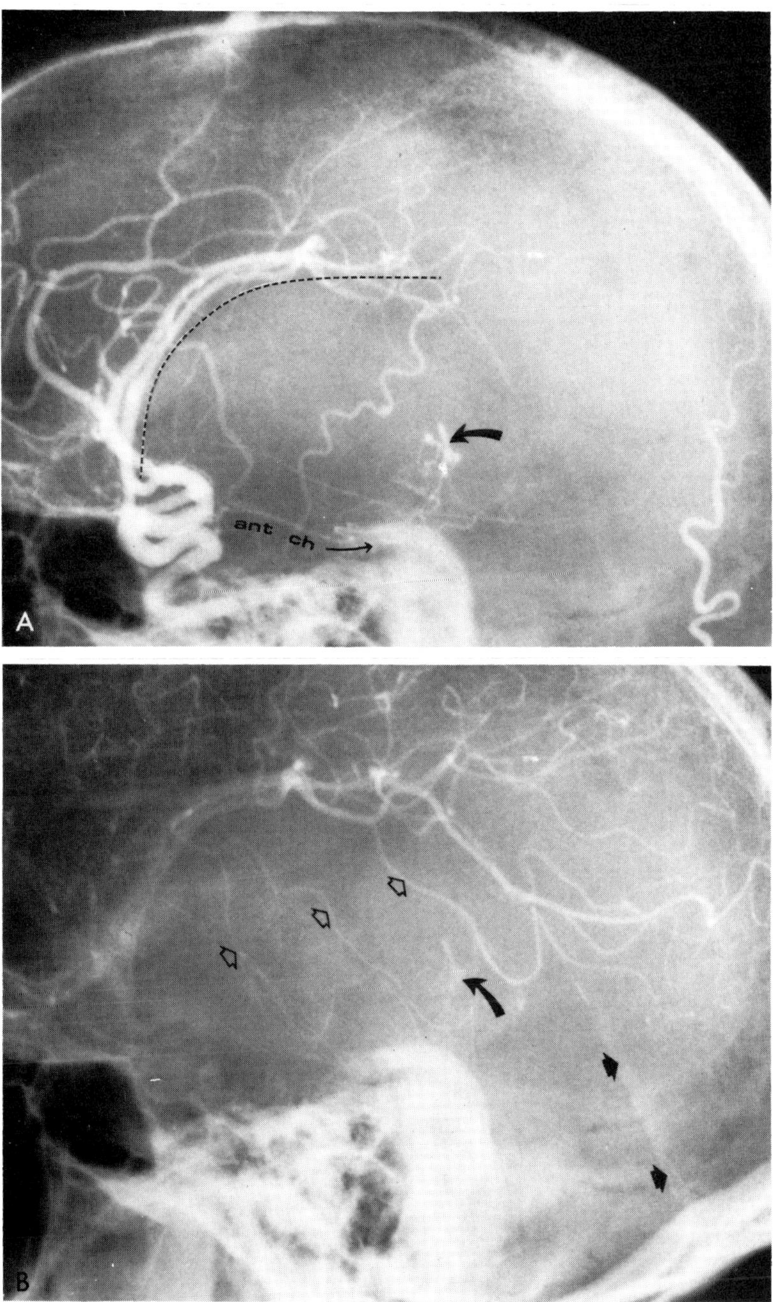

Figure 5–40. *See legend on the opposite page*

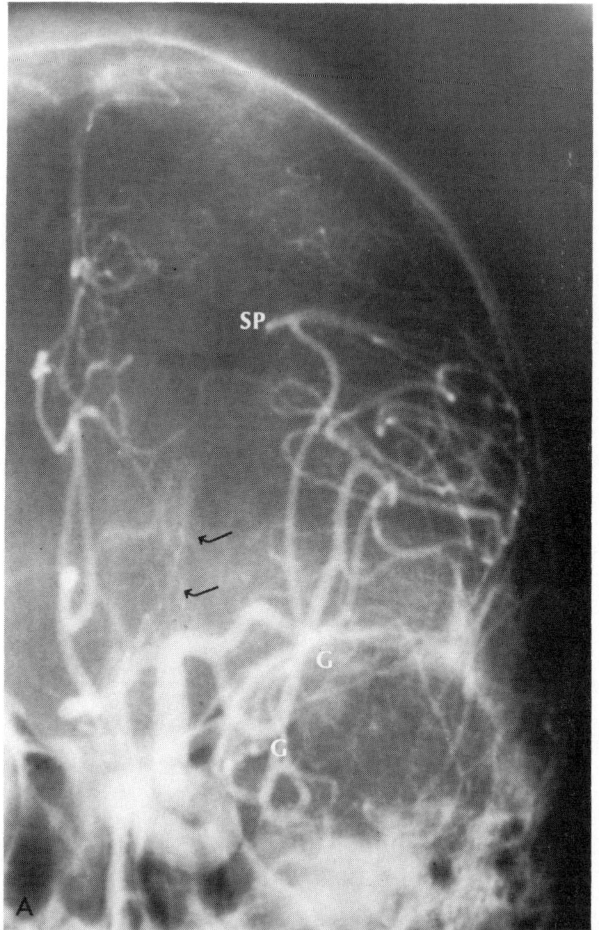

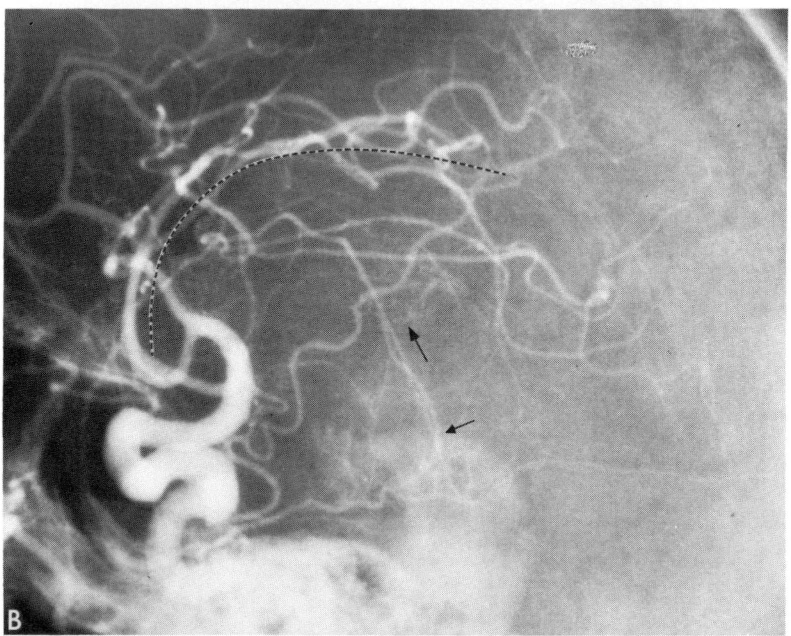

Figure 5–41. *See legend on the opposite page*

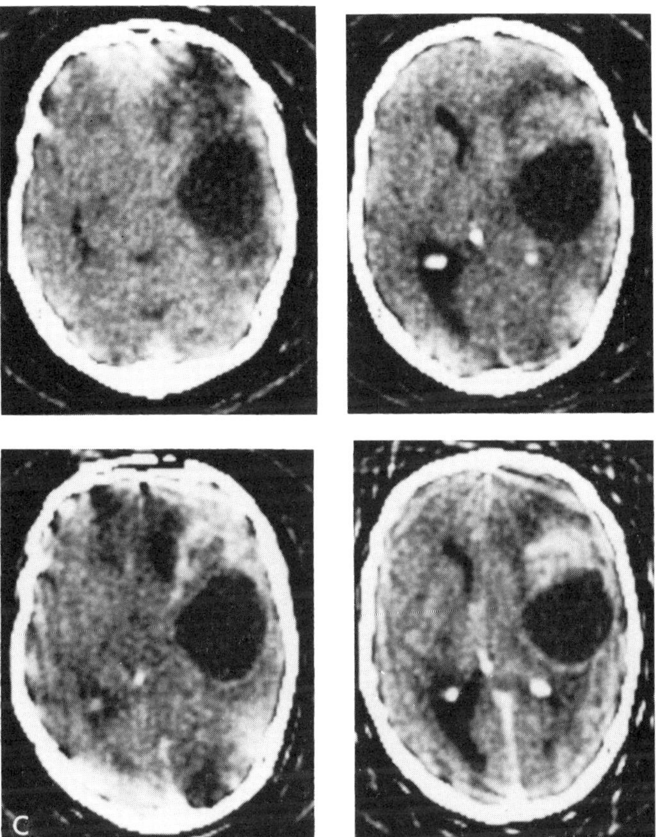

Figure 5–41. TEMPORAL LOBE CYSTIC GLIOBLASTOMA: *A*, The AP angiographic view demonstrates superior and medial displacement of the sylvian point *(SP)* as well as medial displacement of all the branches of the middle cerebral artery. The genu *(G)* of the middle cerebral artery also is displaced medially. The branches of the middle cerebral artery can be seen to reach the inner table of the calvaria. The mass is so large and extends so deep that there is also medial displacement of the lenticulostriate arteries *(small curved arrows)*. There is a proximal and distal shift of the anterior cerebral artery.

B, The lateral view reveals marked elevation of the main branches of the middle cerebral artery *(dashed line)* and draping of the branches of the middle cerebral artery over the mass. The small arrows also indicate multiple small areas of neovascularity, particularly in the anterior temporal region.

C, CT scans show a large cystic lesion occupying the entire right temporal region. The fluid within the cyst is of higher density than CSF, reflecting its high protein content. Anterior to the cyst there is a mass of higher density than normal brain tissue and irregular areas of surrounding edema. The postinfusion scan reveals enhancement of the mass anterior to the cyst and a rim of peripheral enhancement around the tumor itself. There is a shift of the midline to the contralateral side.

Differential diagnosis includes abscess, cystic metastasis, cystic astrocytoma or cystic glioblastoma.

Surgically proved cystic glioblastoma.

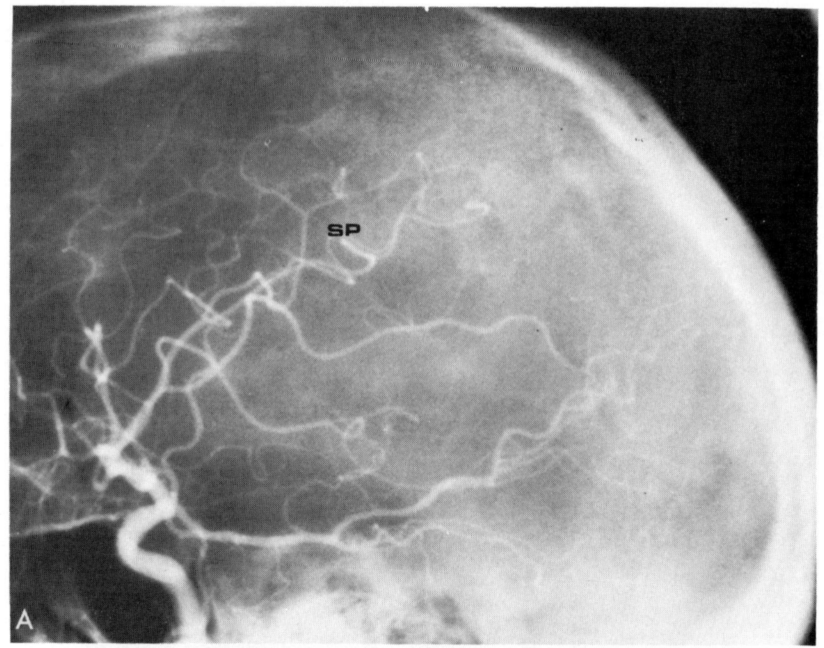

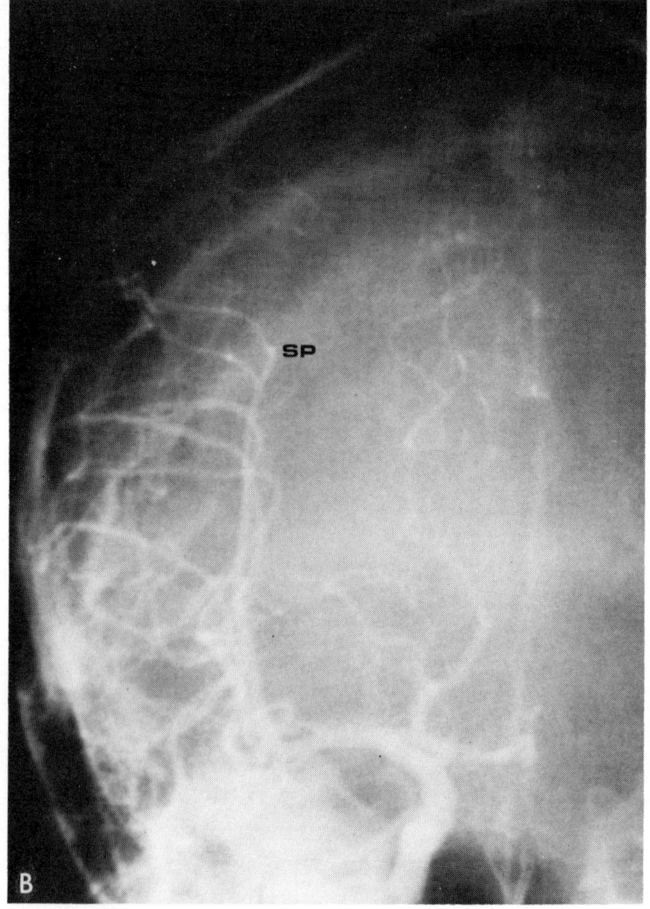

Figure 5–42. *See legend on the opposite page*

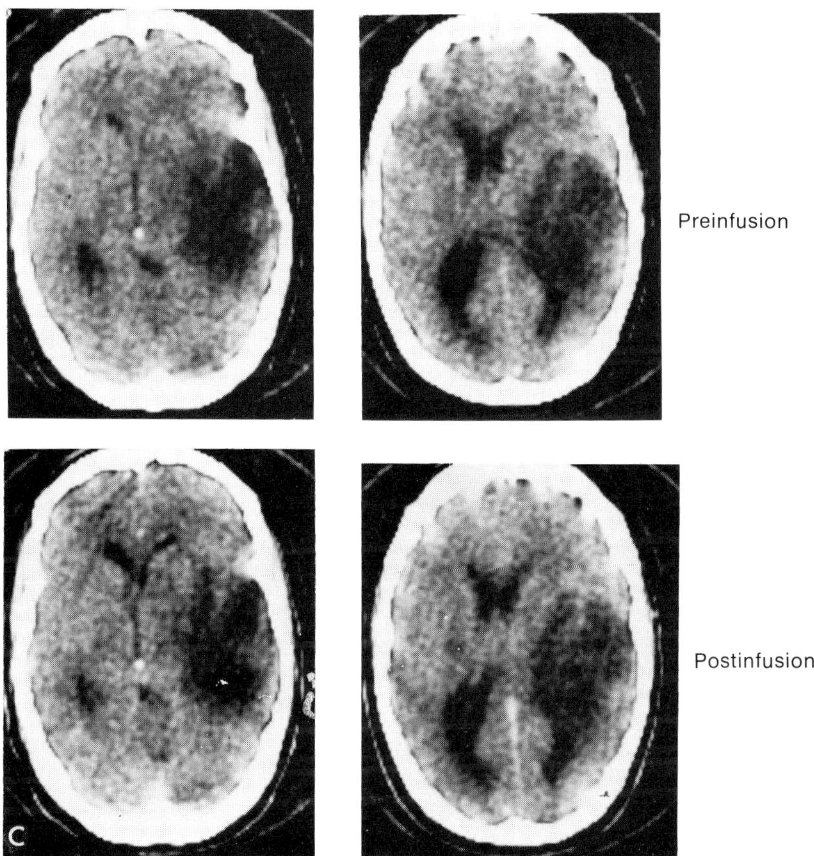

Figure 5–42. TEMPORAL AND BASAL GANGLIA GLIOBLASTOMA: *A*, The lateral view reveals elevation of the sylvian triangle and the sylvian point *(SP)*. There is draping of the middle cerebral vessels over the temporal lobe mass, and a wide separation between the middle cerebral artery and the posterior cerebral artery. The posterior cerebral artery is displaced inferiorly and medially because of transtentorial herniation.

B, The AP view reveals that the sylvian point is displaced superiorly and medially *(SP)*, as are the rest of the vessels of the middle cerebral artery group. The posterior cerebral artery is displaced medially. There is a very slight shift of the anterior cerebral artery to the contralateral side. The lenticulostriate arteries are also displaced medially because the mass extends deep into the basal ganglia.

C, The CT scan reveals a non-enhancing mass in the right temporal lobe. The lesion is irregular in its distribution and extends deep into the right cerebral hemisphere. There is a shift of the midline and compression of the body of the right lateral ventricle. The contralateral ventricle is dilated secondary to the transtentorial herniation.

Differential diagnosis includes a primary brain tumor, an area of infarction that is space-occupying (unlikely), an area of cerebritis and possibly herpes simplex.

Surgically proved glioblastoma.

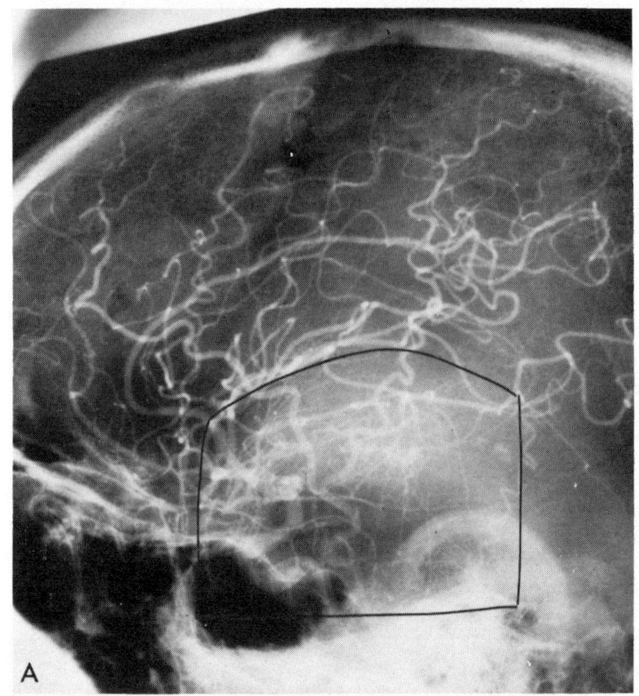

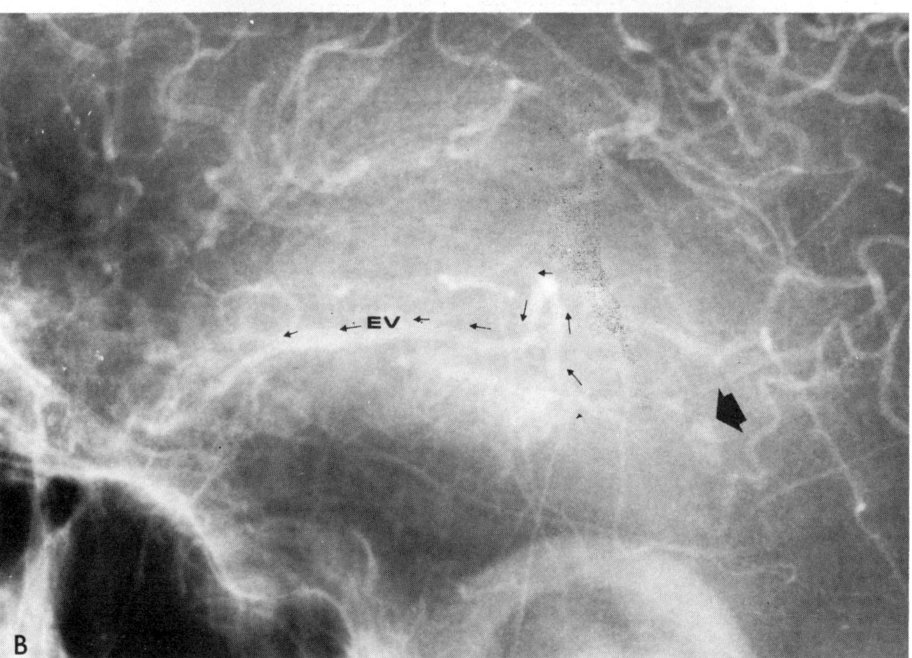

Figure 5–43. TEMPORAL LOBE GLIOMA: The early arterial view *(A)* reveals elevation of the sylvian triangle and multiple, small abnormal-appearing vessels in the temporal region *(black lines)*. The lateral magnification views (*B* and *C*) of the posterior temporal region show the abnormal vessels to better advantage and also demonstrate an early vein *(small arrows)*, which drains into the middle cerebral vein *(EV)*. There is also an abnormal area of puddling of the contrast material in the posterior temporal region *(black arrowhead)*. This puddling of contrast material persists well into the venous phase (*black arrow* in *C*).

D, CT scans from another patient with a similar process demonstrate an enhancing lesion *(open arrows)* in the posterior portion of the left temporal lobe. There is a large amount of irregular edema anterior to the mass, and there is distortion of the retrothalamic cistern *(closed arrow)*. There is marked shift to the contralateral side.

Surgery revealed a glioblastoma in both cases.

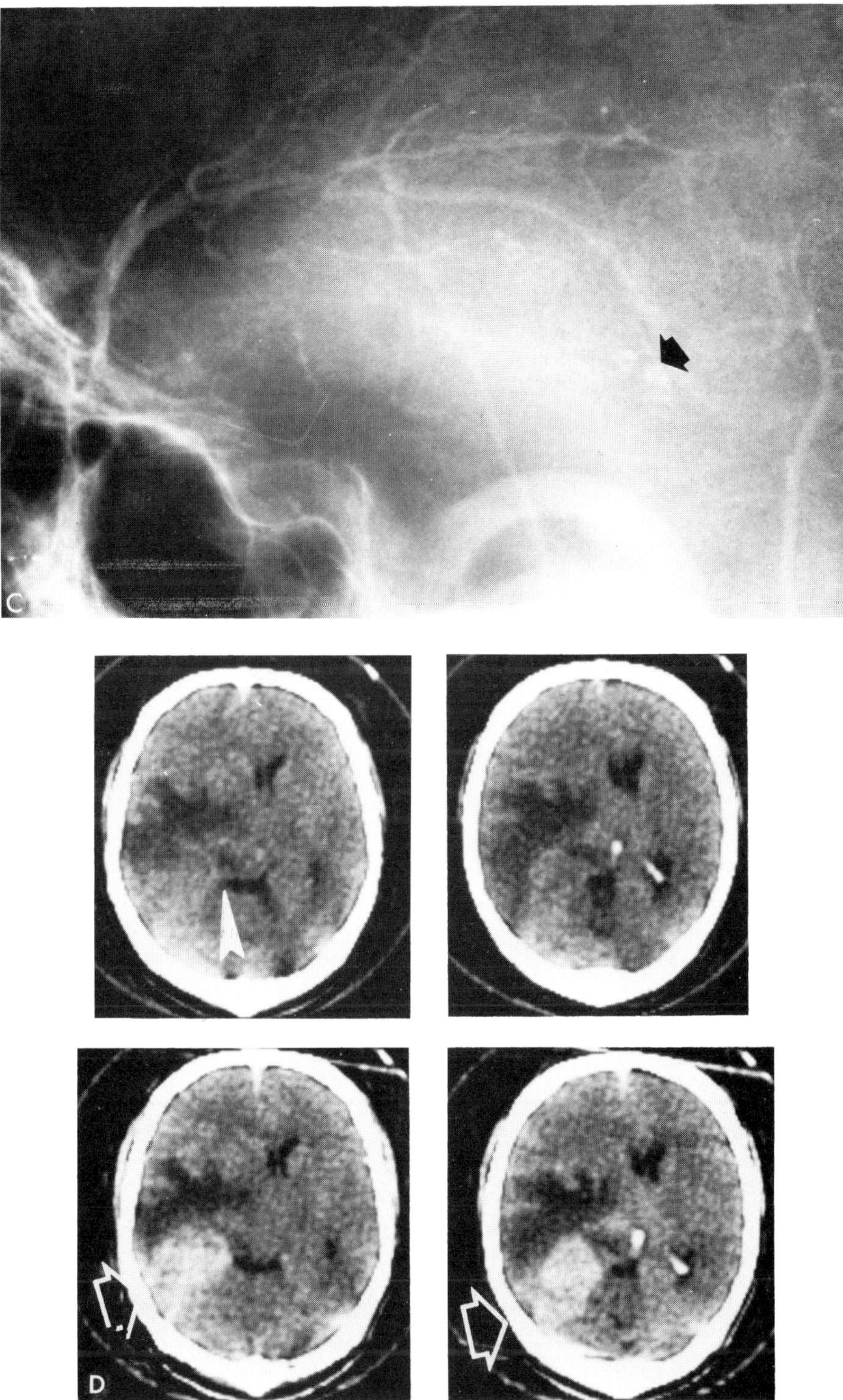

Figure 5–43. *(Continued) See legend on the opposite page*

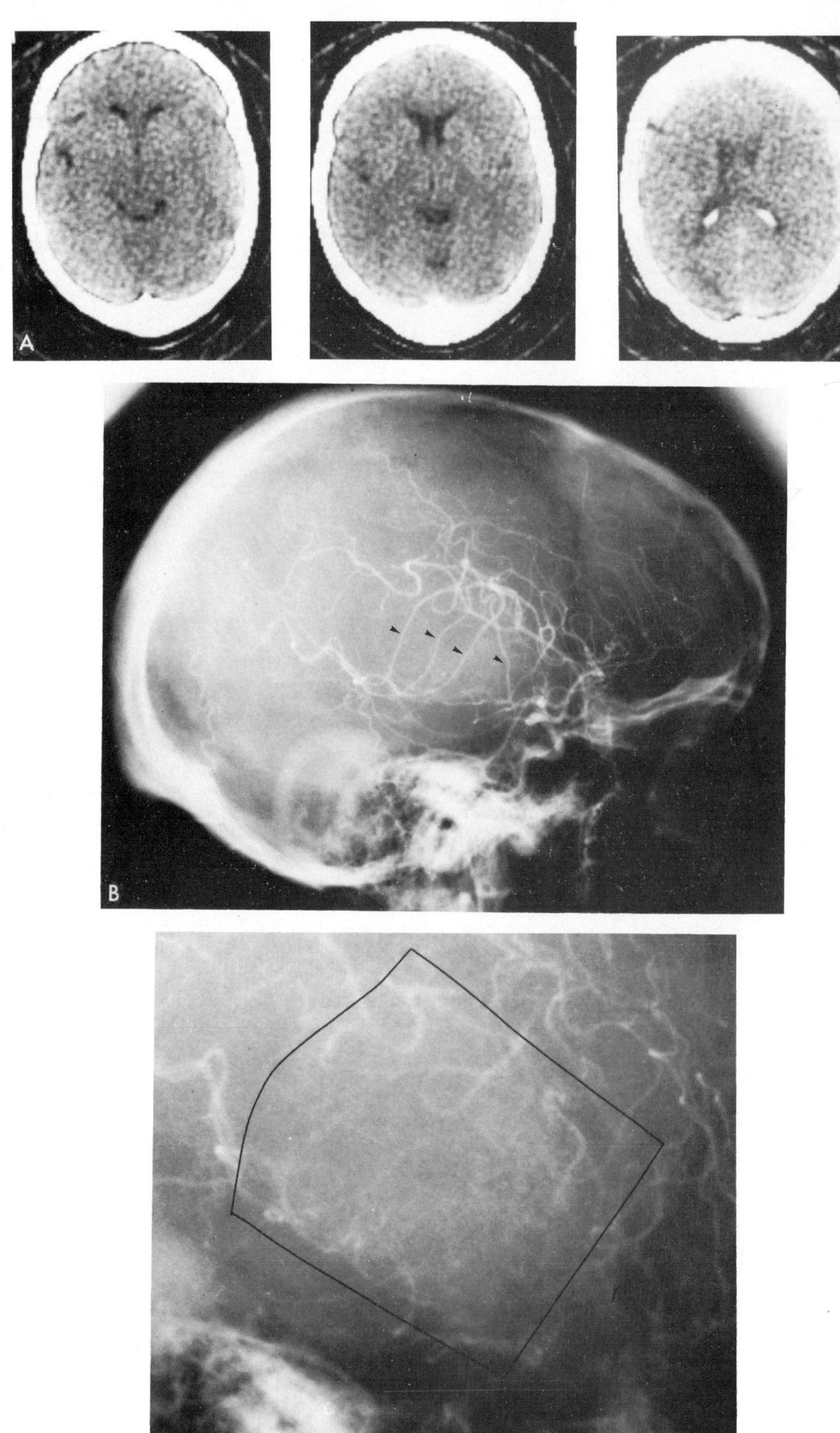

Figure 5–44. *See legend on the opposite page*

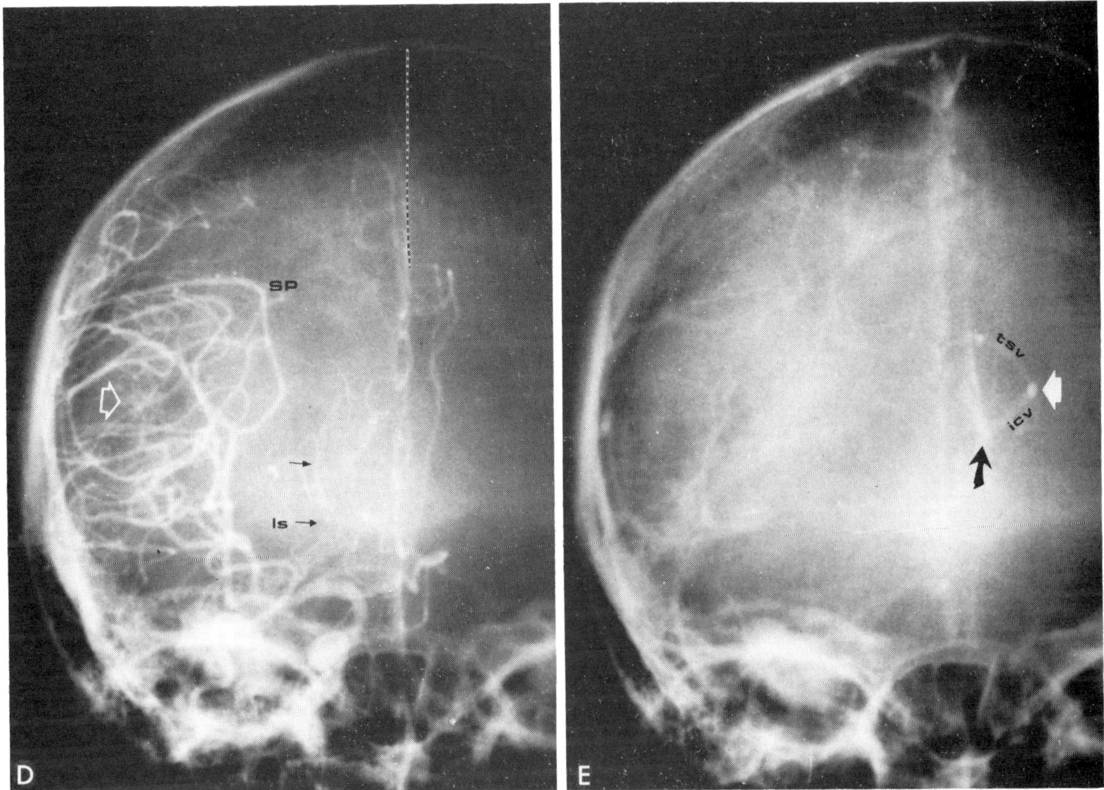

Figure 5–44. TEMPORAL LOBE GLIOBLASTOMA: This patient presented with signs and symptoms of a temporal lobe mass; however, the initial CT scan *(A)* appeared to be within normal limits. A postinfusion scan was not performed at that time, but the angiogram (not shown) was normal.

Two months after the initial study, the patient returned, and a second angiogram was performed. *B*, The lateral view demonstrates stretching of all the vessels in the temporal lobe region *(arrows)*. The opercular vessels are draped over the enlarged temporal lobe, which now contains a mass. The late arterial view *(C)* reveals an area of neovascularity in the temporal region *(black lines)*, and the findings are very typical of glioblastoma.

The AP view *(D)* reveals elevation and medial displacement of the sylvian point *(SP)*. There is a distal shift of the anterior cerebral artery, and medial displacement of the lenticulostriate vessels *(ls)* is evident. The area of abnormal vascularity can be seen in the temporal region on the AP view as well *(open white arrowhead)*.

The AP venous phase *(E)* reveals that the thalamostriate vein is displaced to the contralateral side *(tsv)*, joins the internal cerebral vein *(white arrow)* and then courses inferiorly and posteriorly to join the vein of Galen in the midline *(large black arrow)*.

Illustration continued on the following page

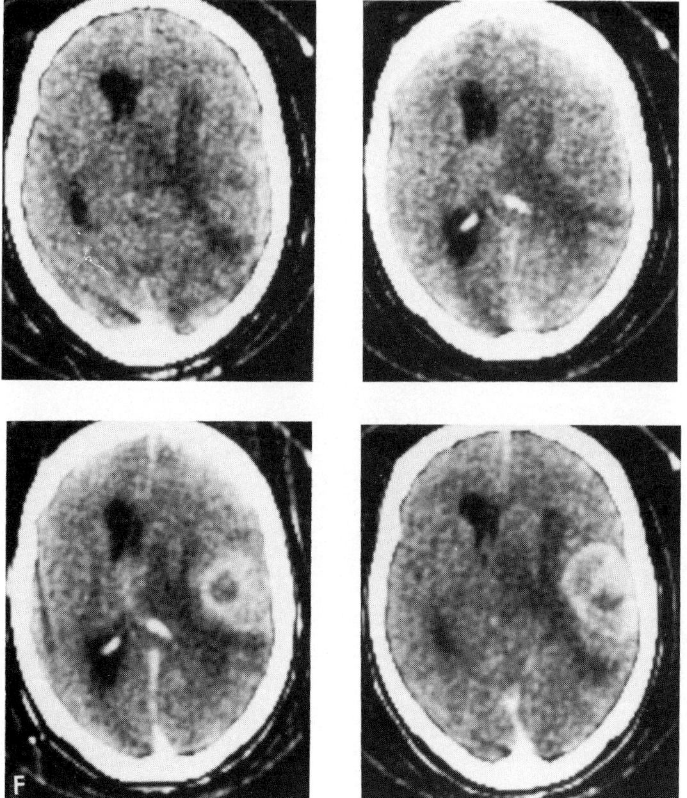

Figure 5–44. *Continued*

F, CT scans taken at this time show a large, thick-walled ring of enhancement in the right temporal region. The tumor has a lobulated appearance and a radiolucent center — consistent with necrosis of the inner portion of the mass. There is a large amount of irregular surrounding edema and a marked shift to the contralateral side.

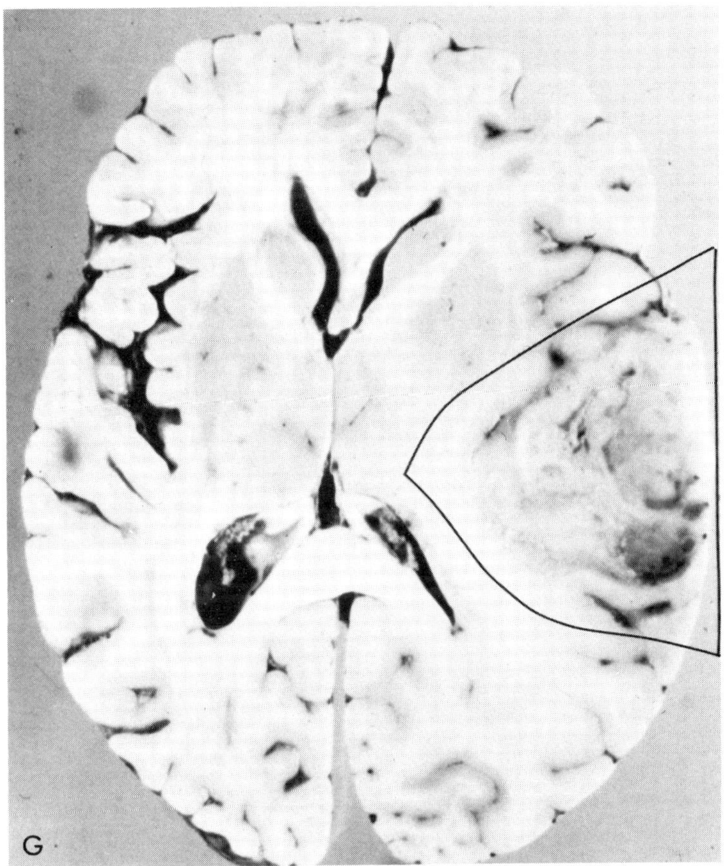

Figure 5–44. *Continued*

G, The pathologic specimen correlates well with the CT scan, demonstrating the tumor with central necrosis in the temporal lobe *(black lines).*

Diagnosis: Glioblastoma multiforme.

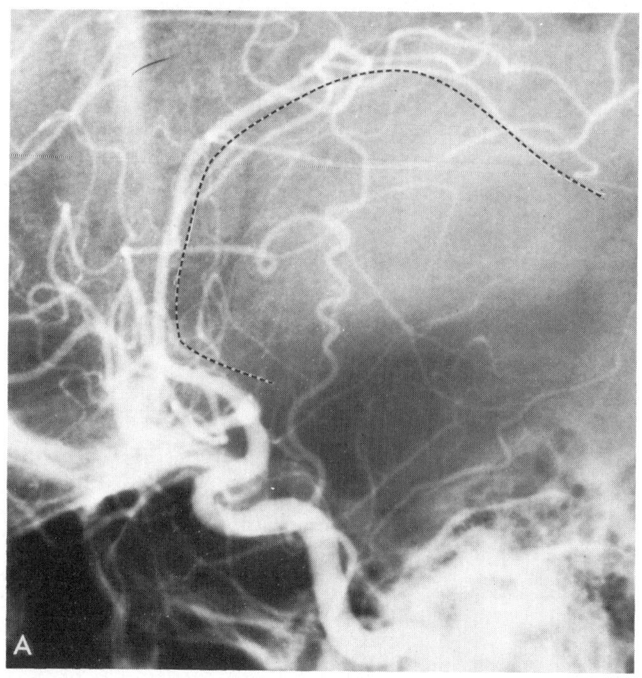

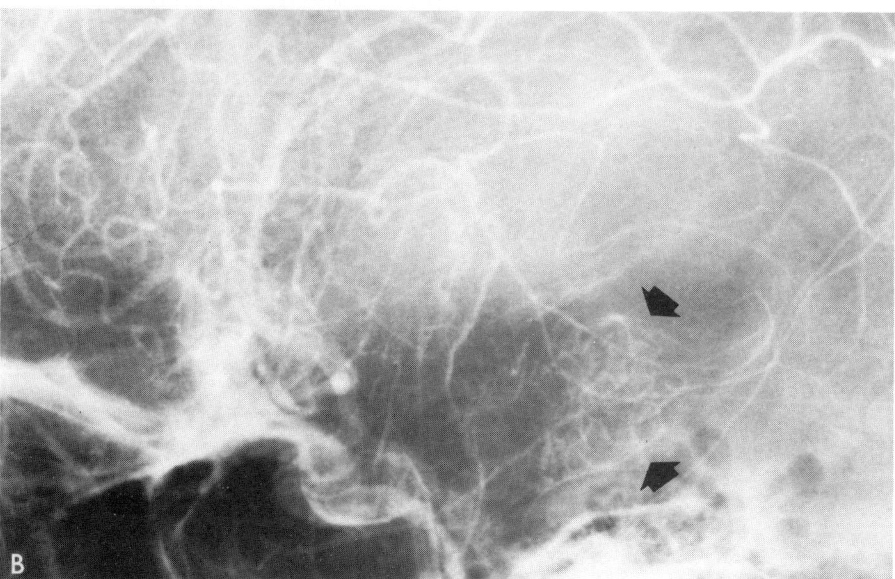

Figure 5–45. TEMPORAL LOBE GLIOBLASTOMA: *A*, The lateral view demonstrates such marked elevation of the middle cerebral branches that they appear to be the anterior cerebral artery *(dotted line)*.

B, The lateral arterial phase shows multiple small tumor vessels and a small separate collection of neovascularity in the posterior temporal region *(arrowheads)* that almost appears to be separated from the rest of the tumor.

C, The AP view of the vertebral angiogram reveals medial displacement of the posterior cerebral artery *(dashed line)* on the right side. The left posterior cerebral artery follows a normal course.

D, CT scans demonstrate a large radiolucent mass with a well defined margin in the right temporal lobe. There is shift to the contralateral side. The middle cut shows a nodule of tumor projecting into the cystic portion of the tumor, which demonstrates enhancement on the postinfusion scan *(narrow arrow)* and is apparently the separate area of neovascularity seen on the angiogram. The postinfusion scan also reveals a solid area of homogeneous enhancement *(wide arrow)* low in the temporal region and a ring of enhancement around the partially cystic and partially solid glioblastoma.

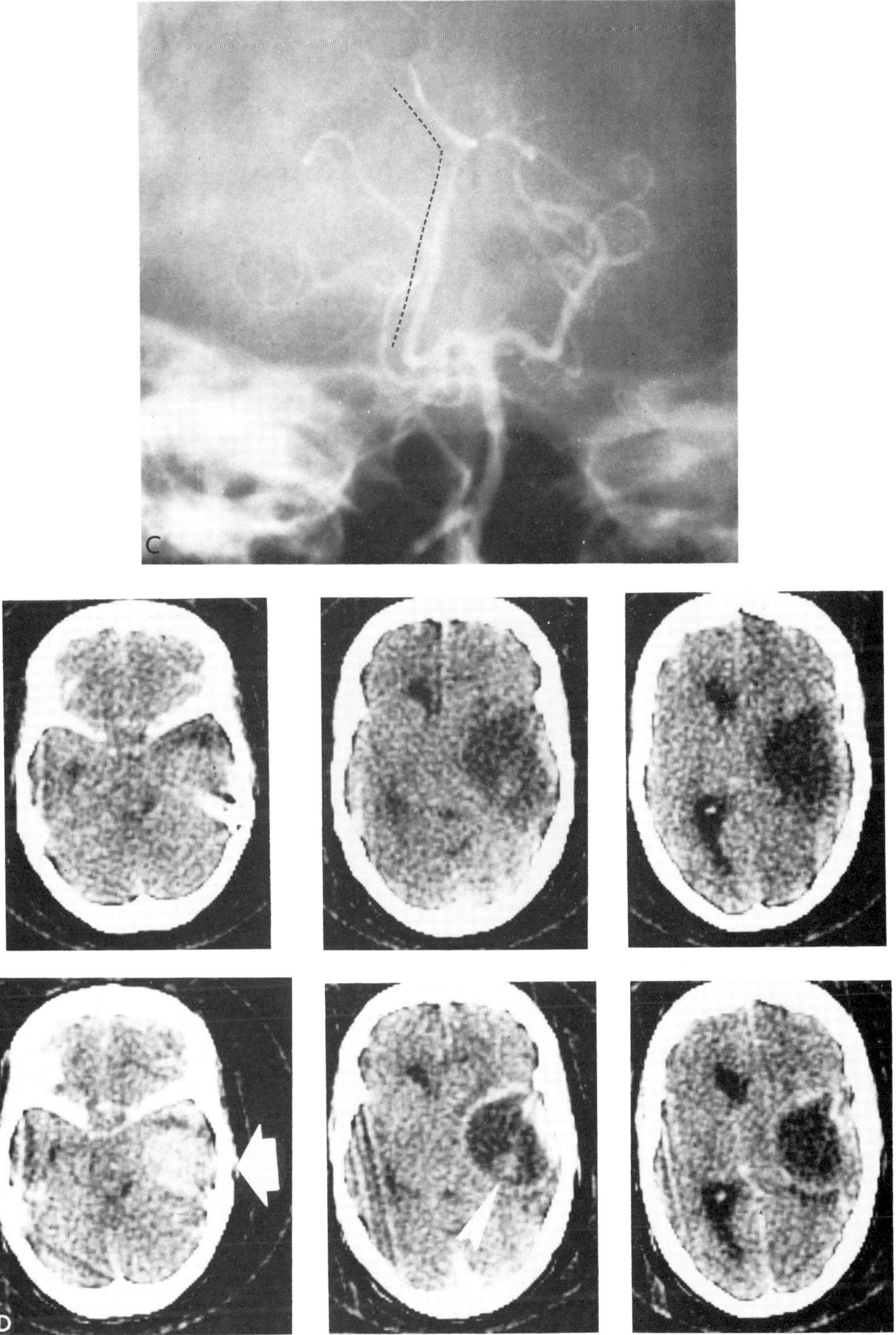

Figure 5–45. *Continued. See legend on the opposite page*

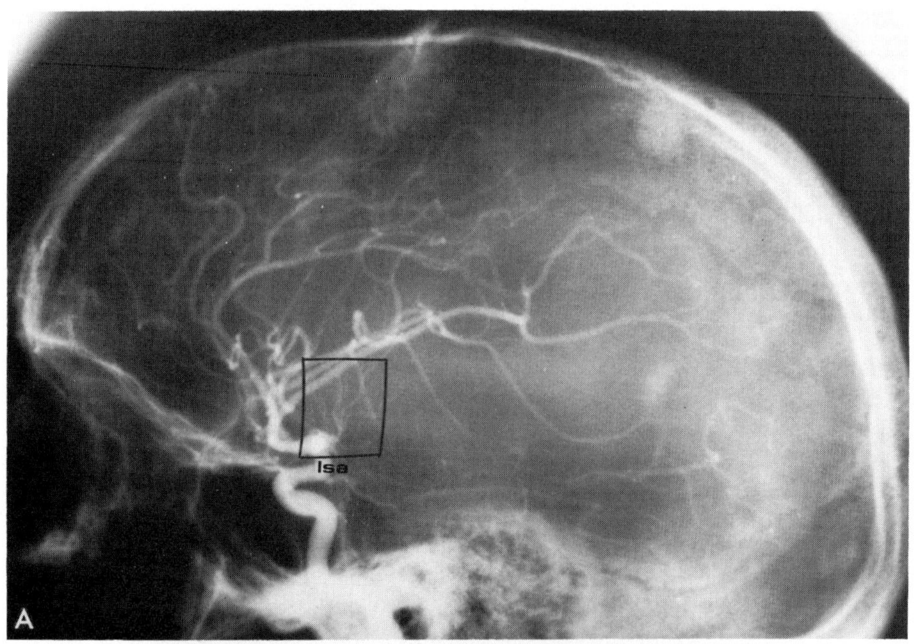

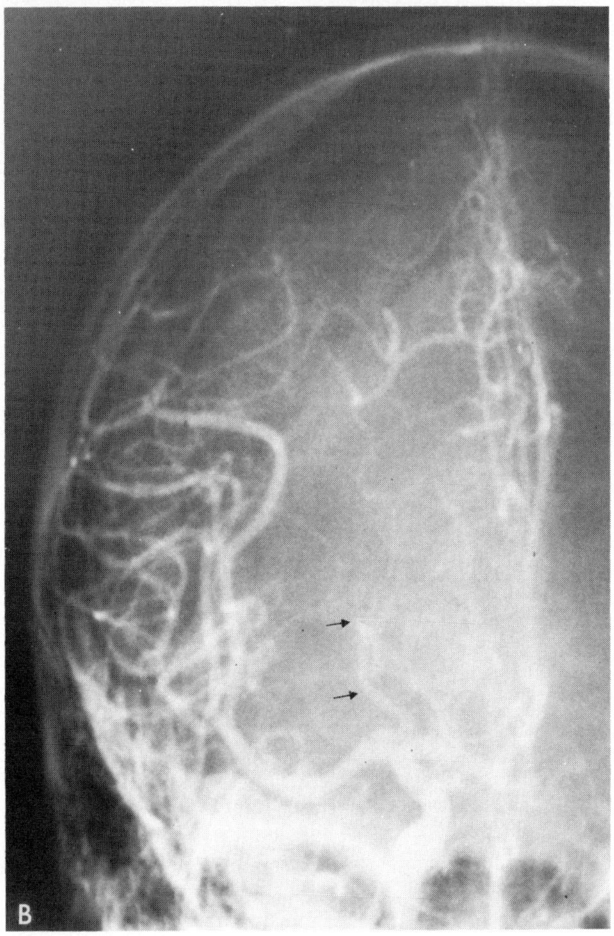

Figure 5–46. *See legend on the opposite page*

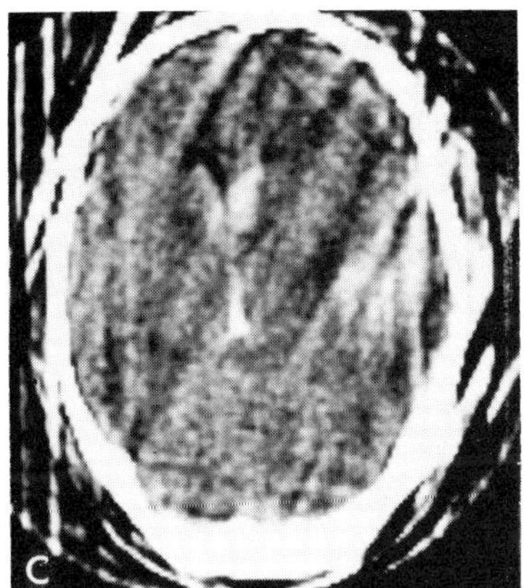

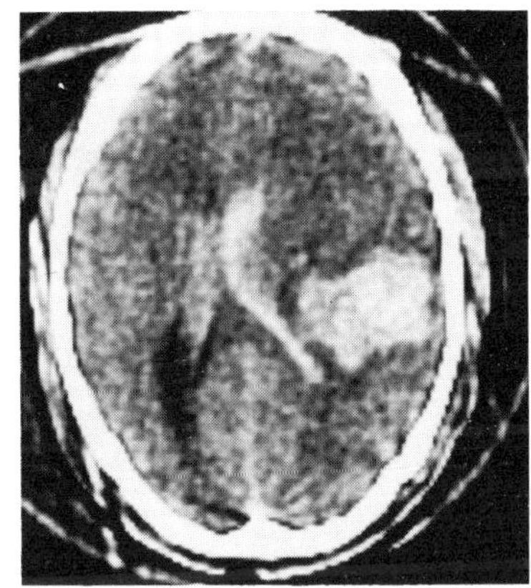

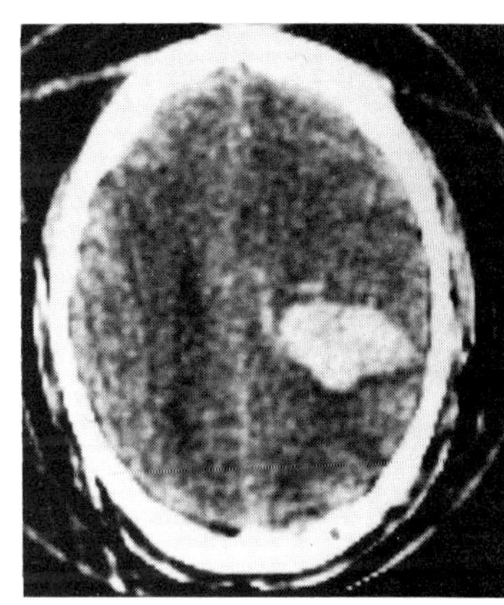

Figure 5–46. TEMPORAL LOBE HEMATOMA: *A*, The lateral view demonstrates elevation of the sylvian triangle and draping of the temporal opercular vessels over an avascular mass in the temporal lobe. Because the middle cerebral artery vessels are elevated, one can visualize the lenticulostriate arteries as they supply the basal ganglia *(black lines; lsa)*. The patchy sclerotic areas over the posterior portion of the skull are "paste" from a preceding electroencephalogram. The anterior choroidal artery is displaced inferiorly.

B, The AP view reveals minimal elevation of the sylvian point; however, there is medial displacement of the anterior choroidal artery and the lenticulostriate arteries *(arrows)*. There is a mild shift of the pericallosal artery to the contralateral side.

C, The CT scan demonstrates a large temporal hematoma that has ruptured into the ventricular system (probably via the temporal horn of the lateral ventricle), resulting in blood accumulation in the lateral and third ventricles. There is a mild shift of the midline, which probably would have been greater had the hematoma not ruptured into the ventricles to create an internal decompression.

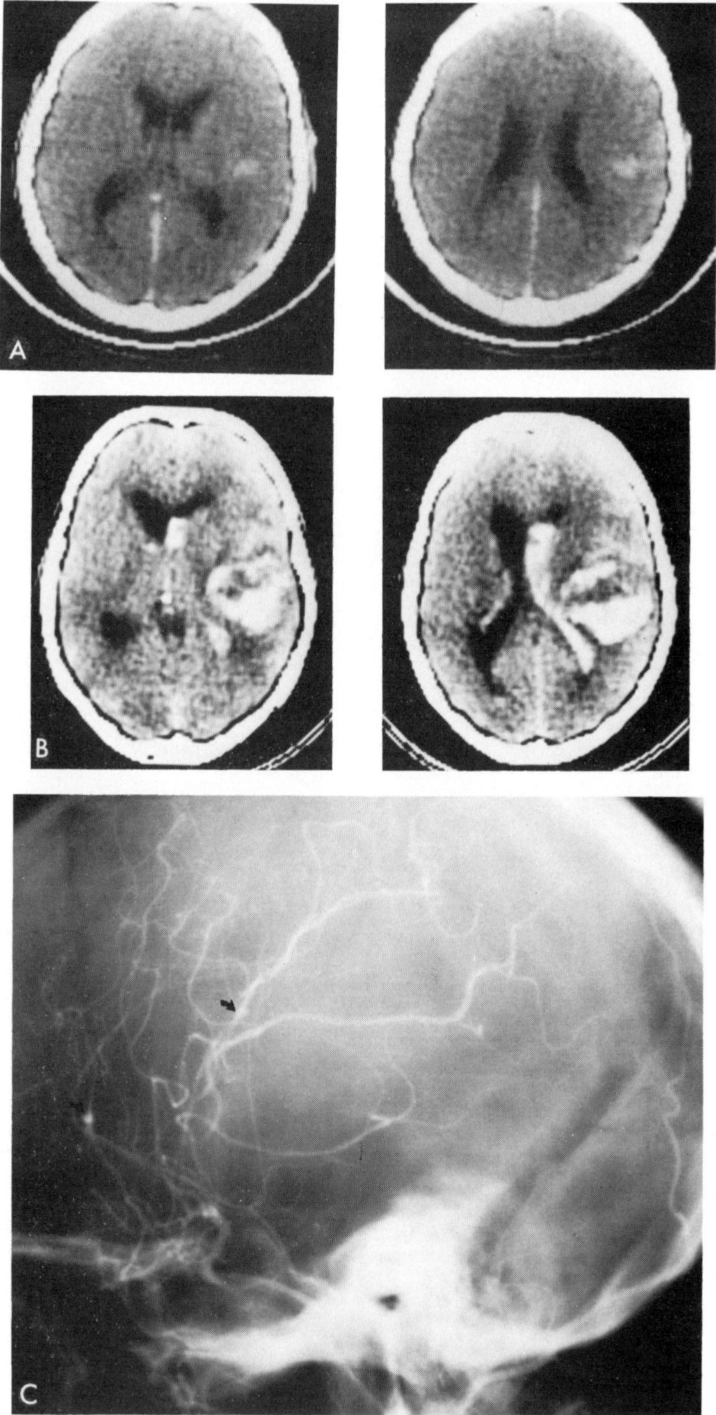

Figure 5–47. MYCOTIC ANEURYSM WITH RUPTURE: Previously, a prosthetic valve had been placed in the aortic valve, and the patient developed bacterial endocarditis.

A, The initial CT scan showed that the lateral ventricles are mildly enlarged and that there is a small area of enhancement deep in the right hemisphere. This probably represents an area of early abscess formation or cerebritis.

B, A CT scan one week later demonstrated a large hematoma in the right temporal lobe region. It has ruptured into the right lateral ventricle and the third ventricle. The scan also reveals a small amount of blood in the dependent portion of the left lateral ventricle.

C, An angiogram performed at the time of the second CT scan showed a large avascular mass in the temporal lobe. There is elevation of the sylvian triangle and draping of the vessels over the

Legend continued on the opposite page

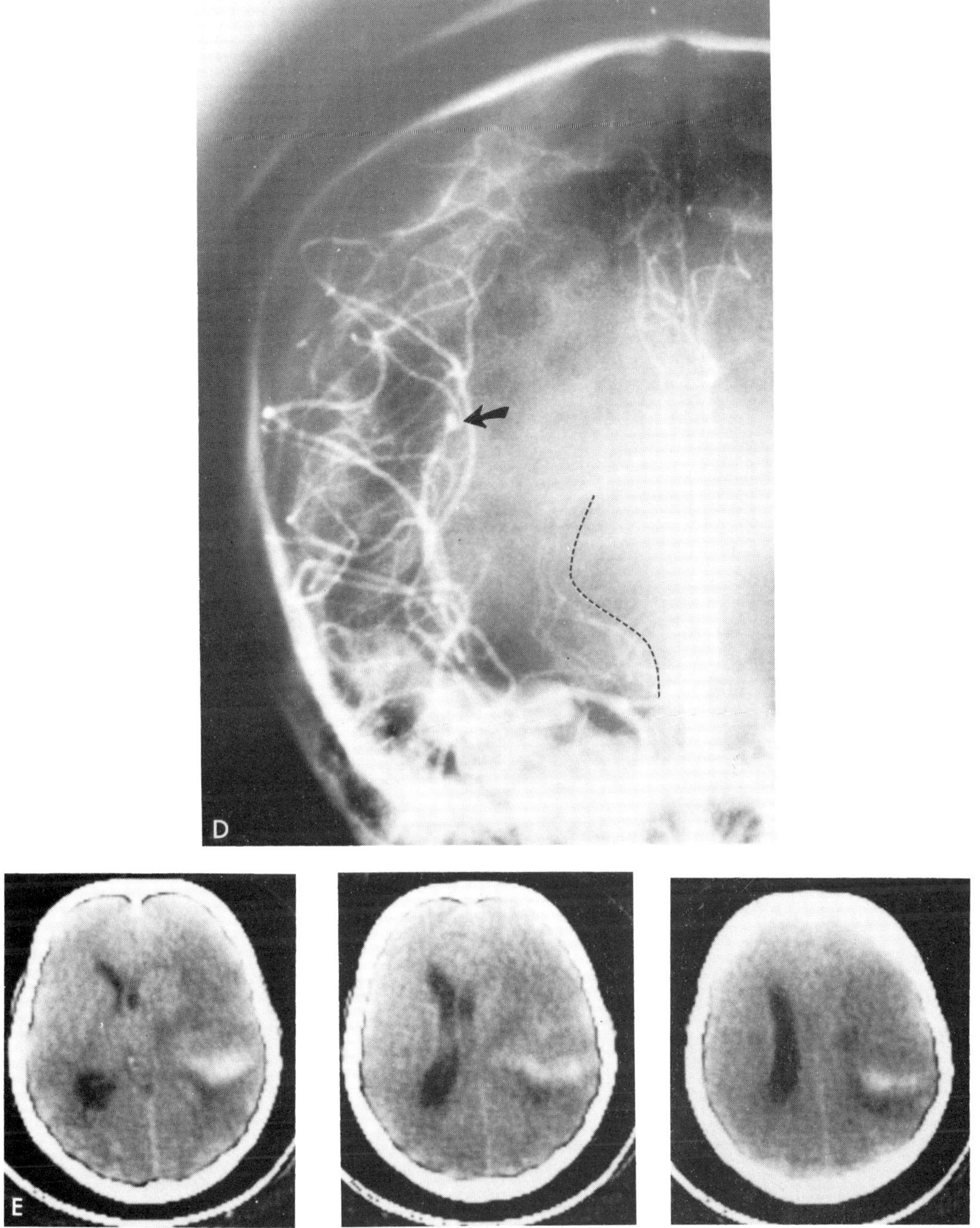

Figure 5–47. *Continued*
temporal lobe. There is spasm of the supraclinoid portion of the internal carotid artery. Two aneurysms involving the distal portions of the middle cerebral artery vessels also are demonstrated *(arrows)*. It is apparently the more superior and posterior aneurysm that has ruptured, leading to the large temporal hematoma.

D, The AP view demonstrates the more posterior aneurysm *(arrow)*. There is superior and medial displacement of the sylvian point and medial displacement of the lenticulostriate arteries *(dashed line)*.

E, A follow-up scan approximately two weeks later reveals partial resorption of the intracerebral hematoma.

IMP: Mycotic aneurysms (infected) with rupture and hematoma formation.

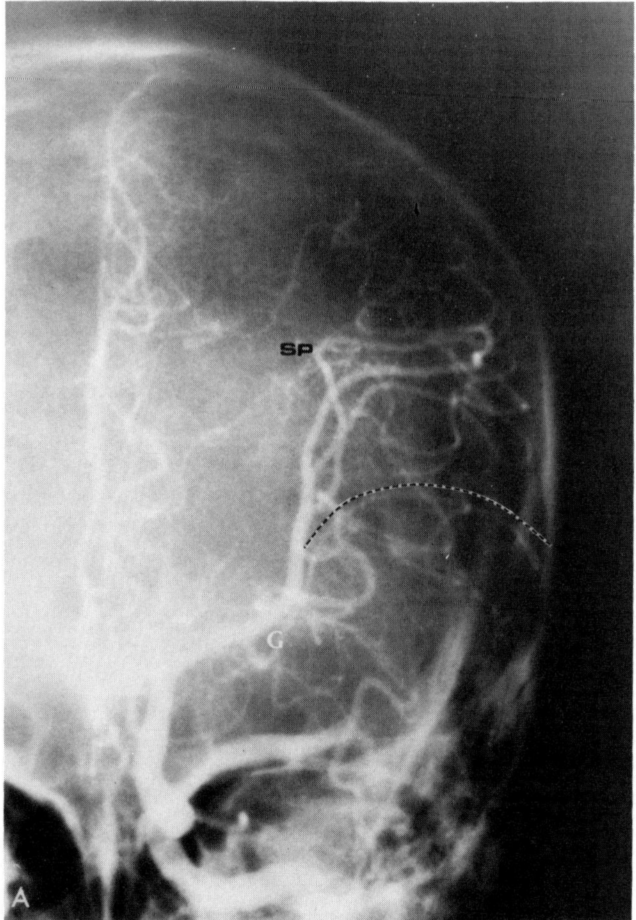

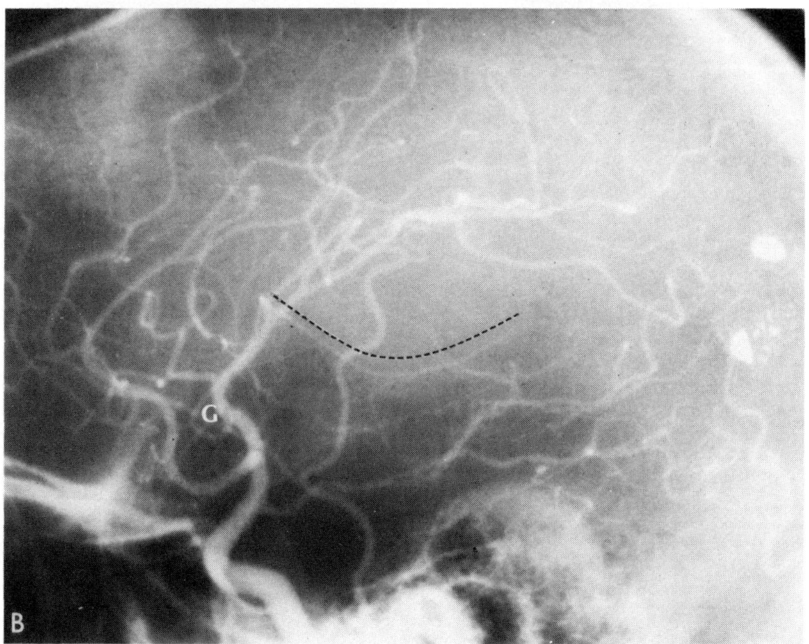

Figure 5–48. *See legend on the opposite page*

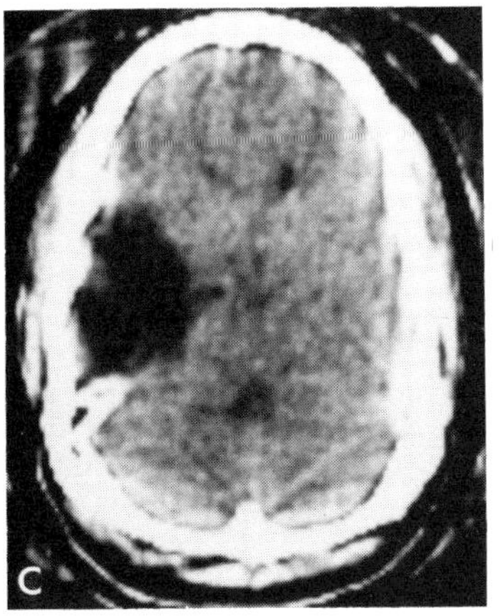

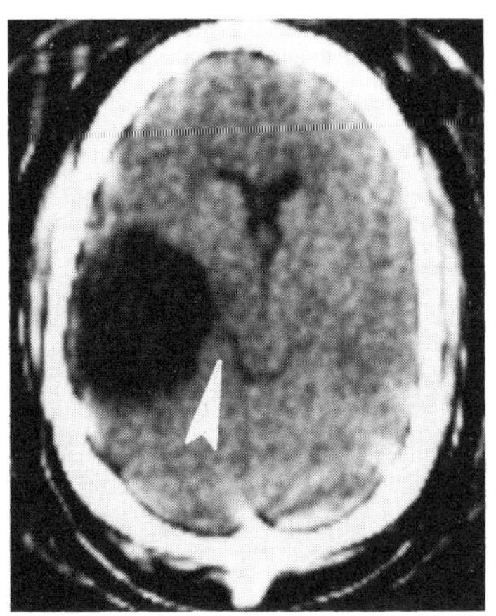

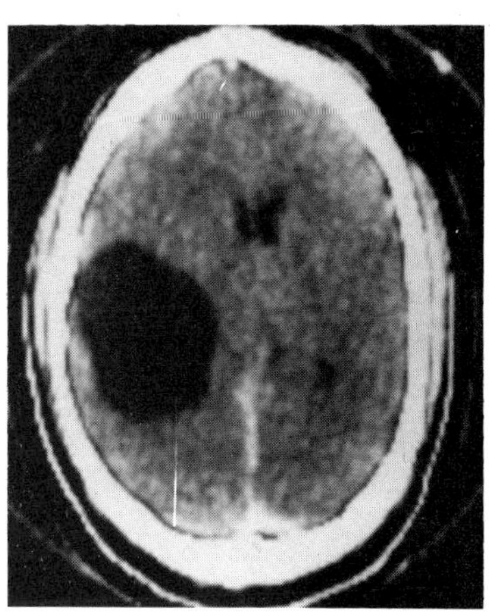

Figure 5–48. TEMPORAL PORENCEPHALIC CYST: The AP *(A)* and lateral *(B)* views of the carotid angiogram reveal elevation and medial displacement of the sylvian point *(SP)* and medial displacement of the other vessels of the middle cerebral artery group. The genu of the middle cerebral artery *(G)* is displaced superiorly and medially. One of the middle cerebral artery branches *(dashed line)* can be seen to course over the large temporal lobe mass. Note that the middle cerebral artery vessels all touch the inner table of the skull.

C, The CT scan reveals a large, well defined, cystic lesion in the left temporal lobe that is surrounded by cerebral tissue. There is a slight shift to the contralateral side. The retrothalamic cistern on the left side is distorted *(arrow)*. The fluid within the cyst was of the same density as CSF. There is no enhancement of the lesion following the infusion of contrast material.

IMP: Temporal porencephalic cyst; etiology probably birth trauma. Not surgically proved.

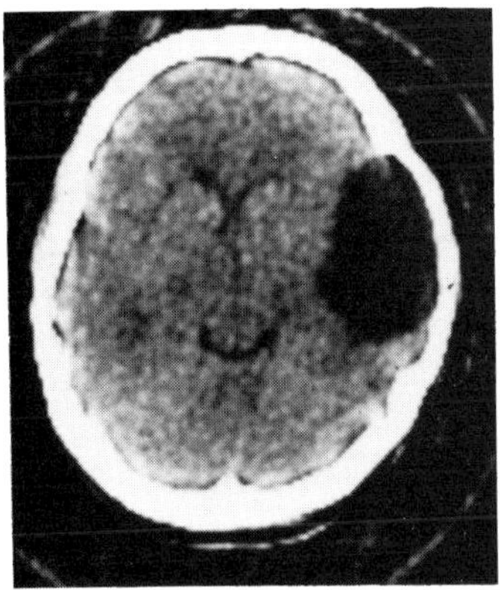

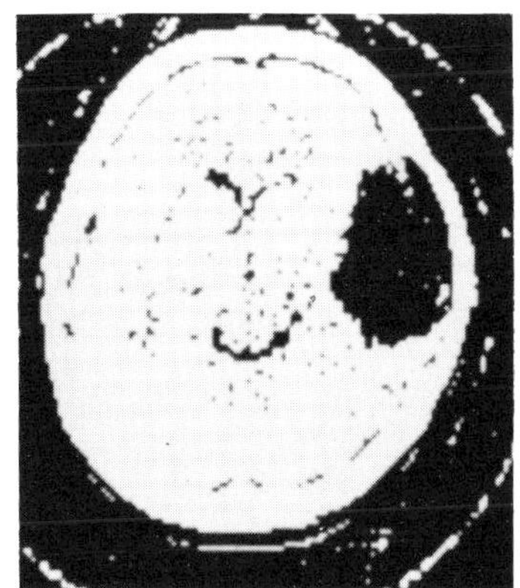

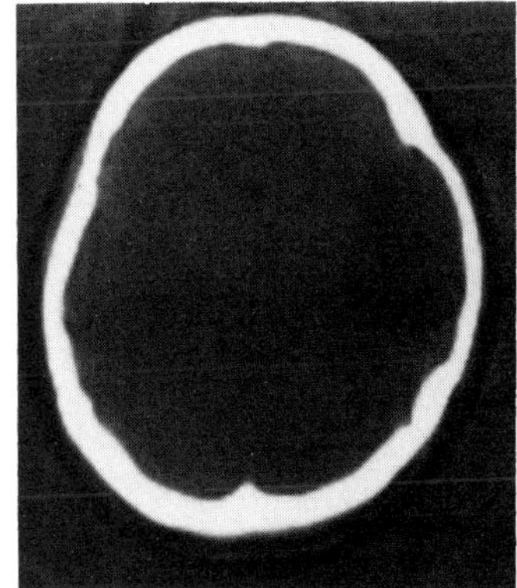

Figure 5–49. TEMPORAL ARACHNOID CYST: The CT scan demonstrates a large, well defined cystic area in the right temporal region. The fluid within the cyst was of CSF density. There is no shift of the midline, but there is evidence of thinning of the bone over the cyst. There is no change following the infusion of contrast material. The appearance is that of a temporal arachnoid cyst.

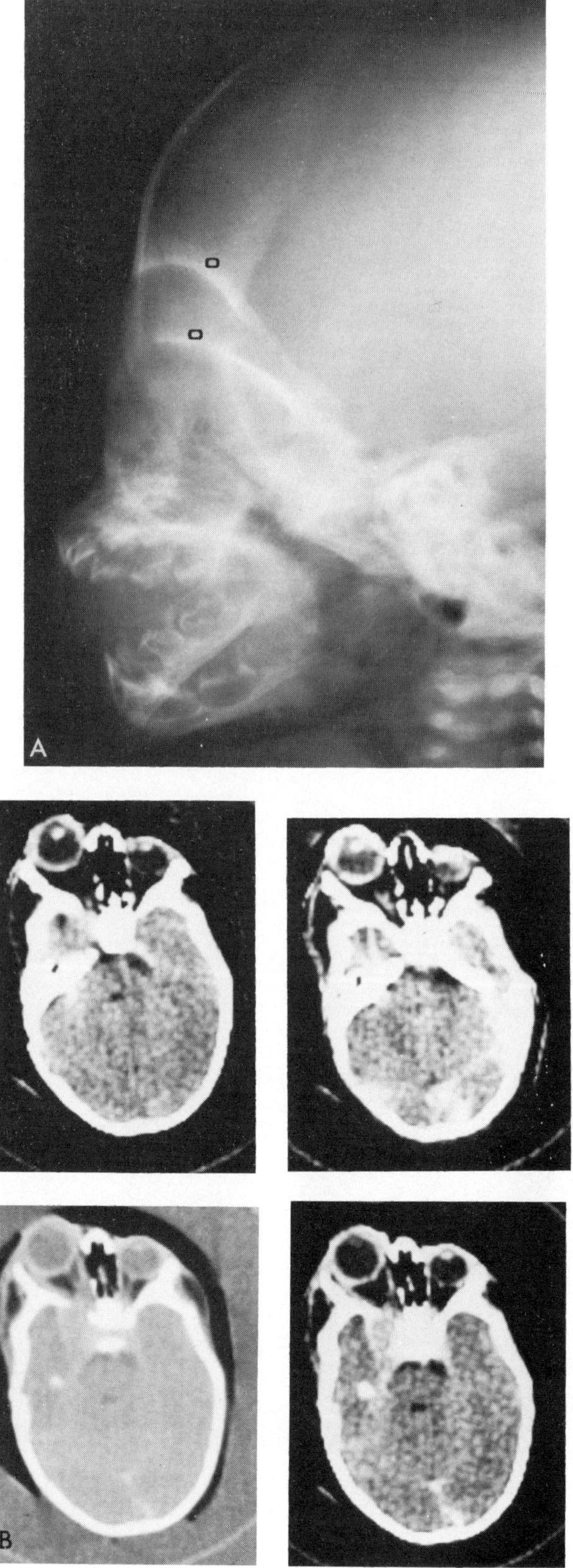

Figure 5–50. *See legend on the opposite page*

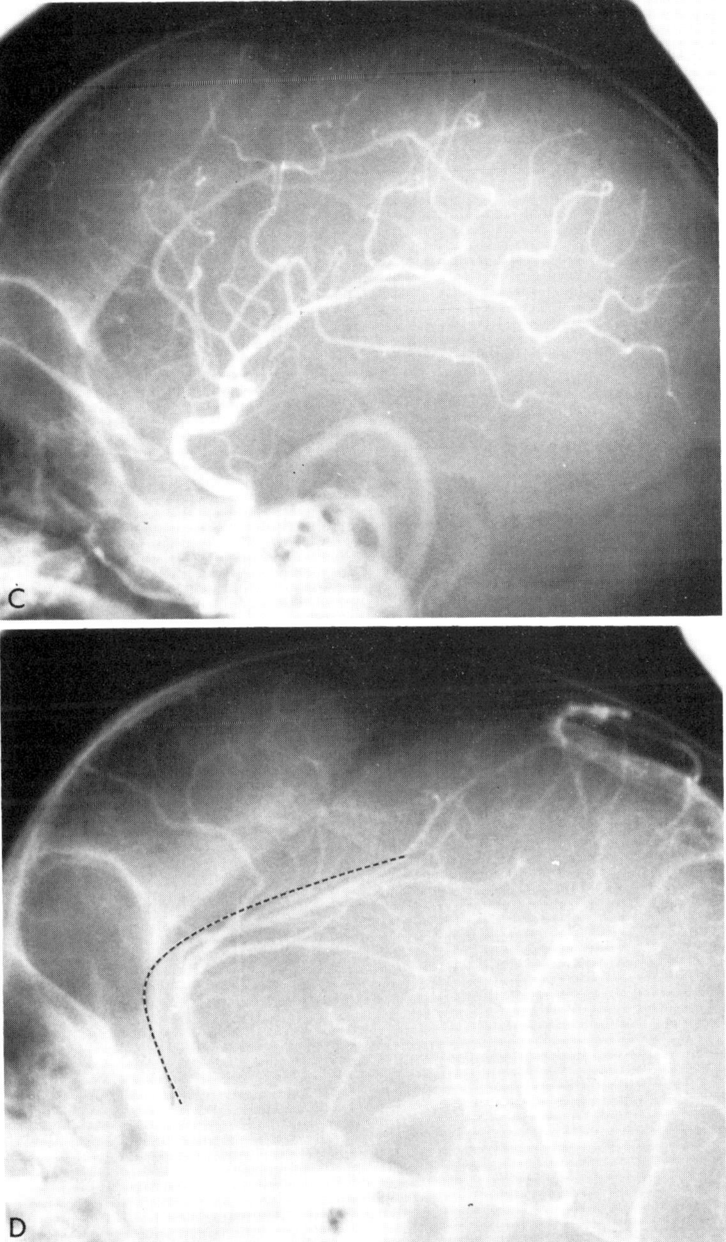

Figure 5–50. MIDDLE CRANIAL FOSSA AND ORBITAL DYSPLASIA SECONDARY TO NEUROFIBROMATOSIS: *A,* On the lateral view of the skull series, the orbital roof on the affected side is much higher than on the opposite side *(O)*, and the greater wing of the sphenoid bone is not seen on the affected side.

B, The CT scan shows the expansion of the left middle cranial fossa, the enlargement of the entire orbit on the left and even a globe larger on the left than on the right. There is no evidence of a mass lesion.

C and *D,* The lateral view in the arterial phase of the carotid angiogram reveals opening of the carotid siphon, elevation of the sylvian triangle and elevation and superior displacement of the middle cerebral veins *(dotted line)* secondary to the enlargement of the temporal lobe.

IMP: Neurofibromatosis; temporal fossa dysplasia.

BASAL GANGLIA MASS LESIONS

Mass lesions in the region of the basal ganglia may be very subtle; not uncommonly there are no abnormal arteriographic findings. In many cases the arteriogram is normal, except for a slight or moderate shift of the internal cerebral vein to the contralateral side. With a mass of sufficient size there is a proximal and distal shift of the anterior cerebral artery of varying degree and a greater shift of the internal cerebral vein. The sylvian point and the other branches of the middle cerebral artery are displaced laterally. Depending on the exact position of the mass there may be an alteration of the position of the lenticulostriate arteries as they feed the region of the basal ganglia. If the mass — usually a hemorrhage — involves the globus pallidus and the medial portions of the basal ganglia, there will be lateral displacement of the lenticulostriate vessels and the anterior choroidal artery. If hemorrhage into the putamen has occurred — and this is by far the most common location — there will be medial displacement of the lenticulostriate and anterior choroidal arteries associated with lateral displacement of the middle cerebral artery branches. The latter pattern is the most common and occurs secondary to hypertensive hemorrhage into the putamen of the basal ganglia; it is secondary to rupture of small aneurysms that involve the lenticulostriate vessels.

If the hemorrhage has ruptured into the lateral ventricles, a resulting ventricular dilatation may displace the thalamostriate laterally and bow the thalamostriate vein in a manner similar to that seen with any other cause of hydrocephalus.

The lateral view usually is normal, but may show stretching of the branches of the middle cerebral artery in the region of the basal ganglia; or, if the hemorrhage extends superiorly, stretching of the opercular branches of the middle cerebral artery in the posterior frontal and anterior parietal regions will be seen.

Included with the section on hypertensive basal ganglionic hemorrhages are several examples of hypertensive brain stem and cerebellar hemorrhages. These cerebellar hemorrhages are not uncommon. Computed tomography is the diagnostic procedure of choice, and early surgical evacuation may be life-saving.

Tumors also may occur in the basal ganglia, although they are uncommon. The angiographic displacements are similar to those caused by hemorrhage, although neovascularity also may be demonstrated.

In summary, the angiographic findings with mass lesions in the basal ganglia area are:

AP View.

1. The angiogram may be entirely normal.
2. There may be a proximal and distal shift of the pericallosal artery to the contralateral side.
3. There may be lateral displacement of the middle cerebral artery vessels.
4. The lenticulostriate vessels will be displaced medially or laterally, depending on the position of the hemorrhage.
5. There may be hydrocephalus secondary to rupture of the hemorrhage into the lateral ventricle.

Lateral View.

6. The lateral view is usually normal, but may show stretching of the vessels in the suprasylvian region.

Mass lesions in the thalamus will give a similar angiographic appearance. If the mass is avascular, its detection may be very difficult. On the venous phase of the angiogram a mass in the region of the thalamus may demonstrate elevation and displacement of the internal cerebral vein and curvilinear displacement of the basal vein of Rosenthal in a posterior and lateral direction. This latter finding may be the only detectable abnormality.

The region of the basal ganglia and thalamus are well demonstrated on the CT scans.

MIDLINE MASS LESIONS

Mass lesions in the midline of the cerebrum are very difficult to detect angiographically. They are best studied by CT scanning, and, in fact, the CT scan has proved to be an ideal method for examining these patients. Angiography of the midline structures requires study of both the carotid and the vertebrobasilar systems.

Hypothalamic lesions provide a "normal" angiogram in most cases. If the mass is of sufficient size, there may be obstruction of the foramen of Monro and resulting hydrocephalus. The vertebral angiogram may demonstrate abnormal vessels supplying the tumor, but this is uncommon.

Pineal tumors demonstrate hydrocephalus because of obstruction of the outlet of the third ventricle and the aqueduct of Sylvius. The hydrocephalus may be the only discernible abnormality seen on the carotid arteriogram. The venous phase at times reveals localized curvilinear elevation of the internal cerebral vein and the vein of Galen as it is displaced around a tumor mass. This finding should be looked for. The vertebral angiogram is more likely to demonstrate abnormal vessels supplying the region of the tumor. The vessels are derived from the medial and lateral posterior choroidal vessels and supply the region of the pineal; in some cases they supply a very vascular area with abnormal vessels and early draining veins, best seen on the lateral view. Even this finding of abnormal vascular supply from the vertebrobasilar system is unusual. In most cases no abnormal vessels can be seen, and the only really abnormal finding is the hydrocephalus.

The CT scan is the ideal method to evaluate midline tumors. With tumors of pineal origin there is evidence of a midline mass lesion, usually of higher density than that of normal brain substance; very commonly, areas of amorphous calcification also are seen. It is of particular interest to note that the normal pineal gland may be calcified and positioned at the midline while an abnormal mass surrounds the pineal and allows the gland to occupy its normal midline position. Therefore, a midline position of the pineal gland on the plain skull films certainly does not rule out the possibility of a pineal tumor. On the other hand, the size of the calcification does not correlate with the size of the pineal tumor because the calcification often either does not occupy the entire bulk of the tumor or is subradiographic. At times the tumor may be asymmetrically calcified, and the calcification may, indeed, lie off the midline. The calcification of the tumor, which is readily demonstrated on the CT scan, is usually *subradiographic*.

COMPUTED TOMOGRAPHY OF PINEALOMAS

A pineal tumor creates distortion of the posterior portion of the third ventricle, and the anterior portion of the ventricle is also distorted in a curvilinear fashion around the mass. There is encroachment upon the wings of the ambient cistern (retrothalamic cistern) and a mass of varying size, which may or may not contain areas of calcification. The postinfusion CT scan demonstrates marked enhancement of the tumor — usually in a homogeneous fashion, although occasional tumors enhance in an irregular fashion. In addition, these pineal tumors are known to spread through the central nervous system axis, and at times the "drop metastasis" to the region of the pituitary may be demonstrated on the postinfusion scan. These metastatic lesions apparently occur from abnormal deposits of cells which travel around the midbrain and proliferate in the suprasellar cistern. These deposits may be asymptomatic; their presence is discovered only by demonstration on the CT postinfusion scan. Spread also may occur to the region of the spinal cord secondary to drop metastases.

Classification of Pineal Tumors. Three histologic tumor types arise from the region of the pineal gland:

1. Pinealomas: either pineoblastoma or pineocytoma.
2. Gliomas.
3. Teratomas.
   a. Typical and teratoid.
   b. Germinoma (most common) or atypical teratoma.

Ectopic pinealomas are similar to the germinomas and occur in the pituitary region.

PITUITARY TUMORS

Plain skull radiographs may reveal enlargement of the sella turcica in the presence of a pituitary tumor. In most cases with clinical evidence of bitemporal hemianopia there will be sellar enlargement and thinning and posterior displacement of the dorsum sellae and the posterior clinoids. (See Chapter 2 for a more thorough discussion.)

The angiogram may be normal if the tumor is small. In fact, one of the primary reasons for performing an angiogram on these patients is to rule out an internal carotid artery aneurysm as the cause of the symptoms. If the tumor is of sufficient size and extends into the suprasellar cisterns, there will be lateral displacement of the cavernous portions of the internal carotid arteries and elevation of the horizontal portions of the anterior and middle cerebral arteries. If the suprasellar extension is only in the midline, there will be elevation only of the horizontal segment of the anterior cerebral artery. Care must be taken in the interpretation of this finding because in the normal individual the horizontal portion of this vessel may be elevated even in the absence of a pituitary tumor.

Lateral magnification views may demonstrate hypertrophy of multiple small branches of the cavernous internal carotid artery supplying the tumor. There may be enlargement of the meningiohypophyseal trunk as well.

When it is of sufficient size to obstruct the foramen of Monro, a pituitary tumor causes obstructive hydrocephalus.

The venous phase demonstrates elevation of the venous angle, the septal vein and the internal cerebral vein if the tumor is of sufficient size. With lateral extension of the tumor into the middle cranial fossa, there is lateral displacement and superior elevation of the anterior portion of the basal vein of Rosenthal. Often this can be readily demonstrated in the lateral view, where the basal vein of Rosenthal is displaced superiorly in a curvilinear fashion as it courses around the lateral extension of the pituitary mass.

With large mass lesions associated with destruction of the dorsum sellae and posterior clinoids, there is posterior displacement of the basilar artery; and, if the mass is of sufficient bulk, the lesion may create superior elevation of the proximal portions of the posterior cerebral arteries in a curvilinear fashion as they course over the posterior-superior portion of the tumor. Posterior displacement of the anterior pontomesencephalic vein is also associated with this change, reflecting posterior displacement of the pons.

COMPUTED TOMOGRAPHY OF THE SELLA

Computed tomography of sellar and suprasellar lesions has met with mixed success. The base cuts of the CT scan will reflect the enlargement of the bony margins of the sella turcica. The more superior cuts will demonstrate the suprasellar cistern and any evidence of obliteration of either the suprasellar cistern or the anterior recesses of the third ventricle. However, even in the presence of an intrasellar mass with suprasellar extension, the CT scan may not reveal the extent or even the presence of a tumor. The postinfusion scan *may* demonstrate enhancement of a mass in the sella with or without suprasellar extension. If, indeed, the CT scan confirms the presence of a mass lesion, the pattern usually will be that of homogeneous enhancement of the tumor. However, it is *very* important to remember that even in the presence of a sellar tumor with suprasellar extension the CT scan may be entirely *normal.* In other words, even with thin cuts, CT scanning of the sella may not be sufficiently accurate to rule out the presence of lesions of the sella even with a normal scan. Coronal cuts through the sella have been suggested; these may be helpful, if available. It is apparent, however, that if there is reason to suspect a sellar or suprasellar tumor and the CT scan is normal, a pneumoencephalogram or Amipaque cisternogram is indicated for full evaluation of the presence and extent of the tumor. This is especially true of cystic tumors, which may not be appreciated on the CT scan.

An empty sella may be suspected if the fluid within the sella is of CSF density and does not change in density after the infusion of contrast material.

AMIPAQUE CISTERNOGRAPHY

Amipaque, introduced in 1978, is a water soluble myelographic contrast material that also may be used for cisternography in conjunction with computed tomography. Evaluations of the sella and suprasellar cisterns are possible after the introduction of this water contrast material into the lumbar subarachnoid space and manipulation of the contrast material into the suprasellar cisterns.

Technique of Amipaque Cisternography. Four to 6 cc of Amipaque in a concentration of 180 mg of I^2 per ml is introduced into the lumbar subarachnoid space and allowed to flow cephalad until the contrast accumulates in the suprasellar and other basilar cisterns. The patient is then kept in the 15° head-down position and placed in the CT scanner. In the normal patient the suprasellar cistern is bathed in the high density of the intracranial solution of Amipaque and demonstrates a pentagonal or five-pointed star configuration. With an "empty sella" the Amipaque will be seen to accumulate within the sella as well as in the suprasellar cisterns. With an intrasellar mass lesion with suprasellar extension, the mass will appear as a radiolucent defect in the center of the Amipaque pool. With a mass of sufficient size, the suprasellar cistern will be obliterated.

In the normal individual the anterior recesses of the third ventricle will be outlined by the Amipaque and will appear as a slitlike low density area in the midline. In the presence of a suprasellar mass the anterior recesses of the third ventricle will be obliterated by the mass. (Note that Amipaque introduced by lumbar tap using the above method does not enter into the ventricular system; therefore, the CSF within the ventricle is of normal density.)

Craniopharyngioma. The vascular displacements seen with a craniopharyngioma are similar to those seen with a pituitary tumor with suprasellar extension, except that the craniopharyngioma may demonstrate abnormal vessels. In addition, craniopharyngiomas frequently are calcified. These calcifications can be demonstrated on plain skull radiographs.

Computed tomography of a craniopharyngioma reveals a cystic lesion in the region of the suprasellar cistern that extends into the sella. The fluid within the cyst is of higher density than CSF fluid and reflects the density of the abnormal material within the cystic tumor. The areas of calcification are within the walls of the craniopharyngioma and are readily detected on the CT scan, even when they are subradiographic.

"PITFALLS' OF ANGIOGRAPHY

Not all masses fit precisely into the categories that have been defined. Masses that are small but occupy two lobes of the brain, or masses that are very large and thus affect multiple areas of the brain, will produce vascular displacements that include changes seen in more than one category of lesion. In fact, a combination of changes will be seen rather than a classic pattern of displacement. By the same token, multiple lesions will also alter the appearance of the angiogram and result in a combination of changes that includes patterns of vascular displacements from two different groups.

The beginning angiographer should commit to memory the various normal positions of the anatomic structures that have standard measurements. Thus, deviations from the normal can be readily evaluated by actual linear measurement. It should be kept in mind, however, that no single measurement should be clung to tenaciously, because a variety of changes may come to play upon the actual vessel displacements. Most important, balancing lesions may be present in both hemispheres, or there may be two separate lesions in the same hemisphere that will alter anticipated vascular displacements.

Initially, when reviewing an angiogram all pertinent information should be at hand to provide help in arriving at an accurate diagnosis. The chart, clinical history and pertinent physical findings should be well known to the angiographer. Any other positive or significant negative test results also should be available for comparison or correlation with the angiographic study. This is true, after all, for the clinician who sees the patient in consultation; and it is of vital importance when evaluating the clinical condition and the angiographic findings. With increasing experience, the clinical history and physical findings may be all one needs to arrive successfully at the correct diagnosis. This knowledge of the clinical situation will also help the angiographer choose an approach to the procedure and decide which vessels are to be studied. For example, if a meningioma of the posterior fossa is suspected, a vertebral angiogram for the posterior fossa must be performed — but it is also important to study the carotid circulation to determine whether there is vascular supply to the tumor from the tentorial artery.

Angiography of Multiple Lesions. With multiple lesions the angiographic picture is not as straightforward as when there is a solitary mass. If multiple lesions are present, there may be a balancing or nearly balancing effect of the masses, and thus no shift of the midline structures. In such a case the mass will be localized by evaluation of the intrinsic displacement of various intracranial vessels and of the displacement of vessels from their anticipated normal position, even in the absence of midline shift. When multiple lesions are present, the CT scan has proved invaluable in demonstrating abnormal areas. Indeed, it is the ideal method for diagnosis of multiple lesions.

Because there is definite morbidity and risk of mortality from angiography, there is little or no room for error. It is important that the *appropriate* angiogram be performed. Great care should be taken to obtain excellent film studies so that an accurate diagnosis can be made and therapy instituted (See Chapter 11).

CHAPTER 6

ARTERIOSCLEROSIS

Recent advances in surgical technique have brought an ever-increasing demand for precise radiographic demonstration of the extracranial vasculature so that needed surgical repair can be undertaken. The many changes that can affect these vessels can be outlined by using a variety of radiologic approaches. The method selected may in some cases be determined by the type of problem that the patient exhibits; in others, the approach may be dictated by the preference or skill of the operator or by the requirements of the referring physician.

Arteriosclerosis, because of its various effects upon the cardiovascular and cerebrovascular systems, is one of the leading causes of death and disability today. Approximately 25 per cent of individuals presenting with signs and symptoms of cerebrovascular disease will have demonstrable extracranial carotid disease. Because this type of vascular change is potentially curable, there is today a greater emphasis on the precise radiologic demonstration of the lesion so that carotid endarterectomy or bypass procedure can be performed. In centers with an active cardiovascular and peripheral vascular surgical group, an increased number of patients are studied because of the possibility of surgically correctable carotid occlusive disease.

Stenosis of the carotid artery at the level of the bifurcation in the neck is quite common and is readily correctable by endarterectomy. Instead of treating these patients as another "standard work-up," each should be approached as if he were unique. Indeed, the many minor variations on the theme of arteriosclerosis in each patient demand an examination tailored to the individual patient's needs. This will better serve both that patient and the referring physician.

Our work-up for patients suspected of having operable extracranial carotid stenosis begins with a right brachial (RBA) and left carotid arteriogram (LCA). The nature of our patient population is such that most individuals have extensive peripheral vascular occlusive disease — thus precluding the use of the femoral arteries and the Seldinger technique. By using the RBA we are able to evaluate the antegrade flow through the right vertebral artery and through the right carotid artery.

Although stenosis of the carotid artery presents a potential technical difficulty in performing carotid angiography, we have not found this problem to be significant in day-to-day practice. The needle puncture should be performed very low in the neck — well below the carotid bifurcation. The skin should be entered approximately 2 cm above the clavicle in the base of the neck and the needle angled slightly cephalad. When free flow of pulsating blood is obtained, the guidewire is advanced beyond the tip of the needle. If resistance is encountered, as from an area of stenosis or an occluded vessel, the wire should not be forced. Utmost care should be exercised at this point. The wire is then pulled back slightly, held immobile and the needle then slightly advanced over the guidewire. The wire is then removed and the obturator placed and the needle immobilized with the Davis rake so that it is not inadvertently advanced into the carotid artery farther than desired. We use a standard brachial technique and allow an 0.5 second delay before beginning filming.

Films are obtained in a biplane fashion. The AP view ranges up to the base of the skull and down to and including the origin of the great vessels as they arise from the arch of the aorta. The lateral view is obtained so that the central ray is at the level of the carotid bifurcation, but it also includes vessels in the neck from the shoulder to the base of the skull. We attempt to "cone-down" the views so that attention is directed toward the vessels, their origins and their bifurcations. The filming sequence is rapid: four films per second for two seconds. If a "steal" is suspected (e.g., retrograde flow down the left vertebral artery), additional films are obtained at a rate of one film per second for an additional six seconds.

A second injection is then made with coned-down views of the intracranial circulation in both the AP and lateral projections. It is obvious that surgical correction of extracranial carotid stenosis will not benefit the patient if additional areas of stenosis exist within the intracranial circulation. I feel strongly that including the neck on a non-coned view of the intracranial circulation for evaluation of extracranial carotid stenosis results in an unsatisfactory examination. It is demonstrated almost daily that biplane studies of the vessels are necessary for accurate evaluation. On one plane the vessel may appear entirely or nearly normal; on the opposite view a severe stenosis or an ulcerated lesion may be identified. Therefore, it behooves the examiner to examine these vessels in at least two projections.

One must remember that more than 50 per cent narrowing of a vessel must occur to produce significant stenosis and that a stenosis greater than 50 per cent must occur to produce a decrease in the blood flow through an area. On the other hand, irregular or ulcerated lesions are more likely to accumulate such debris as fibrin or platelet clots, causing transient ischemic attacks even in the absence of significant stenosis.

A thorough examination of the intracranial circulation is needed for complete evaluation. Occasionally, a patient with a subdural hematoma or a brain tumor — particularly a meningioma, but any tumor may have this effect — may present with minimal symptoms that mimic those of a transient ischemic attack. Therefore, a study of the intracranial circulation is imperative. Finally, other disease entities, such as berry aneurysms, subdural hematomas or unsuspected arteriovenous malformations, may be the cause of the patient's symptoms, rather than extracranial vascular occlusive disease.

In 20 to 25 per cent of individuals the left common carotid artery arises from the innominate artery or has a common origin with the innominate as the vessels arise from the arch of the aorta. In some cases, the force of the injection will also fill the left common carotid artery with sufficient contrast material to outline the vessels for diagnosis. If one is successful in filling the left side, an oblique view should be obtained in biplane projection; alternatively, each patient can be studied initially in the oblique projection. The author prefers the left posterior oblique projection, because when the left carotid artery is in a dependent position it is more likely to fill sufficiently for diagnosis.

FIBROMUSCULAR HYPERPLASIA

Fibromuscular hyperplasia affects the tunica media of the blood vessels, creating a variety of changes, among them fibrosis and stenosis of the vessels. This produces a "stack of coins" radiographic appearance, and often there is much more significant stenosis of the vessel than can be appreciated on the angiogram (Fig. 6–5). A focal area of involvement may mimic the appearance of arteriosclerosis, but a larger area of involvement has a characteristic appearance. Fibromuscular change involves the internal carotid arteries and may be associated with changes in the renal arteries; it rarely involves the intracranial vessels.

STROKE SYNDROME

A variety of approaches may be used in the patient with "stroke" syndrome. Also, there are a number of different schools of thought concerning the timing of the work-up of patients with this syndrome. It is generally agreed, however, that an individual who is experiencing transient ischemic attacks — which, by definition, do not result in permanent neurologic deficit — should have angiography for diagnosis. If a surgically correctable lesion is found, an endarterectomy should be performed.

A patient who is developing an acute stroke and who demonstrates progressive neurologic damage, angiography definitely may aggravate the condition. Therefore, the patient with a "stroke in progress" should be subjected to angiography only after utmost consideration. In an individual with a completed stroke, angiography may demonstrate the abnormality, but the patient may anticipate no benefit from surgery because of permanent neurologic damage.

Occlusive vascular disease may involve the carotid arteries in the neck, and so may be readily amenable to surgery; on the other hand, it may involve the intracranial vascular supply, which is less susceptible to surgical treatment. With occlusion of the middle cerebral artery at its origin or stenosis of the horizontal portion of the middle cerebral artery, selected patients may benefit from a vascular bypass procedure. With recent advances in microsurgical techniques have made possible an anastomosis between superficial temporal artery and the branches of the middle cerebral artery distal to the area of stenosis or occlusion. This is performed by mobilizing the superficial temporal artery and anastomosing this vessel to the middle cerebral artery branches through a small craniotomy defect. With further advances in technique, this procedure probably will increase in popularity.

ANGIOGRAPHIC FINDINGS WITH STROKE SYNDROMES

1. Over 50 per cent of the studies are normal. The involved vessel is so small that the thrombosis or embolus that has occluded the vessel cannot be visualized by angiography.

2. There may be total occlusion of the common or internal carotid artery.

3. There may be a significant (over 50 per cent) stenosis of the implicated carotid artery; or the extracranial vessel may demonstrate an ulcerated or irregular plaque, even in the absence of a significant stenosis.

4. Branch occlusions of the internal carotid artery may occur. These include occlusion of the anterior or, more commonly, the middle cerebral artery — or of any of the terminal branches of these vessels.

5. In approximately 15 per cent of acute stroke cases there will be significant mass effect, resulting in a shift of the midline to the contralateral side.

6. There may be evidence of early venous drainage.

7. There may be retrograde filling of the vessels that are occluded more proximally.

8. The areas of infarction may demonstrate "luxury perfusion."

Luxury Perfusion. Following a stroke a perfusion of small vessels may open into and around the relatively avascular area. This is probably a nonfunctioning area of small vessels around the infarction. Its angiographic appearance is that of a blush or "luxury perfusion" in the abnormal area. There may be localized dilatation of cerebral blood vessels. Early draining veins also may be seen.

Thix phenomenon is visible angiographically immediately after a stroke and for two weeks thereafter. The phenomenon of luxury perfusion is also demonstrable on the CT scans, but appears to be present from approximately 1 week post-insult to 6 weeks after the stroke. Luxury perfusion is visible only on the postinfusion scan.

CT SCANNING OF ACUTE INFARCT

With an acute infarct the CT scan may have an entirely normal appearance. With time, an increasing number of infarcts will be visible on the plain CT scan. Approximately 60 to 70 per cent of acute bland infarcts will be detected by routine CT scan within the first 7 days. On the other hand, a normal CT scan in a patient with an acute stroke can confirm the diagnosis by ruling out other diagnostic possibilities. Such entities as basal ganglionic hemorrhage, hemorrhagic infarct, intracerebral hematoma, subdural hematoma or even primary or secondary brain tumors may present with the clinical appearance of an acute infarct.

The areas of infarction appear as areas of radiolucency that are variable in size. Infarcts resulting from a single small occluded vessel may be quite small. Others may be moderate in size — usually corresponding to a known vascular distribution, such as the middle cerebral artery distribution. Or, the infarct may be very large, resulting in radiolucency of the entire hemisphere. Small or moderate infarcts are most common in the distribution of the middle cerebral artery distribution. In most cases these areas of infarction will be non–space-occupying and will show no evidence of mass effect on the scan. However, in approximately 15 per cent of cases of acute infarct there will be some evidence of mass effect. This evidence may vary from a small local effect to a massive shift of the midline structures, as is seen in a total hemisphere stroke secondary to internal carotid artery occlusion. In cases of infarct that demonstrate mass effect, a postinfusion scan may help to distinguish between an infarct and a tumor with mass effect.

Hemorrhagic Infarcts. Hemorrhagic infarcts are relatively uncommon, and may be difficult or impossible to differentiate from an intracerebral hematoma. Hemorrhagic infarcts, however, tend to occur in a major vascular distribution and are frequently non–space-occupying, causing no or only minimal shift of the midline structure.

POSTINFUSION SCAN OF INFARCTS

The postinfusion scan may reveal no change in the appearance of the infarct. Sometimes the area of infarction may become less apparent; or, uncommonly, the infarct will become more apparent. Occasionally an area of infarction will become visible even though the preinfusion scan was normal. Presumably this occurs because the normal brain tissue takes up the contrast material, whereas the area of infarction does not. Thus, if the patient's clinical appearance suggests an infarct and the initial scan is negative, an infusion of contrast material may be in order for complete evaluation. On the other hand, since the postinfusion scan may reveal no change — especially soon after the acute insult — the infusion study may be academic once an area of hemorrhage has been ruled out. A postinfusion scan gives an added risk of renal damage or allergic reaction to the contrast material. Occasionally on the postinfusion scan a marked uptake of the contrast material will be noted in the area of infarction because of "luxury perfusion." In these cases the preinfusion scan may show an area of infarction or may even have a normal appearance. An angiogram may or may not show an area of vascular occlusion with collateral flow; on the other hand, the luxury perfusion may be visible by CT scan even without evidence of major vascular occlusion on the arteriogram. As noted earlier, this luxury perfusion can first be demonstrated approximately 1 week post-insult and persists for approximately 6 weeks. This area of enhancement usually corresponds closely with the area of lucency on the preinfusion scan and often is quite dense in appearance. Occasionally this enhancement on the CT scan takes the form of dense, finger-like projections of enhancement extending into the brain from the outer convexity with intervening area of radiolucency. Rarely, a "ring" of enhancement similar to that seen with a tumor is seen on the postinfusion scan. Differentiation from tumor may be difficult.

Late Changes. With the passage of time the areas of infarction may disappear, but frequently they leave residual areas of lucency as evidence of their presence. The infarct may leave an area of porencephaly, or it may result in an appearance of hemiatrophy with enlargement of the lateral ventricle and cortical sulci on the side of the stroke.

The study of strokes accounts for a large percentage of patients who are examined with computed tomography. Thorough knowledge of the presentation and of the protean manifestations of infarction is mandatory for accurate interpretation of CT scans.

COLLATERAL CIRCULATION

Subclavian Steal. A variety of "steal" circulations may exist; however, one that is seen frequently and that may result in clinical symptoms of vertebrobasilar insufficiency is the subclavian steal (Fig. 6–21). This syndrome results from an area of narrowing or occlusion of the proximal subclavian artery — usually the left, but the right side also may exhibit this finding—proximal to the origin of the vertebral artery. This results in a deficiency of blood flow to the arm. When the arm is used, the increased demand for blood will cause retrograde blood flow down the vertebral artery and then to the subclavian artery distal to the origin of the vertebral artery. In other words, the arm will "steal" blood from the opposite side and from the vertebrobasilar system by retrograde flow down the vertebral artery on the side where there is stenosis or occlusion of the proximal subclavian artery. This obviously results in a deficient blood supply to the posterior fossa circulation, and these patients may develop syncopal attacks, dizziness and even nystagmus (see Fig. 6–21).

One surgical approach to this disorder is a bypass graft that extends from the carotid artery to the affected subclavian artery. This will increase the blood supply to the arm by taking blood from the carotid system. The carotid artery must be widely patent, or an endarterectomy must first be performed.

External Carotid Artery Collateral Circulation. When there is total occlusion of the internal carotid system one of the main pathways of collateral flow is via the external carotid system. In some individuals there is opening of the collateral pathways behind the globe of the eye, with hypertrophy of the external carotid branches behind the globe that fills the ophthalmic artery and ultimately the intracranial circulation in a retrograde fashion. Clinically, these patients have an ocular bruit because of the increased blood flow through the hypertrophied retro-occular ophthalmic collateral vessels (see Figs. 6–8, 6–9). Vessels that may provide collateral flow are the facial artery, superficial temporal artery, ethmoidal arteries and multiple small arteries and arterial branches.

External Carotid Collateral to Vertebral Artery. Another one of the more common types of collateral circulation involves the carotid and vertebral systems. With occlusion of the common carotid artery below the level of the carotid bifurcation, collateral circulation develops from muscular branches of the vertebral artery and from the thyrocervical trunk. These collateral branches anastomose with the branches of the external carotid artery. Blood then flows retrograde to the level of the carotid bifurcation and then antegrade in the internal carotid circulation or even via ophthalmic collaterals. Similarly, collateral circulation from the external carotid artery may supply a vertebral artery that is occluded or stenotic at its origin.

ANGIOGRAPHY OF COLLATERAL CIRCULATION AND THE STEAL SYNDROMES

The various collateral pathways illustrate the "imagination" of the biologic system in providing for continuous blood flow to critical areas. These collateral pathways usually demonstrate a much slower circulation than do normal anatomic pathways; therefore, when performing angiography to demonstrate abnormal circulation, a prolonged film series is necessary. The author recommends serial filming over at least 8 seconds. The films may be programmed so that they demonstrate both the early arterial and late arterial phases. Films should be obtained in a biplane projection. One possible program would be 2 films per second for 3 seconds and 1 film per second for the next 5 seconds.

MOYAMOYA

This disease was originally described in children, but the author has seen cases in adults secondary to diffuse arteriosclerosis (Fig. 6–19). Of unknown etiology in children, it results in stenosis and progressive occlusion of multiple intracranial vessels and the proliferation of massive collateral circulation from the lenticulostriate and thalamoperforating arteries. This results in a diffuse blush at angiography, giving the appearance of the "puff of smoke" from which the Japanese name originates. I have also seen several cases having the appearance of moyamoya disease in children with sickle cell anemia (Fig. 6–18).

The CT scans are reminiscent of atrophy. The massive collateral vessels do not demonstrate enhancement on the postinfusion scan.

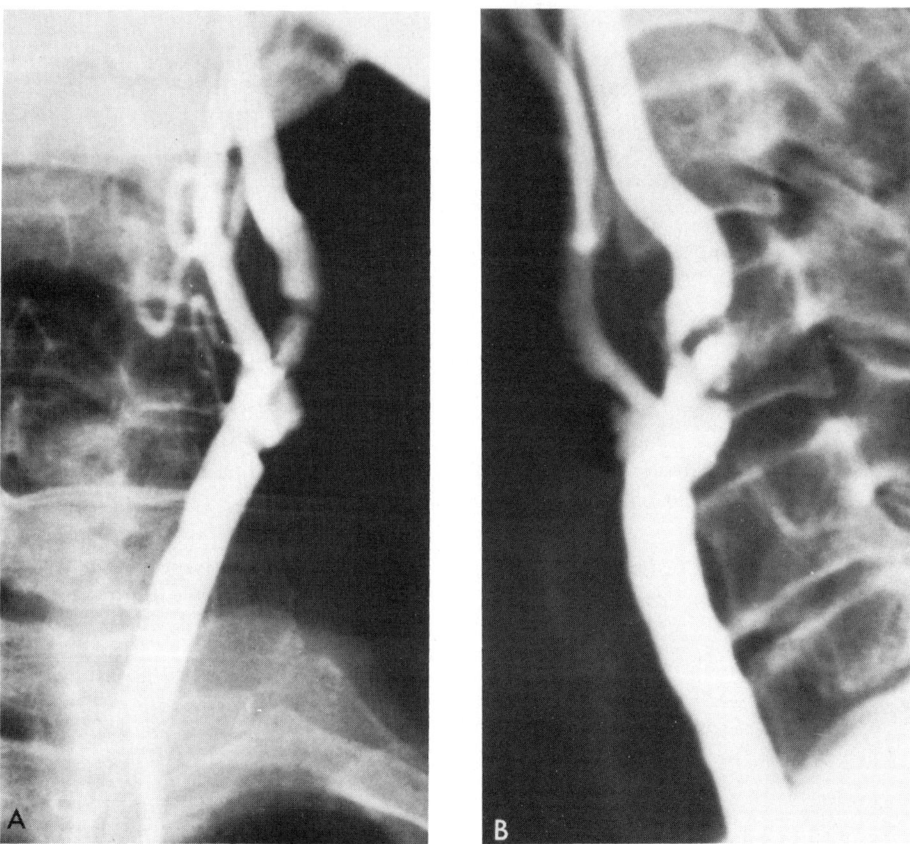

Figure 6–1. ULCERATED PLAQUE WITH STENOSIS SEEN WELL IN ONE PLANE: *A*, The AP view reveals an irregular area of stenosis involving the distal left common carotid artery and the left internal carotid artery. On the lateral (*B*) view, however, the ulcerated plaque with a very high grade stenosis can be more readily appreciated.

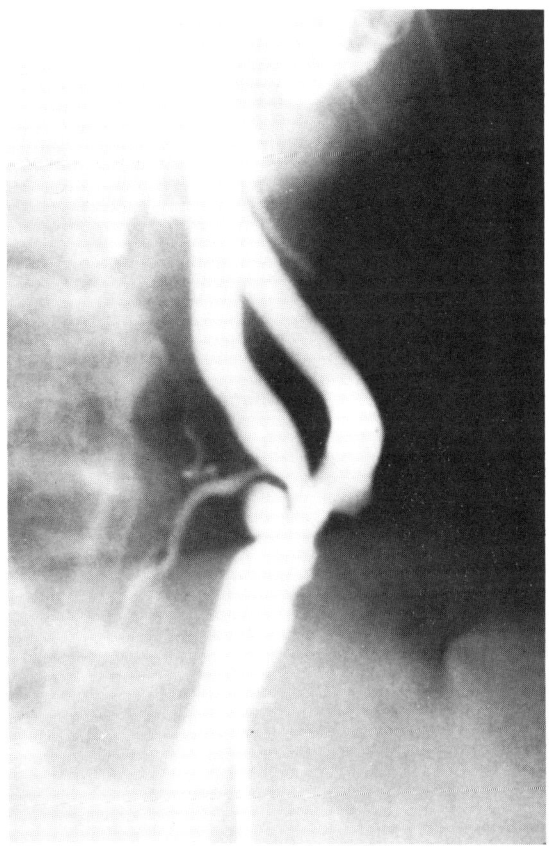

Figure 6–2. ULCERATED PLAQUE WITH STENOSIS: There is an irregular area of stenosis with an ulcerated lesion involving the distal left common carotid artery. The needle is in place well below the bifurcation.

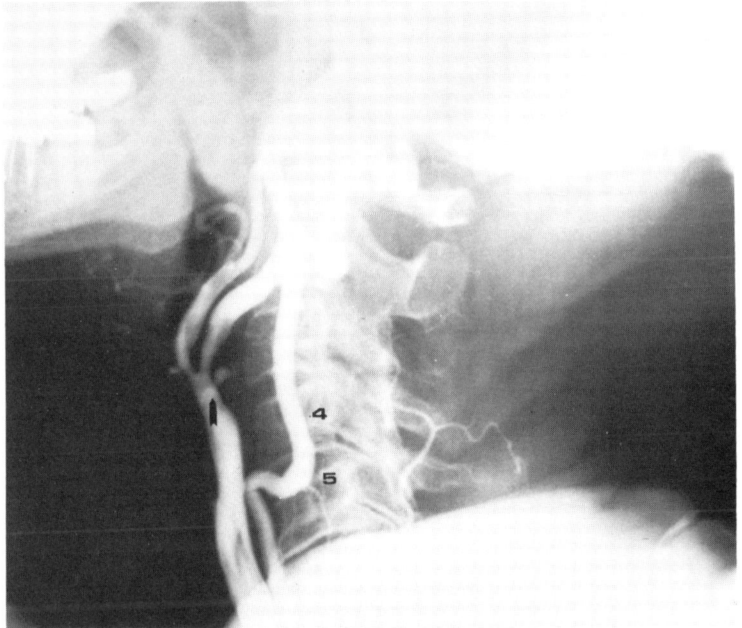

Figure 6–3. ULCERATED PLAQUE: The RBA demonstrates an ulcerated plaque at the origin of the right internal carotid artery (*arrow*). In addition, the vertebral artery enters into the foramina transversaria at the C_4–C_5 level rather than at the level of C_6. This is a normal anatomic variant.

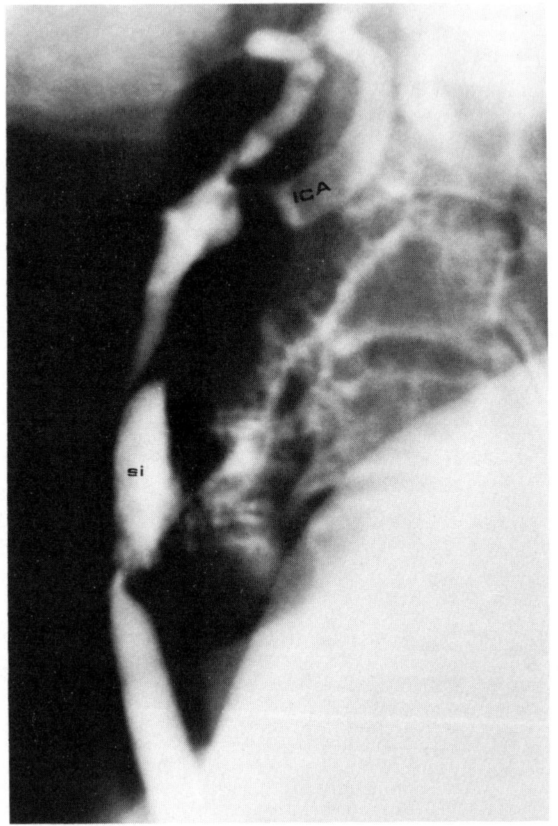

Figure 6–4. CAROTID STENOSIS, SUBINTIMAL INJECTION: The percutaneous carotid arteriogram reveals a large subintimal injection (*si*) associated with areas of stenosis both proximal and distal to the area of subintimal accumulation of contrast material. There is an intraluminal collection of clotted blood in the left internal carotid artery (*ICA*) just distal to the stenosis of the internal carotid artery. In addition, there is a collection of extravasated contrast material in the soft tissues of the neck behind the carotid artery. The extravasation of contrast material probably occurs through the back wall puncture site. There is a large hematoma of the neck with forward displacement of the carotid artery in the neck.

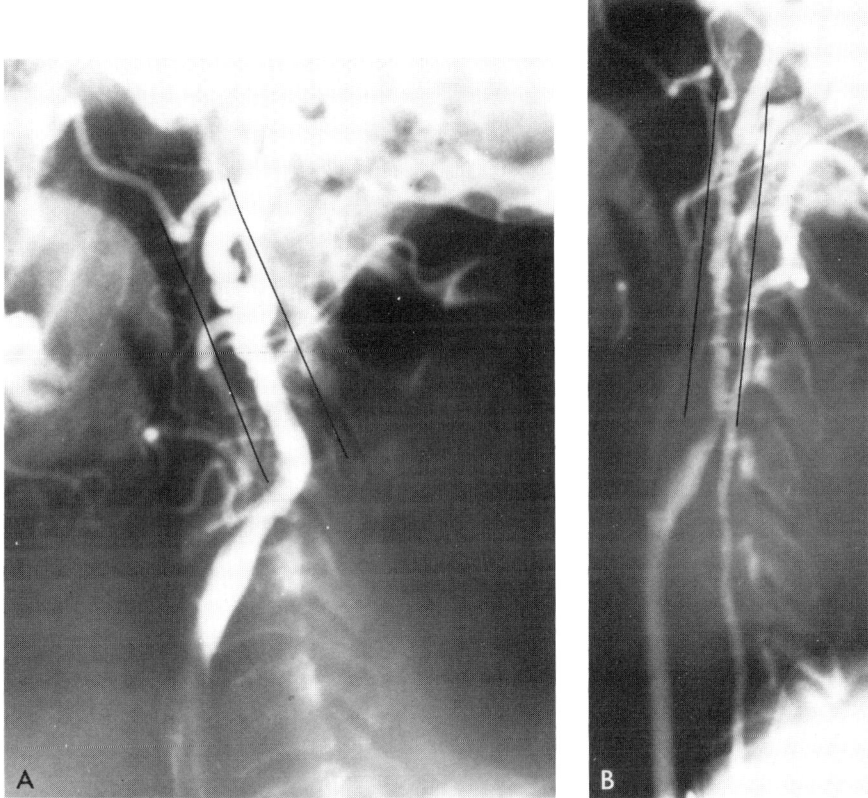

Figure 6–5. FIBROMUSCULAR HYPERPLASIA: *A* and *B*, Both carotid arteriograms demonstrate the "stack of coins" appearance typical of fibromuscular hyperplasia. The internal lumen of the vessel may be much more markedly narrowed than can be appreciated on the arteriogram.

Figure 6–6. EMBOLUS IN THE COMMON CAROTID ARTERY: *A*, The left common carotid arteriogram demonstrates a large embolus in the vessel that causes complete occlusion to the flow of contrast material (*arrow*). The rounded lower end of the thrombus can be identified. Presumably this arises from the heart.

B, The CT scans demonstrated marked lucency involving the entire left hemisphere, associated with mass effect and shift of the midline to the contralateral side. There is sparing of the occipital poles because their blood supply arises from the vertebrobasilar system, consistent with a hemisphere infarct secondary to total occlusion of the internal carotid artery.

C, The pathologic specimen demonstrates an edematous left hemisphere and shift of the midline to the contralateral side.

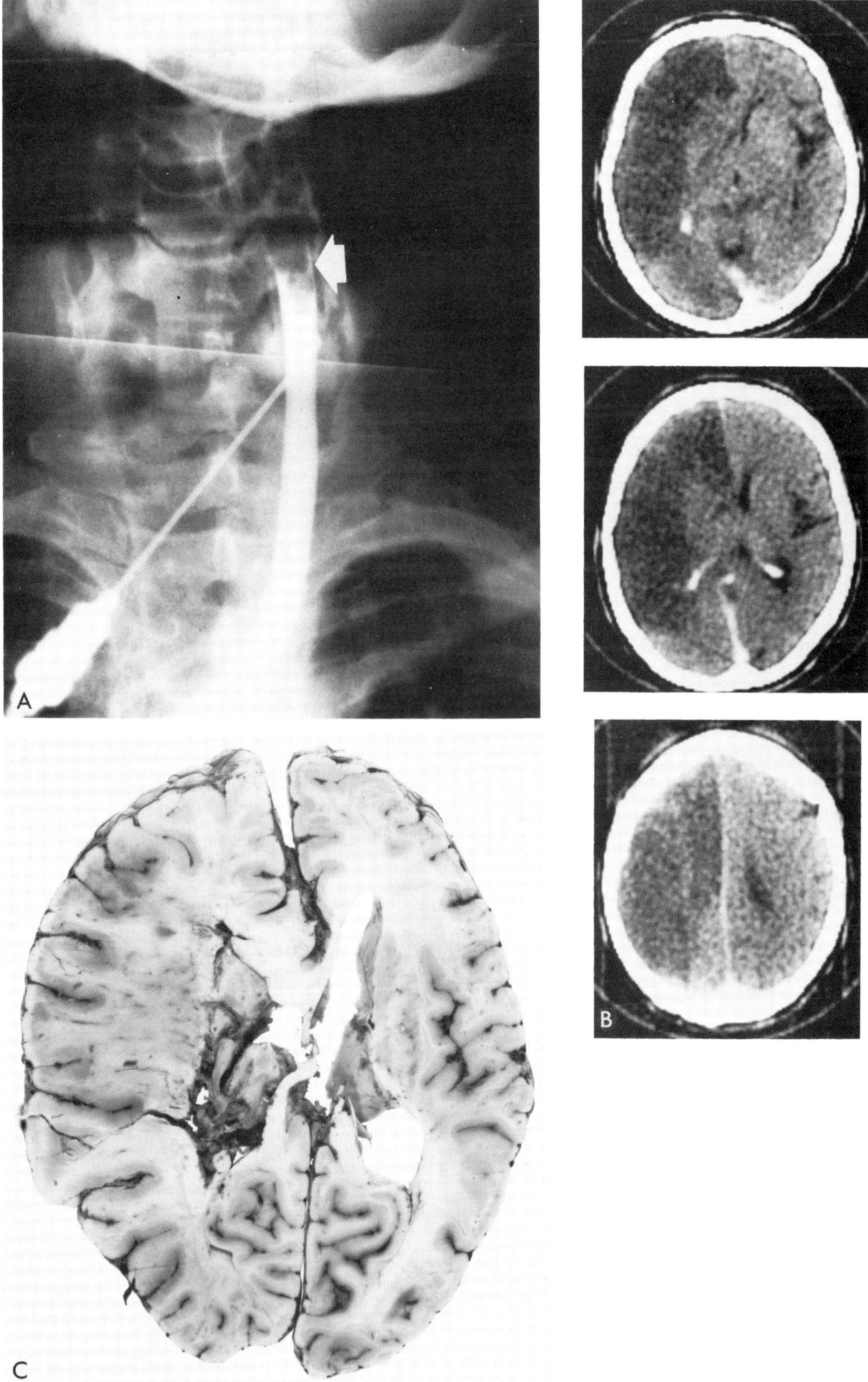

Figure 6–6. *See legend on the opposite page.*

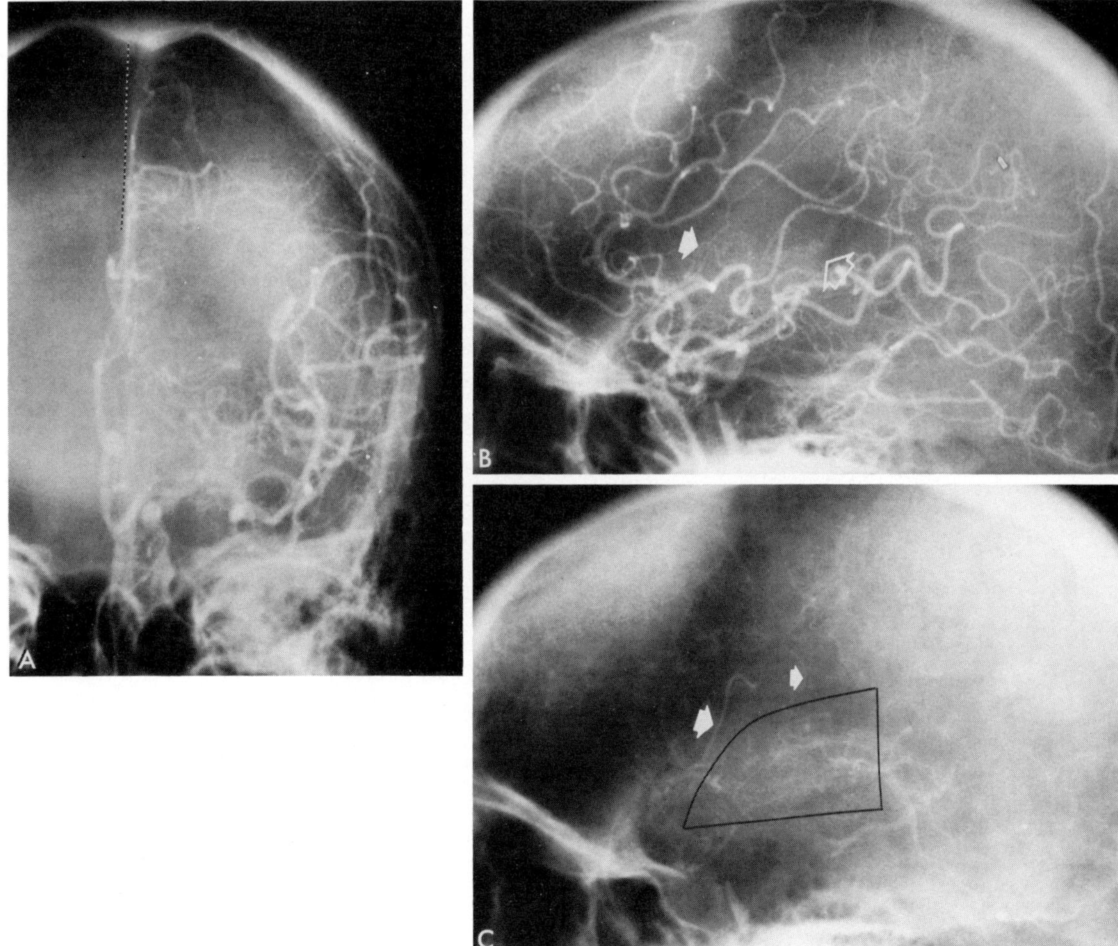

Figure 6–7. ACUTE INFARCT WITH MASS EFFECT: *A,* The AP view of the common carotid arteriogram demonstrates shift of the anterior cerebral artery to the contralateral side. The dashed line indicates the anticipated position of the midline.

B, The lateral view of the arterial phase shows branch occlusions of several of the anterior branches of the middle cerebral artery *(closed arrow);* the open arrow points to an area of luxury perfusion in the region of infarction.

C, The arrowheads demonstrate the occluded vessels filling in a retrograde fashion via collateral circulation. The black lines encircle an area of luxury perfusion.

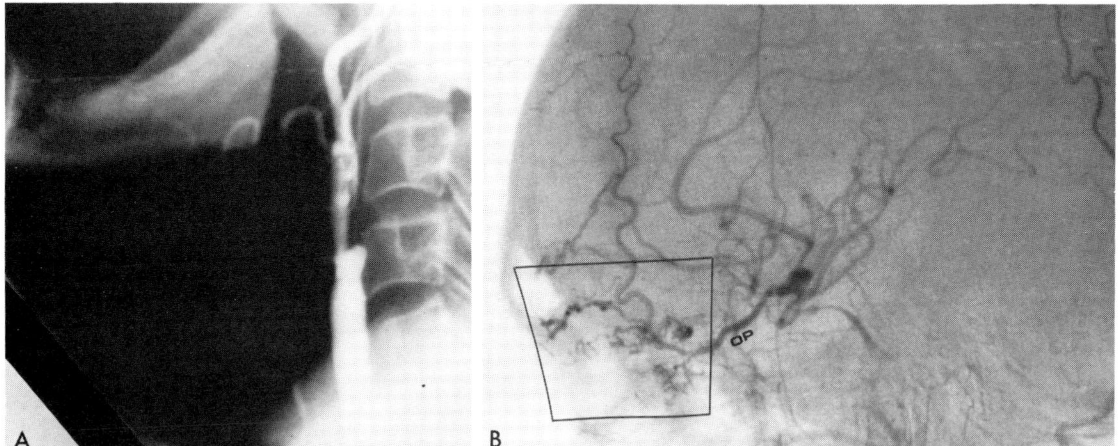

Figure 6–8. OPHTHALMIC COLLATERAL: *A*, There is total occlusion of the internal carotid artery at its origin in the neck. *B*, The external carotid artery is large, and multiple small collateral vessels (*black lines*) may be seen. These eventually fill the ophthalmic artery (*OP*) in a retrograde fashion. The ophthalmic artery then fills the internal carotid artery and the intracranial circulation.

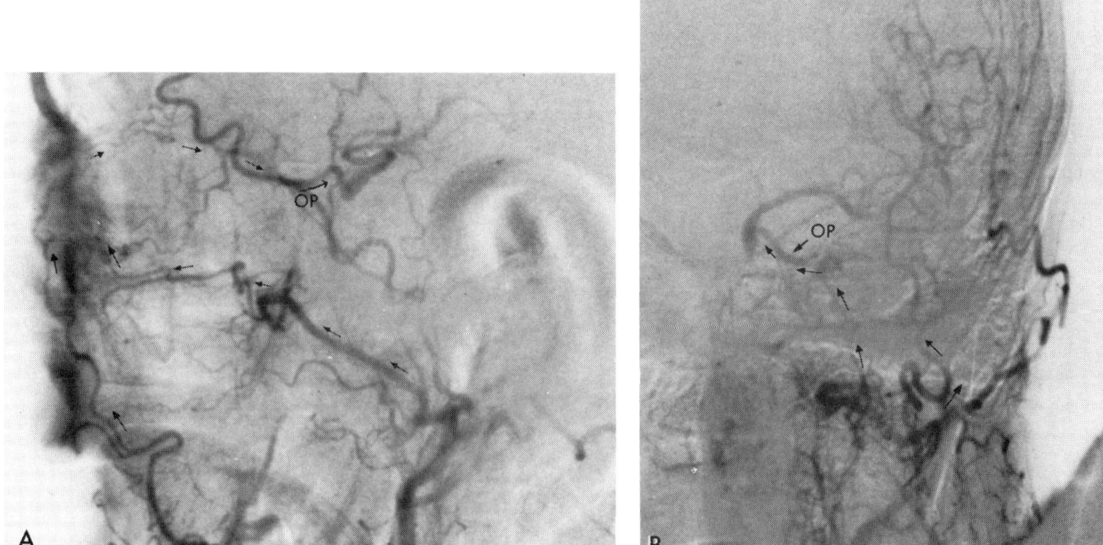

Figure 6–9, ***A*** **and** ***B*****.** OPHTHALMIC COLLATERAL: The internal carotid artery is occluded in the neck at the level of the carotid bifurcation. The branches of the external carotid artery have enlarged and demonstrate extensive collateral flow *(arrows)* through the internal maxillary and facial arteries on the lateral view *(A)* and in the facial artery on the anteroposterior view *(B)*. The flow is ultimately retrograde through the ophthalmic artery (OP) to the internal carotid artery, which supplies the middle cerebral artery distribution.

Subtraction views, as shown here, demonstrate these collateral channels to better advantage.

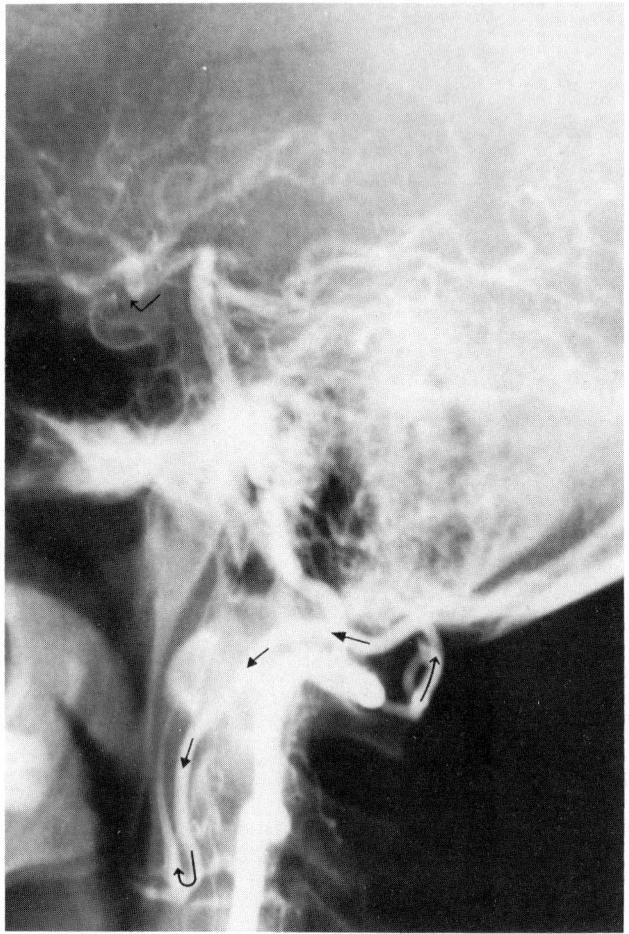

Figure 6–10. COLLATERAL CIRCULATION: The brachial arteriogram demonstrates a total occlusion of the internal carotid artery at its origin in the neck. The vertebral artery gives rise to a large muscular collateral vessel *(arrows)* that communicates with the external carotid artery at the level of the bifurcation, where the external carotid artery and its branches are then noted to fill via this collateral. The intracranial circulation is filling via retrograde flow through the posterior communication artery *(curved arrow)* and then to the anterior and middle cerebral artery circulations.

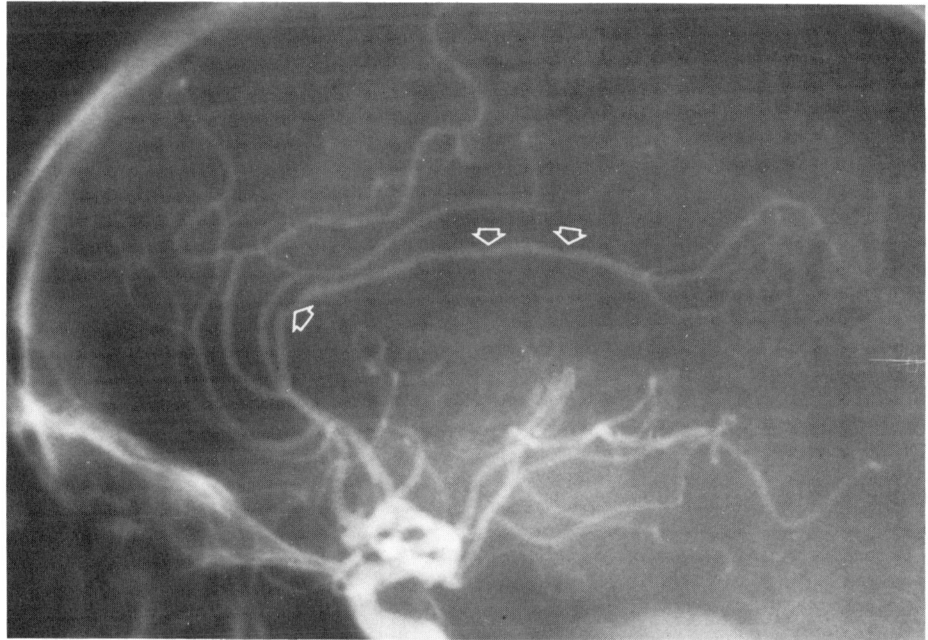

Figure 6–11. The intracranial circulation demonstrates multiple areas of irregular narrowing secondary to diffuse intracranial arteriosclerosis *(arrowheads)*.

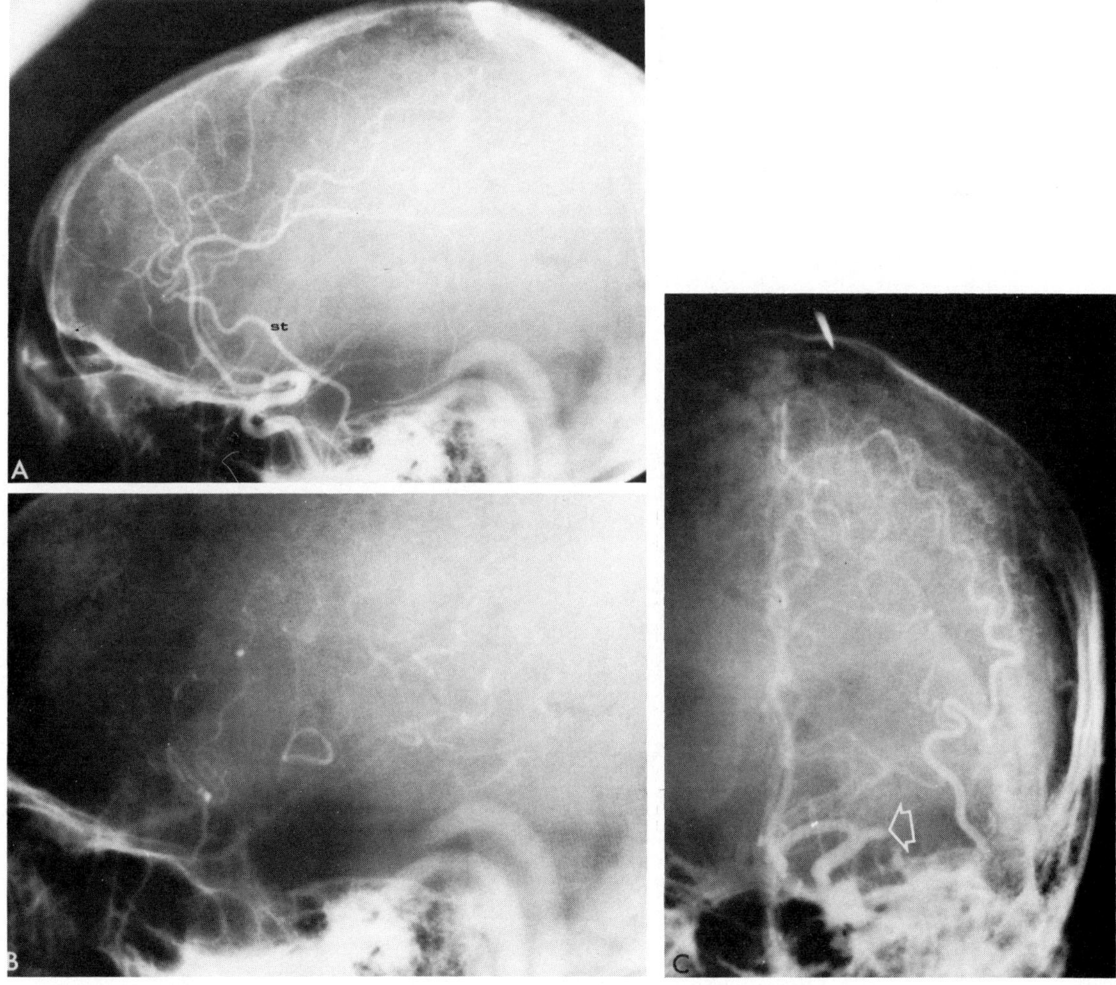

Figure 6–12. MIDDLE CEREBRAL ARTERY OCCLUSION: *A,* The lateral view shows total occlusion of the middle cerebral artery just past the origin of the vessel from the internal carotid artery. The result, therefore, is an anterior cerebral artery arteriogram. The second large vessel seen is the superficial temporal artery (ST).

B, The capillary phase of the arteriogram demonstrates the branches of the middle cerebral artery, which fill in a retrograde fashion.

C, On the AP view, the occluded middle cerebral artery (*arrow*) is seen. The superficial temporal artery projects over the left side of the skull. At times the superficial temporal artery can be mobilized and anastomosed to the middle cerebral artery branches to increase the cerebral blood flow. (The broken tip of a knife blade is seen in the parietal region.)

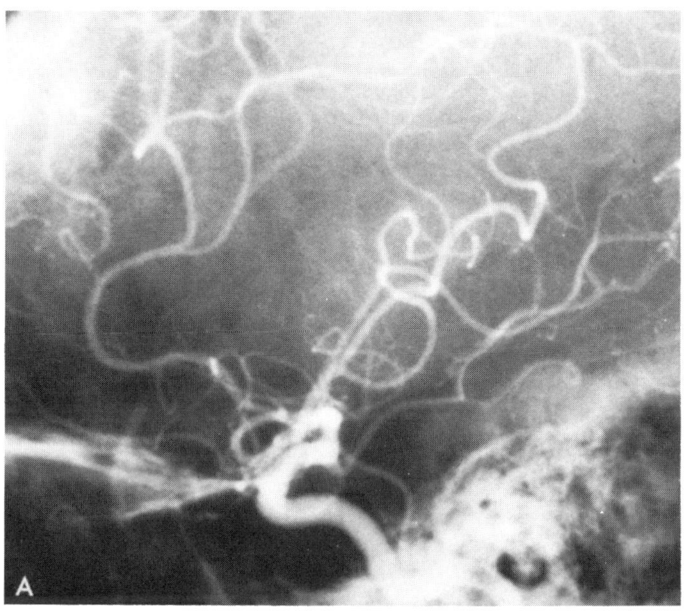

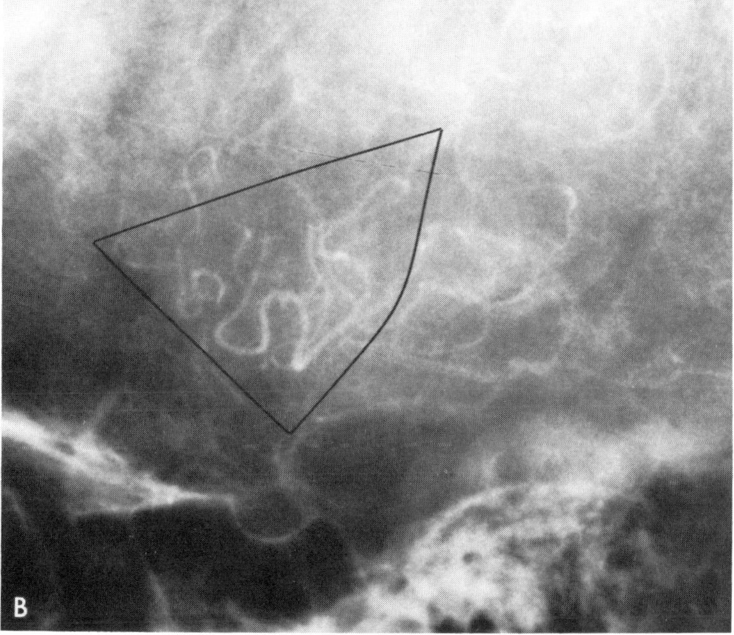

Figure 6–13. BRANCH OCCLUSIONS OF THE MIDDLE CEREBRAL ARTERY: *A*, The early arterial phase demonstrates the multiple branch occlusions involving the middle cerebral artery are present.

B, The capillary phase shows that the branches fill in a retrograde fashion via collateral circulation *(black line)*. Just behind the outlined area there is a faint blush secondary to luxury perfusion in the area of the occluded vessels.

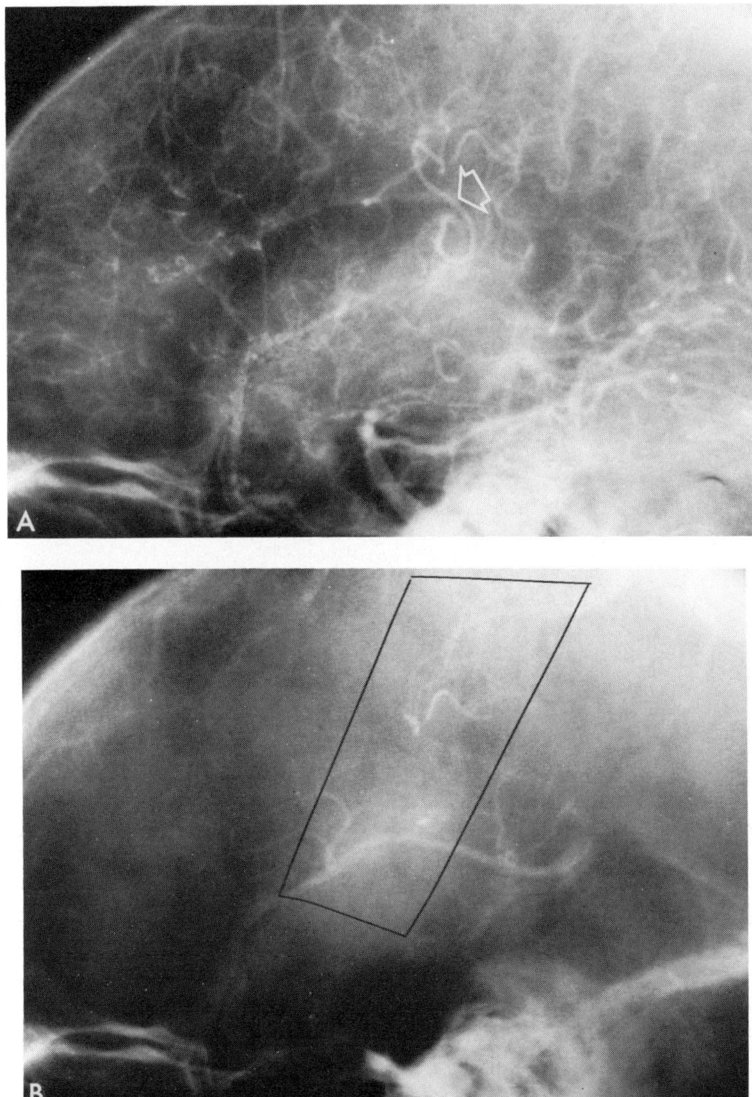

Figure 6–14. BRANCH OCCLUSIONS AND LUXURY PERFUSION: *A*, The late arterial phase demonstrates "hold-up" of the contrast material in one of the branches of the middle cerebral artery group *(arrow)*.

B, The venous phase also demonstrates hold-up of the contrast in the terminal portion of the vessel *(black lines)*.

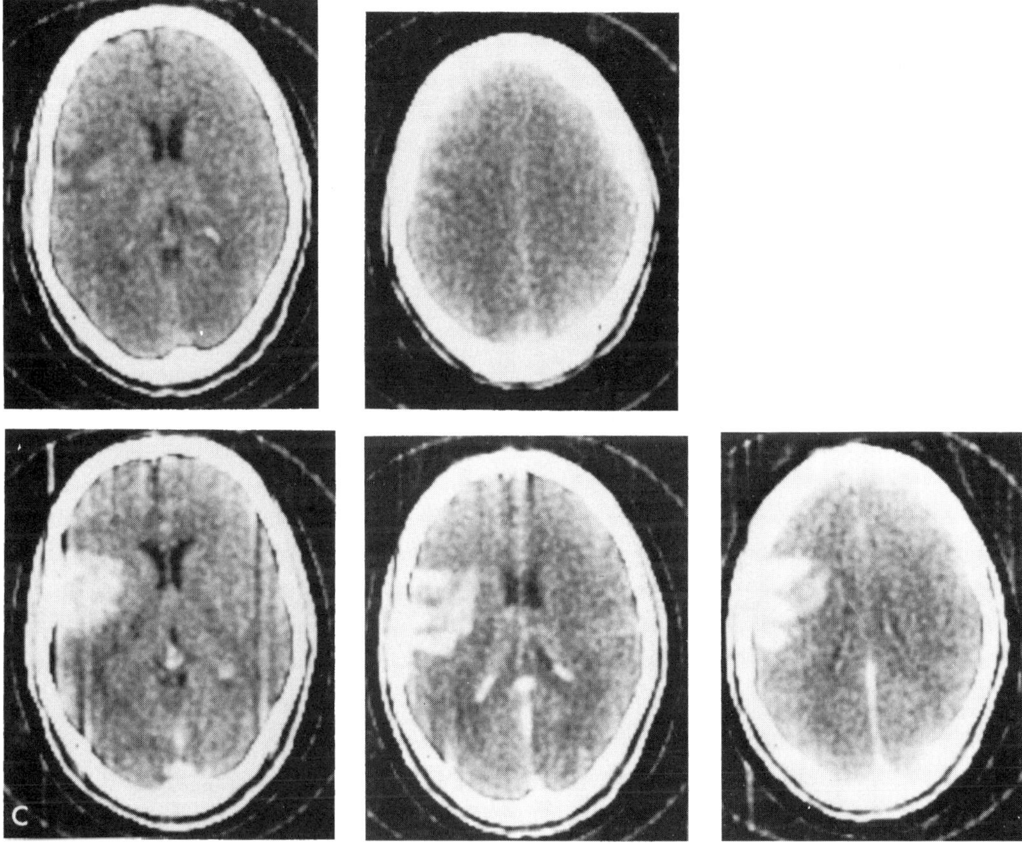

Figure 6–14 *Continued*

C, CT scans reveal an area of radiolucency mixed with areas of slightly increased density; there is marked enhancement following the infusion of contrast material — a classic example of luxury perfusion. There is no mass effect.

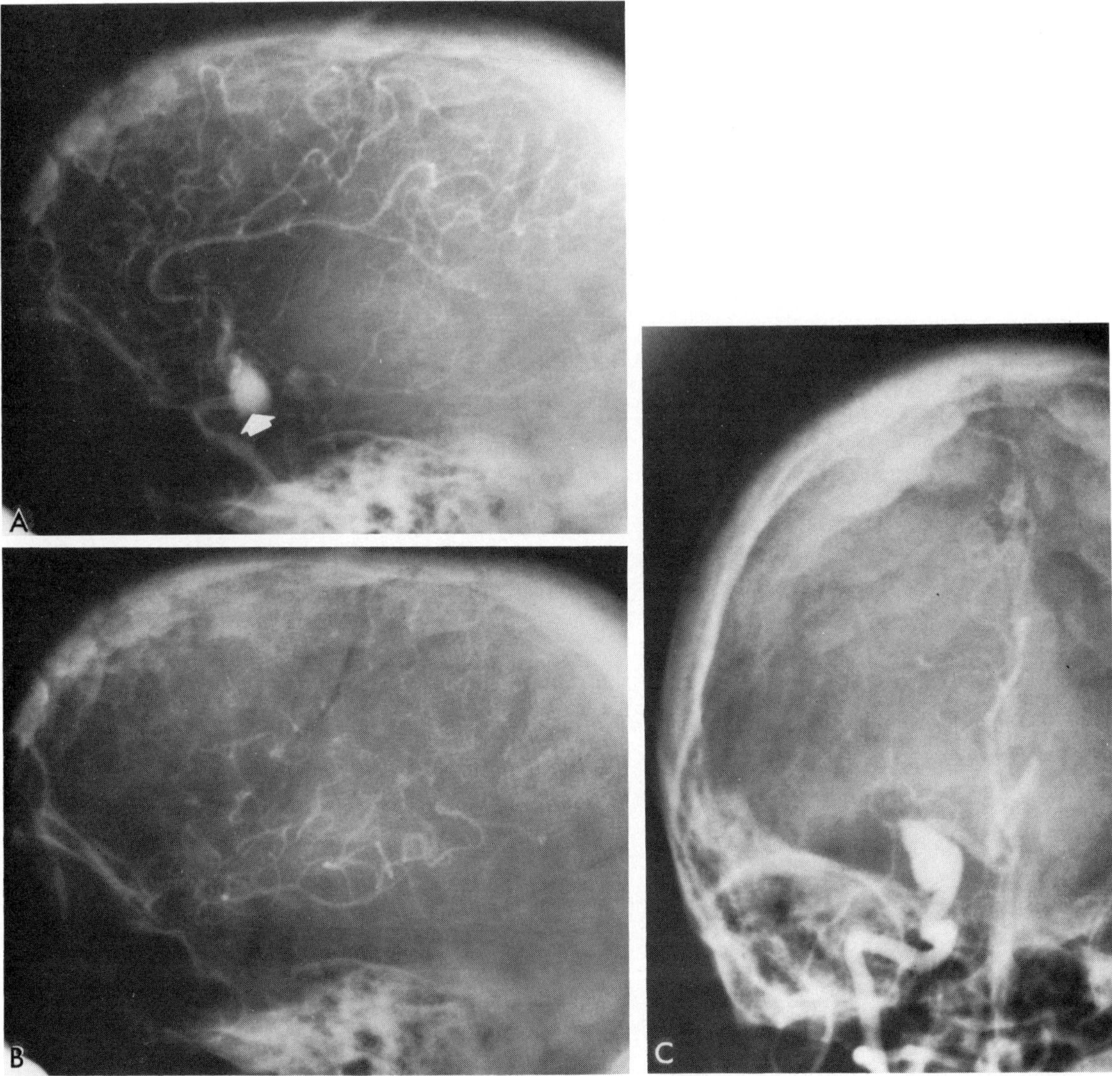

Figure 6–15. MIDDLE CEREBRAL OCCLUSION: *A* and *B,* The arterial and capillary phases of the arteriogram demonstrate a complete occlusion of the middle cerebral artery, which fills later in the capillary phase by collateral flow and retrograde filling. An aneurysm of the internal carotid artery just at the origin of the middle cerebral artery also is evident *(arrow).*

C, The AP view also shows the aneurysm of the internal carotid artery and the total occlusion of the middle cerebral artery at its origin.

Figure 6–16. CEREBRAL INFARCT WITH AN EARLY DRAINING VEIN: The AP *(A)* and lateral *(B)* views of the angiogram show an early draining vein high in the posterior frontal area *(arrows)* in an otherwise normal-appearing angiogram.

C, CT scans demonstrate a small linear area of increased density on the preinfusion scan (etiology? — perhaps a small hemorrhage); the postinfusion scan reveals a wedge-shaped area of enhancement. This is a small infarct with luxury perfusion.

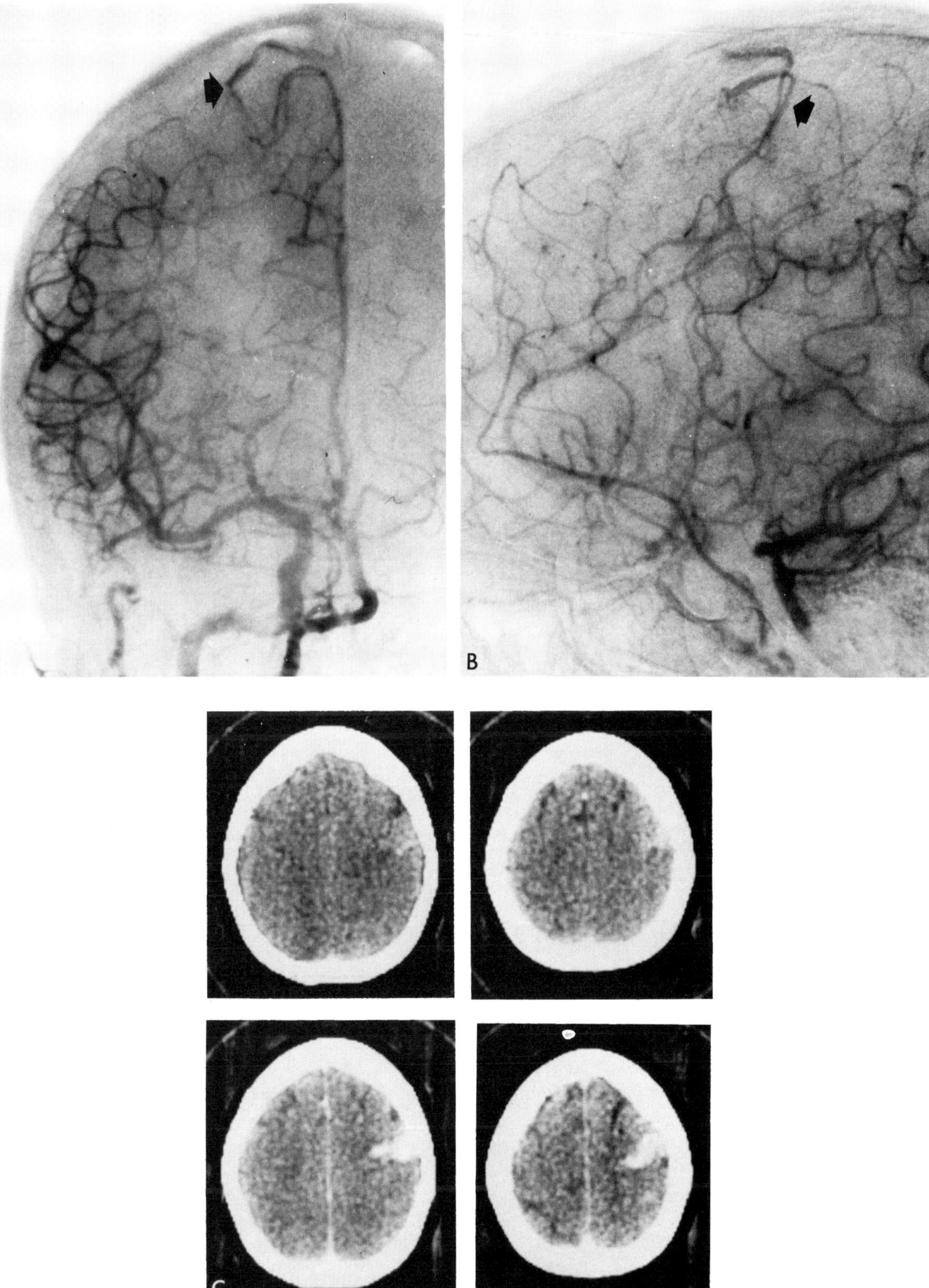

Figure 6–16. *See legend on the opposite page.*

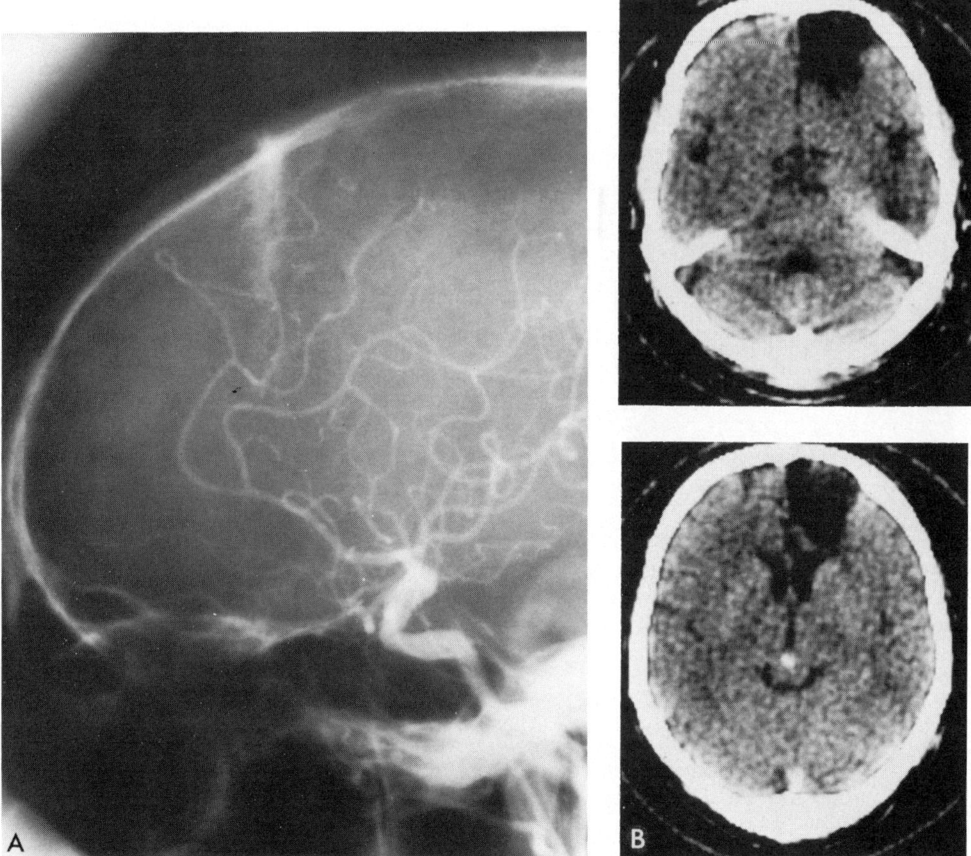

Figure 6–17. PORENCEPHALY SECONDARY TO INFARCTION: The angiogram *(A)* demonstrates an area of avascularity in the frontal pole region; *(B)* the CT scan reveals a porencephalic cyst in the frontal region. The area is filled with fluid of CSF density, has a well defined border and does not demonstrate mass effect. This area of porencephaly was secondary to an infarct of the right frontal region that resulted from occlusion of one of the arterial branches to the frontal pole.

Figure 6–18. MOYAMOYA DISEASE SECONDARY TO SICKLE CELL ANEMIA: *A,* Occlusions and areas of narrowing involving the intracranial vessels are evident. There is marked hypertrophy of the lenticulostriate vessels and a diffuse blush in the region of the middle cerebral artery distribution. In an attempt to provide collateral flow, the meningeal arteries have hypertrophied *(m);* the ophthalmic artery also gives rise to multiple small collateral vessels.

B, The vertebral angiogram also shows the multiple vessel occlusions and dilatation of the thalamoperforate vessels with a diffuse blush in the region of the thalamus. Note the marked enlargement of the posterior meningeal artery *(m)* that also was seen in *A*.

C, The CT scans provide a picture of atrophy, with diffuse enlargement of the lateral ventricles (the left slightly more than the right) and enlargement of the cortical sulci over the left hemisphere. Small areas of radiolucency are also present on the right side — probably secondary to small infarcts. The blush seen on the arteriogram is not seen on the postinfusion CT scan.

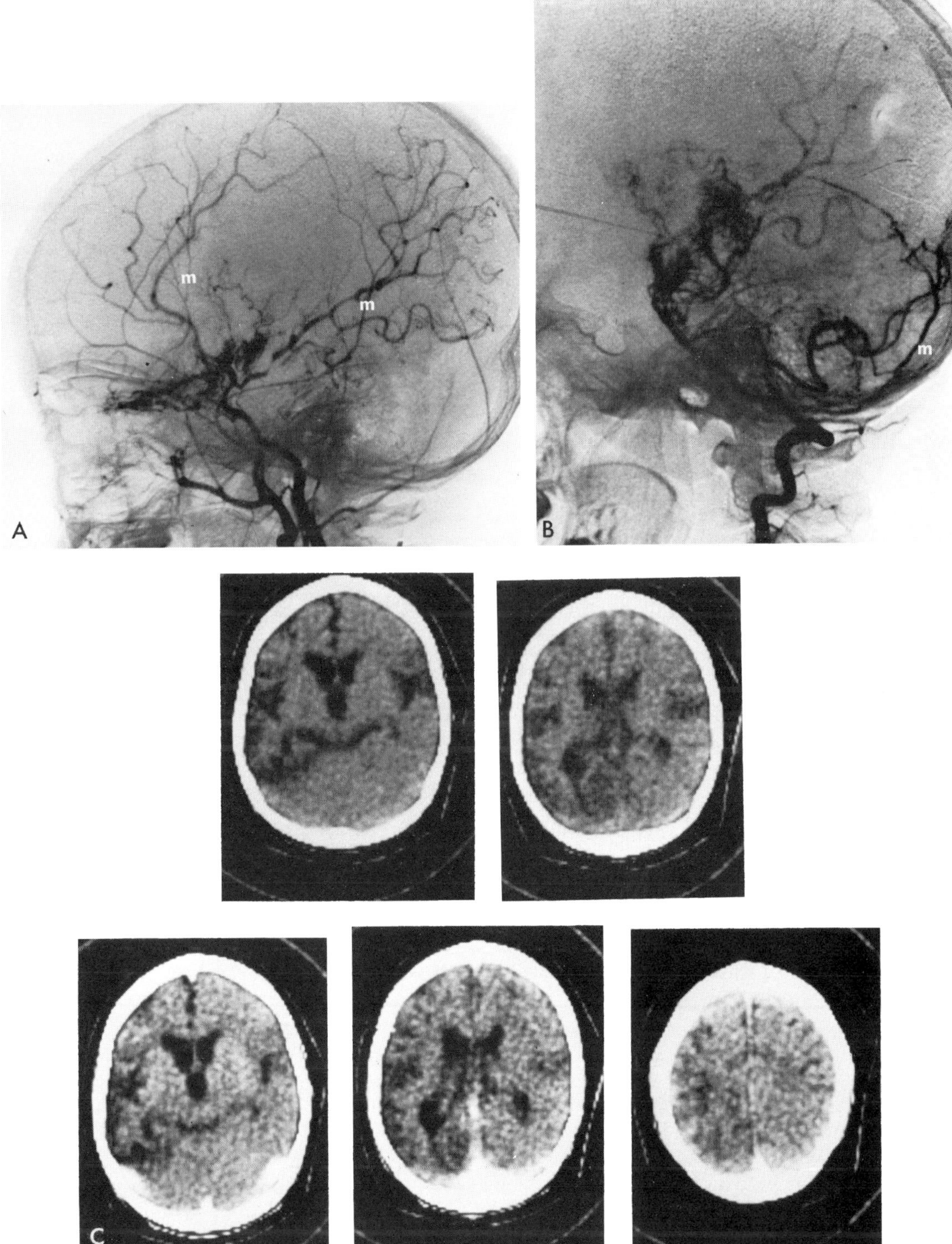

Figure 6–18. *See legend on the opposite page.*

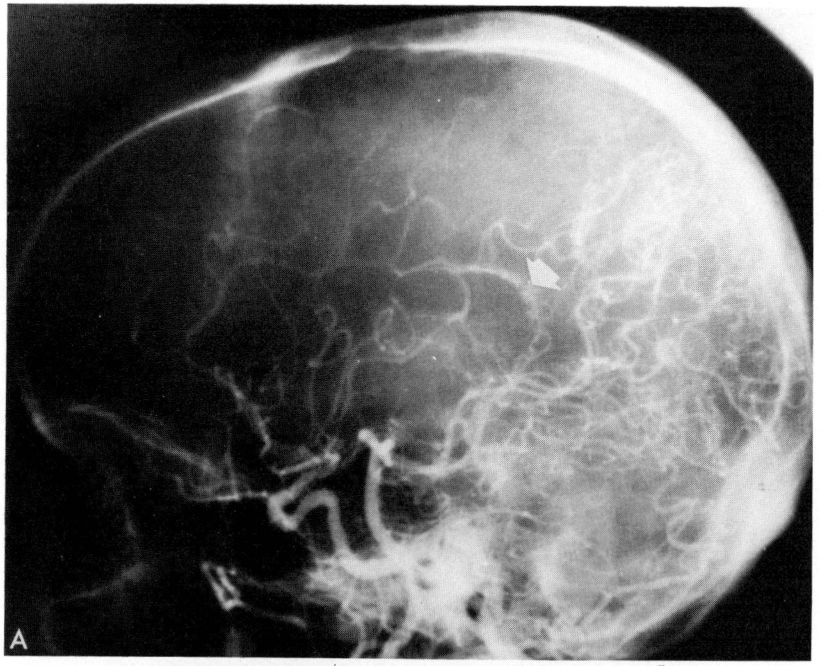

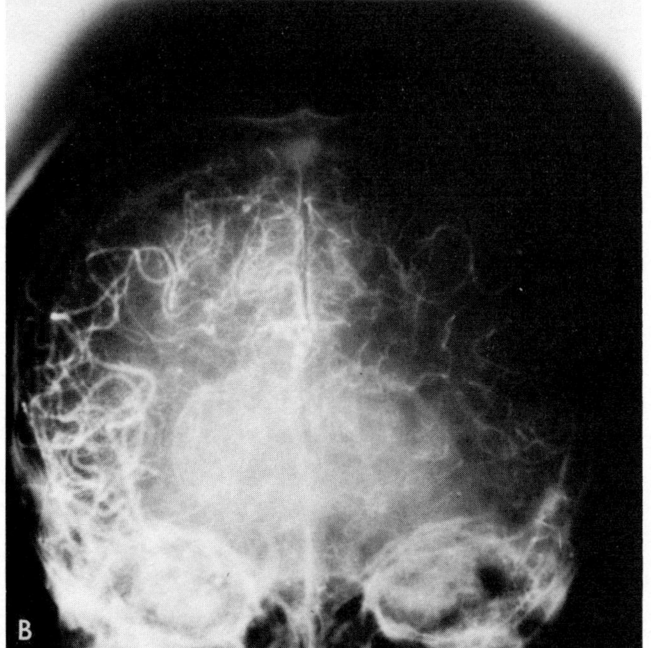

Figure 6–19. "ARTERIOSCLEROTIC MOYAMOYA" DISEASE: *A*, The arteriogram reveals multiple small occlusions of distal branches and marked collateral flow. There is retrograde flow through the posterior pericallosal artery *(arrow)*.

B, The AP view demonstrates a marked blush of the basal ganglia and the thalamus secondary to collateral circulation. This has the appearance of moyamoya disease, and is on the basis of arteriosclerotic vascular occlusive disease.

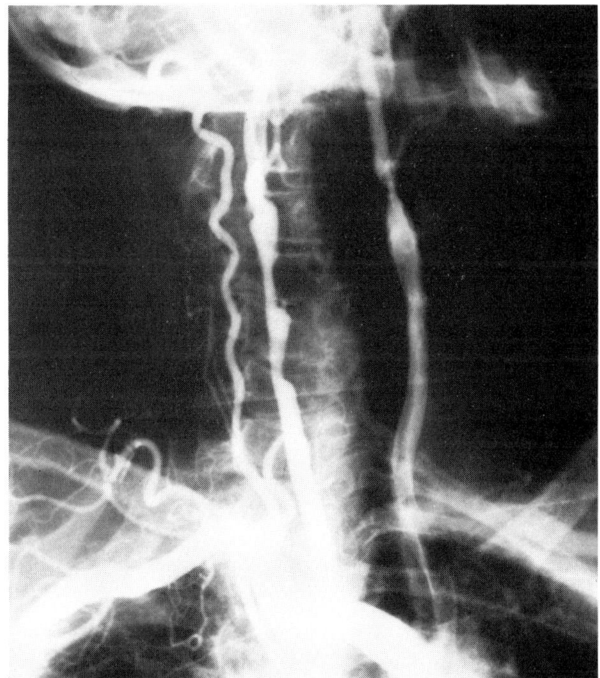

Figure 6–20. DIFFUSE ARTERIOSCLEROSIS: The arch angiogram of this patient reveals total occlusion of the left vertebral artery and marked irregularity of the carotid arteries bilaterally. The curvilinear deformity of the right vertebral artery is secondary to osteophyte formation of the cervical spine.

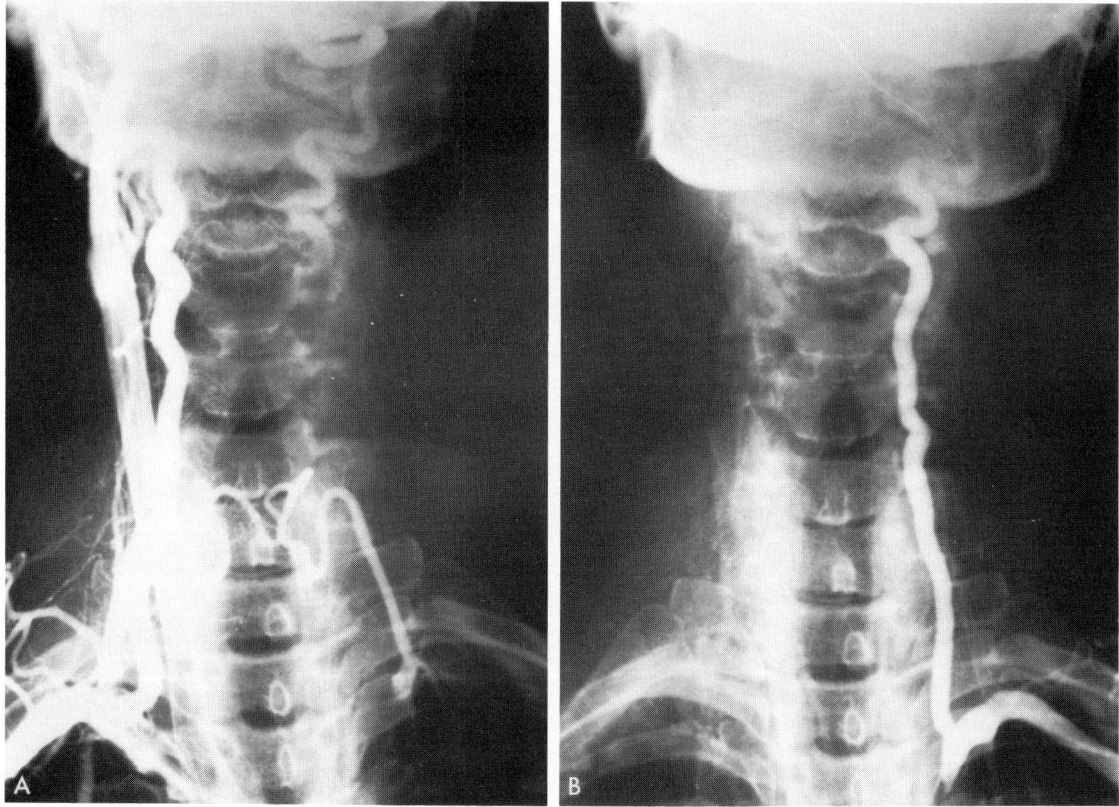

Figure 6–21. SUBCLAVIAN STEAL: *A*, The right brachial arteriogram demonstrates a large right vertebral artery and a normal-appearing right common carotid artery. The inferior thyroid artery is enlarged and extends across the midline to fill the contralateral subclavian artery distal to the origin of the left vertebral artery.

B, The late films show retrograde flow down the left vertebral artery to fill the left subclavian artery. There is total occlusion of the proximal portion of the left subclavian artery.

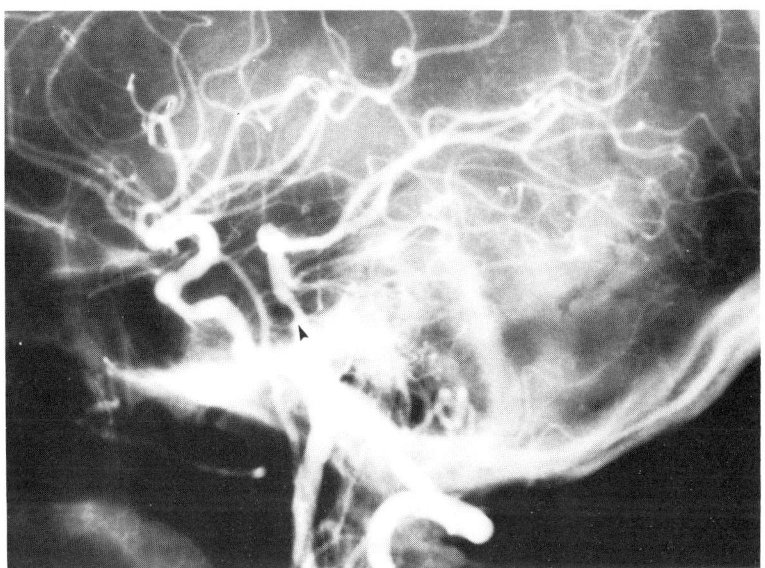

Figure 6–22. BASILAR ARTERY PLAQUE: The lateral view of the right brachial arteriogram demonstrates a well defined plaque at the distal end of the basilar artery *(arrowhead)*. Small arteriosclerotic plaques also are present in the cavernous portion of the carotid artery. On the AP view (not shown) this plaque of the basilar artery may give the false appearance of a fenestrated basilar artery.

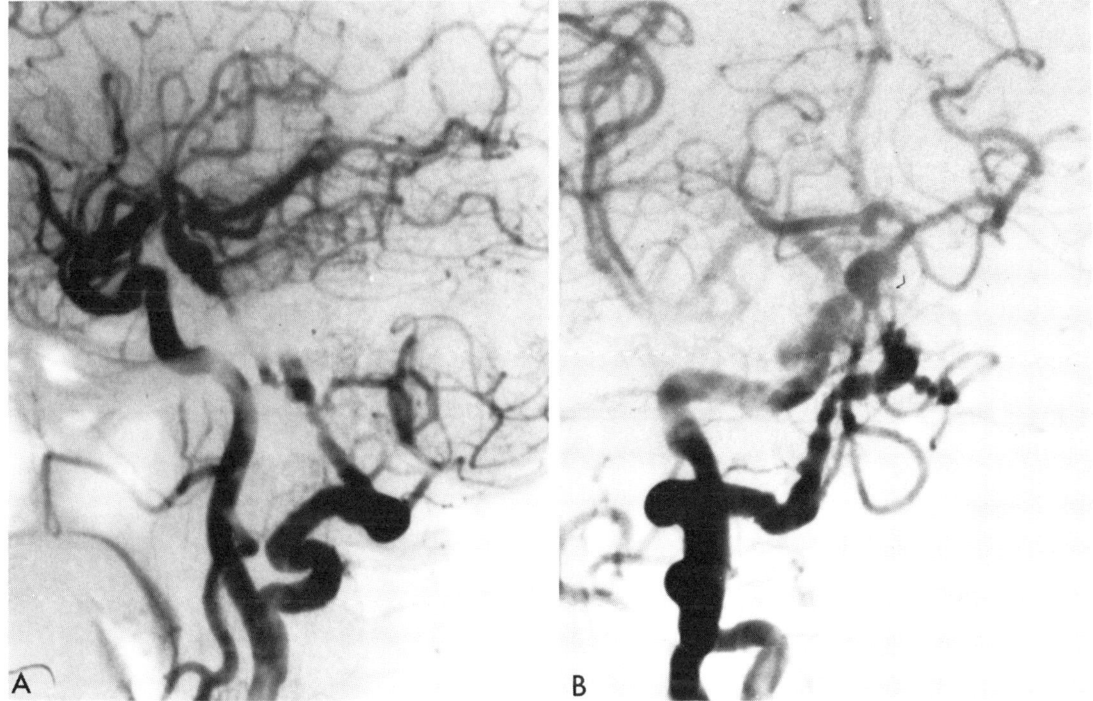

Figure 6–23. VERTEBROBASILAR ARTERIOSCLEROSIS: *A* and *B*, The entire vertebral and basilar artery demonstrates marked irregularity of the vessel walls with areas of dilatation and narrowing. The PICA also demonstrates evidence of irregularity secondary to arteriosclerosis.

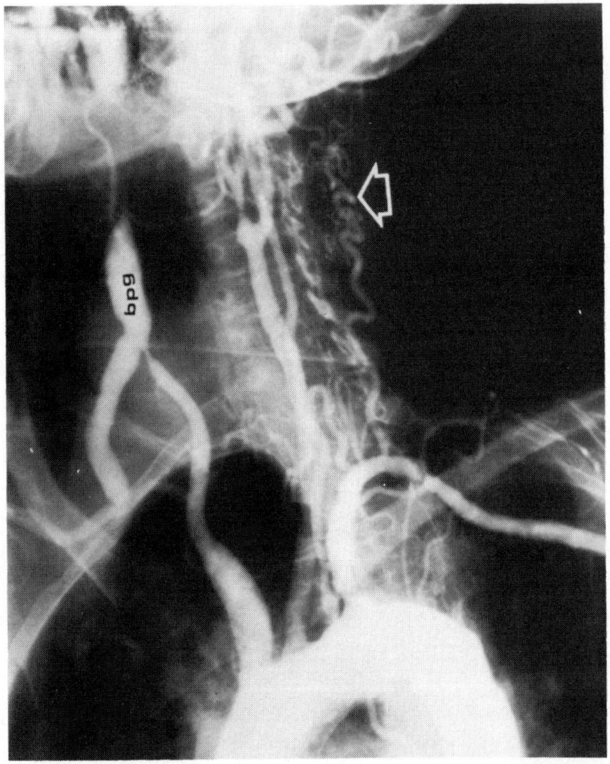

Figure 6–24. BYPASS GRAFT: The arch angiogram with the patient in the RPO position demonstrates marked arteriosclerotic change involving all the great vessels as they arise from the arch of the aorta. The right vertebral artery is totally occluded; the right internal and external carotid arteries also are totally occluded. There is stenosis of the left external carotid artery, and multiple unnamed collateral vessels arise from the thyrocervical trunk to supply the vertebrobasilar system *(arrow)*. There is also a bypass graft *(bpg)* in place that extends from the right common carotid artery to the right subclavian artery. The subclavian artery has a threadlike patency in its proximal portion and is quite small, even distal to the bypass graft.

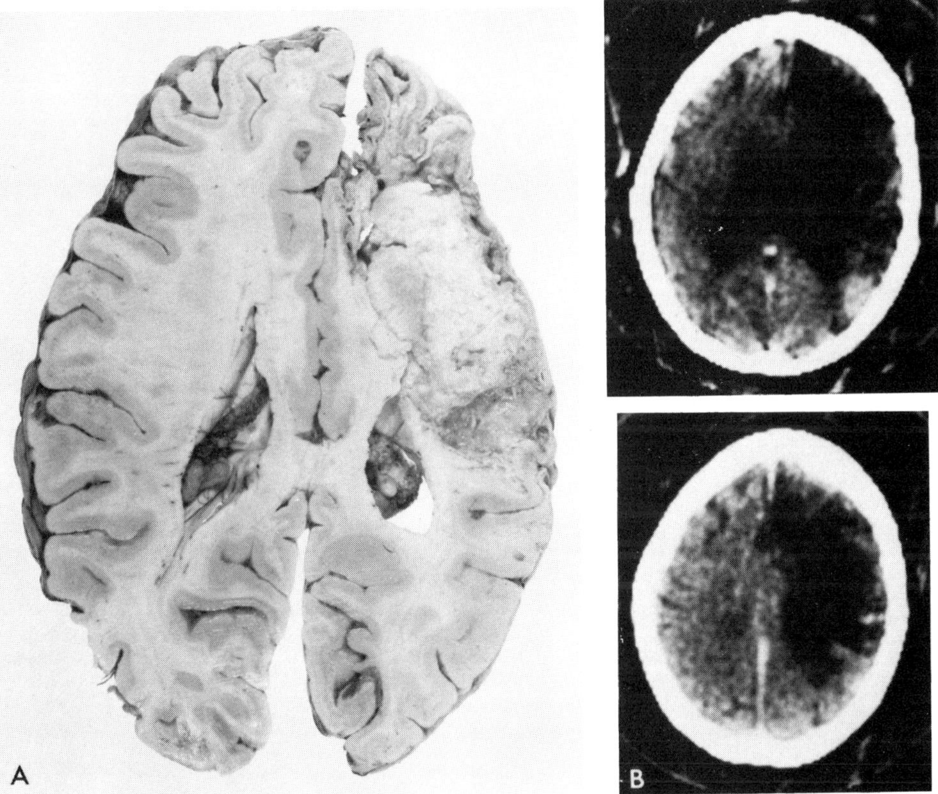

Figure 6–25. OLD MIDDLE CEREBRAL INFARCT: The pathologic specimen *(A)* demonstrates a large area of cystic necrosis involving the right hemisphere. The corresponding CT scan *(B)* reveals a large area of porencephaly secondary to an infarct in the right hemisphere in the region of the right internal carotid artery.

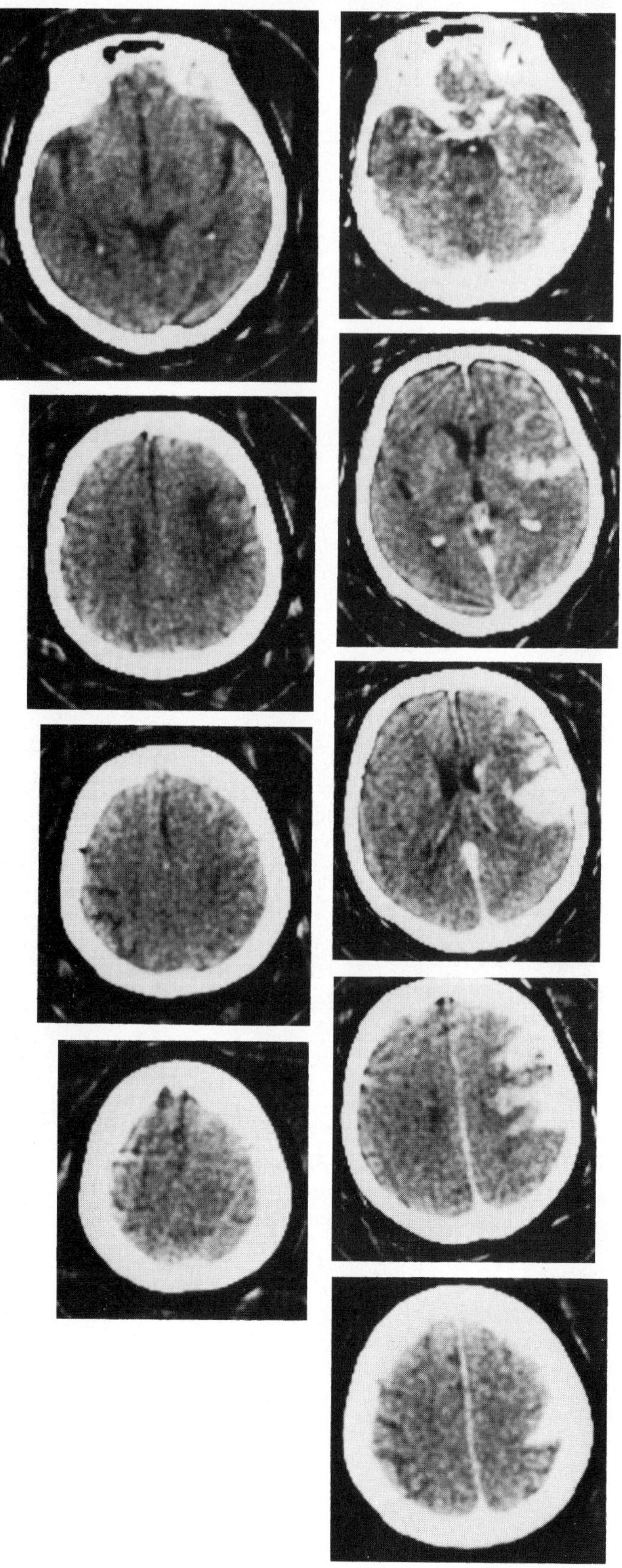

Figure 6–26. *See legend on the opposite page.*

Figure 6–26. INFARCT AND LUXURY PERFUSION: The preinfusion scans in the left column demonstrate an area of radiolucency in the right centrum semiovale. Note that there is obliteration of the cortical sulci on the right side secondary to mild cerebral edema, even though there is no shift of the midline. The postinfusion scans in the right column reveal marked irregular enhancement in the true extent of infarction, which now demonstrates evidence of luxury perfusion.

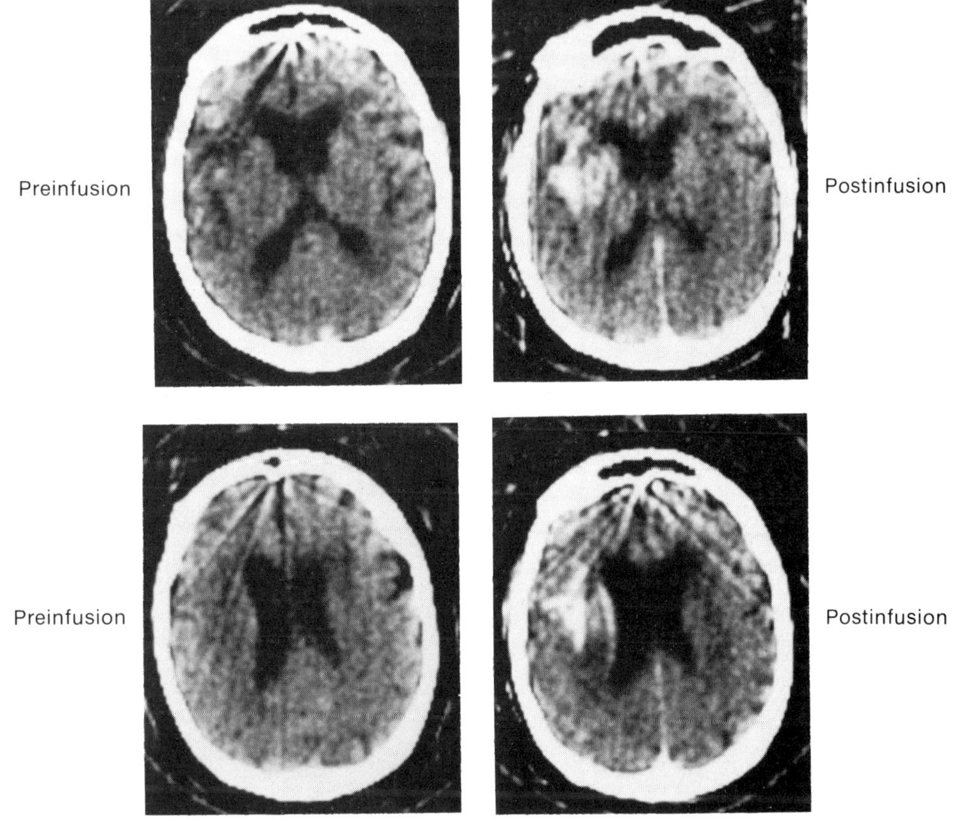

Figure 6–27. INFARCT WITH LUXURY PERFUSION: The preinfusion scan is almost normal-appearing *(left column)* except for mild atrophic change. The postinfusion scan demonstrates a large area of enhancement in the area of infarction, which now demonstrates luxury perfusion *(right column)*.

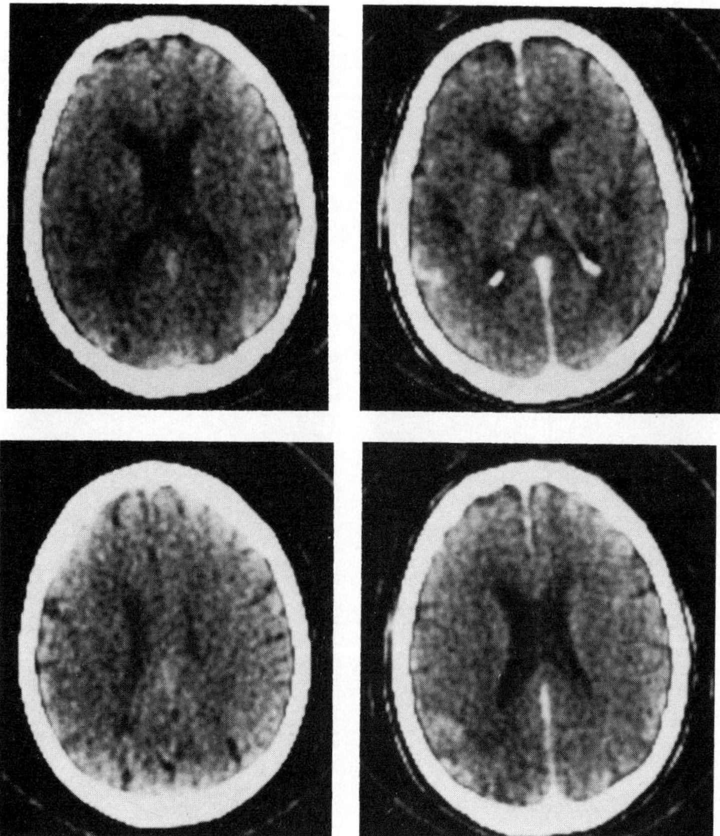

Figure 6–28. INFARCT AND LUXURY PERFUSION: The preinfusion scan is normal, whereas the postinfusion scan demonstrates a small wedge-shaped area of enhancement in the left posterior temporal region consistent with luxury perfusion.

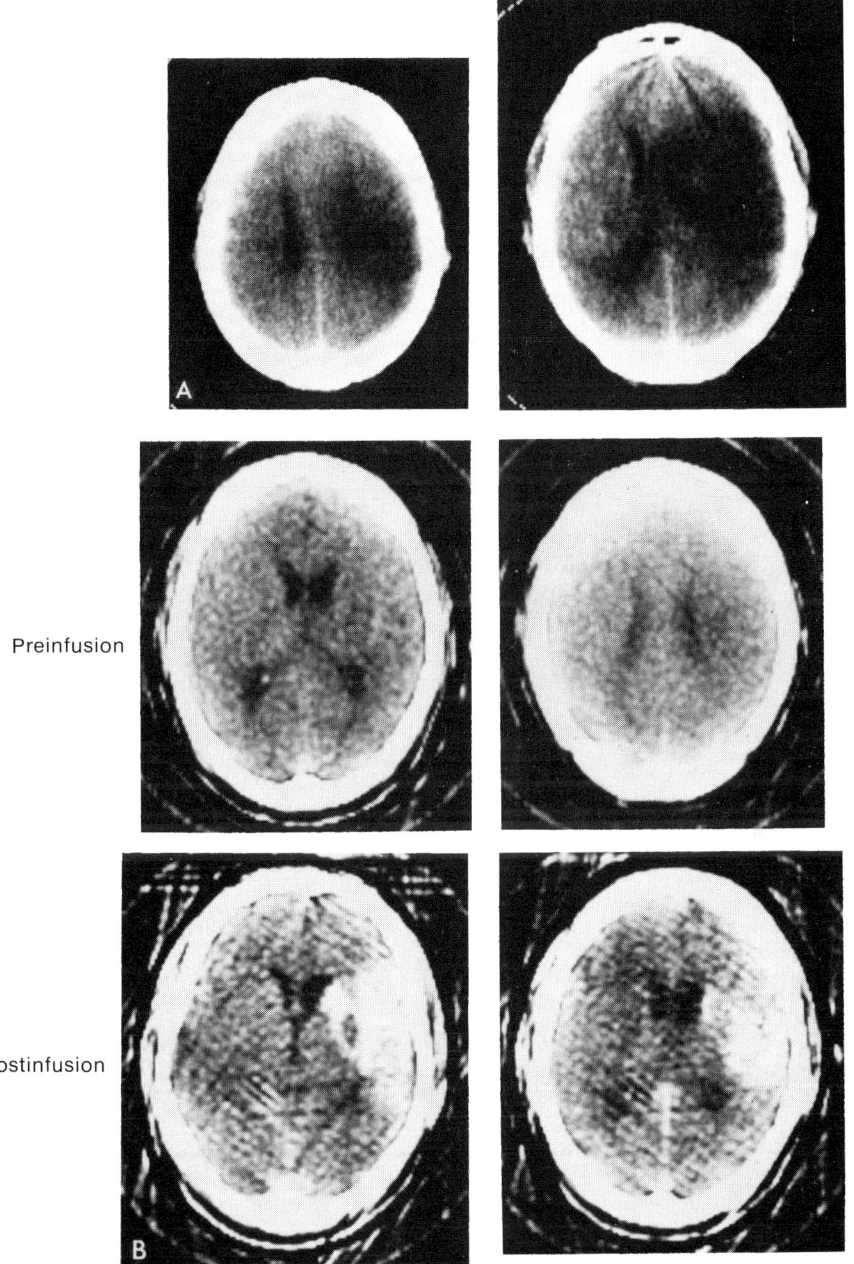

Figure 6–29. INFARCT WITH MASS EFFECT FOLLOWED BY LUXURY PERFUSION: The initial scan *(A)* obtained shortly after a stroke demonstrates a large area of radiolucency in the right hemisphere associated with shift of the midline from right to left.

B, Scans done 20 days later reveal that there is no shift of the midline and only a small area of lucency adjacent to the body of the right lateral ventricle. The postinfusion scan, however, reveals spectacular enhancement in the right hemisphere secondary to luxury perfusion.

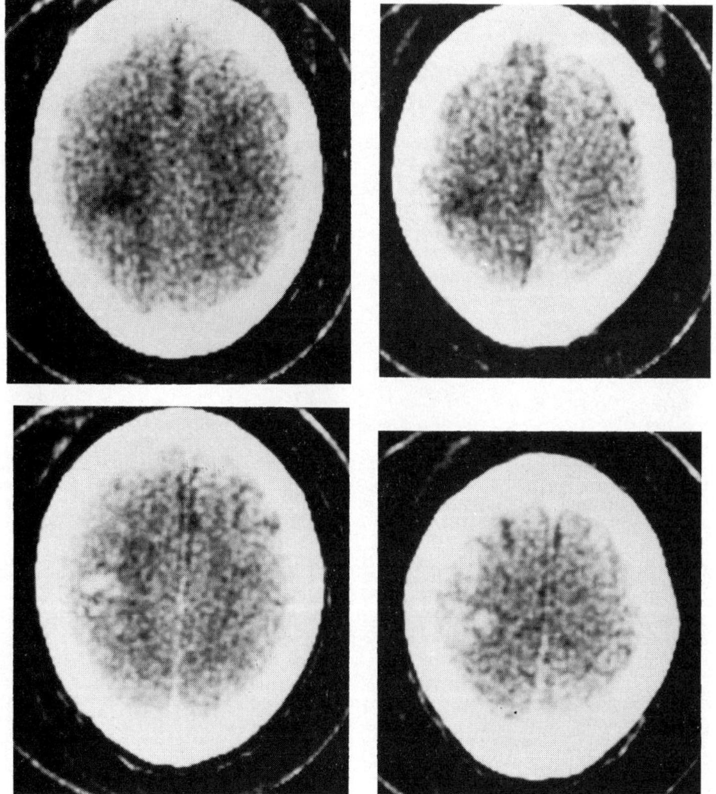

Figure 6–30. INFARCT WITH LUXURY PERFUSION: The preinfusion scan demonstrates poorly defined areas of radiolucency in the left middle cerebral artery distribution. There are small patchy areas of enhancement on the postinfusion scan because of luxury perfusion.

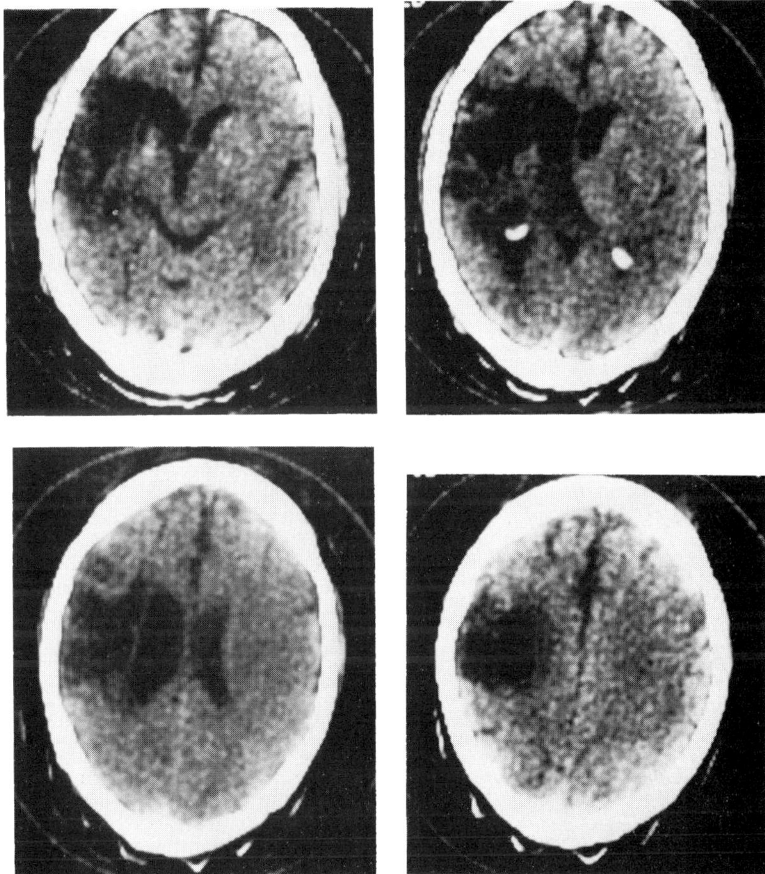

Figure 6–31. INFARCT WITH HEMIATROPHY: A large area of radiolucency can be seen in the left middle cerebral artery distribution; it contains fluid of CSF density. This is an old infarct that has degenerated into multiple cystic areas and may actually be an area of porencephaly. The left lateral ventricle is enlarged, and there is even focal enlargement of the retrothalamic cistern of the left side. The cortical sulci are enlarged more on the left side than on the right. The changes are secondary to an old infarct involving the left middle cerebral artery, which has resulted in left hemiatrophy.

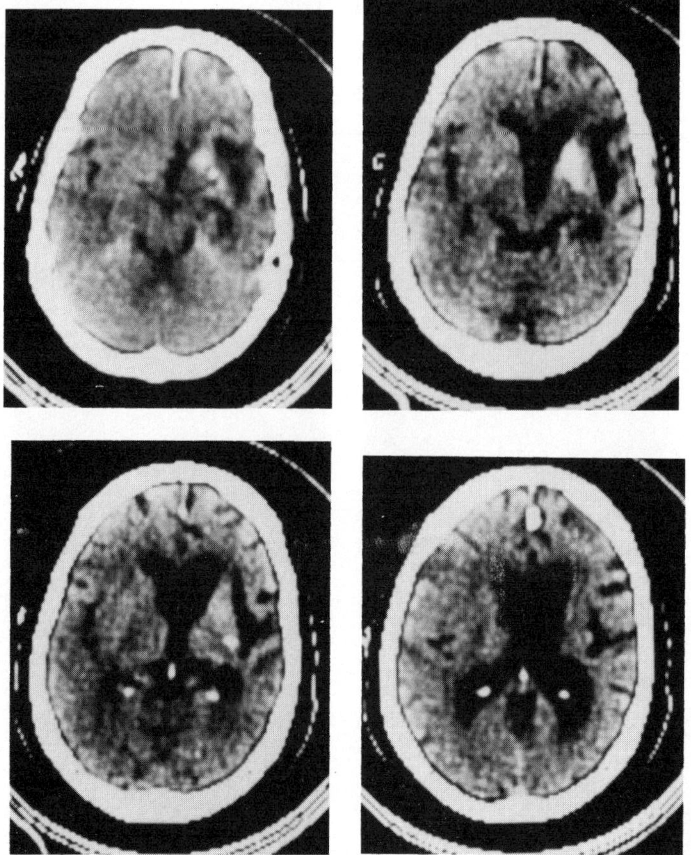

Figure 6–32. CALCIFIED INFARCT, BASAL GANGLIA: There is calcification in the region of the basal ganglia on the right side. In addition, there is enlargement of the sylvian fissure, the right lateral ventricle (including the right temporal horn) and the cortical sulci over the right hemisphere. The findings are consistent with an infarct in the right basal ganglia that has calcified and led to right hemiatrophy.

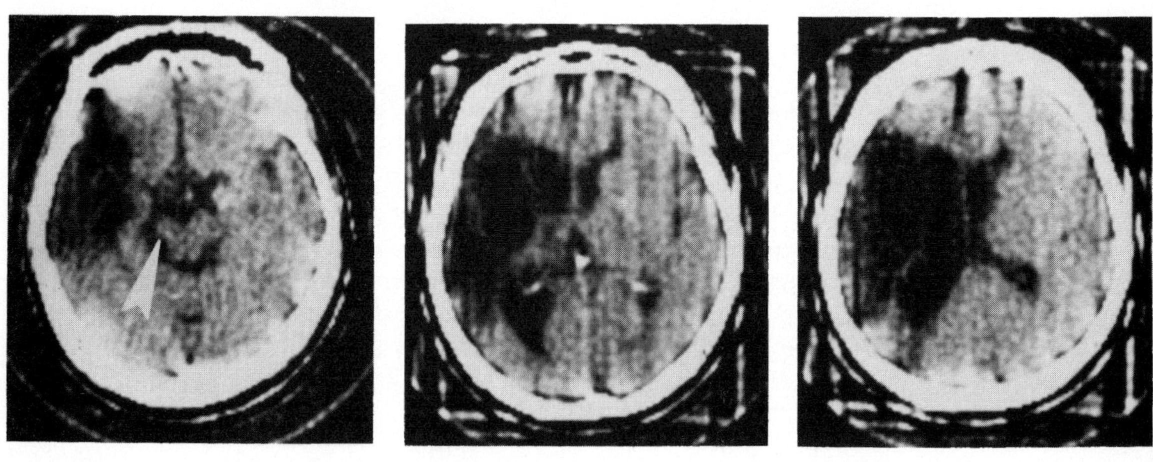

Figure 6–33. LEFT MIDDLE CEREBRAL ARTERY INFARCT WITH PORENCEPHALY: There is evidence of an old left middle cerebral artery infarct that has resulted in a large area of porencephaly on the left hemisphere and dilatation of the left lateral ventricle. Note also the atrophy of the left cerebral pedicle *(arrow)* secondary to atrophy of the descending fiber tracts.

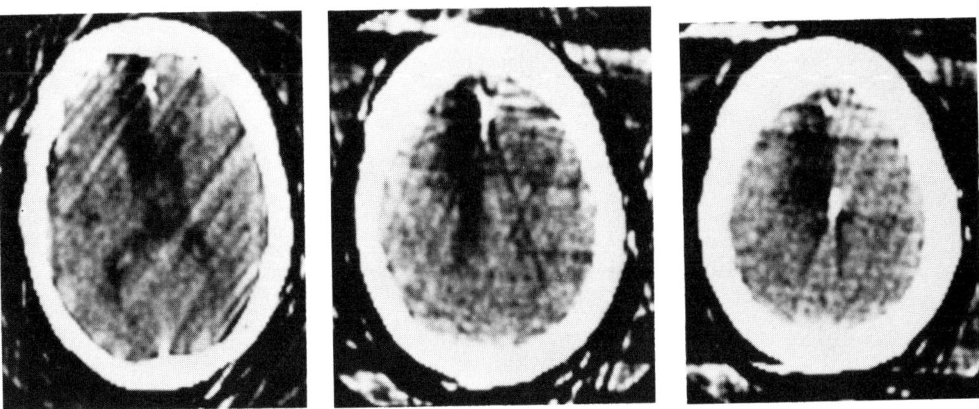

Figure 6–34. ANTERIOR CEREBRAL ARTERY INFARCT: There is an area of radiolucency in the distribution of the left anterior cerebral artery. This is non–space-occupying and is consistent with an area of infarction in the anterior cerebral artery distribution.

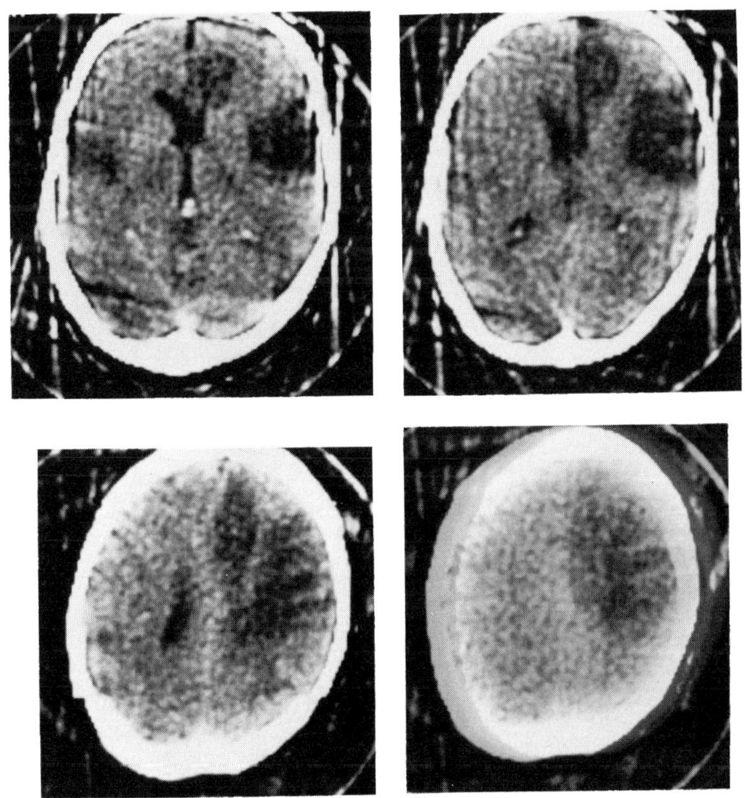

Figure 6–35. INFARCT WITH MASS EFFECT: There are two separate areas of radiolucency. These areas occupy both the anterior and middle cerebral artery distributions. In addition, there is shift of the midline structure to the contralateral side. Obliteration of the body of the right lateral ventricle can be seen. Arteriography demonstrated a complete occlusion of the internal carotid artery on this side. In addition there is a small, poorly defined area of lucency in the distribution of the left middle cerebral artery.

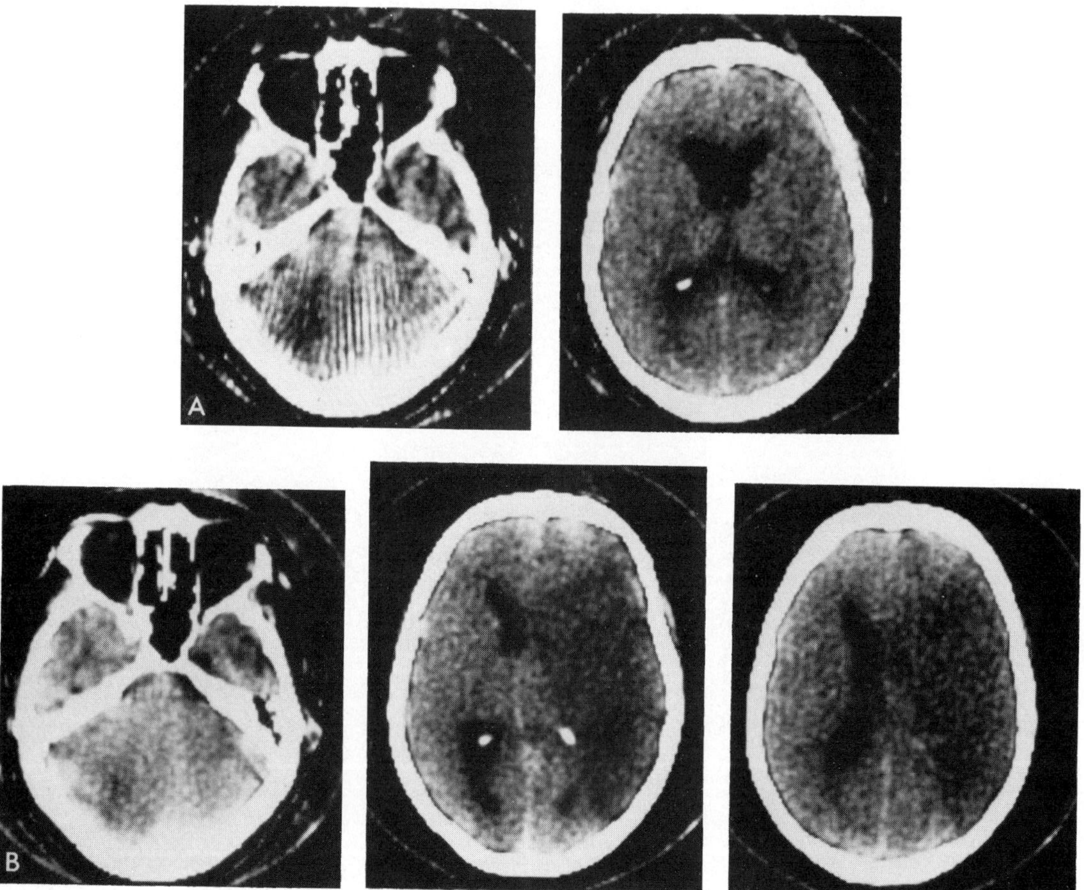

Figure 6–36. PROGRESSION OF INFARCT ON SERIAL SCANS: *A,* Initial scans obtained shortly after the onset of hemiparesis demonstrate an area of radiolucency in the left cerebellum. This probably is an infarct, although the lateral ventricles are mildly enlarged. The cerebral hemispheres are of normal density and are symmetrical.

B, The second scan, obtained two days later, reveals a large area of lucency now involving almost the entire right hemisphere. There is also mass effect, with shift of the midline to the contralateral side and obliteration of the body of the right lateral ventricle. The area of infarction is again seen in the left cerebellum. The findings are consistent with an acute infarct in the right cerebral hemisphere with mass effect.

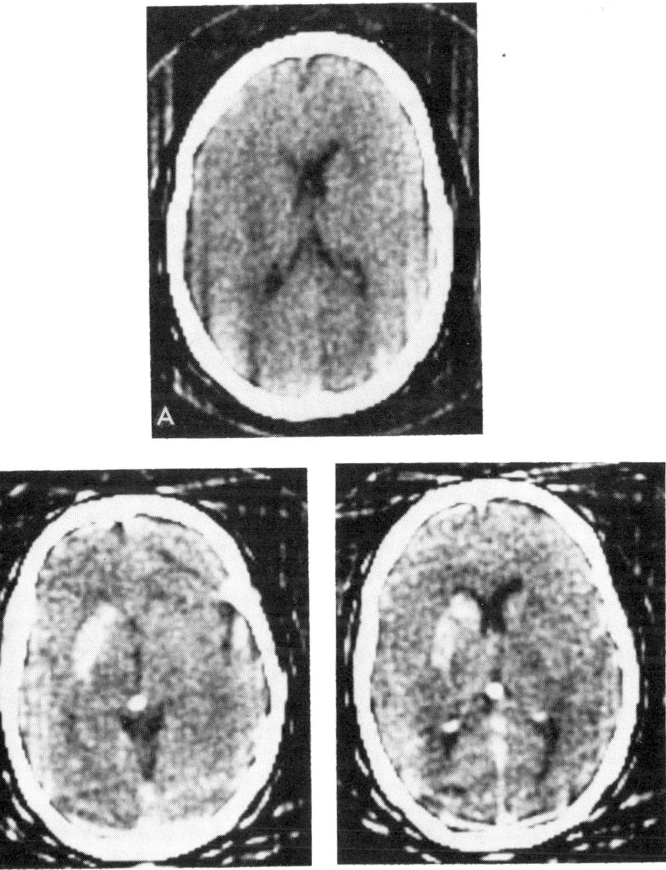

Figure 6–37. PUTAMENAL INFARCT WITH MASS EFFECT AND LUXURY PERFUSION: *A*, The preinfusion scan demonstrates a poorly visualized area of radiolucency in the region of the putamen of the left basal ganglia. There is mild compression of the body of the left lateral ventricle.

B, The postinfusion scans show marked enhancement in the region of the head of the caudate nucleus and the putamen of the left basal ganglia. There is a compression of the frontal horn of the left lateral ventricle.

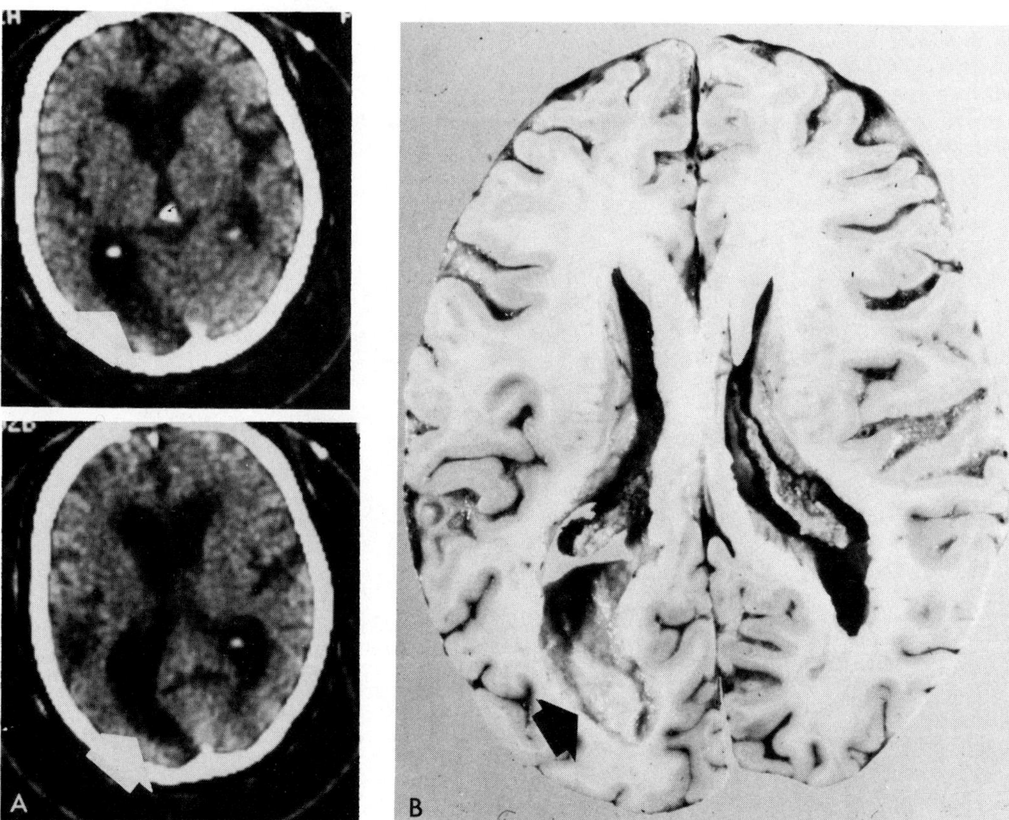

Figure 6–38. LEFT OCCIPITAL INFARCT: *A,* The CT scans demonstrate an area of infarction in the left occipital horn that has resulted in focal dilatation — porencephaly — of the occipital horn of the left lateral ventricle. The infarct is superimposed on cerebral atrophy.

B, The pathologic specimen shows the area of porencephaly involving the occipital horn of the left lateral ventricle and the focal area of encephalomalacia secondary to the infarct.

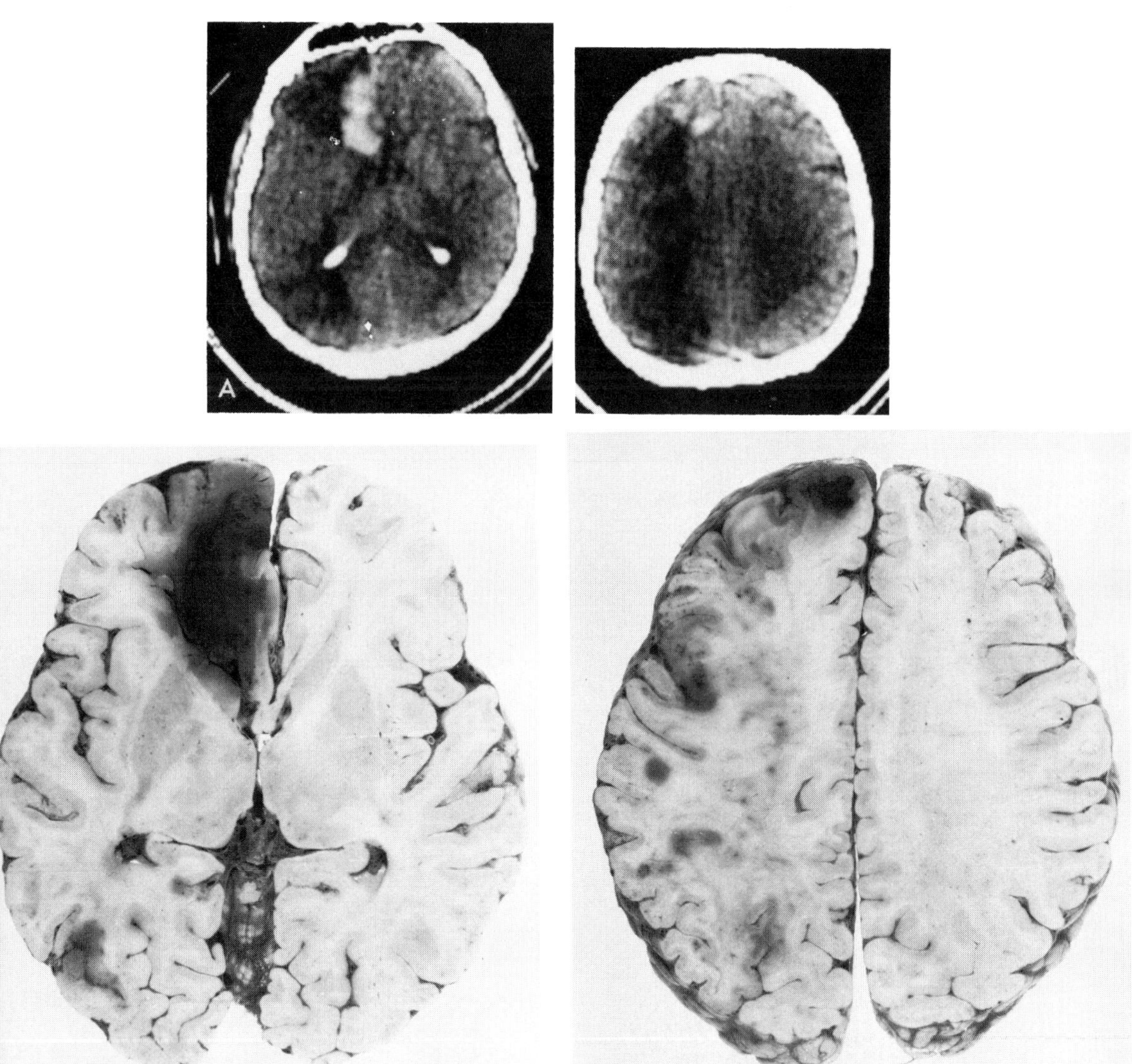

Figure 6–39. HEMORRHAGIC INFARCT: *A*, The CT scan shows a hemorrhagic infarct in the distribution of the left anterior cerebral artery surrounded by an area of radiolucency secondary to edema or a surrounding bland infarct. In addition there are scattered areas of lucency throughout the entire left hemisphere. There is a slight shift of the frontal horns to the right side.

B, The pathologic specimens demonstrated the left frontal hemorrhagic infarct and also small focal areas of hemorrhage throughout the left hemisphere, which presumably developed after the CT scan was obtained. Note the excellent correlation between the CT views and the appearance of the hemorrhage in the pathologic specimen.

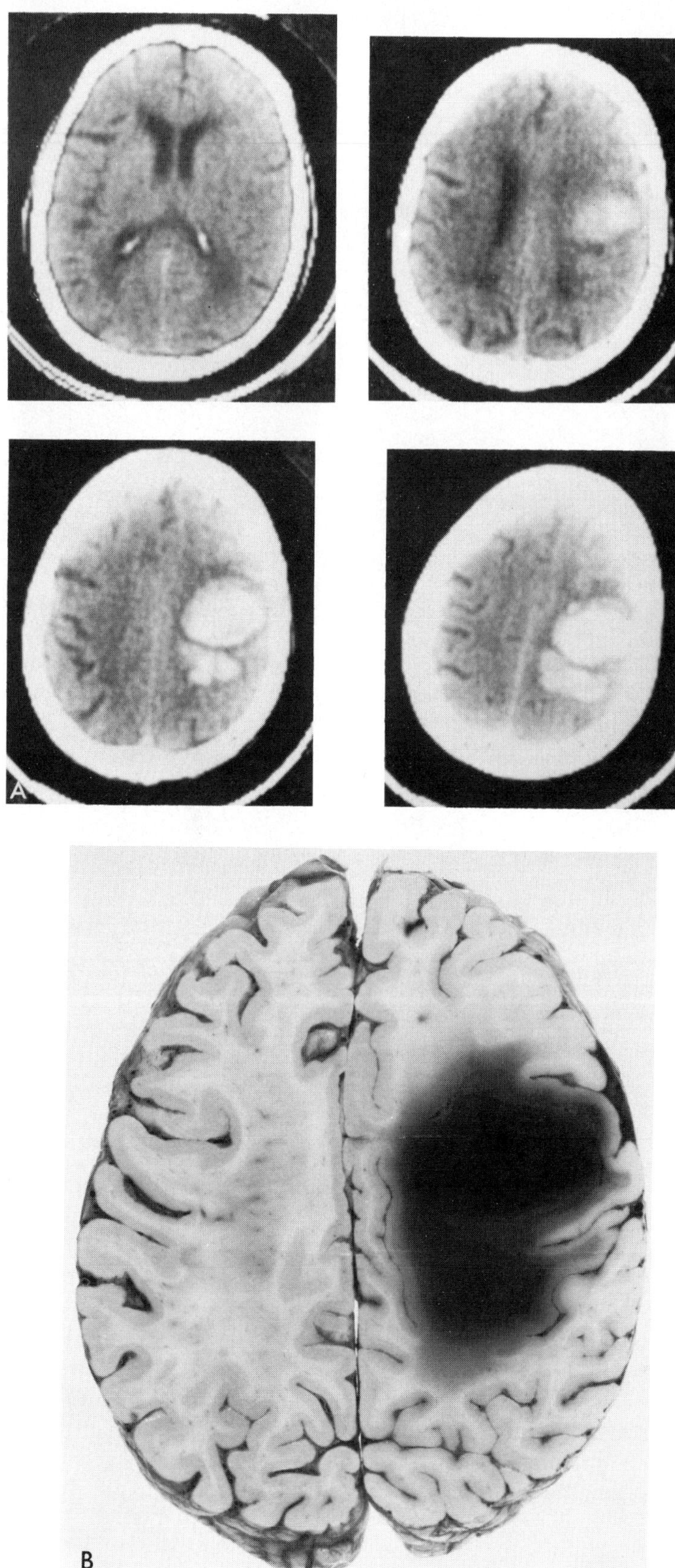

Figure 6–40. *See legend on the opposite page.*

Figure 6–40. HEMORRHAGIC INFARCT: *A*, A large bilobed area of hemorrhage is present in the distribution of the right middle cerebral artery. There is only minimal mass effect with mild compression of the body of the right lateral ventricle; there is focal obliteration of the cortical sulci. Although mild mass effect can be seen, there is much less than one would anticipate with an intracerebral hematoma. The findings are most consistent with a hemorrhagic infarct.

B, The pathologic specimen correlated well with the CT appearance.

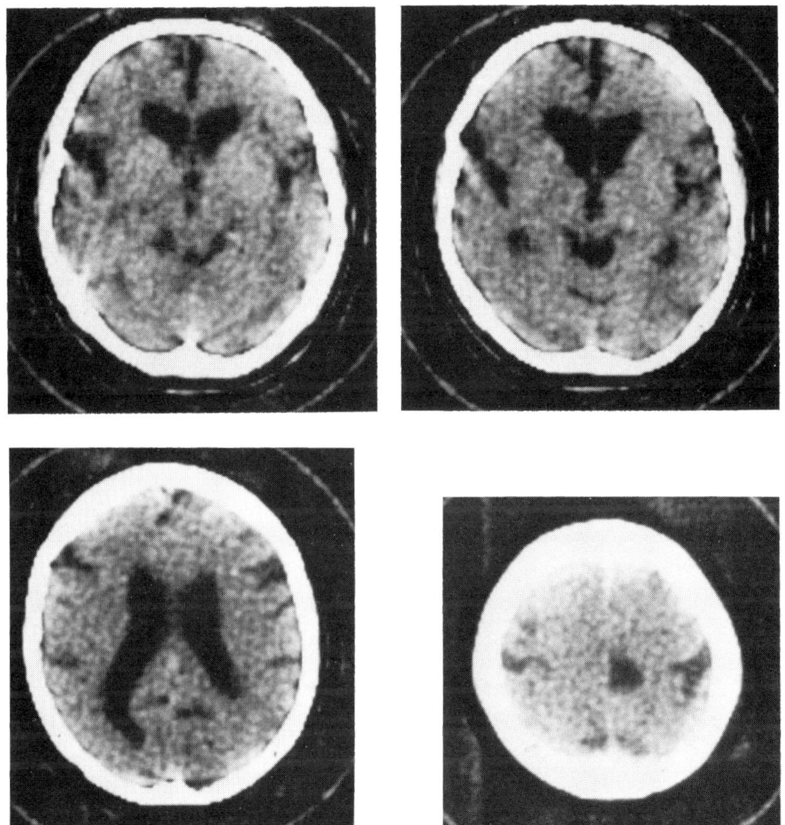

Figure 6–41. MULTIPLE CORTICAL INFARCTS: Multiple small areas of radiolucency are scattered throughout the cerebral cortex. These areas of lucency are consistent with small cortical infarcts superimposed on cortical atrophy.

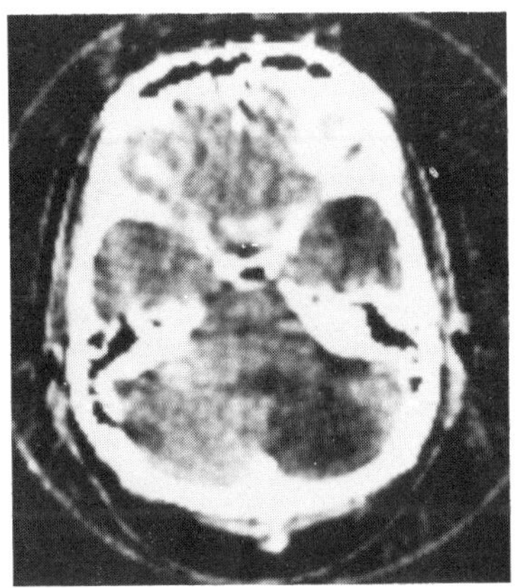

Figure 6–42. PICA INFARCT: An area of lucency can be seen in the distribution of the right posterior inferior cerebellar artery. There is no mass effect — and this is consistent with an area of infarction in the right PICA distribution. This results in Wallenberg's syndrome.

CHAPTER 7

ANEURYSMS

There are many different types of aneurysms. Determination of the etiology and type of aneurysm directs both the clinical course and subsequent treatment. The aneurysm or aneurysms may be developmental, post-traumatic, dissecting, postoperative, mycotic (septic), secondary to neoplastic emboli, venous, syphilitic, microaneurysm of hypertension, arteriosclerotic or berry.

BERRY ANEURYSMS

This chapter deals primarily with berry aneurysms — the type most commonly encountered in the day-to-day practice of neuroradiology. Sometimes these patients present with such focal signs as a unilateral third nerve palsy associated with retro-orbital pain caused by a posterior communicating arterial aneurysm that is resting on the third nerve in the wall of the cavernous sinus. More commonly, the patients arrive at the emergency room following the acute onset of severe headache and decreased cerebral function or coma secondary to subarachnoid hemorrhage. An acute ruptured aneurysm may rapidly lead to death.

These aneurysms may be embedded in cerebral tissue, where their rupture causes an intracerebral hematoma as well as subarachnoid hemorrhage. They may thrombose and occlude or they may result in cerebral emboli and subsequent strokes.

Berry aneurysms are associated with polycystic kidneys and coarctation of the aorta. A congenital defect in the wall of the blood vessel with interruption of the muscular coat and the internal elastic lamina is present at the site of the aneurysm. Berry aneurysms usually occur at bifurcations of the vessels. Although there may be a congenital tendency to develop these aneurysms, they are rarely seen in children.

Age. The aneurysms usually present in the 2nd to 7th decades, with an incidence of 0.5 to 5.0 per cent of the population as judged by autopsy studies.

Location. Ninety to 95 per cent of berry aneurysms occur in the carotid circulation. The remainder are in the vertebrobasilar system.

The most common location for a berry aneurysm is at the middle cerebral artery bifurcation. The most common locations for rupture are the anterior communicating artery and, in order of incidence, the internal carotid, the posterior communicating artery and the middle cerebral artery bifurcation.

Size of Ruptured Aneurysms. Aneurysms 5 to 15 mm in size are most likely to bleed and may demonstrate a small outpouching at the actual site of bleeding, which usually is at the dome of the aneurysm.

MULTIPLE ANEURYSMS

When multiple aneurysms are present, as is true in approximately 20 per cent of cases, it may be difficult to determine the actual site of rupture or which aneurysm has bled. The CT scan may provide a clue to the bleeding site if a small localized hematoma is seen. Localized vascular spasm demonstrated on arteriography may be helpful in localizing the site of bleeding, although vascular spasm may be remote from the actual bleeding site. Evidence of an intracerebral hematoma also may be present, providing further evidence of the bleeding site. In general, if no secondary signs of hemorrhage are present it is assumed that it is the largest aneurysm that has bled. An increase in size of an aneurysm on serial studies is also suggestive of a bleeding aneurysm.

Giant aneurysms are those measuring 2.5 cm or larger.

CT SCANNING WITH ACUTE SUBARACHNOID HEMORRHAGE

The CT scan in a patient with acute subarachnoid hemorrhage (SAH) may be within normal limits. More commonly (in approximately 85 to 90 per cent of cases), the scan demonstrates a diffuse increase in density seen in the basilar cisterns and over the cerebral convexities — a change secondary to blood in the subarachnoid space.

The diffuse increase in density may be very subtle and easily overlooked. Close inspection will show that the usually radiolucent sulci are not seen because they have filled with blood. The blood may even flow retrograde up into the ventricular system, where a "blood–CSF fluid level" will be seen in the dependent portions of the lateral ventricles, or a blood clot cast of the ventricular system may form. The aneurysm may rupture directly into the ventricular system. Occasionally — and I have found this to be of limited help — there will be a focal accumulation of blood within the cerebral substance which is an intracerebral hematoma associated with a ruptured aneurysm. If present, this sign is helpful in defining a bleeding site in a patient without focal findings. On the other hand, an aneurysm may rupture into the brain substance and produce a large intracerebral hematoma. However, this may simulate the appearance of a primary intracerebral hematoma, and only an unusual anatomic location will point to an aneurysm as the true source of bleeding.

In a small percentage of cases the aneurysm may rupture through the arachnoid layer into the subdural space, causing a subdural hematoma. Again, the true source of bleeding may remain obscure — particularly if an angiogram is not performed.

The use of CT for the diagnosis of aneurysm through direct demonstration is, at this point in our technology, inadequate. The *vast* majority of aneurysms are not visualized by CT scan, even after infusion of contrast material. Those aneurysms that are identified on the CT scan usually are quite sizeable and are commonly partially or even completely clotted. They therefore appear as a well defined, rounded area of high density, frequently containing flecks of peripheral calcification. If the aneurysm is not clotted, the enhancement has a homogeneous pattern; if the aneurysm is partially clotted, the areas of enhancement are irregular and correspond to the unclotted portion of the aneurysms. If the aneurysm is completely filled with clotted blood there may be no enhancement — or only peripheral enhancement secondary to the vasa vasorum that supply the walls of the vessels.

Acutely, there may be ventricular dilatation secondary to clotted blood in the ventricles — especially clotted blood in the third and fourth ventricles — which acts as a mechanical obstruction to ventricular function. Later in the clinical course there may be dilatation of the ventricles because of a communicating hydrocephalus that develops when blood in the subarachnoid space interferes with the absorption of CSF by the arachnoid villi.

ANGIOGRAPHY

At one time all patients with subarachnoid hemorrhage and suspected aneurysm underwent emergency angiography to define their anatomic abnormality. However, at the present time there appears to be a general reevaluation and revision of the methodology for work-up of these patients. At our institution the examination begins with an emergency CT scan in an attempt to determine the site of origin of the hemorrhage, to rule out a large intracerebral hematoma and to determine whether the abnormality may actually be a hypertensive basal ganglionic hemorrhage that has ruptured into the ventricular system, resulting in the clinical appearance of a subarachnoid hemorrhage. A lumbar puncture usually is not performed for diagnosis if a CT scan is available.

Standard grading system:

Grade I (minimal bleed): alert; no neurologic deficit.

Grade II (mild bleed): alert; minimal neurologic deficit or third nerve palsy; stiff neck.

Grade III (moderate bleed): drowsy or confused; stiff neck, with or without neurologic deficit.

Grade IV (moderate or severe bleed): semicoma, with or without neurologic deficit.

Grade V (severe bleed): coma and decerebrate movements.

One higher grade is always assigned to patients over the age of 50, or if another major medical problem exists.

When the patient's clinical condition has improved to a Grade II or less, elective cerebral angiography is performed via the femoral approach using the Seldinger technique. The study is begun with examination of the clinically implicated vascular system. If marked spasm is demonstrated, no further injections are made. If there is no spasm or a mild one, a thorough study of each blood vessel's supply is performed. This includes appropriate oblique views or submentovertex views as necessary. Sufficient views are obtained to demonstrate the neck of the aneurysm so that an appropriate surgical approach can be planned. Following this, the remaining vascular supply to the brain is studied sequentially until all the possible sites of aneurysm have been demonstrated. If other aneurysms are found, appropriate views are obtained to demonstrate the neck of the aneurysm.

If an individual vessel cannot be catheterized for technical reasons, the appropriate percutaneous angiogram should be performed while the patient is in the radiology department so that all four vessels are well demonstrated. Failure to do this may result in failure to diagnose an existing aneurysm. In other words, if a vessel has not been adequately demonstrated it cannot be considered as not involved by an aneurysm.

Bilateral carotid angiography will demonstrate approximately 90 per cent of aneurysms present. In double aneurysm cases, if one aneurysm is demonstrated in the supratentorial circulation, there is a 3 to 5 per cent chance of the second aneurysm arising in the posterior fossa.

Arterial spasm following a subarachnoid hemorrhage is maximal between six and 12 days. Rebleeding after the initial insult is most likely to occur at five to seven days after the initial bleed.

ANTERIOR COMMUNICATING ARTERY ANEURYSM

AP, lateral, oblique and submentovertex views are performed as needed. The submentovertex view is often the most helpful in demonstrating the neck of the aneurysm and its relationship to the anterior cerebral arteries.

POSTERIOR COMMUNICATING ARTERY ANEURYSM

AP, lateral and oblique views in both oblique projections are performed as needed.

MIDDLE CEREBRAL ARTERY ANEURYSM

AP, lateral and "through-the-orbit" view — with the middle cerebral artery bifurcation centered in the mid-portion of the orbit — are performed as needed. The "through-the-orbit" view is often most helpful in demonstrating the neck of the aneurysm and its relationship to the middle cerebral artery. This view frequently separates the multiple overlapping vessels around the genu of the middle cerebral artery. On other views they tend to overlap.

POSTERIOR FOSSA ANEURYSMS

AP, lateral, oblique and submentovertex views are performed as needed. The author has found the submentovertex view to be especially helpful in the diagnosis of posterior circulation aneurysms.

On the oblique projections, both AP and lateral or single plane studies are performed as needed. In patients with meningismus secondary to blood in the subarachnoid space, it may be difficult to obtain a submentovertex view.

SEDATION

I have found it helpful to supplement any premedication with intravenous Valium as needed for adequate sedation, and would recommend that the premedication be adjusted for each patient. Valium is then given in 2- to 3-mg doses IV as needed. Often this supplementary medication is given just before an injection of contrast material so that the patient remains immobile for the filming run.

Approximately three quarters of patients with subarachnoid hemorrhage demonstrate an aneurysm as the site of bleeding. Arteriovenous malformations account for another 10 per cent; another 10 per cent are secondary to intracerebral hemorrhage. The remainder are undiagnosed.

RE-EXAMINATION

If no aneurysm is demonstrated after thorough examination of both carotid and both vertebral arteries, the patient is treated medically and then restudied with four-vessel arteriography after approximately one week of medical management. This is necessary because focal spasm may have occluded the neck of the aneurysm on the initial study. A vascular lesion of the spinal cord may present as a subarachnoid hemorrhage, and so a myelogram may be necessary for further evaluation.

The cases that follow represent a variety of aneurysms seen in daily practice. A somewhat greater than usual emphasis is put on the use of CT scanning in the diagnosis of aneurysm. Although I have not found CT scanning to be of great help in the diagnosis of aneurysm, CT scanning is the procedure of choice in the diagnosis of subarachnoid hemorrhage (SAH). CT scanning is also very helpful in evaluating and following any changes in ventricular size that may occur following SAH.

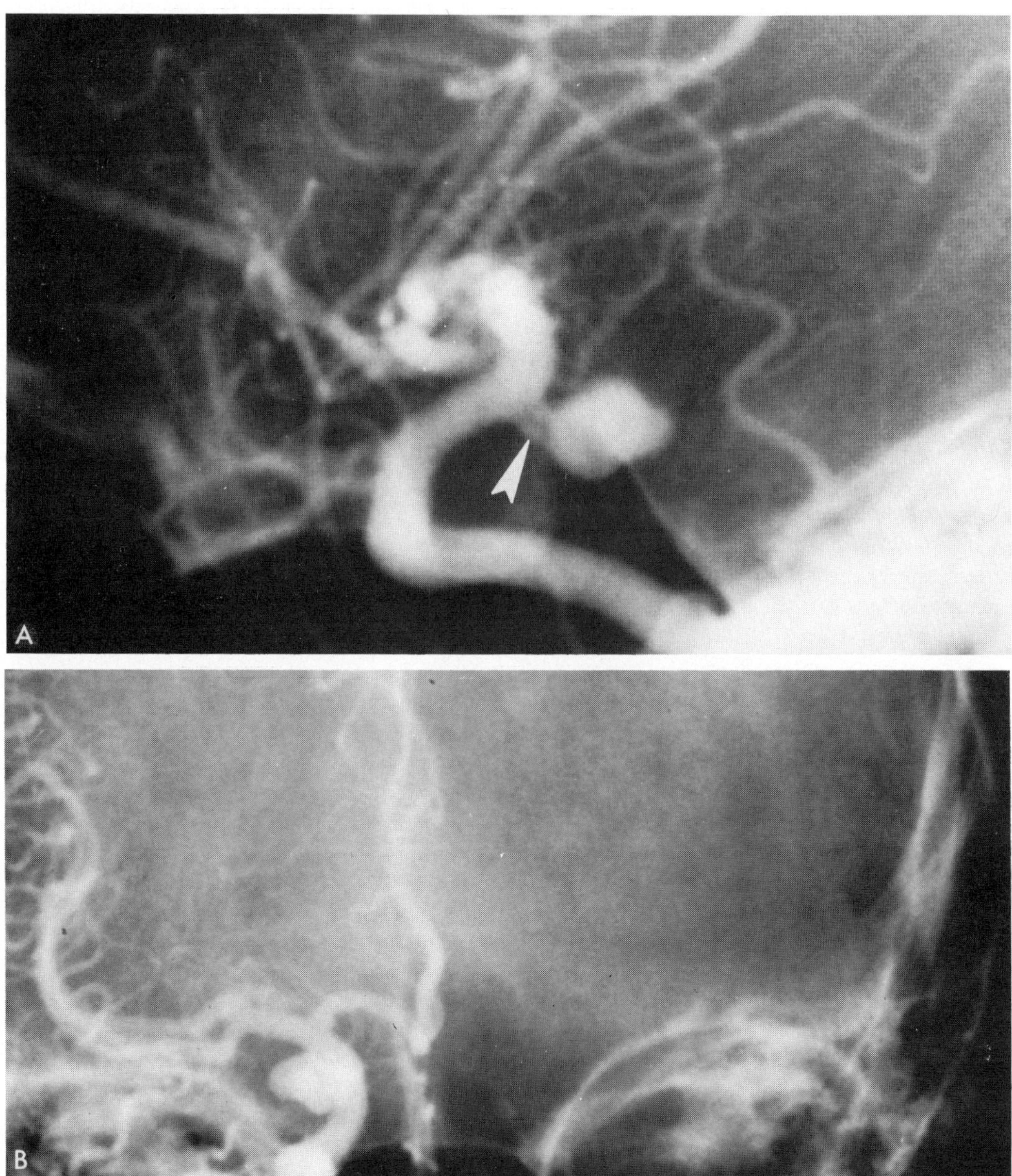

Figure 7–1. POSTERIOR COMMUNICATING ARTERY ANEURYSM: The right common carotid angiogram demonstrates a 1.2 cm aneurysm of the posterior communicating artery. The aneurysm has a well defined neck *(arrow)* and projects posteriorly on the lateral view *(A)*. It is noted to project slightly laterally on the AP view *(B)*, just below the bifurcation of the internal carotid artery. The neck of the aneurysm is hidden behind the internal carotid artery on the AP view.

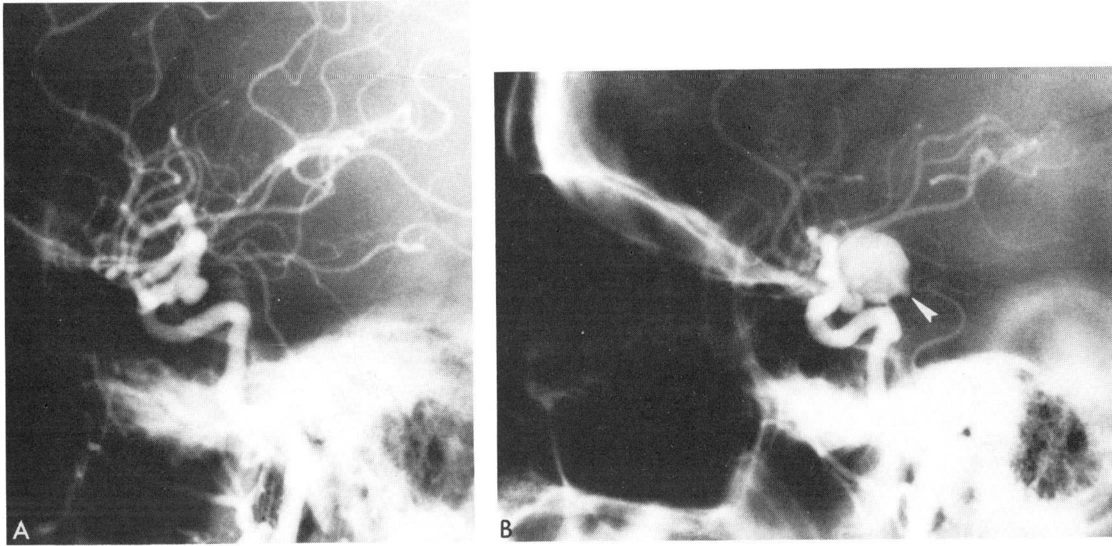

Figure 7–2. BILATERAL POSTERIOR COMMUNICATING ARTERY ANEURYSMS: *A*, On this side, a small, broad-necked posterior communicating artery aneurysm projects posteriorly.

B, On the contralateral side, a large, lobulated aneurysm projects posteriorly and superiorly. The patient presented clinically with a subarachnoid hemorrhage and a third nerve palsy on the side of the larger aneurysm. The small localized bulge posteriorly is probably the actual point of hemorrhage *(arrow)*.

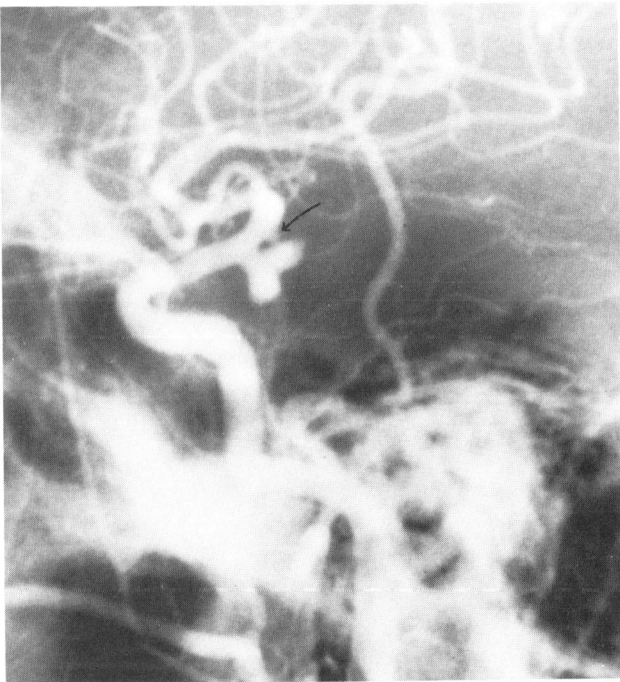

Figure 7–3. BILOBED POSTERIOR COMMUNICATING ARTERY ANEURYSM: A bilobed aneurysm of the posterior communicating artery arises from the internal cartoid artery and demonstrates a small neck. The small dilatation just at the origin of the anterior choroidal artery is an infundibulum of this vessel *(arrow)*.

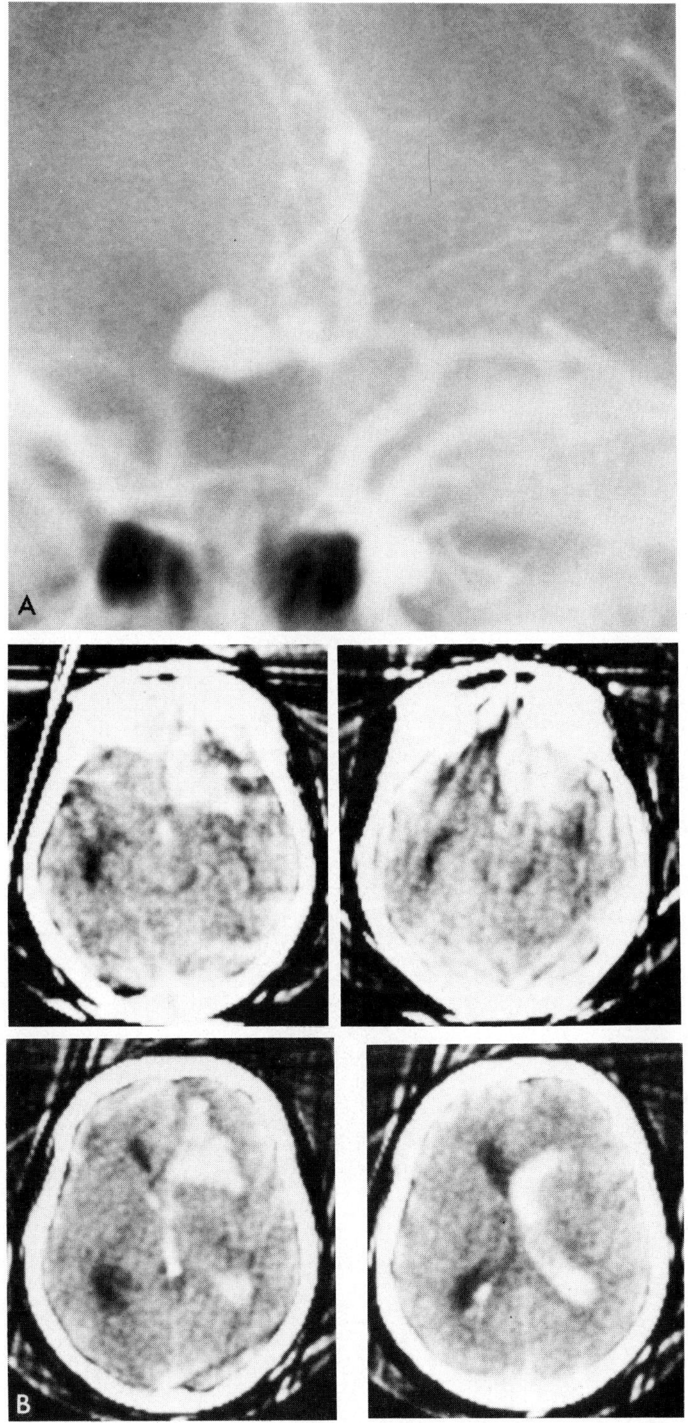

Figure 7–4. *See legend on the opposite page.*

Figure 7–4. ANTERIOR COMMUNICATING ARTERY ANEURYSM: *A*, The AP view reveals a large, lobulated aneurysm of the anterior communicating artery that projects directly toward the contralateral side and demonstrates a narrow neck at its point of origin. The anterior cerebral artery and its branches are displaced around the aneurysm because the rupture has resulted in an intracerebral hematoma as well as a subarachnoid hemorrhage.

B, The CT scan shows a large right frontal hematoma that has ruptured into the right lateral ventricle and the third ventricle. A small amount of blood is seen in the dependent portion of the left lateral ventricle.

The extent of the cerebral hematoma and the ventricular rupture is much better demonstrated on the CT scan than on the angiogram.

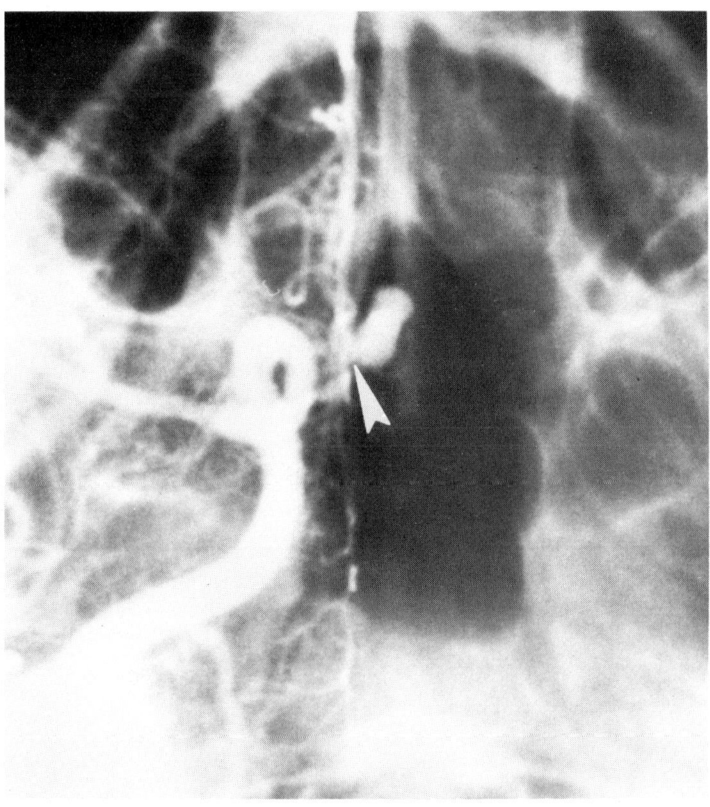

Figure 7–5. SUBMENTOVERTEX VIEW OF AN ANTERIOR COMMUNICATING ARTERY ANEURYSM: The submentovertex view shows the anterior communicating artery aneurysm as it projects across the midline from its point of origin *(arrow)*. The neck is well demonstrated. In general, the submentovertex view is the best for demonstrating anterior communicating artery aneurysms.

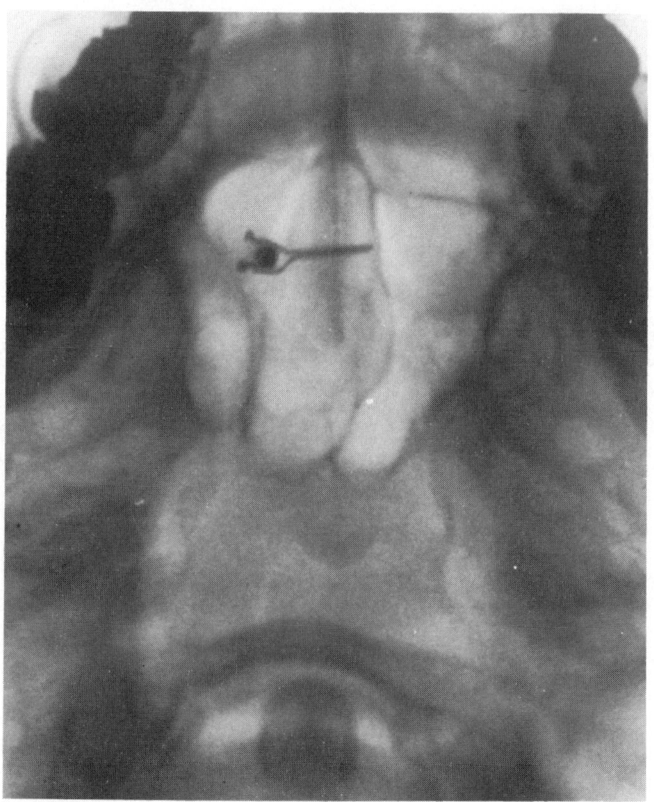

Figure 7–6. ANEURYSM CLIP ON AN ANTERIOR COMMUNICATING ARTERY ANEURYSM: The aneurysm clip is well demonstrated at the level of the anterior communicating artery on the submentovertex view.

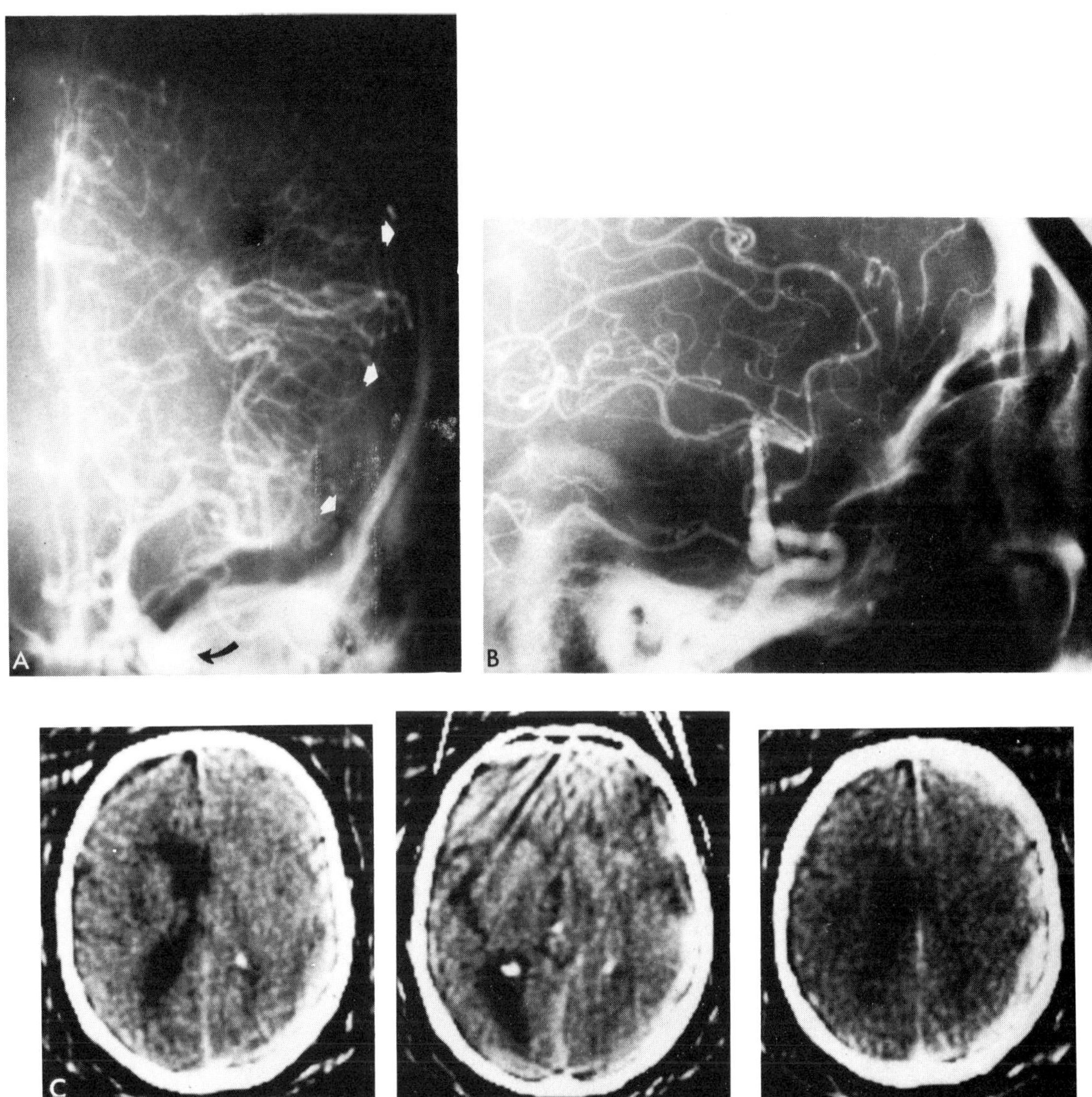

Figure 7–7. POSTERIOR COMMUNICATING ARTERY ANEURYSM WITH AN ASSOCIATED SUBDURAL HEMATOMA: *A* and *B,* A lobulated posterior communicating artery aneurysm is seen on both the AP *(black arrow)* and the lateral view. The supraclinoid portion of the internal carotid artery is straightened and displaced medially, posteriorly and superiorly. In addition, there is a moderate sized extracerebral accumulation of blood that displaces the middle cerebral artery vessels away from the inner table of the skull *(white arrowheads).* This subdural hematoma results when the aneurysm ruptures through the arachnoid membrane into the subdural space.

C, CT scans demonstrate an acute subdural hematoma over the right hemisphere. There is shift of the midline to the contralateral side. The straight sinus and the falx cerebri are more dense than normal because they are outlined by blood in the subarachnoid space. The aneurysm is not seen on the CT scan.

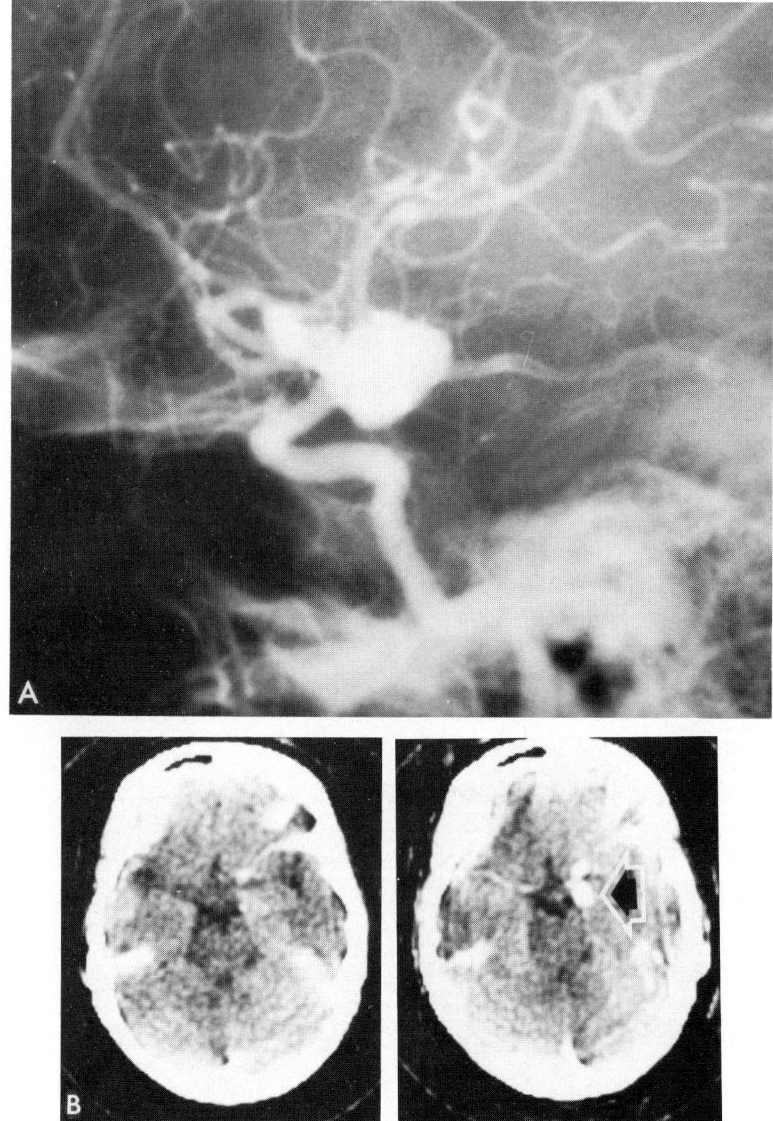

Figure 7–8. POSTERIOR COMMUNICATING ARTERY ANEURYSM DEMONSTRATED ON THE CT SCAN: *A,* The angiogram shows the posterior communicating artery aneurysm. Note that the posterior cerebral artery arises from the aneurysm — a finding that indicates that the patient may have difficulty when the aneurysm is clipped and flow through the posterior cerebral artery is interrupted.

B, The aneurysm is demonstrated in the parasellar area on the postinfusion scan *(arrow).* A small fleck of calcification is visible on the preinfusion scan along the medial side of the aneurysm; the aneurysm itself is not demonstrated.

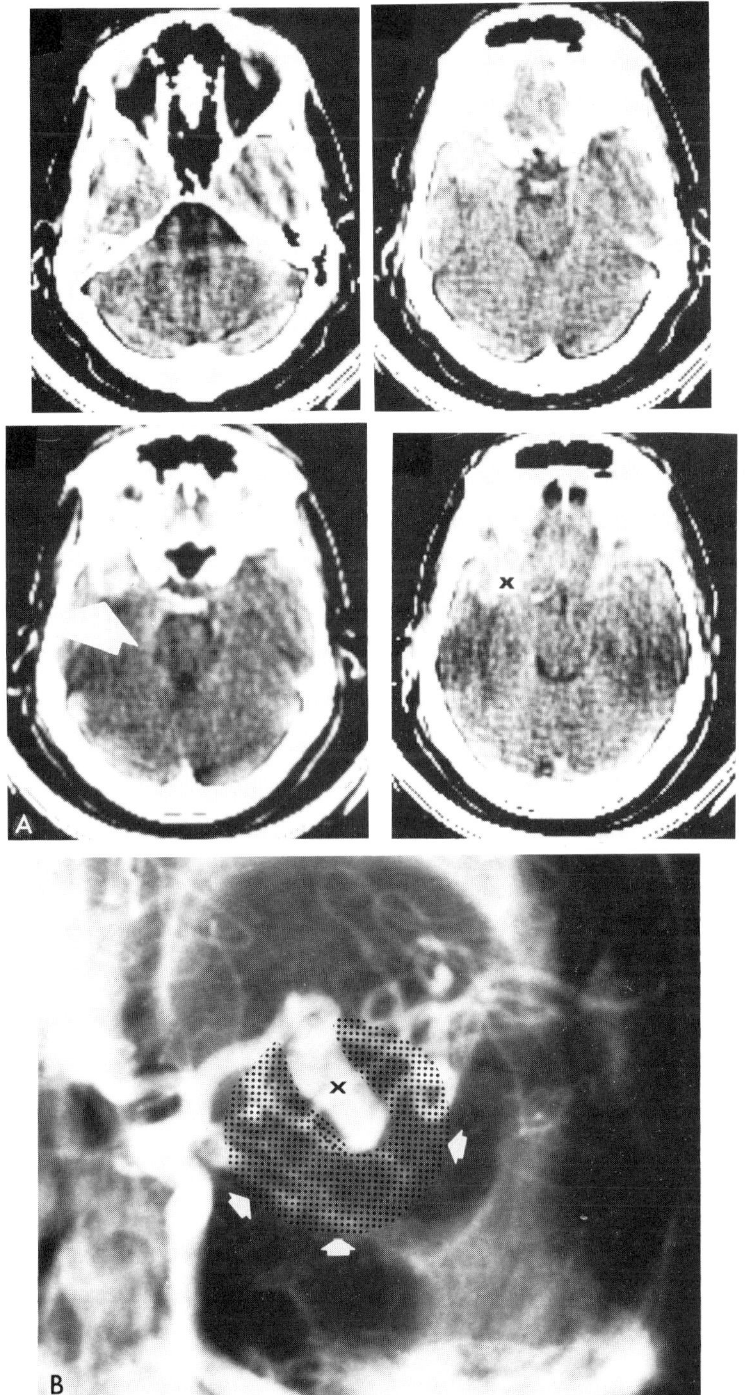

Figure 7–9. MIDDLE CEREBRAL ARTERY ANEURYSM: *A,* The preinfusion scan — upper row — reveals a rounded, fairly well defined area of high density in the anterior margin of the left middle cranial fossa. On the postinfusion scan (lower row), the high density area is again seen *(white arrow).* In addition, there is a small area of enhancement *(x)* more superiorly that was not visible on the preinfusion scan. This is contrast material in the unclotted portion of the aneurysm.

B, The left carotid angiogram demonstrates the unclotted portion of the aneurysm *(X)* that was shown on the postinfusion CT scan. The dotted area *(white arrowheads)* shows the actual size of the aneurysm which was largely clotted on the scan. The aneurysm acts as a mass and elevates the middle cerebral artery.

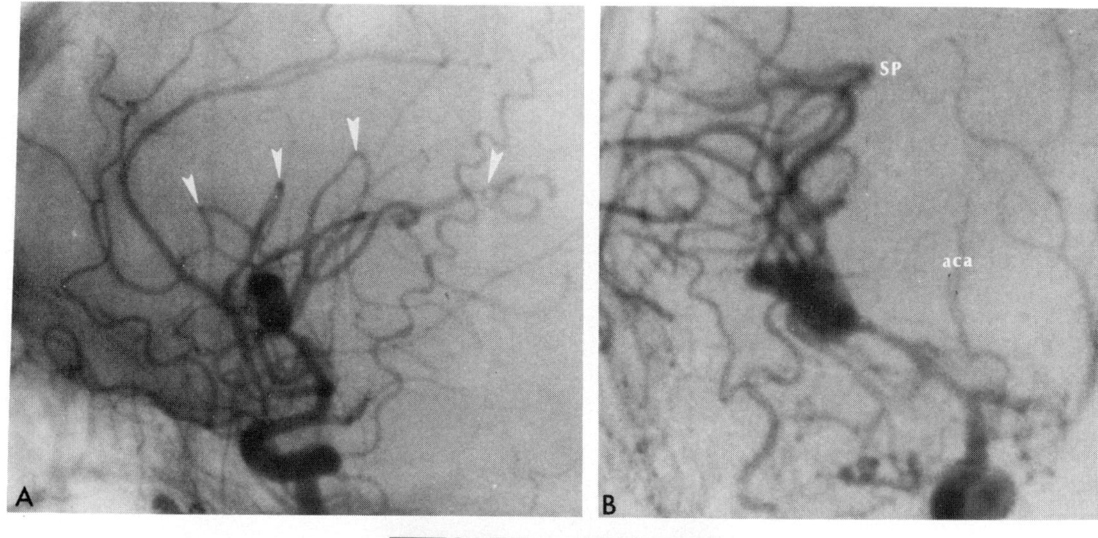

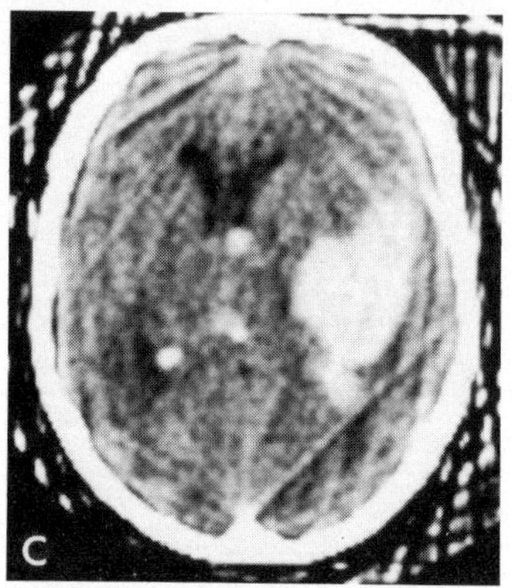

Figure 7–10. RUPTURED TRIFURCATION ANEURYSM: *A,* The lateral view of the carotid arteriogram demonstrates a lobulated aneurysm of the middle cerebral artery. There is spasm of the horizontal portion of the middle cerebral artery, and elevation of the sylvian triangle, which is bowed superiorly in its midportion *(arrowheads).*

B, The AP view reveals medial displacement of the genu of the middle cerebral artery, medial displacement of the sylvian point *(SP)* and medial displacement of the anterior choroidal artery *(aca)* as well as contralateral displacement of the anterior cerebral artery. The aneurysm has ruptured, resulting in a large temporal lobe hematoma.

C, The CT scan shows a large area of hemorrhage deep in the right hemisphere. Blood has accumulated in the lateral ventricle and in the third ventricle — probably because the aneurysm has ruptured into the temporal horn of the lateral ventricle. There is a moderate shift of the midline structures to the contralateral side.

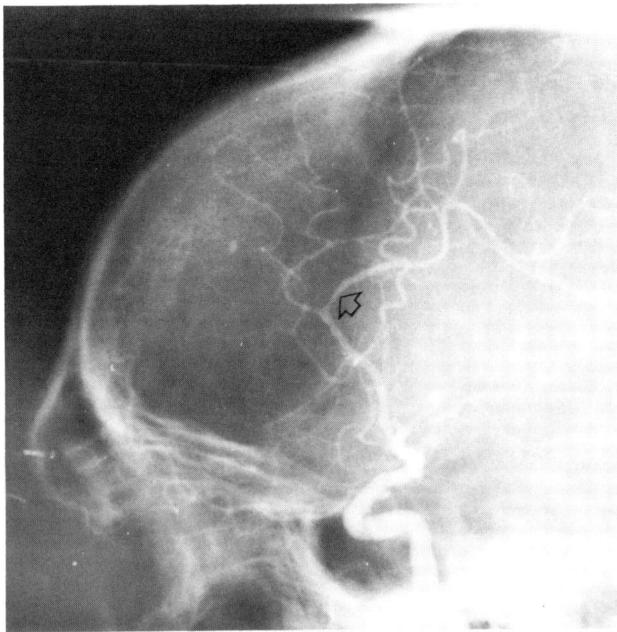

Figure 7–11. SUBARACHNOID HEMORRHAGE WITH ARTERIAL SPASM: This patient had a ruptured anterior communicating artery aneurysm that has resulted in an intracerebral hematoma in the frontal region. The frontal area appears avascular, and the anterior cerebral artery is displaced posteriorly. The aneurysm is not demonstrated, but there is evidence of focal spasm of the anterior cerebral artery *(arrowhead),* which is distal to the site of the aneurysm. There is also diffuse vascular spasm and branch occlusions of the middle cerebral artery group secondary to vascular spasm.

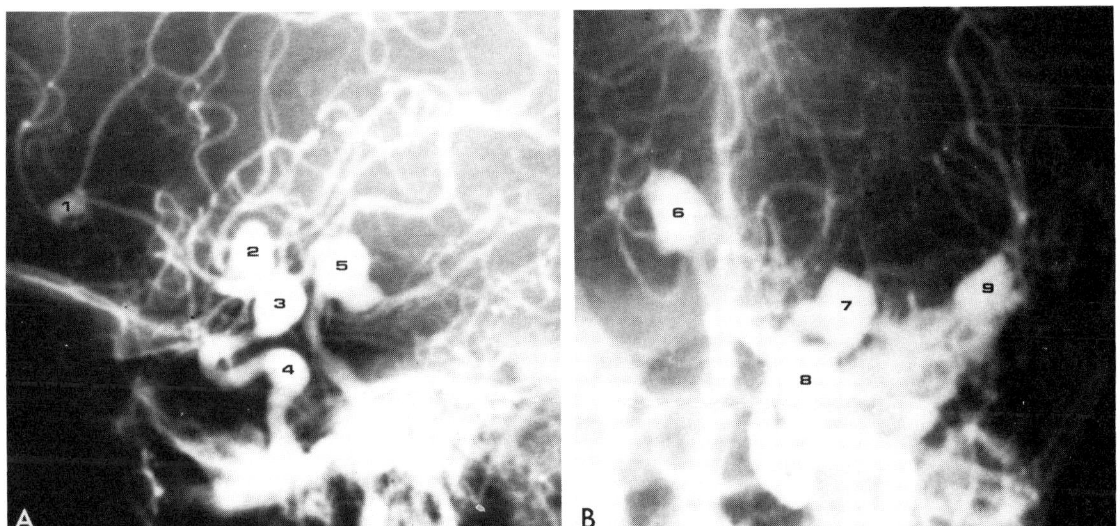

Figure 7–12. MULTIPLE ANEURYSMS: This patient has nine aneurysms visible on this right brachial *(A)*–left carotid *(B)* examination. It is difficult or impossible to judge which aneurysm has bled in this case. (Case courtesy of the Radiology Group at the Carle Clinic.)

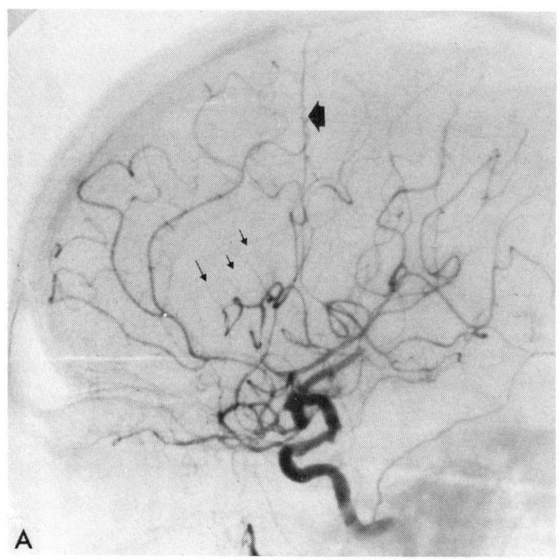

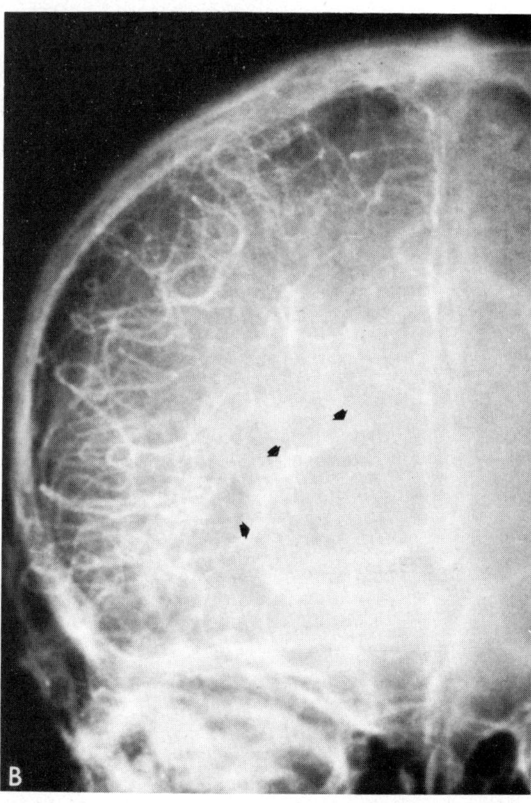

Figure 7–13. SUBARACHNOID HEMORRHAGE: The lateral view *(A)* shows spasm of the supraclinoid portion of the internal carotid artery, and spasm of the middle cerebral artery branches that has resulted in branch occlusions *(small arrows)*, and an enlarged middle meningeal artery *(large arrow)* that attempts to provide collateral circulation.

B, The AP view reveals a marked prominence of the choroidal blush in the temporal horn — also an attempt at collateral flow *(black arrowheads)*.

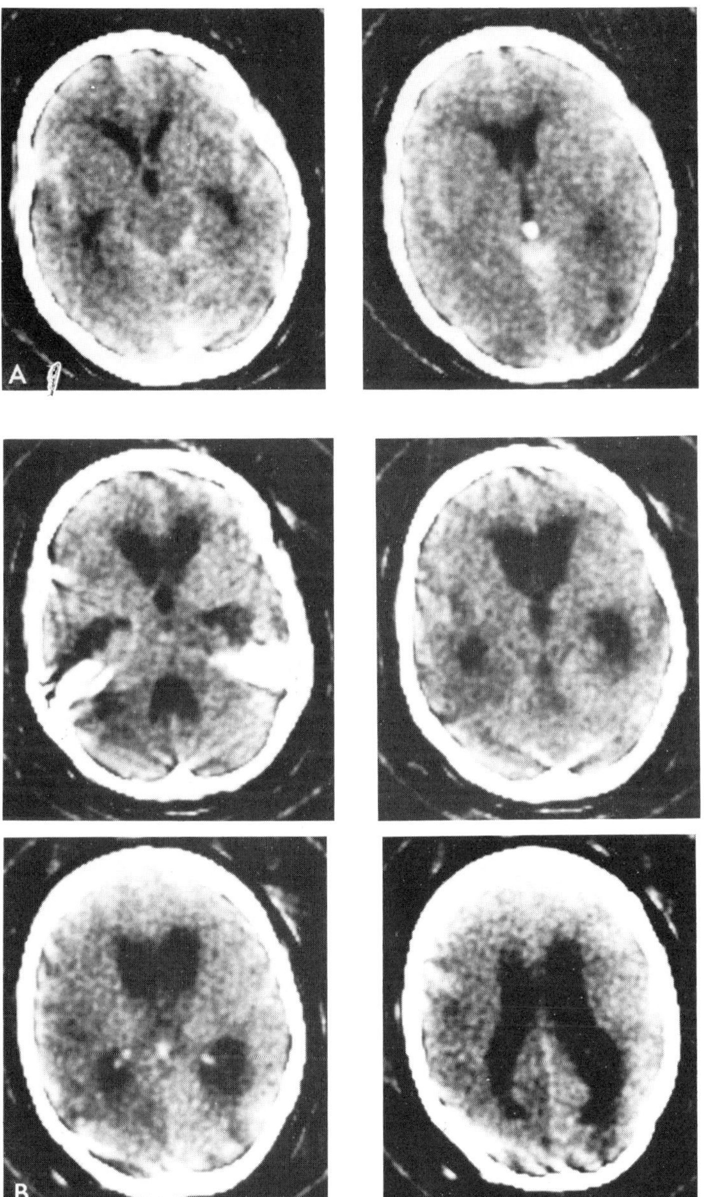

Figure 7–14. CT OF SUBARACHNOID HEMORRHAGE: The initial CT scan *(A)* demonstrates high density material in the cisterns, in the sylvian fissures and in the interhemispheric fissure. This finding is secondary to blood in the subarachnoid space.

B, Follow-up CT scans show diffuse enlargement of the lateral, third and fourth ventricles secondary to a communicating hydrocephalus that developed because of interference with resorption of the CSF by the arachnoid villi. These patients may require a shunting procedure for relief of the communicating hydrocephalus.

Figure 7–15. GIANT INTERNAL CAROTID ARTERY ANEURYSM: *A,* The carotid arteriogram demonstrates a very large aneurysm of the cavernous internal carotid artery.

B, CT scans of the same patient reveal the presence of a much larger aneurysm than was seen on the arteriogram. The aneurysm is very large, extending well into the middle cranial fossa, and demonstrates peripheral calcification. The portion of the aneurysm visualized on the arteriogram enhances on the postinfusion study *(arrow).* Note that it extends into the sella as well as along the left margin of the sella. This giant aneurysm is almost totally clotted.

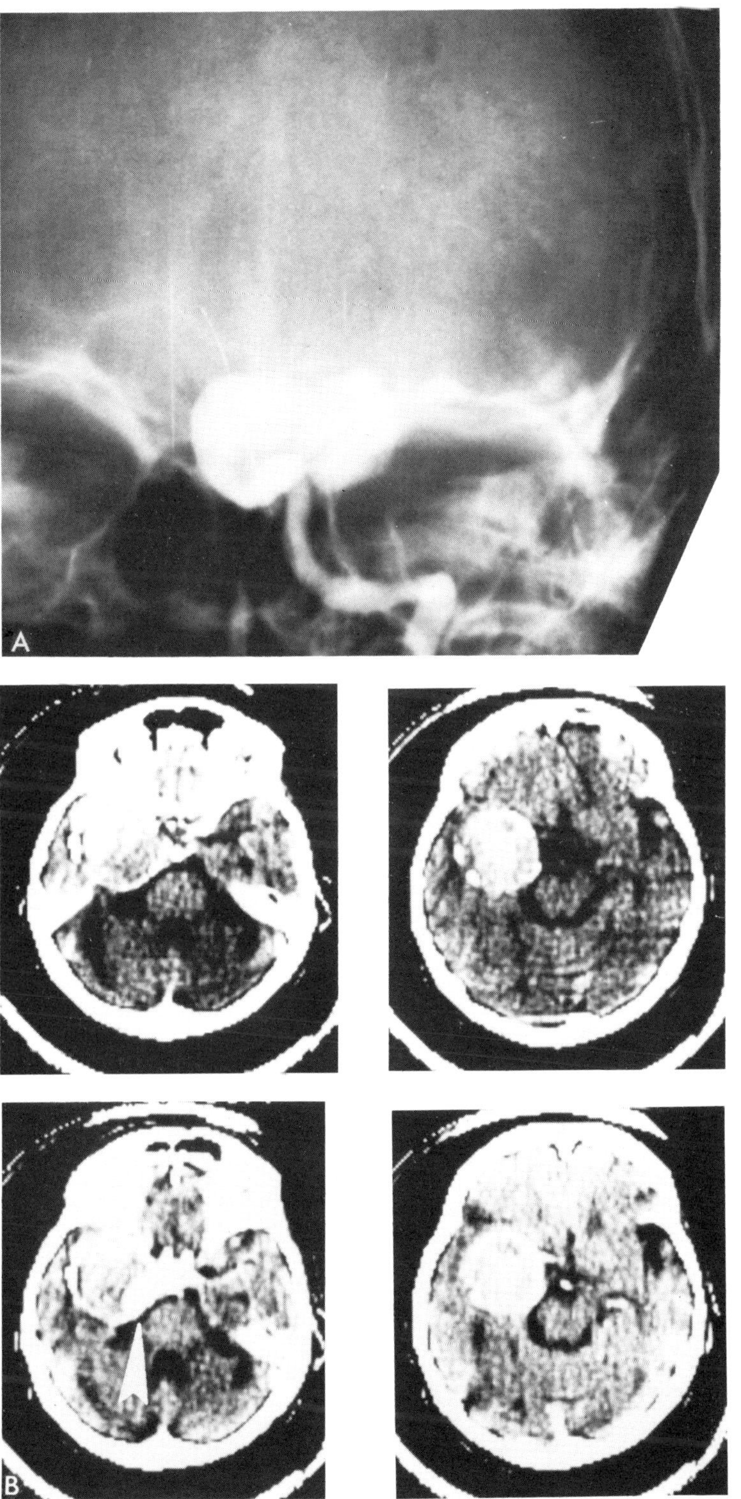

Figure 7–15. *See legend on the opposite page.*

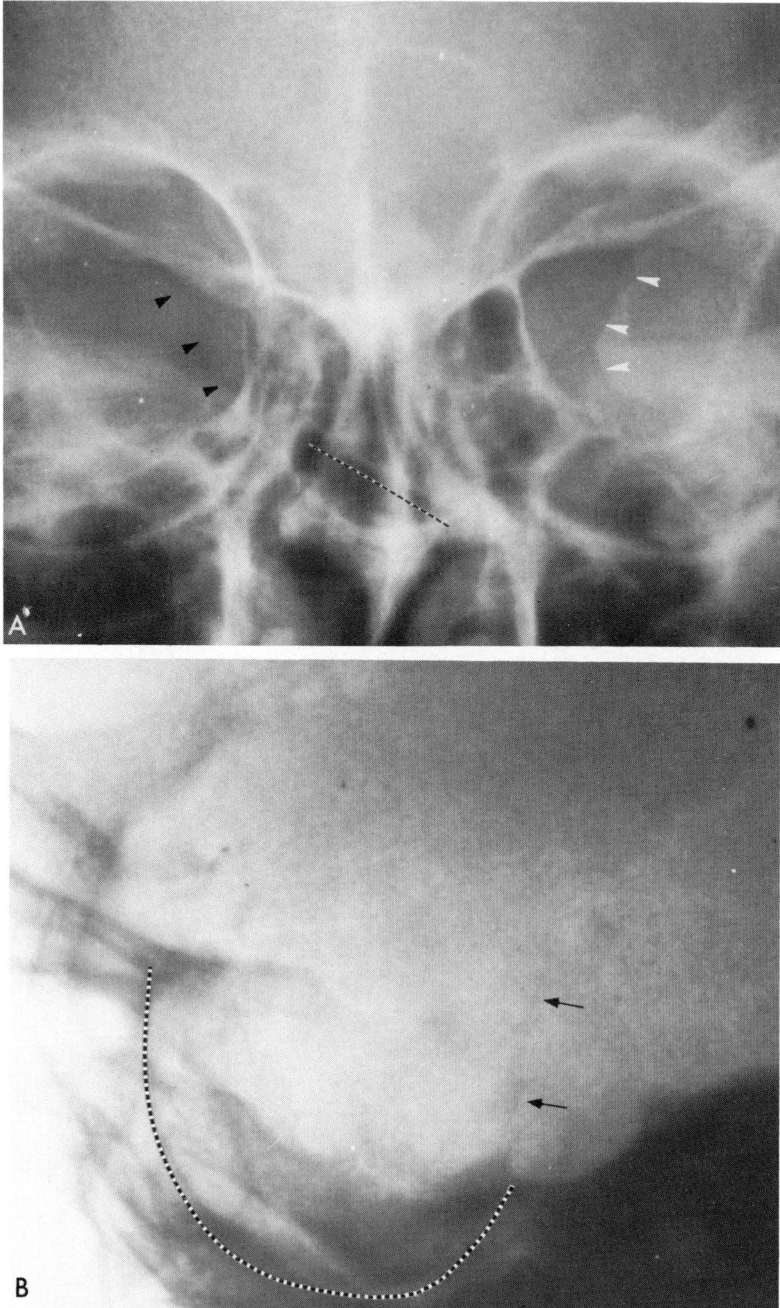

Figure 7–16. CAVERNOUS CAROTID ARTERY ANEURYSM: *A*, The PA view of the skull demonstrates marked erosion and enlargement of the superior orbital fissure on the left side *(white arrows)* compared to the normal-appearing right side *(black arrows)*. Note also the marked slanting of the floor of the sella toward the side of the abnormality *(dashed line)*.

B, The lateral view of the sella reveals that one anterior clinoid is intact, whereas the other has been eroded and is no longer visible. The sella turcica is greatly enlarged, and there is marked depression of the sella on the abnormal side *(dotted line)*. The posterior clinoids and the dorsum sella are thinned and displaced posteriorly *(arrows)*.

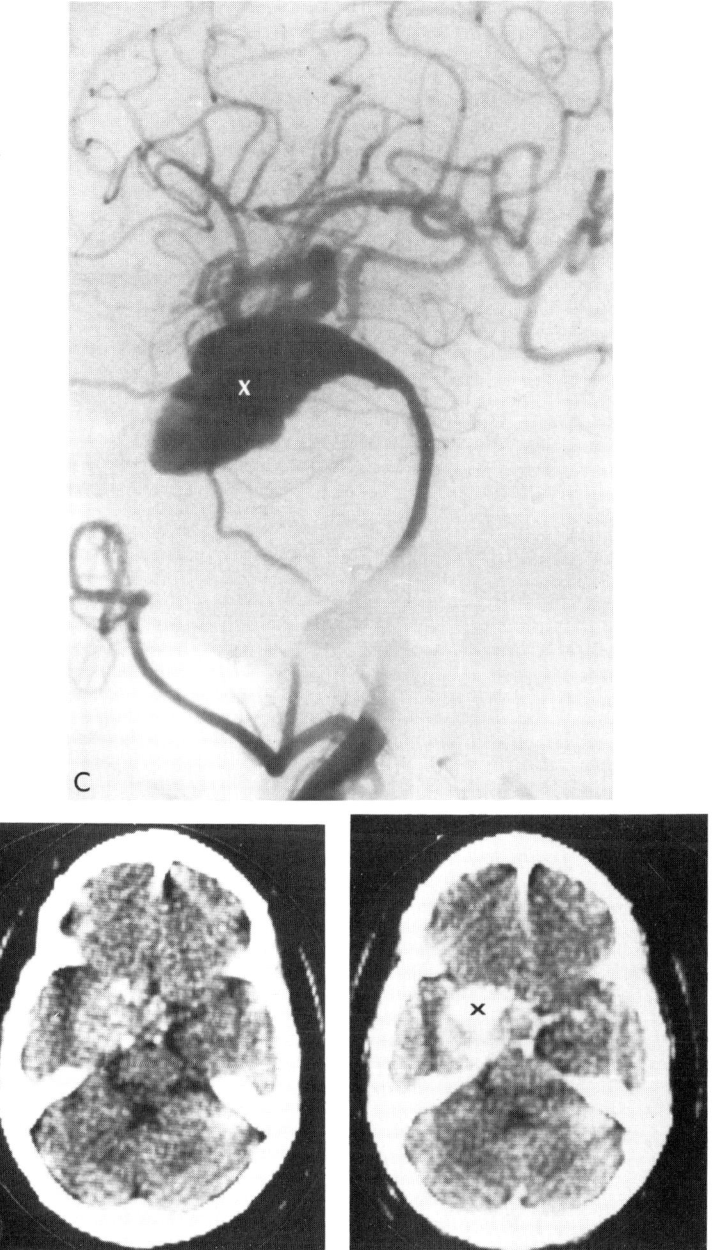

Figure 7–16 *Continued.*

C, The arteriogram reveals the unclotted portion of the aneurysm (X); the internal carotid artery is narrowed by the remainder of the aneurysm.

D, The CT scan reveals the calcified aneurysm in the left parasellar region. Postinfusion, the unclotted portion of the aneurysm (X) demonstrated by angiography enhances with contrast material.

Figure 7–17. GIANT ANEURYSM: *A* and *B*, The patient presented with headache and progressive dementia. The angiogram reveals a large avascular mass lesion in the frontal region. The anterior cerebral artery and its branches are displaced posteriorly and straightened, with minimal displacement to the contralateral side. There is a focal area of dilatation of the anterior cerebral artery at the level of the origin of the callosal marginal artery *(arrows)*, although no actual aneurysm could ever be demonstrated.

C, The CT scan shows a large mass lesion with peripheral calcification, diffusely high density and a somewhat mottled appearance. The lateral ventricles are greatly enlarged, and the frontal horn of the left lateral ventricle is compressed. The mass demonstrated minimal peripheral enhancement on the postinfusion study. Differential diagnosis included: aneurysm, meningioma, brain tumor and osteochondroma. At surgery this proved to be an aneurysm, originating at the bifurcation of the pericallosal and callosal marginal arteries.

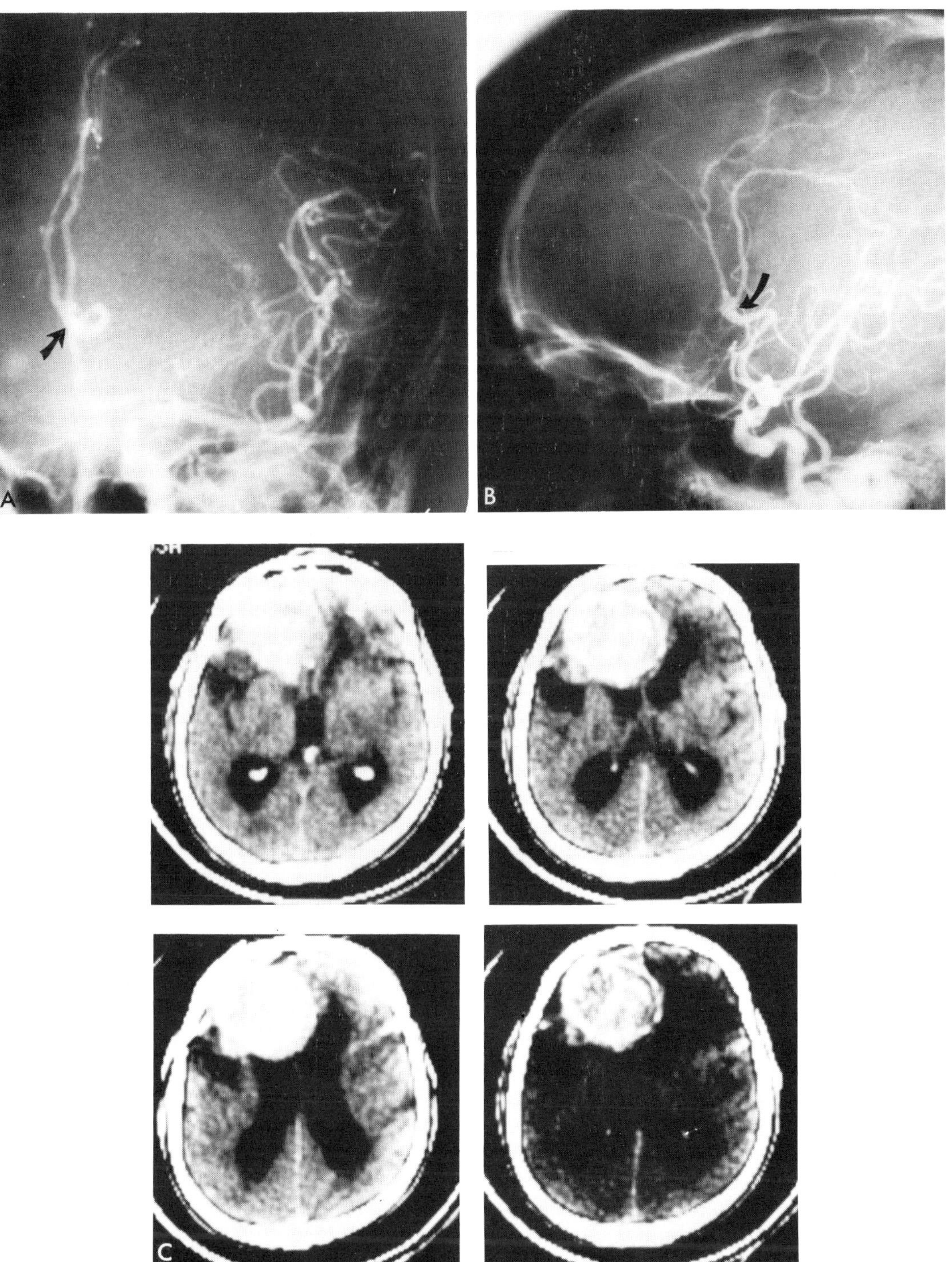

Figure 7–17. *See legend on the opposite page.*

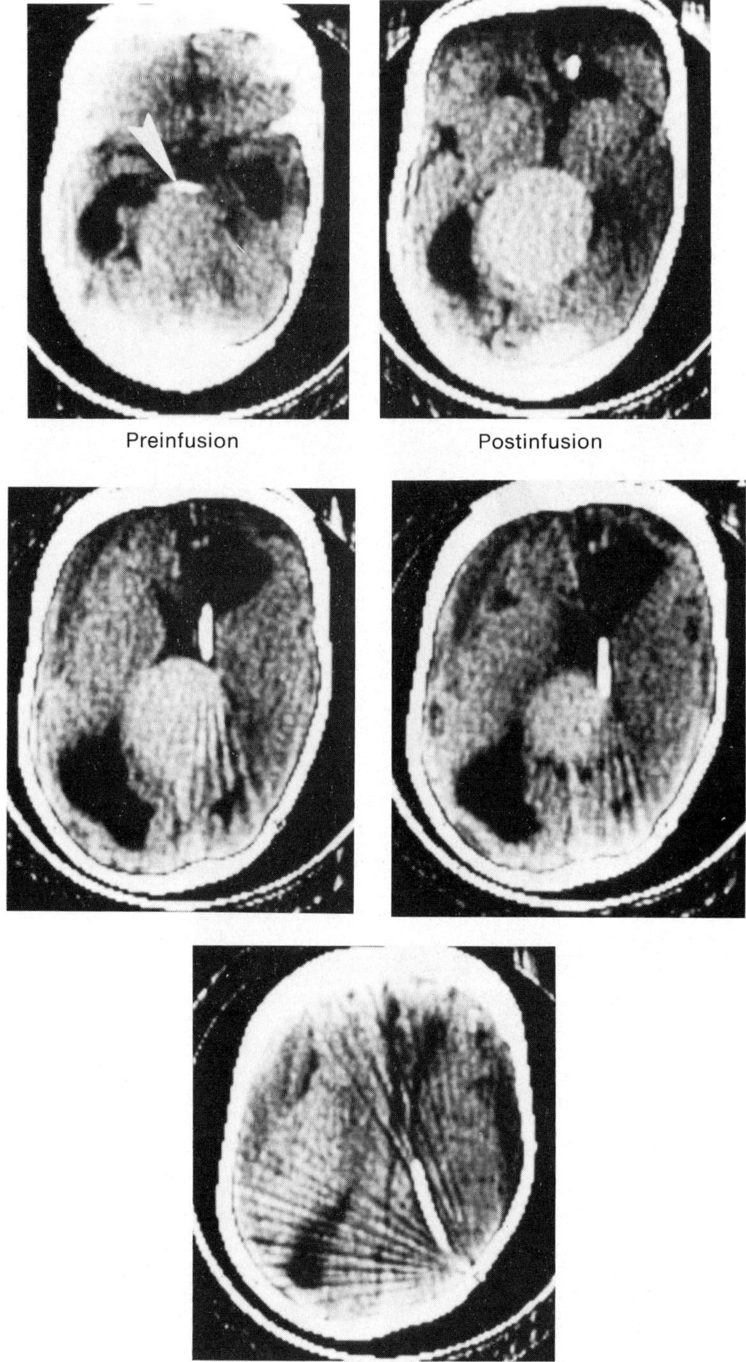

Figure 7–18. ANEURYSM OF THE VEIN OF GALEN: The preinfusion scan shows a large, well defined rounded mass in the midline that exhibits a homogeneous density. There is an area of curvilinear calcification along the anterior margin of the "mass" *(arrowhead).* A shunt tubing device is present on the right side, and there are chronic bilateral subdural hematomas which presumably developed following the shunting procedure. In spite of the shunt tube there is dilatation of the occipital horns of the lateral ventricles. This is a vein of Galen aneurysm, and the homogeneous density in the venous aneurysm is the density of the flowing blood (see Chapter 12).

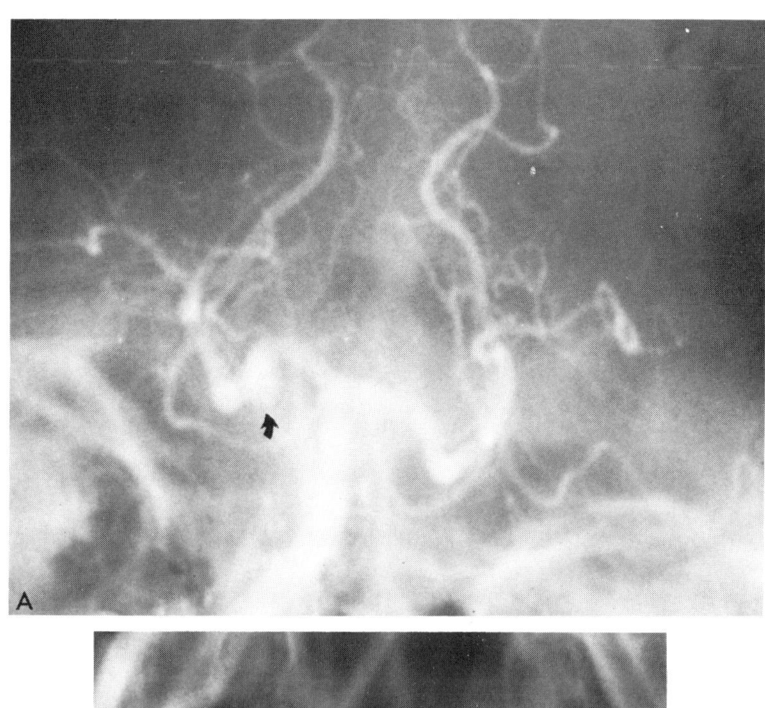

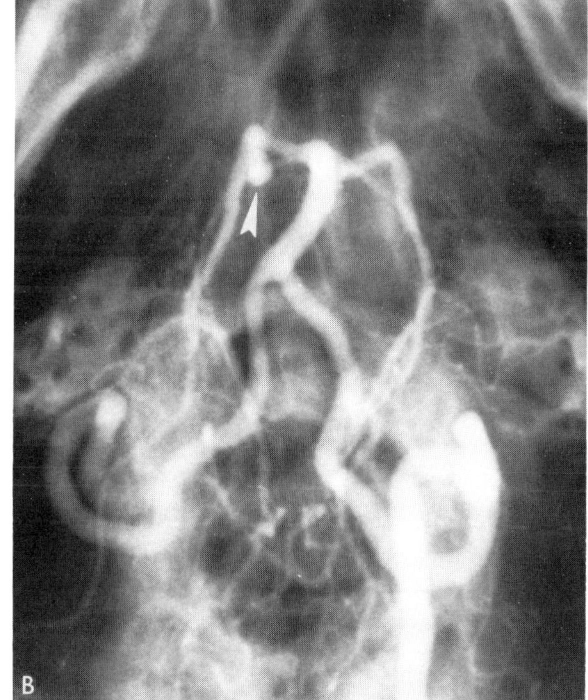

Figure 7–19. POSTERIOR CEREBRAL ARTERY ANEURYSM: *A*, The AP view of the vertebral angiogram shows an aneurysm of the right posterior cerebral artery that appears to arise at the level of the origin of the posterior communicating artery *(arrows)*. There is slight separation of the posterior cerebral arteries and the superior cerebellar arteries secondary to a small localized hemorrhage. This patient also had clinical and CT evidence of a subarachnoid hemorrhage.

B, The submentovertex view demonstrates the aneurysm *(arrow)* to better advantage and reveals that the aneurysm actually projects directly posteriorly from the posterior cerebral artery.

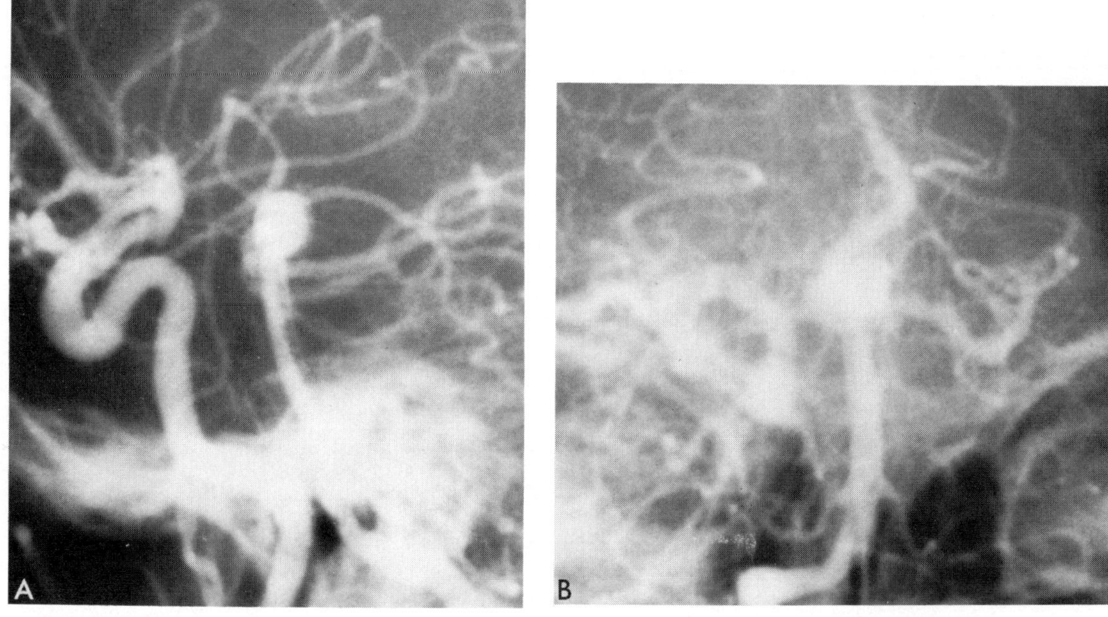

Figure 7–20. BASILAR ARTERY ANEURYSM: The AP *(A)* and lateral *(B)* views demonstrate a lobulated aneurysm involving the tip of the basilar artery. The aneurysm projects directly superiorly. The anterior cerebral artery projects directly over the aneurysm on the AP view.

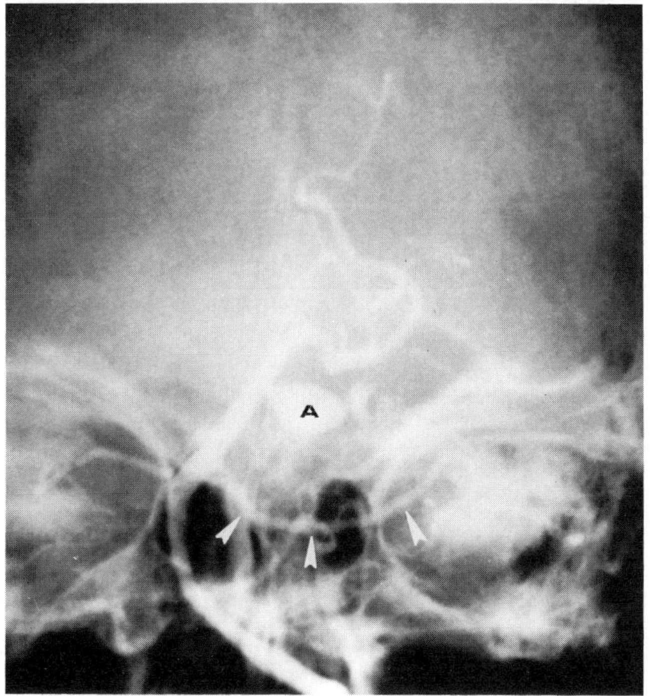

Figure 7–21. The left vertebral arteriogram demonstrates that the basilar artery is displaced to the right side and that there is inferior displacement of the AICA on the left *(arrows)*. A large aneurysm arises from the basilar artery and projects directly toward the left *(A)*. This aneurysm probably arises from one of the pontine perforating arteries and has ruptured along its lateral margin, resulting in a surrounding hematoma that has displaced the AICA and the basilar artery.

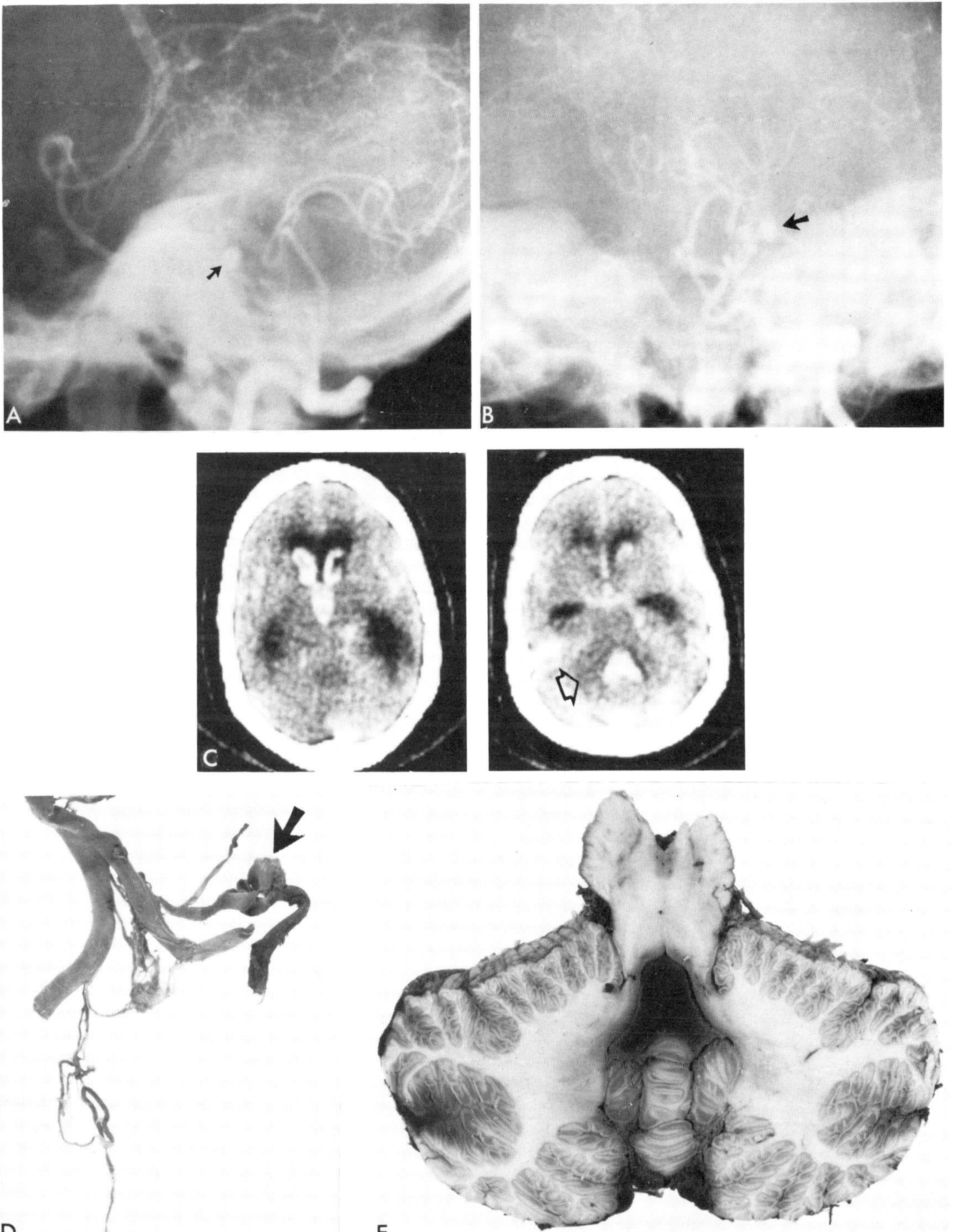

Figure 7–22. PICA ANEURYSMS: *A* and *B*, The lateral and the AP views of the vertebral arteriogram demonstrate an aneurysm of the PICA *(arrows)*, which lies along the course of the posterior inferior cerebellar artery.

C, The CT scan of this same patient reveals that there is clotted blood in the fourth, third and lateral ventricles. In addition, there is an area of radiolucency around the left side of the fourth ventricle — an area of infarction *(arrow)*.

D, The pathologic specimen reveals the aneurysm *(arrow)* along the course of the PICA.

E, The specimen of the posterior fossa structures shows clotted blood in the fourth ventricle.

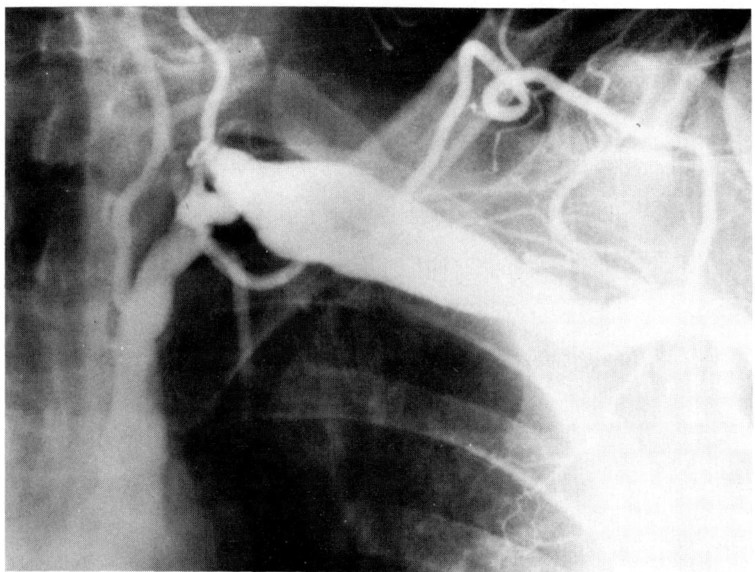

Figure 7–23. SUBCLAVIAN ARTERY ANEURYSM: The left brachial arteriogram demonstrates diffuse dilatation of the entire left subclavian artery. The right subclavian artery had a similar appearance. The etiology of this change is unknown.

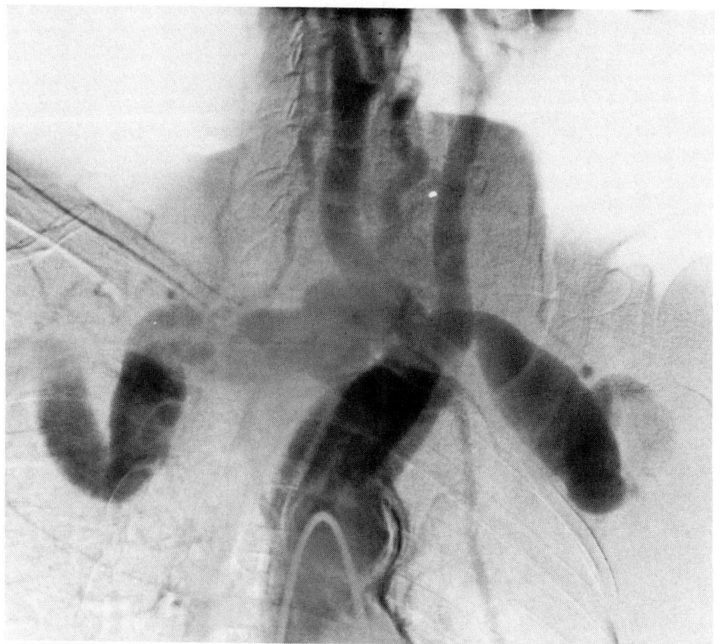

Figure 7–24. ANEURYSMAL CHANGE INVOLVING THE ENTIRE BRACHIOCEPHALIC TRUNK: An arch angiogram in the LPO projection demonstrates diffuse dilatation of all the great vessels as they arise from the arch of the aorta. Although all the vessels are patent, there was marked delay in filling of the intracranial circulation.

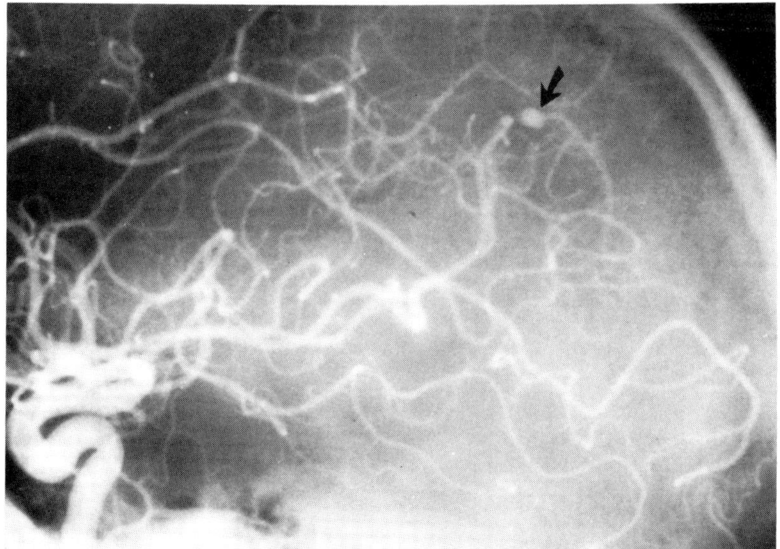

Figure 7–25. MYCOTIC ANEURYSM: The intracranial circulation demonstrates a small aneurysm *(arrow)* along the distal course of one of the middle cerebral arteries. This is an infected aneurysm that developed because of a septic embolus from the affected heart valve in this patient with subacute bacterial endocarditis.

CHAPTER 8

MISCELLANEOUS DEGENERATIVE AND INFLAMMATORY DISEASES

Particularly since the advent of computed tomography, the neuroradiologist has come to play a major role in the diagnosis of degenerative and inflammatory disorders of the nervous system. The following is a list of these diseases as discussed in this chapter. Cases have been chosen that illustrate the great diagnostic usefulness of the CT scan.

1. Atrophy:
   a. Supratentorial.
   b. Infratentorial.
2. Multiple sclerosis.
3. Leukodystrophy.
4. Adrenoleukodystrophy.
5. White matter prominence—undetermined etiology.
6. Meningitis.
7. Ependymal spread of metastatic disease.
8. Radiation necrosis.
9. Benign postoperative enhancement.
10. Carbon monoxide poisoning.
11. Cerebral anoxia secondary to respiratory arrest.
12. Progressive multifocal leukoencephalopathy.
13. Leukoencephalopathy secondary to methotrexate.
14. Cerebral necrosis secondary to perinatal anoxia.
15. Cerebral calcifications.
16. Amphetamine toxicity.

DEGENERATIVE DISEASES

Computed tomography has greatly aided our evaluation of atrophy and other degenerative diseases of the brain. The CT scan provides us with more information than was previously available using other diagnostic methods; at the same time, it causes less discomfort for the patient. Indeed, some abnormalities are easily diagnosed by CT that cannot be evaluated by other methods.

ATROPHY

The demented patient being evaluated for the possible presence of an atrophic process is the ideal candidate for study by computed tomography. In the past, pneumoencephalography was needed to demonstrate enlarged ventricles and enlargement of the cortical sulci greater than 4 mm. In addition, it was necessary to rule out the presence of a mass that might mimic the clinical appearance of dementia. The CT scan readily demonstrates these changes of ventricular and cortical sulcus enlargement; it also rules out the presence of a mass lesion.

It should be recalled that an increase in

size of the ventricles and cortical sulci is a normal process of aging. These changes become more marked in men than in women after 55 years of age. Although absolute values are not yet available, a scan demonstrating enlarged ventricles and sulci might be normal in an individual in the later decades, whereas a similar tomographic appearance in a younger patient would represent atrophy. For this reason, the age of the patient must be kept in mind when interpreting these changes.

Supratentorial. Generalized cerebral atrophy with enlargement of the cortical sulci and lateral ventricles may be seen as part of the normal aging process.

Atrophy is also seen in chronic alcoholics, debilitated patients and in Alzeheimer's and Pick's disease. A similar appearance is noted in patients who have multiple cerebral infarcts in the cortex. Drug abuse and chronic renal failure also may lead to an appearance of atrophy on the CT scan.

Infratentorial. Atrophic changes in the posterior fossa are reflected on the CT scan as enlargements of the fourth ventricle, the prepontine cistern, the cerebellopontine angle cisterns, the superior cerebellar cistern and the cisternae magnae.

Most commonly we see these changes, especially vermian atrophy, with enlargement of the superior cerebellar cistern in patients who are chronic alcoholics.

These changes also may be seen with other diseases that lead to cerebellar atrophy. Among these are cerebello-olivary atrophy, olivopontocerebellar atrophy, dentatorubral atrophy and opticocochleodentate degeneration.

Text continued on page 390

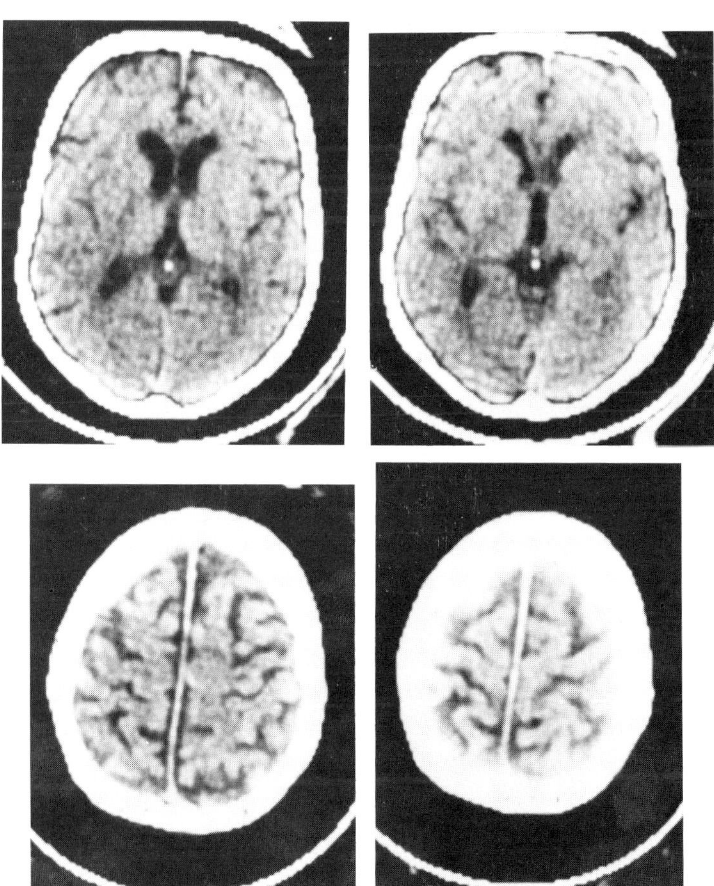

Figure 8–1. ATROPHY: Mild cerebral atrophy with enlargement of the lateral ventricles and cortical sulci.

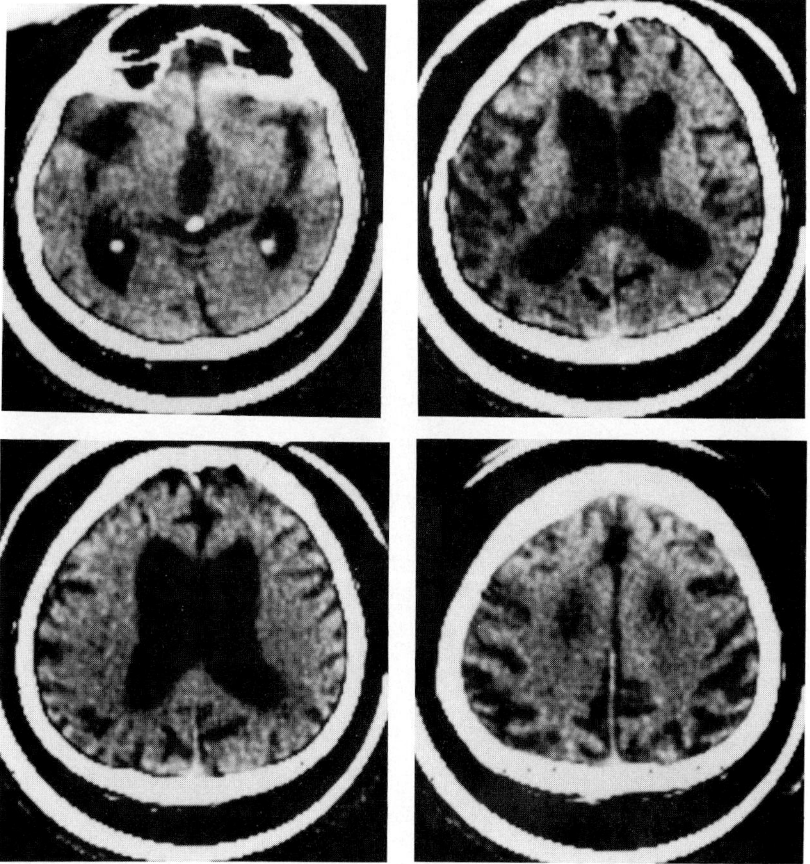

Figure 8–2. ATROPHY: Severe cerebral atrophy with marked enlargement of the lateral ventricles and cortical sulci.

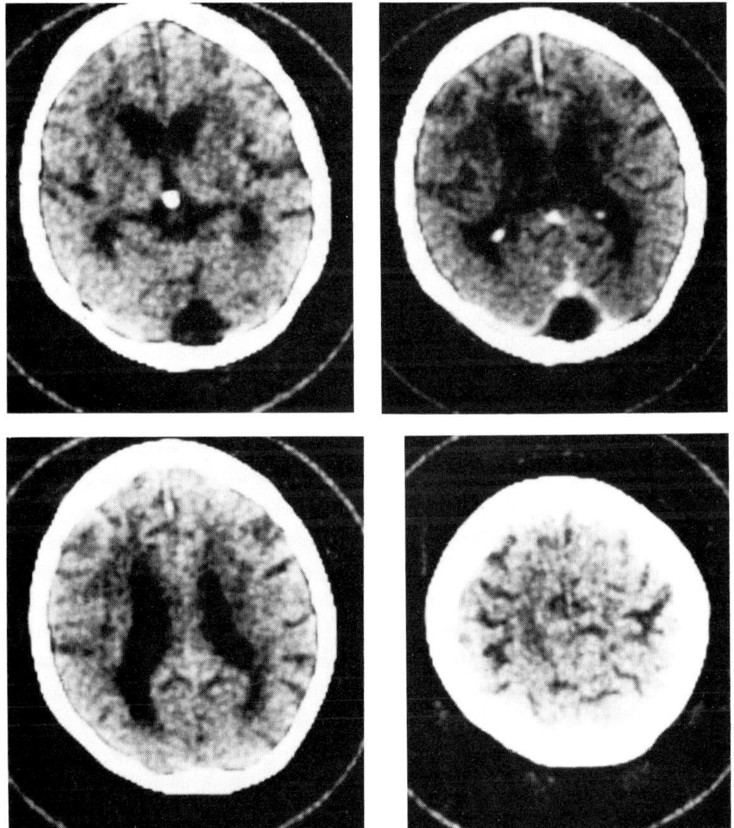

Figure 8–3. ATROPHY AND INFARCTS: Moderate cerebral atrophy with multiple scattered areas of radiolucency secondary to multiple infarcts.

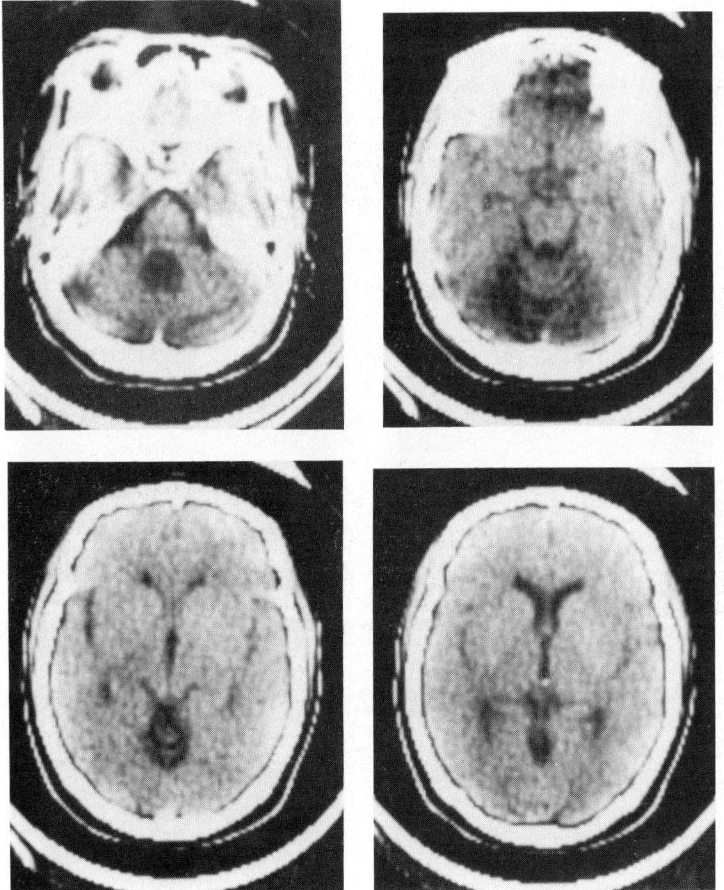

Figure 8–4. POSTERIOR FOSSA ATROPHY: Marked posterior fossa atrophy with enlargement of the fourth ventricle, the prepontine and cerebellopontine angle cisterns and superior cerebellar cistern.

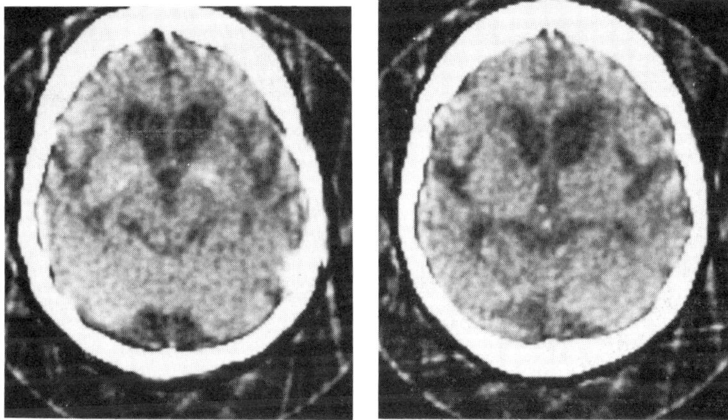

Figure 8-5. ATROPHY: Moderate cerebral atrophy with enlargement of the cisternae magnae secondary to cerebellar atrophy. Great variations in the size of the cisternae magnae are normal.

CHRONIC ILLNESS

Various types of chronic illness appear to be reflected in an appearance of atrophy on the CT scans. Disease states associated with atrophy on the CT scan include *chronic alcoholism* (which may show only vermis or diffuse posterior fossa atrophy), *chronic renal failure, drug abuse, severe heart disease* (especially following multiple operations on the heart) or *cancer*.

INFARCTS

Areas of infarction are also readily identified by CT scanning. Approximately 70 per cent of bland infarcts are identifiable by CT scan within the first seven days post-insult. Of the remaining 30 per cent, a varying number will become apparent after seven days; however, some — particularly the smaller infarcts — never become visible. Multiple small cortical infarcts may result in a CT appearance that mimics atrophy (see Chapter 6).

MULTIPLE SCLEROSIS

Multiple sclerosis is a common demyelinating disease in young adults. The diagnosis is frequently made by the exclusion of other possibilities; in fact, such entities as spinal cord neurofibromas or meningiomas and posterior fossa meningiomas may mimic the clinical presentation of multiple sclerosis.

The CT scan in long-standing multiple sclerosis demonstrates ventricular enlargement with or without cortical sulcus enlargement and without other areas of abnormal density. On the other hand, it is not unusual to see a normal CT scan in a patient with multiple sclerosis.

Patients with multiple sclerosis may demonstrate areas of low density in a periventricular distribution. These areas of demyelinization or plaques usually show no change on the postinfusion scan. When the patient is in an acute phase of multiple sclerosis, these areas of periventricular radiolucency may also demonstrate homogeneous enhancement on the postinfusion portion of the scan. Apparently, these plaques which enhance represent areas of acute demyelinization.

Multiple sclerosis is one of a group of demyelinating diseases. Schilder's disease, a similar process, is seen in children.

Histologically, a series of changes occur in these diseases.

1. There is loss of normal myelin structures, with swelling and breakdown of myelin sheaths.

2. Phagocytosis of the breakdown products occurs, followed by

   a. Inflammatory cellular lesions that are reactive to the parenchymatous lesions.

   b. Catabolism of the phagocytosed material follows, lending to:

   c. Reactive gliosis.

The lesions appear as plaques of demyelination with glioses. Preferentially, these occur in the periventricular regions, along the optic pathways, in the brain stem (especially in the periventricular region), in the central cerebellar white matter and randomly in the spinal cord.

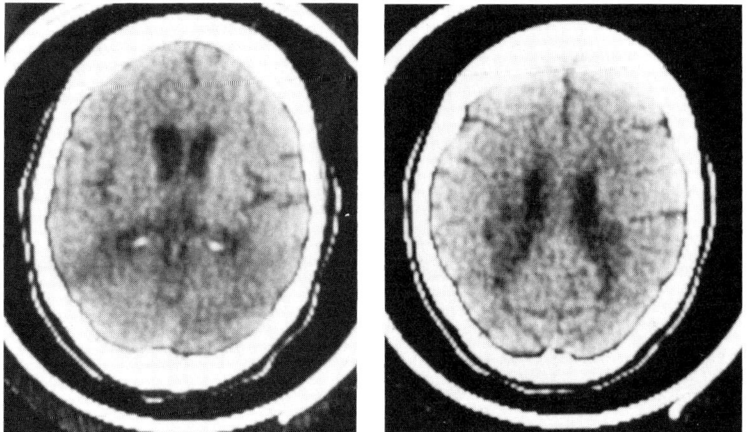

Figure 8–6. MULTIPLE SCLEROSIS: In a 26-year-old woman the CT scan demonstrates an appearance of atrophy, with bilateral areas of periventricular radiolucency that are especially prominent adjacent to the posterior bodies of the lateral ventricles. These are areas of demyelinization.

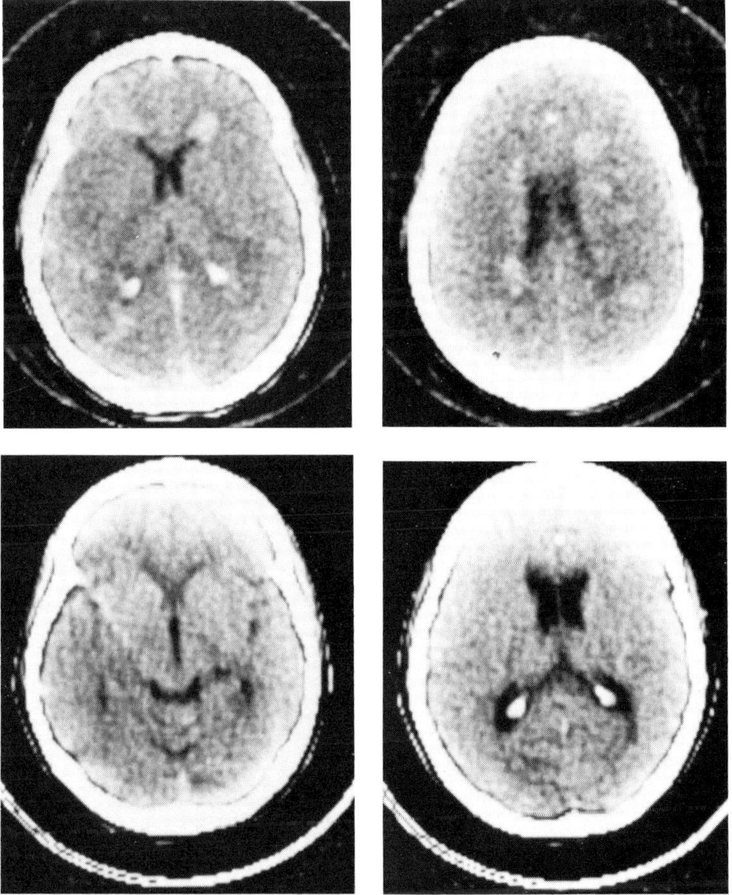

Figure 8–7. MULTIPLE SCLEROSIS: A 23-year-old woman demonstrates multiple scattered areas of enhancement on this postinfusion-only scan. The areas are predominantly periventricular in distribution and are secondary to the acute demyelinization process seen in multiple sclerosis.

A scan obtained two years after the initial study reveals ventricular enlargement, but no evidence of plaque formation or areas of enhancement.

LEUKODYSTROPHIES

All of these poorly understood diseases demonstrate evidence of demyelinization.

Metachromatic leukodystrophy. There is hemispheric demyelinization accompanied by fibrillary gliosis; it is characterized by the presence of nonsudanophilic lipid breakdown products which are metachromatic with cresyl violet and with toluidine blue.

Krabbe's disease. In the areas of demyelinization there are large multinucleated cells accompanied by epithelioid cells.

In the example shown in Figure 8–8, diffuse prominence of the white matter secondary to demyelinization is present. The etiology of Krabbe's disease is unknown, but it is probably a metachromatic leukodystrophy.

ADRENOLEUKODYSTROPHY

This rare demyelinating disease occurs in childhood and leads to mental deterioration and blindness. It is a multisystem disease; however, the nervous system manifestations could be thought of as "pediatric multiple sclerosis." The CT scan usually shows bilateral occipital radiolucencies that may or may not exhibit enhancement.

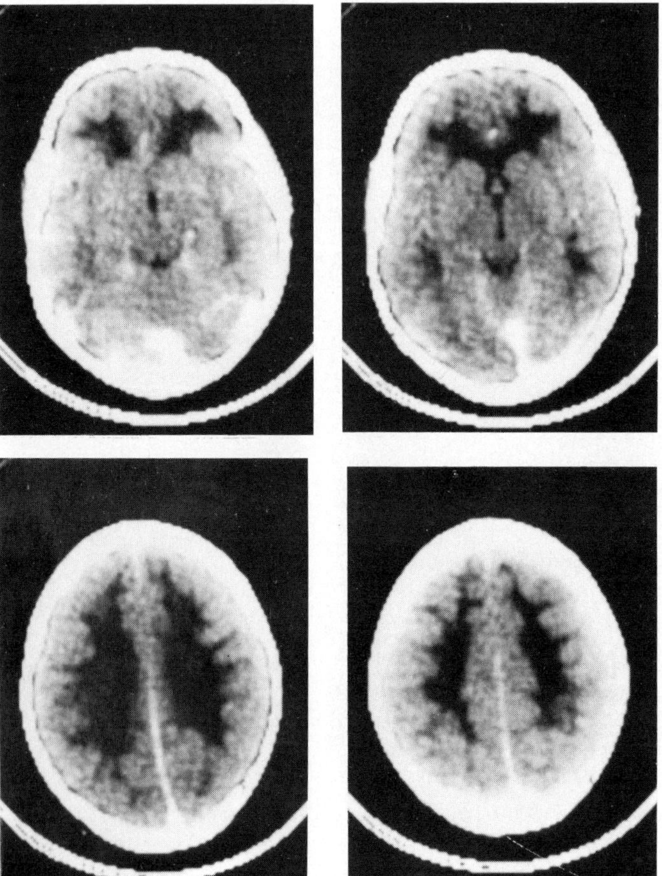

Figure 8–8.

WHITE MATTER PROMINENCE OF UNDETERMINED ETIOLOGY

In Figure 8–9, the preinfusion scan demonstrates a diffuse prominence of the white matter and marked enhancement of the gray matter. Demarcation of gray from white matter is even greater than normal.

The etiology of these changes is not known; however, the author has noted this finding in a large number of patients with a seizure disorder in whom no focal lesion was found.

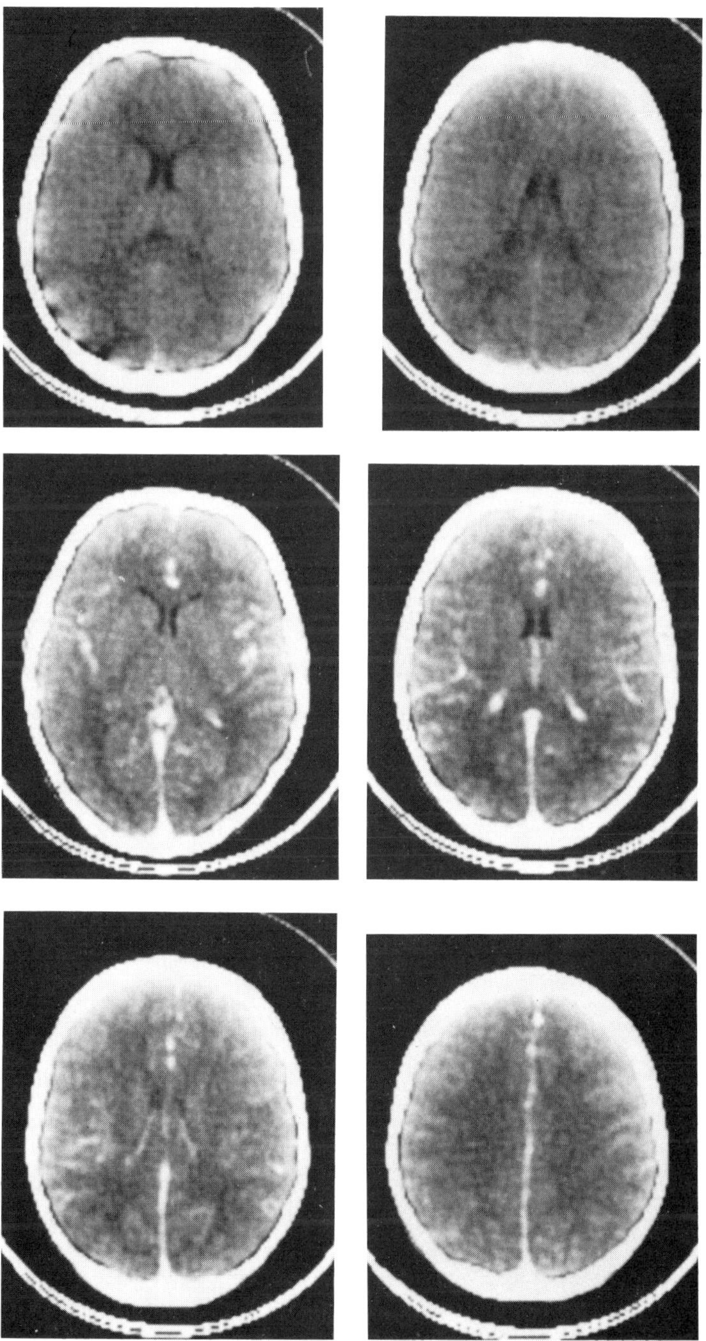

Figure 8–9.

MENINGITIS

The CT scan in these patients may be within normal limits. On the other hand, because all of the central nervous system structures that are bathed by cerebrospinal fluid participate in the infectious process, the scan may demonstrate a variety of abnormalities. A diffuse polymorphic inflammatory cellular infiltrate in the walls of the leptomeningeal arteries and invasion of the ependyma may be seen histologically. These changes can result in the development of thromboses, which lead to areas of cerebral infarction and thus to areas of lucency on the CT scan.

The lateral ventricles may be dilated in a communicating type of hydrocephalus secondary to interference with the resorption of CSF by the arachnoid villi. Or an obstructive hydro- or pyocephalus may result from an obstruction of the outflow of CSF from the ventricles. Subdural empyema also may be seen following meningitis.

Because of the thickening of the meninges, there may be a diffuse enhancement of the meninges on the postinfusion scan.

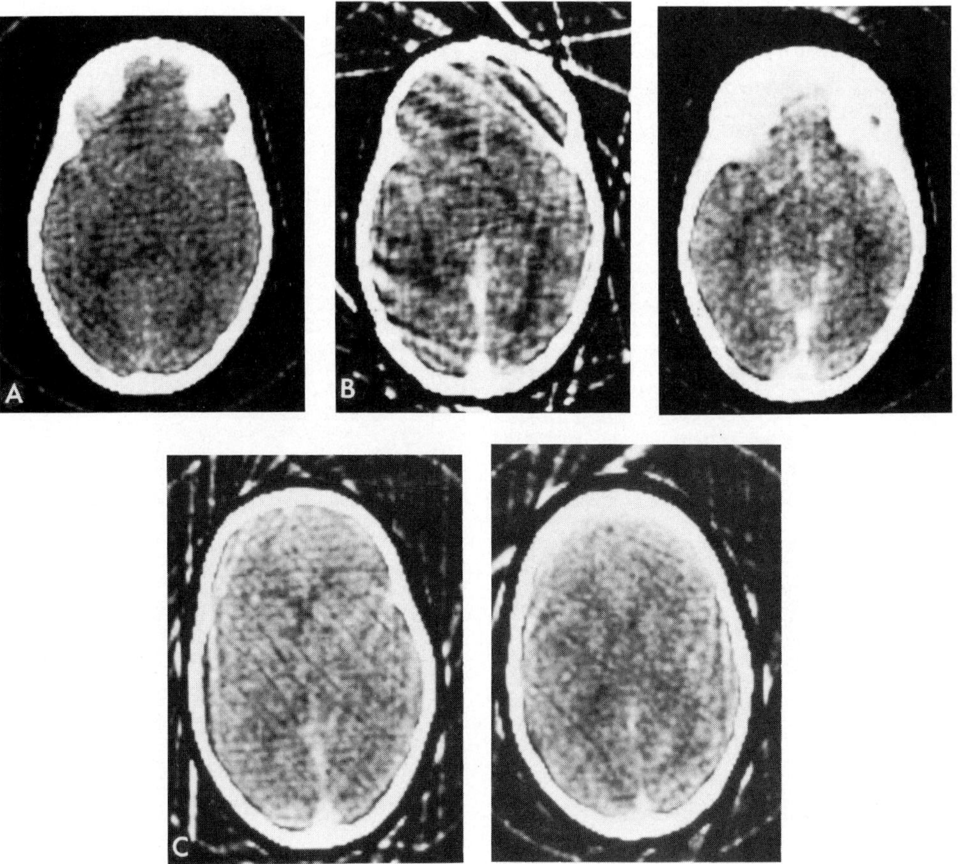

Figure 8–10. MENINGITIS: This example demonstrates an initially normal preinfusion scan *(A)* with marked enhancement of the meninges on the postinfusion scan *(B)*. A follow-up scan after appropriate antibiotic treatment *(C)* no longer demonstrates enhancement of the meninges.

EPENDYMAL SPREAD OF METASTATIC DISEASE

The preinfusion scan in Figure 8–11 demonstrates minimal distortion of the frontal horns of the lateral ventricles; the postinfusion scan reveals spectacular periventricular enhancement. Biopsy revealed metastatic germinoma — probably primary from the region of the pineal gland.

Other types of metastatic disease may spread in a similar fashion throughout the ventricular system.

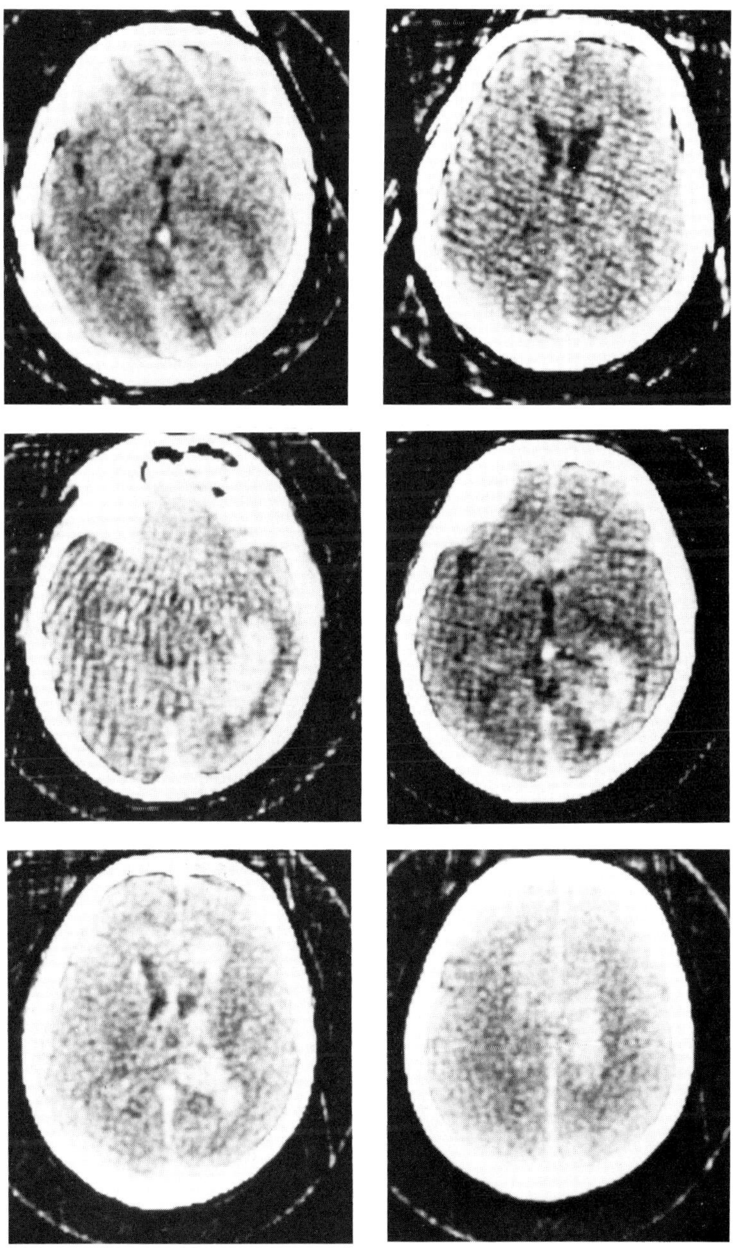

Figure 8–11.

RADIATION NECROSIS

The changes following irradiation to the brain do not appear until months or years after treatment, but they then may progress rapidly to death.

Pathologic evidence of brain swelling is noted. This may produce radiologic evidence of a mass on the angiogram and an area of radiolucency on the preinfusion CT scan. After the infusion of contrast material there may be homogeneous enhancement of these areas of radiation necrosis or a ring of enhancement in the affected area. There may be a mass effect, and if the changes are noted in the bed of a previous tumor differentiation from recurrent or remaining tumor may be difficult without a biopsy.

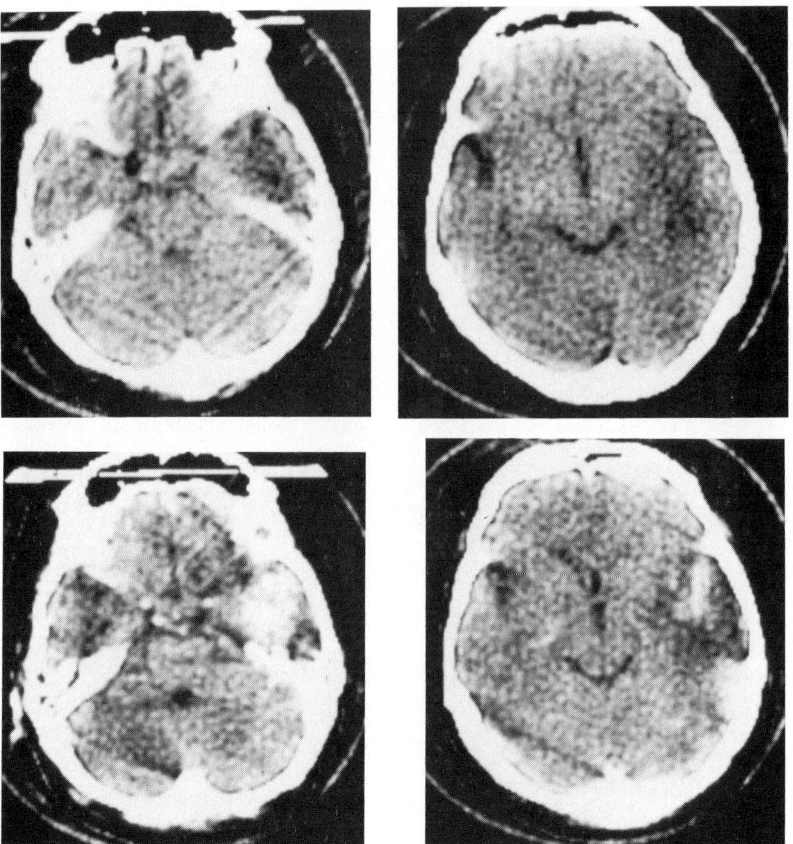

Figure 8–12. RADIATION NECROSIS: There is an area of lucency in the right temporal region, with some mass effect and homogeneous enhancement after the infusion of contrast material. The patient had received radiation treatment to the pituitary gland six years previously. Biopsy revealed radiation necrosis.

BENIGN POSTOPERATIVE ENHANCEMENT

Following surgery there may be an area of enhancement of the image in the bed of the surgery, even in the absence of tumor. In the example shown in Figure 8–13, the patient had had partial removal of a meningioma. Postoperatively, there is an irregular area of enhancement at the surgical site *(arrow)*, which is remote from the tumor.

This type of enhancement also can be seen following needle biopsy, even in the absence of tumor, and perhaps represents a capillary proliferation secondary to operative intervention.

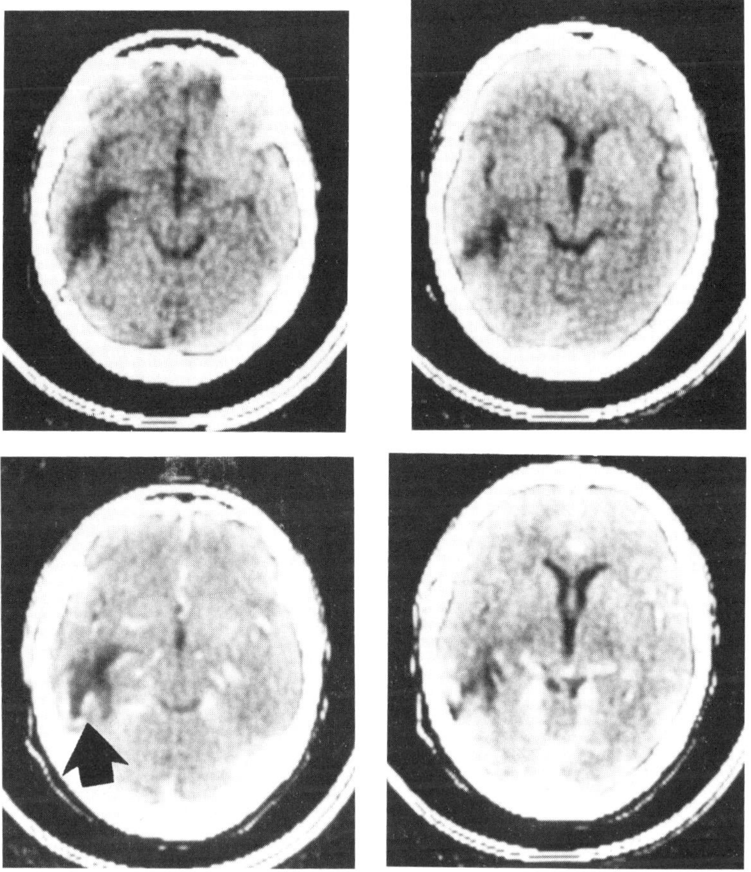

Figure 8–13.

CARBON MONOXIDE POISONING

Classically, necrosis of the globus pallidus occurs with carbon monoxide poisoning. The CT scan in Figure 8–14 demonstrates mild ventricular enlargement and bilateral areas of lucency in the region of the globus pallidus. The patient survived an attempted suicide with carbon monoxide.

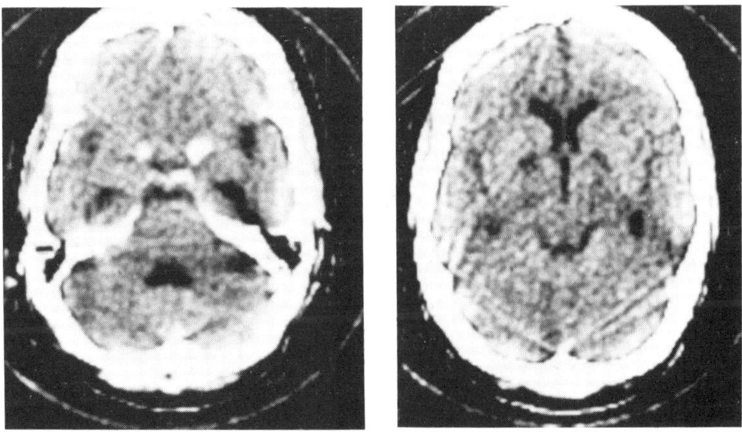

Figure 8–14.

RESPIRATORY ARREST WITH CEREBRAL ANOXIA

A variety of changes can occur with circulatory arrest and cerebral anoxia. The late changes demonstrate necrotic foci with cavities or glial scars. These especially affect Ammon's horn and, in the basal ganglia, the globus pallidus. The white matter is better preserved.

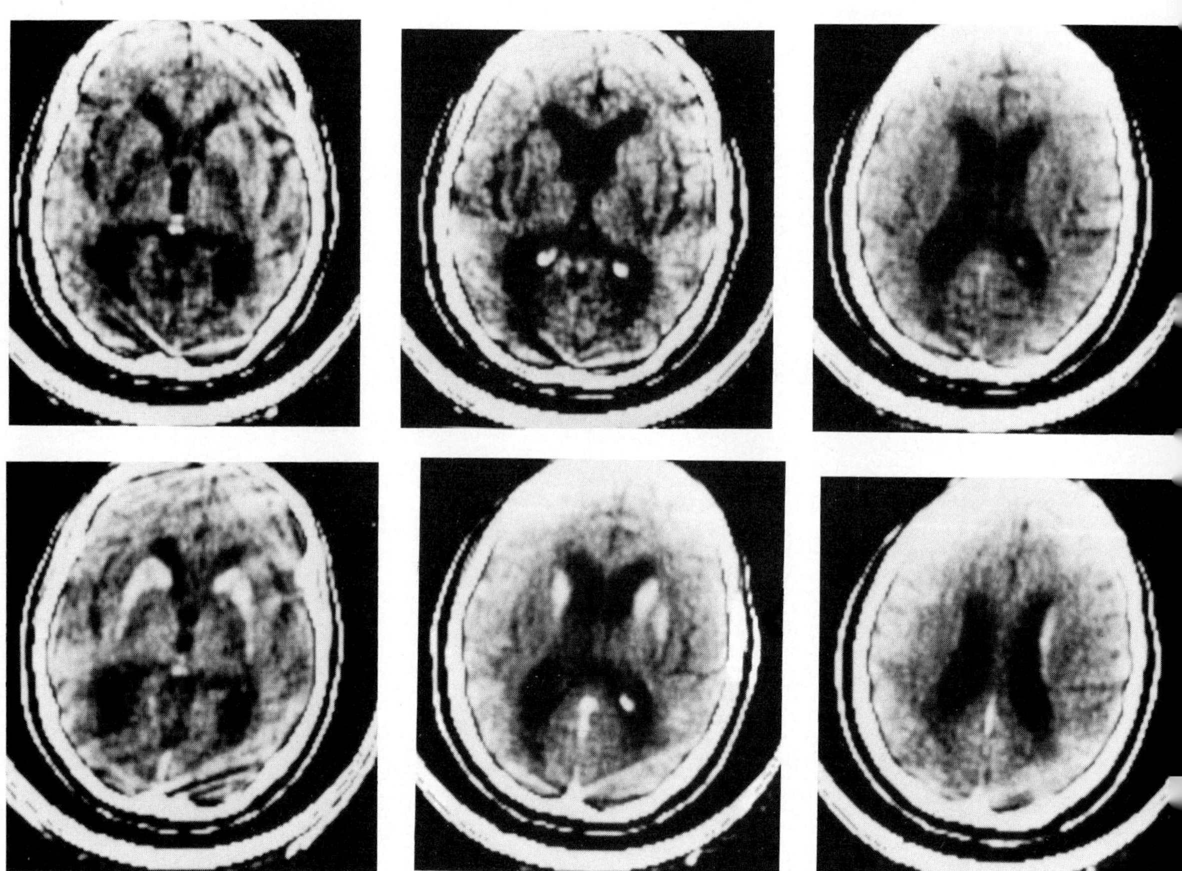

Figure 8–15. CEREBRAL ANOXIA: The CT scan in this 13-year-old girl following cardiorespiratory arrest reveals moderately severe diffuse cerebral atrophy with areas of radiolucency in the basal ganglia bilaterally. The postinfusion scan *(lower row)* shows marked enhancement of the caudate nucleus.

The general appearance is consistent with cerebral anoxia. The etiology of the caudate nucleus enhancement is unknown, but perhaps it represents an attempt at collateral circulation.

PROGRESSIVE MULTIFOCAL LEUKOENCEPHALOPATHY

This entity is frequently seen in patients who have suffered from a pre-existing malignant lymphoproliferative disease such as lymphosarcoma, Hodgkin's disease or lymphatic leukemia or from a variety of other disease processes. There is now evidence that a papovavirus plays an important part in the etiology of the disease.

Pathologic examination reveals cortical atrophy: a finding that is reflected on the CT scan. There are also multiple, sometimes confluent, areas of demyelinization. These usually are in the white matter, but may also affect the gray matter.

The CT scan demonstrates these areas of demyelinization as areas of lucency; on the postinfusion scan there may be multiple scattered areas of enhancement. These changes are present in the example illustrated in Figure 8–16.

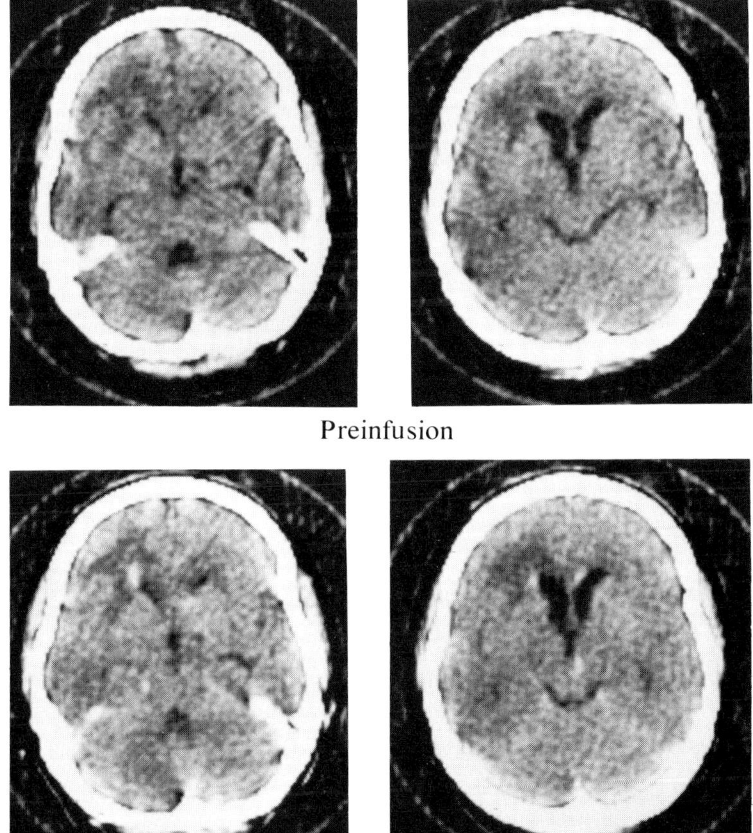

Preinfusion

Postinfusion

Figure 8–16.

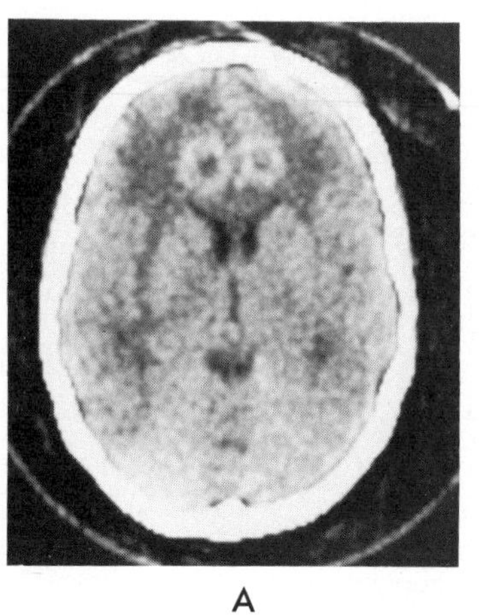
A

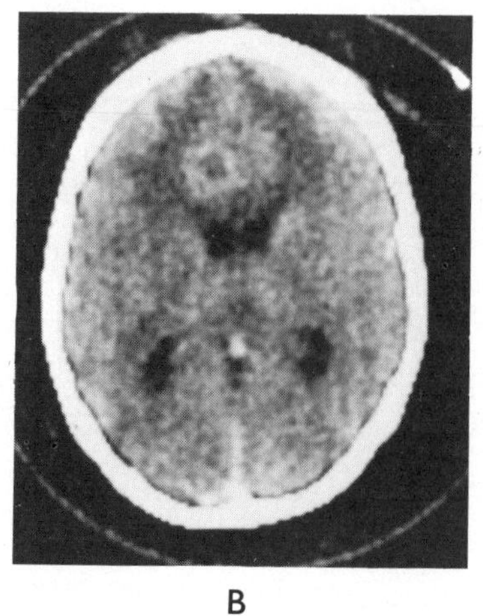
B

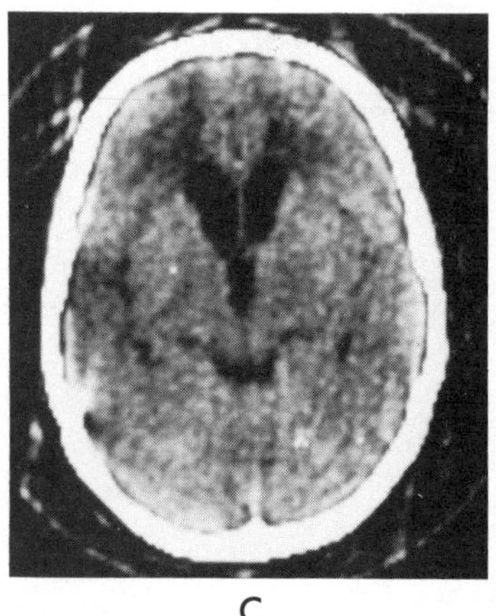
C

Figure 8–17.

LEUKOENCEPHALOPATHY SECONDARY TO METHOTREXATE

Certain chemotherapeutic agents used intrathecally, especially methotrexate, have been implicated in the development of a leukoencephalopathy.

In Figure 8–17, this 13-year-old child had received multiple intrathecal doses of methotrexate for treatment of CNS leukemia. The CT scan after the infusion of contrast material (*A* and *B*) demonstrates two small rings of enhancement deep in the frontal lobes bilaterally just adjacent to the midline and surrounded by a bat-wing pattern of edema. There is some mass effect, with posterior displacement of the frontal horns of the lateral ventricles. The findings are consistent with a leukoencephalopathy (not proved by biopsy).

A follow-up scan (*C*) nine months later demonstrates an atrophic pattern with dilatation of the frontal horns of the lateral ventricles and irregular areas of radiolucency in both frontal lobes secondary to permanent brain damage.

PERINATAL ANOXIA

In premature infants, intraventricular or subependymal hemorrhages from terminal veins are commonly associated with severe asphyxia. These changes are readily identified on the CT scan.

In addition, with perinatal anoxia there may also be extensive neuronal necrosis — a finding reflected on the CT scan as multiple areas of radiolucency resembling infarcts. Clinically, these patients may have an enlarging head size and bulging fontanelle, while the

---

Figure 8–18. CEREBRAL ANOXIA AT BIRTH: *A*, The initial CT scan demonstrates diffuse abnormalities. Multiple areas of radiolucency throughout both hemispheres are distributed in a random fashion. The frontal horns of the lateral ventricles are slitlike structures deep in the midline on the middle cut.

B, In a follow-up scan one week later, the entire brain substance is now low density. Only small bilateral patches of brain substance remain in the temporal regions. Note the relative sparing of structures in the posterior fossa. The postinfusion scan demonstrates enhancement of the falx cerebri.

The appearance is that of diffuse cerebral necrosis secondary to anoxia at birth. Biopsy demonstrated necrotic brain tissue.

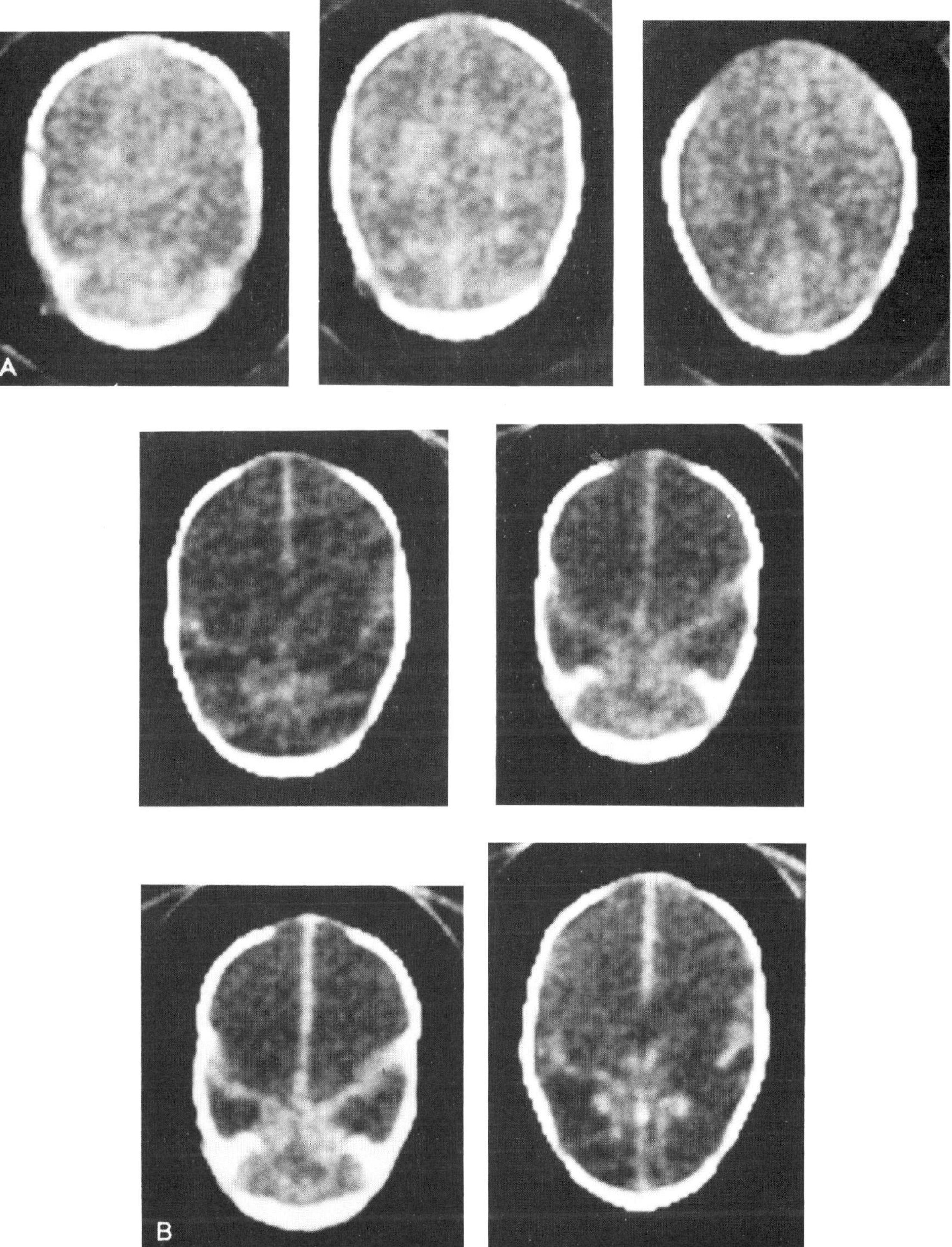

Figure 8–18. *See legend on the opposite page.*

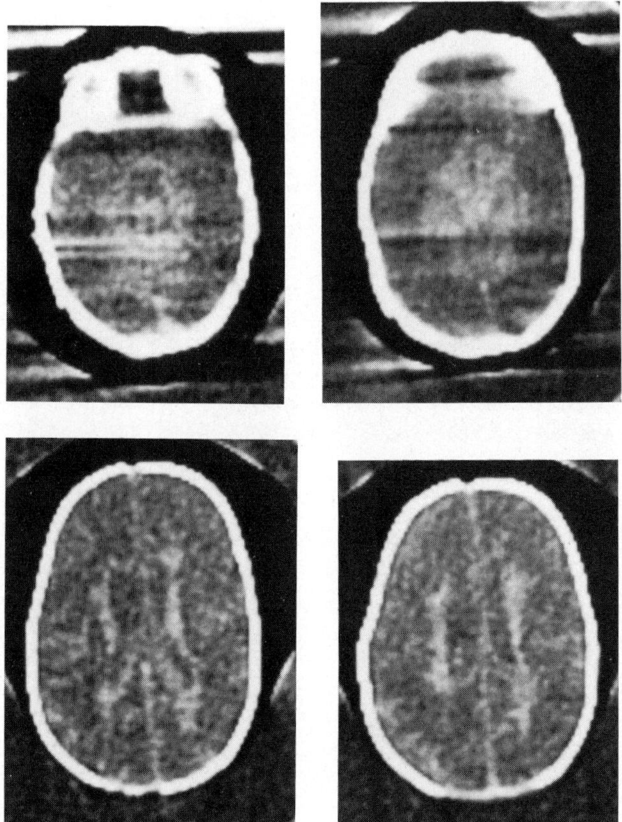

Figure 8–19. CEREBRAL NECROSIS SECONDARY TO ANOXIA: There are diffuse abnormal areas of radiolucency throughout both hemispheres. Small amounts of midline tissue and the structures in the midbrain region have been spared, as has a small amount of tissue in the periventricular region. (Horizontal bands are artifacts of motion.)

CT scan demonstrates varying degrees of abnormality. There may be small to massive areas of lucency, with only small amounts of normal-density brain and compressed lateral ventricles remaining. Not uncommonly, on the CT scan the posterior fossa structures appear to have been spared, and pathologic examination confirms the relative sparing of the cerebellum.

If the infants survive, the appearance on the CT scan following intervals of months to years is that of moderate diffuse cerebral atrophy.

MASSIVE INTRACRANIAL CALCIFICATION

A certain degree of calcification can be seen in the normal individual, particularly in the basal ganglia. These calcifications also may be visible on the plain skull radiographs. Symmetrical calcifications can be seen in a host of other disease processes (see Chapter 2), but occasionally massive symmetrical calcification is demonstrated on the CT scans, as shown in Figure 8–20. The etiology was unknown in this case.

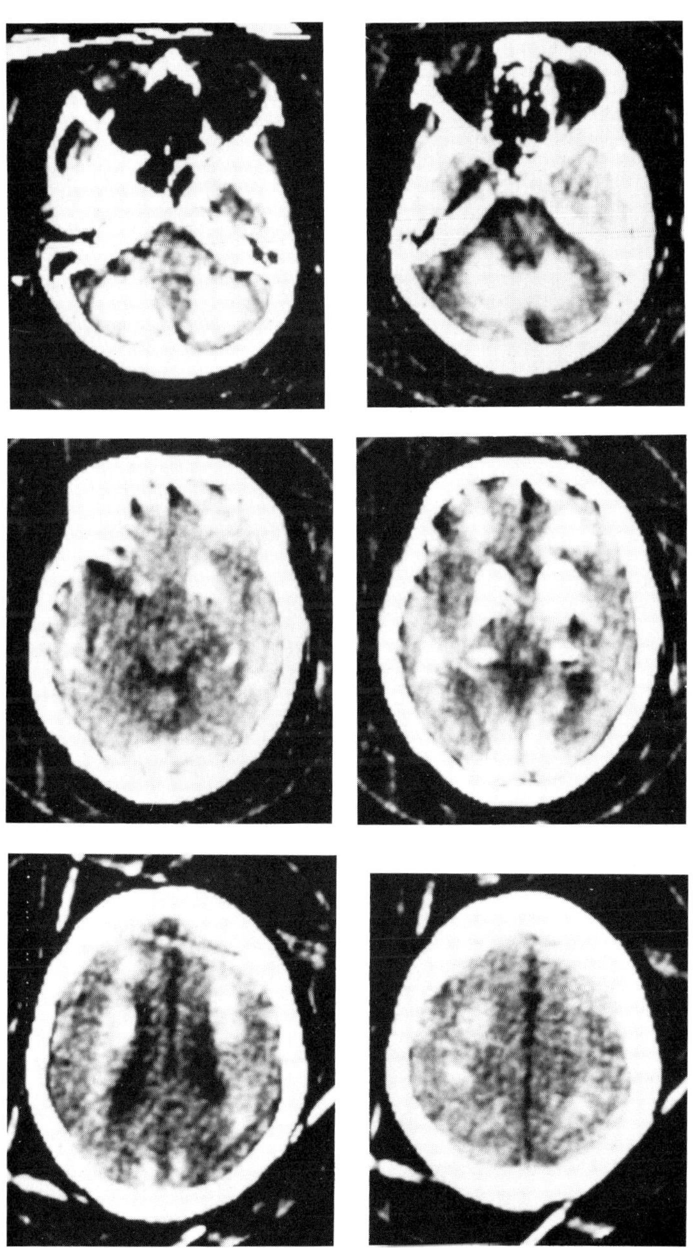

Figure 8–20.

AMPHETAMINE TOXICITY

Drug abuse, particularly the intravenous use of amphetamines, has been shown to create an appearance of intracerebral vascular spasm. The pathophysiology of this change is not precisely understood.

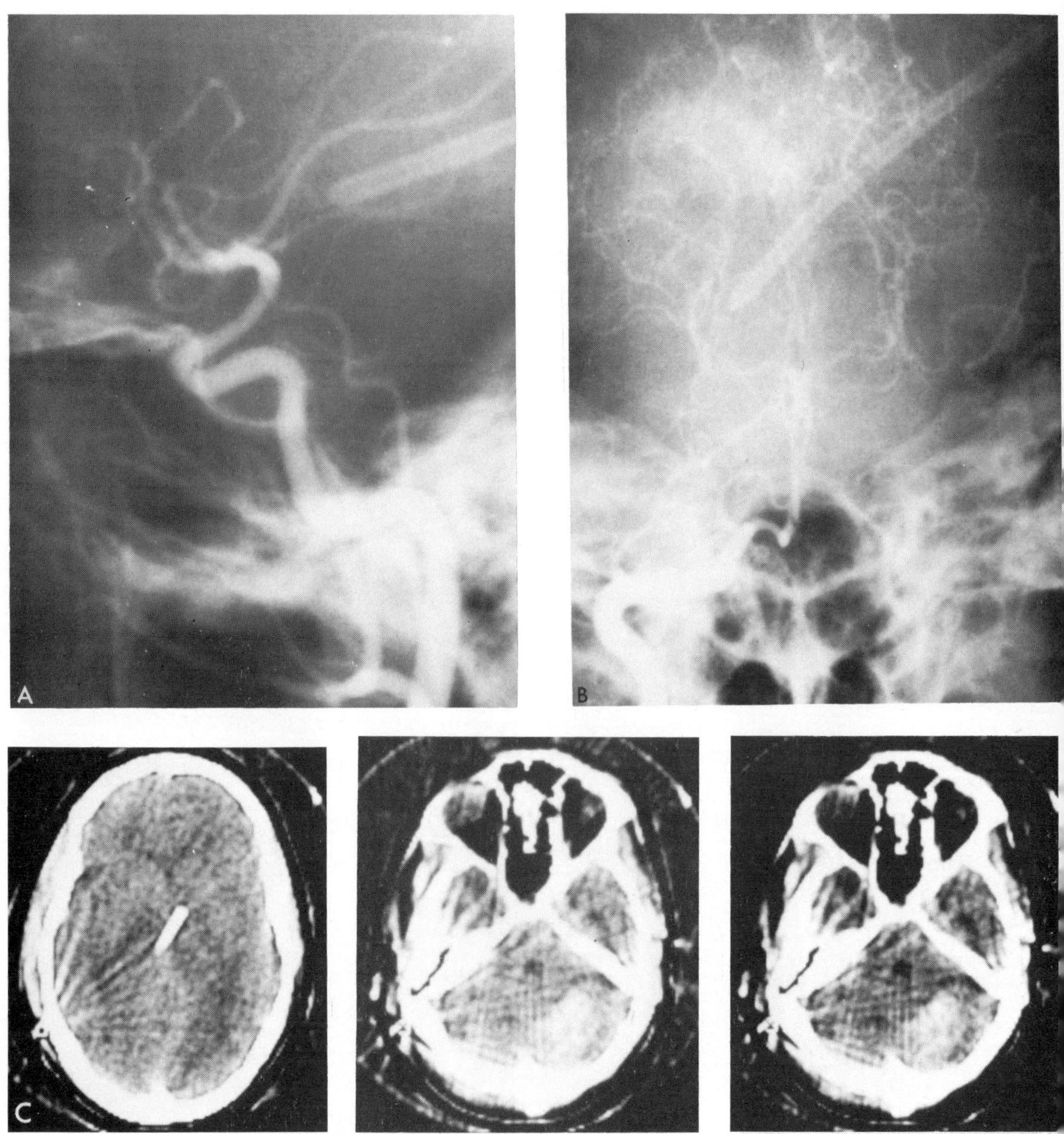

Figdre 8–21. AMPHETAMINE ABUSE: The lateral view of the carotid angiogram *(A)* demonstrates spasm of the supraclinoid portion of the internal carotid artery. The vertebral angiogram *(B)* also shows marked spasm of the vertebral and basilar arteries as well as marked attenuation of all the intracranial branches of the vertebrobasilar system. A shunt tubing device is in place.

C, The CT scan shows the shunt tubing device in place in the lateral ventricles. There are scattered areas of radiolucency, which probably are secondary to infarctions caused by vascular spasm. The low cuts also demonstrate a hematoma in the right cerebellar hemisphere. The etiology of the cerebellar hematoma is unknown.

CHAPTER 9

MENINGIOMAS

Meningiomas are rather unique tumors that arise from the coverings of the brain, the meninges. They are unique in that they may be considered as benign. Meningiomas arise from arachnoid cells imbedded in the dura; consequently, almost all meningiomas have a dural attachment.

Meningiomas can be classified as benign because their *total* removal will result in cure. However, while cure is possible, if the tumor arises in an inaccessible location or if it involves critical structures, total excision often is impossible, resulting in tumor regrowth in its original bed after a varying period of time.

Meningiomas are very rare in the first decade of life. They are seen most commonly in the third to sixth decades. The most common presenting complaint is adult onset of a seizure disorder. Anosmia is a common presenting complaint in patients with a subfrontal meningioma. Older patients may have a history of increasing dementia — particularly those who have frontal meningiomas. With posterior fossa meningiomas, the presenting complaints may be secondary to the patient's obstructive hydrocephalus; there may be nausea and vomiting and ataxia as well as headache. Visual disturbances may develop secondary to medial sphenoid wing, parasellar, diaphragma sella or orbital meningiomas. Exophthalmos also may accompany these orbital meningiomas.

HISTOLOGY

There are three histologic types of meningiomas: (1) endotheliomatous; (2) fibroblastic; (3) angiomatous. Histologic examination of these tumors always reveals arachnoid cells with tonofilament and desmosomes together with a greater or lesser number of collagen fibers. Meningiomas often show whorls of well defined cells and a hyalinized and calcified center; these are termed "psammoma bodies."

PLAIN SKULL CHANGES

Findings very suggestive of meningioma are: (1) "typical" calcification; (2) "typical" vascularity; (3) reactive hyperostosis.

(1) "Typical" calcification implies a well defined area of speckled calcification or even dense calcification in a typical location for a meningioma (see Figs. 9–1, 9–2). This calcification is psammomatous in nature and may be readily demonstrated by CT scanning even when not visible on the plain skull film.

(2) The vascularity seen with meningiomas may be considered "typical" when it reveals enlargement and frequently tortuosity of the grooves of the meningeal arteries as they provide the blood supply to these tumors (see Figs. 9–3, 9–4, 9–5, etc.). The venous grooves may also be enlarged to carry the enlarged veins that drain the tumors.

(3) Reactive hyperostosis is typical of meningioma. The amount of reactive bone does not necessarily correspond to the size of the soft tissue mass. The tumor may extend through the diploë and project into the scalp, creating a palpable mass.

Meningiomas usually are well defined tumors. However, they also may spread along the deeper surface of the dura and tend to invade the overlying bone, resulting in a diffuse homogeneous hyperostosis. These are meningiomas "en plaque."

Meningiomas of the tuberculum sella and planum sphenoidale result in a reactive hyperostosis, causing an appearance of a "blister" of the bone. This blistering is quite typical of meningioma. Rarely, meningiomas cause only bony destruction.

In today's practice meningiomas rarely reach a very large size. With the use of such newer noninvasive techniques as radionuclide scanning and, more recently, computed tomography, meningiomas — and brain tumors in general — are being diagnosed earlier. These bony changes may be apparent only on close inspection of the plain skull films and CT scans of the calvaria. If these changes are mild, their significance may only be appreciated in retrospect after the diagnosis has been established.

In addition, other changes secondary to the meningioma may occur, such as shift of the pineal gland or enlargement or erosions of the sella turcica secondary to long standing increased intracranial pressure (see Fig. 9–1, etc.).

There have been reports of extracranial metastases of meningiomas, usually in patients who have had an operative procedure upon the primary brain tumor.

ANATOMIC LOCATION

There are certain locations where meningiomas are more commonly seen. Although the list of locations is quite substantial, these tumors exhibit a definite preference for some locations over others. Particular areas and their incidence of occurrence are listed below:

Location	*Incidence (%)*
Convexity	50
Sphenoid wing (either medial or lateral position)	40
Parasellar	
Olfactory groove	
Posterior fossa	10
a. From the tentorium (origin may be from either the upper or lower surface)	
b. Cerebellopontine angle	
c. Clivus	

Uncommonly, intraventricular meningiomas occur in and arise from the choroid plexus. These meningiomas do not have a dural attachment.

COMPUTED TOMOGRAPHY

Computed tomography of the brain using contrast enhancement is very helpful and is diagnostic in over 95 per cent of cases of meningiomas.

PREINFUSION

Because meningiomas contain psammomatous calcification, they frequently are visible on the preinfusion scan as an area of increased density. This increased density may be faint, involving the entire bulk of the meningioma, or there may be some increase in density but also multiple scattered areas of punctate or amorphous calcification. In other cases we have seen small areas of calcification within the bulk of the tumor that do not outline the extent of the lesion. In many cases the meningioma is isodense with normal brain substance, and its presence is identified only by mass effect and/or surrounding edema. Meningiomas may be of lower density than normal brain tissue. Rarely, they may be cystic.

Of particular note is the high parasagittal meningioma, which is not seen unless very high cuts are obtained tangentially through the cerebral convexities (see Fig. 9–6). In these cases the edema "below" the meningiomas will be visible before the tumor itself is apparent on the tangential cuts through the convexities.

Edema. The amount of accompanying edema is variable. In some cases there is marked surrounding edema; in others, there is little or none. When edema is present it may be asymmetric in distribution.

Mass. Some cases reveal evidence of the meningioma with surrounding edema and a marked shift to the contralateral side. In other cases, and not uncommonly, the mass is readily visualized but there is little (and in some cases no) shift of the midline structures. It appears in these cases that the tumor grows so slowly that local pressure atrophy of the brain takes place at a rate similar to that of tumor growth — thus, there is no mass effect. In most cases the mass effect is seen to be secondary to a combination of both the tumor mass and the surrounding edema.

POSTINFUSION

Marked homogeneous enhancement of the tumor is usually seen after the infusion of contrast material. If the lesion is incompletely calcified, the true extent of the tumor will become apparent on the postinfusion scan. Meningiomas that are isodense with brain tissue are readily demonstrated on the postinfusion examination, and full appreciation of both the tumor and the surrounding edema is possible. Rarely, meningiomas may show a "ring" of enhancement. This ring is much more common with gliomas.

Findings of increased density of the tumor combined with a typical location, surrounding edema and homogeneous enhancement are pathognomonic of many cases of meningioma.

Skull Changes with CT

When a meningioma has invaded the bony calvaria at its point of origin or when there is reactive hyperostosis, it is necessary to examine the bony calvaria closely. In fact, it is recommended that in every case of suspected meningioma a thorough inspection of the calvaria be done. Review of the areas of bony density should be performed at standard-window width and window level. Following this, the examination should be continued with the unit on the lowest window width, and the window level should be varied to allow accurate examination of the bone. Examination should also be performed when the window width is very high — 400 — and at varying window levels. Bony changes may become apparent only after this type of inspection of the CT scan with varying window widths and window levels. The CT findings will correlate with the plain skull films, but subtle changes may be more apparent on the CT scan.

VASCULAR SUPPLY

Most commonly, meningiomas take their blood supply from the meninges. This vascular supply may derive from any of the blood vessels that normally serve the coverings of the brain. The internal maxillary artery, one of the branches of the external carotid artery, in turn gives rise to the middle meningeal artery. From its origin from the internal maxillary artery, the middle meningeal artery courses laterally and slightly anteriorly below the base of the skull until it enters and passes through the foramen spinosum. The vessel then turns laterally to lie in a groove in the inner table of the skull — the middle meningeal artery groove (see Fig. 9–6). This groove is not seen in children; it develops with age, and normally is apparent only in adults. The middle meningeal artery bifurcates most commonly into two main divisions — the anterior and posterior branches. The anterior branch ascends in a groove at or near the coronal suture. The posterior branch runs posterosuperiorly in the squamosal portion of the temporal bone; because of its very straight course, it may simulate a fracture.

Although most meningiomas receive their blood supply from the external carotid circulation, falx meningiomas and parasagittal meningiomas may be supplied by the terminal portion of the pericallosal artery or terminal branches of the middle cerebral artery. Because the blood supply is usually from the external carotid artery, it is often quite helpful to perform a selective external carotid arteriogram to achieve better definition of the area of tumor involvement. It also may be desirable to perform a selective internal carotid arteriogram or a common carotid arteriogram so that the relationship between the two circulations can be evaluated independently. With common carotid arteriography the overlap between the internal and external carotid circulations may make it difficult to evaluate the area of tumor involvement as accurately as with the selective external carotid injection. When using the femoral approach and the catheter technique, the external carotid artery can be selectively catheterized in a large majority of cases. Under fluoroscopic control, the catheter is placed in the common carotid artery and then slowly advanced until its tip reaches the external carotid. In most cases, the external carotid artery courses anteriorly and medially relative to the internal carotid at the level of the bifurcation. Because of this, the curved tip of the catheter should be directed anteriorly and medially to facilitate correct placement. The use of a guidewire can help in selective catheterization. The wire may be introduced into the external carotid and the catheter then advanced over the wire until it rests in the vessel. At this time, a test dose of contrast material should be instilled under fluoroscopic control to confirm the positioning in the external carotid artery. During visualization of the branches of the external carotid artery, the patient will experience a good deal of discomfort from the injection because the contrast flows to the mucosal surface of the oral cavity. To achieve patient cooperation, a preliminary warning of this discomfort should be given before the examination.

This manipulation of the external carotid artery and contrast injection may result in localized spasm of the artery at the time of arteriography. If spasm should occur, there will be poor filling of the external carotid circulation and "wash-out" of the contrast material down into the internal and common carotid systems. When this problem does not occur, the examination can be facilitated by the fact that the external carotid system often is enlarged if a meningioma is present. Similarly, an enlarged foramen spinosum should be looked for in any patient with a suspected meningioma. This foramen is readily visualized on the submentovertex view of the skull. It should also be noted that normal variations in the size of the foramen spinosum occur; therefore, the presence of an enlarged foramen or a variation in its size is not absolute proof of meningioma — only further confirmatory evidence.

If a percutaneous arteriogram has been performed, it sometimes is possible to catheterize the external carotid artery selectively by elevating the tip of the needle and advancing the needle forward into the vessel. Successful catheterization of the external carotid artery will be confirmed when a test injection elicits a feeling of pain and burning in the patient's teeth and tongue. It is also possible to use a short wire and Davis needle (see Chapter 4) manipulated in the neck to provide more exact control of needle tip placement. With this method, a short wire is passed through the needle in the carotid artery and well beyond the tip of the needle into the carotid artery. Firm pressure is then applied to the carotid artery at, above and below the puncture site. The needle is then removed and the wire left in place. Then, under fluoroscopic control, the Davis polyethylene catheter needle is advanced over the wire that is resting in the carotid artery (a technique is similar to the standard Seldinger technique). After the Davis needle has been inserted through the wall of the vessel and into the arterial lumen, the guidewire is removed. The in-dwelling Davis needle can then be occluded with a firm inner cannula or hooked to a flushing device. Again under fluoroscopic control, contrast material can be injected; the tip of the pliable Davis needle can then be positioned in the external carotid artery. Although standard fluoroscopy in the anteroposterior direction can be used, it is advantageous to use lateral fluoroscopy if it is available. This method is particularly helpful in older patients with peripheral vascular disease where femoral catheterization is impossible, or in those cases where a previously unsuspected meningioma is discovered at the time of carotid arteriography.

In patients with arteriosclerotic changes involving the carotid bifurcation with narrowing of the vessel lumen particular care must be taken that the narrowed lumen is not occluded by the needle or catheter.

Because these tumors originate from the meninges, arteriography will reveal changes secondary to an extracerebral mass lesion. In the case of a supratentorial meningioma, the routine common carotid arteriogram reveals that the cerebral convexity blood vessels fail to reach the inner table of the skull because of the presence of the tumor over the convexity of the brain (see Fig. 9–2). Instead, the vessels will be seen to course around the mass lesion and to be "draped" over the mass rather than separated by it. This change is readily apparent in the presence of a sphenoid wing meningioma, where the tumor is visible in the AP projection as a mass with medial displacement of the vessels of the middle cerebral artery away from the inner table of the skull (see Fig. 9–10).

Often one can also see the enlarged middle meningeal vessel as it feeds the tumor. The lateral view is also quite characteristic in this case, frequently demonstrating the typical blush of the meningioma.

Commonly, the stain of the meningioma has a "sunburst" pattern. With this appearance it will be seen that the meningeal vessel feeding the tumor is enlarged and tortuous; upon reaching the tumor itself it branches into myriad very tiny vessels that appear to begin at a central point and to branch out in a sunburst pattern (see Figs. 9–10 and 9–13).

The blush seen with meningioma often is described as "cloudlike" (Fig. 9–5) because of its dense appearance, which persists into the venous phase. This cloudlike blush is to be distinguished from that of glioblastoma multiforme, in which the tumor blush appears quite early but then fades quickly as it is washed out by unopacified blood. Multiple early draining veins can be seen with meningioma, but this finding is not common.

PARIETAL CONVEXITY MENINGIOMA

The classic parasagittal meningioma presents a typical arteriographic picture. In these cases, however, it is unlikely that the radionuclide scan and the computed tomogram will not have strongly suggested the diagnosis before arteriography. The carotid arteriogram reveals downward displacement of the sylvian triangle by the suprasylvian mass and displacement of the branches of the anterior cerebral and middle cerebral artery away from the inner table of the skull. The middle meningeal artery will be seen to be enlarged and to become even larger and more tortuous in its distal segment. In many cases the distal meningeal vessels will develop a "corkscrew" appearance. The tumor itself demonstrates the typical sunburst pattern of vascularity, with vessels radiating out from the center of the tumor. The typical cloudlike blush remains throughout the venous phase of the arteriogram (see Figs. 9–12 and 9–13). When this very typical pattern is seen it is safe to make a diagnosis of meningioma.

Parasagittal convexity meningiomas frequently invade the superior sagittal sinus. If this is the case, the venous phase of the arteriogram will demonstrate absence of filling of the sinus at the level of the meningioma. This may be better demonstrated by using subtraction techniques. This invasion of the superior sagittal sinus makes surgical removal more difficult.

MENINGIOMAS OF THE ANTERIOR CRANIAL FOSSA

Olfactory groove and other subfrontal meningiomas and meningiomas of the anterior cranial fossa are common. When an anterior cranial fossa meningioma is present, one can frequently identify an enlarged anterior falx artery or an enlarged anterior meningeal artery. This vessel enters the cranial vault through the cribriform plate. Like other abnormal meningeal vessels, this one will be seen to become enlarged, tortuous and to demonstrate a "corkscrew" appearance. This anterior falx or anterior meningeal artery may be noted in many normal arteriograms, but it is seen more frequently when there is enlargement secondary to a meningioma. The enlargement of the anterior meningeal artery as it arises from the ophthalmic artery is not always readily appreciated and should be specifically looked for when a meningioma of the anterior cranial fossa is suspected.

On occasion myriad small meningeal vessels may be seen to arise from an enlarged ophthalmic artery and to supply the tumor in the subfrontal area. These small vessels enter the cranial vault through the cribriform plate.

In addition to the standard arteriogram, magnification views and subtraction techniques will make possible a better evaluation of the vascular supply to the tumor and the extent of the tumor mass. The typical "cloudlike" blush seen with meningiomas in other locations is also seen with these tumors.

Olfactory groove meningiomas and other subfrontal meningiomas produce backward displacement of the pericallosal artery and the vessels that supply the frontal lobes. The pattern of vessel displacement is that of an extracerebral mass lesion. The anterior cerebral artery vessels will be seen to be displaced up and away from the orbital roofs, frequently outlining the tumor location (see Fig. 9–8).

The typical "cloudlike" blush will be seen in the subfrontal area. Subfrontal and olfactory groove meningiomas often rest close to the midline of the cranial vault; consequently, there may be little if any shift of the anterior cerebral and pericallosal arteries across the midline. This finding is also consistent with any extracerebral mass lesion, whereas mass lesions within the frontal lobe shift the anterior cerebral artery and its branches across the midline.

Meningiomas of the planum sphenoidale typically promote hyperostosis of the bone, causing a "blistered" appearance.

Tumors of the "clinically silent" areas — such as the frontal region — may be quite sizable when first examined.

PARASELLAR AND SUPRASELLAR MENINGIOMAS

Parasellar meningiomas are not uncommon and are frequently supplied by myriad small meningeal vessels that arise from the cavernous portion of the carotid. There may also be hypertrophy of the meningohypophyseal trunk as it arises from the internal carotid at the entrance of the cavernous sinus. Depending upon the location of the tumor, there may be opening or closing of the carotid siphon; there may be medial or lateral displacement of the cavernous and supraclinoid portions of the internal carotid artery.

Magnification and use of subtraction techniques allow better demonstration of the vascular supply and the typical blush of the meningioma.

Meningiomas also may originate from the diaphragma sellae. Their blood supply is similar to that noted above (see Fig. 9–13).

TENTORIAL AND POSTERIOR FOSSA MENINGIOMAS

When meningiomas of the posterior fossa are present, there will frequently be an enlarged posterior meningeal artery arising from the vertebral artery at the level of the entrance of the vertebral artery into the cranial vault through the foramen magnum. In addition, with tentorial meningiomas and some other posterior fossa meningiomas—particularly those that originate from the clivus or cerebellopontine angle — one may see an enlarged tentorial artery. The tentorial artery, also known as the artery of Bernasconi and Cassonari, originates from the internal carotid artery at the level of its entrance into the cavernous sinus. It should be noted that the vessel is present normally, but that it becomes enlarged in the presence of a tumor or arteriovenous malformation that arises from the meninges. As the name implies, this small blood vessel is one of the sources of supply to the meninges and can be seen normally—particularly when lateral magnification technique is used. The meningohypophyseal trunk arises from the internal carotid artery just at the level of its entrance into the cavernous sinus; it may also supply a posterior fossa meningioma or give rise to the tentorial artery.

In the presence of a posterior fossa meningioma, the tentorial artery becomes enlarged and tortuous to supply the tumor, producing the typical sunburst and/or cloudlike blush seen with meningiomas in the supratentorial compartment. The presence of such a vessel strongly suggests the possibility of a meningioma (see Fig. 9–16).

Note: The persistent trigeminal artery also has its origin from the internal carotid artery at this point, and a small trigeminal artery may resemble the tentorial artery.

Posterior fossa meningiomas may cause obstructive hydrocephalus. Cerebellopontine angle meningiomas present clinically with a cerebellopontine angle syndrome, but usually with little or no hearing loss.

ORBITAL MENINGIOMAS

Intraorbital meningiomas are occasionally seen. They may arise intracranially or from within the orbit from the dural extension of the meninges that follows the optic nerve into the orbit. They may or may not cause exophthalmos, and usually there is interference with vision. Plain film examination may reveal reactive hyperostosis around the optic canal. Orbital meningiomas are well demonstrated by computed tomography (see Chapter 15), but do not present pathognomonic findings.

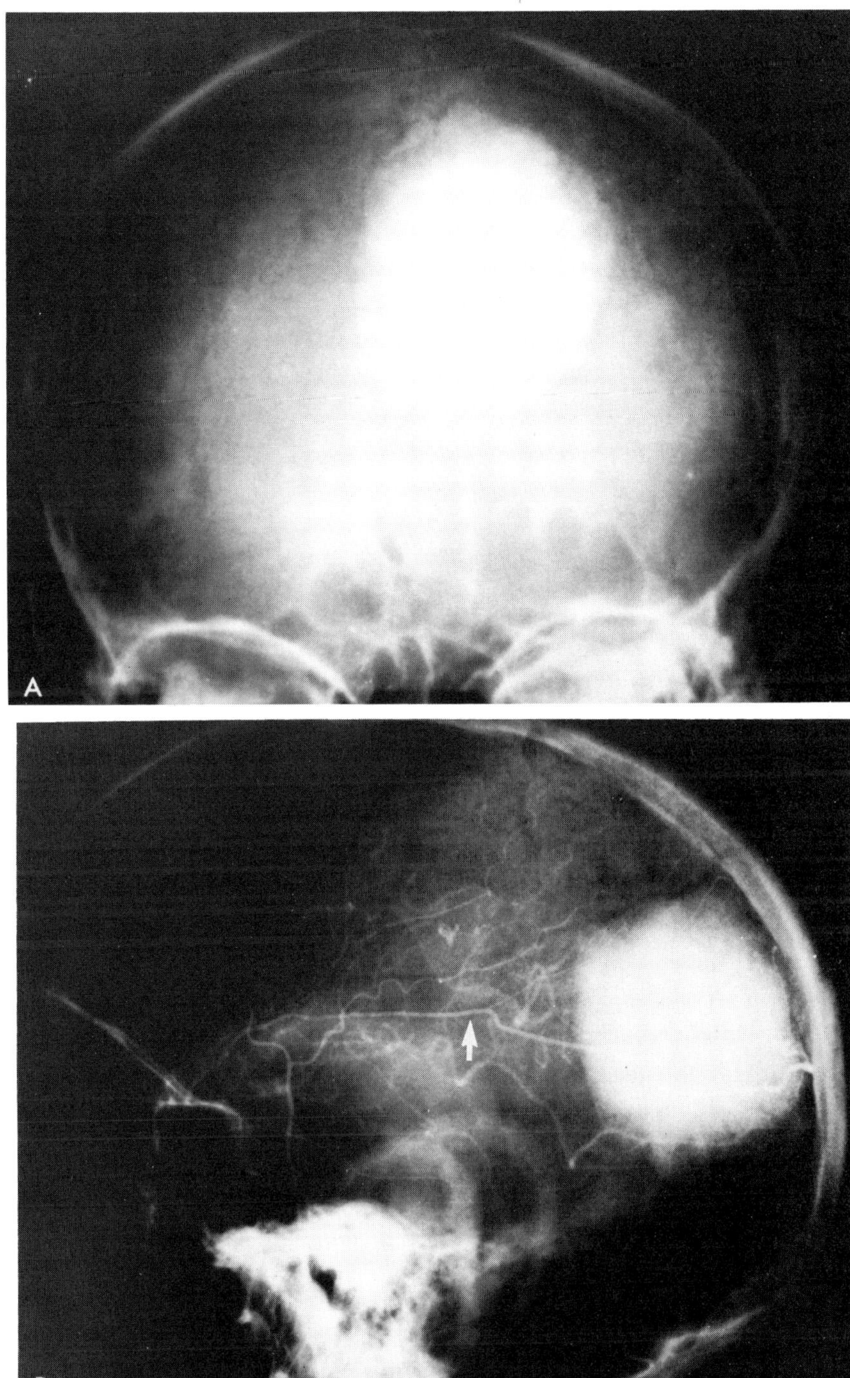

Figure 9–1. DENSELY CALCIFIED FALX MENINGIOMA: *A,* This patient has a densely calcified meningioma that appears to arise from the falx cerebri posteriorly. The tumor rests just above the level of the tentorium and extends on either side of the falx — but mainly off to the left side. Because of pressure atrophy of the adjacent brain tissues from these slow growing tumors, only a small amount of mass effect may be noted arteriographically.

B, The selective external carotid arteriogram shows the posterior branch of the middle meningeal artery (*white arrow*) as it courses posteriorly. It becomes enlarged distally and provides the blood supply to the meningioma. (Case courtesy of Dr. Robert Chandley.)

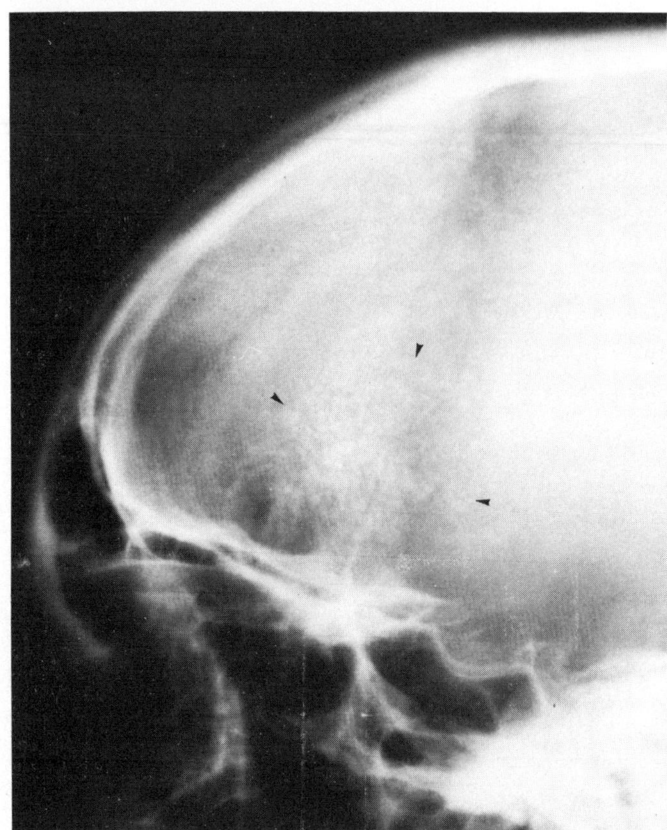

Figure 9–2. CALCIFIED SUBFRONTAL MENINGIOMA: The small black arrows outline the fine amorphous calcification of the subfrontal meningioma. Note the reactive hyperostosis of the planum sphenoidale beneath the meningioma. Also note the truncation of the dorsum sellae and posterior clinoids secondary to nonspecific changes of increased intracranial pressure. This is a very classic appearance of a meningioma.

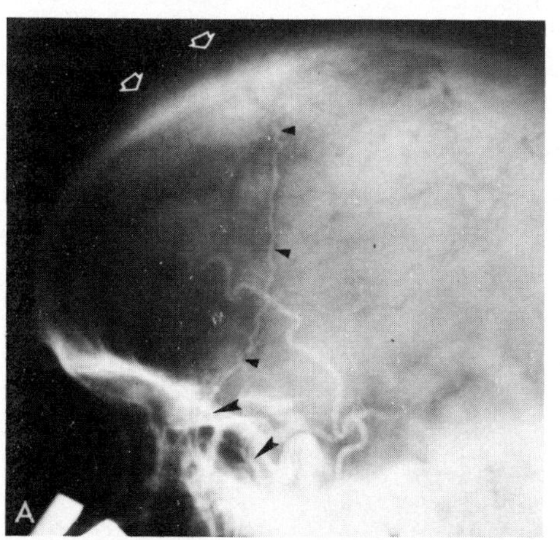

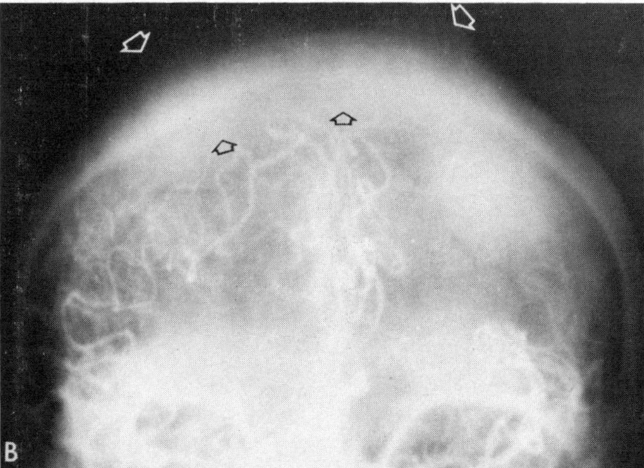

Figure 9–3. LARGE FRONTAL MENINGIOMA WITH SPECTACULAR REACTIVE HYPEROSTOSIS: Marked hyperostosis of the frontal bone extends across the midline and through the outer table of the skull (*open white arrows*).

A, The lateral view of the selective external carotid arteriogram reveals an enlarged and tortuous middle meningeal artery (*black arrows*) coursing superiorly to feed the meningioma.

B, The AP view of the internal carotid arteriogram performed with cross compression reveals the displacement away from the inner table of the skull caused by the mass of the tumor (*open black arrows*). This type of extensive hyperostosis secondary to meningioma is seldom seen in today's practice. (Courtesy of Dr. G. Dobben and O. Sugar of the University of Illinois.)

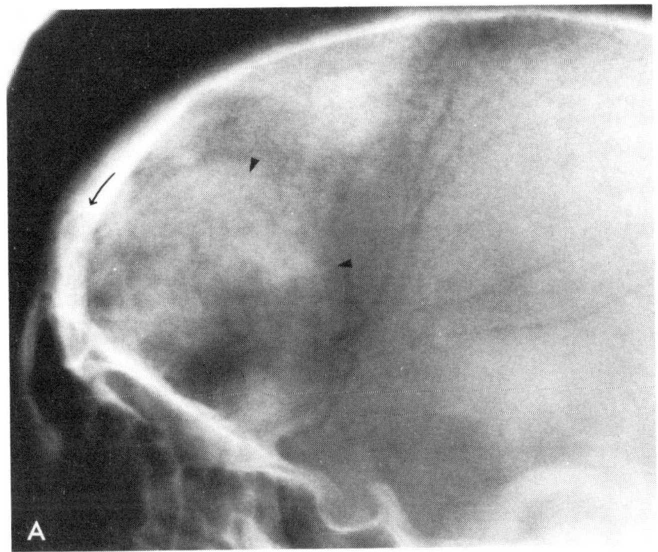

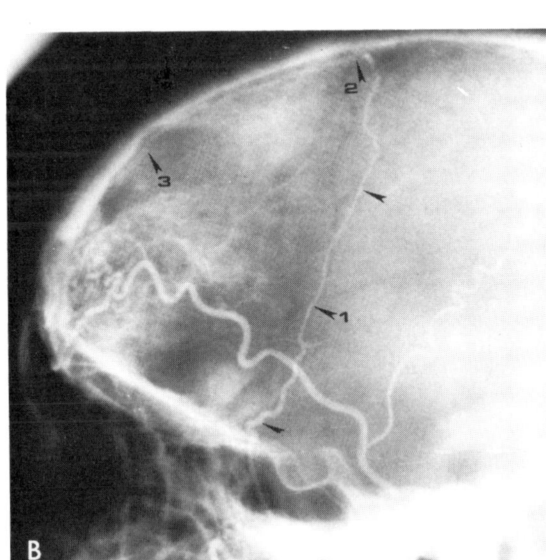

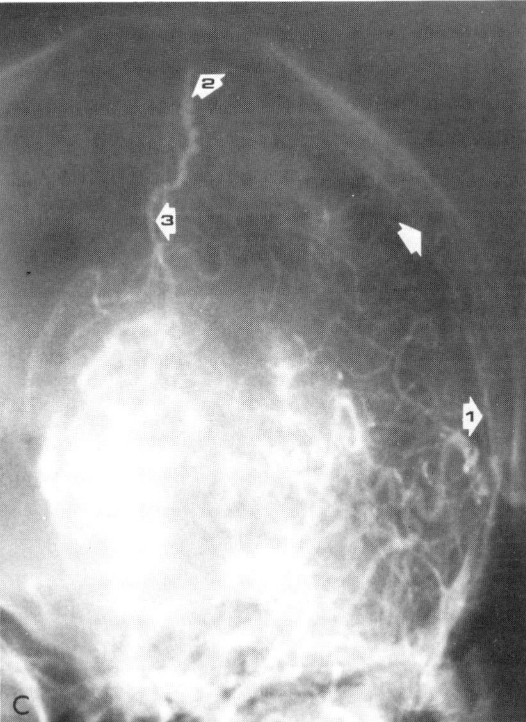

Figure 9–4. SUBFRONTAL MENINGIOMA WITH EARLY DRAINING VEINS: *A*, The lateral skull radiograph shows faint calcification of the large subfrontal meningioma *(small arrowheads)*. There is a small local area of bony destruction (*long arrow*) of the frontal bone just above the frontal sinus.

B, The selective external carotid arteriogram demonstrates the enlarged middle meningeal artery, which becomes more prominent as it goes superiorly and then makes a right-angle turn and courses anteroinferiorly to supply the meningioma. The corresponding points of the middle meningeal artery are numbered on the AP and lateral views. The large tortuous vessel is an enlarged branch of the superficial temporal artery, which also supplies the tumor where it invades the cranial vault.

C, The AP view of the common carotid arteriogram reveals a large area of tumor staining, which extends across the midline. Multiple small early draining views also are present. The course of the middle meningeal artery is numbered to correlate with *B*.

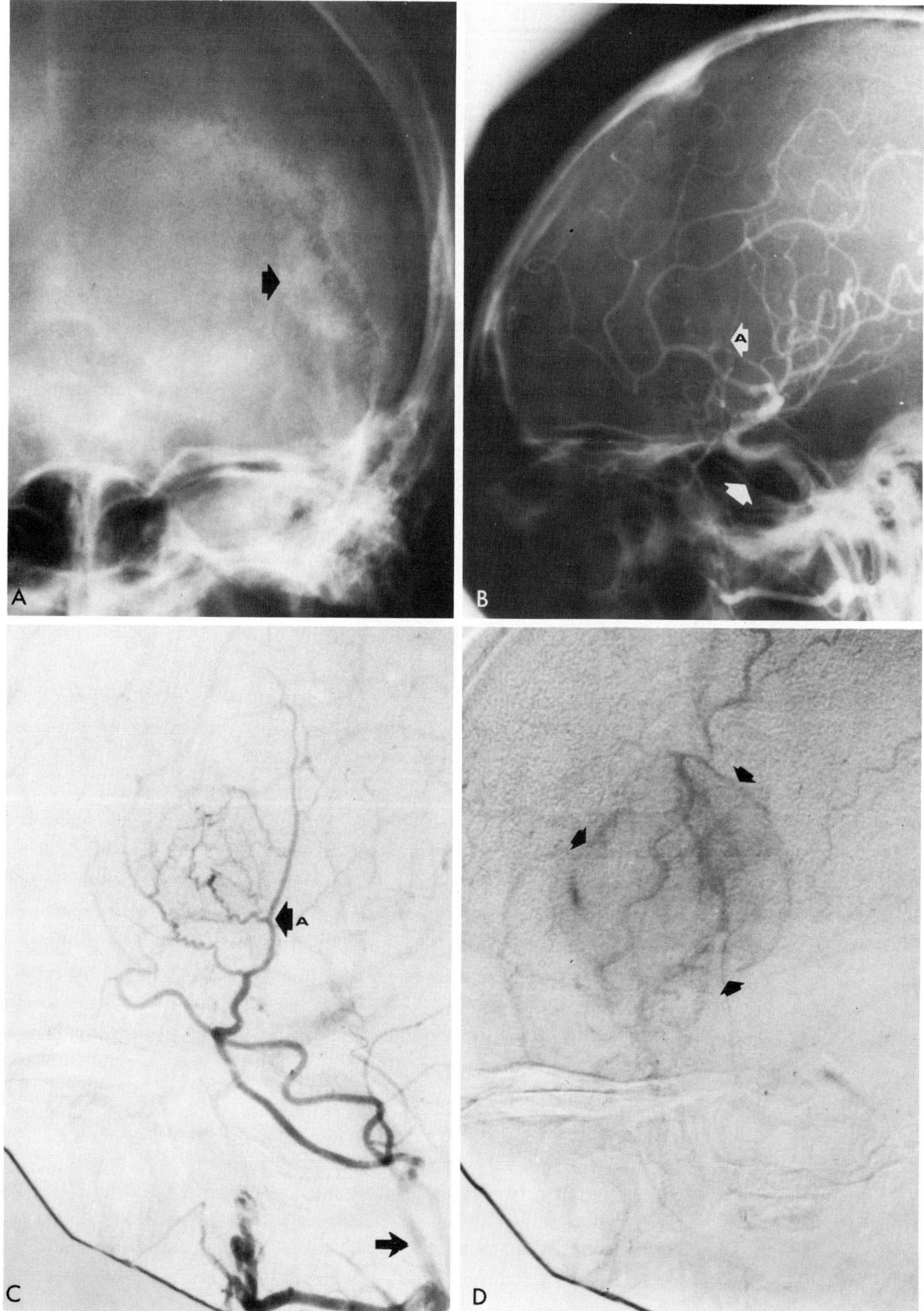

Figure 9–5. *See legend on the opposite page.*

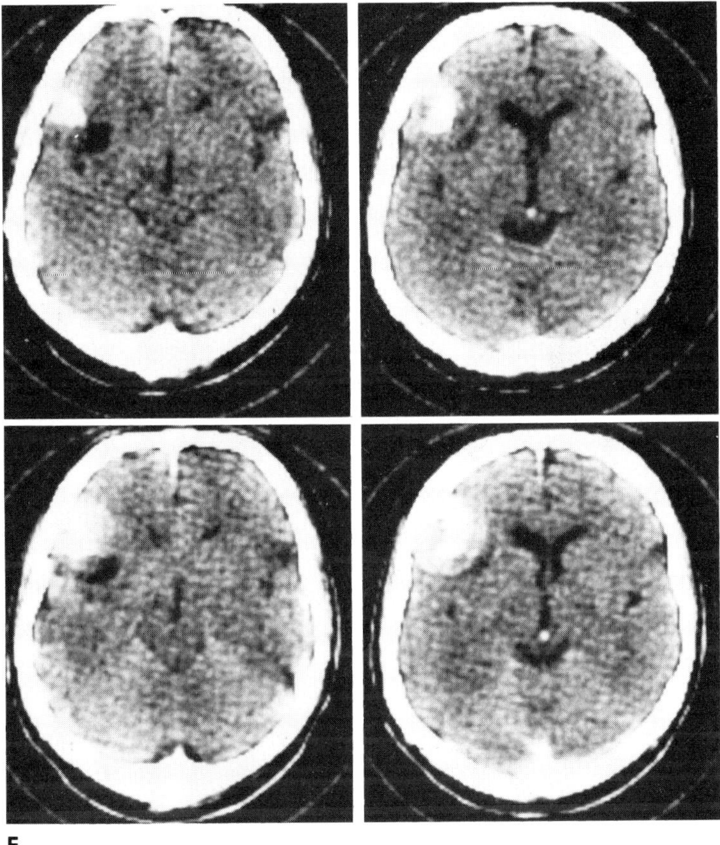

E

Figure 9–5. POSTERIOR FRONTAL MENINGIOMA: *A*, the AP skull radiograph reveals a calcified tumor that projects deep in the cerebral substance (*black arrow*). The tumor actually lies adjacent to the inner table of the calvaria; however, because of the narrow width of the frontal region relative to the biparietal diameter, it appears to lie deep in the brain.

B, The lateral view of the common carotid arteriogram demonstrates stretching of the branches of the middle cerebral artery in the region of the anterior aspect of the sylvian triangle. An enlarged meningeal vessel (*white arrows* and Point "A") courses toward the area of calcification. The unlettered arrow indicates the more proximal point of the vessel.

C and *D*, The selective external carotid arteriogram with subtraction technique better demonstrates this meningeal vessel (*large black arrow*). The smaller arrowhead (Point "A") shows the meningeal vessel at a point similar to that shown in Figure 9–5, *B*. There are multiple small corkscrew vessels which supply the tumor. The venous phase (*D*) demonstrates the "cloudlike blush" (*black arrows*) so typical of meningioma.

E, The preinfusion scan (*upper*) shows a densely calcified mass adjacent to the inner table of the skull in the posterior frontal region on the left side. Postinfusion (*lower*) this is surrounded by an area of enhancement, which reveals that the extent of the tumor is actually larger than the calcified portion of the mass.

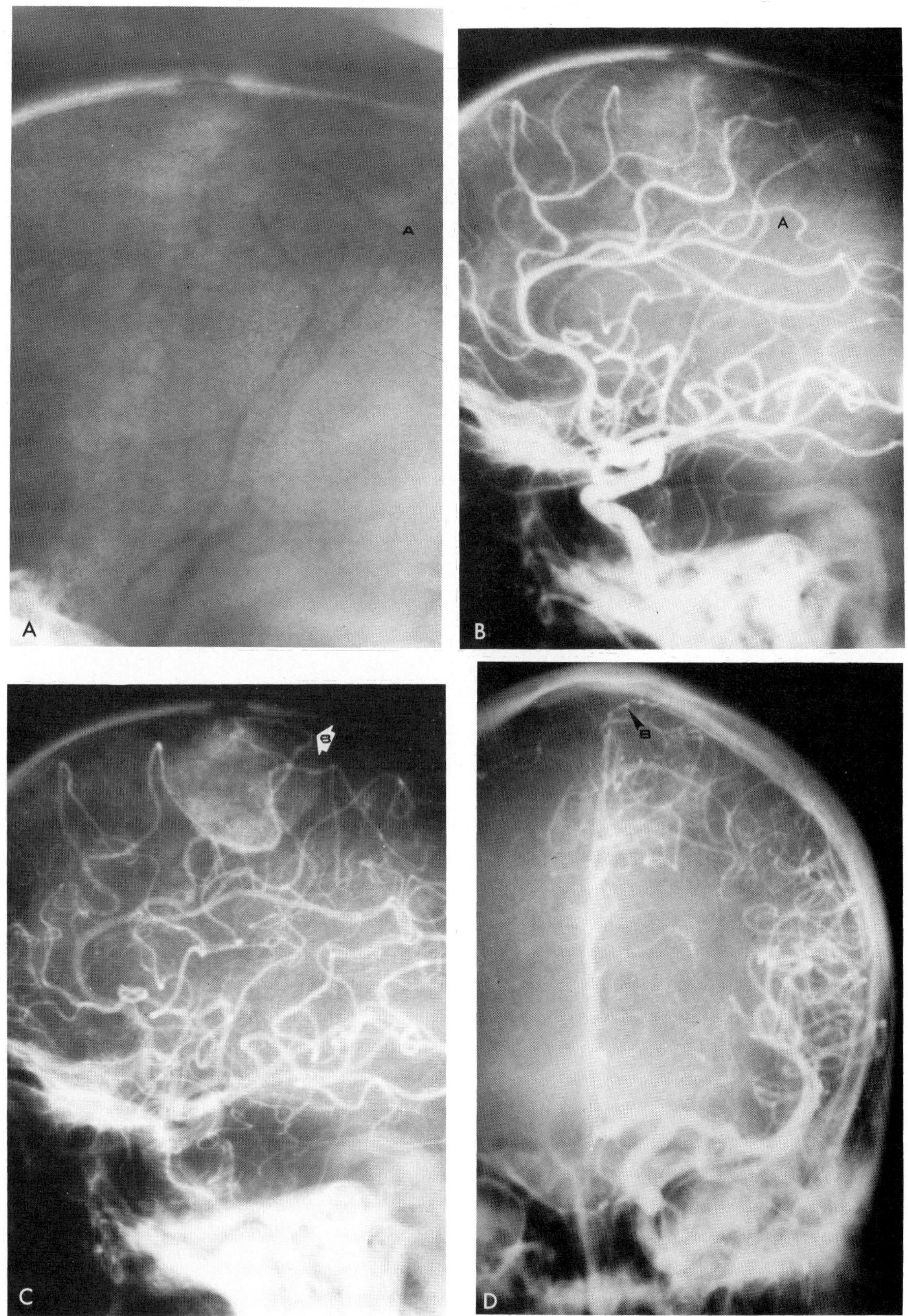

Figure 9–6. *See legend on the opposite page.*

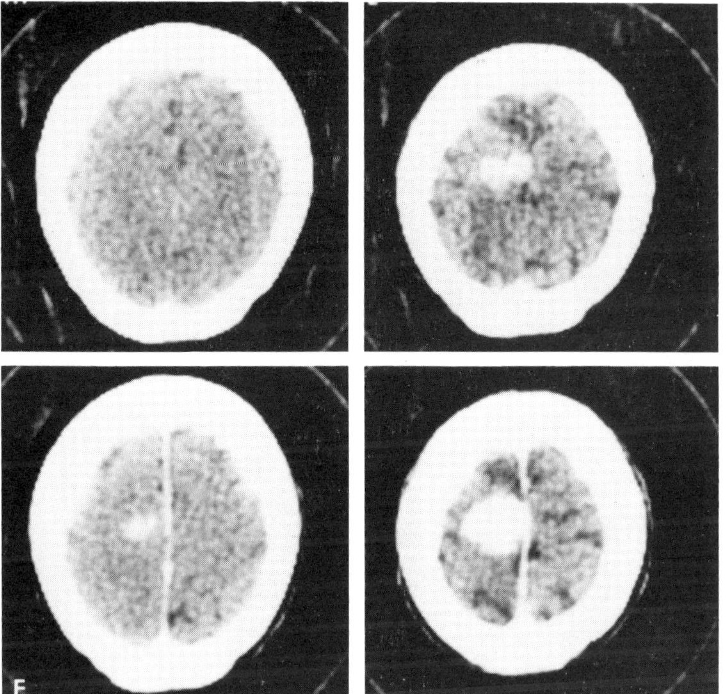

Figure 9–6. PARASAGITTAL MENINGIOMA: *A*, The skull radiograph shows enlargement of both middle meningeal artery grooves. Point "A" marks a bend in the middle meningeal artery. (This point is also marked on the common carotid arteriogram.) Similar changes were noted on the contralateral side. Note the small area of bony erosion along the inner table of the skull just anterior to the coronal suture above the meningioma.

B, The common carotid arteriogram reveals the prominent middle meningeal artery and the very early staining of the meningioma, which is better demonstrated on the later arterial film, *C*.

C, the white arrow and the "B" indicate the turn of the middle meningeal artery. This is also well demonstrated on the AP view, *D*.

E, Preinfusion CT scans reveal a small bilobed area of calcification in the left parasagittal area. Postinfusion, there is homogeneous enhancement of the meningioma. Note that the tumor is larger than the area of calcification. (This is not the same case demonstrated in the arteriogram.)

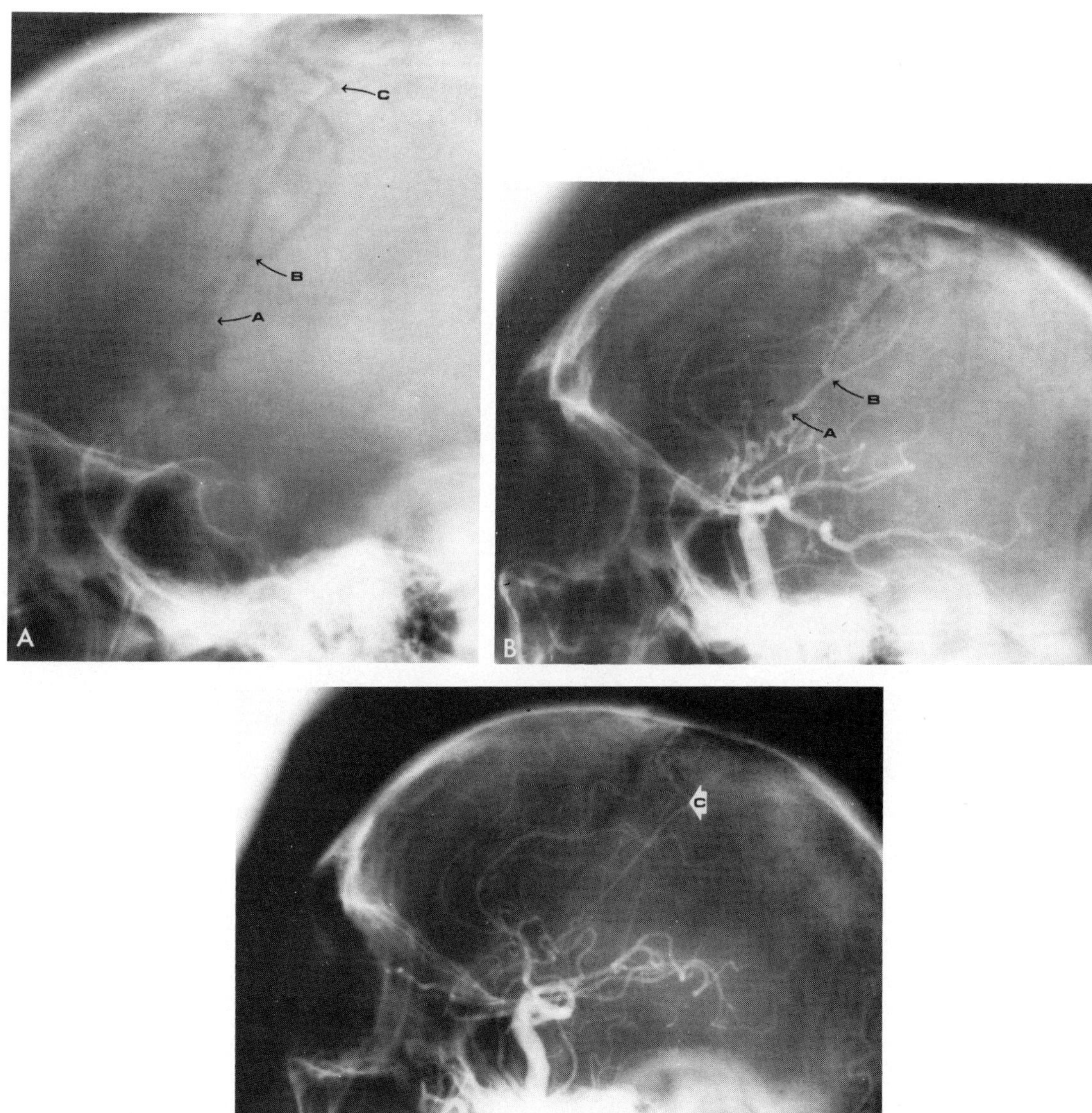

Figure 9–7. PARASAGITTAL MENINGIOMA: The skull radiograph reveals tortuosity and enlargement of the middle meningeal artery grooves bilaterally (Point "B").

B, On the arteriogram, "A" and "B" mark two points along the course of one of the middle meningeal arteries. Note the unusual course of the internal carotid artery at the level of the cavernous sinus. This is a normal anatomic variation.

C, Point "C" marks the curve of the contralateral meningeal artery as it runs in its groove on the opposite side.

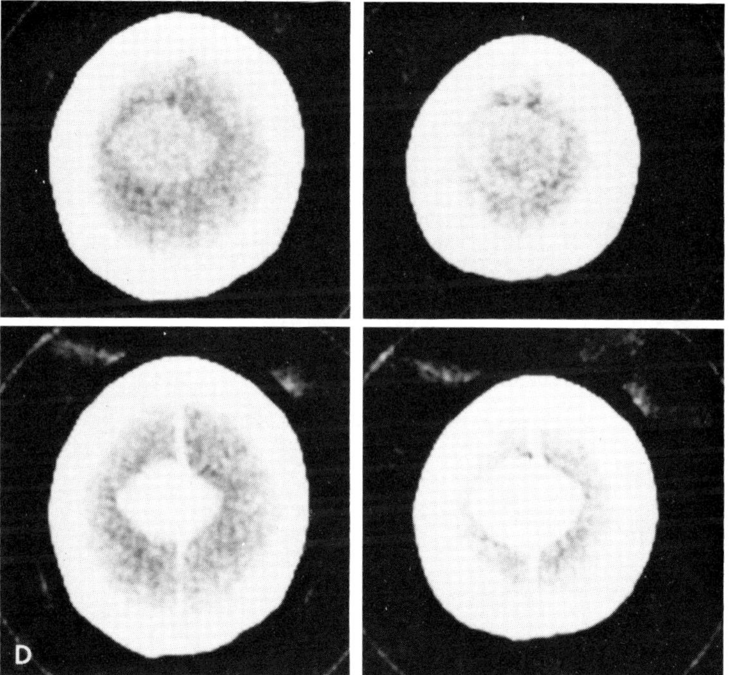

Figure 9–7 *Continued.*

D, The preinfusion CT scan *(upper row)* reveals a dense parasagittal tumor mass that is larger on the left side. The postinfusion scan shows typical dense homogeneous enhancement of the parasagittal meningioma. Invasion of the superior sagittal sinus occurs frequently in high parasagittal convexity meningiomas.

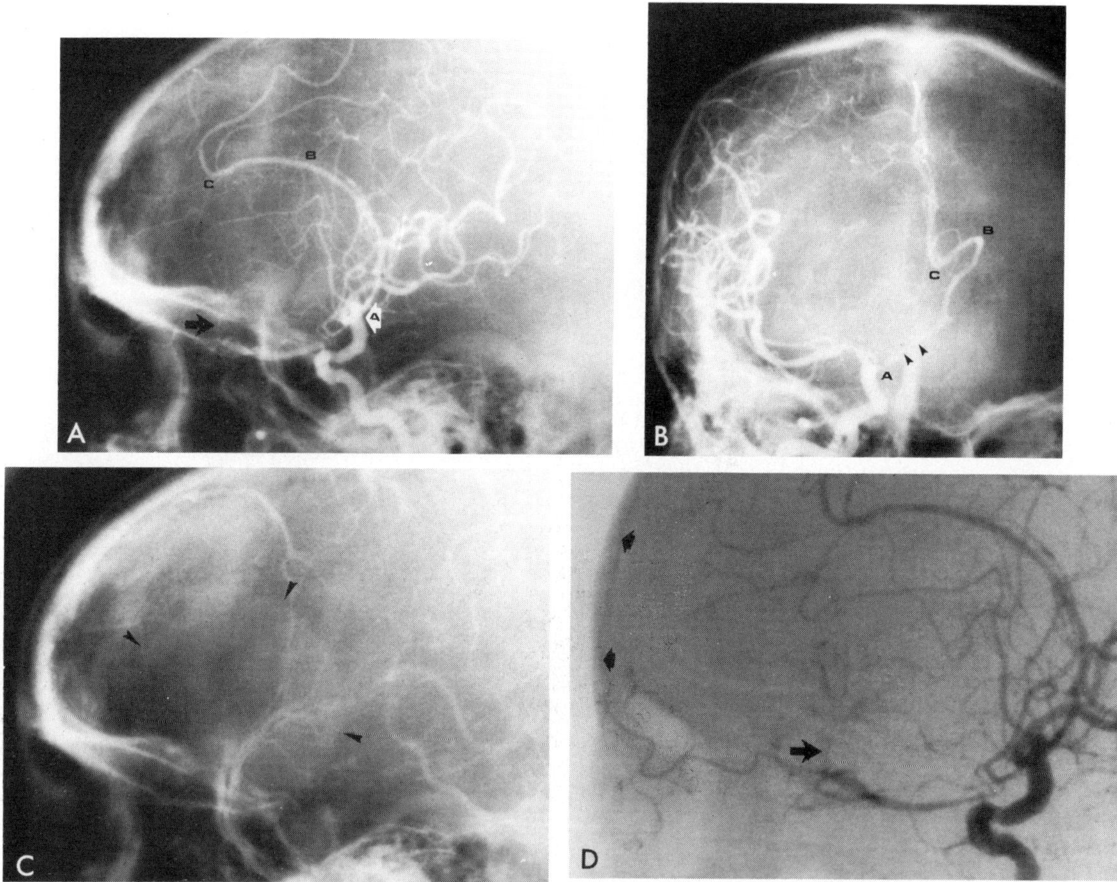

Figure 9–8. SUBFRONTAL MENINGIOMA: *A* and *B*, The lateral and AP views of the selective internal carotid arteriogram reveal marked posterior displacement of the anterior cerebral artery, which is also bowed upward and around a large mass positioned below the frontal lobes bilaterally. The corresponding points of the anterior cerebral artery are marked on both the AP and lateral views. The small arrowheads in *B* identify the irregularly narrowed horizontal portion of the anterior cerebral artery—perhaps secondary to encasement by tumor. The AP view also reveals a shift toward the left side, demonstrating that the tumor is larger on the right side.

C, There is a homogeneous stain that remains well into the venous phase (*arrows*).

D, The subtraction view demonstrates the enlarged ophthalmic artery and the treelike branch that courses directly upward through the cribriform plate to provide blood supply to the tumor (*large arrow*). A large anterior meningeal artery also arises from the terminal portion of the ophthalmic artery and courses along the inner table of the skull (*small arrows*).

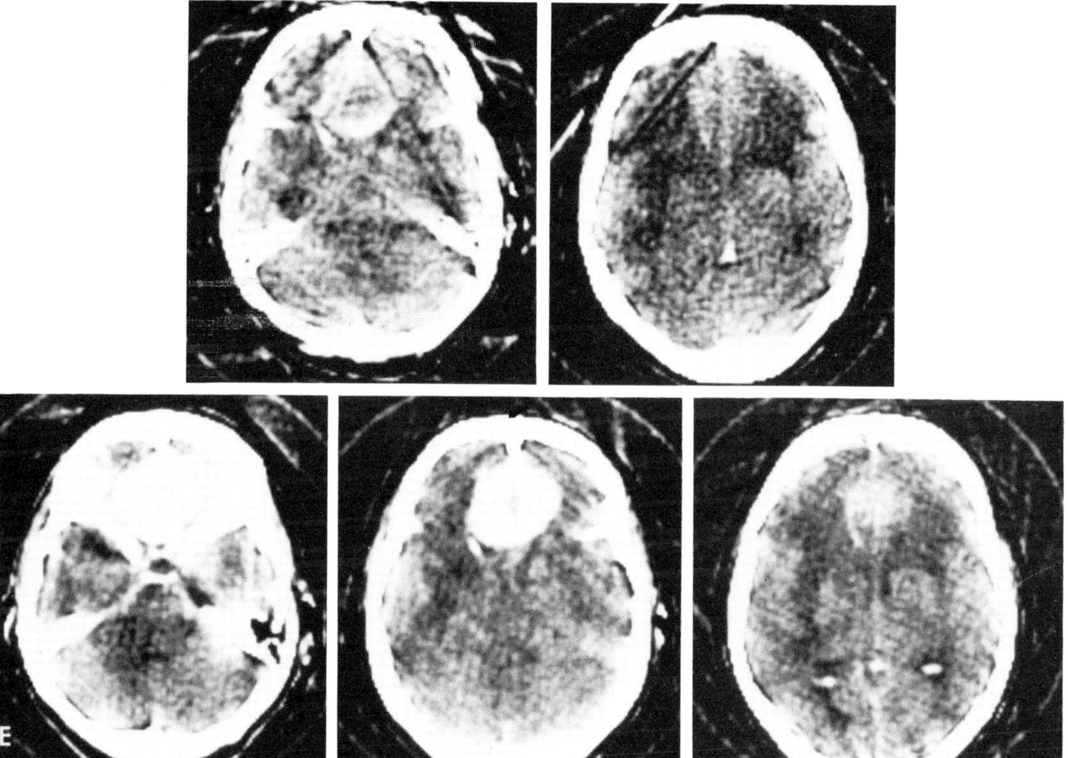

Figure 9–8 *Continued.*

E, The preinfusion scan reveals a large dense tumor mass in the midline arising from the floor of the middle cranial fossa. The mass is surrounded by large scalloped areas of cerebral edema. Postinfusion there is marked homogeneous enhancement of the tumor. The frontal horns of the lateral ventricles are displaced posteriorly and splayed apart.

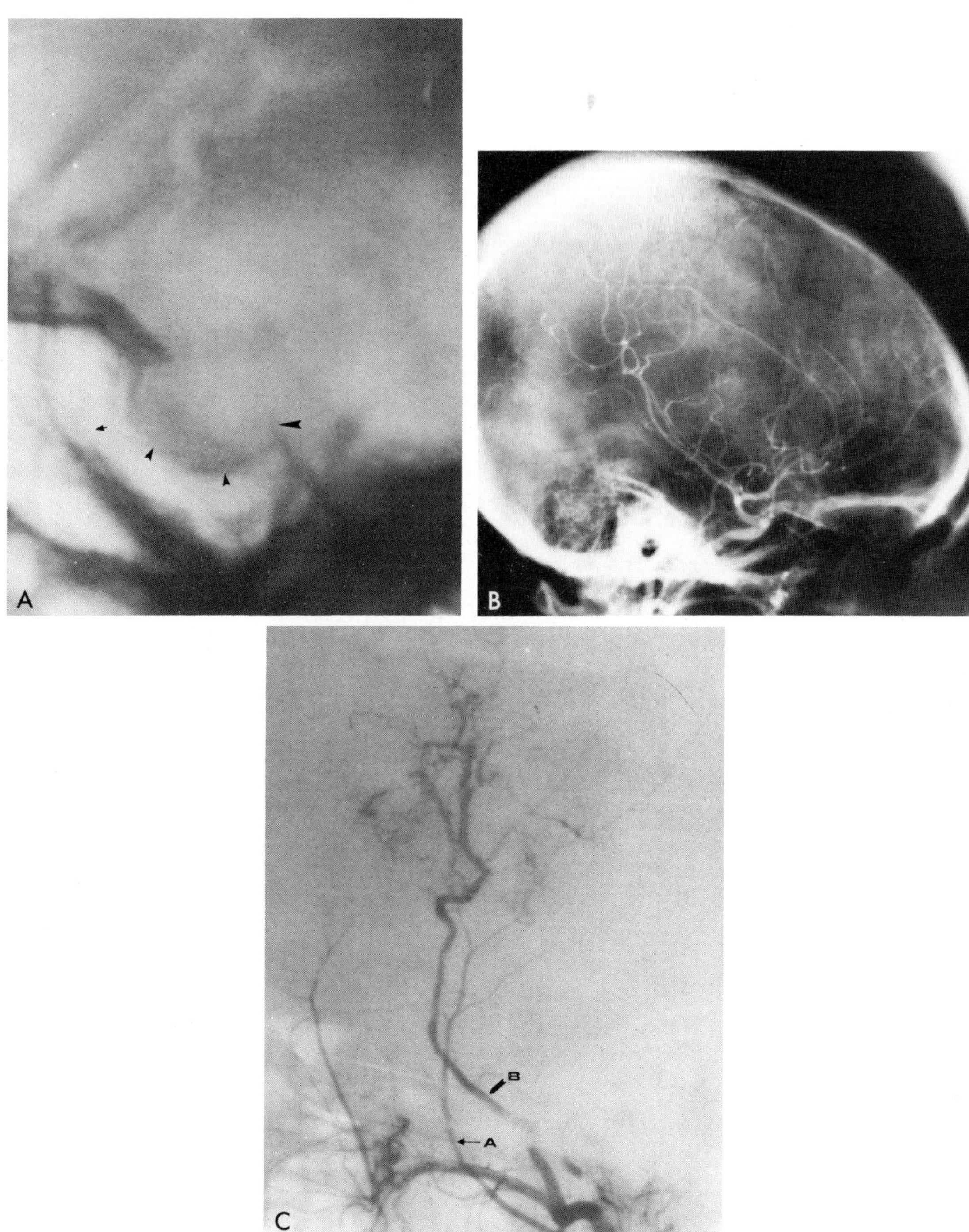

Figure 9–9. *See legend on the opposite page.*

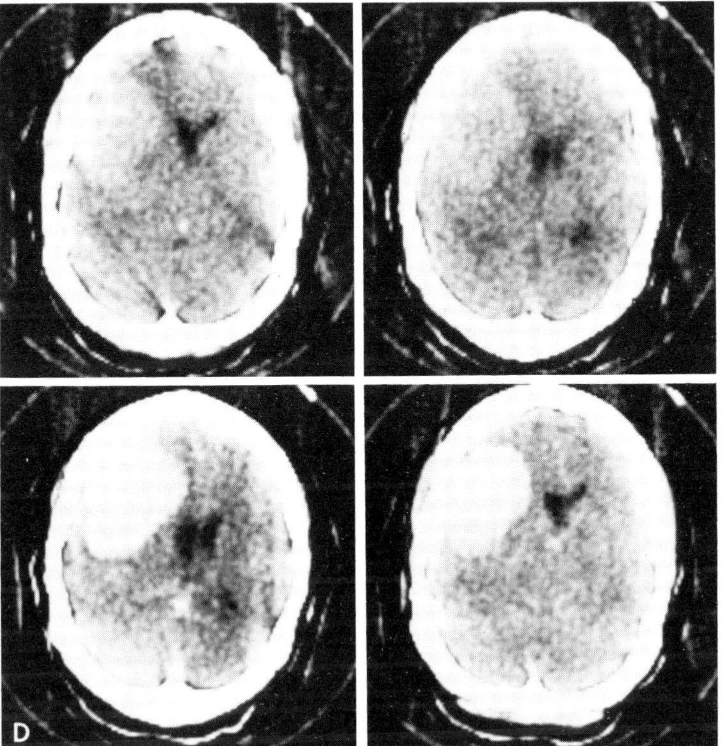

Figure 9–9. CONVEXITY MENINGIOMA: *A*, The skull radiograph reveals erosion and destruction of the posterior clinoids and the dorsum sellae as well as demineralization and thinning of the floor of the sella *(arrows)*. These changes are secondary to chronic increased intracranial pressure.

B, The common carotid arteriogram reveals downward displacement of the sylvian triangle and stretching of the opercular branches of the middle cerebral artery. A large middle meningeal artery is seen to become more tortuous and enlarged distally in order to provide blood supply to the tumor.

C, Selective external carotid arteriography with subtraction technique demonstrates that both the middle meningeal artery (Point "A") and an accessory meningeal artery (Point "B") supply the meningioma. These arteries enlarge distally and demonstrate a tree-branching pattern with multiple, small twiglike vessels seen frequently with meningioma.

D, The preinfusion CT scan shows a large tumor mass of higher density than normal brain substance. There is no surrounding edema, but marked shift from left to right is evident. The tumor appears to rest against the inner table of the skull in the left posterior frontal region. Postinfusion, there is marked homogeneous enhancement of the tumor.

Figure 9–10. FRONTAL CONVEXITY MENINGIOMA: *A*, The common carotid arteriogram shows proximal and distal shift of the anterior cerebral artery with medial and posterior displacement of the anterior portion of the middle cerebral arteries.

B, The lateral view reveals total disruption of the anterior portion of the sylvian triangle with posterior telescoping of the posterior branches of the triangle. A large meningeal vessel supplies the tumor, which demonstrates the sunburst pattern of vascular staining seen with meningioma.

C and *D* are subtraction views of the selective external carotid arteriogram. Corresponding points are marked on the AP and lateral views. "A" is the point of origin of the vessel from the internal maxillary artery. "B" is thc point where the vessel enters the cranial vault via the foramen spinosum—which would be expected to be enlarged in this case. "C" demonstrates the vessel as it grooves into the bony calvaria along the inner table of the skull. The vessel enlarges distally and demonstrates a symmetric sunburst pattern of vascularity that appears to originate from point "D". The small black arrowhead in *C* marks a smaller meningeal vessel that appears to enter the base of the skull via the foramen ovale.

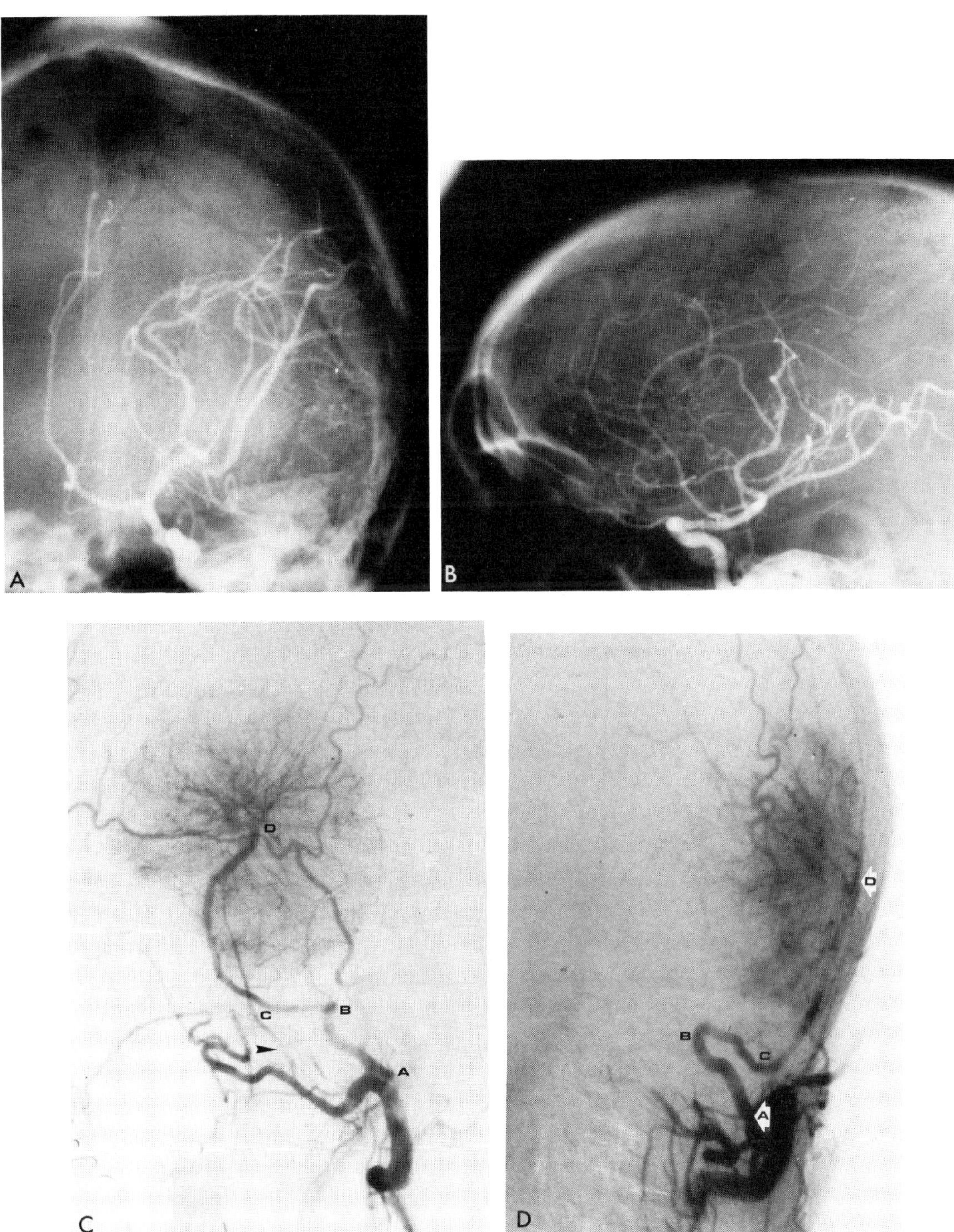

Figure 9–10. *See legend on the opposite page.*

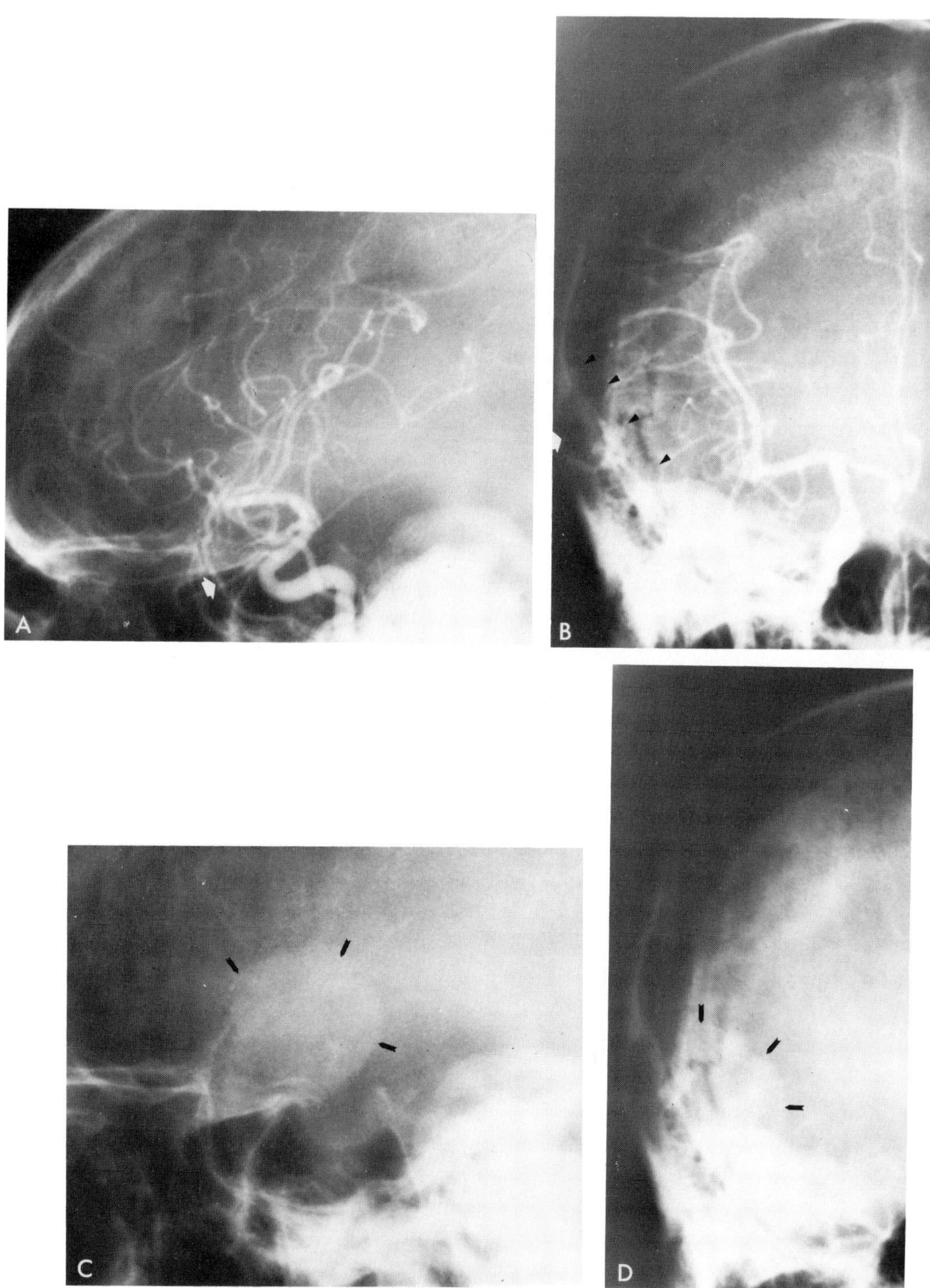

Figure 9–11. *See legend on the opposite page.*

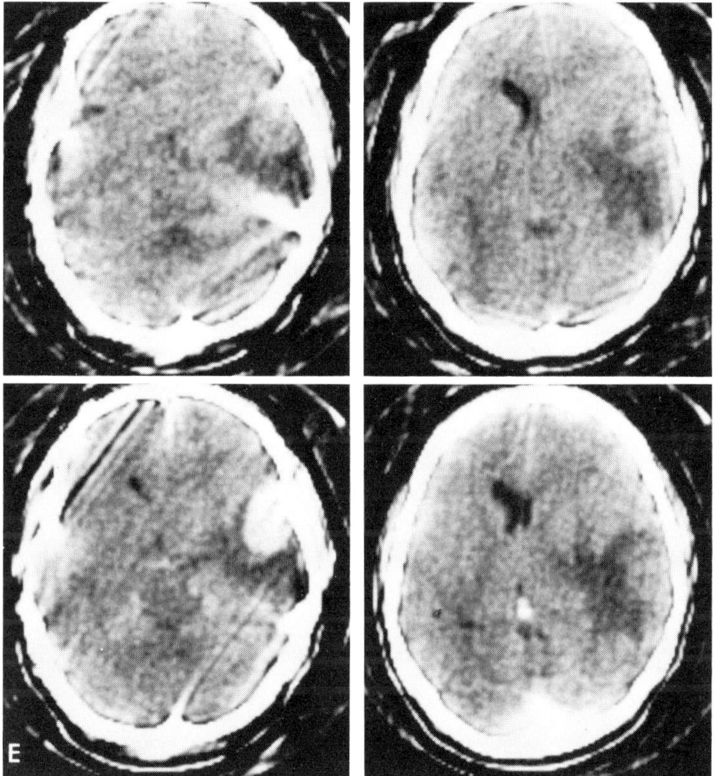

Figure 9–11. SPHENOID WING MENINGIOMA: *A*, The lateral view of the common carotid arteriogram reveals upward displacement of the sylvian triangle and an enlarged middle meningeal artery *(white arrowhead)*. *B*, Medial displacement of the genu of the middle cerebral artery and the sylvian point and a proximal and distal shift of the anterior cerebral artery are seen on *B*. The branches of the middle cerebral artery (*small black arrowheads in B*) are displaced away from the inner table of the skull by the mass of the meningioma resting against the bone and outside the cerebral tissue.

C, The typical cloudlike blush of the meningioma is seen on the capillary phase. *D*, The blush is also demonstrated on the AP view *(arrows)*.

E, The preinfusion scan reveals that the tumor is isodense with the brain and surrounded by asymmetric edema. This edema appears to account for the rather marked mass effect seen on the arteriogram even though the tumor itself is quite small. There is mild shift to the contralateral side. The postinfusion scan reveals homogeneous enhancement of the right sphenoid wing meningioma.

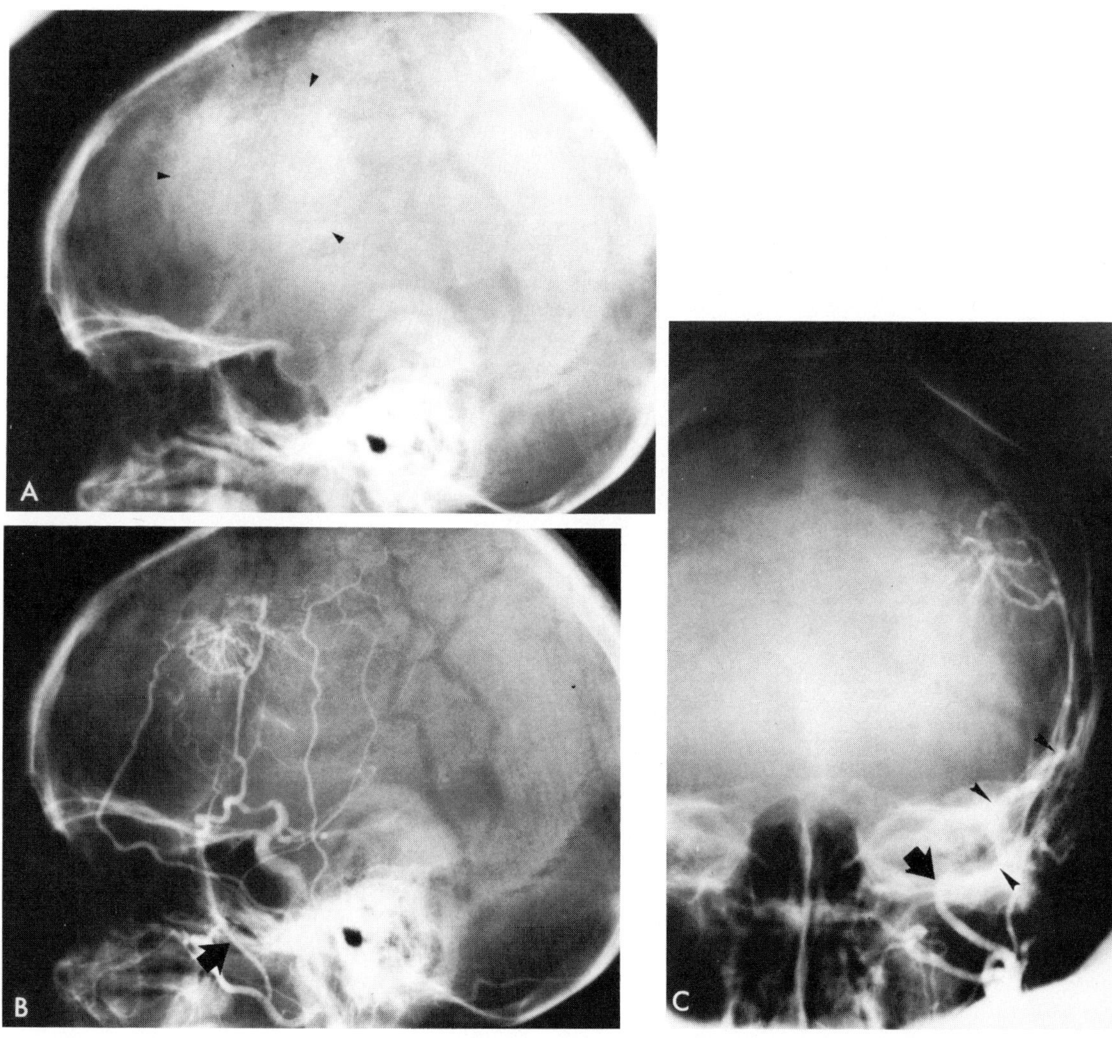

Figure 9–12. FRONTAL CONVEXITY MENINGIOMA: *A*, The skull radiograph reveals the faint outline of a meningioma that became apparent after arteriography.

B and *C*, Selective external carotid arteriography demonstrates the enlarged tortuous middle meningeal artery, which becomes even more dilated in its distal portion and gives rise to multiple branches that have a "corkscrew" appearance. The point of entrance into the base of the skull through the foramen spinosum is identified on the AP and lateral projections (*large arrow*).

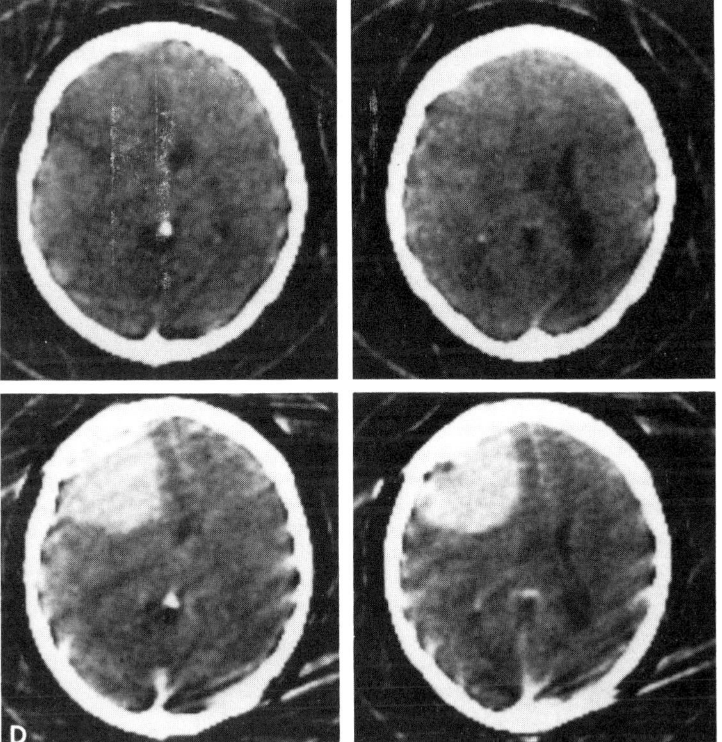

Figure 9–12 *Continued.*

D, The preinfusion CT scan shows a large tumor that is isodense with brain substance and surrounded by a thin rim of edema. There is marked shift from left to right. Homogeneous enhancement is evident after the infusion of contrast material.

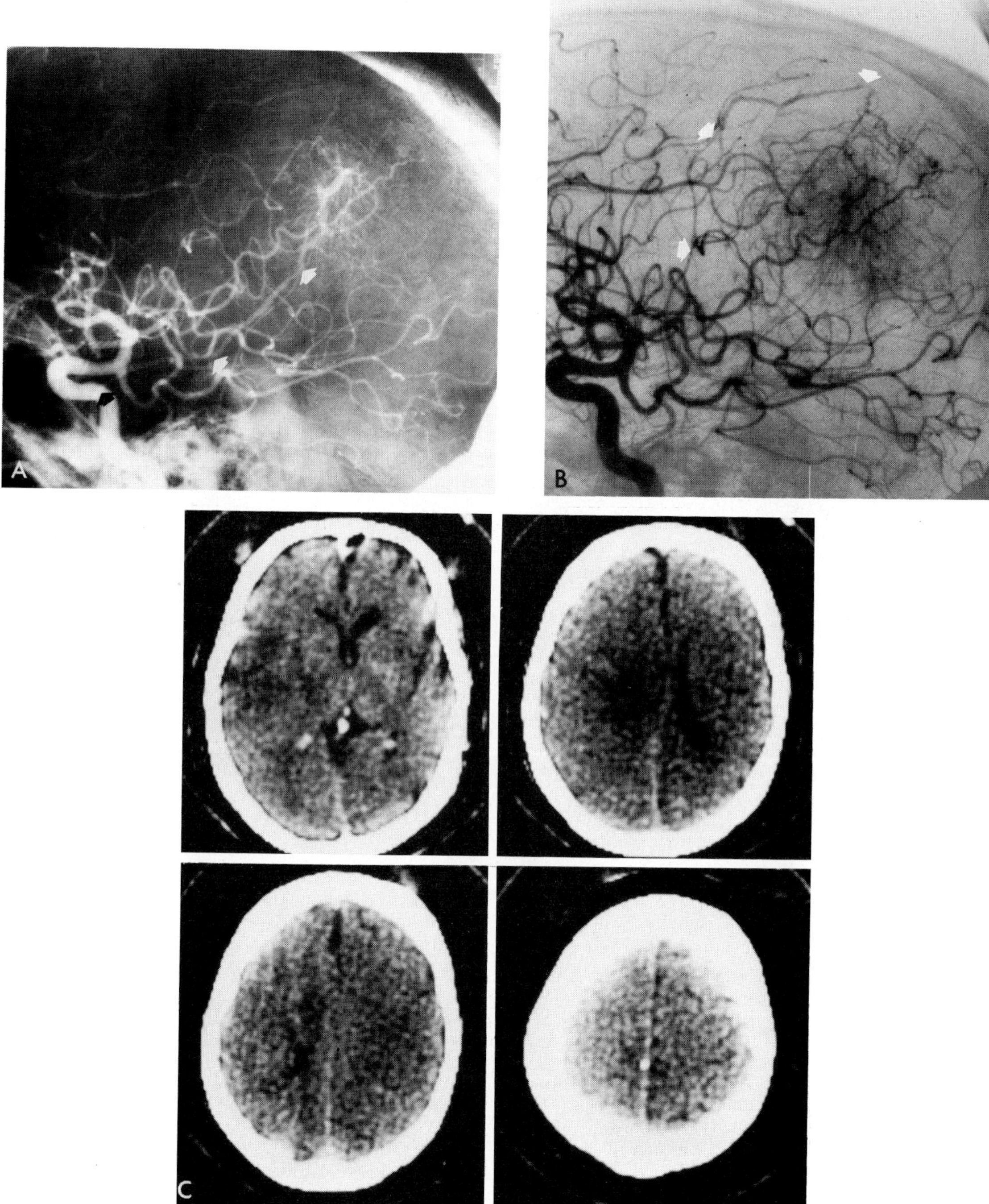

Figure 9–13. *See legend on the opposite page.*

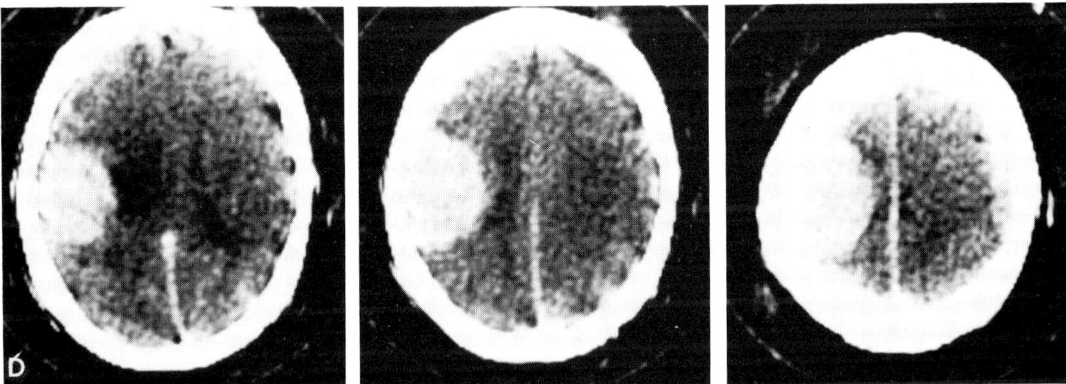

Figure 9–13. PARIETAL CONVEXITY MENINGIOMA: *A*, The common carotid arteriogram reveals downward displacement of the sylvian triangle and a large posterior branch of the middle meningeal artery, which becomes enlarged and more tortuous in its distal portion (*arrows*). The artery supplies a large tumor in the midparietal convexity region.

B, A later arterial phase shows the anterior branch of the middle meningeal artery as it courses posteriorly to provide additional blood supply to the tumor (*arrows*). This subtraction view better demonstrates the sunburst pattern of vascularity.

C, The preinfusion scan shows a tumor that is isodense with brain tissue and surrounded by a thin rim of edema. There is only minimal shift of the midline structures. The slow growth of the tumor probably has resulted in pressure atrophy of a portion of the brain, since only a modest shift to the right is seen.

D, Postinfusion, the tumor enhances in a homogeneous fashion.

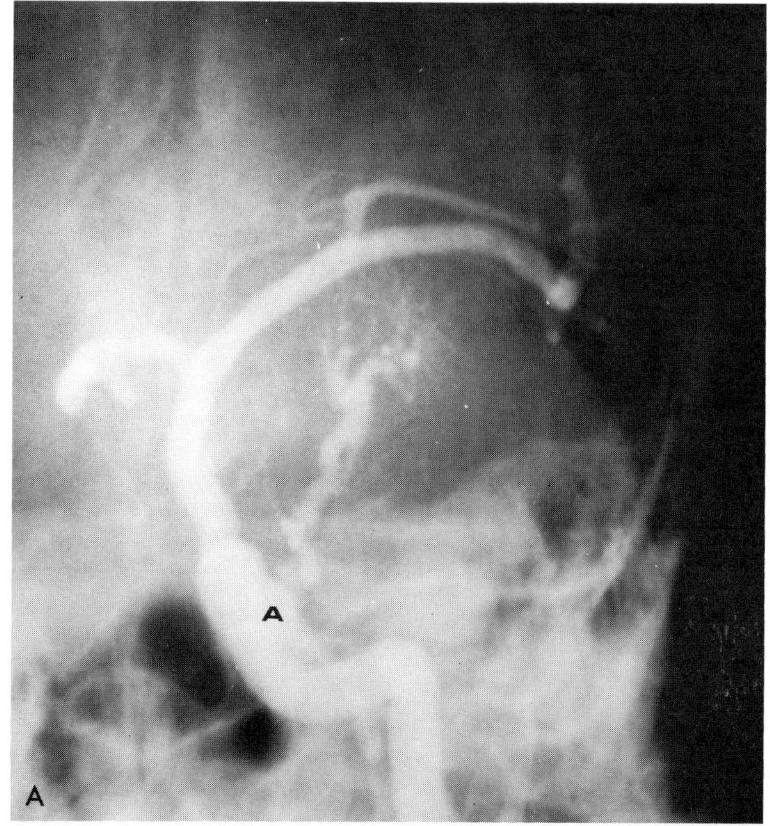

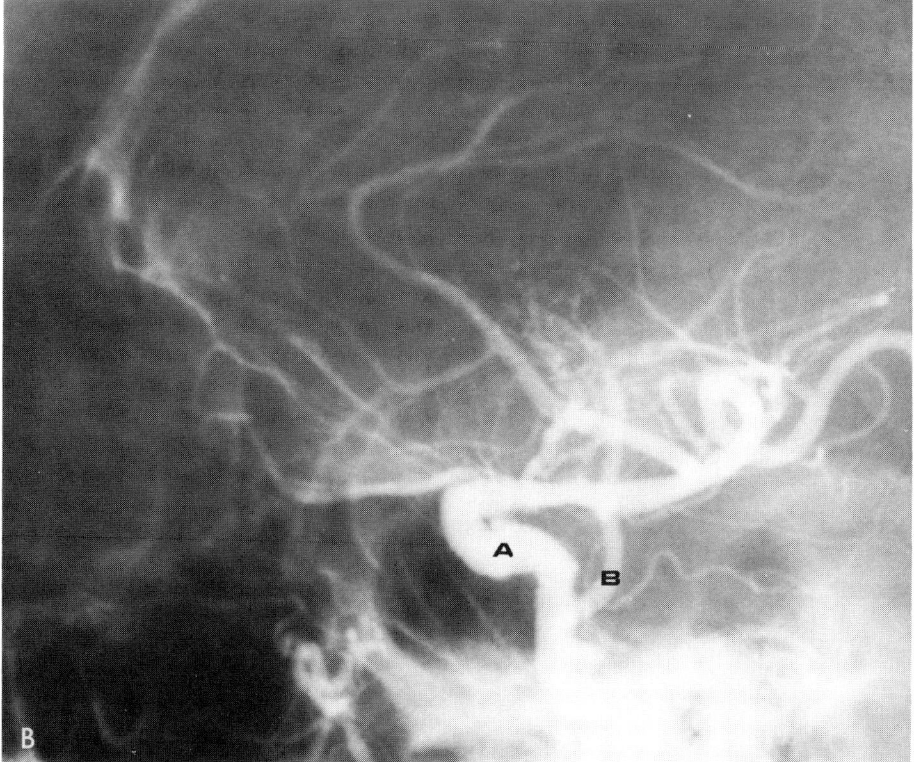

Figure 9–14. *See legend on the opposite page.*

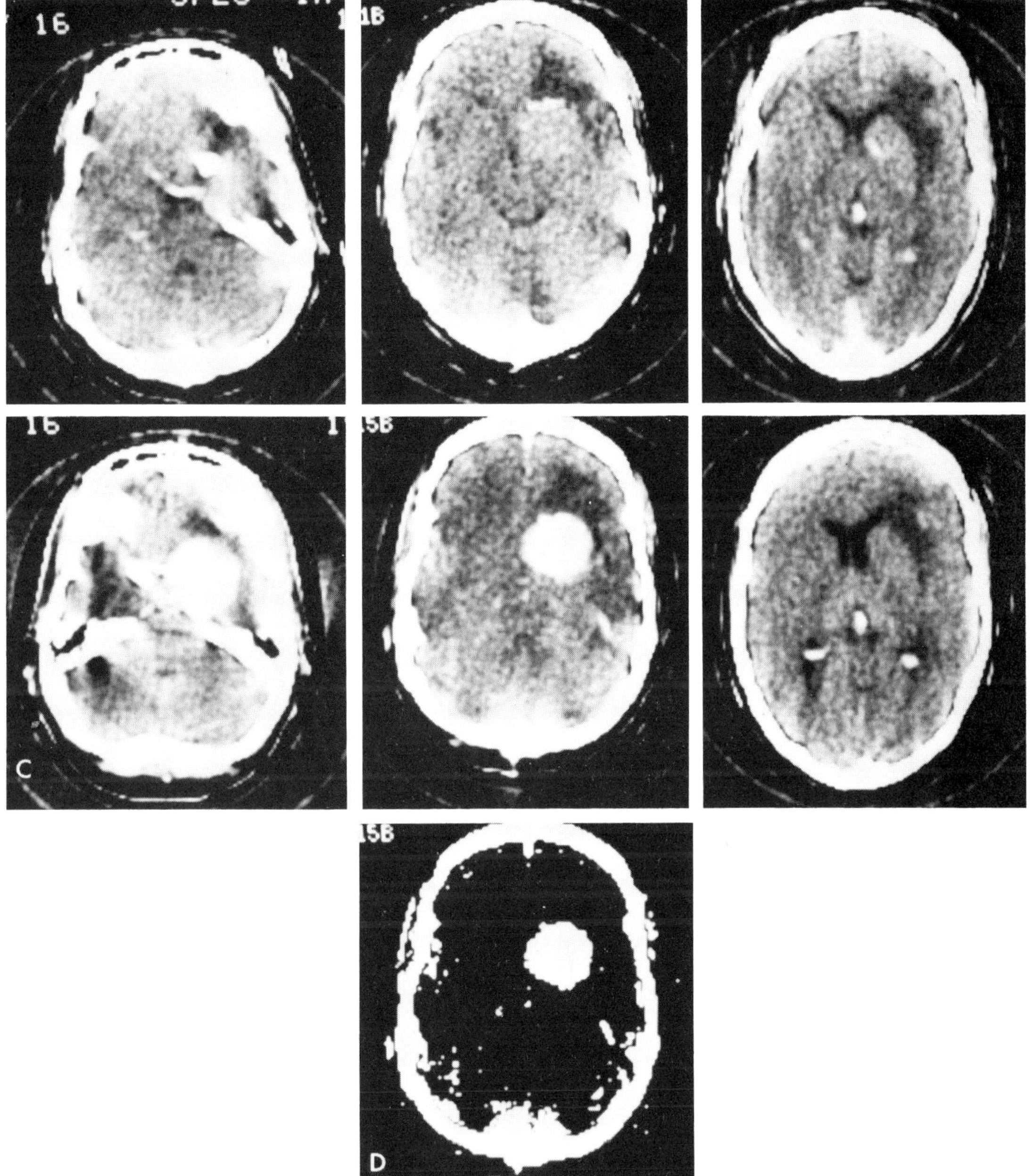

Figure 9–14. PARASELLAR MENINGIOMA: *A* and *B,* Marked elevation of the horizontal portion of the middle cerebral artery and medial displacement of the internal carotid artery are seen as they follow a curvilinear course around the tumor. This meningioma arises from the medial aspect of the sphenoid wing and may be accompanied by hyperostosis of the greater wing of the sphenoid around the superior orbital fissure. If hyperostosis is present, this may strongly resemble fibrous dysplasia. Point "A" on the AP and lateral views marks the origin of an unnamed meningeal vessel at its point of origin from the internal carotid artery. This large vessel becomes even larger and more tortuous as it projects superiorly and posteriorly to supply the tumor. Point "B" is a large superficial temporal artery that could be seen in the soft tissues on the AP view.

C, The preinfusion scan reveals that the tumor is isodense with brain tissue and is surrounded by a rim of edema. There are a few scattered areas of calcification around the periphery of the tumor. Postinfusion there is homogeneous enhancement. Differentiation from an aneurysm may be difficult.

D, On the measure mode the meningioma is readily identified as a high density area of enhancement.

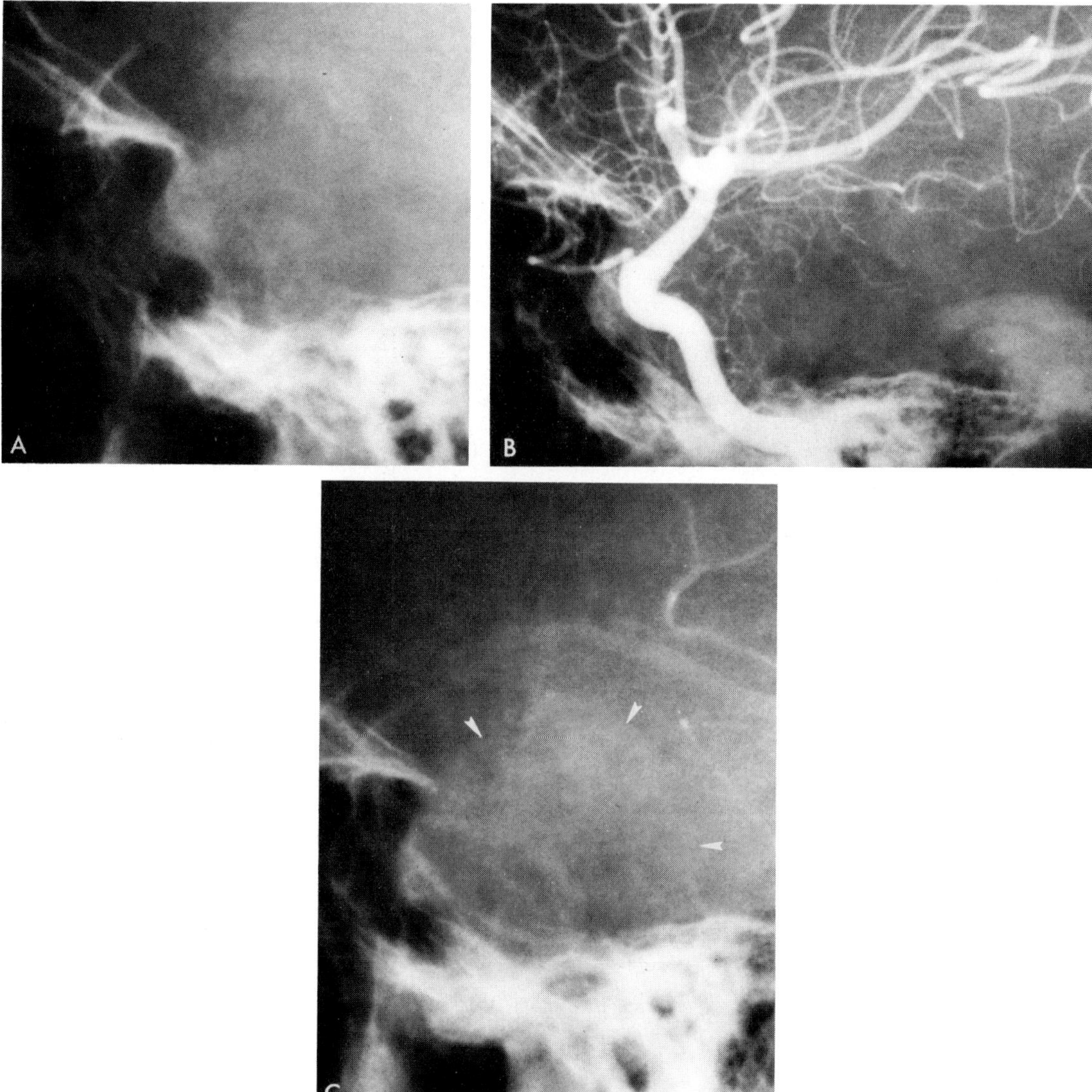

Figure 9–15. PARASELLAR MENINGIOMA: *A*, The skull radiograph reveals apparent destruction of the floor, the anterior clinoids and the dorsum sella and posterior clinoids.

B, The internal carotid artery appears to be suspended at the level of the carotid siphon. Opening of the siphon and elevation of the supraclinoid position of the internal carotid artery are seen. Myriad small vessels arise from the internal carotid artery at the level of the siphon to provide the blood supply of the meningioma.

C, A late blush (*white arrowheads*) outlines the extent of the meningioma.

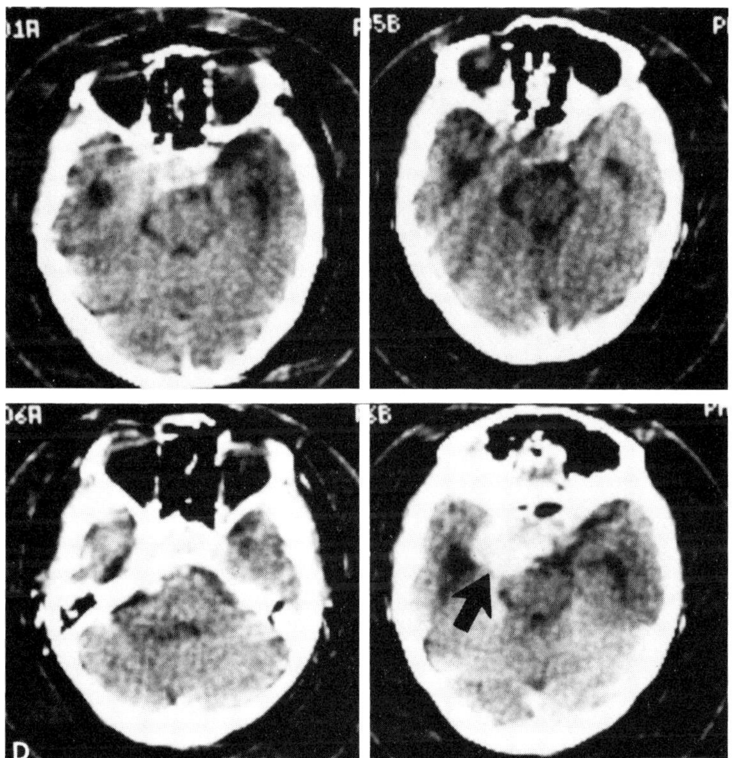

Figure 9–15 *Continued.*

D, The preinfusion CT scan reveals that evidence of destruction of the sella is most marked along the left side. Although the dorsum sella appeared to be destroyed on the skull film, it can be readily identified on the CT scan. It is displaced posteriorly, especially along the left side, and is thinned.

The postinfusion scan reveals homogeneous enhancement of the meningioma. The tumor extends laterally into the middle cranial fossa as well as superiorly (*large black arrow*).

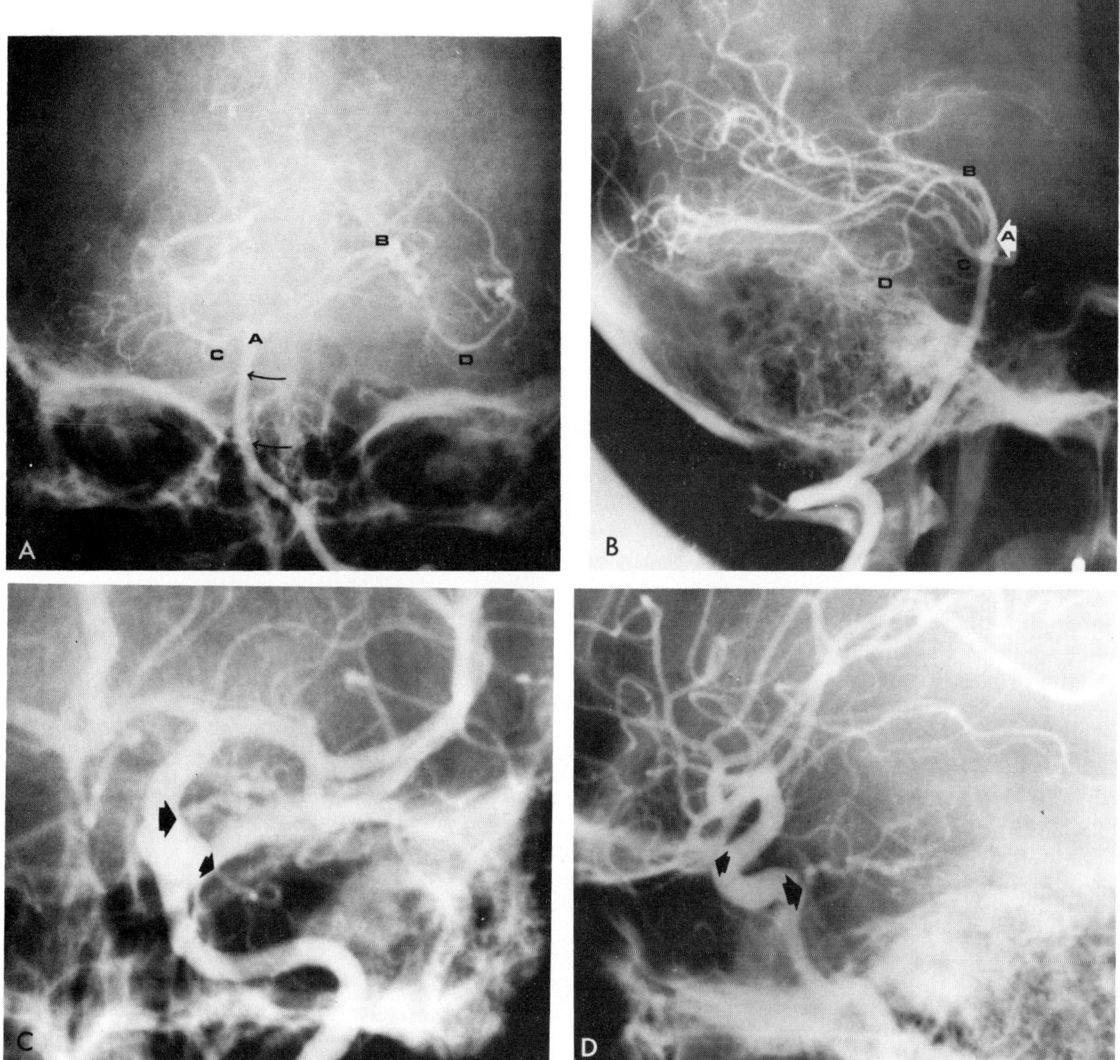

Figure 9–16. TENTORIAL MENINGIOMA: *A* and *B*, AP and lateral views marked as follows: "A" is the origin of the left posterior cerebral artery; "B" is the uppermost point of the left posterior cerebral artery as it is displaced over the tentorial meningioma just below it; "C" is the lowest point of the normally positioned right posterior cerebral artery; "D" is the lowest point of the abnormal left posterior cerebral artery as it is displaced laterally and posteriorly. There is such gross distortion of the left posterior cerebral artery that both the normal and abnormal positions can be readily demonstrated. The basilar artery is displaced to the right *(arrows)*.

C and *D*, the left internal carotid arteriogram reveals a large tentorial artery — the artery of Bernasconi and Cassonari — which provides the main blood supply to the tumor (*large arrowhead)*. The ophthalmic artery is also visualized on both the AP and lateral views (*small arrowhead)*.

E, A subtraction view reveals the ophthalmic artery (*small arrowhead*), the tentorial artery of Bernasconi and Cassonari (*large arrowhead)* and the blush of the meningioma in the posterior fossa and along the free edge of the tentorium as it is supplied by myriad small vessels (*open arrowheads)*.

F, The preinfusion CT scan shows the tumor along the edge of the petrous bone on the left side, extending medially just across the midline and superiorly to the left of the third ventricle. The posterior portion of the third ventricle is thinned and displaced to the right. The tumor is of higher than normal brain density and contains small areas of calcification. There is moderate obstructive hydrocephalus. Postinfusion there is homogeneous enhancement of the tumor, providing a beautiful illustration of the exact location of the mass.

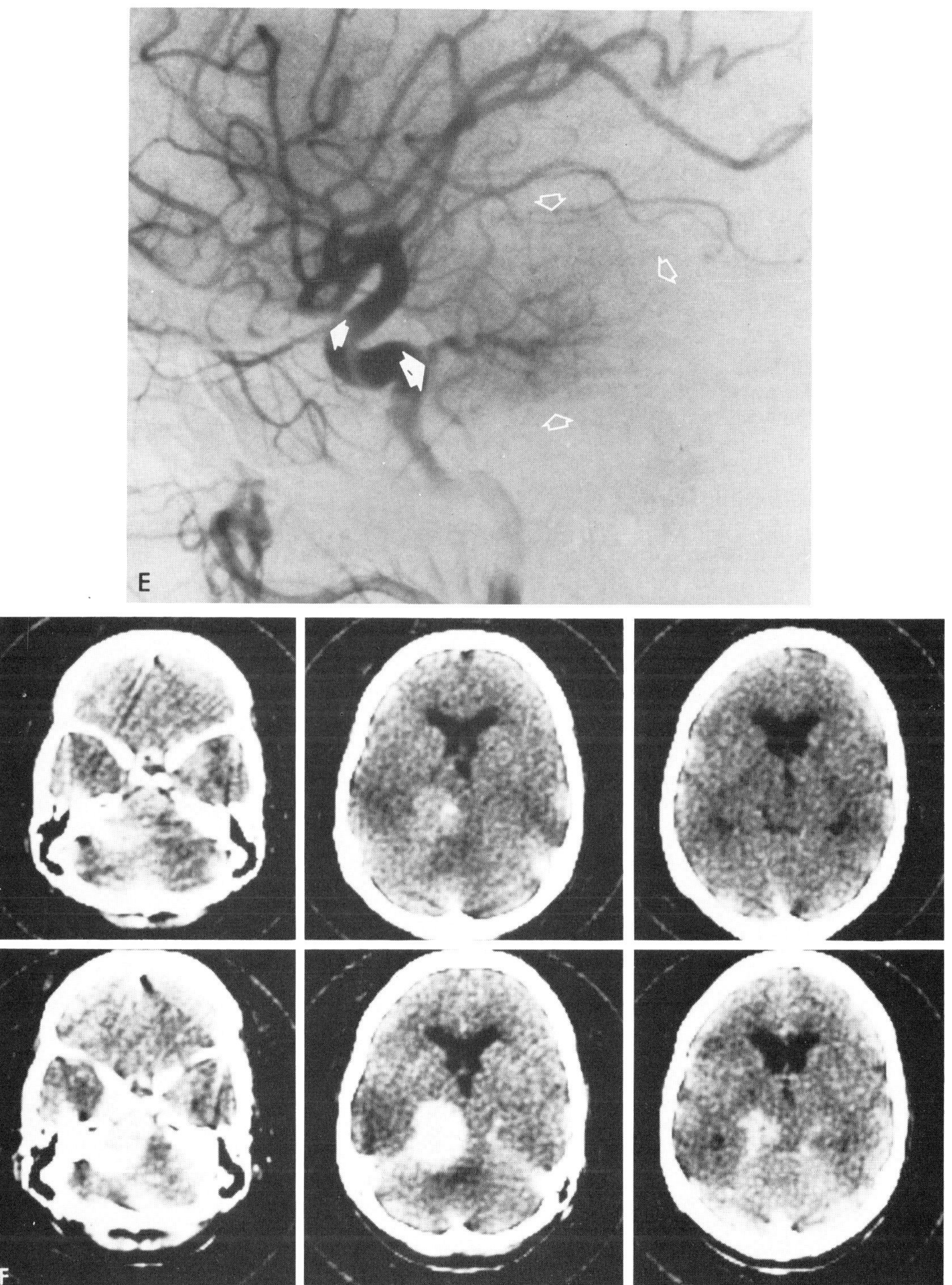

Figure 9–16. *See legend on the opposite page.*

Figure 9–17. TENTORIAL MENINGIOMA: *A*, the left carotid arteriogram reveals a large anomalous meningeal vessel that arises from the cavernous portion of the left internal carotid artery and courses posteriorly and superiorly along the free edge of the tentorium (*arrows*). The vessel becomes slightly larger and more tortuous distally, breaking up into myriad small vessels that provide the blood supply to the meningioma, which is situated at the top of the tentorial notch. There is widening of the sweep of the pericallosal artery because of moderate obstructive hydrocephalus.

B, The preinfusion scan reveals moderate obstructive hydrocephalus. The tumor is isodense with normal brain tissue. There is also artifact from a shunt tubing device. Postinfusion there is homogeneous enhancement of the meningioma (*arrow*), which rests at the level of the juncture of the falx cerebri and the straight sinus and the vein of Galen.

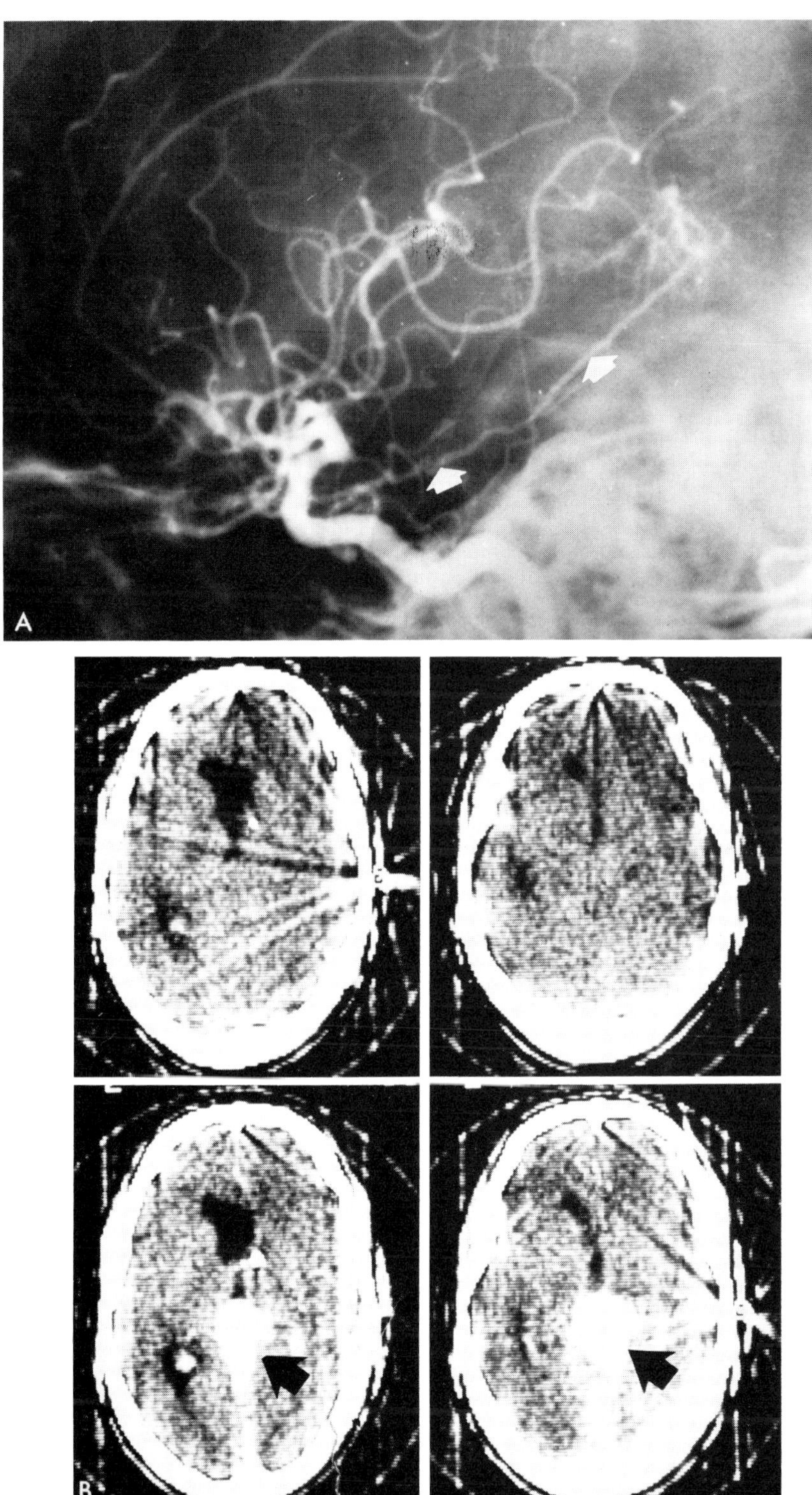

Figure 9–17. *See legend on the opposite page.*

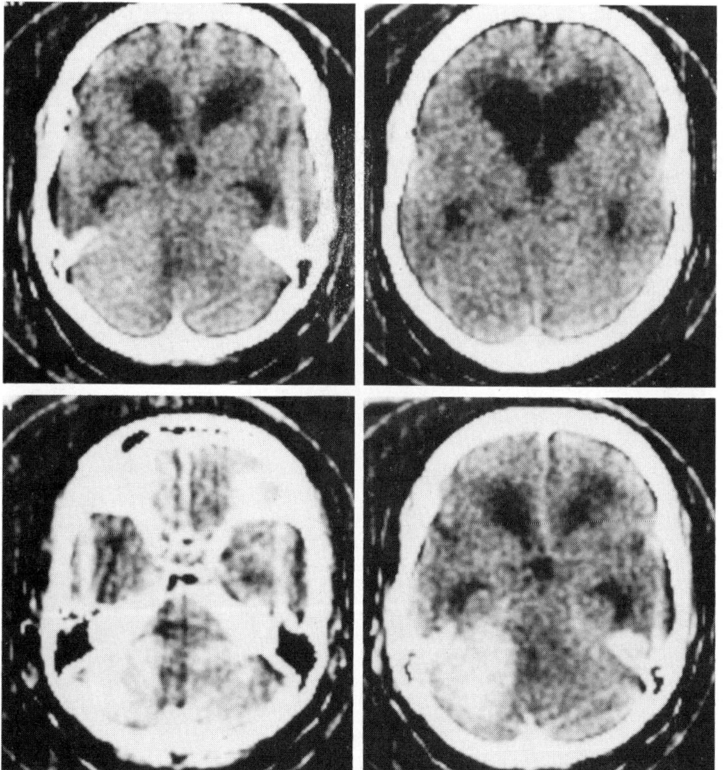

Figure 9–18. TENTORIAL MENINGIOMA: The preinfusion scan reveals severe obstructive hydrocephalus. The fourth ventricle could not be visualized. The large posterior fossa tentorial meningioma is isodense with normal brain substance. Postinfusion there is marked homogeneous enhancement of the meningioma where it is suspended from the midportion of the tentorium on the left side and extends into the posterior fossa. This case illustrates the value of the postinfusion scan.

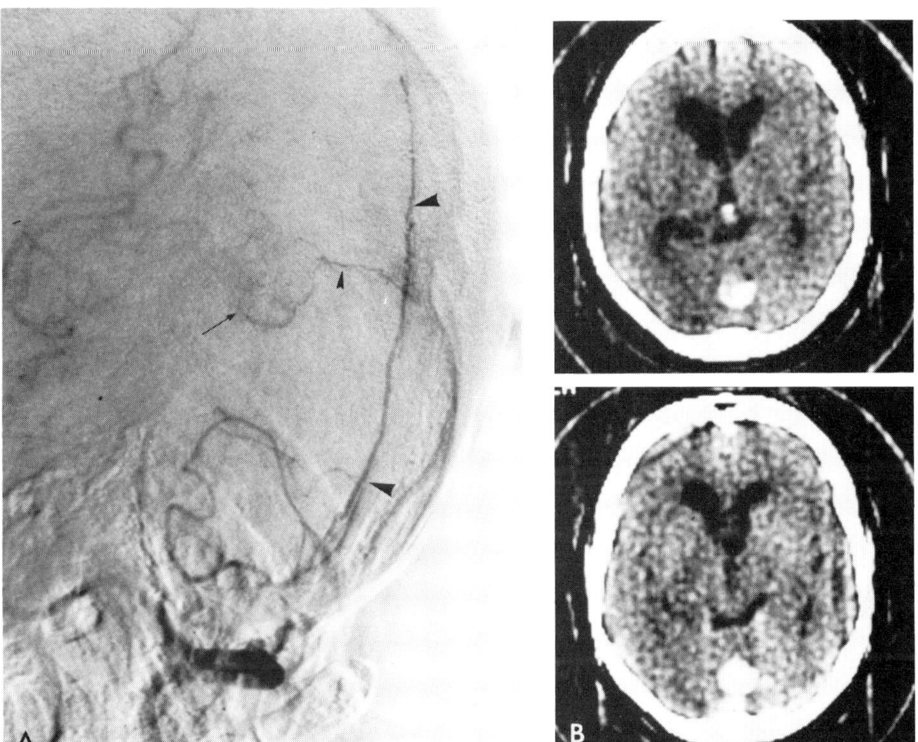

Figure 9–19. SMALL TENTORIAL MENINGIOMA: *A*, The lateral subtraction view (using magnification technique) of the left vertebral arteriogram demonstrates a large posterior meningeal artery (*large arrowheads*) and a smaller branch (*small arrowhead*) that supplies a small tentorial meningioma that projects inferiorly from the tentorium at the midline (*black arrow*).

B, The CT scan reveals a dense area of calcification in the midline in the posterior fossa. Post-infusion (not illustrated), there was only minimal enhancement of the meningioma.

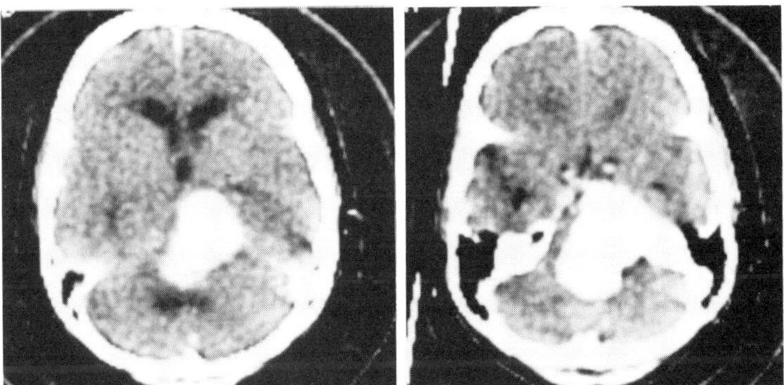

Figure 9–20. DENSELY CALCIFIED CEREBELLOPONTINE ANGLE MENINGIOMA: The CT scan reveals a densely calcified meningioma wrapped around the petrous apex on the right side. The fourth ventricle is flattened and displaced posteriorly. There is moderate obstructive hydrocephalus. No change was noted on the postinfusion scan. This is what is known as a "brain stone" because of its very dense calcification.

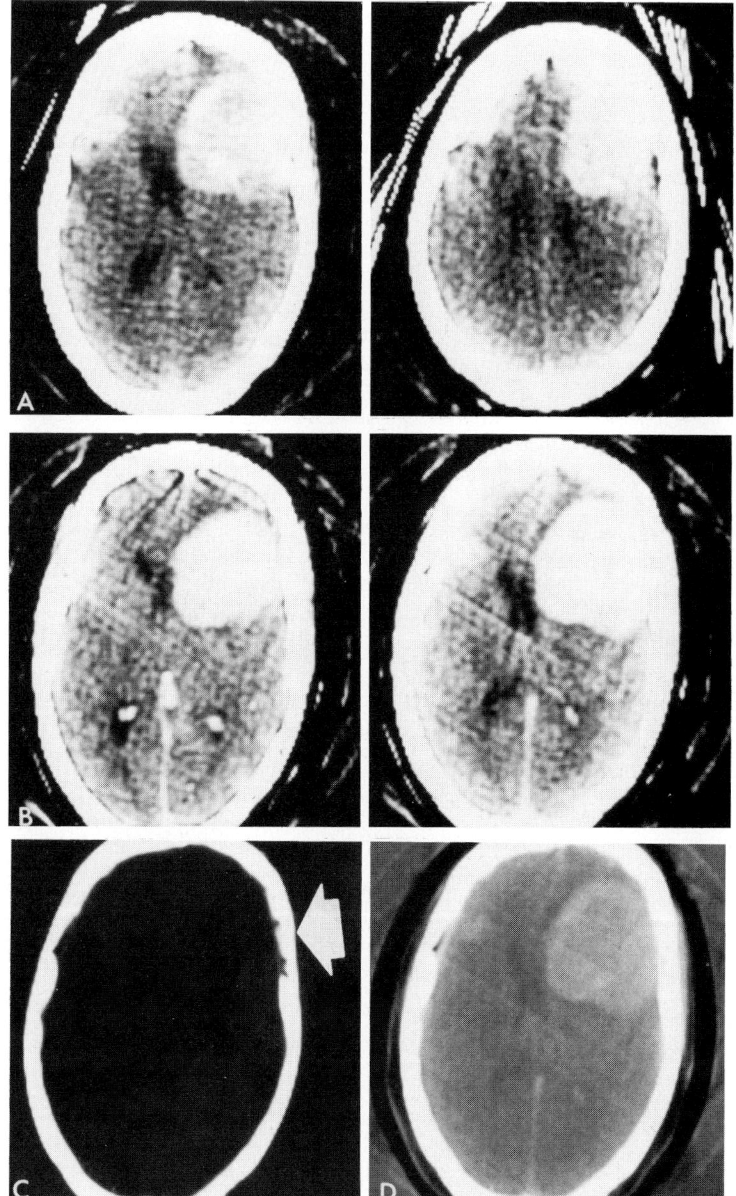

Figure 9–21. CONVEXITY MENINGIOMA WITH BONY INVOLVEMENT: *A*, Preinfusion, the tumor is noted to be very densely calcified. There is distortion of the right frontal horn and anterior body of the right lateral ventricle. There is a slight shift of the midline. Slow growth of the tumor probably has resulted in pressure atrophy of the brain. Note that there appears to be a smaller meningioma in a similar anatomic location on the opposite side.

B, Postinfusion, there is homogeneous enhancement of the tumor, which appears slightly lobulated.

C, On the "measure" mode there is evidence of invasion of the inner table of the skull (*white arrow*) at the level of attachment of the tumor.

D, On a high window width and window level the tumor continues to be visible, but the area of bony involvement is seen only faintly.

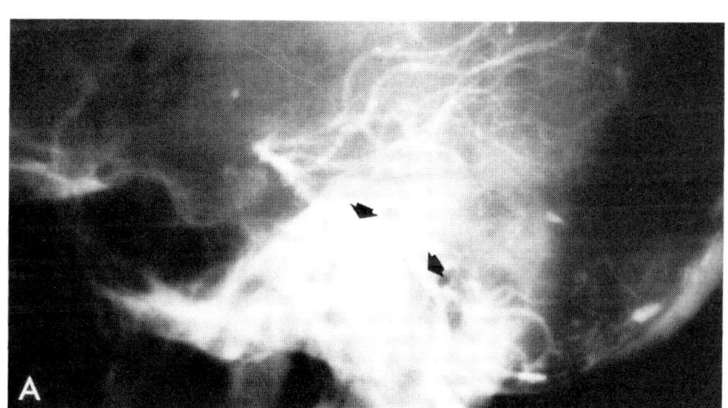

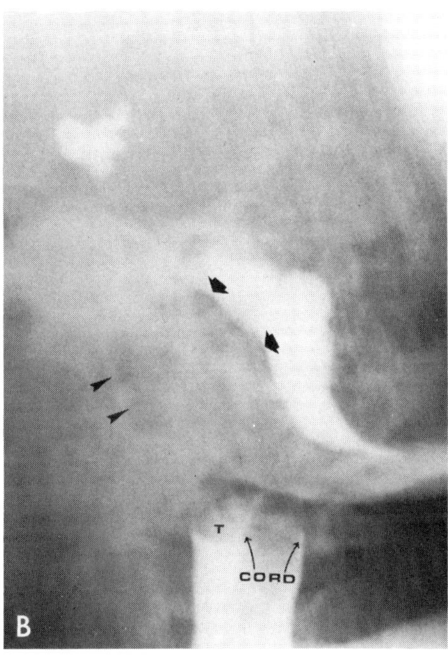

Figure 9–22. CLIVUS MENINGIOMA: *A*, The vertebral arteriogram demonstrates posterior displacement of the vertebral and basilar arteries away from the clivus (*arrowheads*).

B, On the posterior fossa myelogram, the contrast material can be seen as it flows around the tumor (*wide arrowheads*) and the amount of displacement away from the clivus (*thin arrowheads*) is apparent. There is tonsilar herniation *T*, and the tonsil is visible bathed in Pantopaque below the level of the foramen magnum. The cervical spinal cord is displaced to the right.

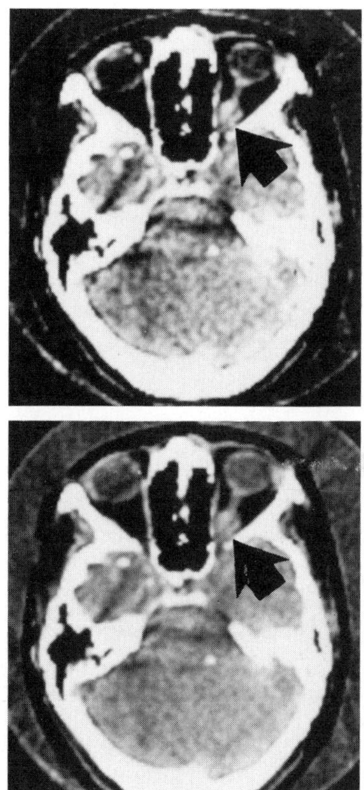

Figure 9–23. CT scans of the orbits reveal a mass lesion wrapped around the optic nerve on the right side. This is an optic nerve meningioma. There are no absolute distinguishing features to differentiate orbital meningiomas from any other orbital mass lesion.

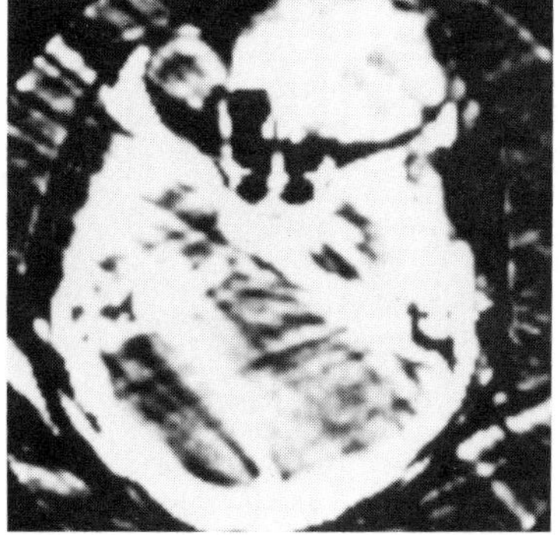

Figure 9–24. The postinfusion scan reveals a large mass in the right orbit. This was proved to be a meningioma.

CHAPTER 10

DEEP HEMISPHERE AND MIDLINE LESIONS

Masses that arise in the midline in the supratentorial compartment are difficult to demonstrate by angiography. In fact, even in the presence of relatively large lesions, the angiogram may demonstrate hydrocephalus but may otherwise be uninformative. Angiography usually does not characterize the lesion or identify its exact position. Abnormal vascularity, if demonstrated, can of course reveal the extent of the mass; however, it is not uncommon to find that the mass is avascular.

Pneumoencephalography, necessary for evaluation before the availability of CT, is no longer required. In fact, CT reveals the position and configuration of the mass better and more precisely than does any other diagnostic method.

Midline lesions outside the sella include:

1. Pinealoma.
2. Teratoma.
3. Hypothalamic glioma.
4. Vein of Galen aneurysm.
5. Colloid cyst of the third ventricle.

Lesions within and immediately adjacent to the sella include:

1. Ectopic pinealoma.
2. Pituitary adenoma.
3. Aneurysm of internal carotid artery.
4. Craniopharyngioma.
5. Empty sella.
6. Meningioma of diaphragma sellae or medial sphenoid wing.
7. Optic glioma.
8. Basal ganglionic hematoma.

BASAL GANGLIONIC HEMATOMA

Hemorrhages that occur in the region of the basal ganglia are secondary to the rupture of small aneurysms arising from the lenticulostriate arteries. These basal ganglia hemorrhages most commonly are seen in hypertensive patients and are especially prevalent among the black population. The clinical presentation is dramatic, with the sudden onset of severe headaches, a dense contralateral hemiplegia and decreased sensorium and/or coma. Complete recovery from a large hemorrhage is rare, and many patients die following a basal ganglia hemorrhage.

Because these hemorrhages can rupture into the ventricular system, their clinical appearance may mimic a subarachnoid hemorrhage. With rupture into the ventricular system, a lumbar puncture will reveal bloody cerebrospinal fluid. In the past, angiography was necessary to rule out an aneurysm as the cause of the bloody CSF. With basal ganglionic hemorrhage, angiography may also be helpful and diagnostic. On the other hand, the angiogram may be normal or may demonstrate only a shift of the internal cerebral vein to the contralateral side. Other abnormalities that may be seen are displacement of the lenticulostriate arteries (either medially or laterally, depending on the position of the hemorrhage), a widened distance between the anterior cerebral artery and the laterally displaced middle cerebral artery group and, in some instances, a shift of the anterior cerebral artery to the contralateral side.

Since the availability of CT scanning, the diagnosis of basal ganglionic hemorrhage can be made with near 100 per cent accuracy. In most instances no other diagnostic tests are necessary.

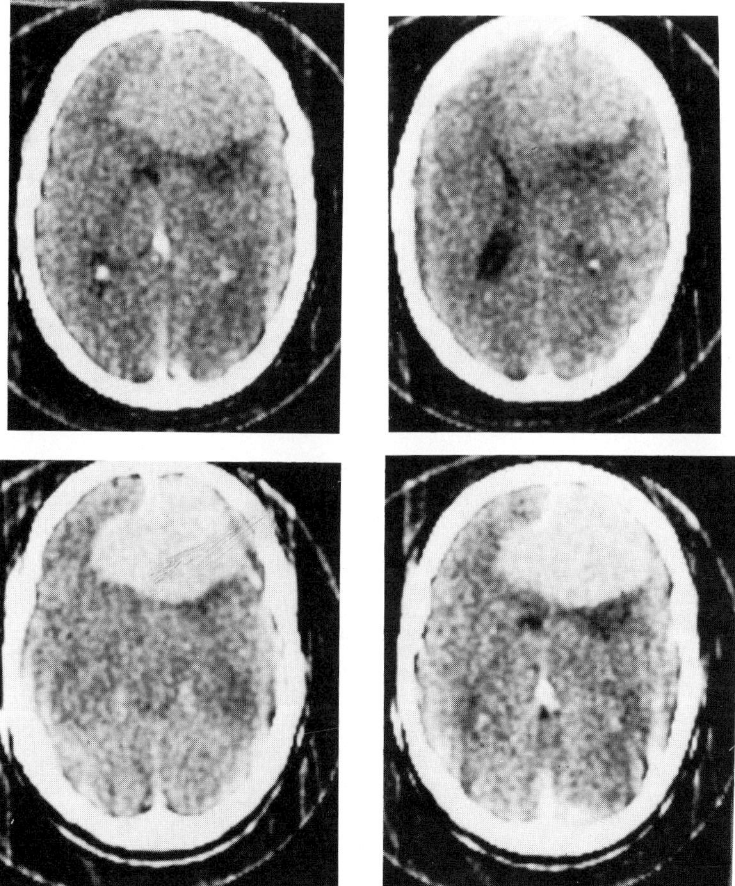

Figure 10–1. BIFRONTAL GLIOBLASTOMA: The CT scan demonstrates a mass in the right frontal region that extends across the midline to the contralateral side via the genu of the corpus callosum. The tumor is of higher than normal brain density on the preinfusion scan, and it enhances homogeneously on the postinfusion scan. There is a small amount of surrounding edema; because the tumor is larger on the right side, there is a shift from right to left. The angiogram on this patient is in the "frontal lobe section."

Surgically proved glioblastoma.

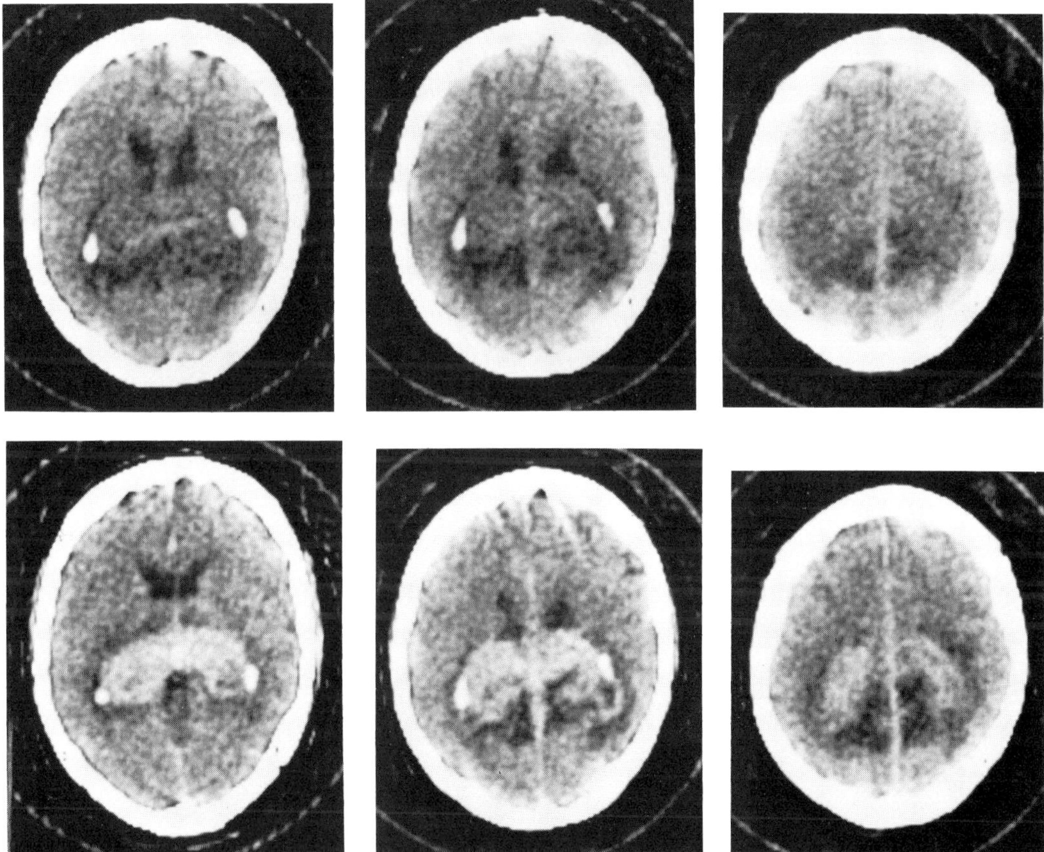

Figure 10–2. BUTTERFLY GLIOBLASTOMA: The pre- and postinfusion scans demonstrate a large enhancing mass deep in the cerebral hemispheres. It exhibits a mixed pattern of high and low density on the preinfusion scan. The tumor extends from one hemisphere to the other via the corpus callosum in a classic "butterfly" distribution.

These tumors may be very difficult to demonstrate by angiography unless they exhibit neovascularity; however, they are beautifully outlined by the CT scan.

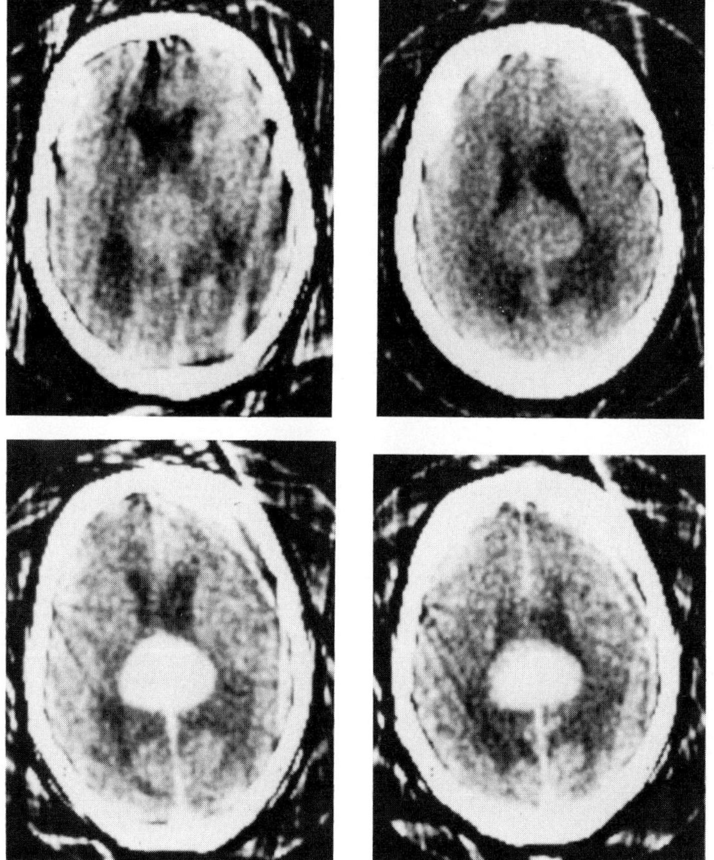

Figure 10–3. CORPUS CALLOSUM GLIOMA: The CT scan reveals a large, well defined, homogeneously enhancing mass in the region of the splenium of the corpus callosum. There is a "bat-wing" pattern of surrounding edema. Mild to moderate obstructive hydrocephalus is present.

Surgically proved corpus callosum glioma.

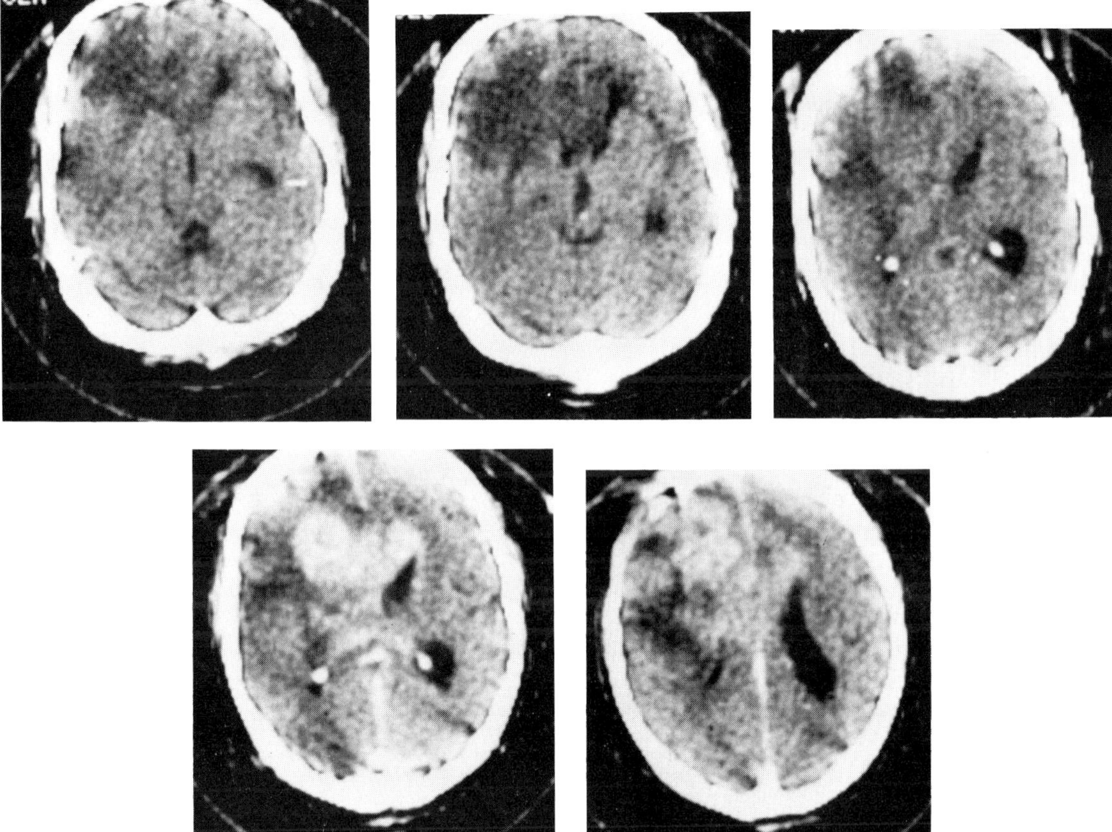

Figure 10–4. BIFRONTAL TUMOR: The CT scan demonstrates a large area of radiolucency in the left frontal lobe that extends across the midline via the corpus callosum to involve the right side as well. The frontal horns of the lateral ventricles are splayed apart by the tumor mass. There is marked homogeneous enhancement of the tumor of the postinfusion scan. This demonstrates a bifrontal distribution with extension via the corpus callosum. Postoperative changes are present in the left frontal convexity region. The tumor is surrounded by a moderate amount of edema.

Surgically proved metastatic breast carcinoma.

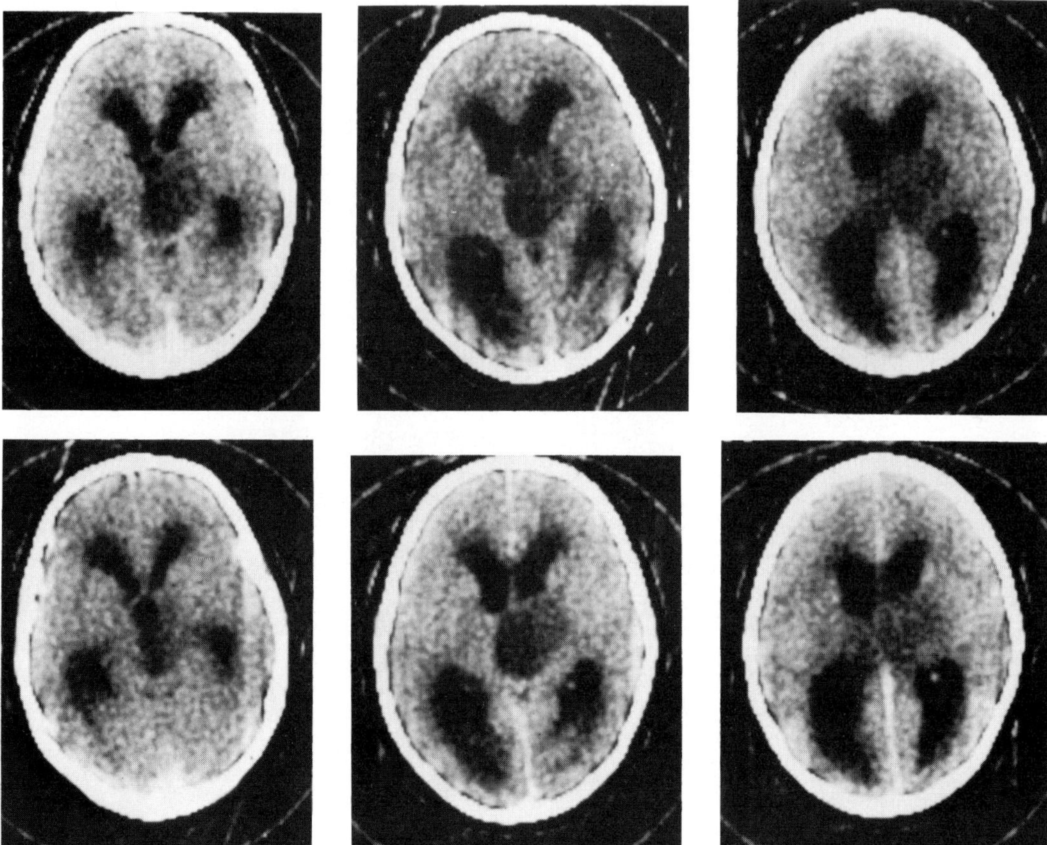

Figure 10–5. MIDLINE GLIOMA: The CT scan demonstrates a low density cystic tumor in the region of the third ventricle that extends to the right of the midline. There is moderate obstructive hydrocephalus. No change in the appearance of the tumor is evident following the infusion of contrast material. The fluid within the tumor measured higher than CSF in density.

Surgically proved cystic glioma.

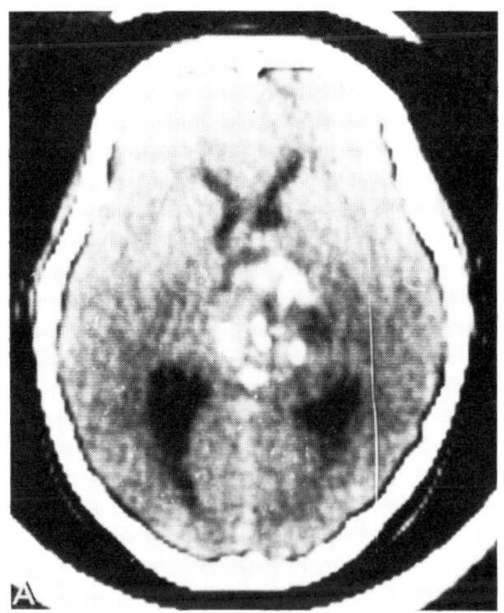

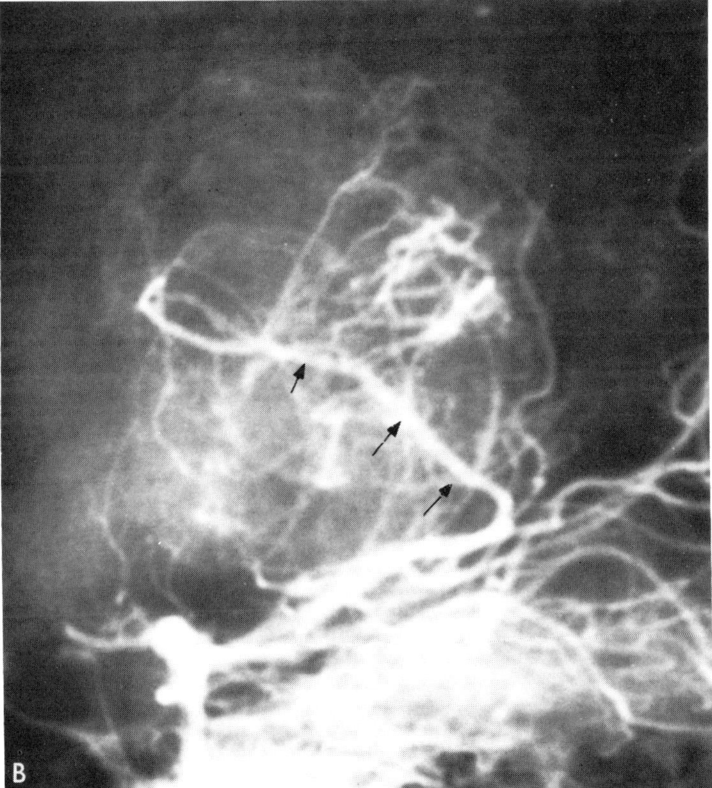

Figure 10–6. EPENDYMOMA: *A,* The CT scan demonstrates an irregularly calcified mass arising in the region of the third ventricle and off to either side — slightly more on the right than the left. There are areas of both peripheral and central calcification. The third ventricle is compressed, and a curvilinear portion of the third ventricle projects just anterior to the mass. The frontal horns of the lateral ventricles are distorted by the mass, and there is mild obstructive hydrocephalus.

B, The lateral view of the vertebral angiogram reveals marked enlargement of the medial posterior choroidal vessels *(arrows)* and multiple small abnormal vessels that extend from this vessel to supply a large area of abnormal vascularity. There was no blood supply to the tumor from the carotid artery system.

Surgically proved ependymoma arising from the third ventricle. Differential diagnosis includes pinealoma, teratoma, astrocytoma or oligodendroglioma. (Case courtesy of Dr. Gregory I. Shenk.)

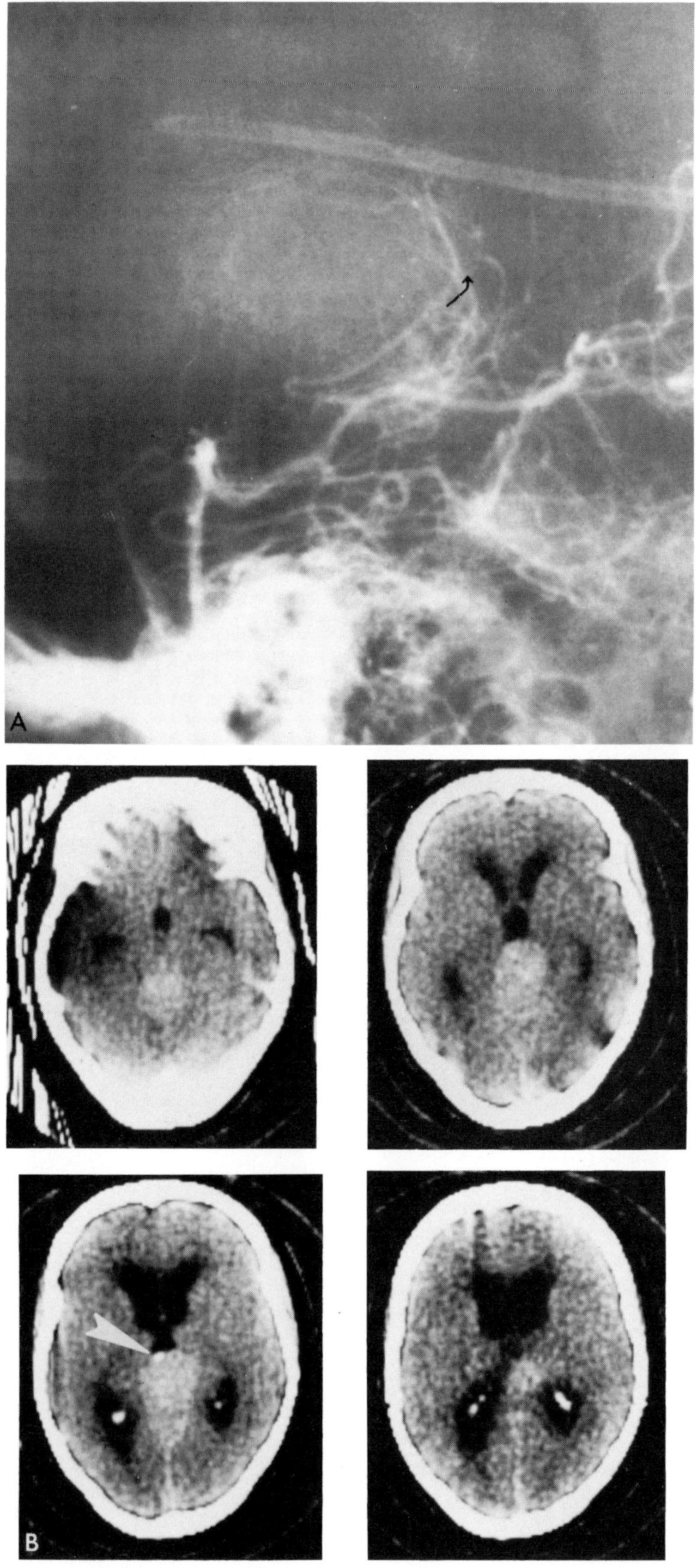

Figure 10–7. *See legend on the opposite page.*

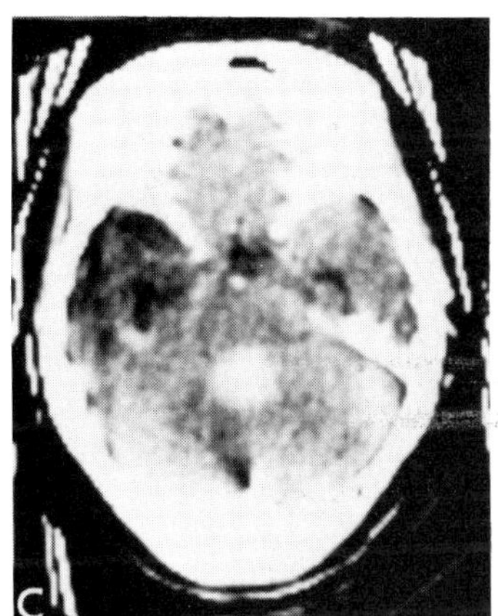

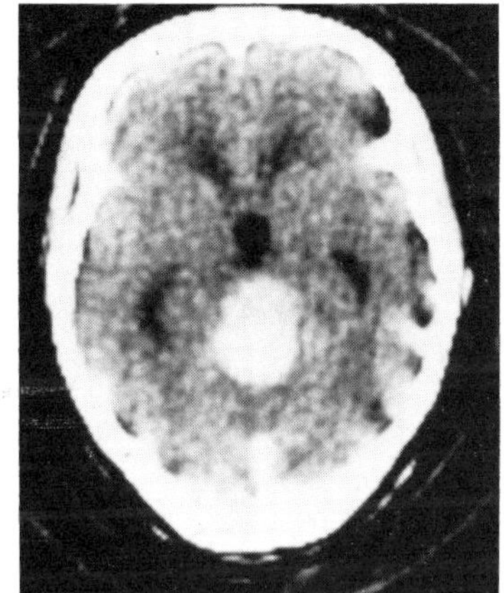

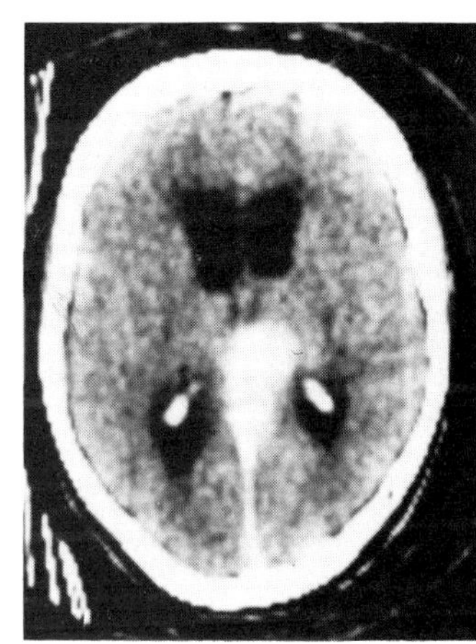

Figure 10–7. PINEALOMA: *A*, The lateral view of the vertebral angiogram reveals enlargement of the medial posterior choroidal artery, which courses in a curvilinear fashion around the tumor mass (*arrow*). A very faint tumor blush is seen anterior to this vessel. The carotid angiogram revealed hydrocephalus but was otherwise unremarkable. A shunt tubing device is seen in place.

B, The preinfusion CT scan reveals a fairly well defined mass in the region of the pineal gland that appears to displace the calcified pineal anteriorly (*arrow*). The mass appears to extend into the posterior fossa at the level of the tentorial notch.

C, There is marked homogeneous enhancement of the tumor on the postinfusion scan. There is moderate obstructive hydrocephalus.

Differential diagnosis includes pinealoma, aneurysm of the vein of Galen (unlikely) or metastasis.

Surgically proved pinealoma.

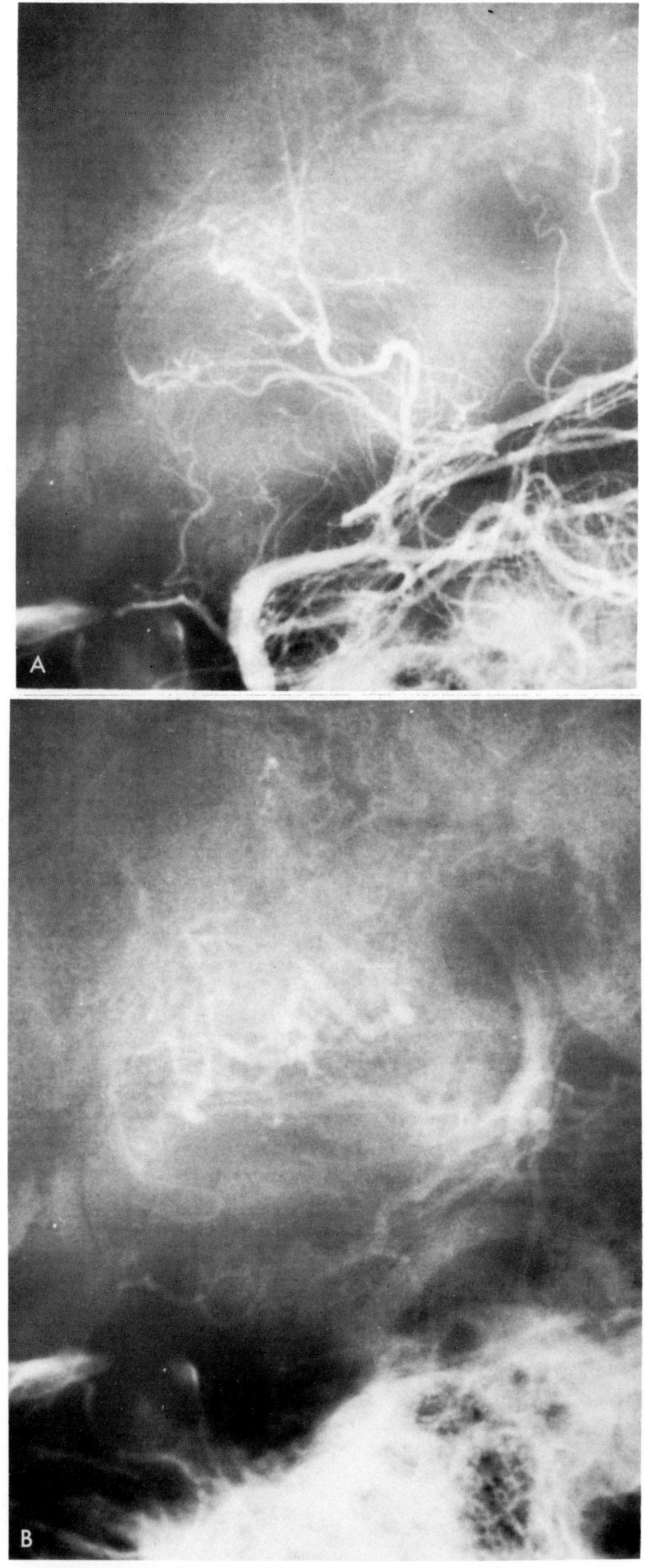

Figure 10–8. *See legend on the opposite page.*

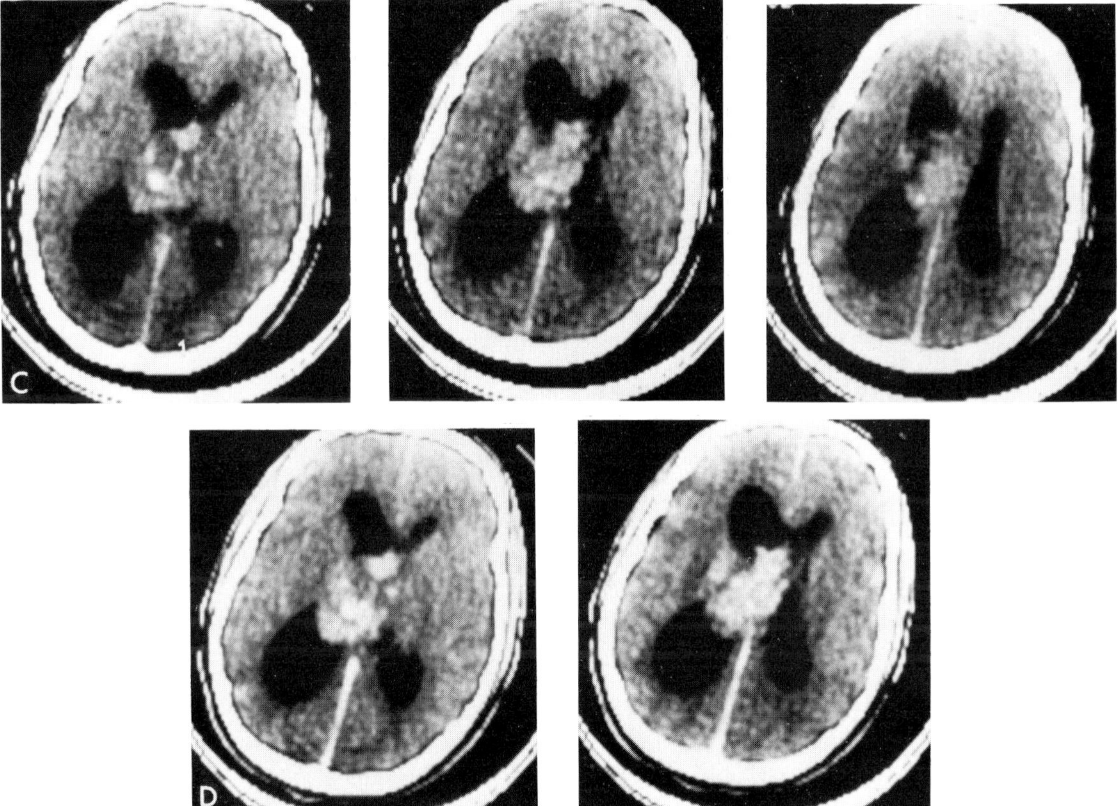

Figure 10–8. PINEALOMA: *A* and *B*, The arterial phase of the vertebral angiogram demonstrates enlargement of the lateral posterior choroidal artery. This vessel gives rise to multiple small abnormal tumor vessels in the region of the mass. The anterior thalamoperforating arteries as they arise from the posterior communicating artery are also enlarged and course superiorly to supply the tumor. The venous phase demonstrates a dense tumor stain and multiple tortuous abnormal veins which were noted to fill prematurely on the serial angiogram. Note the diffuse demineralization of the sella turcica secondary to increased intracranial pressure.

C, The CT scan demonstrates a large, lobulated, irregularly calcified mass in the midline that extends to the left of the midline.

D, There is only moderate enhancement of the tumor on the postinfusion scan.

Differential diagnosis includes pinealoma, ependymoma, glioma and metastases.

Surgically proved pinealoma.

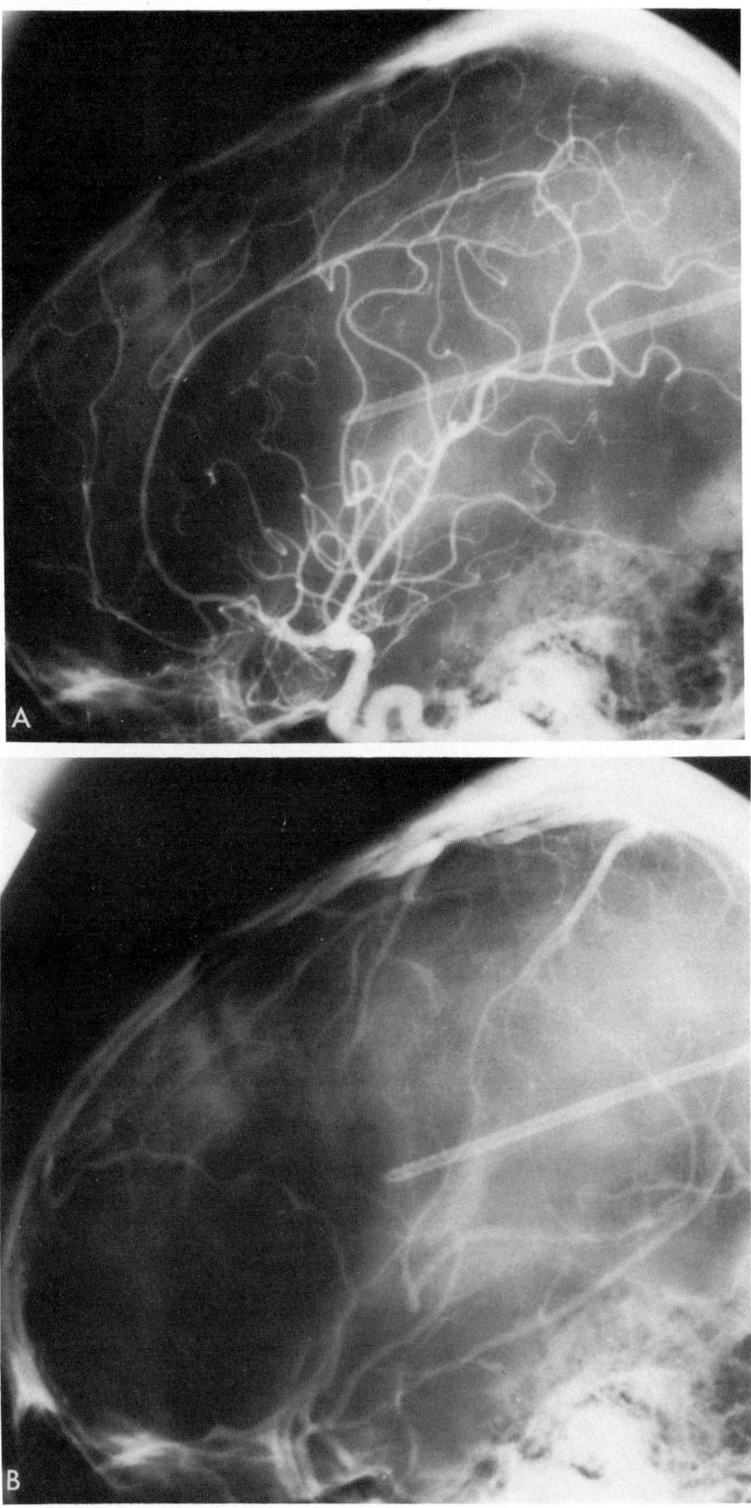

Figure 10–9. *See legend on the opposite page.*

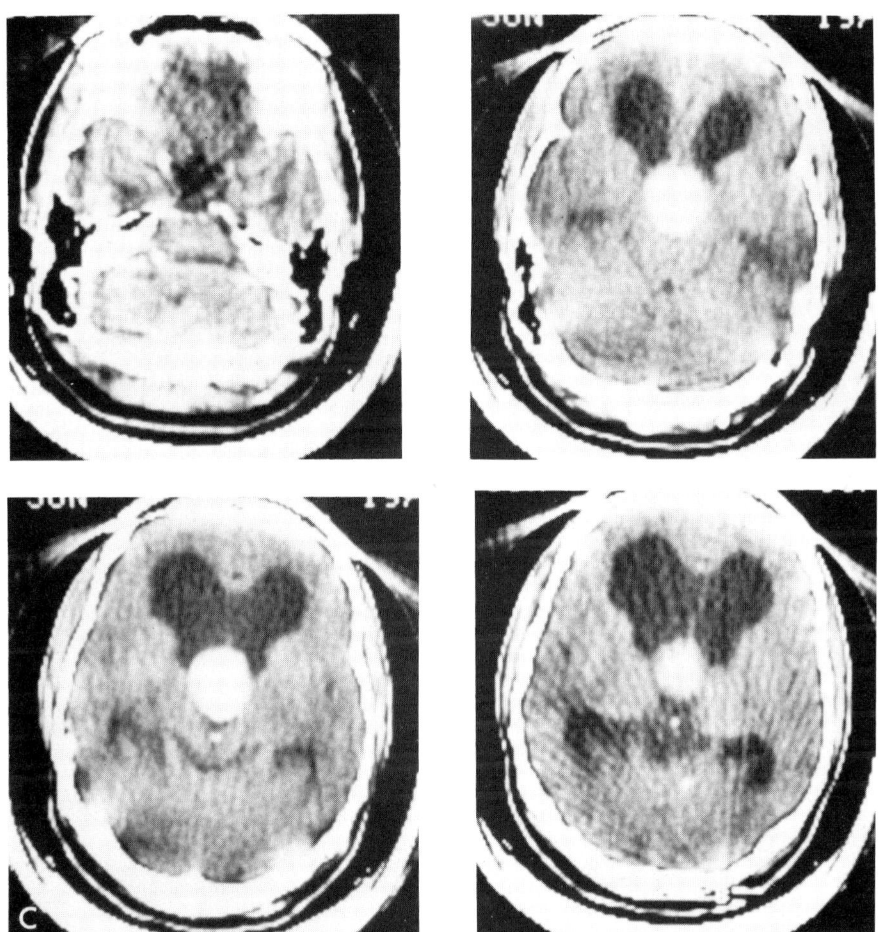

Figure 10–9. COLLOID CYST OF THE THIRD VENTRICLE: Colloid cysts that arise in the anterior third ventricle have been shown to develop from residual epithelial cells of the paraphysis in the anterior portion of the third ventricle. The arterial *(A)* and venous *(B)* phases of the carotid angiogram reveal marked hydrocephalus, but are otherwise unremarkable. The venous phase AP (not shown) demonstrated that the internal cerebral veins are displaced apart by the large mass lesion growing between them.

C, The preinfusion CT scan reveals a large high density mass in the midline occupying the position of the third ventricle and leading to obstructive hydrocephalus secondary to bilateral blockage of the foramen of Monro. There is marked obstructive hydrocephalus.

Choroid plexus papillomas also may develop in the third ventricle and may at times cause unilateral occlusion of the foramen of Monro as it leads into the lateral ventricles. Patients with choroid plexus papillomas may have positional headache because of an intermittent obstruction of the foramen of Monro that leads to ipsilateral hydrocephalus when the patient assumes a certain position.

Illustration continued on the following page.

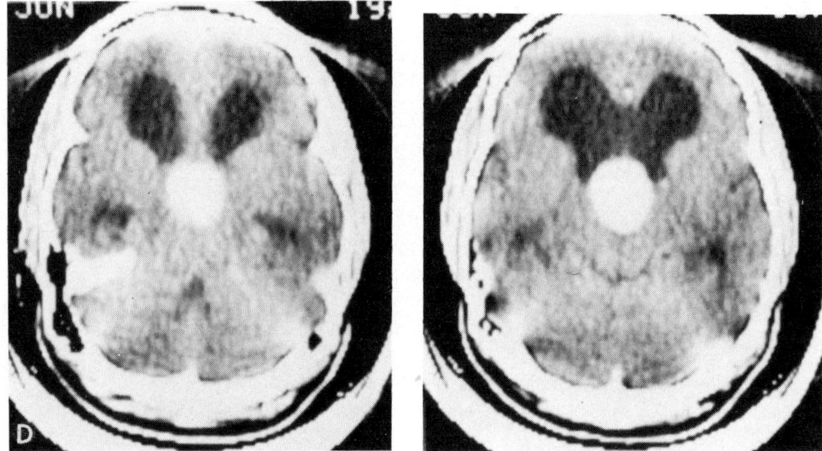

Figure 10–9 *Continued.*
D, No change is seen following the infusion of contrast material.

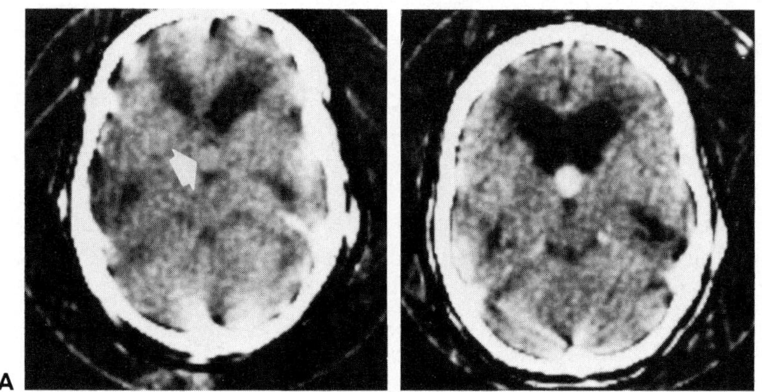

Figure 10–10. *See legend on the opposite page.*

B

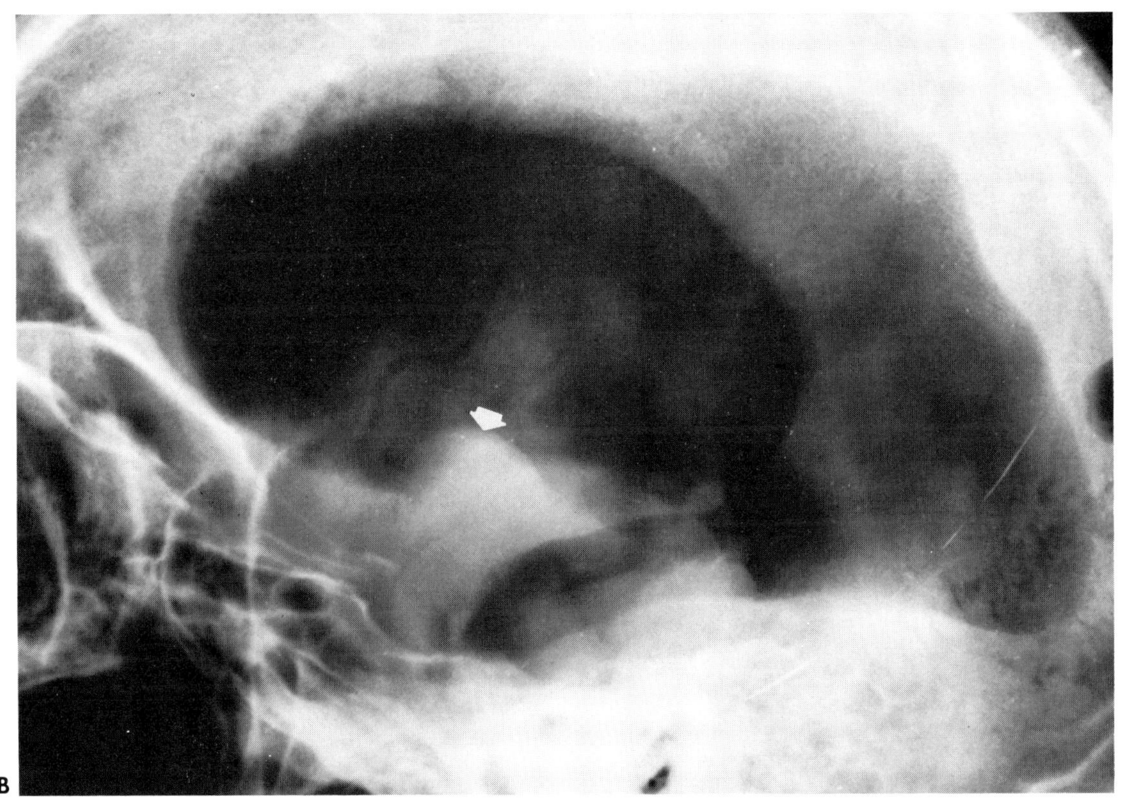

Figure 10–10 *Continued.* Surgically proved colloid cyst of the third ventricle.

Differential diagnosis incudes aneurysm, teratoma, hemorrhage (unlikely) or hemorrhagic primary or secondary brain tumor.

A, The CT scan demonstrates an isodense mass in the anterior portion of the third ventricle that reveals homogeneous enhancement on the postinfusion scan. Obstructive hydrocephalus is also present. Colloid cysts may be of higher density than normal brain substance or isodense on the preinfusion scan.

B, The pneumoencephalogram in another patient demonstrates a mass in the anterior portion of the third ventricle (*white arrowhead*) that is associated with marked hydrocephalus secondary to obstruction of the foramen of Monro bilaterally.

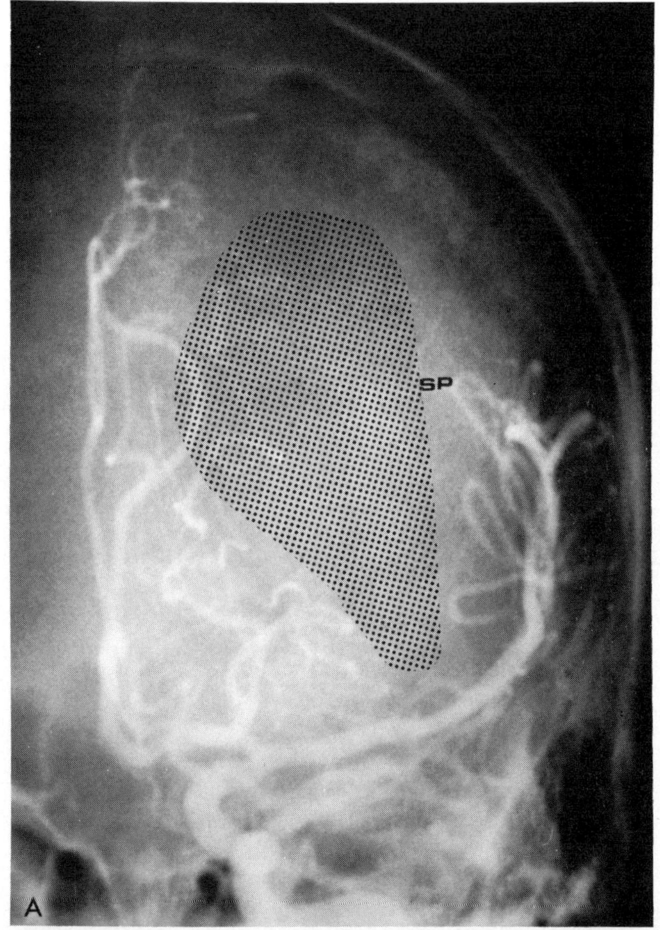

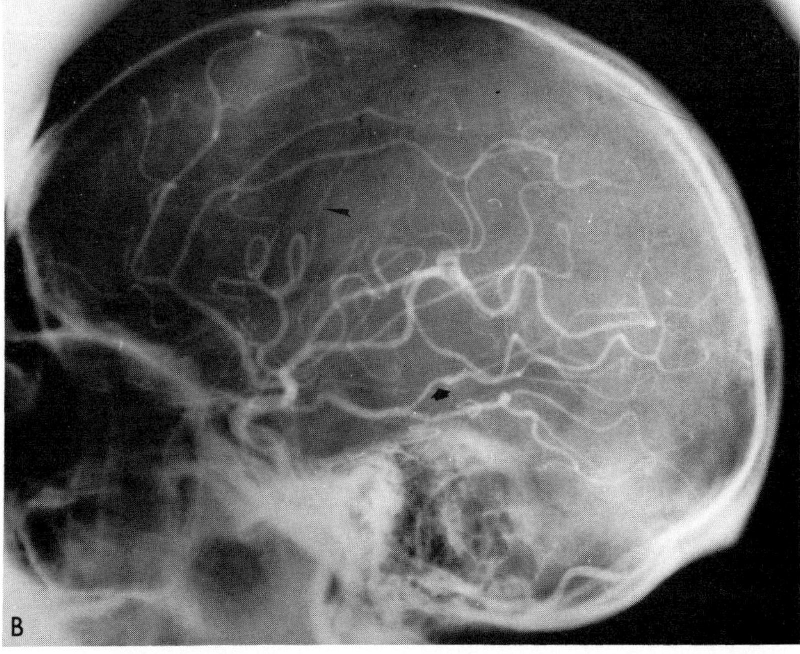

Figure 10–11. *See legend on the opposite page.*

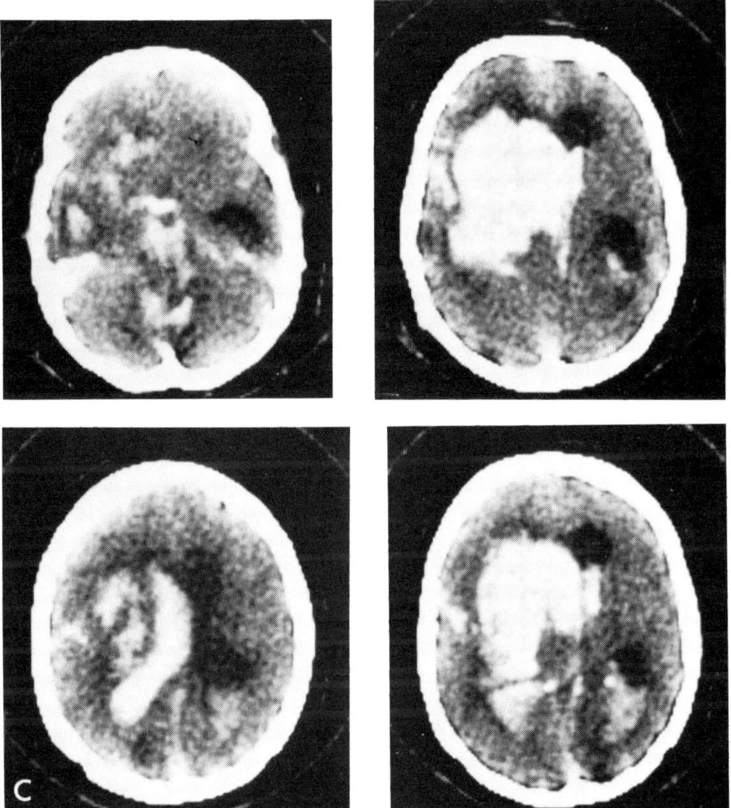

Figure 10–11. BASAL GANGLIONIC HEMORRHAGE: *A*, The AP view of the carotid angiogram reveals shift of the anterior cerebral artery to the contralateral side, more marked in the mid- and distal portions than in the proximal. The sylvian point and the middle cerebral artery branches are displaced laterally (*SP*); the shaded area outlines the approximate position of the bulk of the basal ganglionic hemorrhage.

B, The lateral view demonstrates widening of the sweep of the pericallosal artery. The sylvian triangle appears to be in a relatively normal position. Branches of the middle cerebral artery and the posterior cerebral artery show areas of focal spasm secondary to blood in the subarachnoid space (*arrows*).

C, The CT scan demonstrates a large left basal ganglionic hematoma. In addition, there is rupture into the ventricular system, with blood in the lateral, third and fourth ventricles. There is blood in the dependent portions of the lateral ventricles, giving the appearance of blood/CSF fluid levels. The hemorrhage has also ruptured into the subarachnoid space and can be seen outlining multiple cortical sulci.

Figure 10–12. BASAL GANGLIONIC HEMORRHAGE: *A*, The AP view of the carotid angiogram reveals both proximal and distal shift of the pericallosal artery. There is lateral displacement of the sylvian point and the remaining branches of the middle cerebral artery as they run in the isle of Reil. The shaded area outlines the approximate position of a large avascular mass in the region of a putamen of the basal ganglia. The lenticulostriate arteries are displaced medially by the mass.

B, The subtraction view of the angiogram better demonstrates the lenticulostriate arteries and the large avascular area in the region of the putamen. There is spasm of the distal horizontal portion of the middle cerebral artery.

C, The lateral view demonstrates downward displacement of the midportion of the sylvian triangle (*dashed line*) and stretching of all the opercular branches of the middle cerebral artery in the posterior frontal and anterior parietal regions *(arrows)*. The mass extends high up to affect these vessels. The meningeal artery is quite prominent, probably because of excessive filling of the external carotid artery system secondary to increased intracranial pressure.

D, The CT scan demonstrates a large intracerebral hematoma in the region of the putamen of the right basal ganglia. The isle of Reil is poorly visualized but is displaced laterally. The hematoma has ruptured into the ventricular system and demonstrates a blood/CSF level in the dependent portion of the left lateral ventricle. There is shift from right to left and dilatation of the left lateral ventricle.

IMP: Classic hypertensive basal ganglionic hemorrhage.

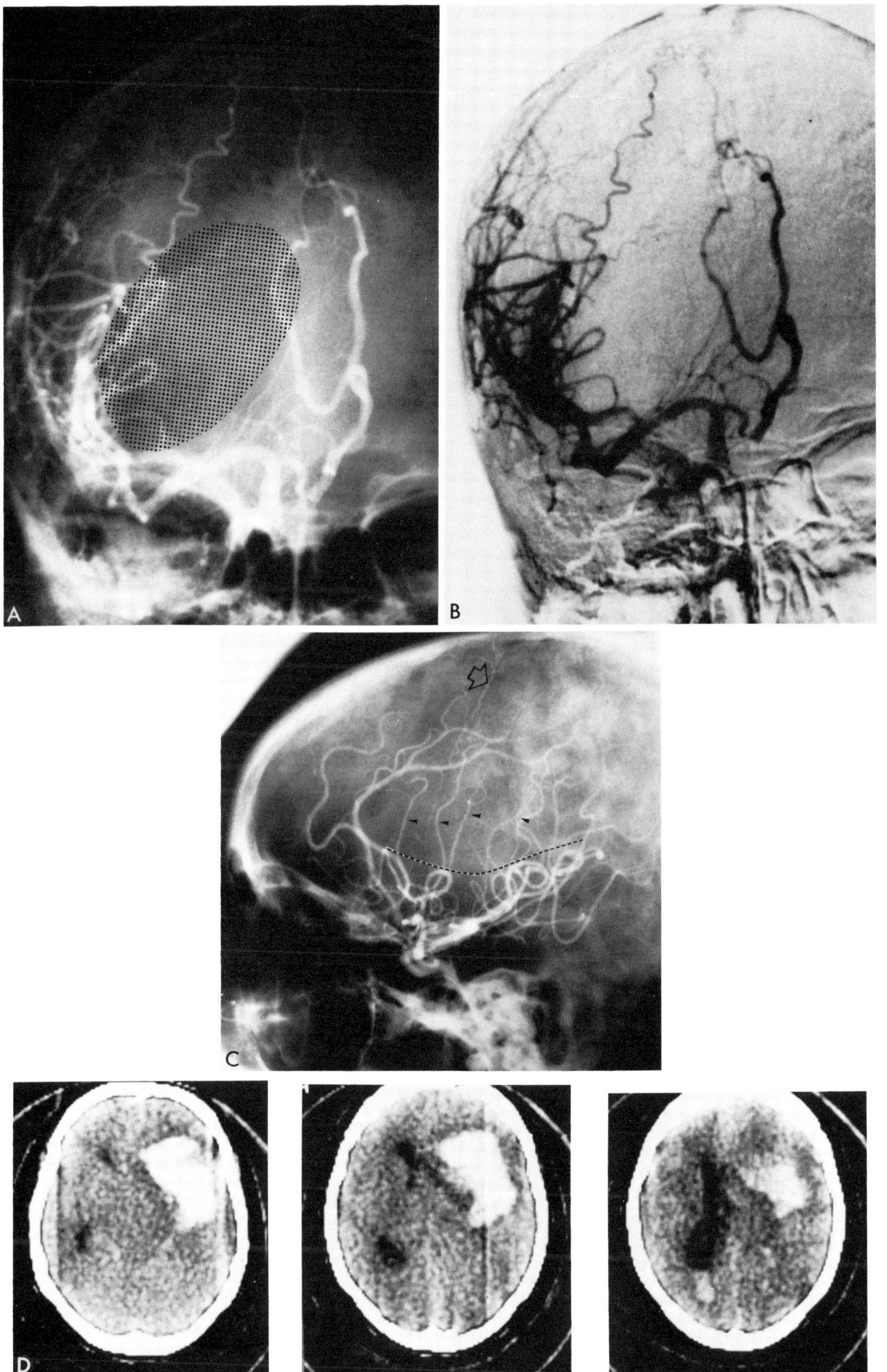

Figure 10–12. *See legend on the opposite page.*

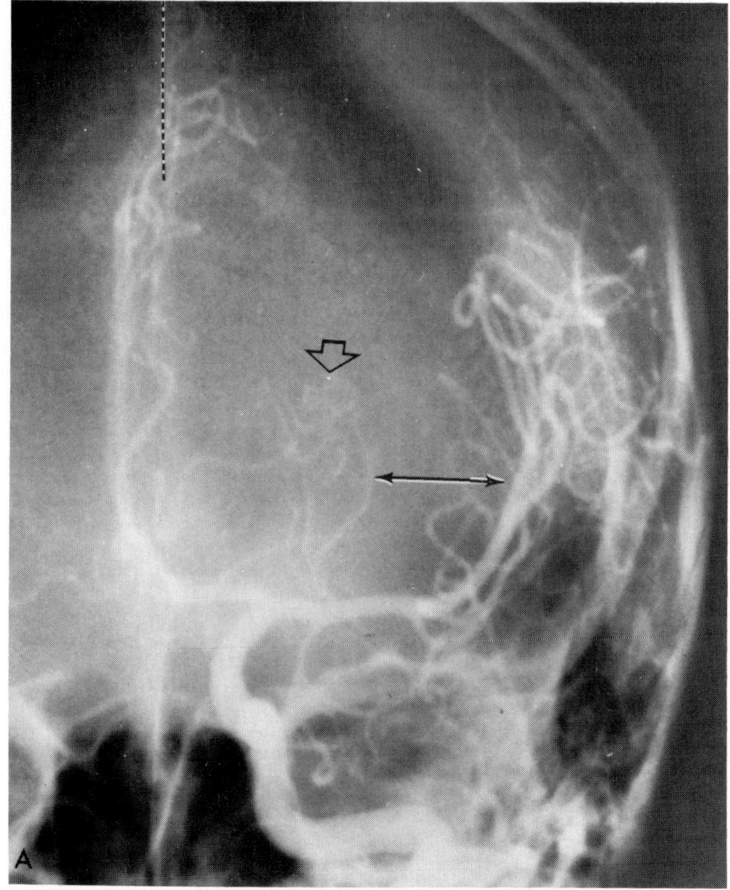

Figure 10–13. BASAL GANGLIONIC HEMORRHAGE: *A*, The AP view of the angiogram reveals an increased distance between the anterior cerebral and middle cerebral arteries as well as medial displacement of the lenticulostriate arteries *(double-headed arrow)*. There is a proximal and distal shift of the anterior cerebral artery and its branches. The distal portions of the lenticulostriate arteries appear to be dilated and tortuous *(open arrow)*, perhaps reflecting small aneurysm formation thought to be responsible for these hypertensive basal ganglionic hemorrhages. Dotted line marks the normal falx.

B, The CT scan shows a large basal ganglionic hemorrhage on the left side that has ruptured into the ventricular system. Clotted blood is also present in the fourth ventricle.

C, The pathologic specimen demonstrates a classic basal ganglionic hemorrhage.

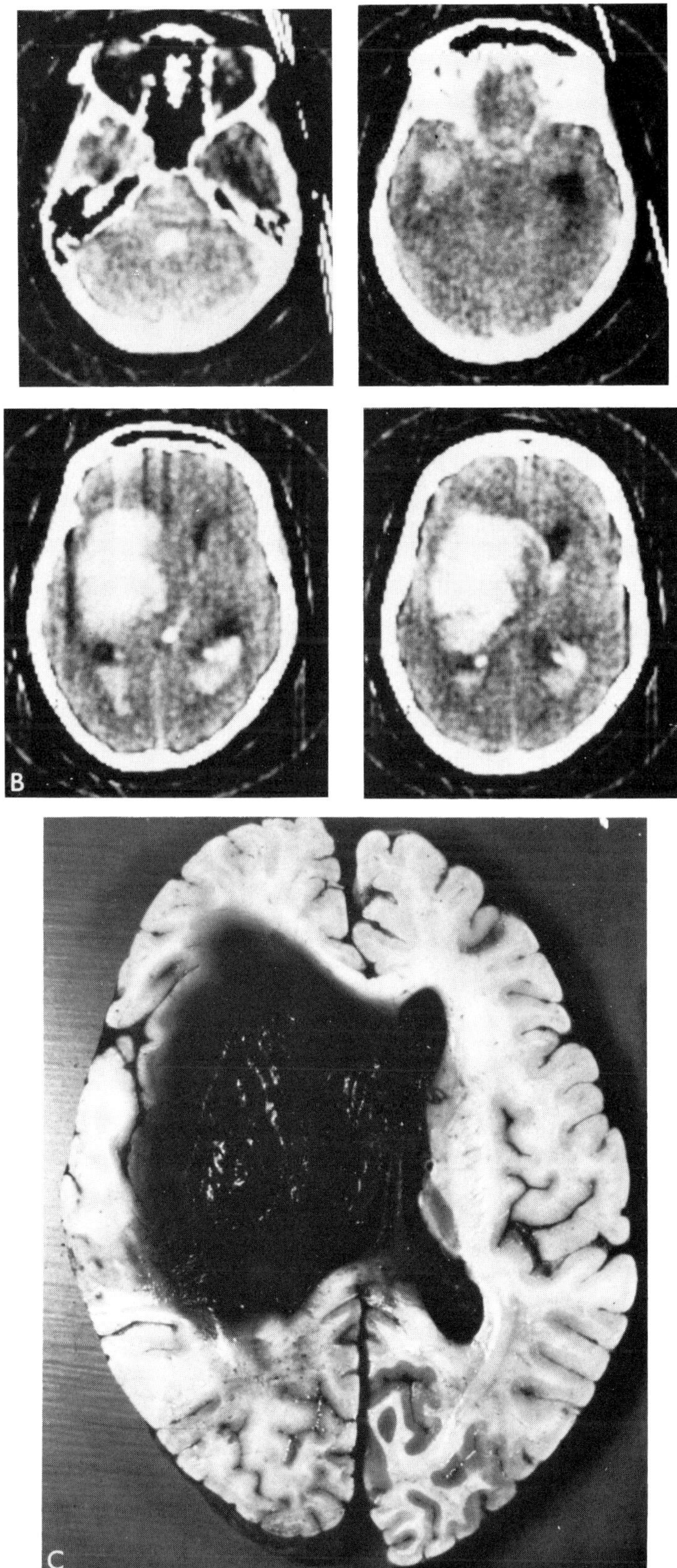

Figure 10–13 *Continued.*

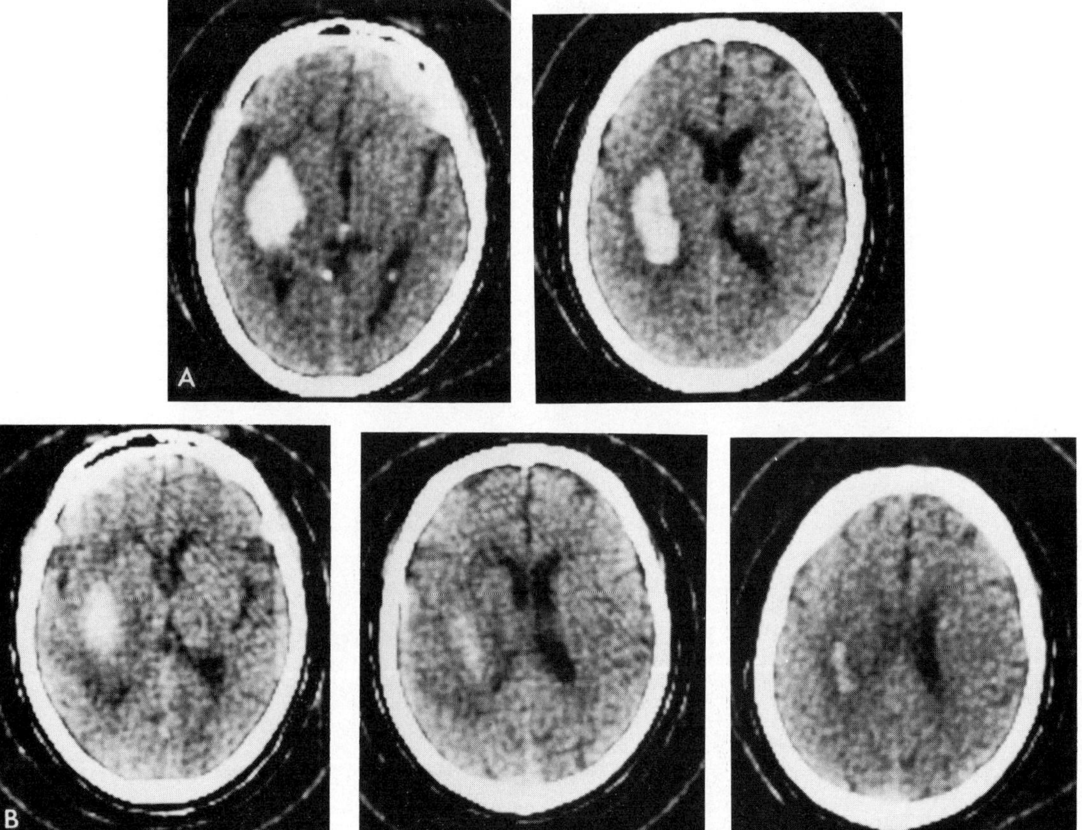

Figure 10–14. BASAL GANGLIONIC HEMORRHAGE: *A*, The initial CT scan demonstrates a moderate sized hemorrhage in the region of the putamen of the basal ganglia on the left side. A slight shift from left to right and obliteration of the normal cisterns and sulci on the side of the hemorrhage are seen.

B, A follow-up scan obtained two and one half weeks later reveals partial resorption of the hemorrhage, more surrounding edema and a greater shift than present on the initial scan.

IMP: Resolving basal ganglionic hemorrhage.

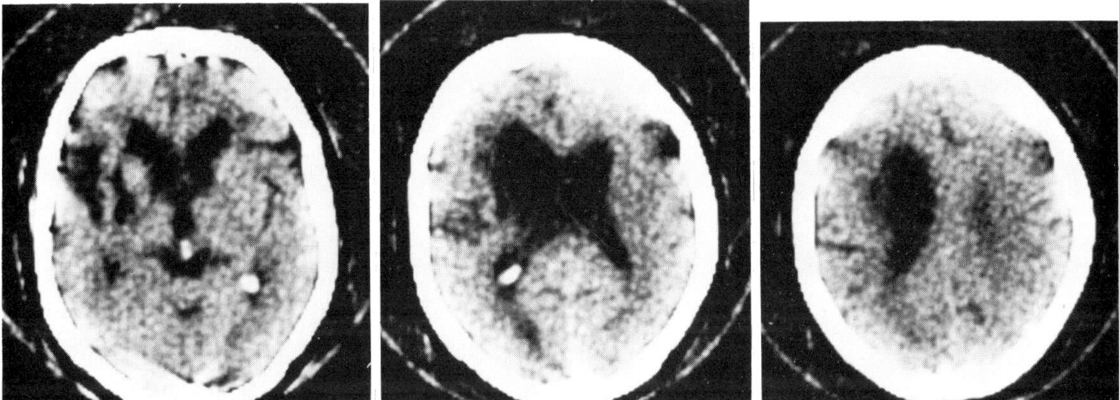

Figure 10–15. OLD BASAL GANGLIONIC HEMORRHAGE: With time, the hemorrhage ultimately absorbs and may lead to the development of a closed porencephalic cyst in the bed of the hematoma. In this example there is also enlargement of the left lateral ventricle and cortical sulci on the side of the hematoma, secondary to atrophy.

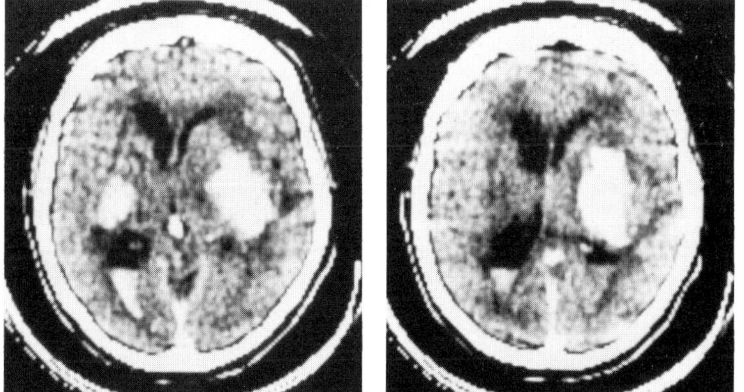

Figure 10–16. BILATERAL BASAL GANGLIONIC HEMORRHAGE: The CT scan demonstrates bilateral basal ganglionic hemorrhages slightly larger on the right than on the left. There is rupture into the ventricular system on the left side, with a blood/CSF level in the dependent portion of the left lateral ventricle. (Case courtesy of Dr. David Neer.)

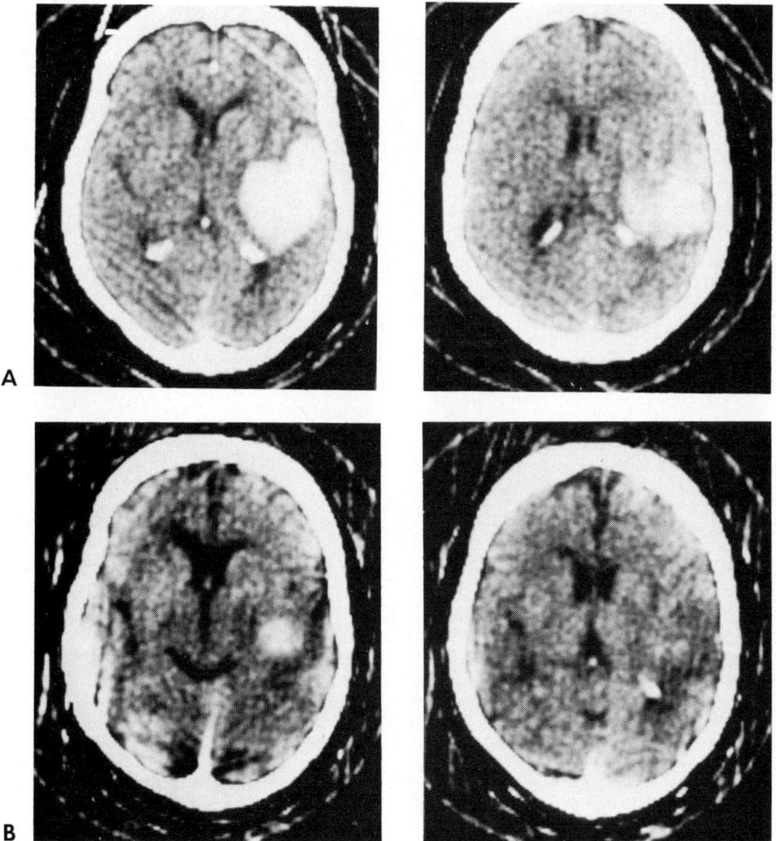

Figure 10–17. RESOLVING BASAL GANGLIONIC HEMATOMA: *A*, The CT scan initially reveals a large basal ganglionic hemorrhage in the right hemisphere. *B*, Approximately three and one half weeks later there is nearly complete resorption of the hematoma. The lateral ventricles have increased in size on the follow-up study.

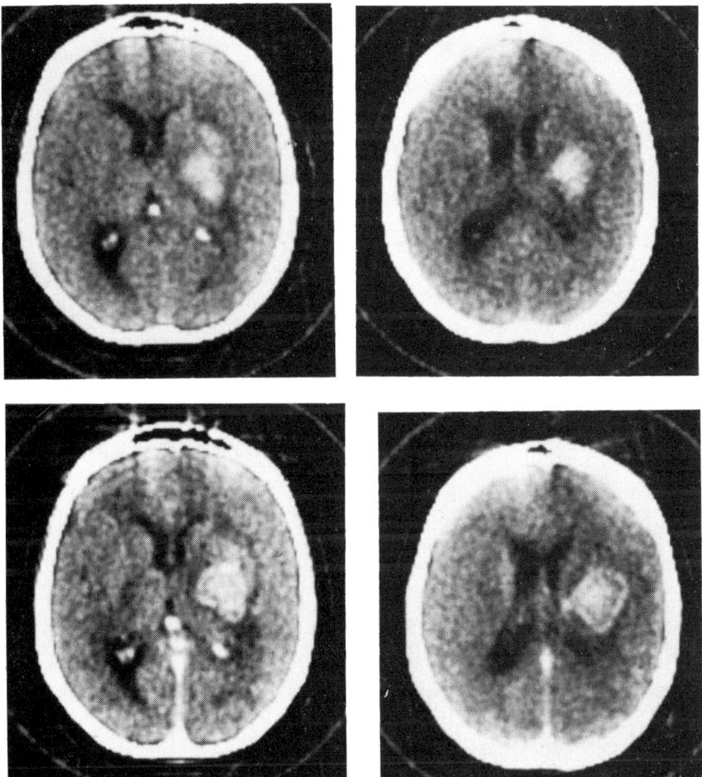

Figure 10–18. RESOLVING BASAL GANGLIONIC HEMATOMA: The CT scan reveals a partially resorbed basal ganglionic hematoma on the right side. There is a small amount of surrounding edema and slight compression of the body of the right lateral ventricle. The postinfusion scan demonstrates a ring of enhancement around the hematoma — a finding not uncommonly seen with resorbing hematoma.

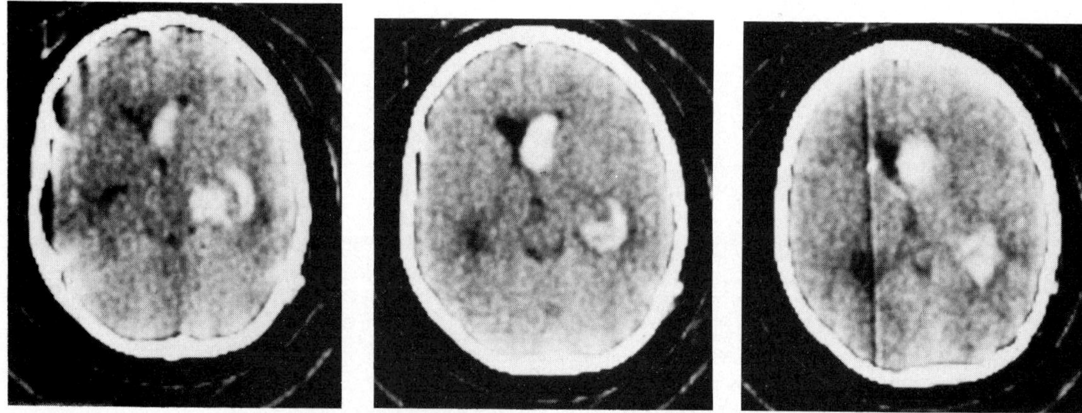

Figure 10–19. THALAMIC HEMORRHAGE WITH VENTRICULAR RUPTURE: The CT scan reveals a small rounded area of hemorrhage into the lateral aspect of the right thalamus. The hematoma has ruptured into the ventricular system, and blood forms a cast of the frontal horn and the temporal horns of the right lateral ventricle.

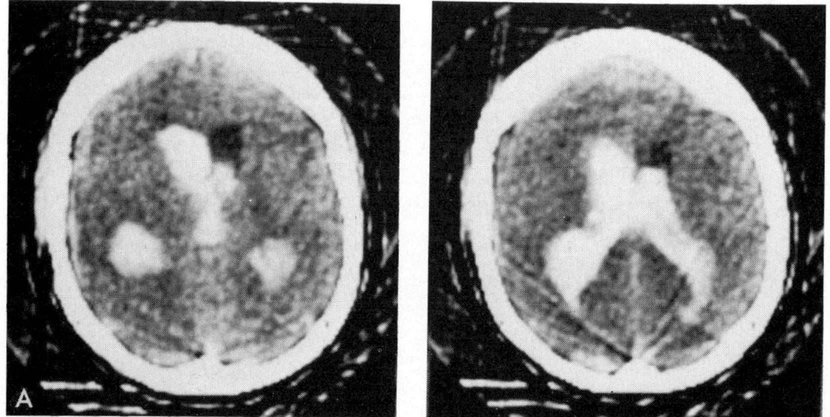

Figure 10–20. INTRAVENTRICULAR HEMORRHAGE: *A*, The CT scan reveals that the entire ventricular system is filled with clotted blood secondary to hemorrhage into the ventricles. This finding may be secondary to a subarachnoid hemorrhage or to rupture of a subependymal vein in the wall of the lateral ventricle.

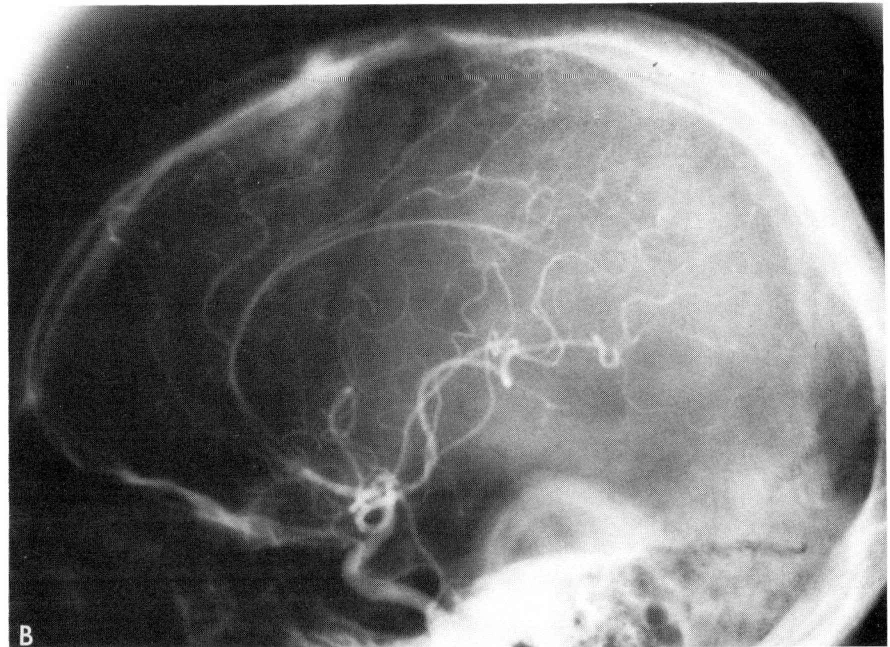

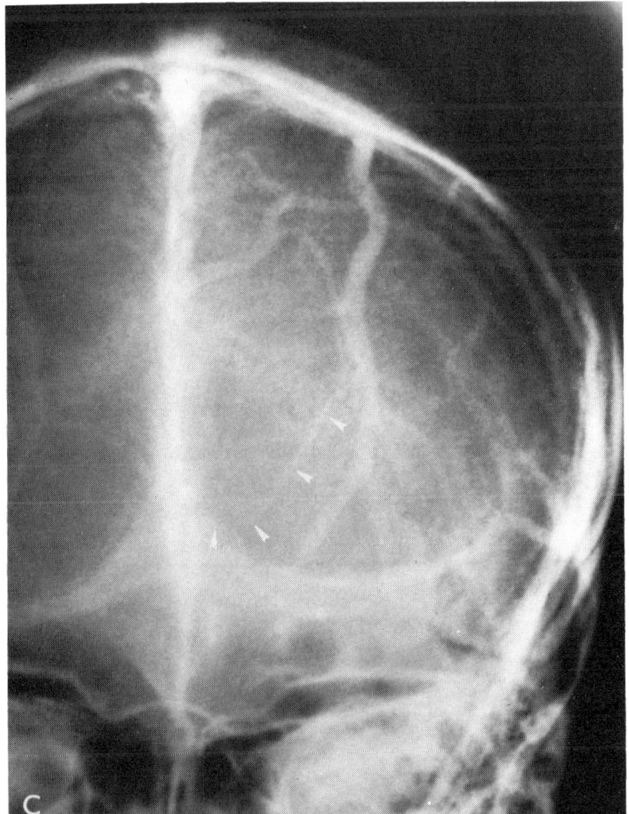

Figure 10–20 *Continued.*

B and *C*, The arterial and venous phase of the angiogram demonstrates a widened sweep of the pericallosal artery and lateral displacement of the thalamostriate vein (*arrows*) secondary to the dilatation of the ventricular system by the blood.

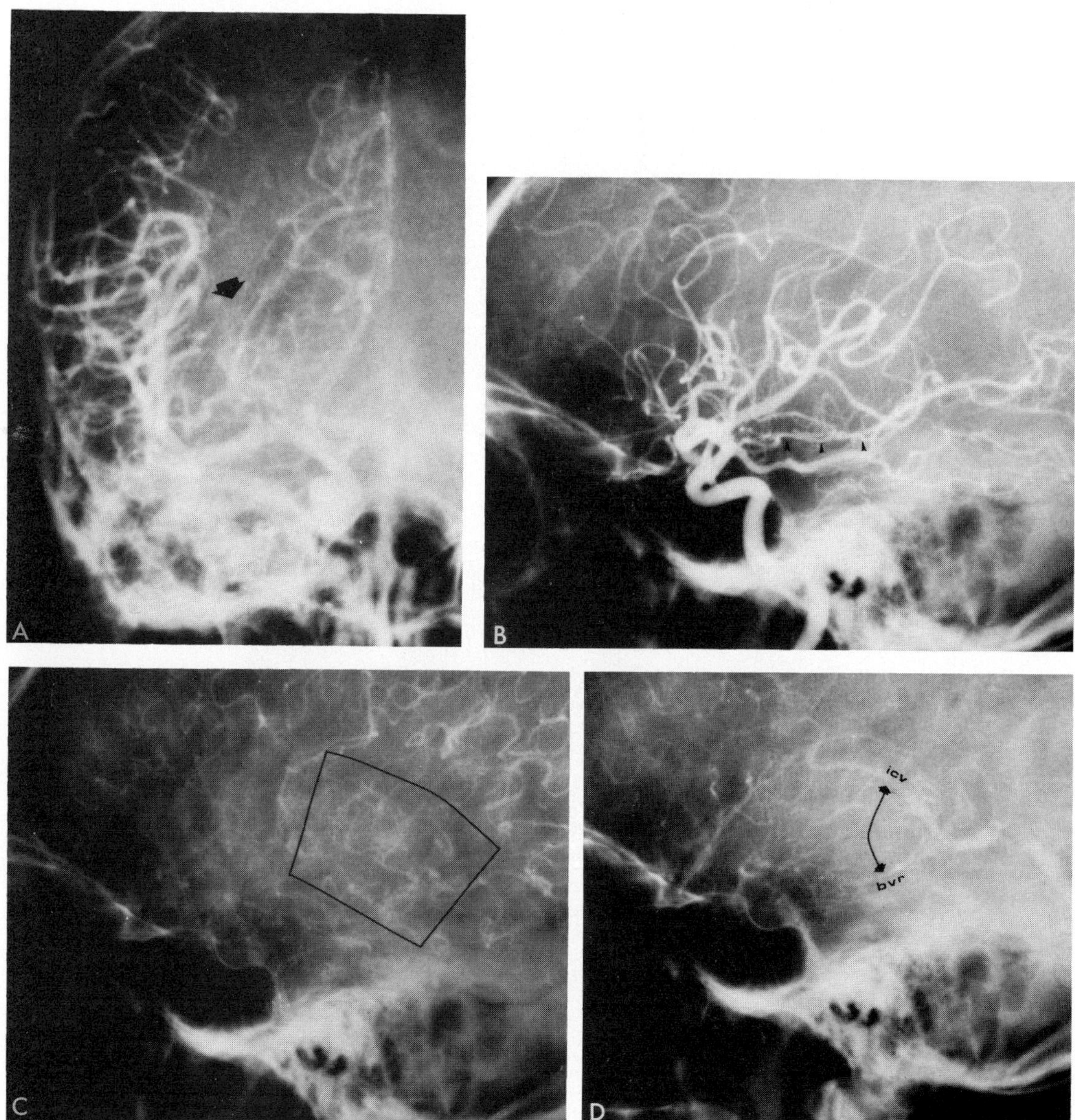

Figure 10–21. THALAMIC GLIOMA: *A,* The AP angiographic view reveals an enlarged anterior choroidal artery (*arrow*) that courses posteriorly and medially to supply a tumor in the region of the right thalamus.

B, The lateral view reveals the anterior choroidal artery supplying the tumor (*black arrows*) but otherwise demonstrates no real vascular displacement.

The capillary phase (*C*) reveals a faint tumor blush in the region of the thalamus (*black lines*); the venous phase (*D*) demonstrates a widening of the distance between the internal cerebral vein and the basal vein of Rosenthal by the tumor mass in the region of the thalamus (*double-headed arrow*).

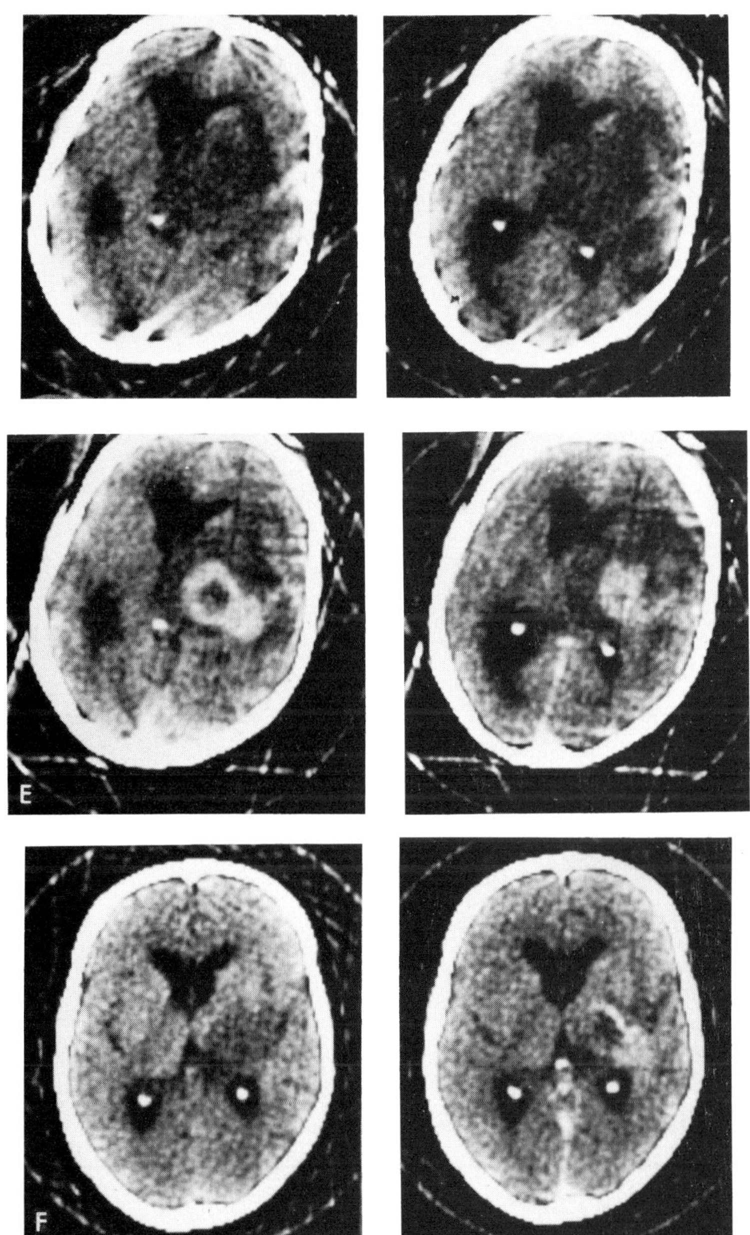

Figure 10–21 *Continued.*

E, The CT scan reveals a large lucent lesion in the region of the right thalamus; an enhancing mass with surrounding edema is seen on the postinfusion scan. The tumor enhanced with both a ring and a solid portion. There is slight shift from right to left and compression of the body of the right lateral ventricle.

F, A follow-up scan obtained following radiation therapy demonstrates marked regression of the tumor.

Biopsy-proved thalamic glioblastoma.

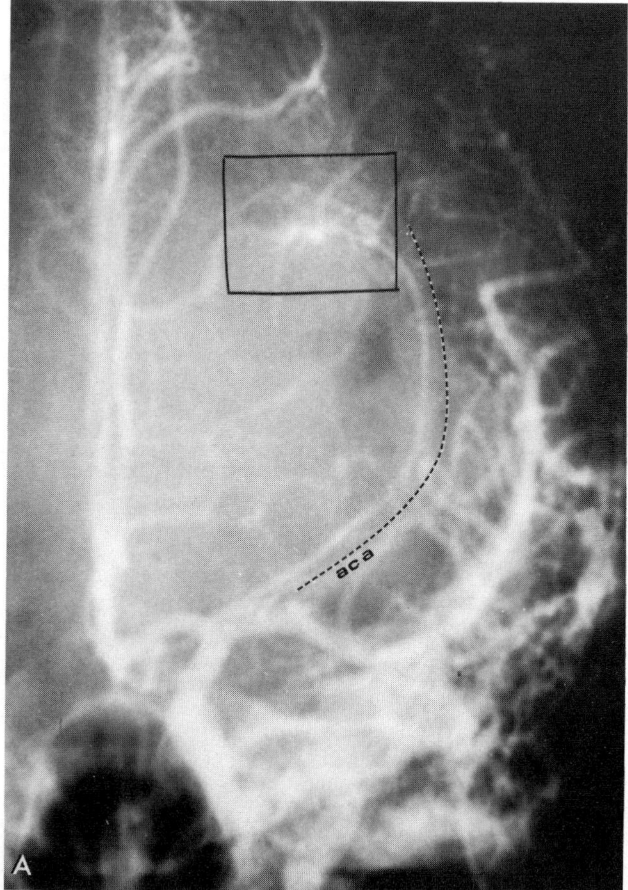

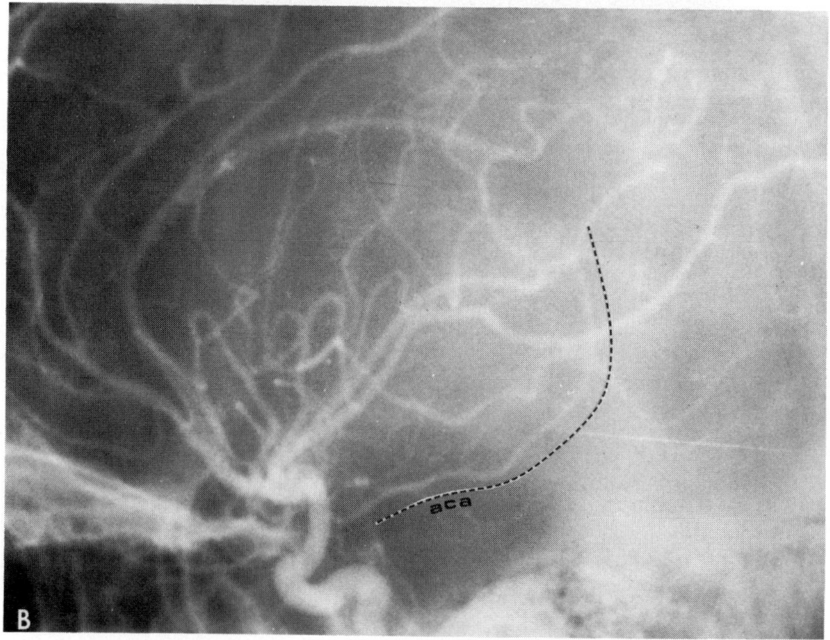

Figure 10–22. *See legend on the opposite page.*

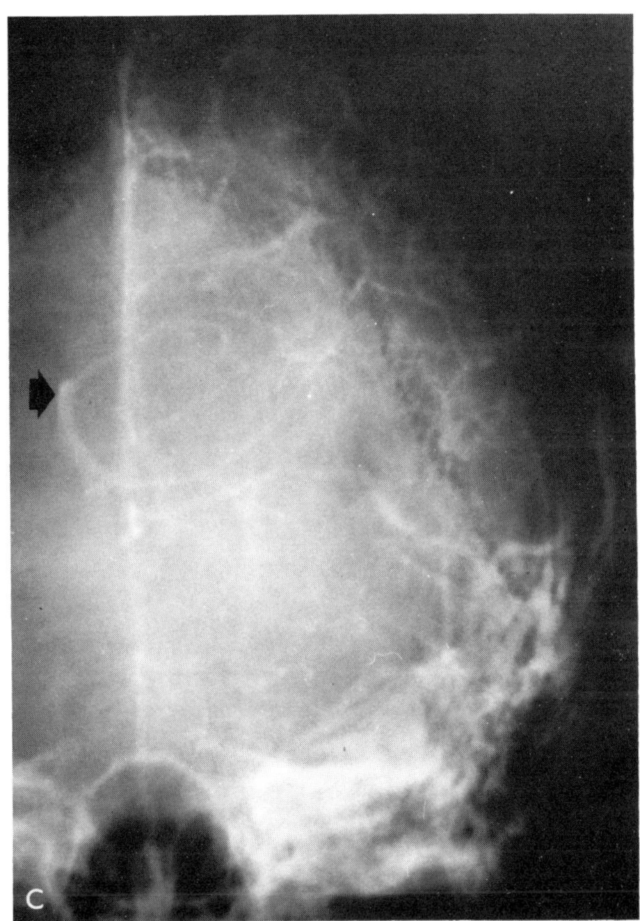

Figure 10–22. THALAMIC GLIOMA: *A* and *B*, The AP and lateral views of the carotid angiogram reveal a greatly enlarged anterior choroidal artery (*aca*) that supplies an area of tumor blush in the superior aspect of the right thalamus (*black lines*). There is obstructive hydrocephalus; the anterior cerebral arteries are closely applied to the midline, and the middle cerebral artery branches in the isle of Reil are displaced laterally by the dilated temporal horn as well as by the mass. The AP venous phase (*C*) demonstrates a marked shift of the internal cerebral vein (*arrow*).

Biopsy: Thalamic glioma. (Case courtesy of Drs. Oscar Sugar and Glen Dobben.)

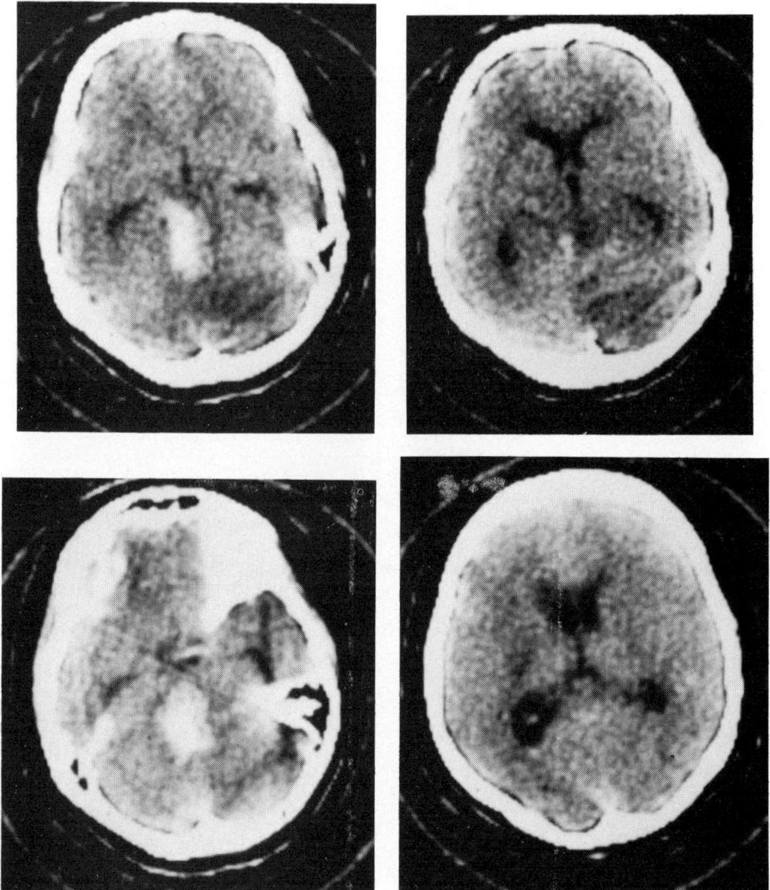

Figure 10–23. PONTINE HEMORRHAGE: The CT scan demonstrates a large area of hemorrhage in the pons that extends superiorly to involve the left cerebral peduncle. There is a small amount of blood in the dependent portions of the lateral ventricles, creating blood/CSF levels. There is moderate obstructive hydrocephalus.

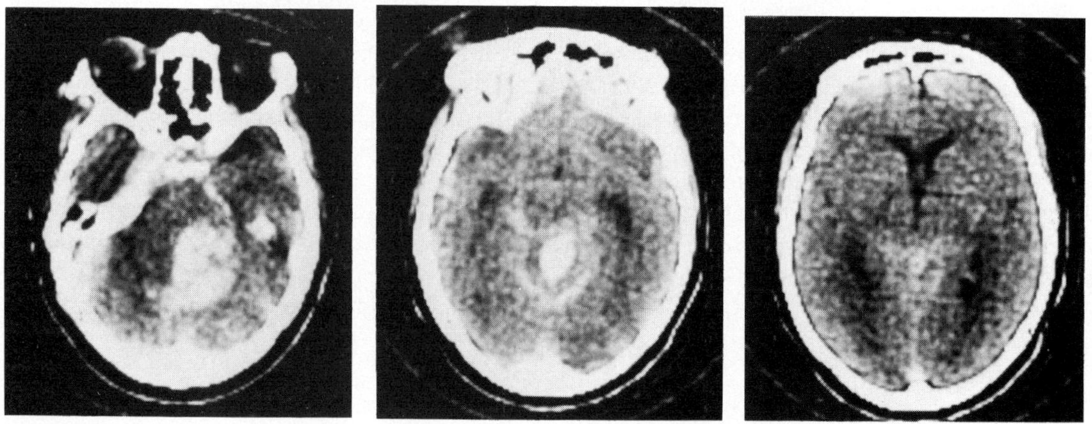

Figure 10–24. PONTINE AND CEREBELLAR HEMORRHAGE: The CT scan shows a large area of hemorrhage in the right cerebellum and the right side of the pons. The blood also has entered the subarachnoid space; it outlines the basilar cistern in the posterior fossa and fills the cerebellar folia.

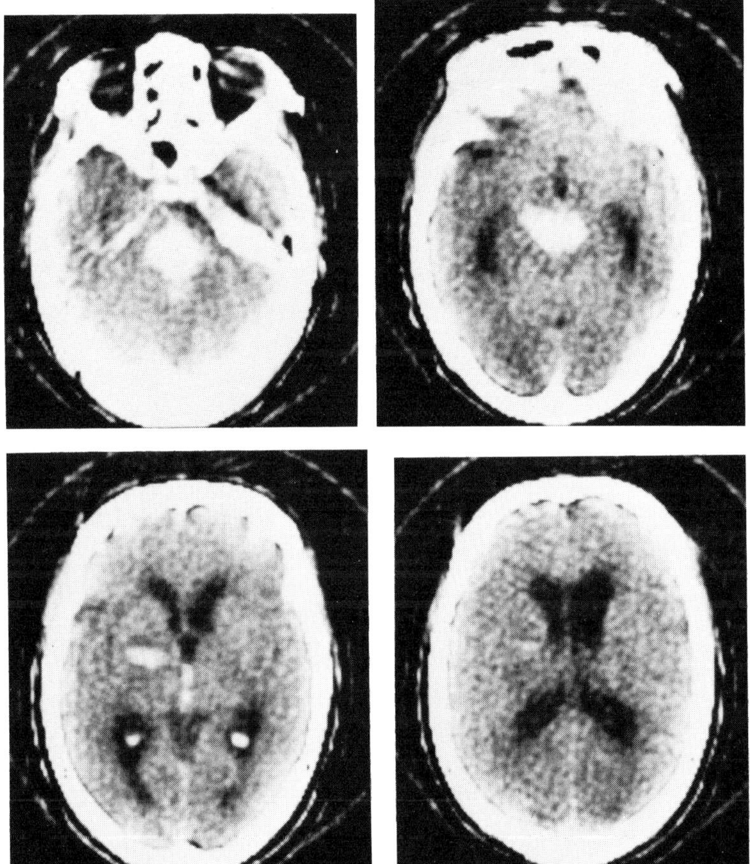

Figure 10–25. PONTINE HEMORRHAGE: There is a large area of hemorrhage in the pons and in the left cerebral peduncle. A small amount of blood in the third ventricle and evidence of hemorrhage into the basal ganglia on the left side are seen. Moderate obstructive hydrocephalus is present.

Figure 10–26. HYPERTENSIVE CEREBELLAR HEMORRHAGE: *A*, The CT scan demonstrates a large right cerebellar hematoma. The hemorrhage has ruptured into the fourth ventricle, and clotted blood is also present in the third and lateral ventricles. There is moderately severe obstructive hydrocephalus. The pathologic specimen (*B*) shows the precise correlation between the CT scan and the pathologic anatomy.

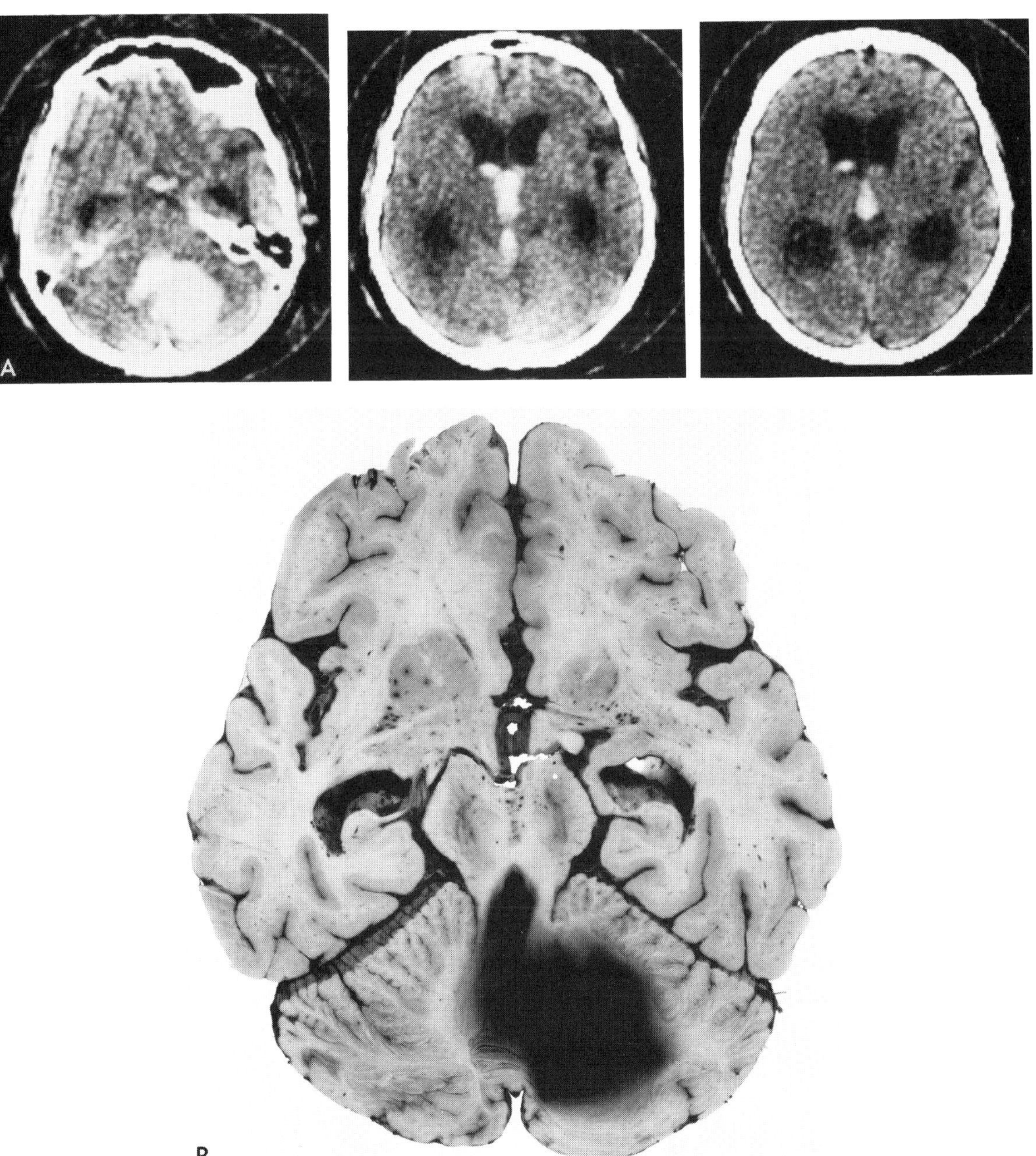

Figure 10–26. *See legend on the opposite page.*

Figure 10–27. SUPERIOR SAGITTAL SINUS THROMBOSIS: *A,* The initial CT study appears within normal limits. One week later (*B*), a second CT scan demonstrates an irregular area of hemorrhage in the left posterior parietal region and large areas of radiolucency throughout both hemispheres — slightly more marked on the right side than on the left. The falx is displaced in a curvilinear fashion toward the left side.

C, The pathologic specimen reveals large areas of hemorrhage in the high parietal regions bilaterally as well as marked edema of both cerebral hemispheres. There was also evidence of superior sagittal sinus thrombosis and bilateral cortical vein thrombosis. The areas of hemorrhage occur in the distribution of the occluded cortical veins, resembling a hemorrhagic infarct.

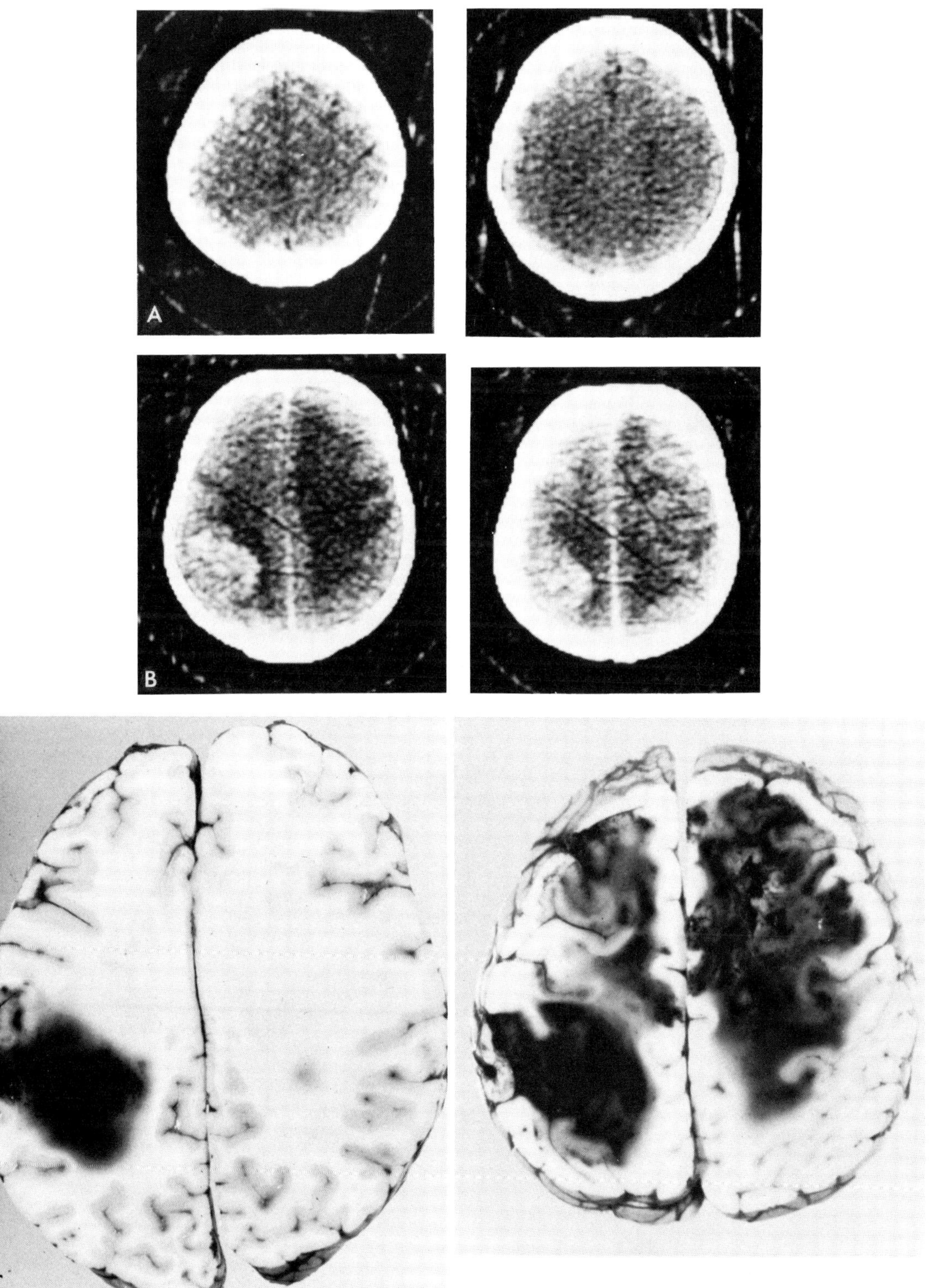

Figure 10–27. *See legend on the opposite page.*

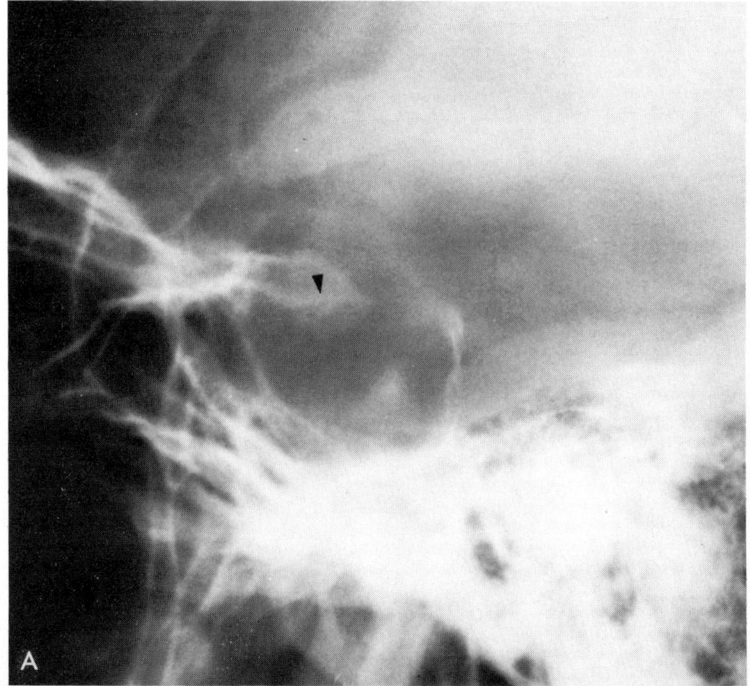

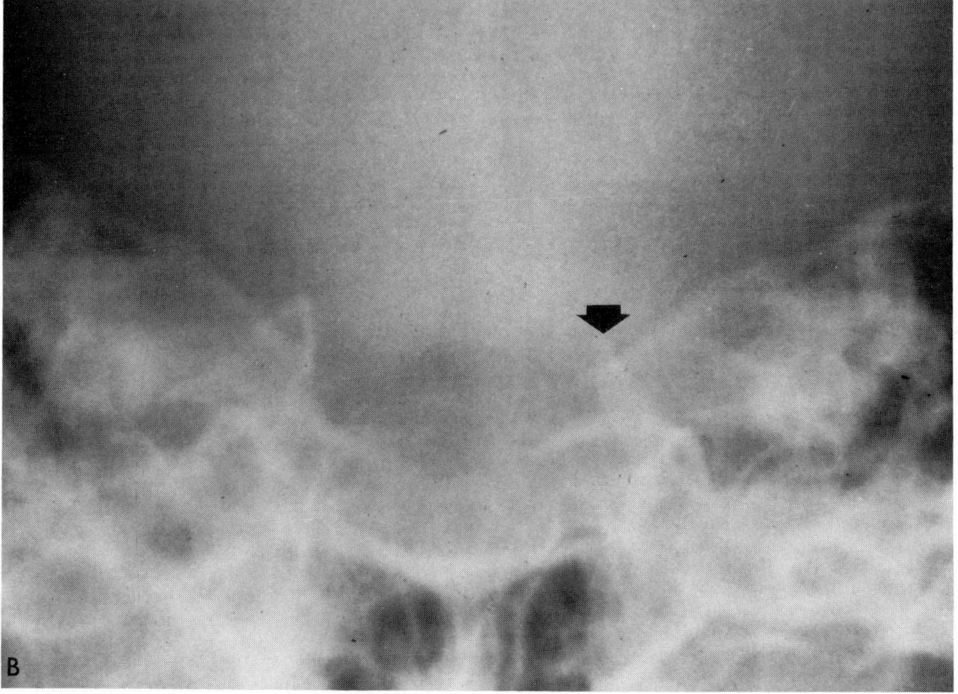

Figure 10–28. PITUITARY ADENOMA: The lateral and AP views (*A* and *B*) of the sella reveal that the sella turcica is enlarged and that the posterior clinoids and the dorsum sella are thinned and displaced posteriorly. Undercutting of one of the anterior clinoids is seen on both views (*arrows*). Both anterior clinoids are also thinned along their medial margins secondary to the enlarging intrasellar tumor.

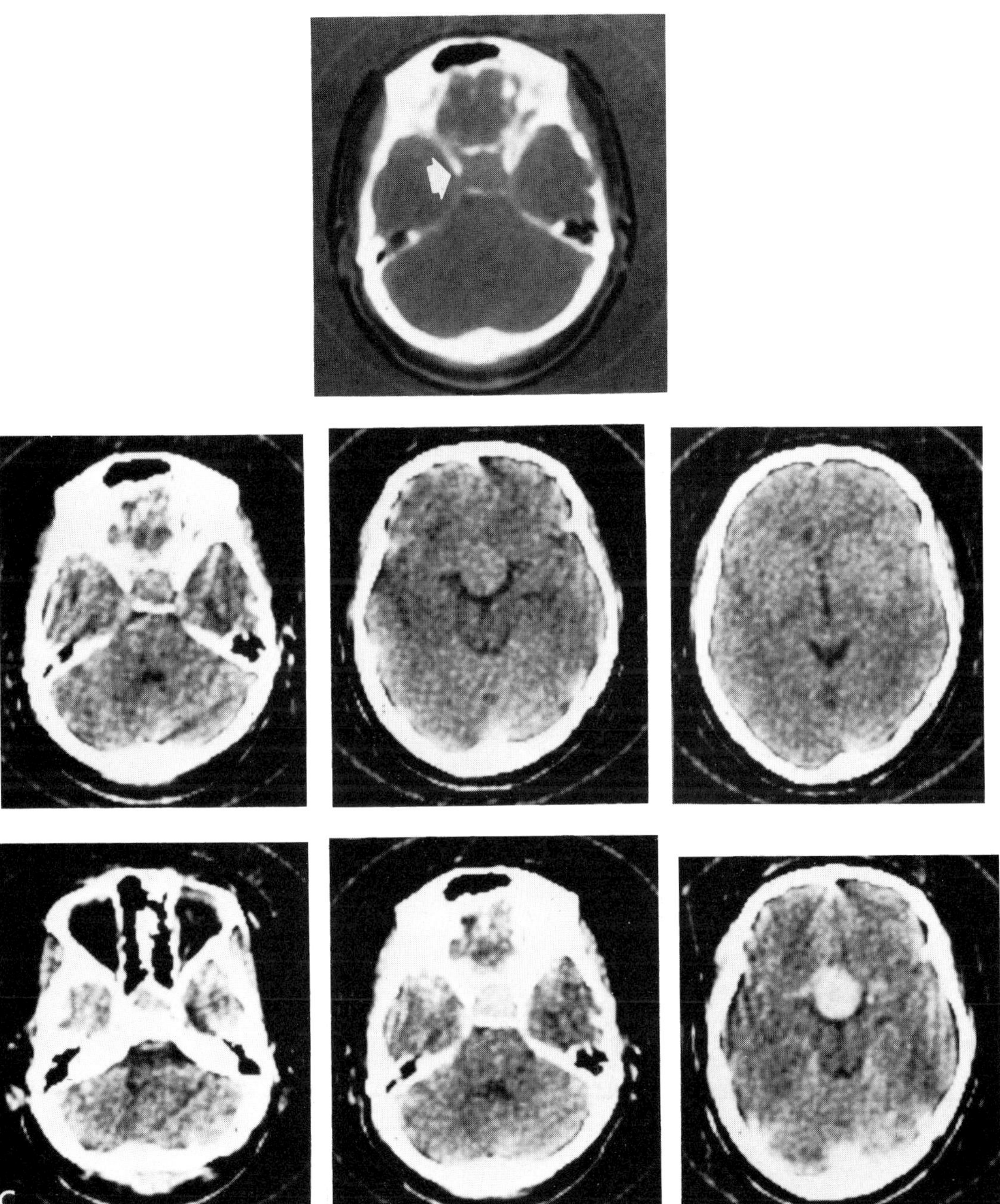

Figure 10–28 *Continued.*

C, CT scans of the region of the bony sella show the enlargement of the sella; they also confirm the presence of erosion of the medial side of the left anterior clinoid process (*arrow*). A mass is visible in the region of the sella; it extends up into the suprasellar cistern, which is obliterated. The postinfusion scan demonstrates marked enhancement of the tumor in a homogeneous fashion.

Surgically proved chromophobe adenoma of the pituitary.

Figure 10–29. PITUITARY ADENOMA: *A,* The carotid angiogram demonstrates opening of the carotid siphon (*arrows*). No abnormal vessels are seen.

B and *C*, AP and lateral views of the vertebral angiogram show the enlarged sella and: (*1*) tip of basilar artery; (*2*) highest portion of the superiorly displaced posterior cerebral artery on the right side; (*3*) the normal course of the posterior cerebral artery on the left side.

On the right side, the pituitary tumor has grown into the suprasellar cistern and posteriorly to such an extent that it affects the posterior cerebral artery, which passes in curvilinear fashion up, over and around the adenoma.

D, The lateral view of the venous phase demonstrates the marked superior displacement of the anterior and midportions of the basal vein of Rosenthal (*bvR*) as it courses over the lateral extent of the tumor on the right side. The internal cerebral vein is also superiorly displaced (*icv*). Both veins join to form the vein of Galen (*VG*).

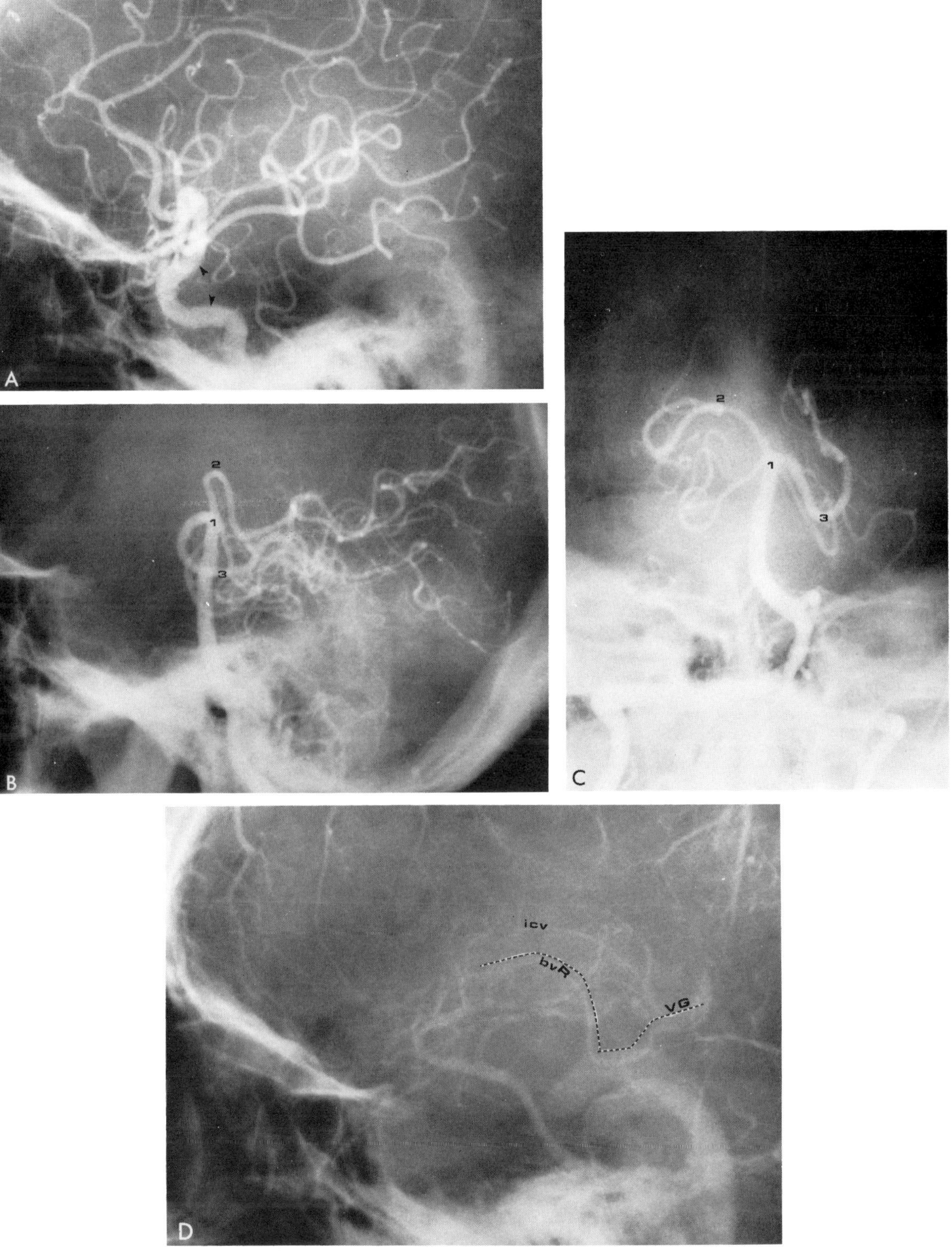

Figure 10–29. *See legend on the opposite page.*

Illustration continued on the following page.

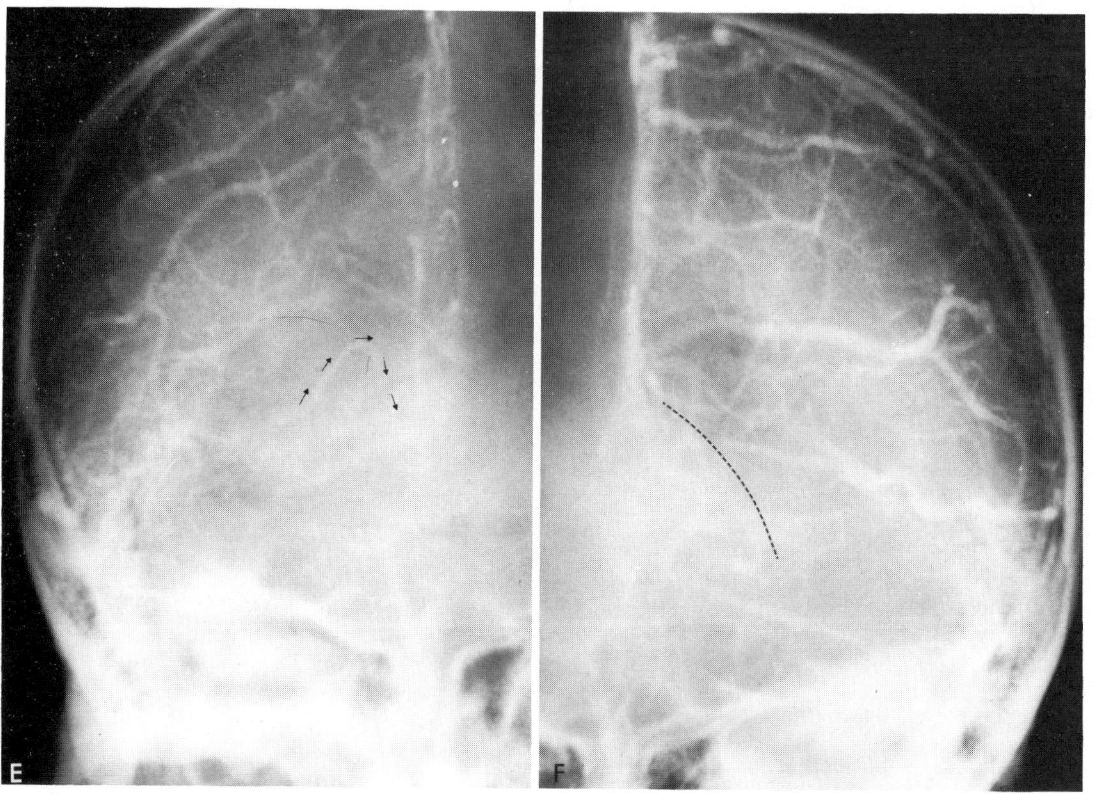

Figure 10–29 *Continued.*

E and *F*, The AP views also demonstrate the superior displacement of the basal vein of Rosenthal on the right side (*small arrows*) and the normal course of the basal vein on the left side (*dashed line*).

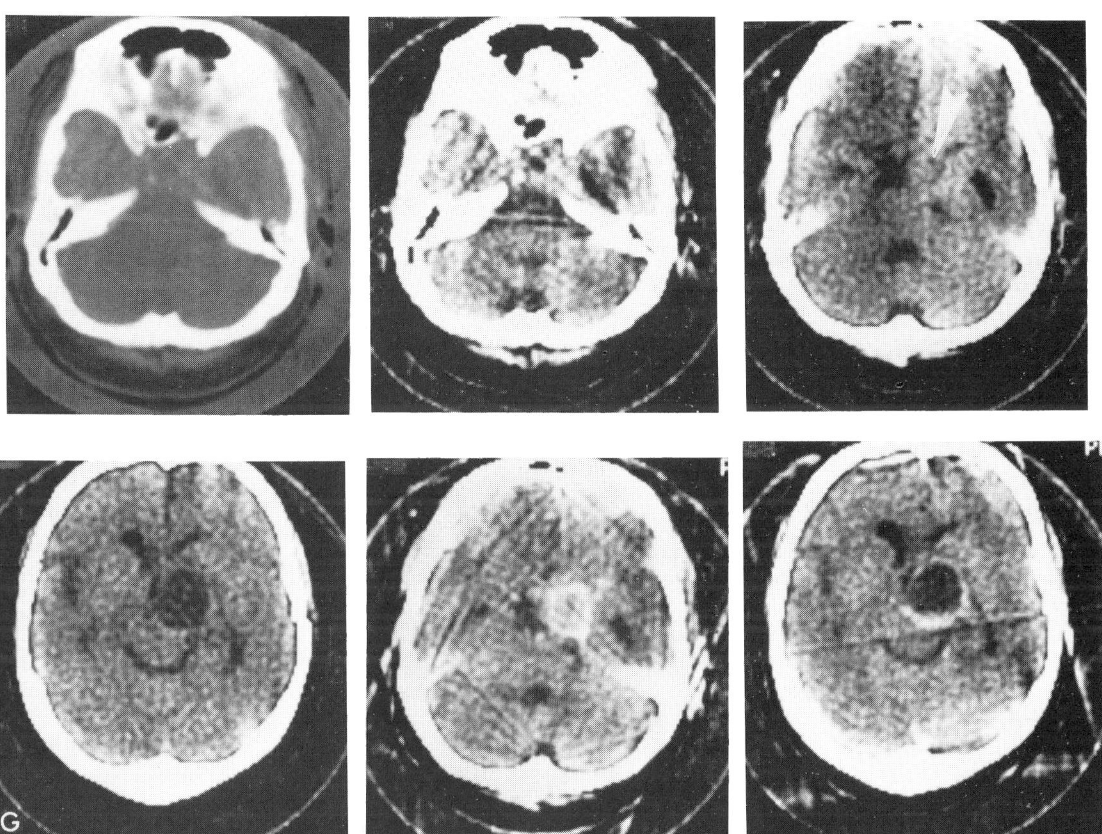

Figure 10–29 *Continued.*

G, CT scans of the region of the sella confirm the presence of a large sella and show evidence of a tumor mass in the region of the sella that is both solid (*white arrow*) and cystic in its superior portion and larger on the right side than on the left. The third ventricle is displaced to the left. The postinfusion scan demonstrates homogeneous enhancement of the solid portion of the tumor and a ring of enhancement around the cystic mass on the right side.

Surgically proved partially cystic chromophobe adenoma.

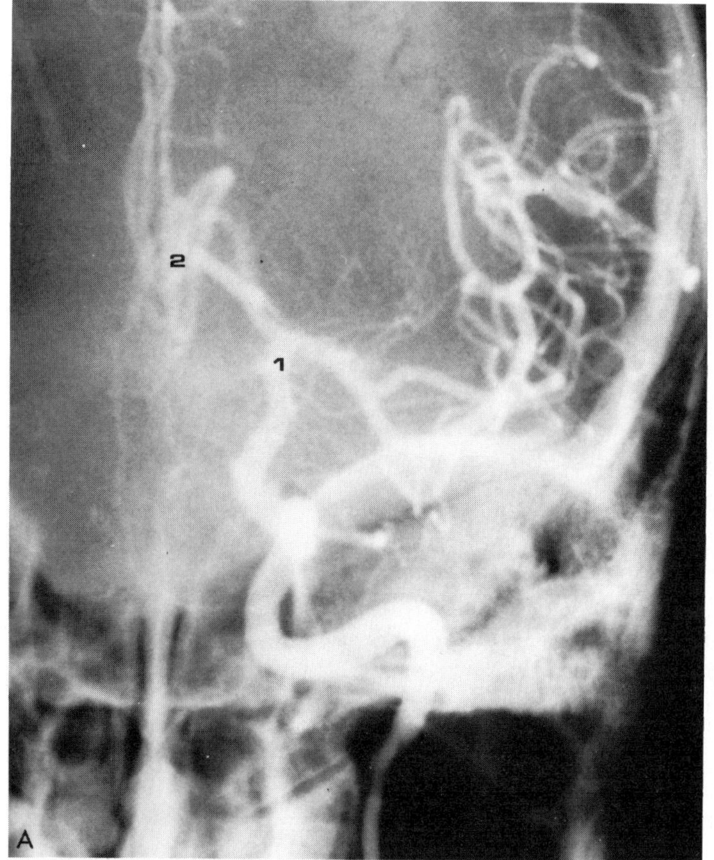

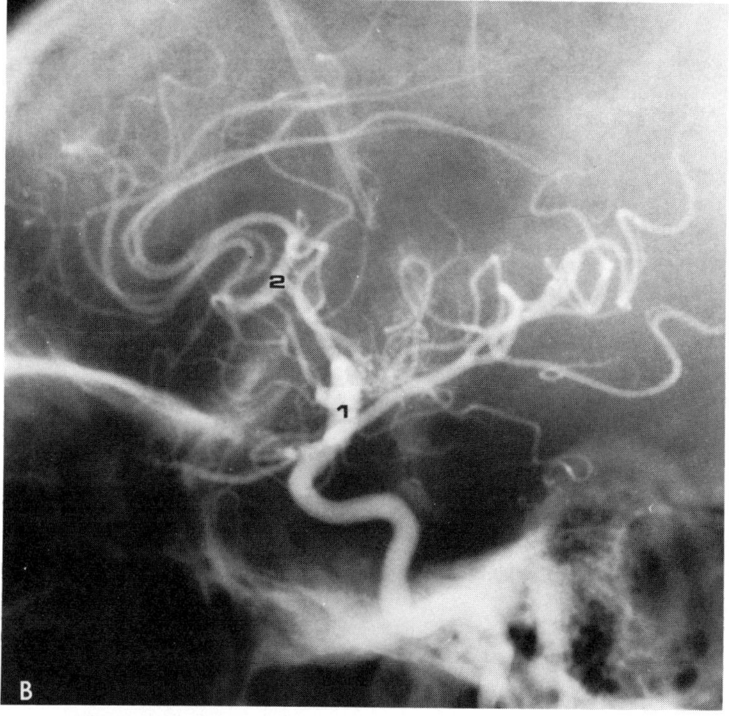

Figure 10–30. *See legend on the opposite page.*

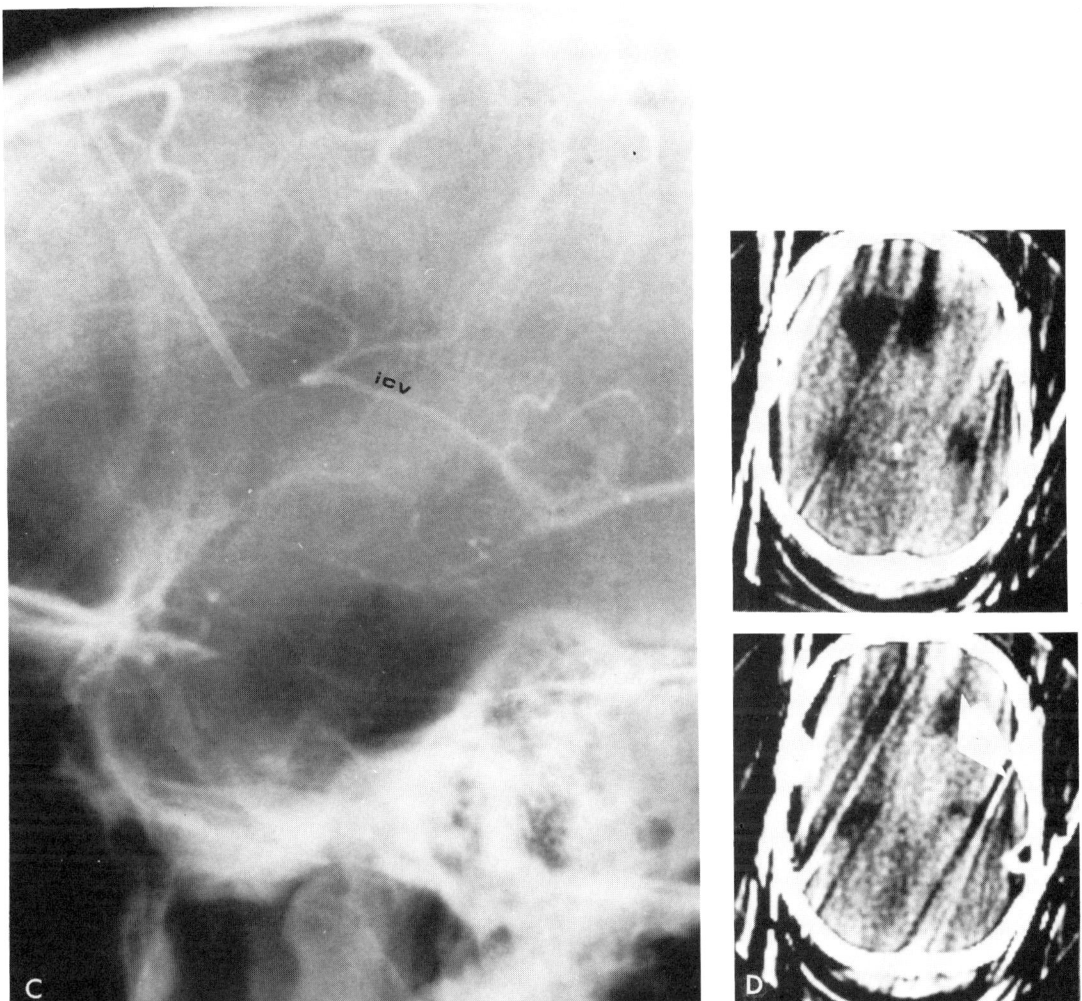

Figure 10–30. PITUITARY ADENOMA WITH OBSTRUCTIVE HYDROCEPHALUS: *A*, The AP view of the carotid angiogram demonstrates lateral displacement of the cavernous portion of the internal carotid artery, superior displacement of the supraclinoid portion of the internal carotid artery and superior displacement of the proximal portion of the middle cerebral artery. Elevation of the anterior cerebral artery is more marked medially. Point *1* marks the bifurcation of the internal carotid artery; Point *2* is the level of the anterior communicating artery.

B, The lateral view demonstrates a "floating" cavernous internal carotid artery.

C, The lateral view of the venous phase shows superior displacement of the internal cerebral vein (*icv*) and the enlarged sella turcica. The angiographic findings are those of a large intrasellar mass with suprasellar extension. There is obstructive hydrocephalus secondary to blockage of the foramen of Monro, and the shunt tubing device can be seen in place.

D, The CT scan is degraded by patient motion artifact, but nevertheless demonstrates a mass in the midline (*arrow*) that is of higher density than normal brain tissue. There is moderately severe obstructive hydrocephalus.

Surgically proved chromophobe adenoma.

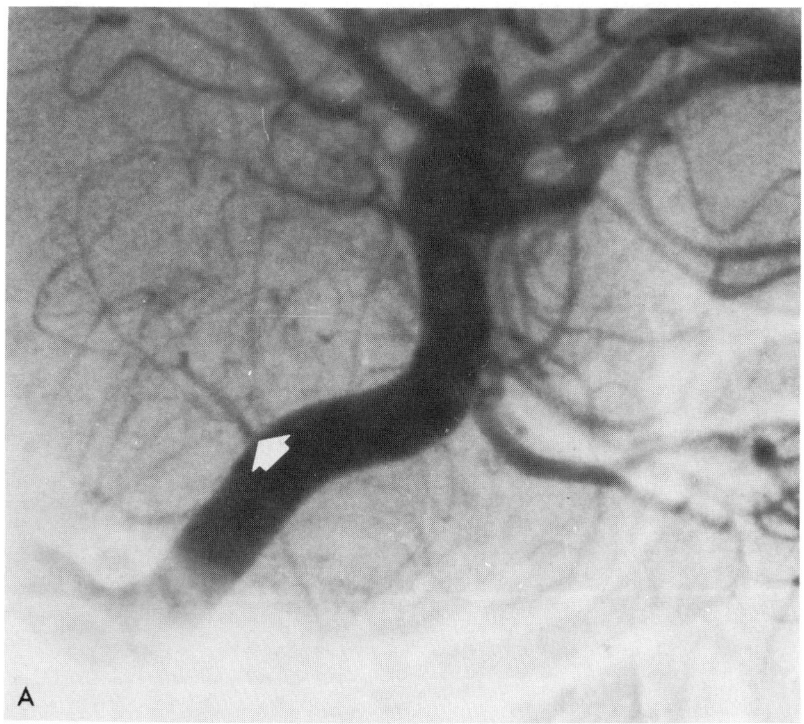

Figure 10–31. PITUITARY ADENOMA: *A*, Using magnification and subtraction techniques, the lateral view of the carotid angiogram demonstrates opening of the carotid siphon and an enlarged meningohypophyseal trunk that has multiple small vessels distributed in a curvilinear fashion around the pituitary tumor (*white arrow*).

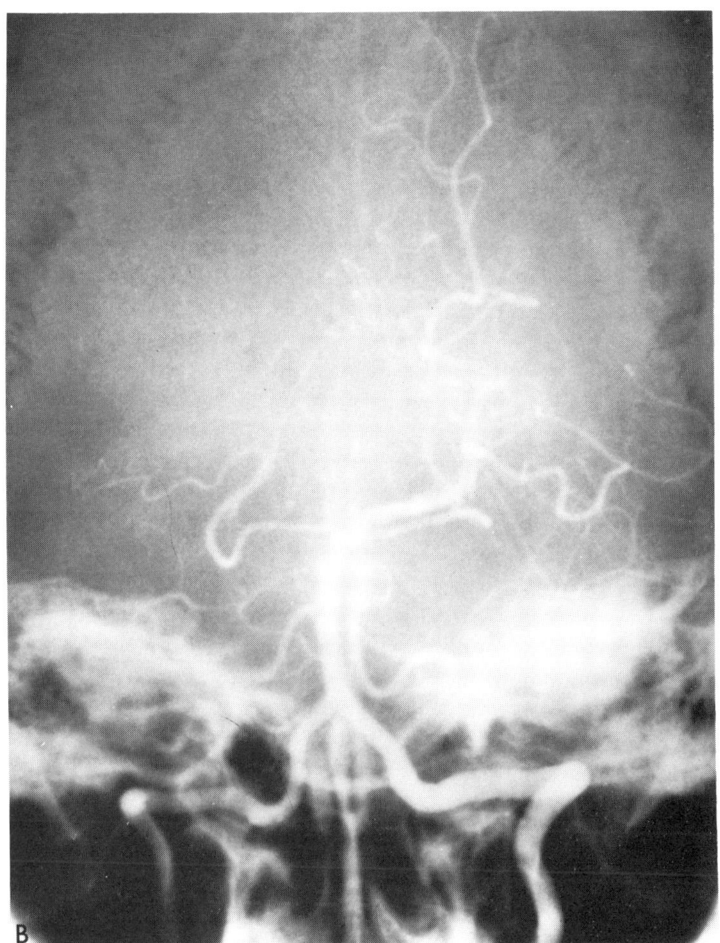

Figure 10–31 *Continued.*

B, The AP view of the vertebral angiogram reveals that the basilar artery is displaced to the right side; there is slight elevation of the superior cerebellar and posterior cerebral arteries on the left side.

Illustration continued on the following page.

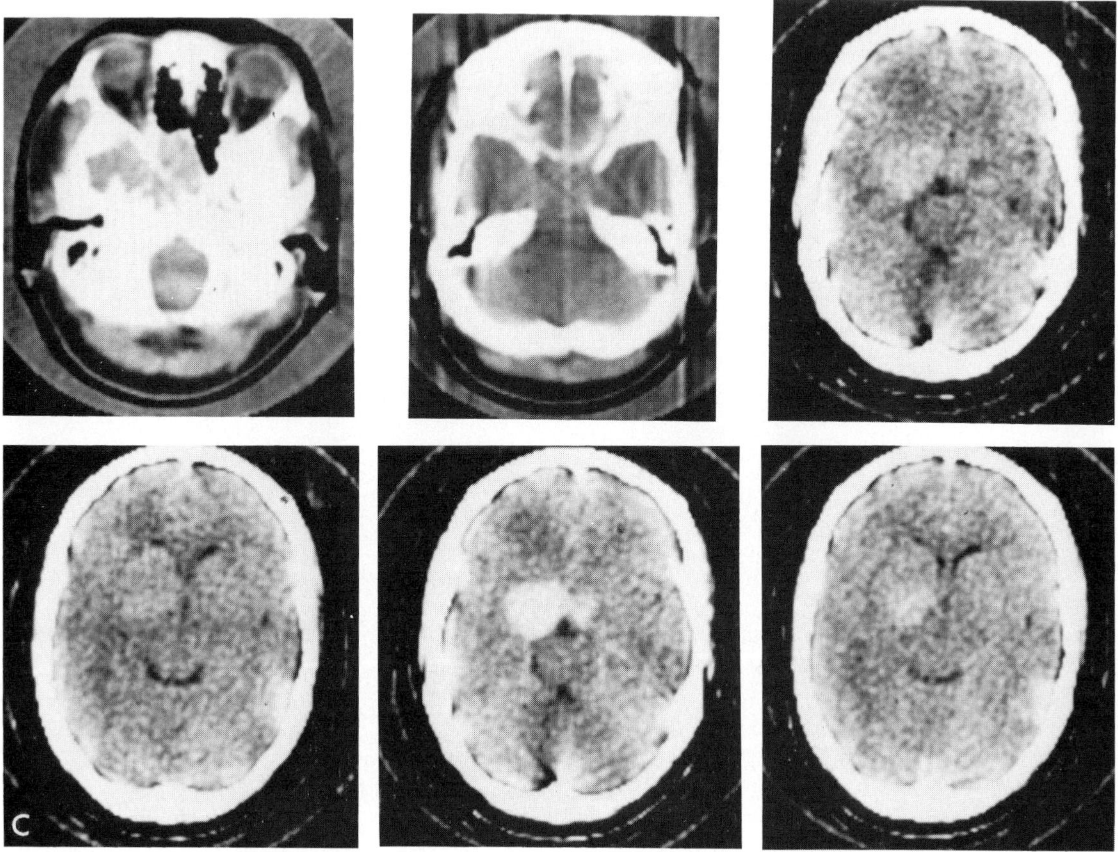

Figure 10–31 *Continued.*

C, The CT scan shows the enlarged sella turcica, which is larger on the left side than on the right; there is a well defined, bilobed rounded mass in the region of the sella that extends to the left of the sella. The mass is higher than normal brain density on the preinfusion scan. Postinfusion, there is marked homogeneous enhancement of the bilobed tumor, which extends up into the suprasellar cisterns.

Illustration continued on the following page.

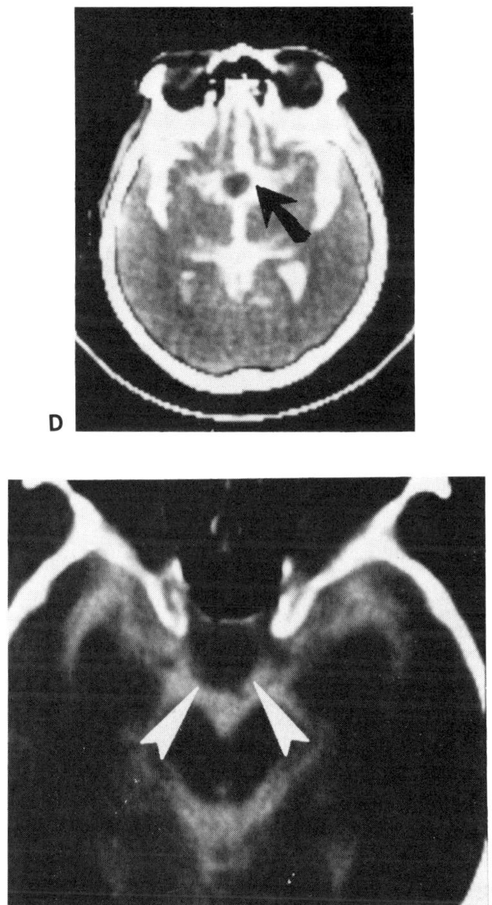

Figure 10–31 *Continued.*

D, This CT scan from another patient was obtained after the instillation of 5 cc of 180 mg of I/cc solution of Amipaque. The CT scan demonstrates a mass lesion (*arrow*) extending up into the suprasellar cistern.

E, The adenoma appears as a lucent lesion bathed by the higher density Amipaque in the suprasellar cistern.

Differential diagnosis includes meningioma as well as pituitary adenoma. Surgically proved chromophobe pituitary adenoma.

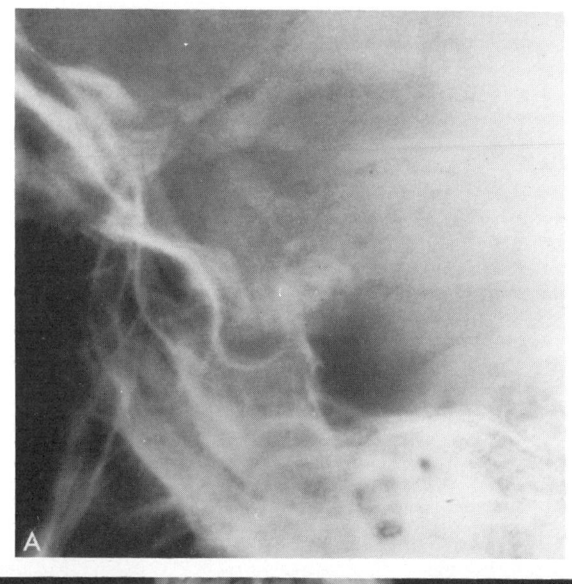

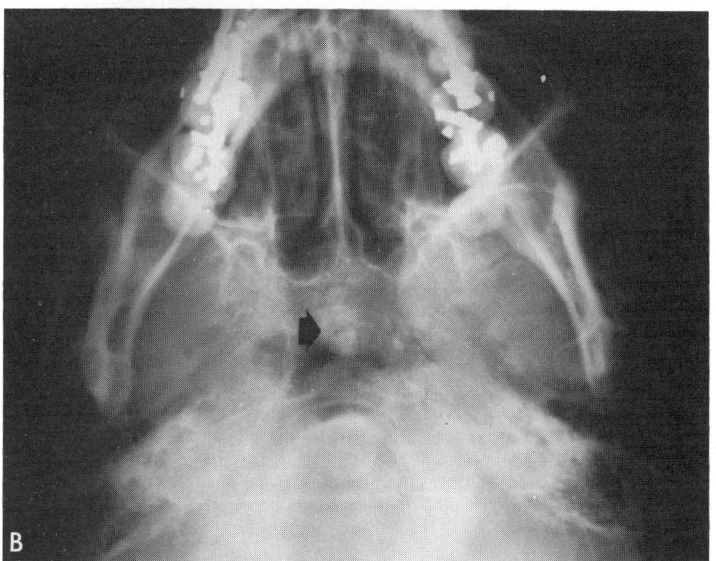

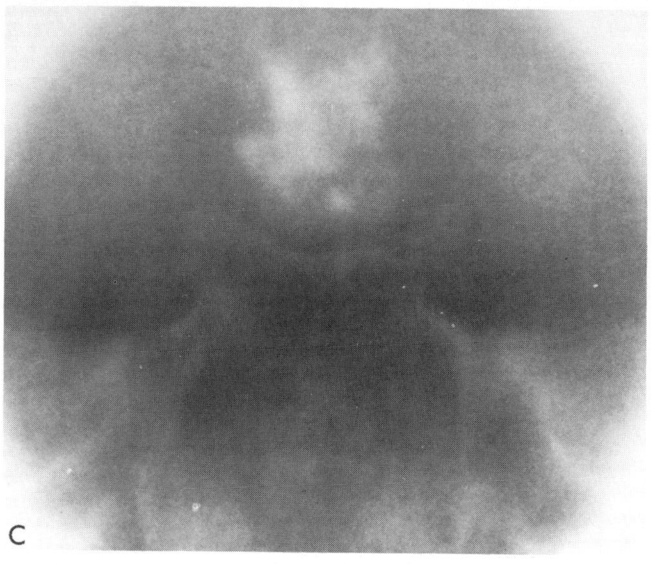

Figure 10–32. *See legend on the opposite page.*

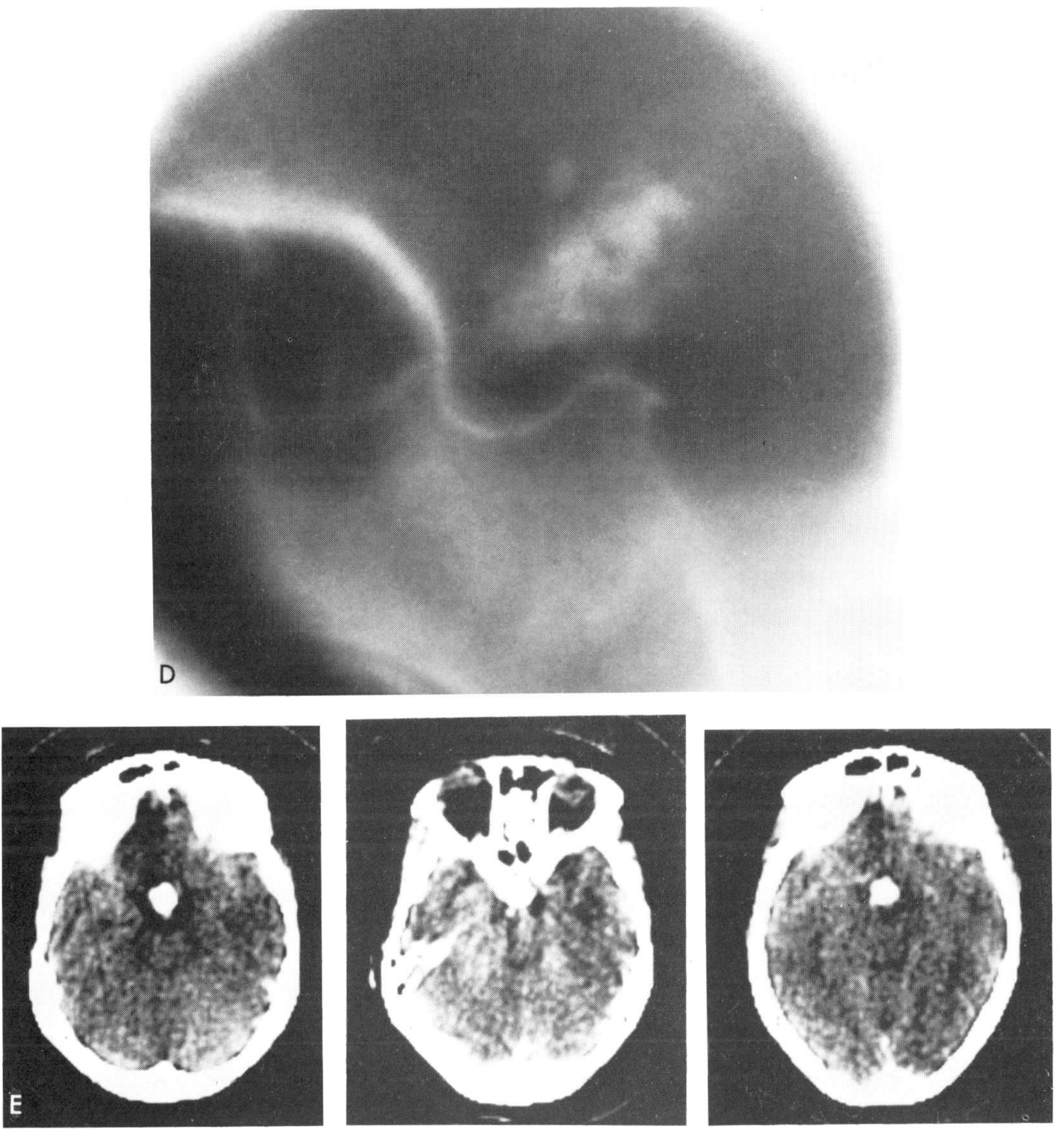

Figure 10–32. CRANIOPHARYNGIOMA: *A,* The lateral view of the skull reveals a densely calcified mass in the sella that extends into the suprasellar cisterns.

B, The calcification is also seen on the submentovertex view of the skull (*arrow*).

C, The AP tomographic view demonstrates the area of calcification just superior to the dorsum sella in the midline.

D, The lateral view also shows the calcified mass, which is in the suprasellar cistern but extends into the sella.

E, The CT scan confirms the presence of a densely calcified mass in the suprasellar cistern and extending into the sella.

The appearance is that of a calcified craniopharyngioma. These tumors are usually cystic.

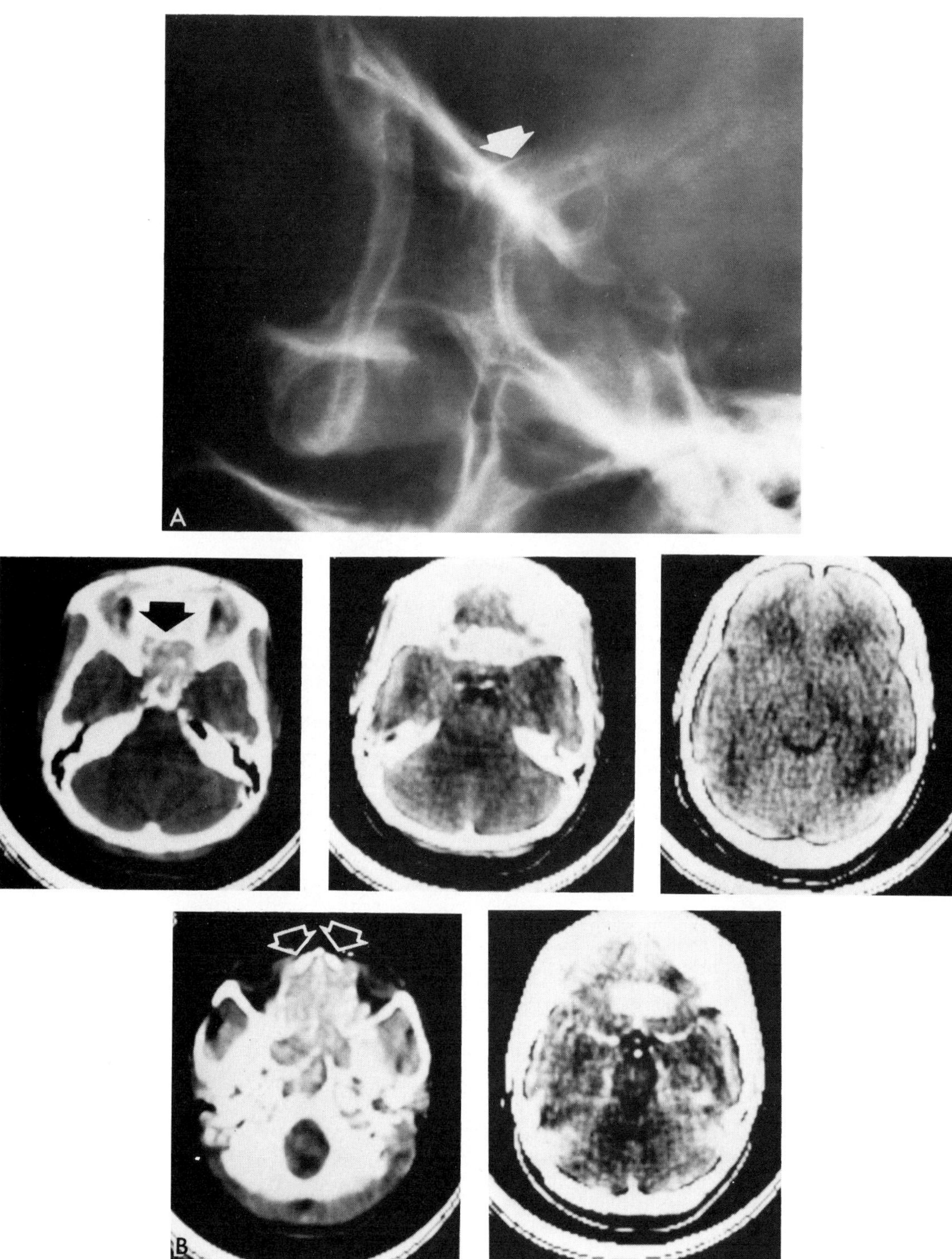

Figure 10–33. *See legend on the opposite page.*

Figure 10–33. MUCOCELE OF THE SPHENOID SINUS: *A*, The lateral view of the skull demonstrates destructive changes and irregular opacification of the sella. The planum sphenoidale is displaced superiorly and is markedly thinned (*arrowhead*). There is obviously an expanding lesion in the region of the sphenoid sinus.

B, CT scans demonstrate an area of increased density in the region of the expanded sphenoid sinus (*black arrow*) and the superiorly displaced planum sphenoidale. The third ventricle appears to be normal in size and position.

The lower cuts through the nasal cavity reveal an extensive soft tissue mass throughout the nasal cavity (*open arrows*); physical examination disclosed multiple nasal polyps. There is no change on the postinfusion scan.

Surgically proved mucocele of the sphenoid sinus.

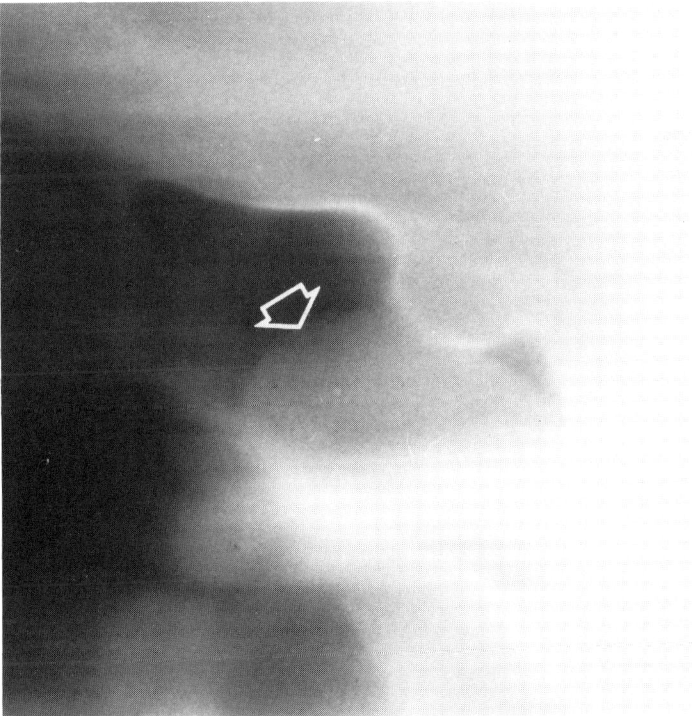

Figure 10–34. RETENTION CYST OF THE SPHENOID SINUS: The lateral view of the midline tomographic cut through the region of the sphenoid sinus demonstrates a broad based retention cyst in the floor of the sphenoid sinus (*arrow*).

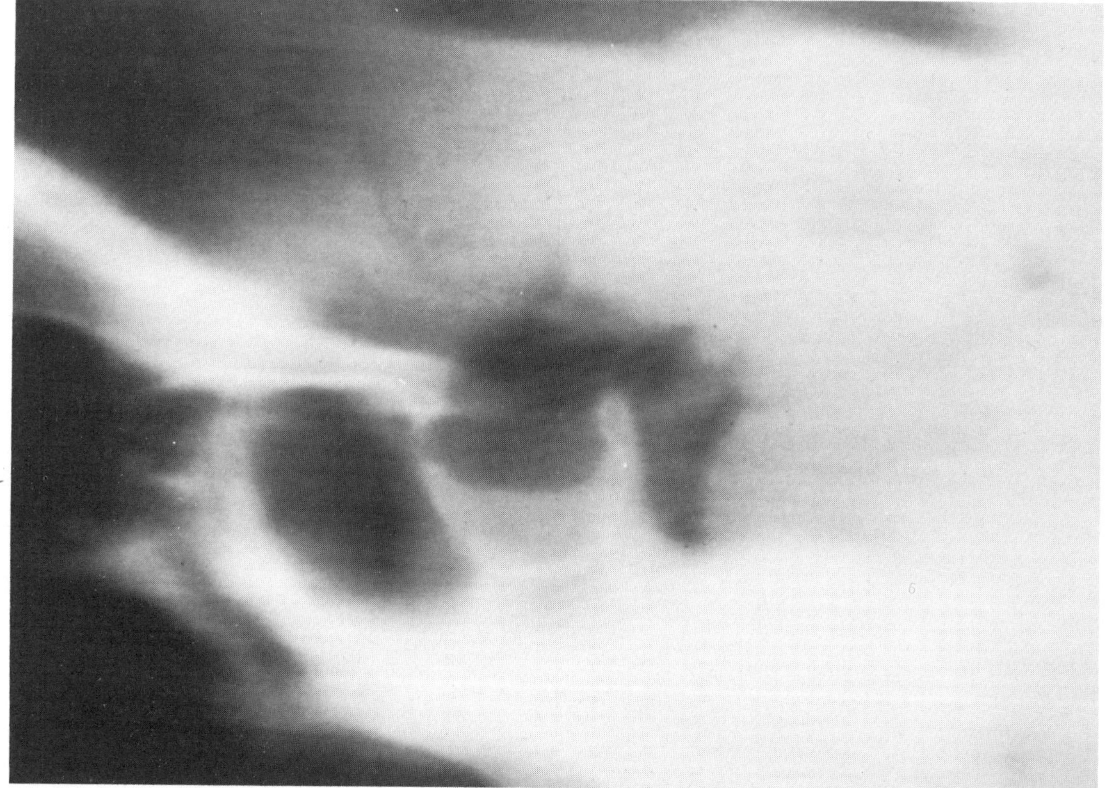

Figure 10–35. EMPTY SELLA SYNDROME: This syndrome is usually seen in women. The clinical symptoms are headache and, occasionally, visual difficulties. The sella is usually enlarged. Air will enter the sella during pneumoencephalography.

The size of the sella is slightly enlarged in this patient. A midline tomogram with the patient in the inverted position demonstrates that the sella turcica fills with air, although a small amount of pituitary tissue remains in the floor of the sella.

Amipaque cisternography also can be used to demonstrate this entity. The contrast material can be seen to enter the sella, and this can be readily demonstrated on the CT scan. The significance of these radiographic findings has not yet been clearly defined.

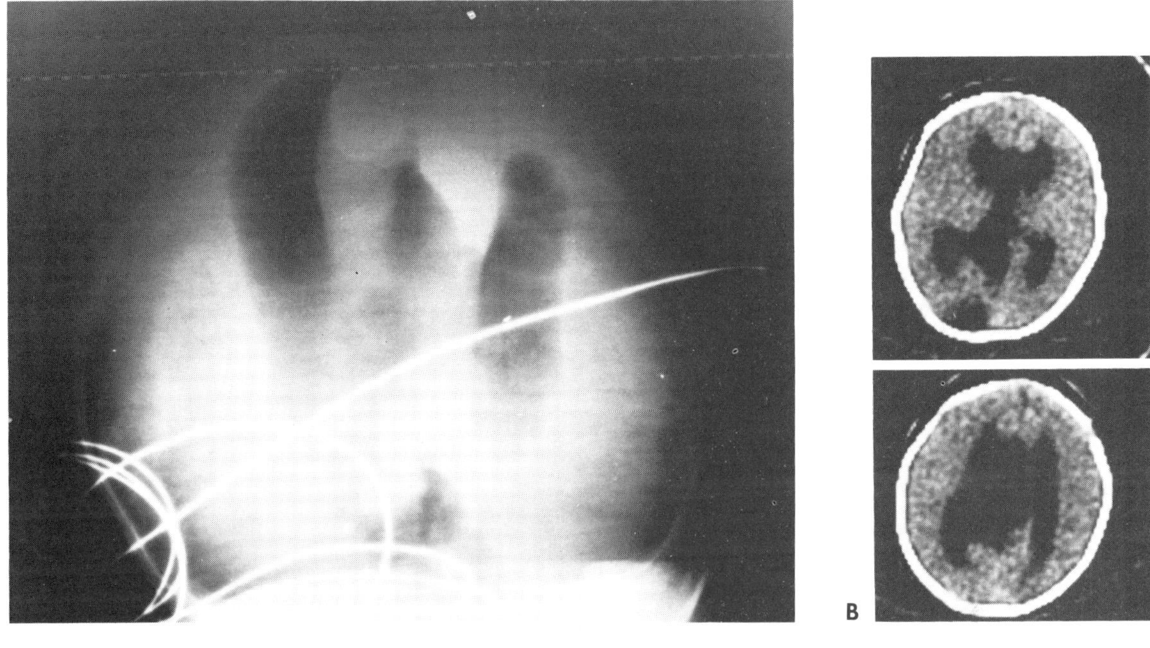

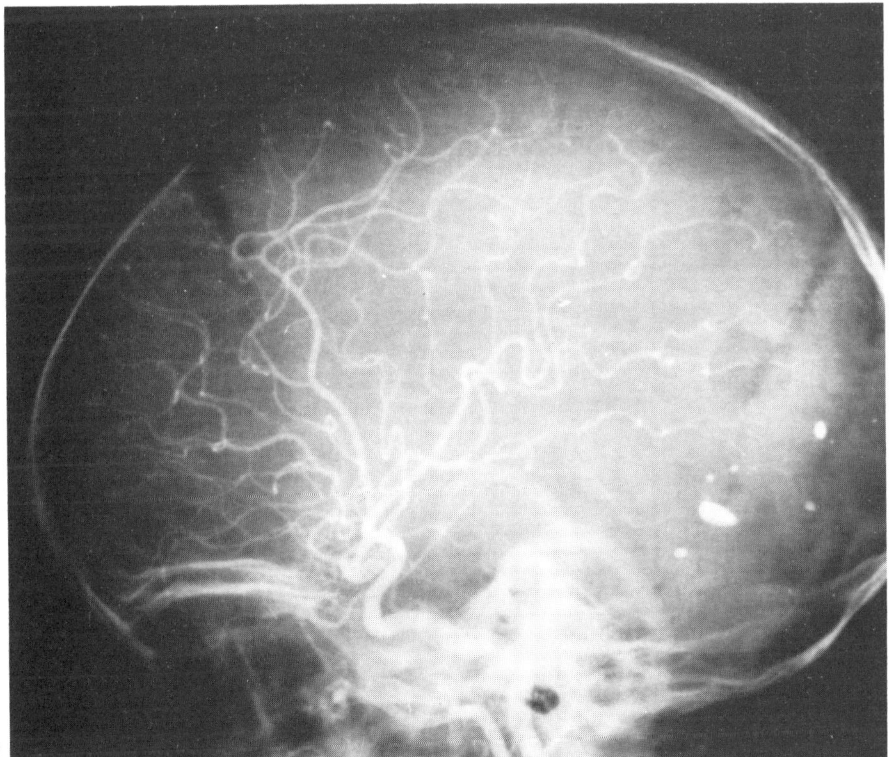

Figure 10–36. AGENESIS OF THE CORPUS CALLOSUM: The pneumoencephalogram (*A*) demonstrates that the lateral ventricles are wide-spread and that the third ventricle pushes superiorly between the lateral ventricles. The CT scan (*B*) confirms those findings, and the appearance is quite typical for an agenesis of the corpus callosum.

C, The angiogram reveals a straightened and meandering course of the pericallosal artery — another finding typical of agenesis of the corpus callosum.

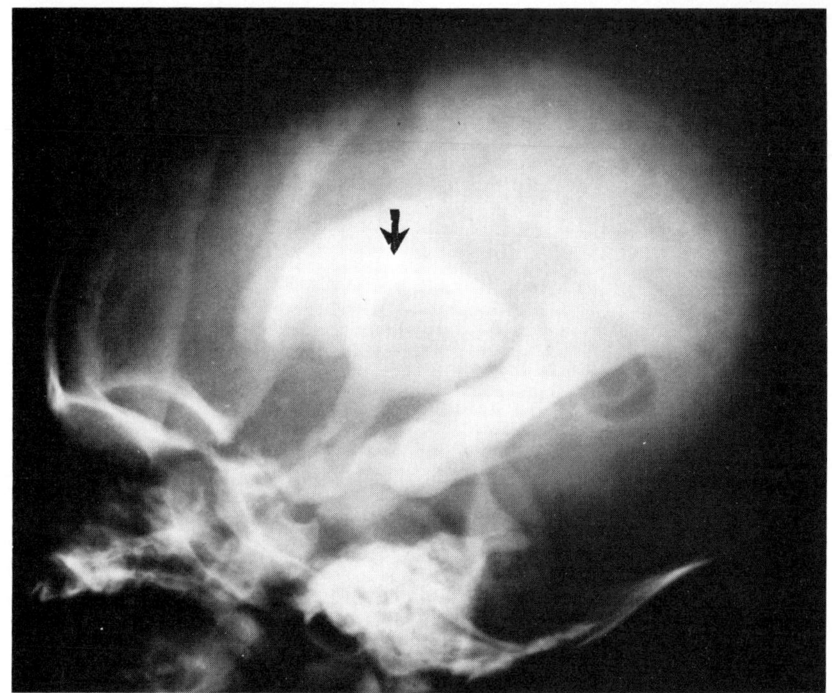

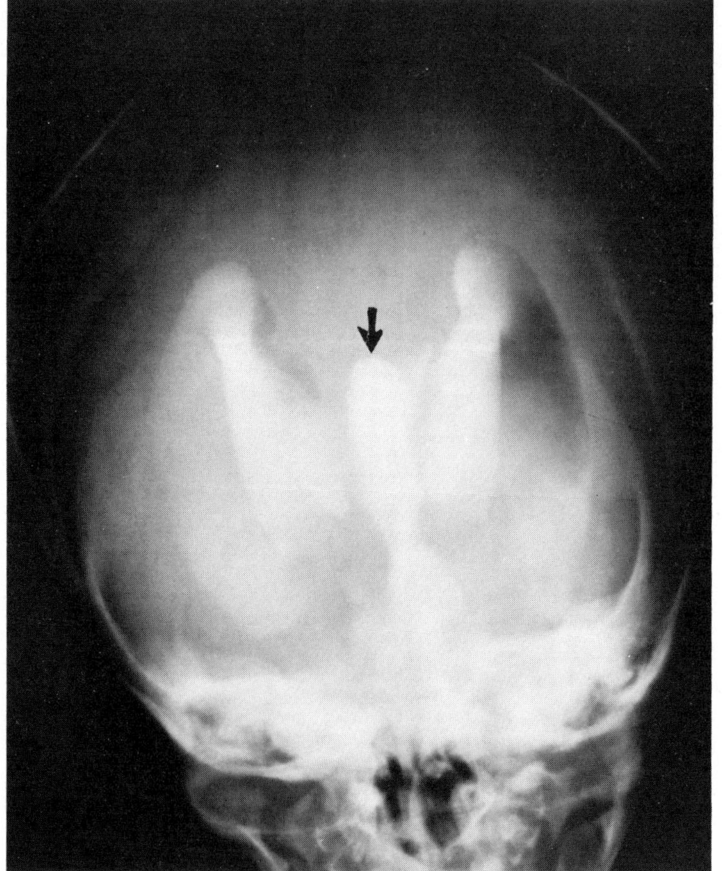

Figure 10–37. AGENESIS OF THE CORPUS CALLOSUM: The wide-spread lateral ventricles and high-riding third ventricle are well demonstrated by these Conray ventriculograms. The arrowheads demonstrate the top of the third ventricle in the lateral and AP projections.

CHAPTER 11

HYDROCEPHALUS, PORENCEPHALY AND METASTASES

HYDROCEPHALUS

There is no better examination than the CT scan for the initial work-up of hydrocephalus. If CT scan facilities are not available, the work-up will require the use of plain skull radiographs, angiography, pneumoencephalography and ventriculography.

The term "hydrocephalus" implies the presence of large ventricles, but these may or may not be associated with increased head size. An obstructive hydrocephalus usually is secondary to a mass lesion that obstructs the ventricular system. This obstruction can be at any level — e.g., at the foramen of Monro because of a colloid cyst of the third ventricle; at the cerebral aqueduct because of a pinealoma or aqueduct stenosis; or at the fourth ventricle because of an ependymoma. The obstruction causes enlargement of the ventricle and an enlarging head size in children; in adults, there is changed or increased intracranial pressure.

In a "communicating" hydrocephalus there is no mass lesion. Rather, one finds interference with the absorption of CSF by the arachnoid granulations secondary to a subarachnoid hemorrhage or interference with the normal flow of CSF through the tentorial notch because of adhesions following meningitis.

With an atrophic process such as that seen with toxoplasmosis or cytomegalic inclusion disease, there will be large lateral ventricles but a small head size.

Several examples of hydrocephalus associated with the Arnold-Chiari malformation and aqueduct stenosis are illustrated in this chapter. Examples of many other types of hydrocephalus are presented elsewhere in this book.

AQUEDUCT STENOSIS AND INSUFFICIENCY

Aqueduct occlusion may be a congenital finding in some cases. At birth or shortly thereafter the child's head begins to enlarge. It is not clear why the head does not grow large in utero — although in some cases it may be large even at birth. The aqueduct may be forked, having two blind ends along its more cephalad portion. The distal end of the aqueduct will be closed and will not communicate with either limb of the proximal aqueduct. In this case the slightly dilated proximal aqueduct can be visualized on the autotomogram of the ventriculogram; the distal aqueduct is subsequently demonstrated by a pneumoencephalogram.

In addition to forking of the aqueduct, there may be a gliosis about the aqueduct that ultimately leads to its occlusion.

If there is narrowing of the aqueduct without total occlusion, the subsequent development of a meningitis may cause enough reactive fibrosis to occlude the small opening totally.

In some patients with aqueduct insufficiency, the fluid pathway may be sufficiently patent so that enlargement of the head does not develop during the pediatric period. Indeed, some of these patients may live into adulthood and even to old age before their abnormality is discovered. In these cases it seems that the lateral ventricles enlarge very slowly over a long period of time because their borderline aqueduct sufficiency allows only minimal flow of CSF out of the ventricular system. However, an episode of meningitis or subarachnoid hemorrhage may be all that is needed to create occlusion or critical insufficiency of the pathway, and the patient develops the signs and symptoms of hydrocephalus. In these older patients it is of the utmost importance to be certain that it is not a tumor that is creating the problem. Care must be taken to rule out tumor because adult aqueduct insufficiency is only possible, not common.

A CT scan with contrast enhancement is sufficient in most cases to rule out the presence of a mass lesion as the cause of obstructive hydrocephalus.

Plain Skull. Because increased intracranial pressure is so insidious in its onset and often long standing, its secondary changes often are reflected in the sella turcica. There is enlargement of the sella turcica and erosion of the dorsum sellae and posterior clinoids associated with demineralization and destruction of the sella. These changes occur because of the marked dilatation of the third ventricle, which continues to pound down on the dorsum sella with each transmitted pulsation secondary to heartbeat and respiration. There may also be an increase in the digital markings of the calvaria because of the increased intracranial pressure.

If the aqueduct stenosis is associated with the Arnold-Chiari malformation, there may be an associated small posterior fossa because of the inferior displacement of the posterior fossa structures into the cervical region.

ARNOLD-CHIARI MALFORMATION

The Arnold-Chiari malformation is a developmental abnormality of the hindbrain. With this congenital abnormality, alterations in the growth of the brainstem, midbrain and cerebrum lead to characteristic alterations in the posterior fossa structures. The main feature of this abnormality is the displacement of the cerebellar tonsils into the region of the cervical canal. This appears to be related in part to the failure of the pons to flex during its course of development. In addition to low-lying cerebellar tonsils, the Arnold-Chiari malformation also may be associated with abnormal development of the spinal cord, resulting in meningoceles or myelomeningoceles and spinal dysraphia. One theory of the development of the malformation is that the meningomyelocele holds the spinal cord in the lumbar region, resulting in the downward displacement of the tonsils. This traction theory does not, however, explain all cases of this abnormality because the hindbrain malformation may occur without a meningomyelocele.

Arnold described the displacement of the cerebellar tonsils into the upper cervical canal; Chiari described the downward protrusion of the medulla and fourth ventricle into the cervical spinal canal, which causes the primitive cervical flexure of the embryo to be retained and the medulla to lie dorsal to the cervical spinal cord in the region of the cervical spinal canal.

There are four types of Arnold-Chiari malformation:

Type I. This is a variable downward displacement of the tonsils and inferior cerebellum into the cervical canal. This type of Arnold-Chiari malformation is not associated with a meningomyelocele. There may be an associated basilar impression and platybasia. Although an aqueduct stenosis may be present, it appears that these patients — who may live into adulthood without difficulty — suffer from a "foramen magnum syndrome" with resulting failure of CSF to circulate out of the fourth ventricle and over the cerebral hemispheres, where resorption recurs, leading to hydrocephalus.

Type II. There is downward displacement of the cerebellar tonsils into the cervical canal, but these patients also exhibit caudad displacement of the lower pons and medulla. The fourth ventricle is also displaced inferiorly and can be identified on the pneumoencephalogram as an elongated and distorted air shadow in the cervical region. In addition to the hindbrain malformation, a myelomeningocele is also present in Type II Arnold-Chiari malformation. Derek Harwood-Nash and Fitz consider the Type II malformation to be the classic abnormality seen in neuroradiologic practice. This malformation becomes apparent at birth or shortly thereafter. Hydrocephalus develops early in the clinical course and is secondary to the aqueduct stenosis or occlusion present in every case. This stenosis is secondary to forking, compression or inflammatory gliosis, and occlusion may occur by intracerebral hemorrhage or infection.

Although a simple meningocele may be present in the absence of the Arnold-Chiari malformation, a meningomyelocele is always associated with the malformation. However, the malformation may have either a meningocele or meningomyelocele. The pneumoencephalographic findings include a large massa intermedia and a pointed floor of the lateral ventricles. An accessory commissure may be present in the region of the lamina terminalis, and, of course, the elongated aqueduct and the inferiorly positioned fourth ventricle will be seen in the region of the cervical canal.

Type III. This is a displacement of the medulla and fourth ventricle and all of the cerebellum into an occipital and high cervical encephalomeningocele. Type III Arnold-Chiari malformation may come to the radiologist's attention if arteriography is performed to determine how much of the cranial contents are contained in the encephalocele. If a ventriculogram is performed, ventricular connections with the encephalocele may be demonstrated.

Type IV. Aplasia of the cerebellar hemispheres, the vermis and the pons is associated with a small, funnel-shaped posterior fossa. Usually the third and lateral ventricles are not enlarged. There is marked dilatation of the fourth ventricle and the cisternae magnae. The pons has a "pigeon-breast" shape. This is an uncommon malformation, and some believe that it does not fall in the category of Arnold-Chiari malformations.

CT Scan. The CT scan reveals a varying degree of obstructive hydrocephalus. The lateral and third ventricles will be noted to be enlarged, while the fourth ventricle is very small. Frequently there is differential enlargement of the occipital horns of the lateral ventricles as compared to the frontal horns. This appears to be secondary to a dysplastic development of the ventricular system. In some cases the fourth ventricle is not seen in the posterior fossa. This is because of the inferior displacement of the aqueduct and fourth ventricle into the cervical canal.

At the present time most patients with the Arnold-Chiari malformation have a CT scan for initial evaluation, are given a ventriculoperitoneal shunt and then followed by CT scanning. The vast majority require no further diagnostic work-up beyond the CT scan.

COMMUNICATING HYDROCEPHALUS

A "communicating hydrocephalus" implies that there is *no* evidence of a mass blocking the ventricular system. This may also be called a "low-pressure hydrocephalus" — meaning that the pressure of the fluid in the lumbar or ventricular system is not increased. This variety of hydrocephalus may develop from a variety of causes.

One cause is meningitis. It appears that a communicating hydrocephalus develops from meningitis because of apparent interference with the absorption of CSF by the arachnoid villi. Not all patients with meningitis develop a communicating hydrocephalus.

Another cause is subarachnoid hemorrhage. This communicating hydrocephalus is thought to develop because the blood in the subarachnoid space over the cerebral convexities interferes with the absorption of CSF by the arachnoid villi. It should be remembered that an acute obstructive hydrocephalus may develop following a subarachnoid hemorrhage from the accumulation of clotted blood in the aqueduct and fourth ventricle.

A communicating hydrocephalus also

may develop in the presence of excess CSF production, as seen with choroid plexus papilloma.

Chronic subdural hematomas also have been associated with ventricular enlargement and the picture of a communicating hydrocephalus. In the case of patients with chronic extracerebral accumulations of fluid it is felt that the local pressure over the cerebral convexities interferes with the reabsorption of CSF and results in ventricular enlargement.

Idiopathic low-pressure hydrocephalus develops for unknown reasons. It is associated with dementia, incontinence and difficulty in walking.

Hydrocephalus ex vacuo refers to fluid accumulations following brain atrophy. This term is now obsolete and should not be used.

All the varied causes of communicating hydrocephalus produce enlargement of the lateral ventricles without significant enlargement of the cortical sulci. With cerebral atrophy the cortical sulci also are enlarged. This diagnosis can be readily suggested by computed tomography.

SUBARACHNOID HEMORRHAGE

The blood vessels that feed the cerebral tissues are carried by the pia mater of the leptomeninges. Following a ruptured aneurysm, the blood accumulates in the subarachnoid space. In addition, the aneurysm may rupture into the cerebral tissue, producing an associated intracerebral hematoma. The hemorrhage usually is associated with severe headache, nausea and vomiting and frequently with a syncopal episode. Localizing physical findings may or may not be observed following the episode of hemorrhage. The patient develops a stiff neck secondary to the irritation of the meninges by the blood in the subarachnoid space. The CT scan of a subarachnoid hemorrhage without an intracerebral hematoma reveals areas of increased density in the basilar cisterns, sylvian fissures and interhemispheric fissure and over the cortical sulci. The blood in the subarachnoid space appears white on the CT scan, whereas the normal scan reveals areas of radiolucency in these distributions.

In addition, subarachnoid hemorrhage may even result in the appearance of blood in the ventricular system. It seems that the blood in these cases enters the fourth, third and lateral ventricles via the foramen of Luschka and Magendie and then through the aqueduct and foramen of Monro into the lateral ventricles. It is this free circulation of blood in the subarachnoid space that results in the accumulation of blood in the lumbar subarachnoid space that is found at the time of lumbar tap.

Acutely there may be an obstructive hydrocephalus because of clotted blood in the fourth ventricle and cerebral aqueduct that acts as a mechanical obstruction to the flow of CSF. This hydrocephalus may resolve after the dissolution of the clot. On the other hand, the ventricles may never return to normal size.

Following the acute hemorrhage, a communicating hydrocephalus may develop as soon as the first week after the initial insult. A simple and probably incomplete explanation of the development of this communicating hydrocephalus after a subarachnoid hemorrhage is that the blood in the subarachnoid space over the cerebral cortex interferes with the normal function of the arachnoid villi to reabsorb the circulating CSF. Although the progression of hydrocephalus from initial obstruction to communicating may be a continuum, there may be no evidence of acute obstructive hydrocephalus but a later development of a communicating or low-pressure hydrocephalus.

A communicating hydrocephalus develops over a highly variable period of time. In addition, not all patients who develop large ventricles and apparent communicating hydrocephalus become symptomatic. Patients who do become symptomatic will be improved by the placement of a shunt tubing device.

The presence and development of hydrocephalus can be readily followed by CT scans or, if a scanner is not available, by angiography.

Text continued on page 516

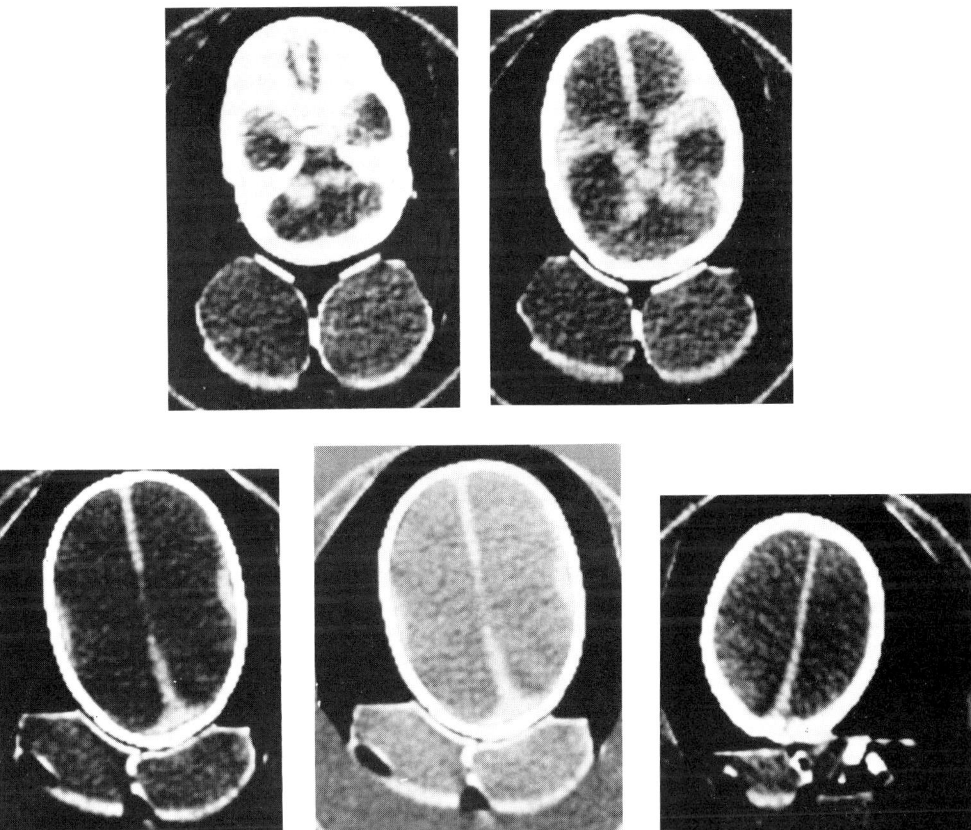

Figure 11–1. MASSIVE HYDROCEPHALUS: The lateral ventricles are greatly dilated, with only a thin rim of cerebral tissue remaining. The third ventricle is also dilated. The cerebellum appears to be very hypoplastic, with a large cisterna magna and poor development of the cerebellum. The exact etiology of the abnormality in this case is uncertain, but is probably congenital.

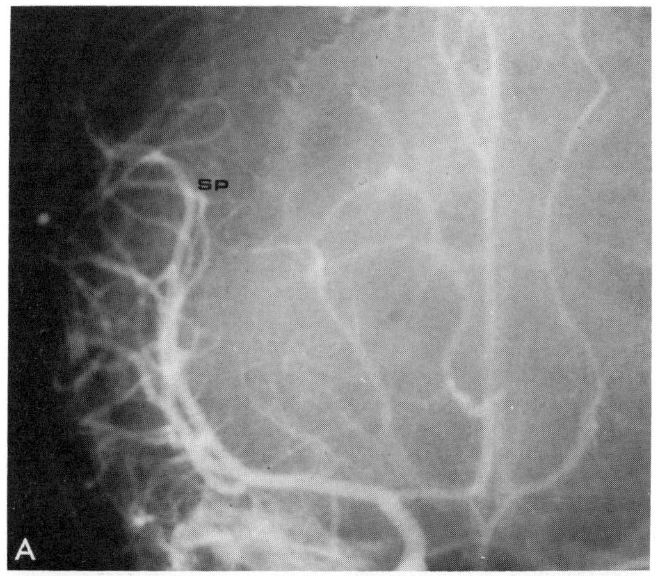

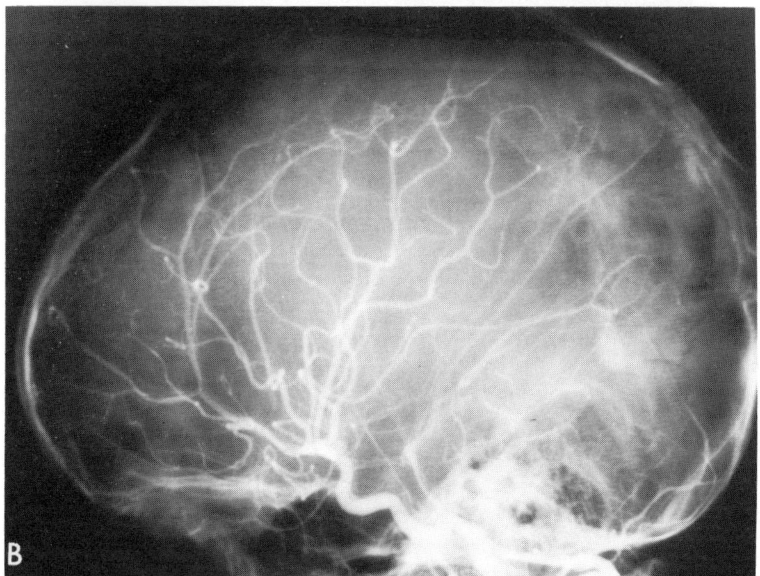

Figure 11–2. ANGIOGRAPHIC APPEARANCE OF HYDROCEPHALUS: Carotid angiography: *A*, The AP view of the arterial phase demonstrates that the anterior cerebral artery and its branches are straightened and closely applied to the midline. They show no undulations.

The sylvian point *(SP)* and all the middle cerebral artery branches in the isle of Reil are displaced laterally by the dilated temporal horn. This results in a widened distance between the anterior and middle cerebral artery group.

B, The lateral view demonstrates a widened sweep of the pericallosal artery. There is elevation of the sylvian triangle secondary to dilatation of the temporal horn.

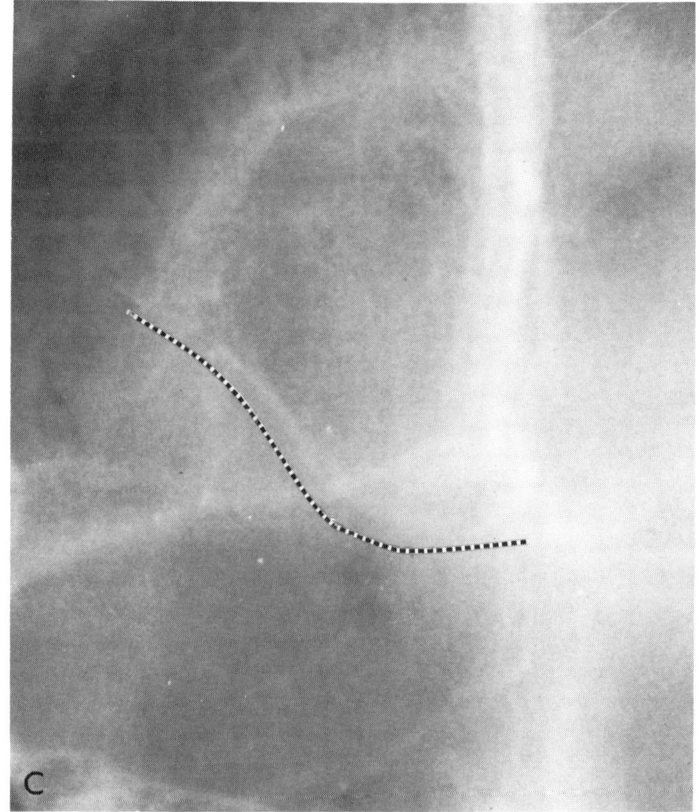

Figure 11–2 *Continued*

C, The AP view of the venous phase demonstrates a widened sweep of the thalamostriate vein secondary to dilatation of the lateral ventricle (*dotted line*).

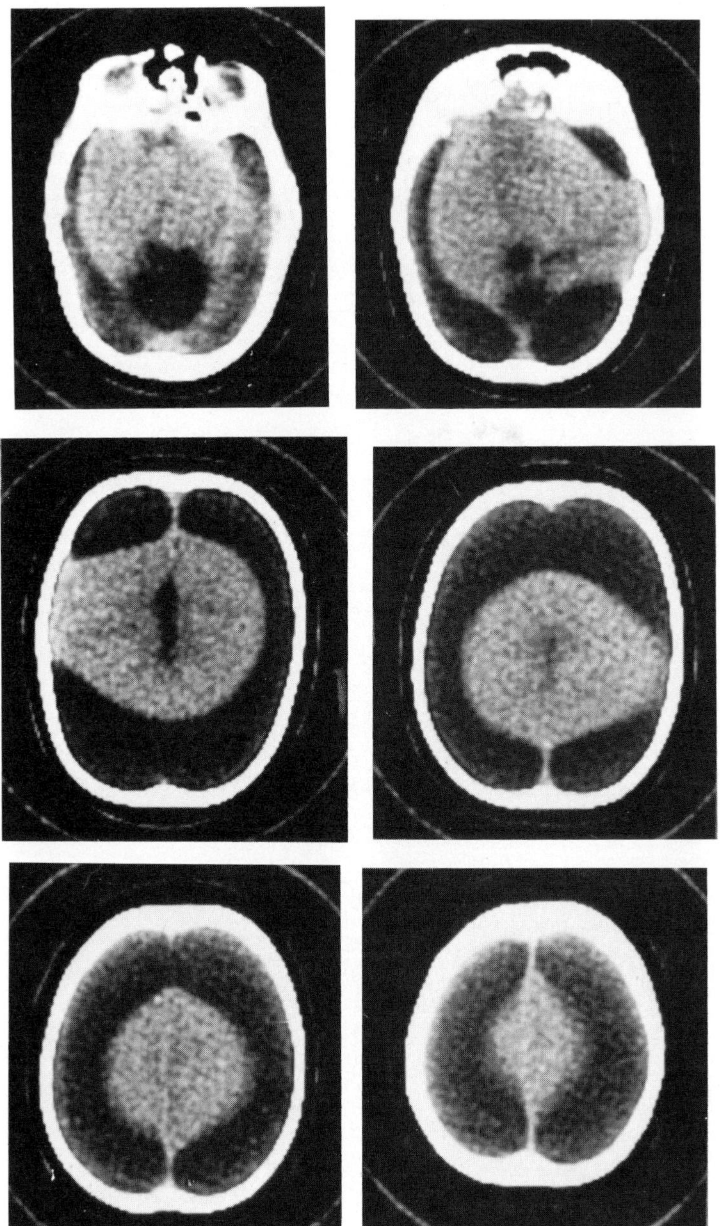

Figure 11–3. CONGENITAL MALFORMATION OF THE BRAIN: The cranial contents have a diffusely abnormal appearance. There is a slitlike radiolucency in the anticipated position of the lateral ventricles and large accumulations of lucent material over the cerebral hemispheres bilaterally. A large cystic accumulation of fluid can be seen in the anticipated position of the fourth ventricle. Presumably, the changes were caused by a massive germ plasm abnormality that has resulted in abnormal development and no recognizable cranial contents.

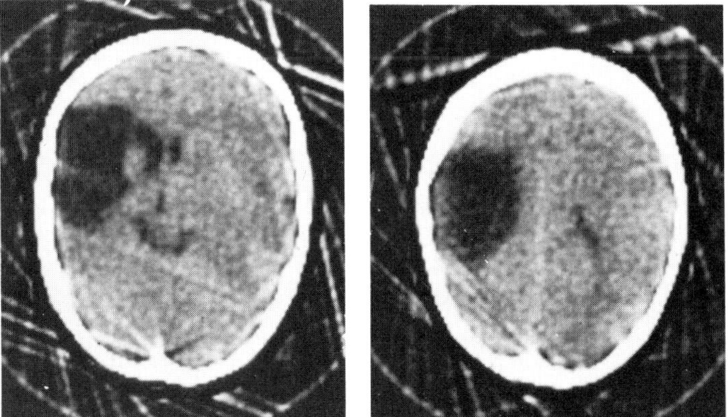

Figure 11–4. There is a large, well defined radiolucent area in the distribution of the left middle cerebral artery. Dilatation of the left lateral ventricle and shift to the midline toward the left side are evident. The retrothalamic cistern is also enlarged on the left side. The appearance is that of left hemiatrophy, which frequently is the result of a germ plasm defect or head trauma at birth.

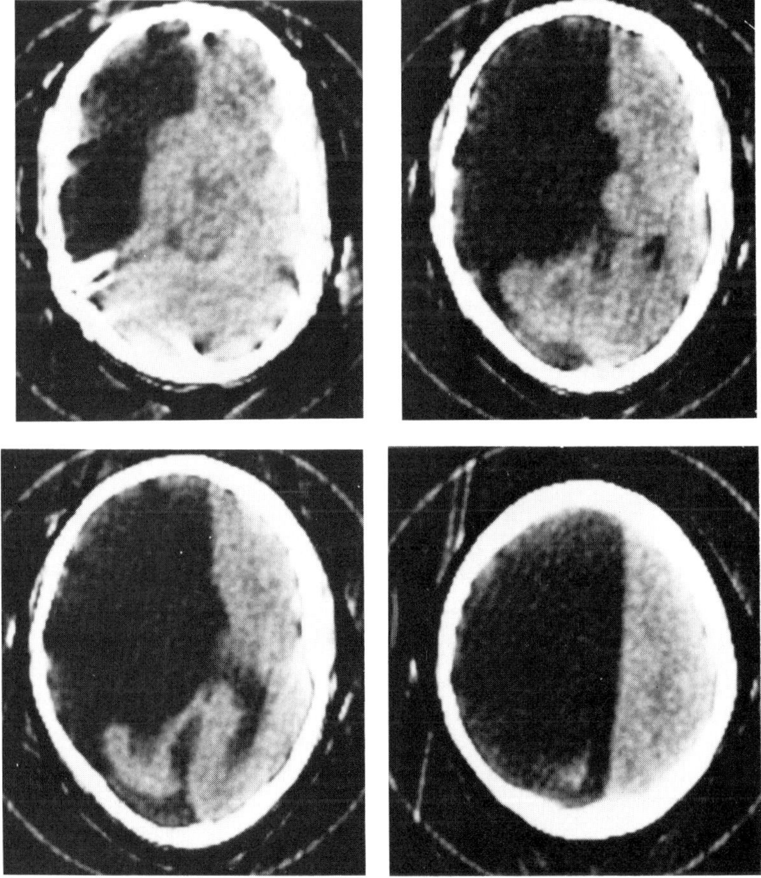

Figure 11–5. CEREBRAL APLASIA: The entire left cerebral hemisphere is replaced by fluid of CSF density. There is some evidence of preservation of the midline tissues at the base of the brain. The lateral ventricles are maldeveloped. There appears to be a small amount of brain tissue in the region of the left occipital lobe. The etiology of these changes is uncertain, but presumably was a massive germ plasm defect.

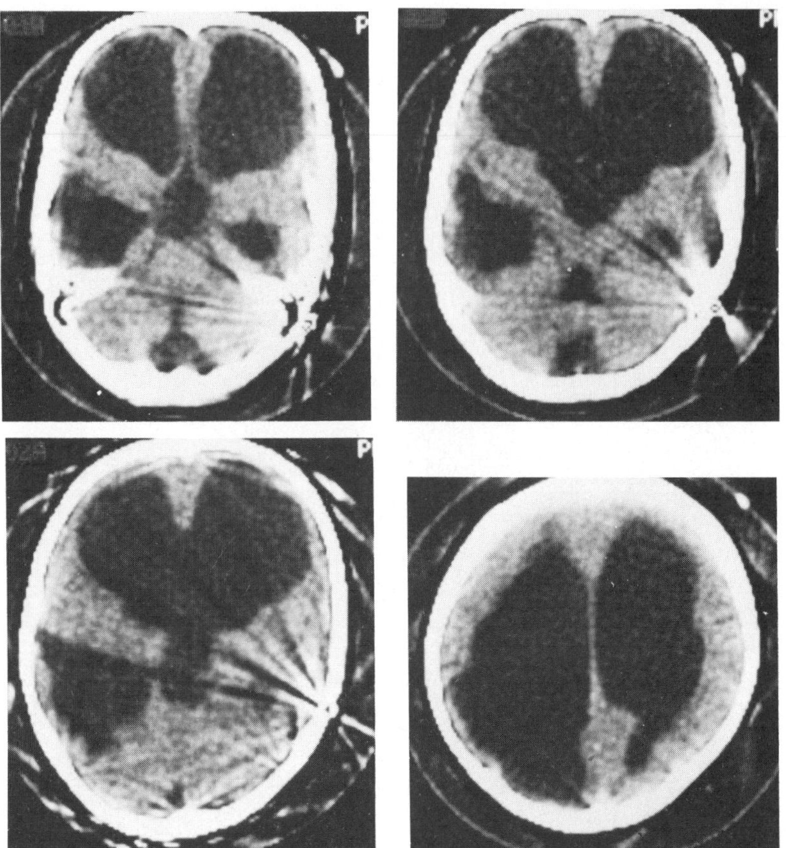

Figure 11–6. AQUEDUCT STENOSIS: Marked enlargement of the lateral and third ventricle is evident. The fourth ventricle is larger than one would normally anticipate, but the enlargement is not marked. These findings are secondary to aqueduct stenosis. An artifact is present secondary to the metallic portion of a shunt tubing device.

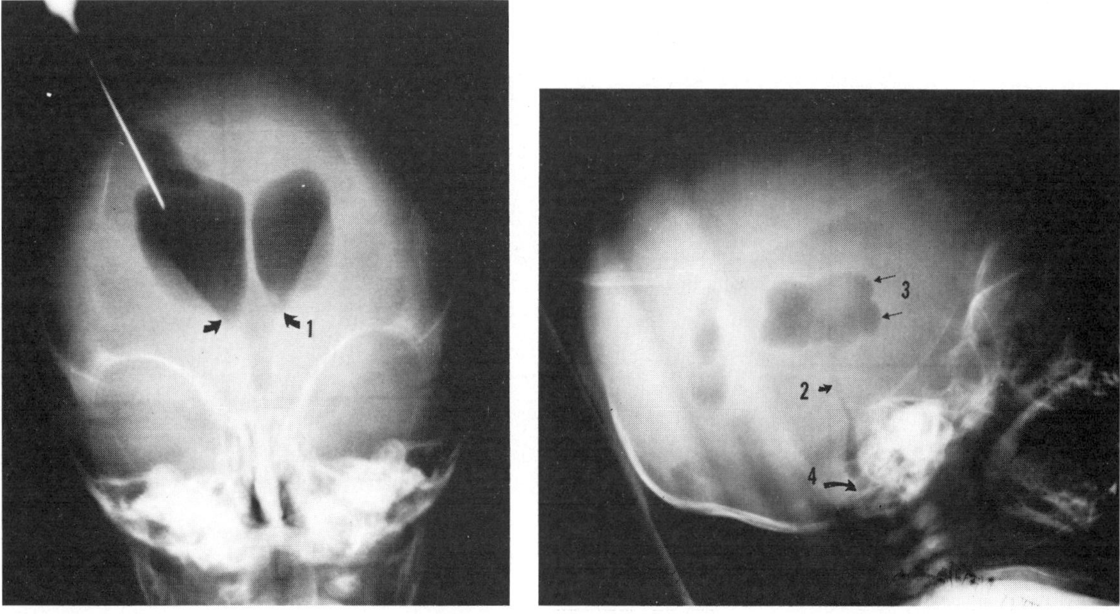

Figure 11–7. ARNOLD-CHIARI MALFORMATION: *1,* Pointed floors of the lateral ventricles; *2,* Elongated aqueduct of Sylvius; *3,* Deformed anterior margin of the third ventricle; *4,* Fourth ventricle displaced into the upper cervical region.

All the findings illustrated here are typical of the Arnold-Chiari malformation.

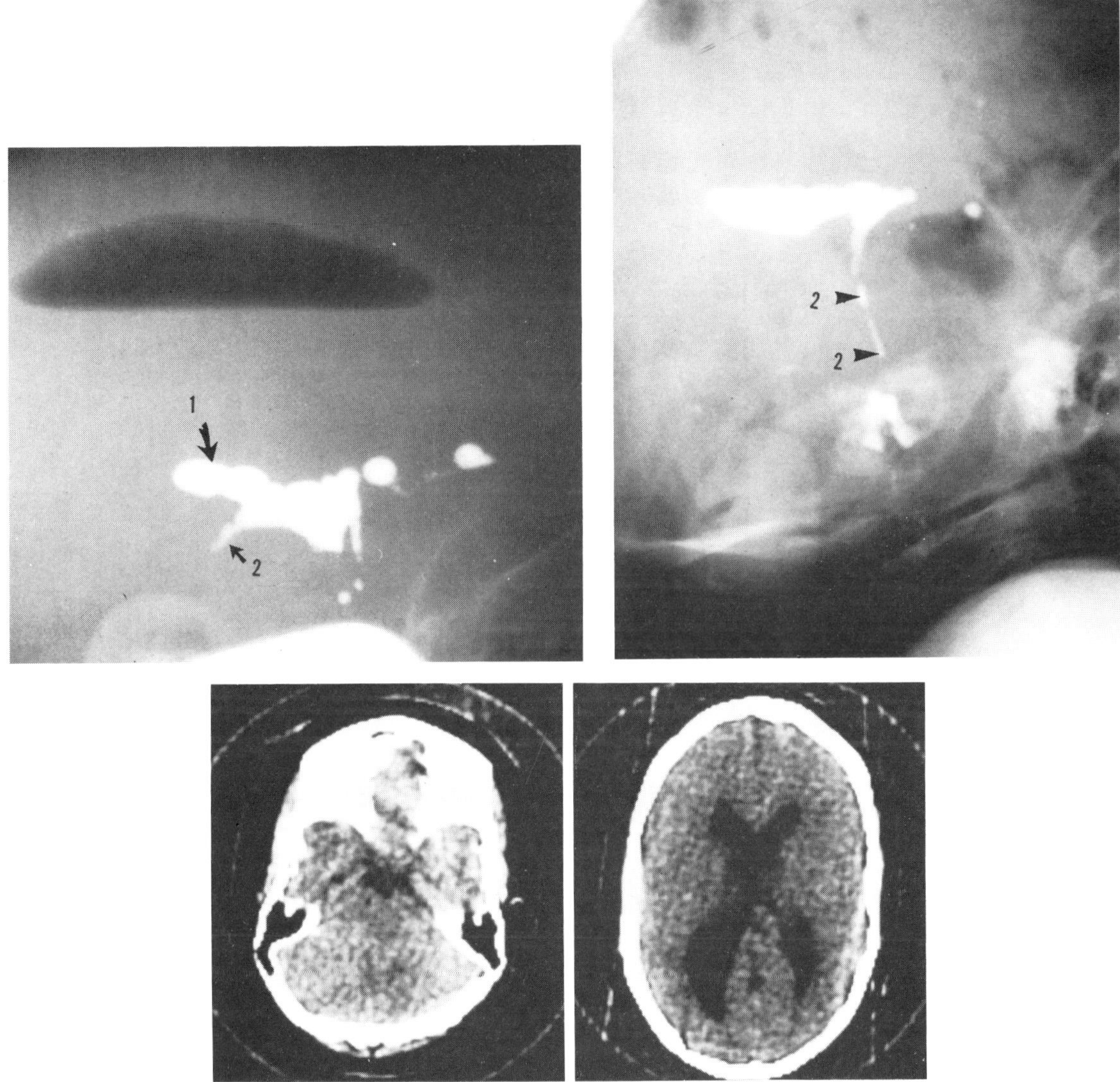

Figure 11–8. ARNOLD-CHIARI MALFORMATION: *1*, Suprapineal recess; *2*, Narrowed sylvian aqueduct (Pantopaque ventriculogram).

The suprapineal recess is enlarged secondary to hydrocephalus. The sylvian aqueduct is narrowed, and the fourth ventricle is displaced inferiorly. The lower cut of the CT scan shows that the fourth ventricle is never seen because it is inferiorly displaced. The lateral ventricles are moderately enlarged. Typically, this enlargement involves the occipital horns more than the frontal horns.

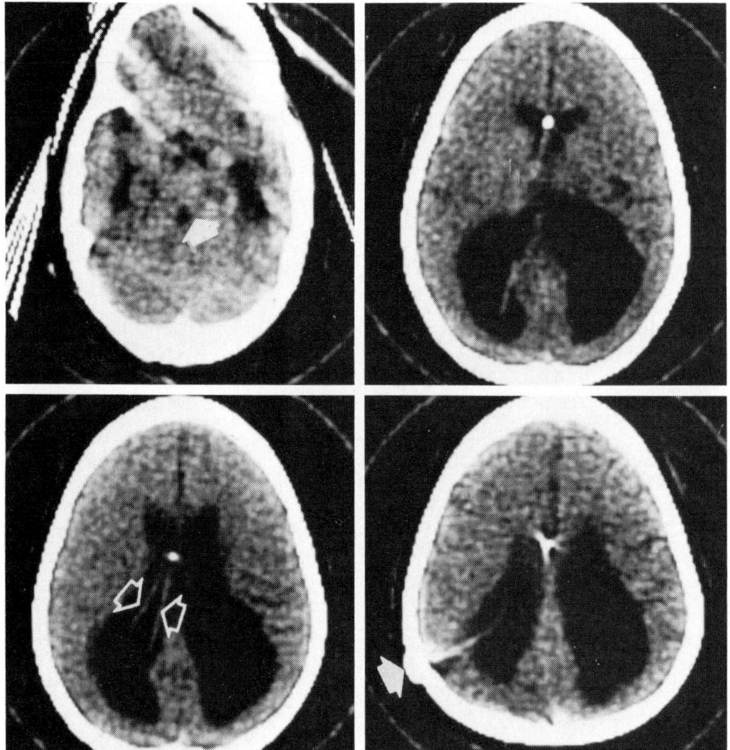

Figure 11–9. ARNOLD-CHIARI MALFORMATION: The white arrowhead indicates the dilated aqueduct of Sylvius. The fourth ventricle is displaced inferiorly into the upper cervical region. The upper sections demonstrate the greater enlargement of the occipital horns compared to the frontal horns. The open arrowheads show two shunt tubes in place in the lateral ventricle. The closed arrowhead indicates the extracranial component of the shunt tubing device.

Figure 11–10. AQUEDUCT STENOSIS ASSOCIATED WITH THE ARNOLD-CHIARI MALFORMATION: There is massive ventricular dilatation, with only a thin mantle of remaining cerebral tissue detectable in the frontal regions. Some preservation of the deep midline structures and the posterior fossa structures can be seen. The sutures and fontanelles are widely patent. The fourth ventricle is never seen; it is displaced inferiorly because of the Arnold-Chiari malformation and lies in the upper cervical region. An associated aqueduct stenosis has resulted in the marked ventricular enlargement.

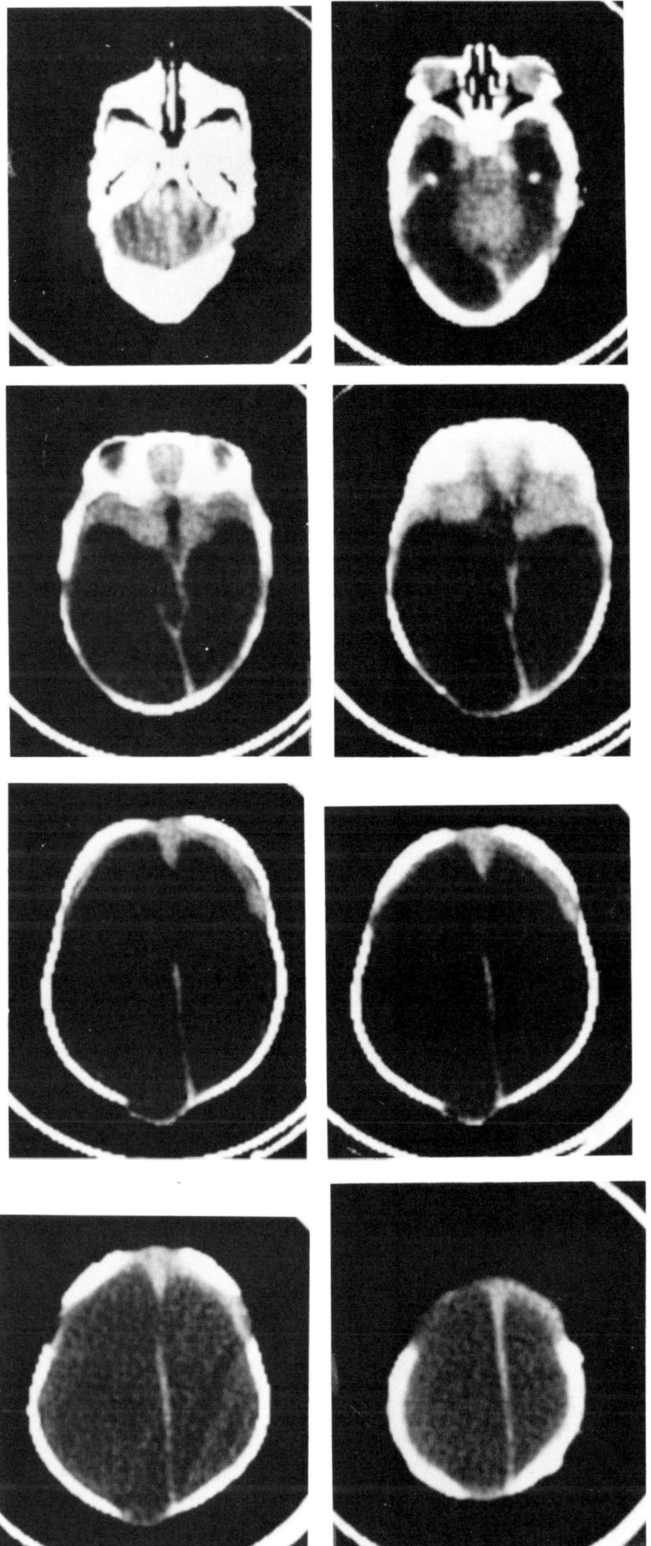

Figure 11–10 *See legend on the opposite page*

Figure 11–11. COMMUNICATING HYDROCEPHALUS: The ventriculogram (*A*) allows visualization of the lateral, third and fourth ventricles. However, the ventricles are greatly enlarged. This finding is not uncommon following a subarachnoid hemorrhage; it may be seen following head trauma or meningitis.

B, The CT scan in another patient demonstrates evidence of a recent subarachnoid hemorrhage with blood in the sylvian fissures, in the third ventricle and in the dependent portions of the lateral ventricles. There is mild hydrocephalus secondary to mechanical obstruction of the ventricular system; however, a communicating hydrocephalus eventually may develop secondary to interference of the function of the arachnoid villi by the blood in the subarachnoid space and failure to resorb the CSF.

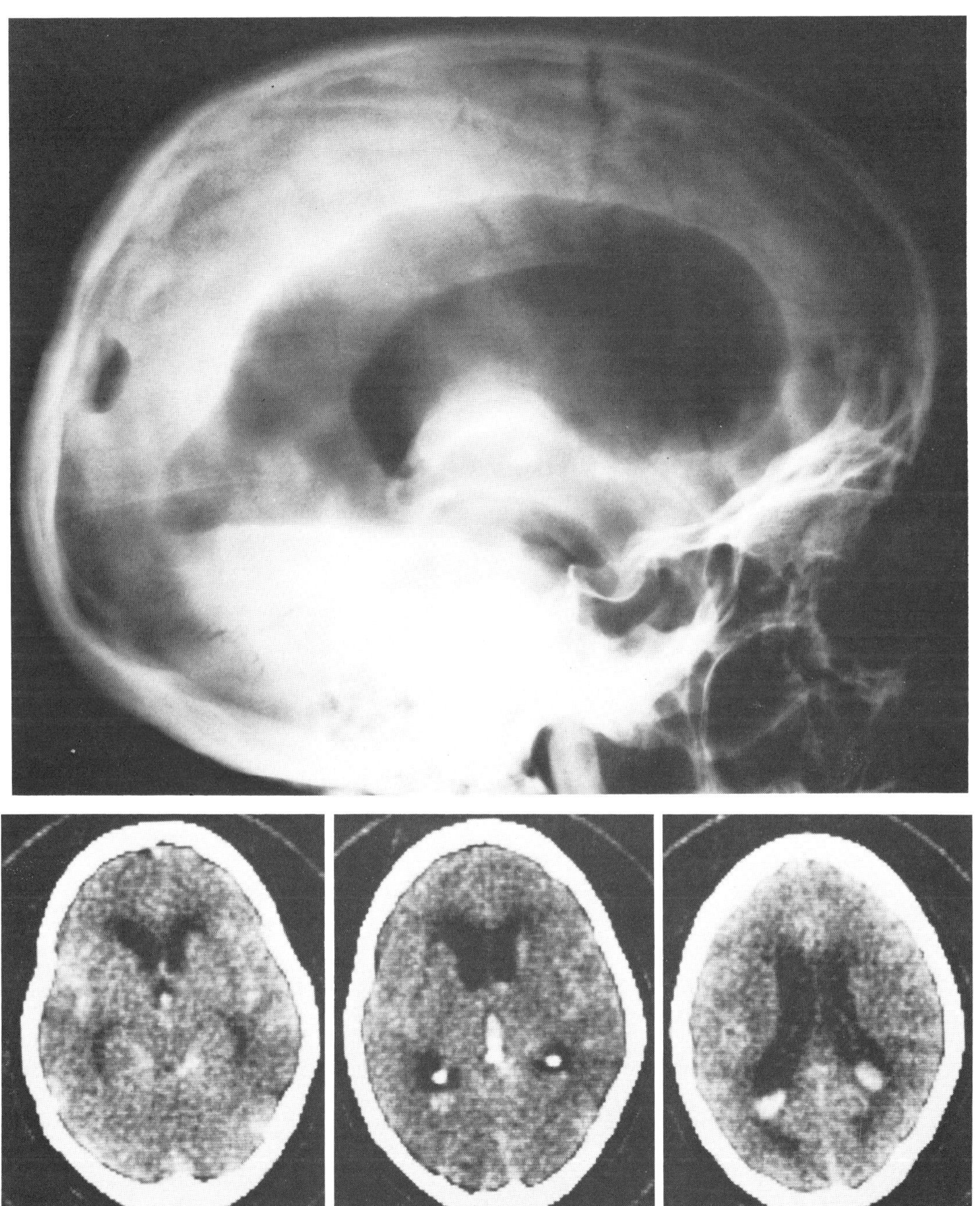

Figure 11–11 *See legend on the opposite page*

PORENCEPHALY

Areas of porencephaly are readily identified on CT scans. They have a well defined border, contain fluid the same density as cerebrospinal fluid and do not change in density following the use of contrast material. Before the advent of CT scanning, the diagnosis of porencephaly depended on a combination of plain radiographic findings, angiography, pneumoencephalography and ventriculography. However, even with all these techniques, the radiographic appearance was that of any space occupying lesion, and surgery was required for definite diagnosis. Since the development of CT, it usually is possible to diagnose the abnormality and treat the patient without additional diagnostic work-up.

The term "porencephaly" was coined by Heschl in 1859, who defined it as a "pore" in the brain. The term "porencephalic cyst" implies a lesion that has an ependymal lining and communicates with the lateral ventricles or subarachnoid cyst. A broader definition of porencephalic cyst also includes "closed" porencephaly, which does not communicate with either the ventricular system or the subarachnoid space. By any diagnostic examination other than CT, these areas of closed porencephaly would appear as a mass lesion. The examples illustrated here include some porencephalic cysts and a variety of other CSF-containing lesions.

Areas of porencephaly may have a variety of etiologies:

1. Germ plasm defects.
2. Intrauterine cerebrovascular accidents.
3. Birth trauma.
4. Vascular thrombosis or embolism.
5. Postinflammatory changes.
6. Focal atrophy.
7. Hemorrhage.
8. Postsurgical changes.

Care must be taken not to mistake a cystic neoplasm for a porencephalic cyst. However, when a tumor is present, the fluid within the cyst is of higher density than CSF, and usually a ring or solid area of enhancement is noted after the infusion of contrast material.

Post-traumatic hematomas, spontaneous hematomas and infarcts have all been observed to progress to areas of porencephaly on serial CT scans. The areas of postsurgical porencephaly are readily correlated with the surgical procedure. Usually no further diagnostic tests are necessary to determine the correct diagnosis.

These patients may be neurologically intact, or they may demonstrate seizure disorders, mental retardation or hemi- or monoparesis.

Text continued on page 524

Figure 11–12. ENCEPHALOMALACIA PROGRESSING TO PORENCEPHALY: The initial CT scan (*A*) reveals scattered areas of radiolucency throughout both hemispheres. A scan one week later (*B*) demonstrates a large area of radiolucency occupying the entire right hemisphere, apparently secondary to infarction (etiology — probably cerebral anoxia).

A follow-up scan (*C*) two weeks later showed an area of irregular enhancement in the region of the right middle cerebral artery secondary to luxury perfusion. The final scan (*D*) several months later shows that this area of infarction has progressed to a large area of porencephaly occupying almost the entire right hemisphere.

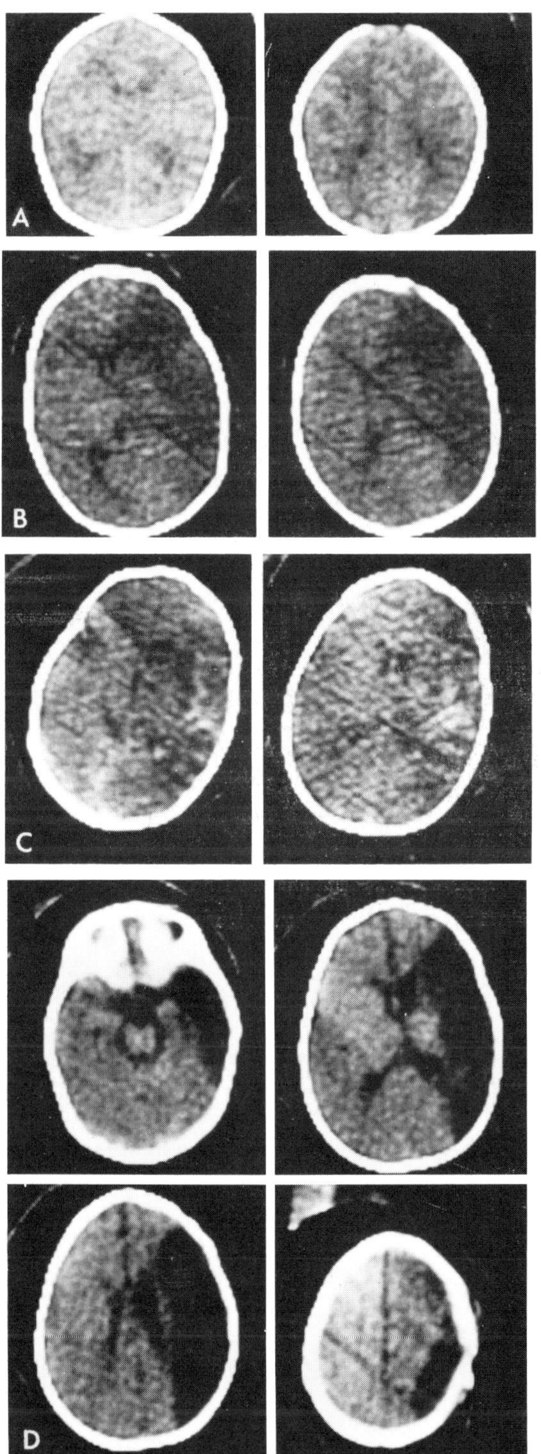

Figure 11–12 *See legend on the opposite page*

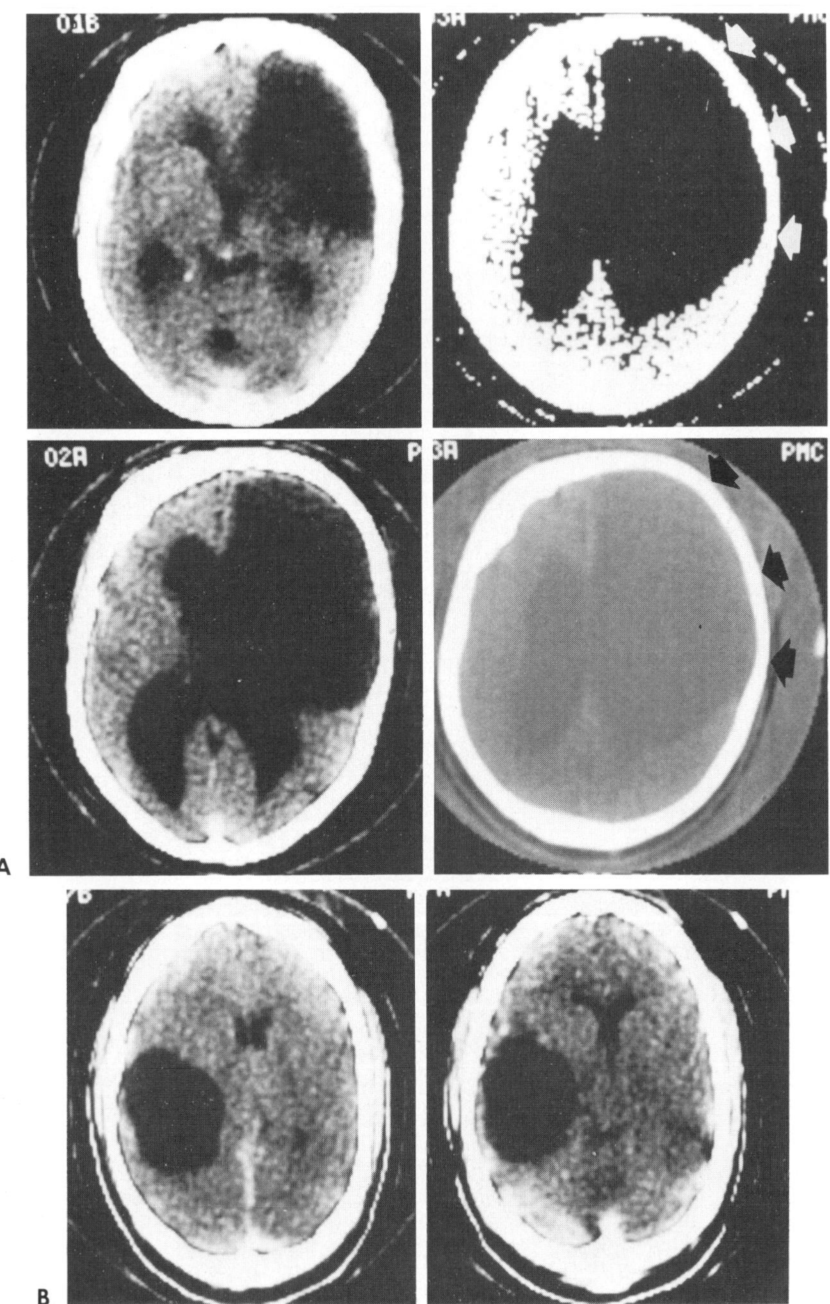

Figure 11–13. PORENCEPHALY: *A*, There is a large area of porencephaly in the right hemisphere that communicates with the right lateral ventricle. There is bulging of the bony calvaria over the porencephalic cyst. The bone is also thinned in the area of the cystic lesion *(arrows)*. The fluid within the cyst is of CSF density. This porencephalic cyst is probably secondary to birth trauma.

B, A large left temporal porencephalic cyst probably communicates with the left temporal horn (another patient).

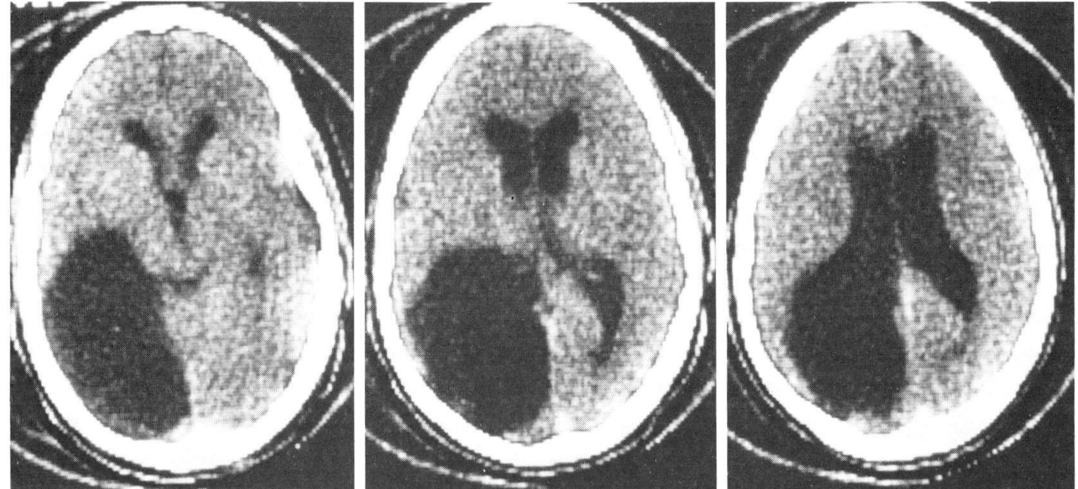

Figure 11–14. PORENCEPHALY SECONDARY TO BIRTH TRAUMA: *A*, There is a large left occipital porencephalic cyst. Although the cyst appears to communicate with the occipital horn of the lateral ventricle, there may be a thin ependymal lining separating the two.

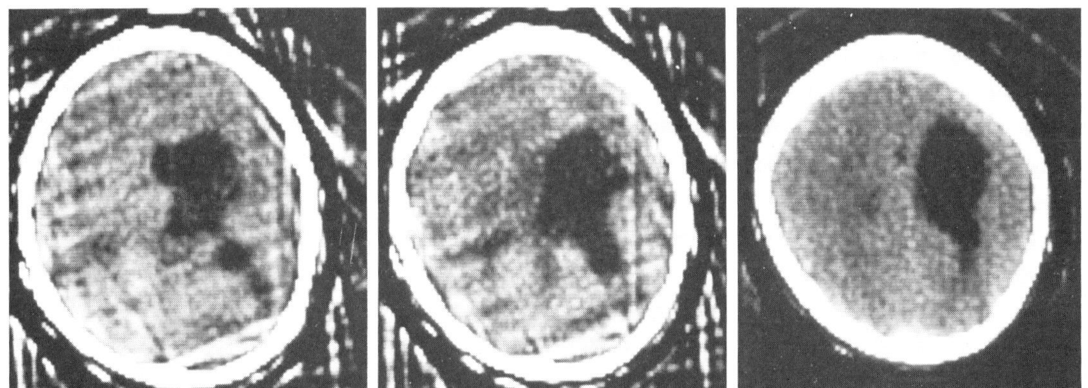

Figure 11–15. PORENCEPHALY OF UNKNOWN ETIOLOGY: This patient had a clinical diagnosis of cerebral palsy. The CT scan demonstrates an irregular porencephalic cyst that extends from the frontal horn and body of the right lateral ventricle.

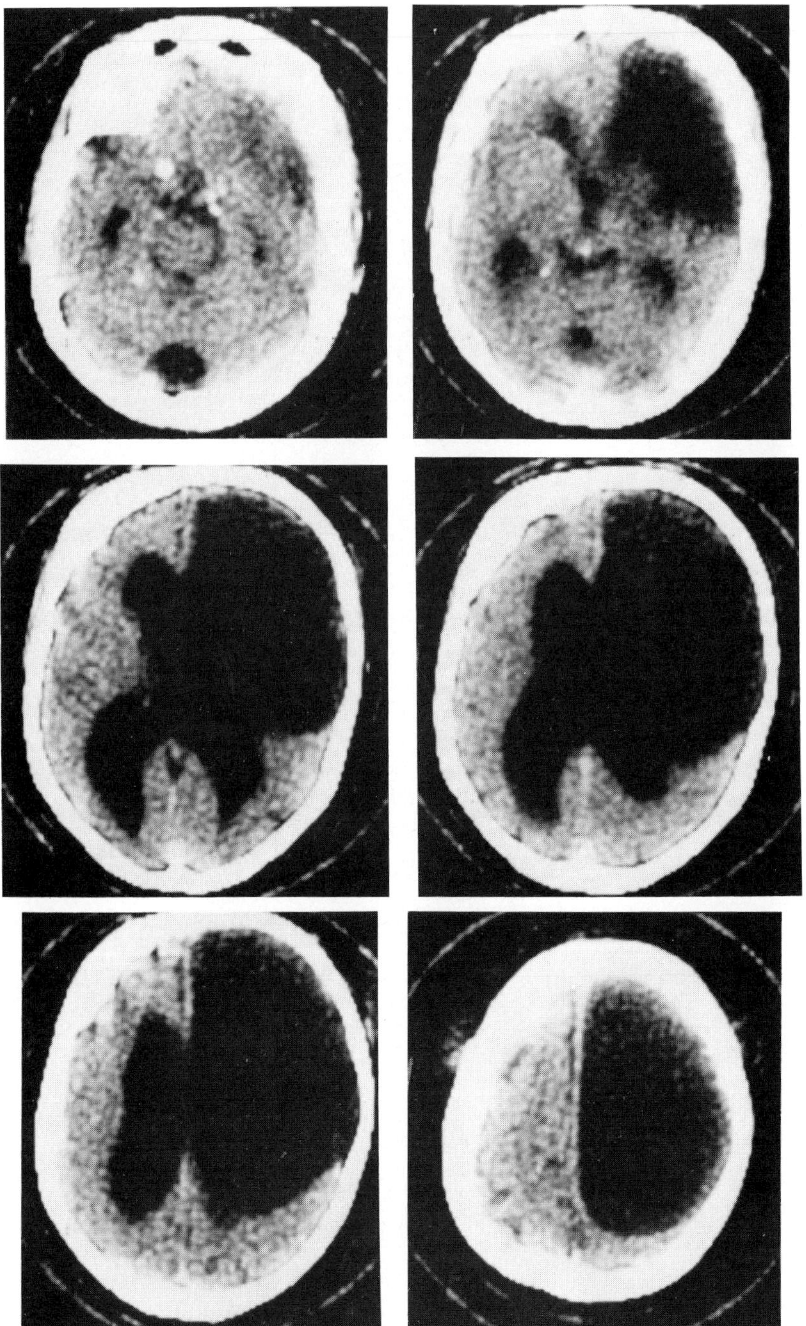

Figure 11–16. LARGE PORENCEPHALIC CYST: Both of the lateral ventricles are large, and a large cystic extension of the right lateral ventricle extends to the high convexity region, thinning the overlying bony calvaria. The fluid measures of CSF density and represents porencephalic dilatation of the right lateral ventricle. The patient shown is an adult who has exhibited left hemiatrophy since birth. The changes presumably are secondary to a germ plasm defect or to birth trauma. Although it appears that the right lateral ventricle communicates freely with the cyst, pathologic studies show that there may be a thin ependymal lining between the cyst and the ventricle.

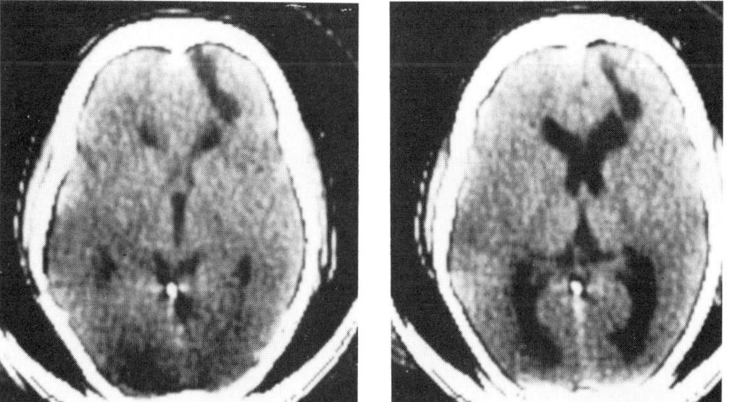

Figure 11–17. POSTSURGICAL PORENCEPHALY: An area of radiolucency can be seen in the right frontal region; it is well defined, non–space-occupying and contains fluid of CSF density. The lateral ventricles are mildly dilated. The right frontal lesion is a porencephalic cyst that developed after placement of a catheter for ventriculography.

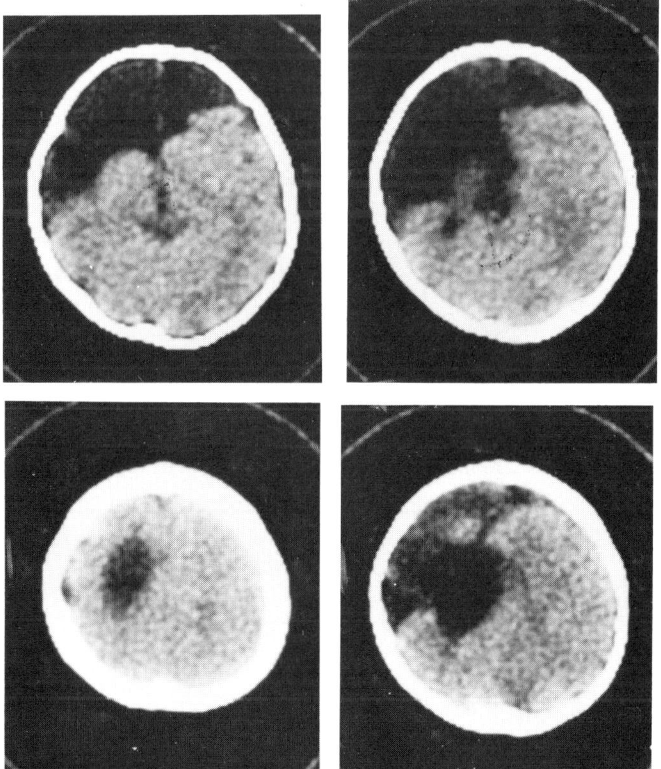

Figure 11–18. PORENCEPHALY AND HEMIATROPHY: The left lateral ventricle is dilated in the fashion of a porencephalic cyst. There is also a large accumulation of radiolucent fluid over the left frontal and parietal regions and a small accumulation of fluid over the right frontal region. Presumably the extracerebral accumulations are chronic subdural hematomas, and there is an associated left hemiatrophy.

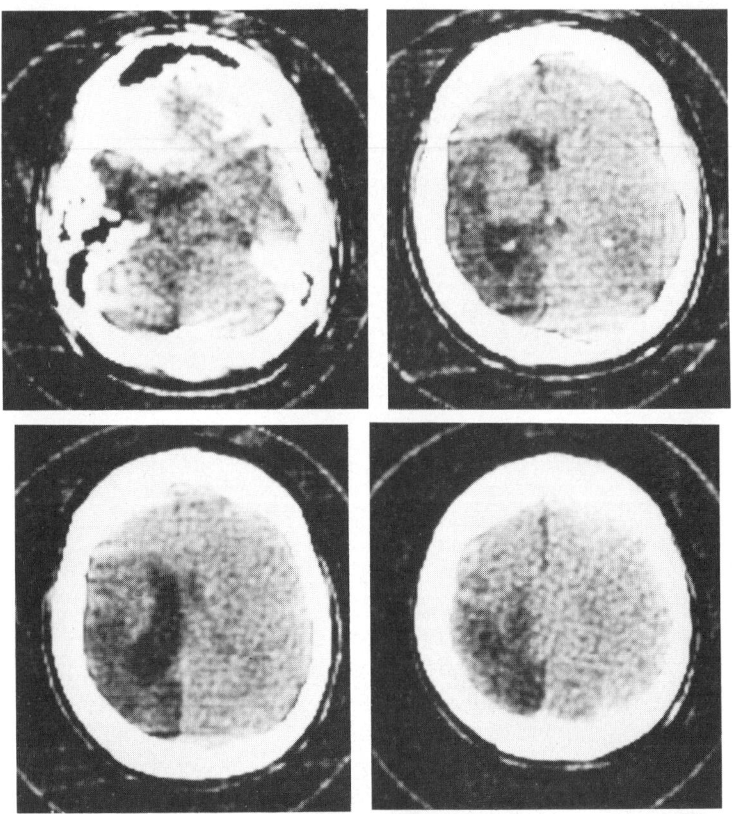

Figure 11–19 *See legend on the opposite page*

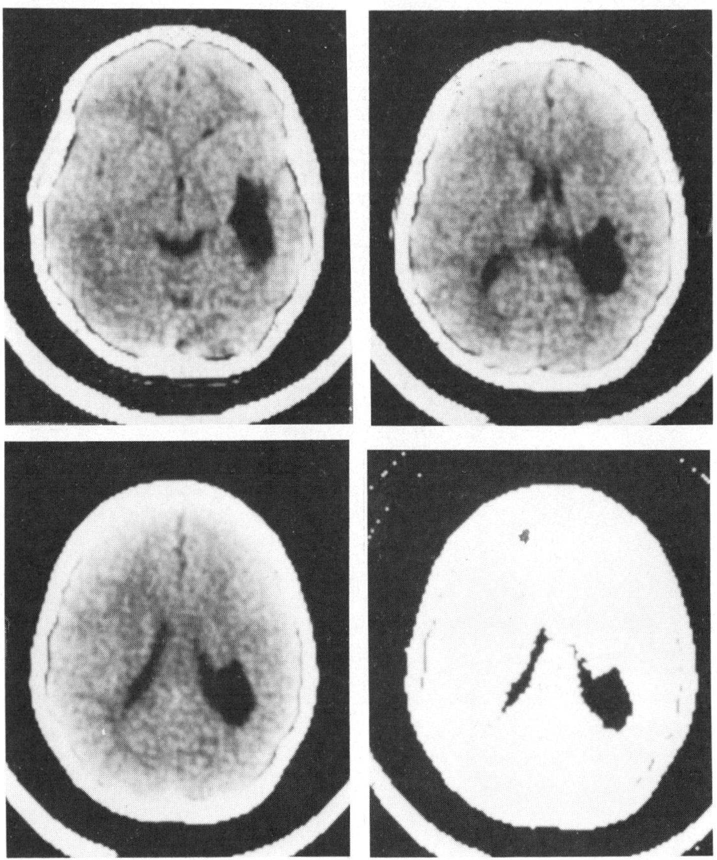

Figure 11–20 *See legend on the opposite page*

Figure 11–19. HEMIATROPHY: There is dilatation of the left lateral ventricle as compared to the right. Shift toward the atrophic left side and atrophy of the hemisphere on the left side with areas of radiolucency over the left hemisphere also are seen. There is thickening of the bony calvaria of the left hemisphere. The appearance is that of classic left hemiatrophy.

Figure 11–20. PORENCEPHALY: The CT scan demonstrates a small porencephalic cyst in the region of the atrium of the right lateral ventricle. The lesion has a well defined margin, and contains fluid of CSF density. No change is seen following the infusion of contrast material. The area of porencephaly is probably secondary to birth trauma.

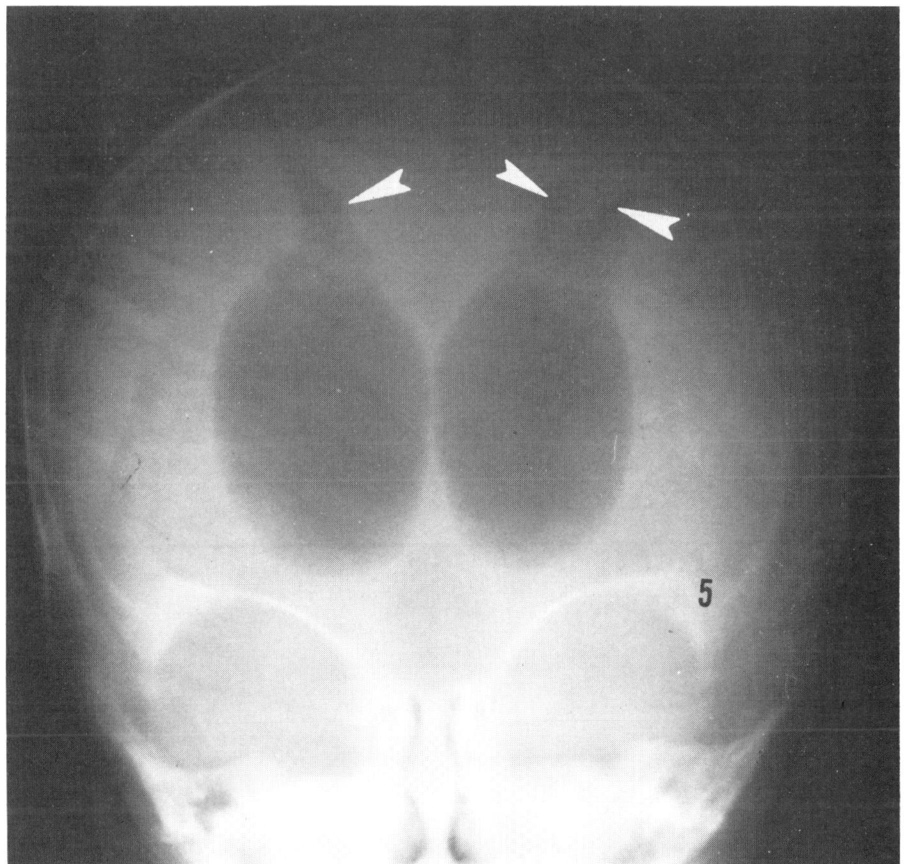

Figure 11–21. AREAS OF PORENCEPHALY SECONDARY TO VENTRICULAR TAPS: The white arrowheads demonstrate areas of porencephaly bilaterally that develop following brain injury secondary to ventricular taps.

METASTASES

Now that CT scanning is available, it can be stated that the CT scan with infusion of contrast material is the diagnostic procedure of choice for cerebral metastases. It is recommended that at the time of initial work-up each patient should first have a preinfusion scan, followed by infusion of contrast material and another scan. For follow-up examination, only a postinfusion scan may be performed if there is no suspicion of intracerebral hemorrhage.

There is no doubt that, of all the tests available, the CT scan provides the most accurate evaluation of the presence or absence of metastases. The CT scan will detect lesions as small as 1 cm in diameter. Because the scan can have a normal appearance before infusion of contrast material, a postinfusion scan is essential. Most metastatic lesions are space-occupying; however, even sizable metastases may be present without significant mass effect, or there may be symmetrical bilateral metastases that result in no shift of the midline. Most metastases demonstrate contrast enhancement on the postinfusion study.

Multiple metastatic lesions occur frequently; however, a certain number of patients have only one intracranial metastasis. The patients' symptoms reflect the position of the lesion, although it is not uncommon to have a patient present with a clinical history consistent with transient ischemic attacks. CT with infusion is much more sensitive than the radionuclide scan for diagnosing metastatic lesions — especially those located in the midbrain and posterior fossa.

Both routine and postinfusion studies are useful for treatment planning for radiation therapy and for estimating response to treatment with radiotherapy or chemotherapy.

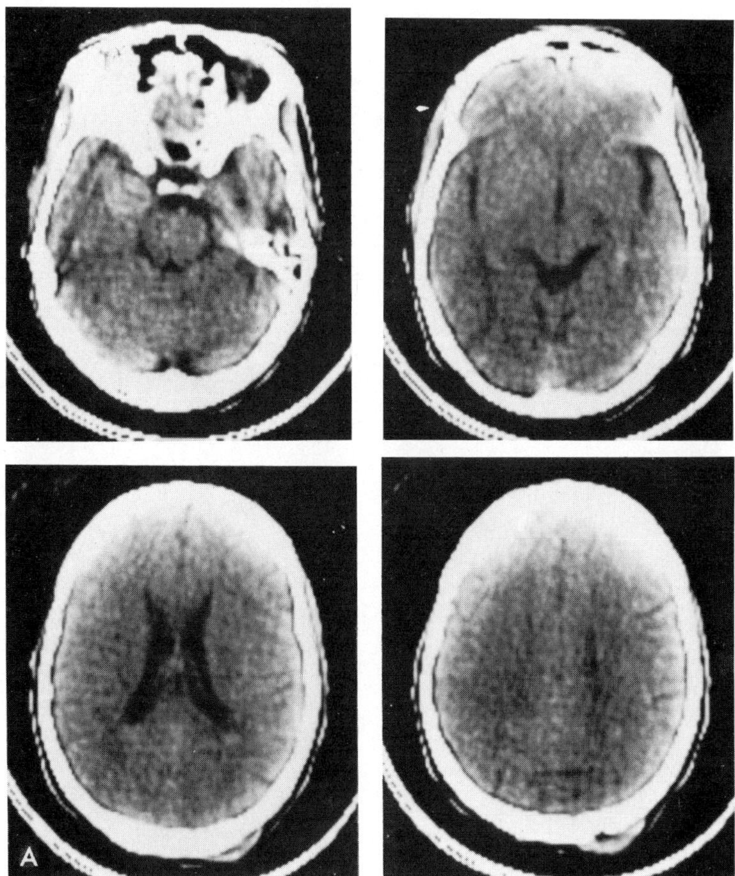

Figure 11–22. *See legend on the opposite page*

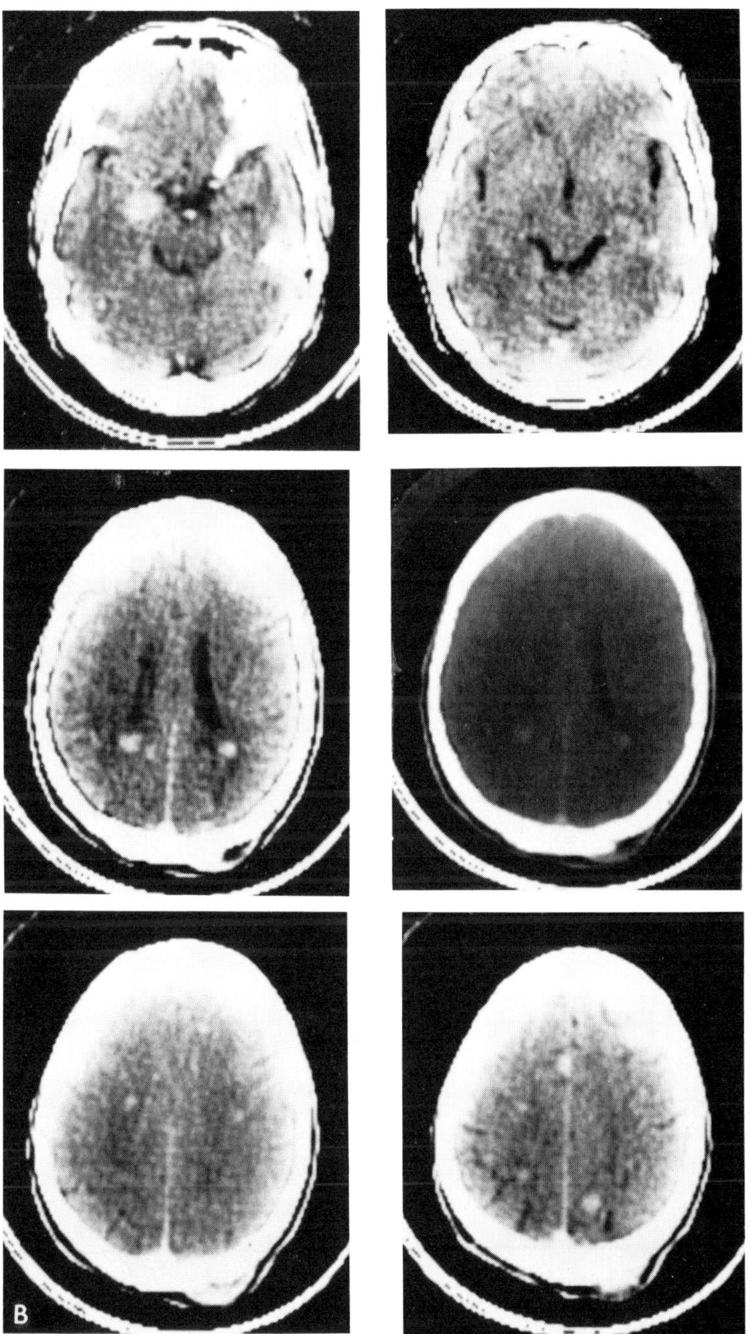

Figure 11–22. METASTASES: *A*, The preinfusion scan demonstrates questionable areas of higher than normal brain density scattered throughout the cerebral substance. There is a well rounded lesion of higher than normal brain density in the left parasellar region. This is noted to enhance on the postinfusion scans. *B,* Following the infusion of contrast material there is evidence of multiple bilateral enhancing lesions of varying sizes scattered throughout both hemispheres. Because the lesions are symmetric and bilateral, there is no shift of the midline structures. There is also a bony metastasis in the right parietal region associated with an extracranial soft tissue component.

IMP: Multiple metastases; primary breast cancer.

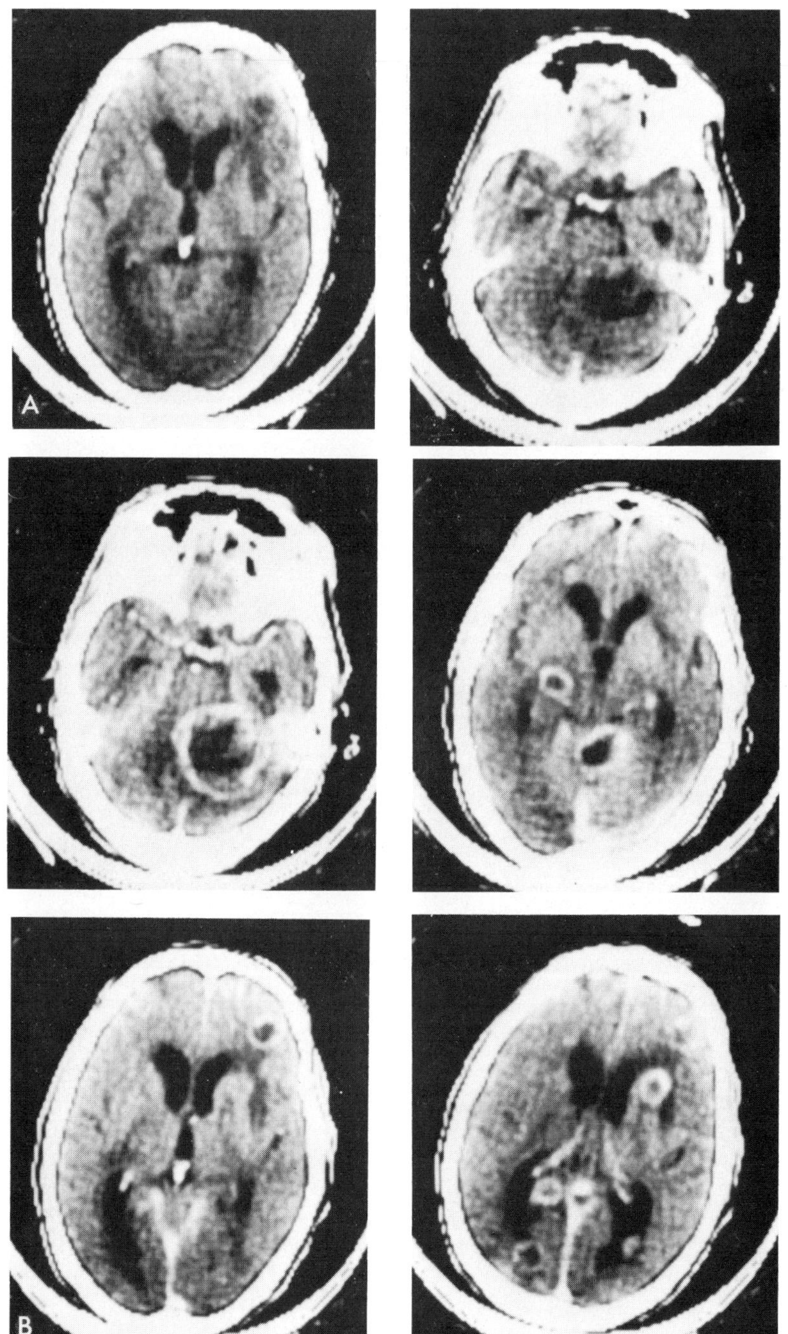

Figure 11–23. MULTIPLE METASTASES, SUPRA- AND INFRATENTORIAL: *A*, The preinfusion scan reveals multiple areas of radiolucency in both hemispheres and in the infratentorial region. There is mild obstructive hydrocephalus. Because the lesions are balancing, there is no shift of the midline.

B, The postinfusion scan reveals that the lesions enhance in a ring-shaped fashion; all are surrounded by varying amounts of cerebral edema.

IMP: Multiple metastases; primary lung cancer.

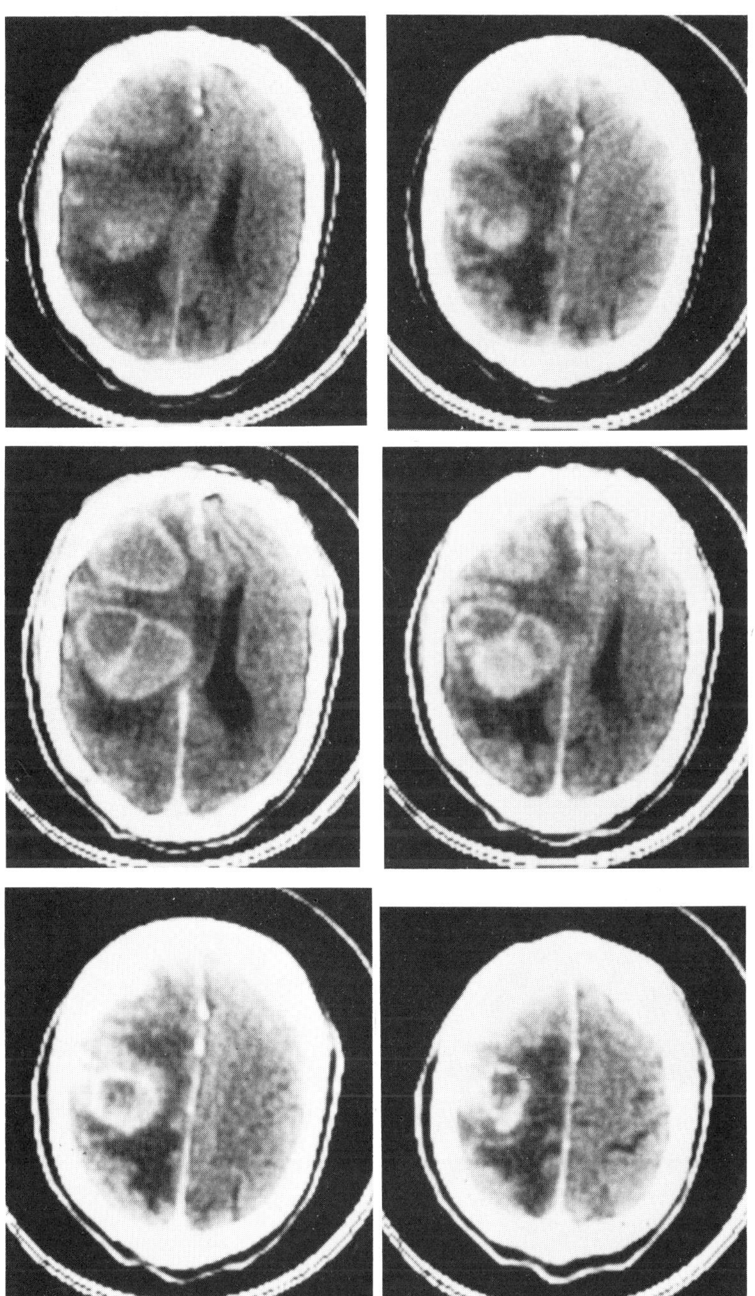

Figure 11-24. METASTASES: The CT scan demonstrates multiple enhancing lesions in the left hemisphere with marked surrounding edema and both rings and areas of solid enhancement. There is marked shift from left to right and curvilinear shift of the falx cerebri as well. Obliteration of the cortical sulci is seen on the side of the metastases.

IMP: Multiple metastases; primary lung cancer.

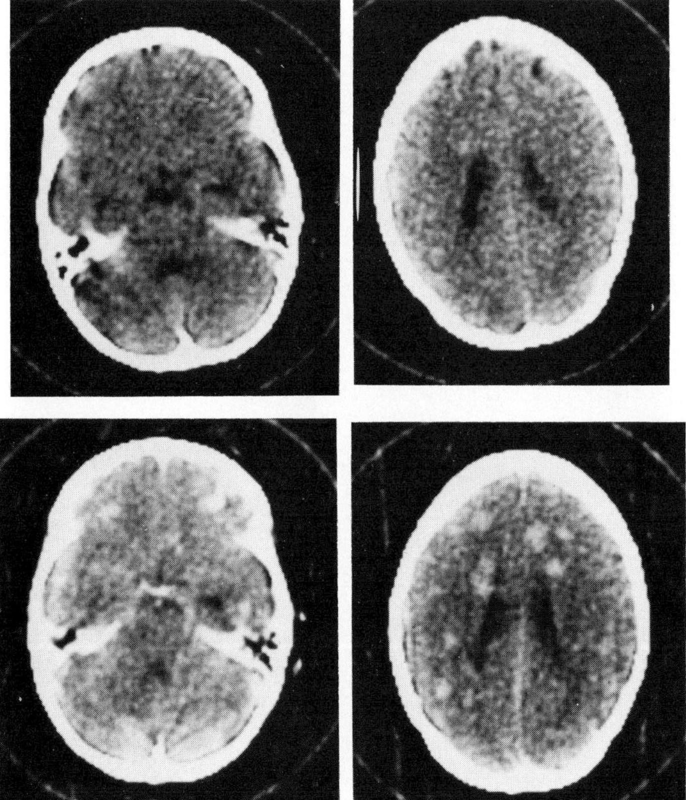

Figure 11–25. MULTIPLE METASTASES: The preinfusion scan appears essentially normal; however, after the infusion of contrast material there are multiple small metastatic lesions throughout both hemispheres. The possibility of progressive multifocal leukoencephalopathy also should be considered in this case.

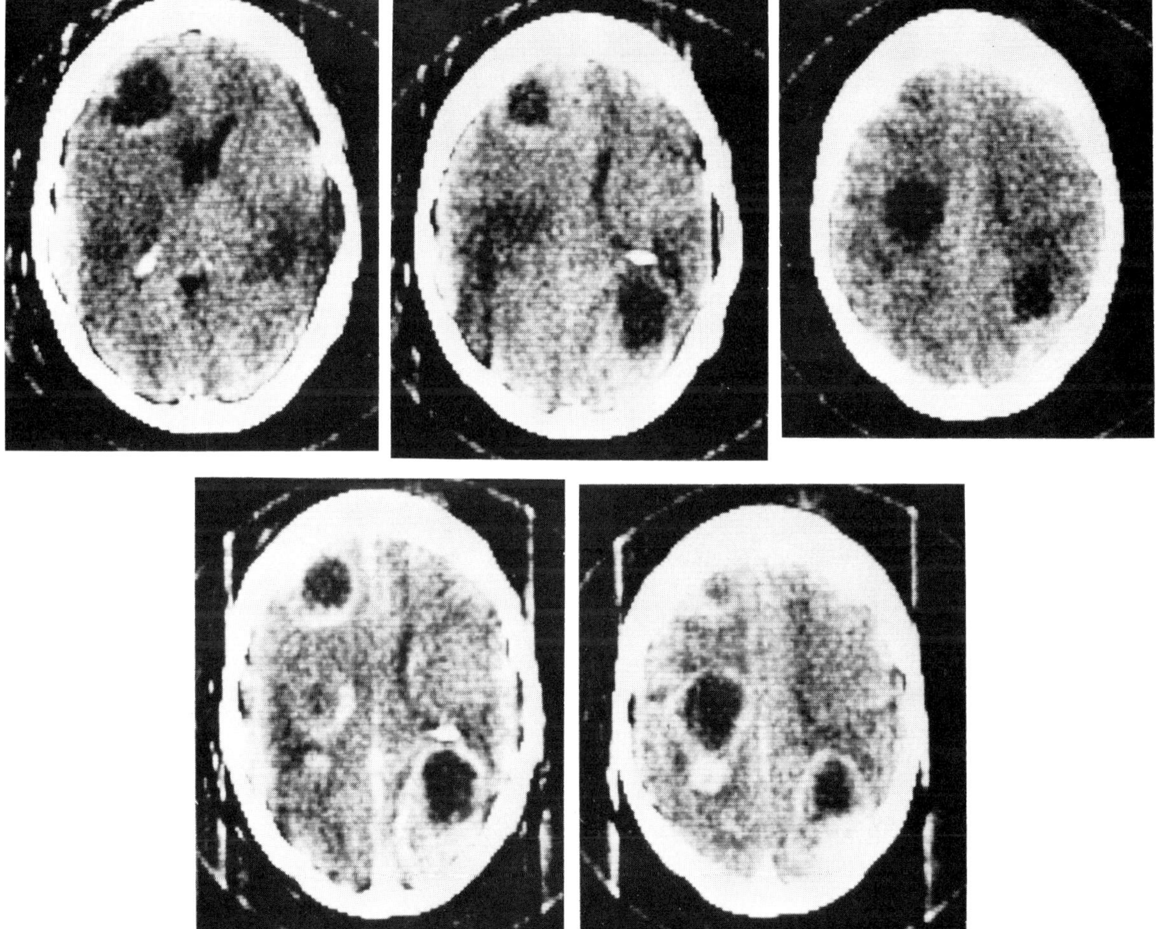

Figure 11–26. MULTIPLE METASTASES: There are multiple metastases throughout both hemispheres. They enhance with rings and solid areas of enhancement. Many of the masses appear to have necrotic centers.

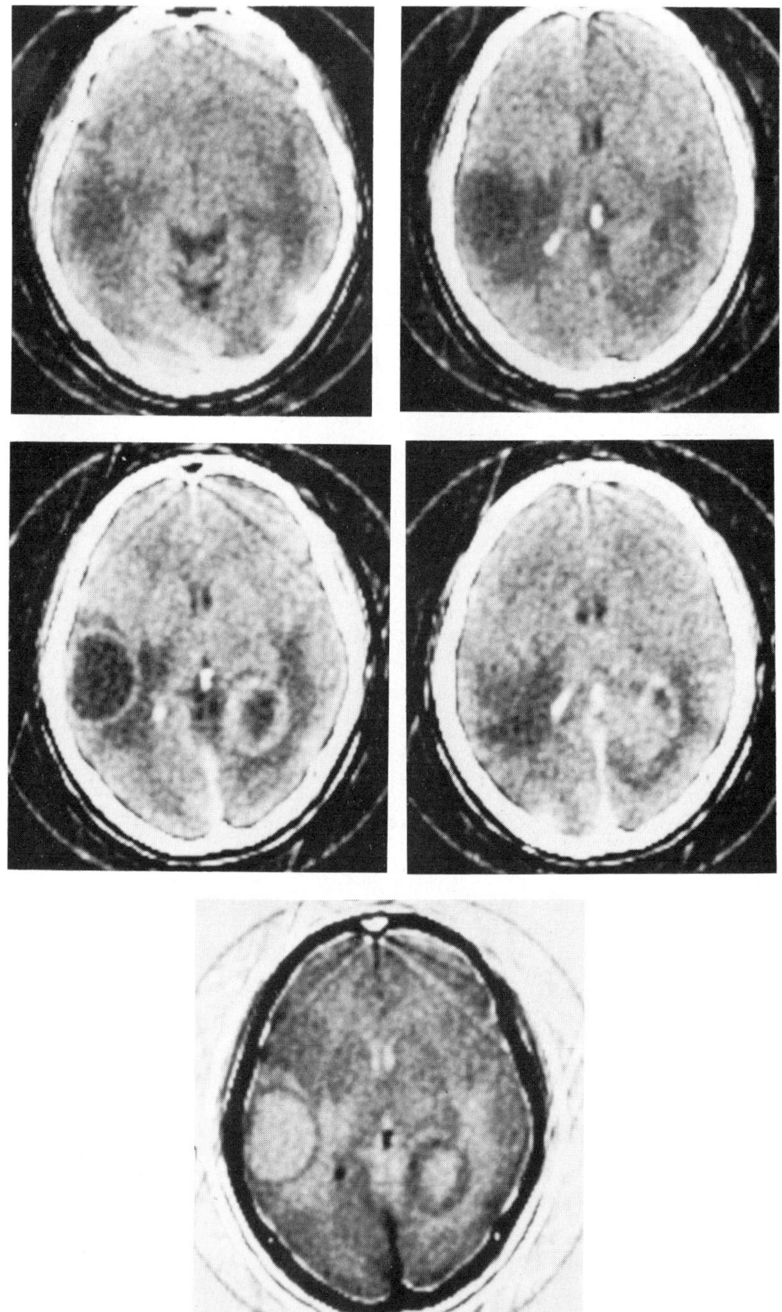

Figure 11–27. MULTIPLE METASTASES: Large bilateral metastases with surrounding edema have caused compression of both lateral ventricles, which now appear very slitlike and compressed on the midline.

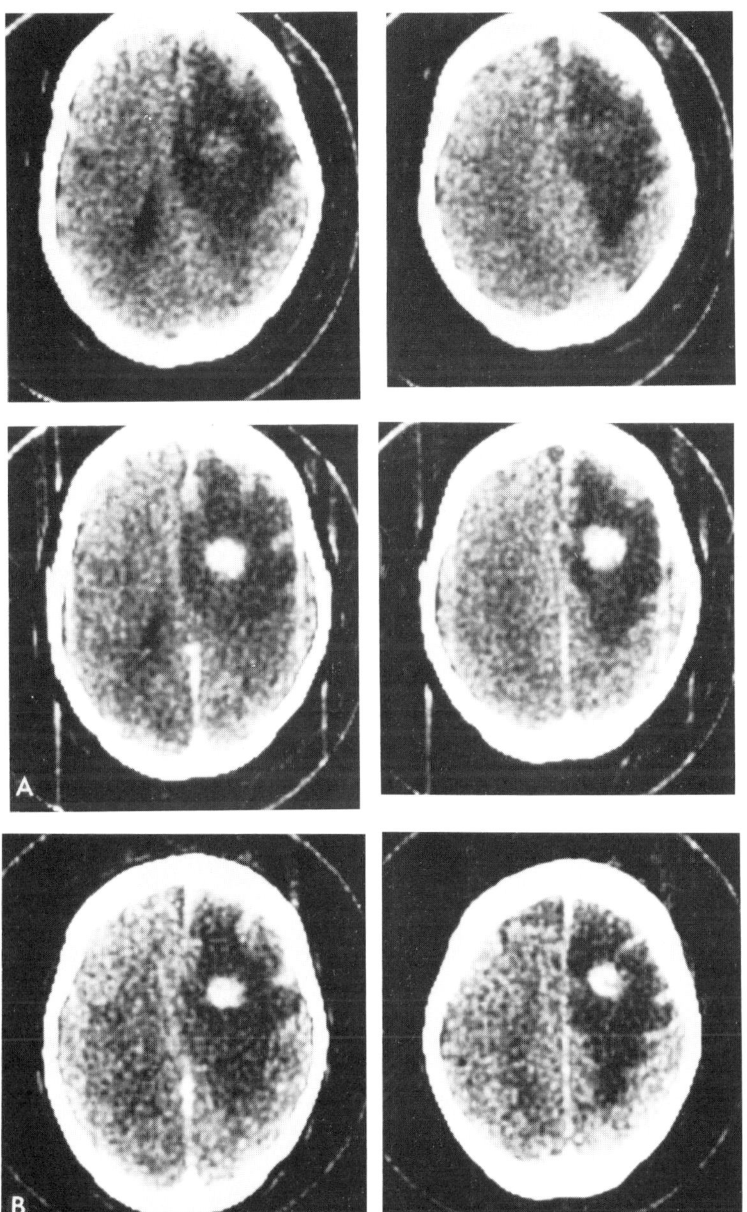

Figure 11–28. SOLITARY METASTASIS; MARKED EDEMA: *A,* There is a solitary metastatic lesion in the right hemisphere that exhibits spectacular surrounding edema.

B, A follow-up scan approximately five months later reveals a slight decrease in the size of the lesion following treatment.

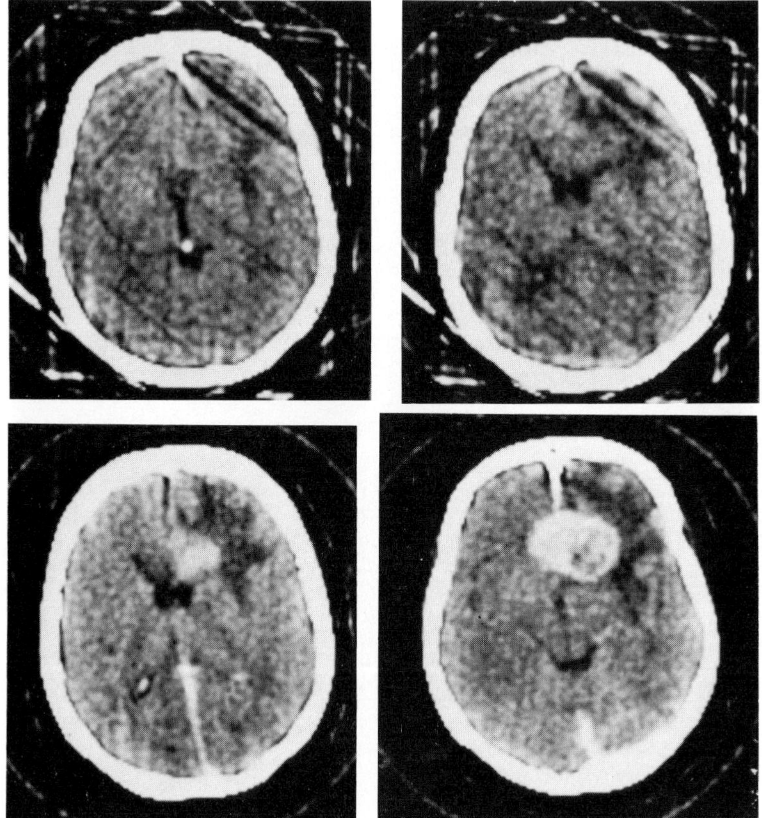

Figure 11–29. BREAST CANCER METASTATIC TO CORPUS CALLOSUM: A large solitary lesion is seen in the genu of the corpus callosum. It is larger on the right side than on the left and demonstrates surrounding edema (greater on the right) and marked enhancement with a varying pattern on the postinfusion scan.

IMP: Metastatic breast cancer extending through the corpus callosum.

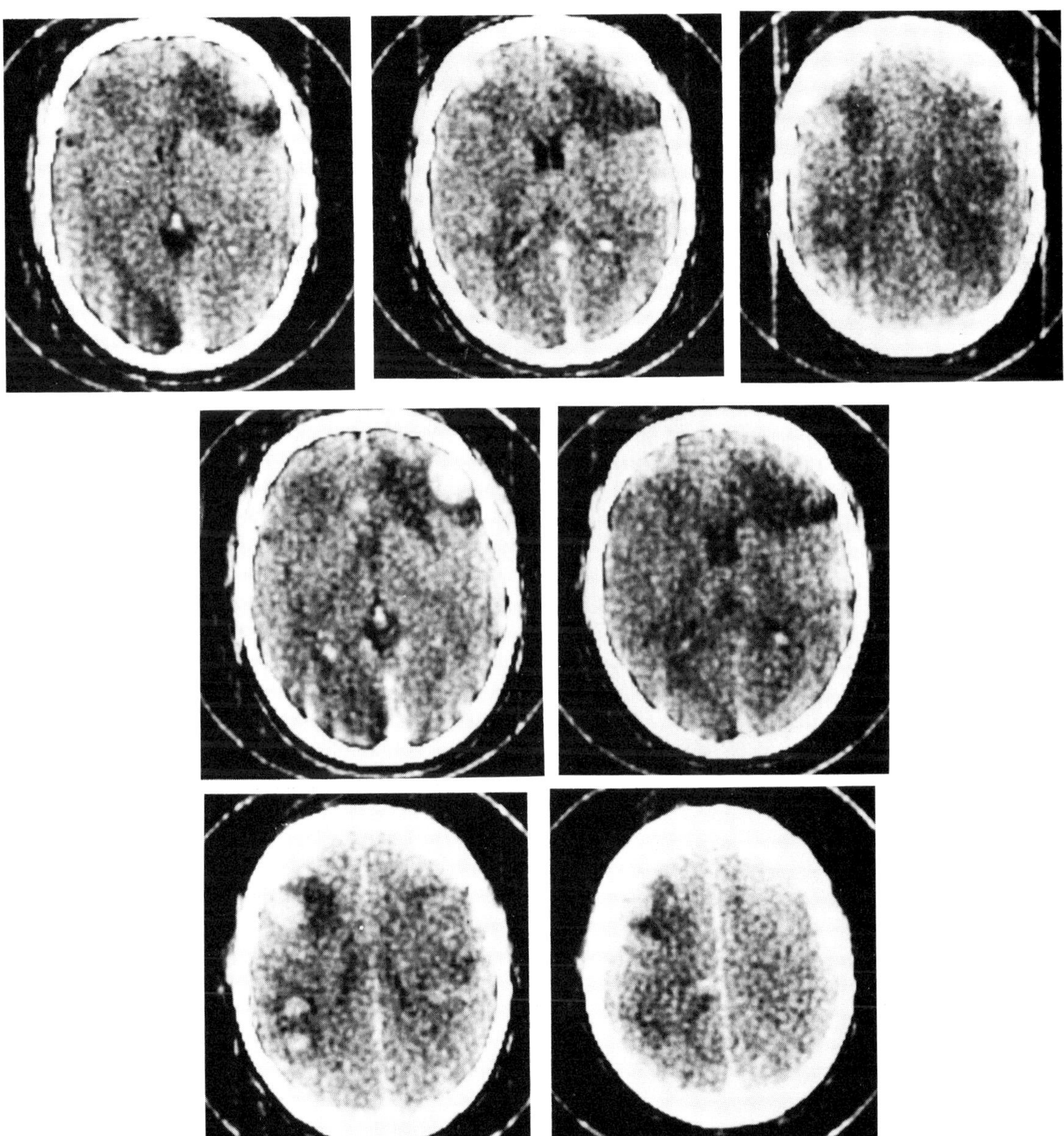

Figure 11–30. METASTATIC MELANOMA: The preinfusion scan reveals scattered high density lesions throughout both hemispheres. The postinfusion scan reveals marked homogeneous enhancement of the lesions. This appearance is quite typical of metastatic melanoma, which often is very vascular and therefore of high density on the preinfusion scan; it enhances greatly on the postinfusion scan. Scans in metastatic melanoma may also demonstrate that the metastatic nodules are hemorrhagic.

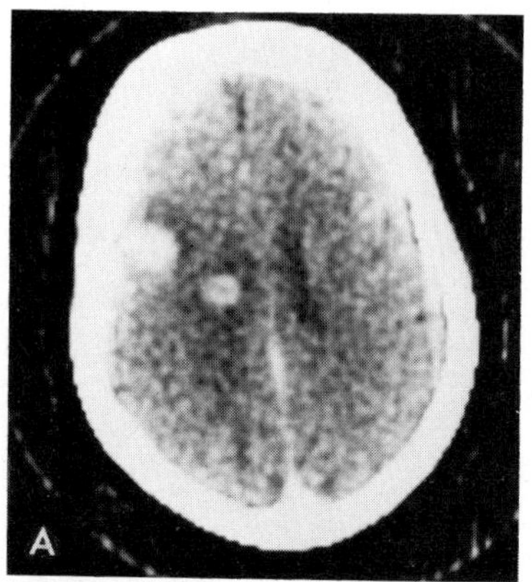

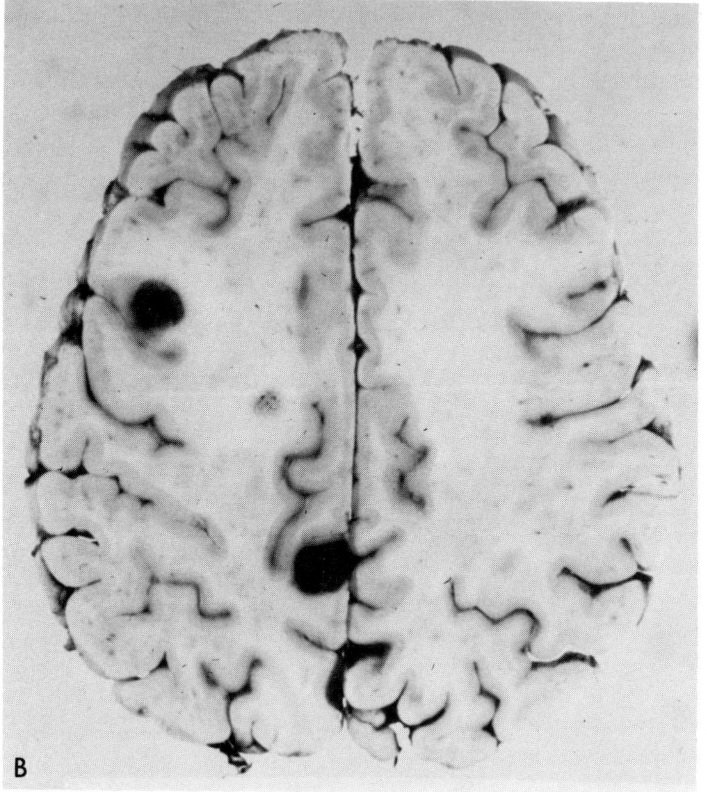

Figure 11–31. The CT scan (*A*) and the pathologic specimen (*B*) demonstrate two metastatic lesions. The smaller is approximately 1 cm in size, the larger is approximately 1.5 cm.

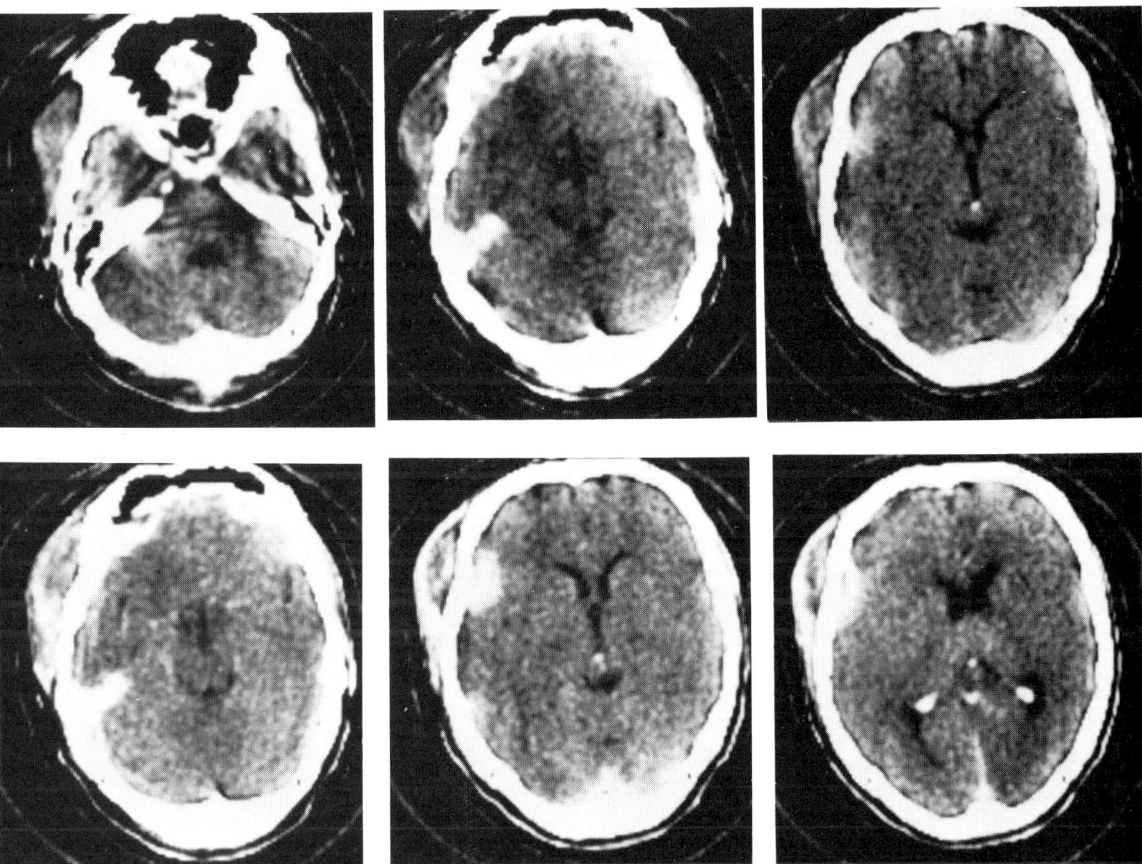

Figure 11–32. METASTATIC RENAL CARCINOMA: A large soft tissue metastasis is apparent on the left side of the calvaria in the posterior frontal region. The postinfusion scan demonstrates enhancement of the lesion and also reveals an intracranial component of the tumor. The plain skull films demonstrated a large lytic lesion in the bony calvaria at this level.

CHAPTER 12

ARTERIOVENOUS MALFORMATIONS

PATHOLOGY

Arteriovenous malformations (AVMs) — blood vessel abnormalities in which there is an abnormal communication between the arterial and venous circulations — are formed by a tangle of abnormal vessels. These vessels have thickened, malformed walls that make it difficult to identify them as either arteries or veins.

Consideration of their various angiographic and pathologic features suggests one method of classification that divides the vascular malformations into:

1. Cavernous angioma;
2. Racemose angioma
   a. Capillary ectatic angioma or capillary telangiectasis,
   b. Capillary-venous calcifying angioma (Sturge-Weber disease),
   c. Arteriovenous angioma.

These malformations may be supplied by one or more enlarged feeding arteries and drained by one or more (commonly multiple) large venous channels. The venous channels may drain either superficially or into the deep venous system. These latter arteriovenous malformations are the type most commonly seen in daily practice (c).

The vast majority of these lesions will be found in the supratentorial circulation — approximately 86 per cent. Of the remainder, approximately 6 per cent are in the infratentorial circulation; the remaining 8 per cent occur in the extracranial circulation. Arteriovenous malformations are less common than aneurysms.

CLINICAL SYMPTOMS

The presenting complaints of these patients are quite varied (see Table 12–1). Symptoms include grand mal seizures, syncopal attacks, transient ischemic attacks and finally the catastrophic events associated with hemorrhage of the malformations, such as dense hemiplegias and/or coma. When hemorrhage occurs, these lesions may present in a fashion similar to that seen with subarachnoid hemorrhage or intracerebral hematoma secondary to other causes.

PLAIN SKULL

The plain skull films may reveal areas of either curvilinear or punctate calcification that outline a portion or all of the malformation. The areas of curvilinear calcification may resemble those seen with an aneurysm. Frequently, areas of calcification can be identified on the CT scan that cannot be seen on radiographs of the skull. There may be enlargement of the vascular grooves of the skull — particularly if the malformation involves the meningeal coverings of the brain.

If the malformation is associated with

obstructive hydrocephalus, as seen with vein of Galen aneurysms, changes may be noted in the sella turcica secondary to the hydrocephalus and to continued pressure on the sella from the dilated third ventricle, with enlargement of the sella and truncation of the dorsum sella and the posterior clinoids.

With carotid cavernous fistulas, the superior orbital fissure may be enlarged secondary to pressure erosion.

COMPUTED TOMOGRAPHY OF AVMs

The routine preinfusion CT scan appears to be normal in approximately 25 per cent of cases. In the remainder there may be areas of increased density secondary to the deposition of calcium in the walls of the vessels of the malformation. Focal areas of radiolucency secondary to local atrophy may be seen; there may be evidence of hemiatrophy of the hemispheres either ipsilateral or contralateral to the malformation. A mild mass effect secondary to the malformation may be noted, with shift to the contralateral side.

Postinfusion, there is marked enhancement of the malformation, which may have a wedge-shaped appearance that is broad-based superficially. More commonly, there is a "bag of worms" appearance of the malformation, with enhancement of the individual tortuous vessels. In other cases, both the individual feeding arteries and the draining veins can be identified.

The position of the malformation relative to areas of atrophy can be readily identified on the scan.

When the malformation is accompanied by hemorrhage, an area of increased density corresponding to the area of hemorrhage is superimposed on any other findings on the CT scan. If recent hemorrhage has occurred, the infusion of contrast material usually causes no change. With a resorbing hematoma, a ring of enhancement may be seen.

Aneurysms of the great vein of Galen often will be seen as a well defined area of increased density. This type of malformation may cause obstructive hydrocephalus of varying degree. Vein of Galen aneurysms produce marked enhancement of the vein. The rest of the malformation may or may not be identified.

CT scan may be diagnostic in some cases, but arteriography is necessary for final diagnosis and evaluation. It should be mentioned that when an AVM is suspected the computed tomogram should be performed both without and with infusion of contrast material.

INCIDENCE AND LOCATION BY CT SCANNING

The exact incidence of these malformations is unknown because patients may be asymptomatic. In a review of over 10,000 computed tomograms performed over a three-year period, 23 AVMs were identified (Table 12–1). All were subsuquently proved by arteriography. Of these 23 patients with arteriovenous malformations, only six presented with a catastrophic event; three patients had intracerebral hematomas and three had cerebrovascular accidents. The remainder had presenting complaints similar to those mentioned above, i.e., syncopal attacks, dizziness or adult onset of grand mal seizures (see Table 12–3). The low incidence of hemorrhage in this series probably can be attributed to the fact that the computed tomogram represents a noninvasive diagnostic procedure that can be performed in minimally symptomatic patients without the dangers inherent in invasive procedures. With CT, more of the relatively asymptomatic or minimally symptomatic patients with previously unsuspected AVMs are diagnosed. In our series, seven patients had normal preinfusion CT scans (Table 12–2). In

TABLE 12–1 23 ARTERIOVENOUS MALFORMATIONS — PRESENTING SYMPTOMS

Seizures	
Generalized	6
Focal	2
"CVA" (3 hemorrhages)	6
Transient ischemic attack	1
Syncope	1
Visual hallucinations	1
Miscellaneous	5
Asymptomatic (calcifications on skull film)	1

TABLE 12–2 FINDINGS PREINFUSION

Shift or mass effect	Definite	4
	Equivocal	3
Calcification		5
Hemorrhage		3
Focal atrophy		1
Increased density		6
Decreased density		12
Hydrocephalus		2
Normal preinfusion		7

TABLE 12–4 23 ARTERIOVENOUS MALFORMATIONS

	Right	*Left*
Parietal	5	6
Basal ganglia	4	2
Frontal	1	3
Occipital	2	0
Tentorial	0	1

this group of seven patients, the symptoms were similar to those of any other group of patients sent for study (see Table 12–3).

Table 12–4 shows the anatomic positions of the 23 malformations. It is interesting to note that, in spite of the fact that the parietal lobe is the smallest lobe anatomically, most of the malformations were located predominantly in the parietal lobe.

RADIONUCLIDE STUDIES

Although the subject is beyond the scope of this text, it should be mentioned that radionuclide scanning is very helpful in the diagnosis of arteriovenous malformations. The radionuclide scan is positive in a large percentage of these cases and classically reveals a pattern of early blush on the arteriogram phase of the radionuclide scan followed by rapid wash-out of the radionuclide on subsequent films.

The computed tomogram has proved to be very helpful in the diagnosis of these abnormalities and is positive in a high percentage of cases. It is, however, entirely possible that a small, superficially placed cortical AVM could be missed by the CT scan because of the partial volume phenomenon with the adjacent inner table of the bony calvaria. Therefore, a normal CT scan does not rule out the presence of AVM with absolute assurance. It would appear, however, that if both the radionuclide scan and the CT scan are normal the patient is very unlikely to have an arteriovenous malformation.

TABLE 12–3 CLINICAL SYMPTOMS OF THE 7 PATIENTS WITH NORMAL PREINFUSION SCANS

Seizures	2
"CVA"	2
Visual hallucination	1
Transient ischemic attack	1
Asymptomatic (calcifications seen on skull film)	1

ARTERIOGRAPHY

Because of an increased incidence of aneurysms in patients with AVMs, it is advantageous to study these abnormalities by the femoral approach, using selective catheterization of all the great vessels arising from the arch. At the time of fluoroscopy for catheter placement, the carotid and/or vertebral vessels may be noted to be far larger than normal.

The amount of blood flow through the malformation usually far exceeds normal; therefore, an increase in the amount of contrast material injected may be necessary for adequate evaluation. In addition, the arteriovenous circulation time is frequently very rapid, necessitating a more rapid filming technique than ordinarily is used. Instead of the routine two films per second for the first three seconds, it may be necessary to increase this to four or even six films per second for the first three seconds in order to evaluate arterial feeding and venous drainage. This, of course, must be varied for each case. The timing becomes most important when one is attempting to outline the arterial supply and the venous drainage in order to facilitate surgical intervention. In many cases it is also necessary to perform multiple vessel studies to evaluate all the feeding vessels. This serves a dual purpose of ruling out the presence of an aneurysm. It should be noted that malformations in the parietal lobe may feed from the middle cerebral artery on the ipsilateral side while stealing blood from the contralateral side. In these cases, the cross-over from the other side results in a "steal phenomenon" from the contralateral hemisphere; indeed, these patients may become symptomatic from the relatively anemic hemisphere contralateral to the malformation. We have seen one case where the CT scan revealed apparent atrophy with enlargement of the cortical sulci on the side contralateral to the malformation, angiography revealed that there was evidence of a "steal" from the atrophic hemisphere.

The diagnostic and frequently pathognomonic arteriographic criteria include enlarged feeding arteries, the malformation itself — which appears as a tangle of blood vessels ("bag of worms") — and early draining veins (see Figs. 12–1 and 12–2). The mass is typically non–space-occupying, except in those cases where hemorrhage has occurred. The malformation may be relatively small, and often is obscured by overlying large feeding arteries and draining veins.

Arteriovenous malformations often first become symptomatic at the time of hemorrhage. The hemorrhage is readily diagnosed by CT scanning, which reveals an area of increased density of variable size that measures between 45 and 90 Hounsfied units. If the hemorrhage is acute there will be no change in the density following infusion of contrast material. An unusual position of the hemorrhage should raise the index of suspicion that the hemorrhage is not hypertensive but may be related to another bleeding source, such as aneurysm or arteriovenous malformation. In those cases, arteriography will be necessary to evaluate the presence of an AVM. Blood in the cerebral tissue or the subarachnoid space is very irritating to the blood vessels; besides the associated intracerebral hematoma, one may also see marked vascular spasm (Fig. 12–5) at arteriography.

In addition, there are occasions of "occult" malformations that hemorrhage, resulting in total obliteration of the precipitating blood vessel abnormality. These appear as areas of hemorrhage on the CT scan and as an avascular mass lesion at arteriography. The true nature of the lesion is discovered only at surgery, when the typical histologic appearance of the malformation is discovered.

Rarely, a very malignant glioblastoma multiforme may simulate the appearance of an arteriovenous malformation. In occasional rare cases of glioblastoma there is enlargement of the feeding arteries and early draining veins, making differentiation from an AVM difficult. It should be remembered, however, that glioblastomas are space-occupying lesions, whereas AVMs, in the absence of hemorrhage, are non–space-occupying.

TREATMENT

Surgical correction of these blood vessel abnormalities can be attempted, but has met with only limited success. Follow-up arteriography often reveals that new feeding channels have opened following closure of the original vessels.

In addition to the surgical treatment, instillation of plastic pellets, gelfoam, muscle or dura into the feeding arteries has been performed in an attempt to obliterate the malformation or to make it more amenable to a surgical approach. When attempting this method, an arteriogram is first performed for baseline evaluation; then repeat arteriography is performed after each successive instillation of single or multiple pellets. "Superselective" catheterization of the vessel to be embolized is desirable. It is also necessary to monitor the patient's clinical neurologic status carefully during this type of procedure. Balloon catheters also have been used to occlude the arteries in order to prevent materials from moving retrograde out of the vessel and being embolized incorrectly.

CAROTID CAVERNOUS FISTULA

An additional malformation sometimes seen is the carotid cavernous fistula. This abnormality implies an abnormal direct communication between the internal carotid artery and the cavernous sinus. Although these carotid cavernous fistulas can develop spontaneously, they are seen most often after severe head trauma — apparently when there is tearing of the internal carotid artery at the level of the cavernous systems. In most cases, this traumatic development of a fistula results in almost immediate symptoms. Rupture of a berry aneurysm at the level of the cavernous portion of the carotid artery also may result in a carotid cavernous fistula with similar findings. The author has seen one case of a spontaneous carotid cavernous fistula in a 23-year-old woman with fibromuscular hyperplasia of the blood vessels.

The clinical findings with a carotid cavernous fistula are a pulsating exopthalmos and an annoying bruit that the patient can hear. The conjunctiva become injected and chemosis may develop. Extraocular muscle palsies and blindness may occur. These changes may be ipsilateral or bilateral; rarely, they involve only the contralateral eye.

Diagnosis is made and/or confirmed at the time of carotid arteriography. The pattern of venous drainage varies from patient to patient, but very commonly involves retrograde filling of the superior ophthalmic vein (Figs. 12–7 and 12–8). This vein may become so greatly distended that it results in erosion and enlargement of the bony margins of the superior orbital fissure (Fig. 12–7). The retrograde flow into the venous system also can go up into the middle cerebral venous system and to the cerebral convexity to drain into the superior sagittal sinus.

As with studies of any other rapid flow system, films should be shot in quick sequence — usually at a rate of four or, preferably, six films per second for the first three seconds. An increased volume of contrast material is also recommended in many cases for better delineation. The rapid filling of the cavernous sinus and, subsequently, of the superior ophthalmic vein becomes readily apparent at the time of the study.

These C-C fistulas frighten and discomfort the patient and are a difficult surgical problem. Ligation of the carotid has met with limited success. Obliteration of the cavernous sinus with a balloon catheter has been successful in some cases.

We have seen one unusual case of a carotid venous fistula that drained primarily into the venous structures of the cerebellopontine angle and posterior fossa (Fig. 12–9). This patient presented with a history of tinnitus in the left ear. The plain films revealed enlargement of the internal auditory canal on the side of the fistula. The carotid venous fistula was discovered during the course of work-up for a cerebellopontine angle tumor.

VEIN OF GALEN ANEURYSM

This arteriovenous malformation is seen in children; it often presents at birth or in the very young age group as high output congestive heart failure. These vein of Galen aneurysms are actually deep-seated AVMs that drain into the vein of Galen and produce enlargement of the vein because of excessive blood flow (Figs. 12–11 and 12–12). This enlargement of the vein of Galen results in obstruction of the aqueduct of Sylvius and the outlet of the third ventricle and consequently in obstructive hydrocephalus. In these cases, "aneurysm of the vein of Galen" is actually a misnomer, but it has become deeply entrenched in our terminology. These AVMs usually are fed by the posterior cerebral arteries. The surgical approach may be very difficult, and the prognosis for these patients is usually very poor.

DURAL ARTERIOVENOUS MALFORMATIONS

Malformations that involve the dural covering of the brain (Fig. 12–6) also may be seen. These dural malformations are fed by the meningeal vessels, and are similar histologically to other malformations. When dural malformations involve the tentorium, arteriography should include study of the carotid arteries in an attempt to visualize an enlarged tentorial artery where it arises from the internal carotid artery at its entrance into the cavernous sinus and proceeds to the free edge of the tentorium. As noted in Chapter 9, enlargement of this vessel is also seen in tentorial meningiomas. Visualization of these vessels helps the surgeon to plan an operative approach.

SCALP ARTERIOVENOUS MALFORMATIONS

Arteriovenous malformations of the scalp may be congenital or may develop secondary to trauma (Fig. 12–16). These malformations also may develop following craniotomy. In acquired lesions, one usually can obtain a history of injury, following which a compressible soft tissue mass developed and large draining vessels became visible over the cranial vault. The arteriographic appearance is quite typical, with feeding vessels from the external carotid and enlarged draining veins. Occasionally these scalp malformations can reach a spectacular size (Fig. 12–16). In smaller malformations, bright-lighting the soft tissues over the cranial vault will help to differentiate the supplying and draining vessels from intracranial vessels.

Of course, selective internal and external carotid injections with filming in the AP and lateral projections will serve to outline the vascular pattern most accurately. Direct puncture and injection of the scalp malformation has been suggested, but would seem less desirable than selective internal and external carotid injection.

SPINAL CORD ARTERIOVENOUS MALFORMATIONS

Arteriovenous malformations of the spinal cord do occur (see Chapter 17). The malformation itself usually is small and is drained by multiple enlarged veins that are visible on the dorsal aspect of the cord. They most frequently are supplied by the artery of Adamkewicz, which arises from one of the intercostal vessels of the lower thoracic or upper lumbar aorta, but most frequently at the D_{12} level on the left side. Selective catheterization and injection of this vessel will outline the malformation and the draining veins. Care must be taken that the artery is not occluded by the catheter, as this may lead to paralysis of the lower extremities. Paralysis also may occur secondary to a toxic reaction to the contrast material.

It may be necessary to catheterize each of the intercostal vessels in turn. Magnification and subtraction techniques also should be used. Meticulous care should be taken during injection of these vessels to prevent untoward reactions.

Flush aortography is also useful to outline any enlarged vascular supply that may be present. Spinal arteriography is a time-consuming procedure and sometimes is difficult for both the patient and the physician.

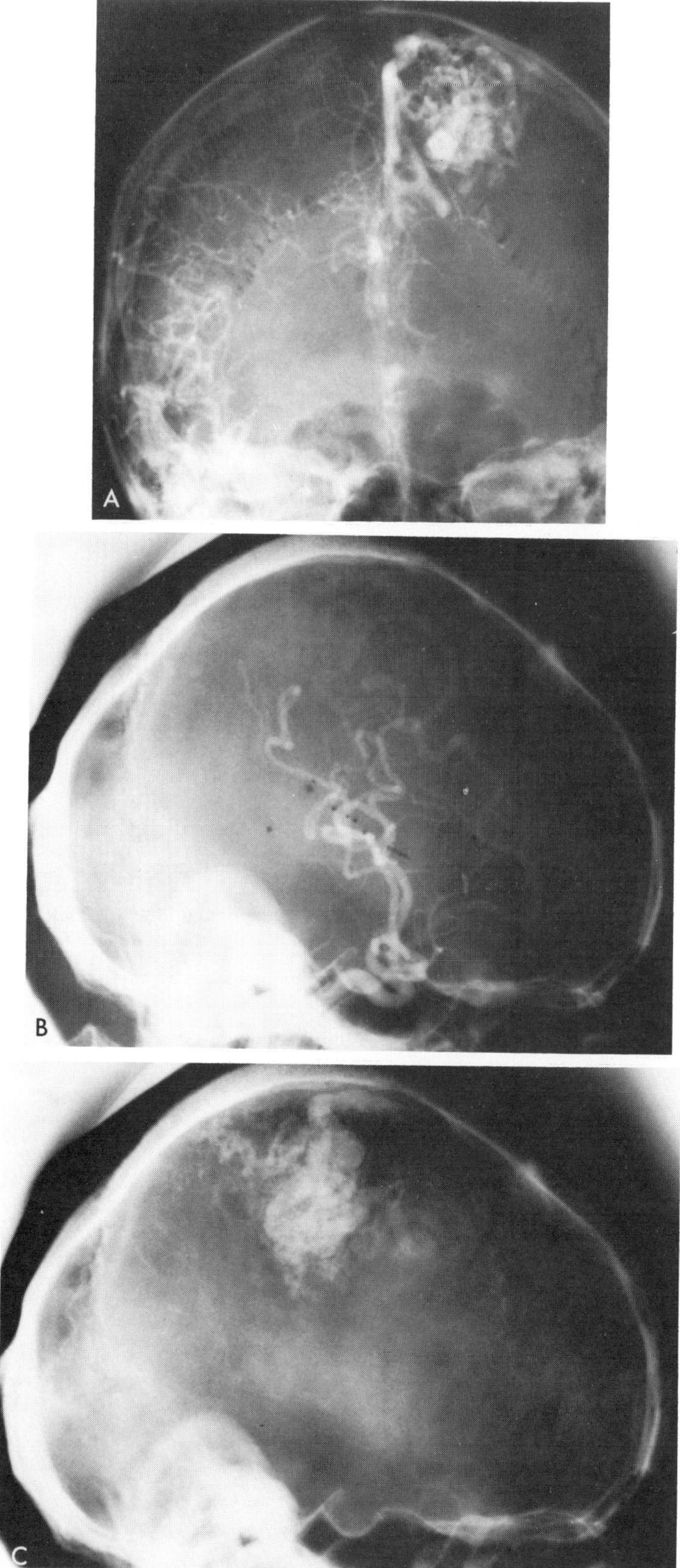

Figure 12–1 *See legend on the opposite page*

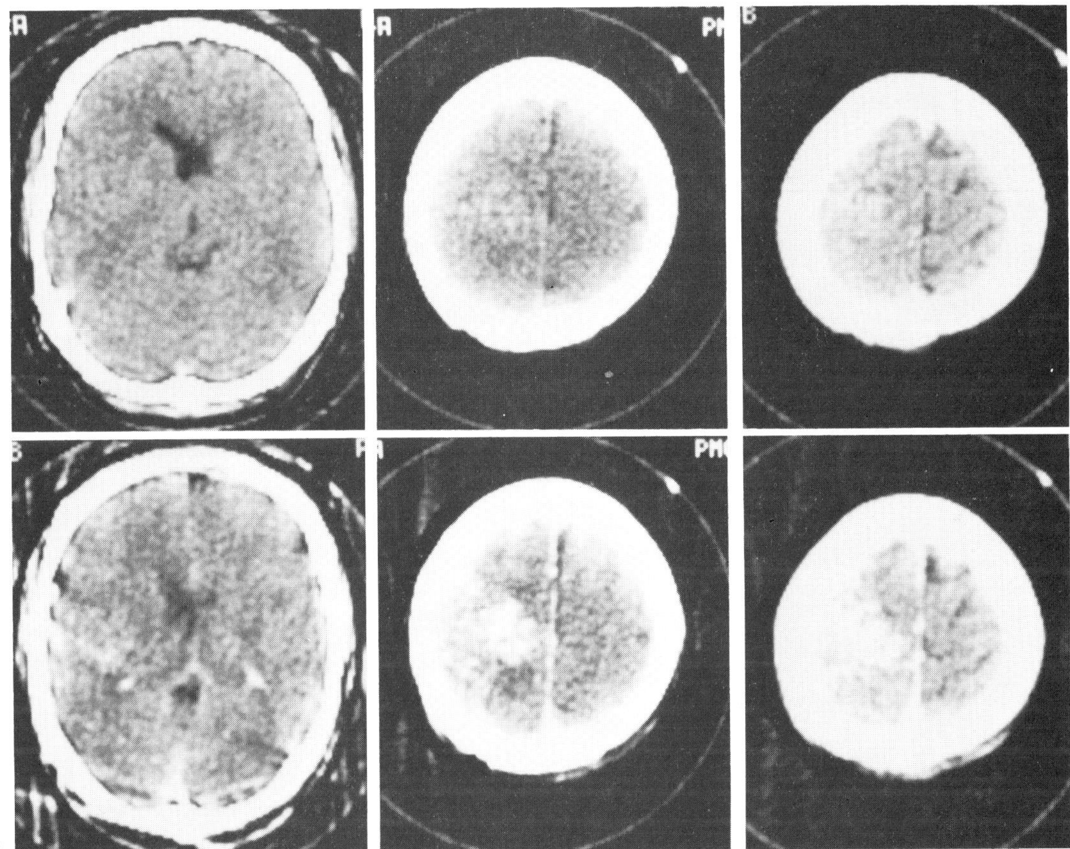

Figure 12–1. This patient presented with a history of the adult onset of seizures. *A*, The left parietal malformation fills from the anterior cerebral arteries on both the right and the left sides. The malformation acts in the same way as an intentional "cross compression," drawing the opacified blood over from the right carotid arteriogram to fill the left parietal malformation from the left anterior cerebral artery.

B and *C*, The early and late arterial phases of the left carotid arteriogram reveal enlarged feeding arteries from the middle cerebral artery on the left side; the malformation itself; and the early draining veins, which drain to the superior sagittal sinus.

D, The CT scan reveals asymmetry of the frontal horns of the lateral ventricles with enlargement of the left frontal horn — possibly secondary to slight atrophy on the left side. A faint increase in the left parietal region on the preinfusion scan enhances postinfusion in the "bag-of-worms" fashion seen frequently in arteriovenous malformations. Note that there appears to be enlargement of the cortical sulci on the right side, contralateral to the malformation. This cortical atrophy is perhaps secondary to "stealing" of the blood supply to the contralateral hemisphere.

Note the absence of shift of the midline structures on both the arteriogram and CT scan. This absence of mass effect is very typical of arteriovenous malformations.

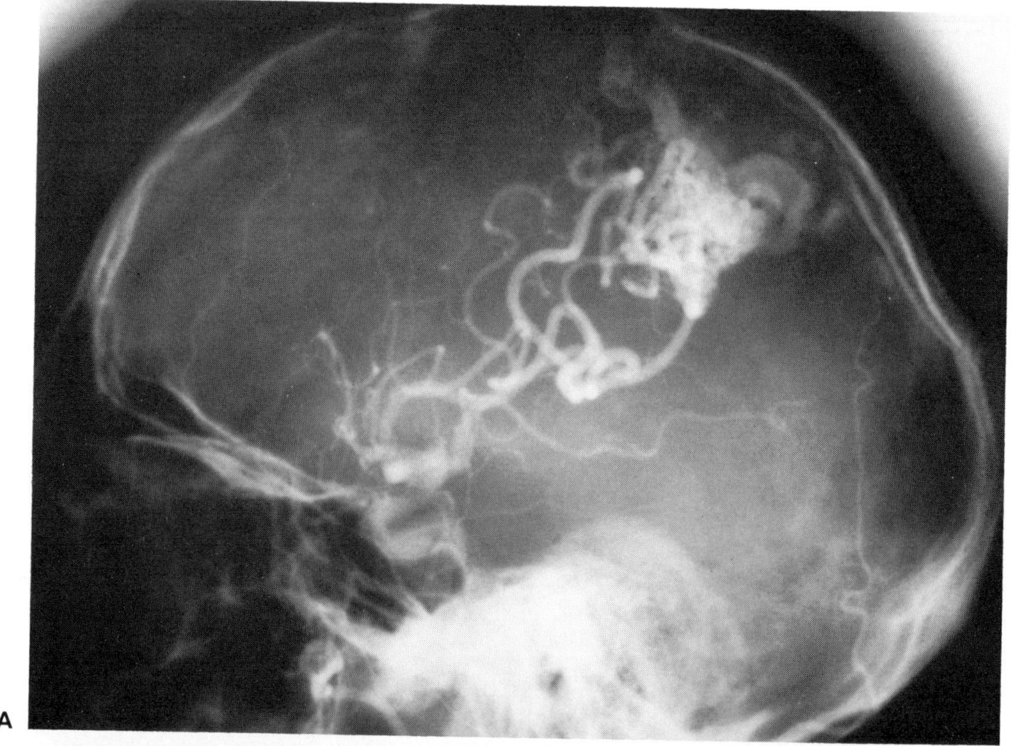

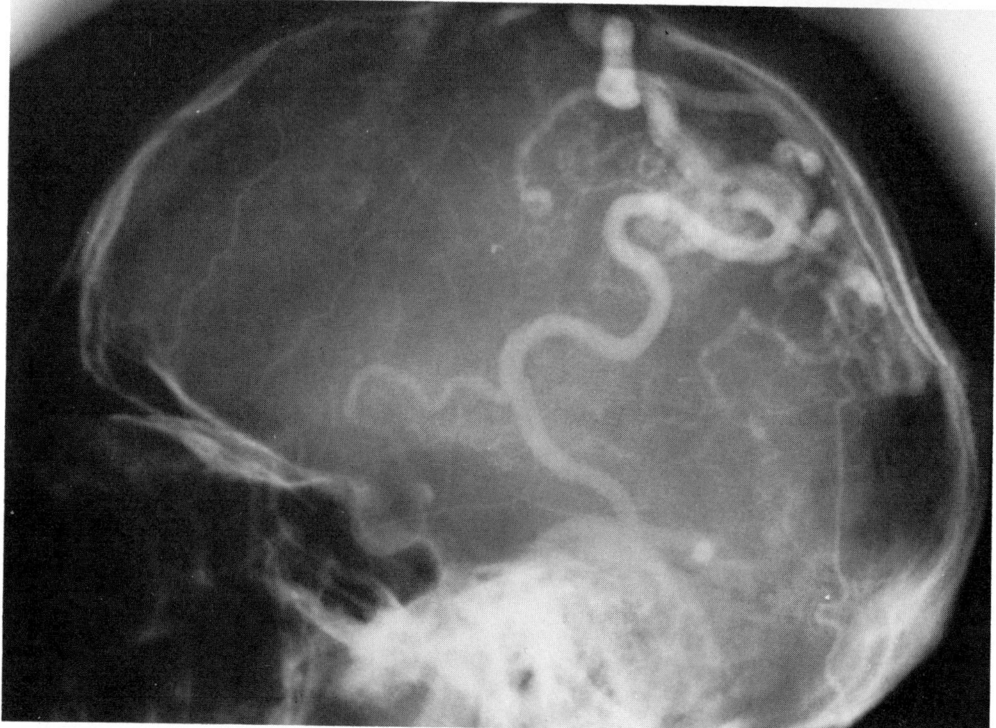

Figure 12–2 *See legend on the opposite page*

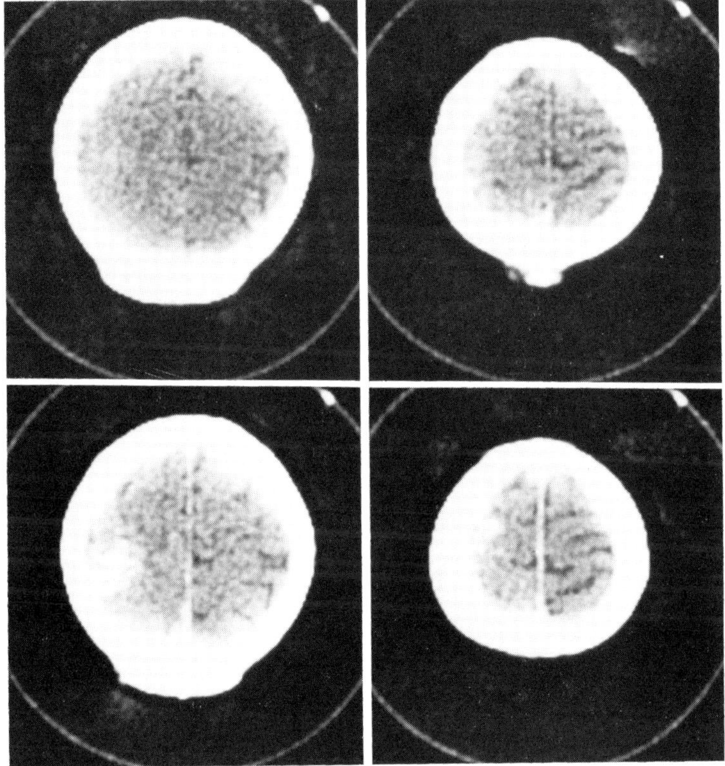

Figure 12–2. This is a "classic" case of a left parietal malformation fed by enlarged feeding vessels of the left middle cerebral artery (*A*) and drained by multiple early draining veins (*B*). Note that the veins drain to both the superior sagittal sinus and to the other cortical veins, which drain inferiorly to the transverse sinus and the region of the middle cerebral vein.

C, The CT scan reveals a faint area of increased density in the left parietal region, which enhances in the "bag-of-worms" appearance typical of AVMs. Note the enlargement of the cortical sulci in the contralateral hemisphere — perhaps secondary to "steal" from the contralateral hemisphere by the malformations. There is no shift of the midline structures.

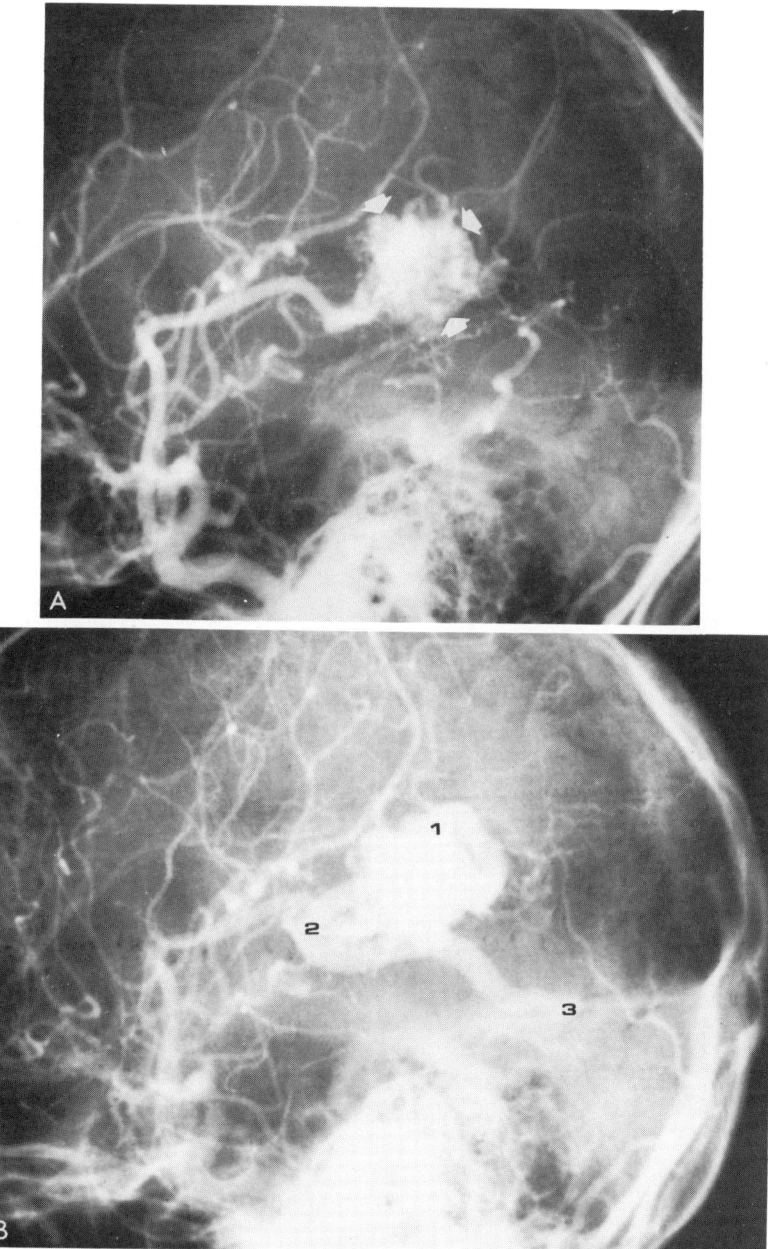

Figure 12–3. This 11-year-old boy presented with a history of flashing lights in the right visual field. *A* and *B,* The arteriograms reveal an arteriovenous malformation (*white arrows*) in the posterior temporal parietal region on the left side. It is fed by one enlarged vessel from the middle cerebral artery and drains into the enlarged vein of Labbé.

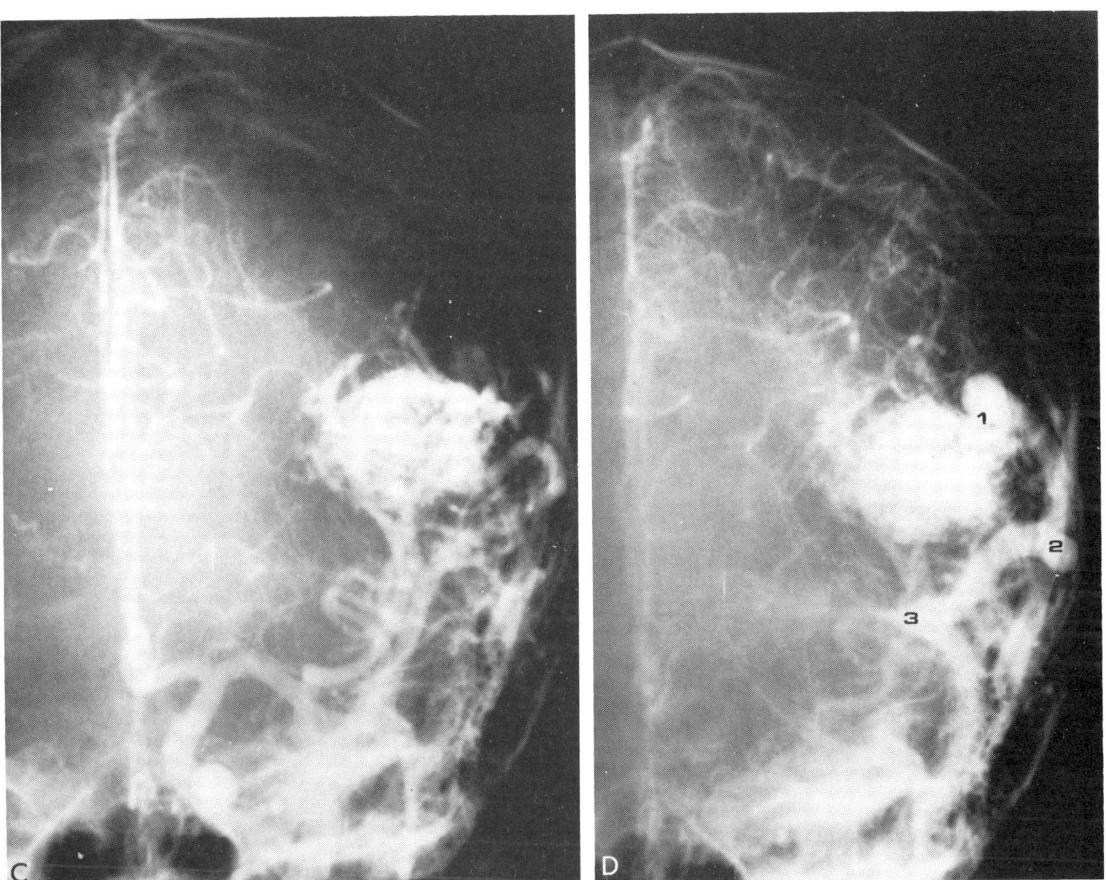

Figure 12–3 *Continued.*

C and *D*, The anteroposterior views demonstrate the malformation and the enlarged vein of Labbé. The vein of Labbé is marked (*1*) at its origin in the malformation; this correlates with the lateral view (*B*), which is marked in a corresponding fashion. (*3*) is the point of entrance of the vein of Labbé into the transverse sinus. The transverse sinus then drains into the sigmoid sinus and ultimately into the internal jugular vein.

Illustration continued on the following page

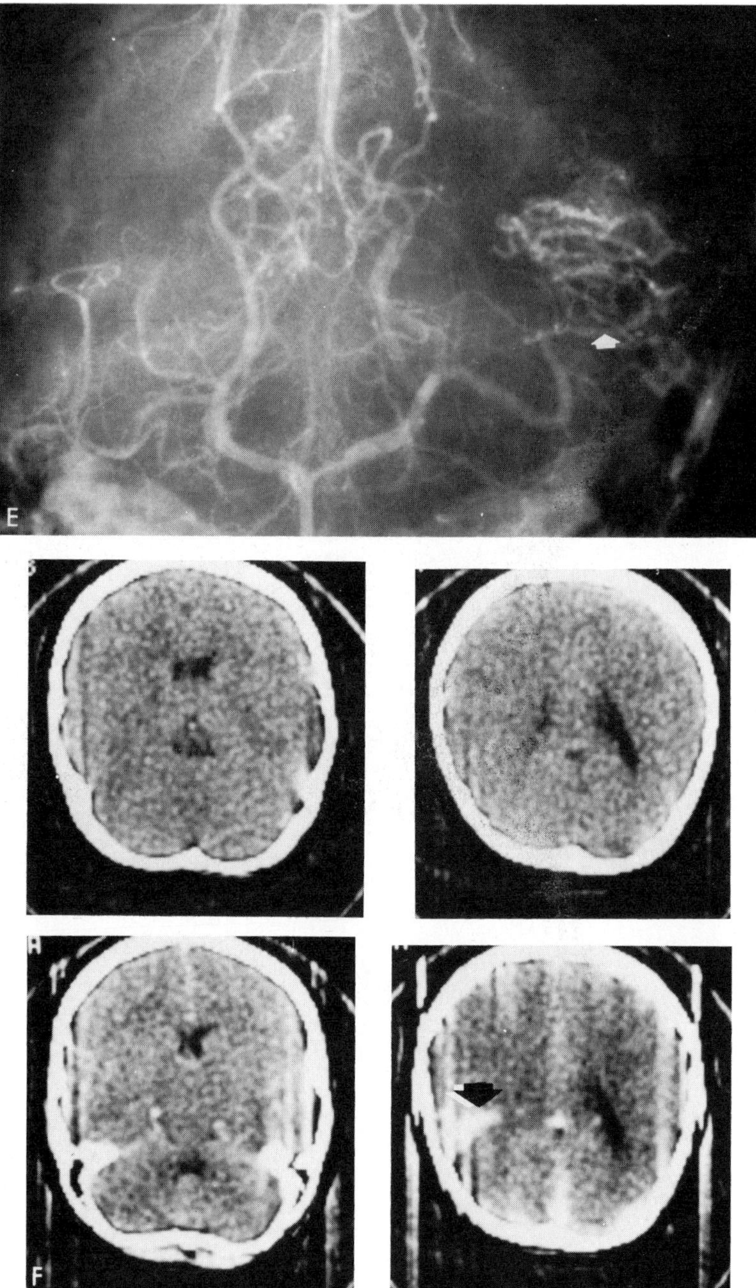

Figure 12–3 *Continued*

E, A small portion of the malformation was seen to fill from the posterior temporal branch of the left posterior cerebral artery *(white arrow).*

F, The preinfusion CT scan is essentially normal; a wedge-shaped area of enhancement is noted on the postinfusion scan (*arrow*). Care must be taken not to confuse the wedge of enhancement with the petrous pyramid on the left side.

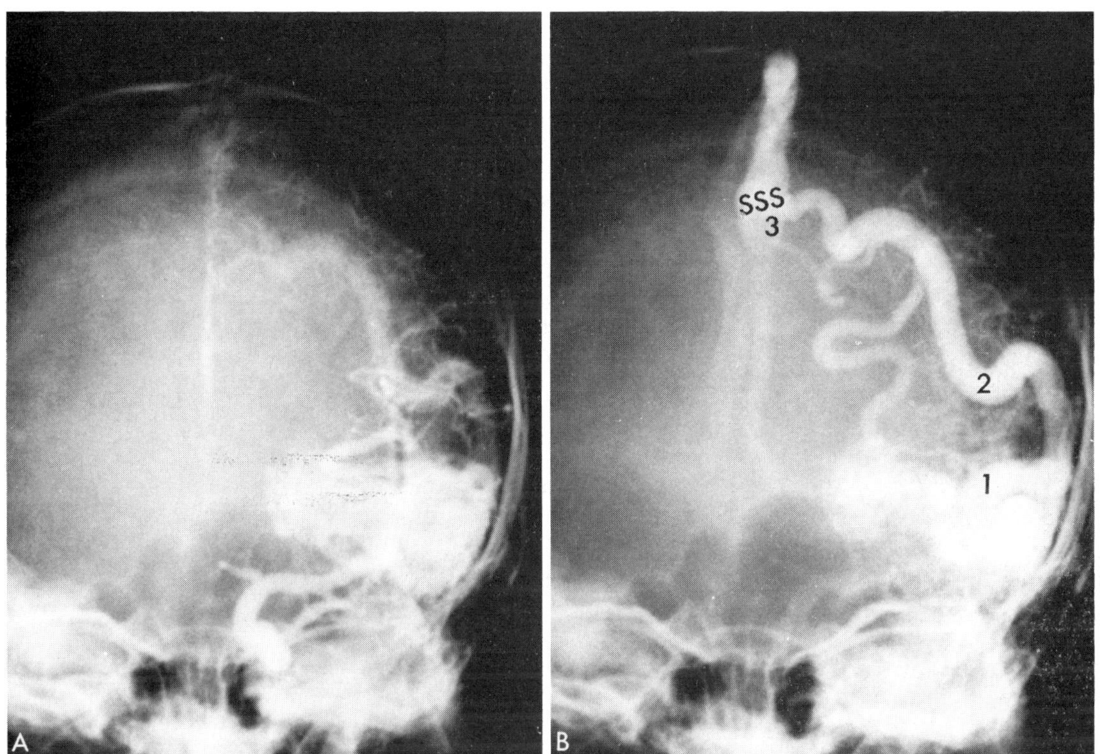

Figure 12–4. This 11-year-old presented with a history of one grand mal seizure. The anteroposterior view (A) of the left carotid arteriogram reveals filling only of the left middle cerebral artery, which is seen on both this and the lateral (C) view to have one large middle cerebral artery feeder to the deep frontal malformation. The anterior cerebral artery does not fill because the malformation is "pulling" unopacified blood from the right side to the left hemisphere. Multiple large draining veins are noted to drain into the superior sagittal sinus as well as inferiorly into the region of the cavernous sinus (*B* and *D*). Corresponding points are labeled on the anteroposterior and lateral views of the large draining vein which drains to the superior sagittal sinus. (1) is the point of origin, (2) is one of the large curves of the vein over the cortex of the brain and (3) is the point that the vein enters into the superior sagittal sinus (*sss*).

A small medial portion of the malformation was demonstrated to fill from the right carotid arteriogram.

E, The preinfusion scan reveals a poorly defined area of increased density deep in the left frontal lobe region. This enhances on the postinfusion scan in an irregular, nearly wedge-shaped pattern that is broad-based superficially. Again, note the lack of midline shift.

Illustration continued on the following page

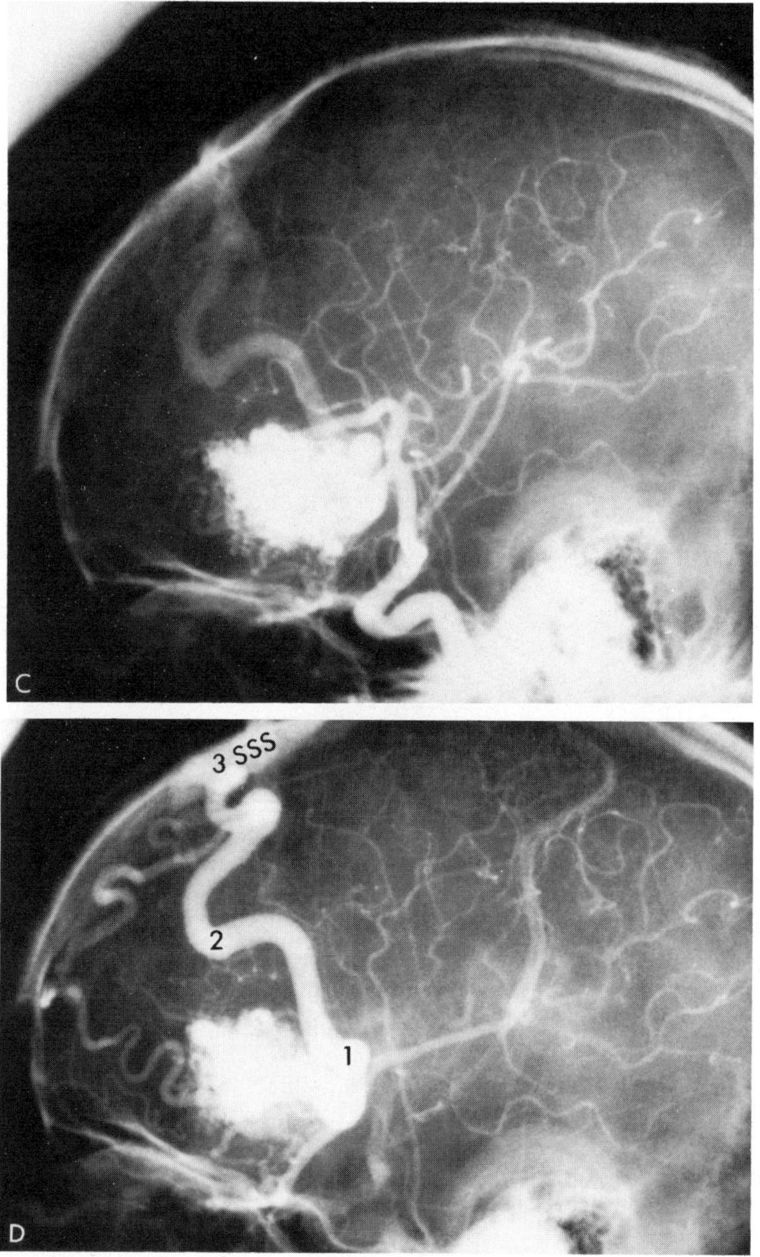

Figure 12–4 *Continued*

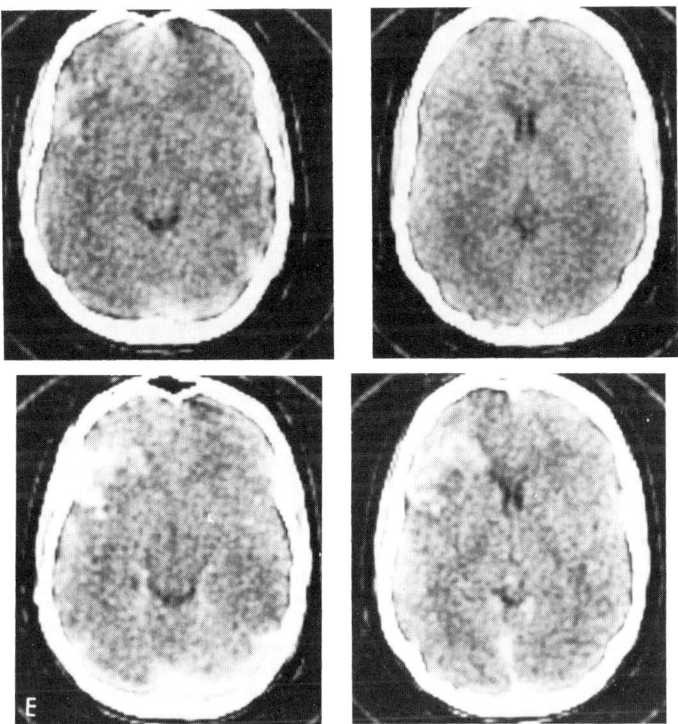

Figure 12–4 *Continued*

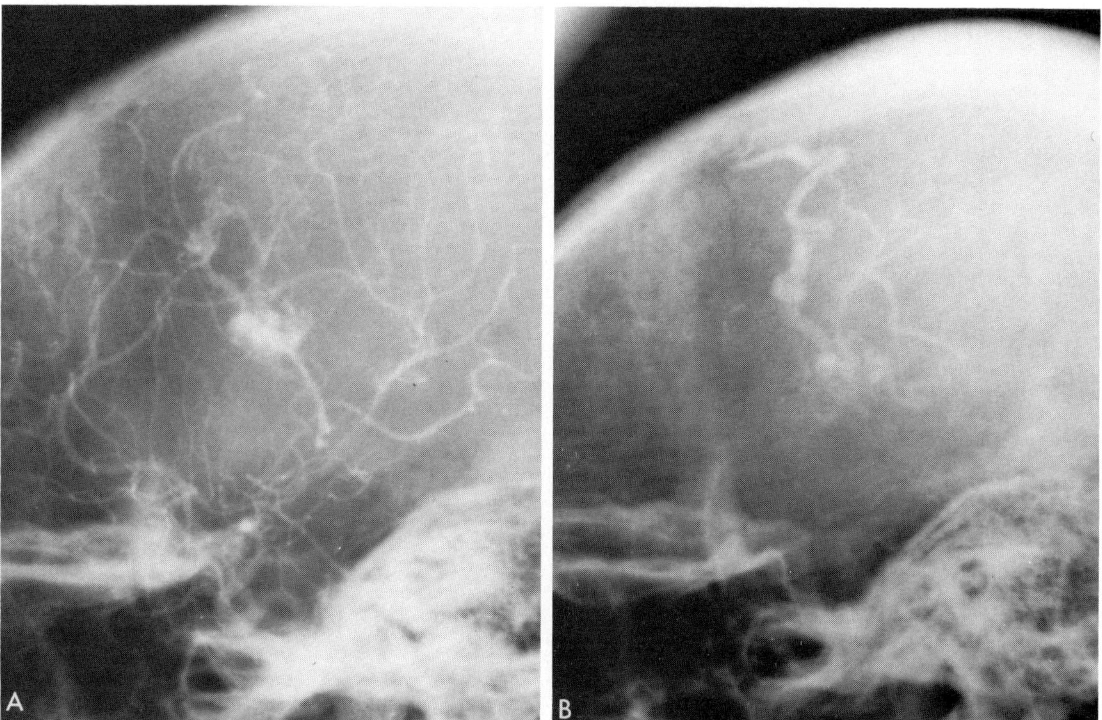

Figure 12–5. This 36-year-old woman presented with a sudden onset of unconsciousness and a left hemiparesis. *A* and *B*, The arterial and capillary phases of the arteriogram reveal a small arteriovenous malformation just above the midportion of the sylvian triangle. The malformation is supplied by one moderate sized middle cerebral artery vessel and drained by several cortical veins. It is surrounded by an avascular area, resulting in stretching of the opercular branches of the middle cerebral artery and downward placement of the sylvian triangle. These findings are consistent with an AVM that is surrounded by an area of hemorrhage. In addition, the vessels exhibit diffuse narrowing secondary to arterial spasm because of irritation by the adjacent blood.

C, The AP view reveals shift of the anterior cerebral artery to the contralateral side and medial displacement of the sylvian point (*arrow*).

D, The postoperative arteriogram shows that the malformation has been obliterated. The branches of the middle cerebral artery have returned to a more normal caliber, and there is less stretching of the opercular branches of the middle cerebral artery because the hematoma has been evacuated. Some downward displacement of the midportion of the sylvian triangle remains *(arrows)*.

E, The CT scan reveals a small intracerebral hematoma adjacent to the cortex on the right side. There is shift from right to left. There was no change following the infusion of contrast material.

An arteriogram was performed because the hematoma was not in the anticipated position of a hypertensive hemorrhage. This revealed the arteriovenous malformation.

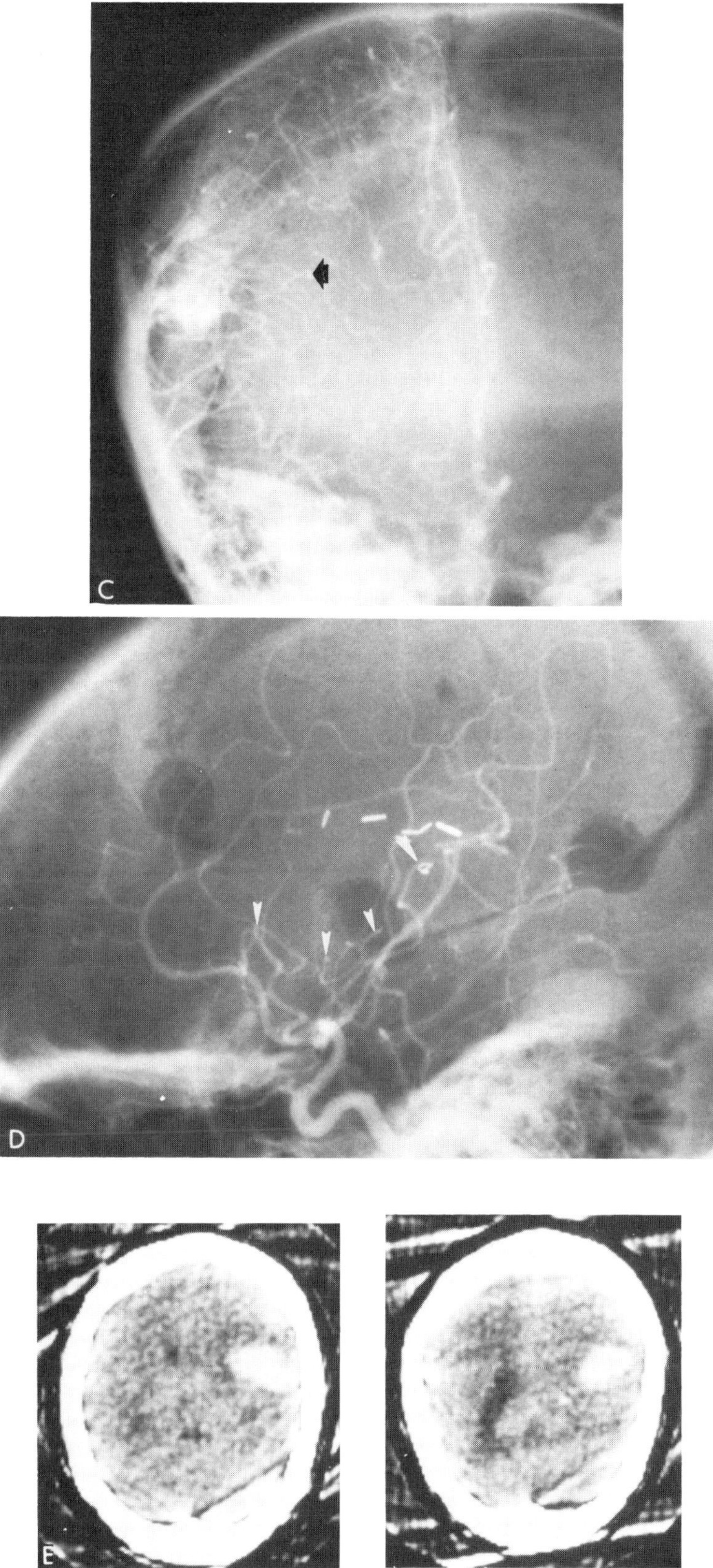

Figure 12–5 *Continued*

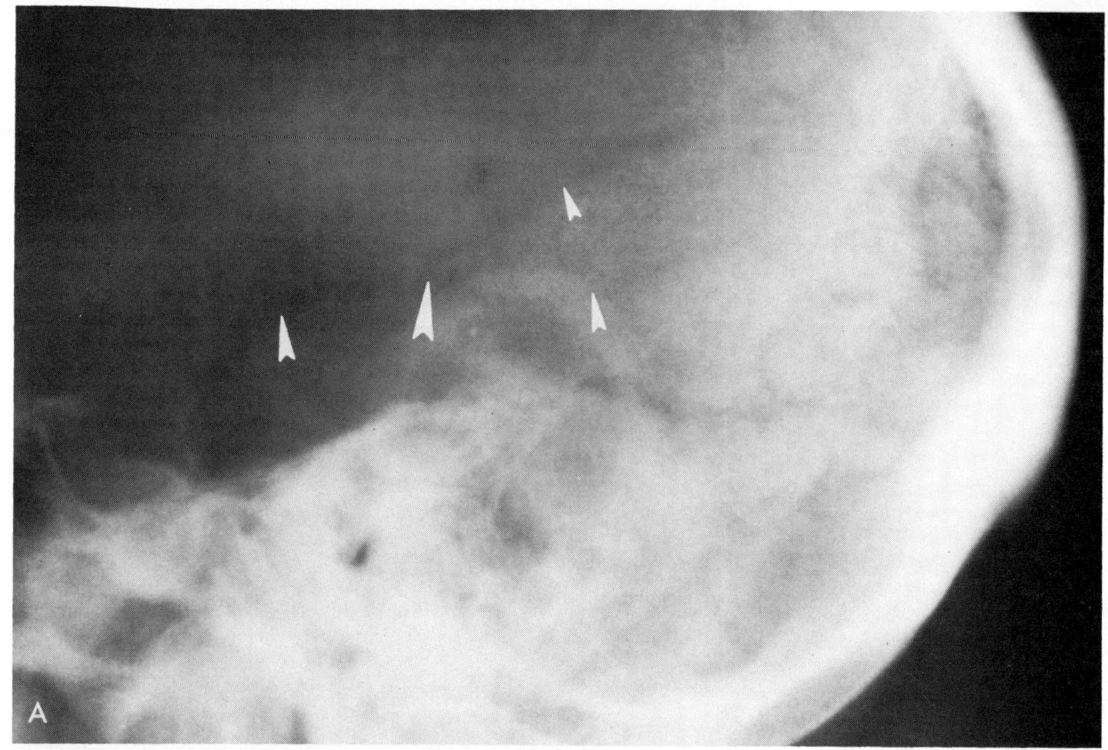

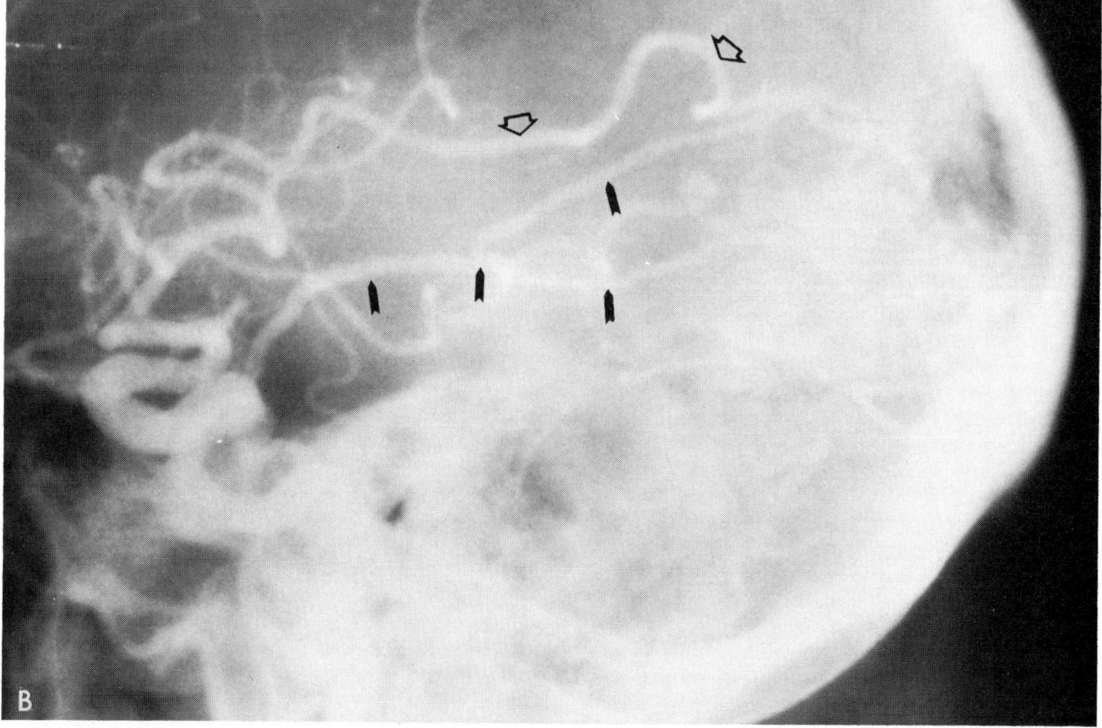

Figure 12–6. TENTORIAL ARTERIOVENOUS MALFORMATION: *A*, The plain skull films reveal enlarged vascular grooves that carry the enlarged branches of the posterior meningeal artery (*white arrows*) as they course posteriorly to supply the tentorial malformation.

B, The left carotid arteriogram shows the branches of the meningeal artery (*black arrows*) as they lie in the vascular grooves noted on the skull film. In addition, an enlarged branch of the left middle cerebral artery (*open arrows*) is also noted to supply the malformation.

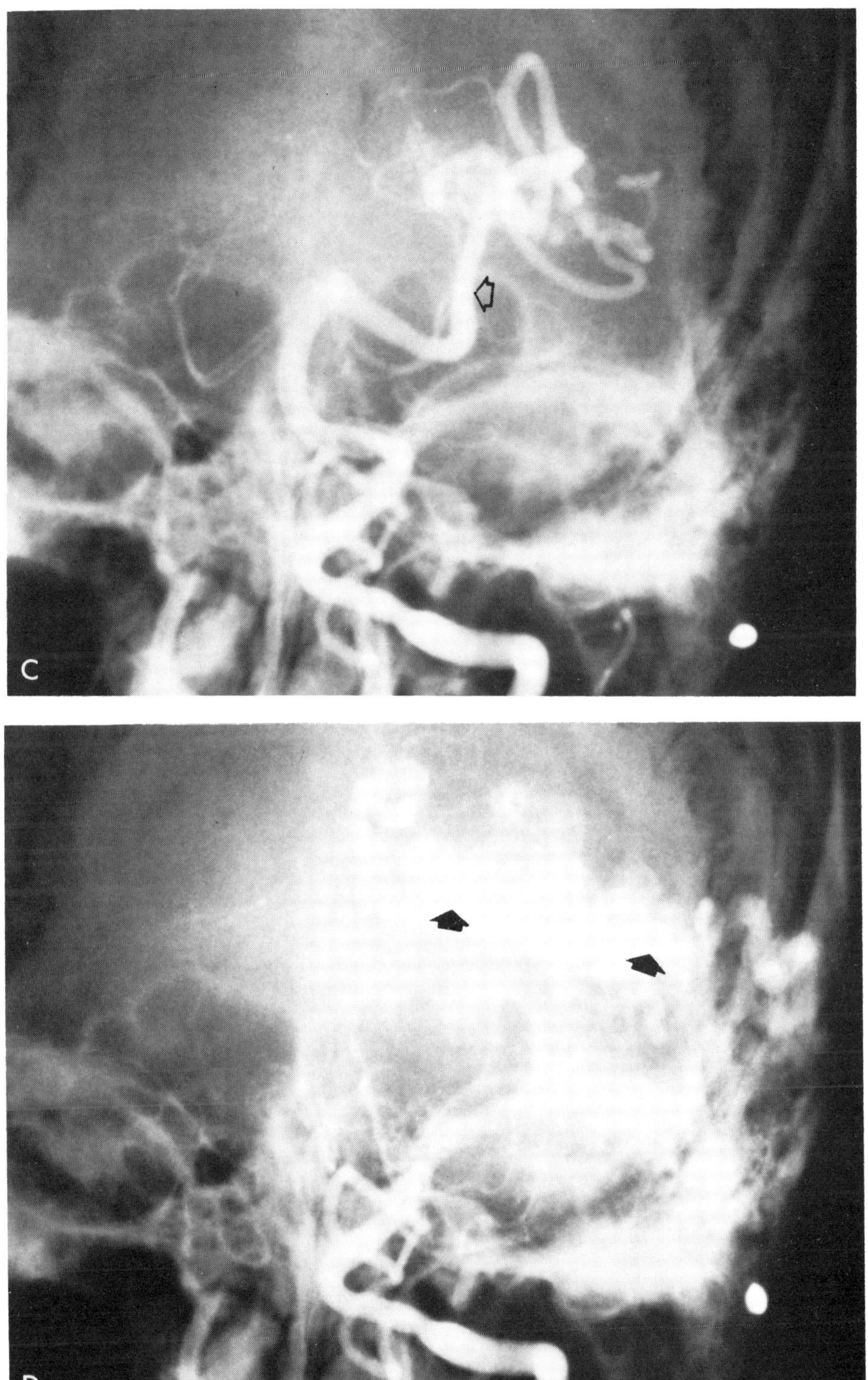

Figure 12–6 *Continued*

C, The left vertebral arteriogram reveals an enlarged left posterior cerebral artery (*open arrow*) that courses posteriorly to supply the malformation.

D, A later arterial film of the left vertebral arteriogram shows a large tangle of vessels resting on top of the tentorium cerebelli and extending from the midline to the region of the sigmoid sinus (*black arrows*).

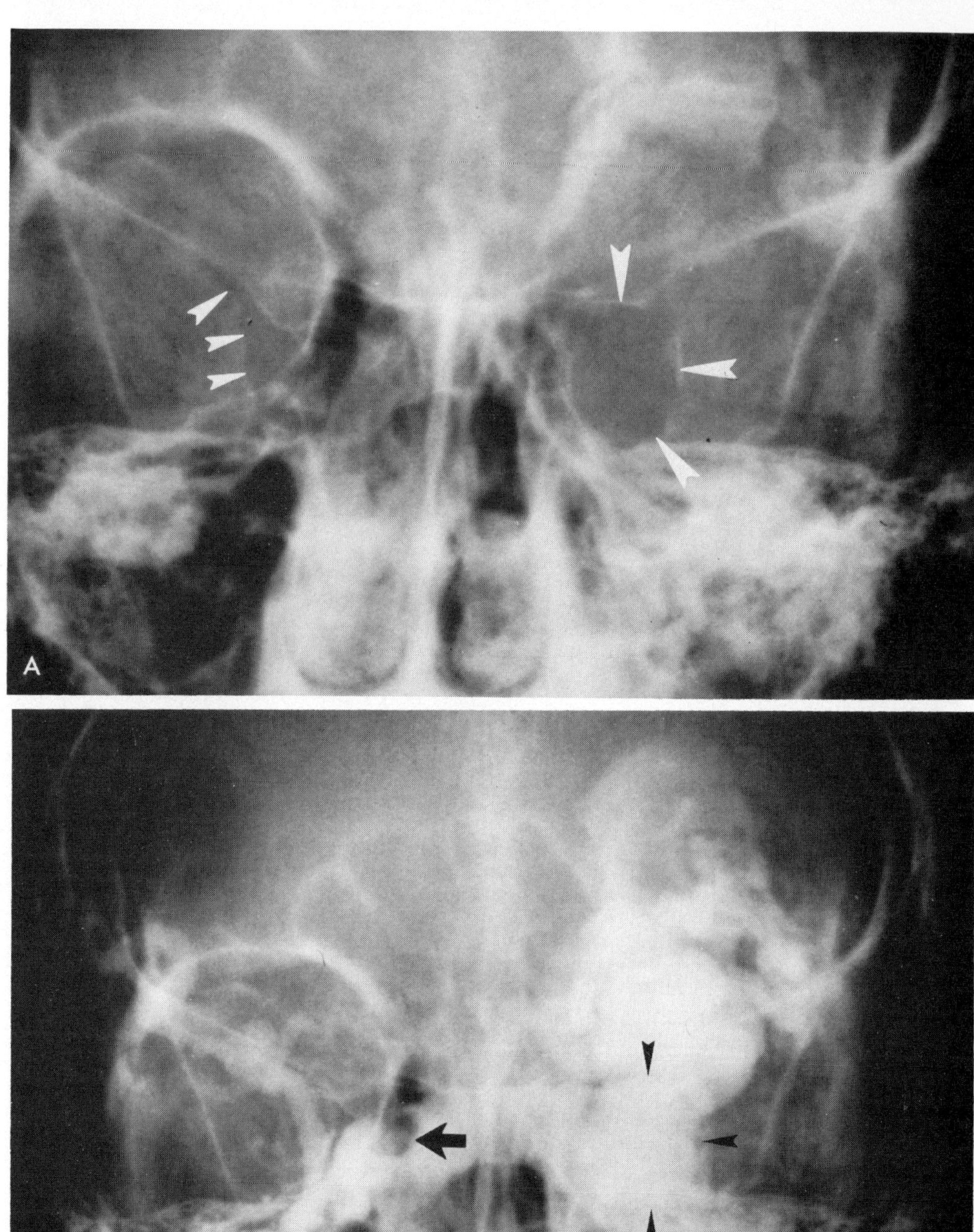

Figure 12–7. CAROTID CAVERNOUS FISTULA: *A,* The plain film reveals marked pressure erosion and enlargement of the superior orbital fissure on the left side. The erosion is secondary to the pressure of the markedly enlarged superior ophthalmic vein (*large white arrows*). The normal superior orbital fissure is demonstrated on the right side (*small arrows*).

B, The left carotid arteriogram reveals the rapid shunting of the blood into the venous system. The markedly enlarged superior ophthalmic vein is marked by the small black arrows. The cavernous sinus is filled and extends in a curvilinear fashion to the opposite side, where the right internal carotid artery is demonstrated (*large black arrow*) as a negative shadow in the contrast-filled cavernous sinus. The right internal carotid artery is visualized because it is filled with unopacified blood.

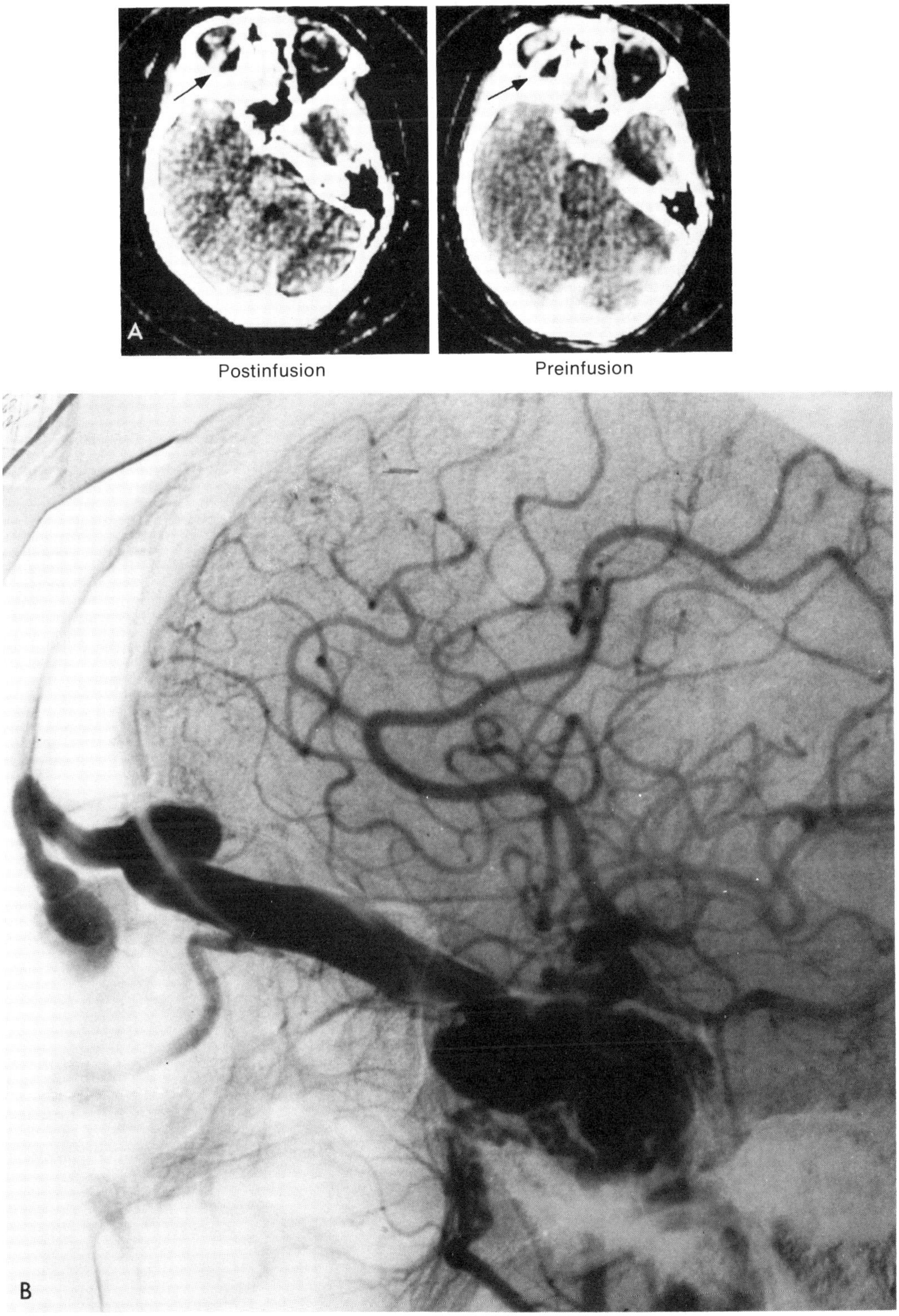

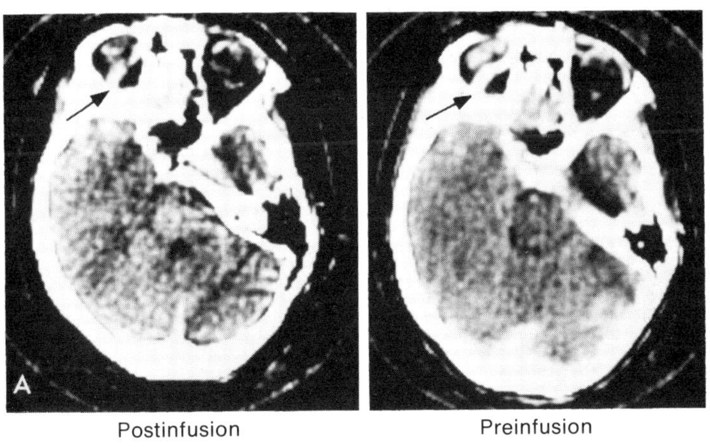

Figure 12–8. CAROTID CAVERNOUS FISTULA: *A*, The CT scan of the orbit reveals exophthalmos on the left side. In addition, a dense curvilinear structure extends obliquely across the upper portion of the orbit on the left (*small arrow*). After the infusion of contrast, this structure enhances greatly. It was shown to be the dilated superior ophthalmic vein on the left carotid arteriogram.

B, The left carotid arteriogram shows a carotid cavernous fistula with retrograde flow into the greatly enlarged superior ophthalmic vein on the left side. It is the superior ophthalmic vein that is demonstrated on the CT scan.

Figure 12–9. CAROTID VENOUS FISTULA: *A*, The left carotid arteriogram reveals a large carotid artery in the cervical portion of the carotid artery and immediate filling of the venous plexus at the base of the skull. In addition, there is marked engorgement of the petrosal sinus and the tributary veins of the posterior fossa.

B, The AP view demonstrates the marked enlargement of the veins of the posterior fossa, filling of the petrosal veins on the contralateral side and filling of enlarged veins that drain into the vein of Galen and the straight sinus (*arrows*).

C, The preinfusion scans, levels 1B and 2A, reveal areas of increased density that appear to be intimately related to the petrous bone. On the 2A cut the area of increased density appears to be well rounded and to contain a small punctate area of increased density. This well defined area of increased density is consistent with the dilated veins seen on the arteriogram. The postinfusion scan (8B) reveals marked enhancement of these structures, including the dilated veins in the parasellar area (*arrow*).

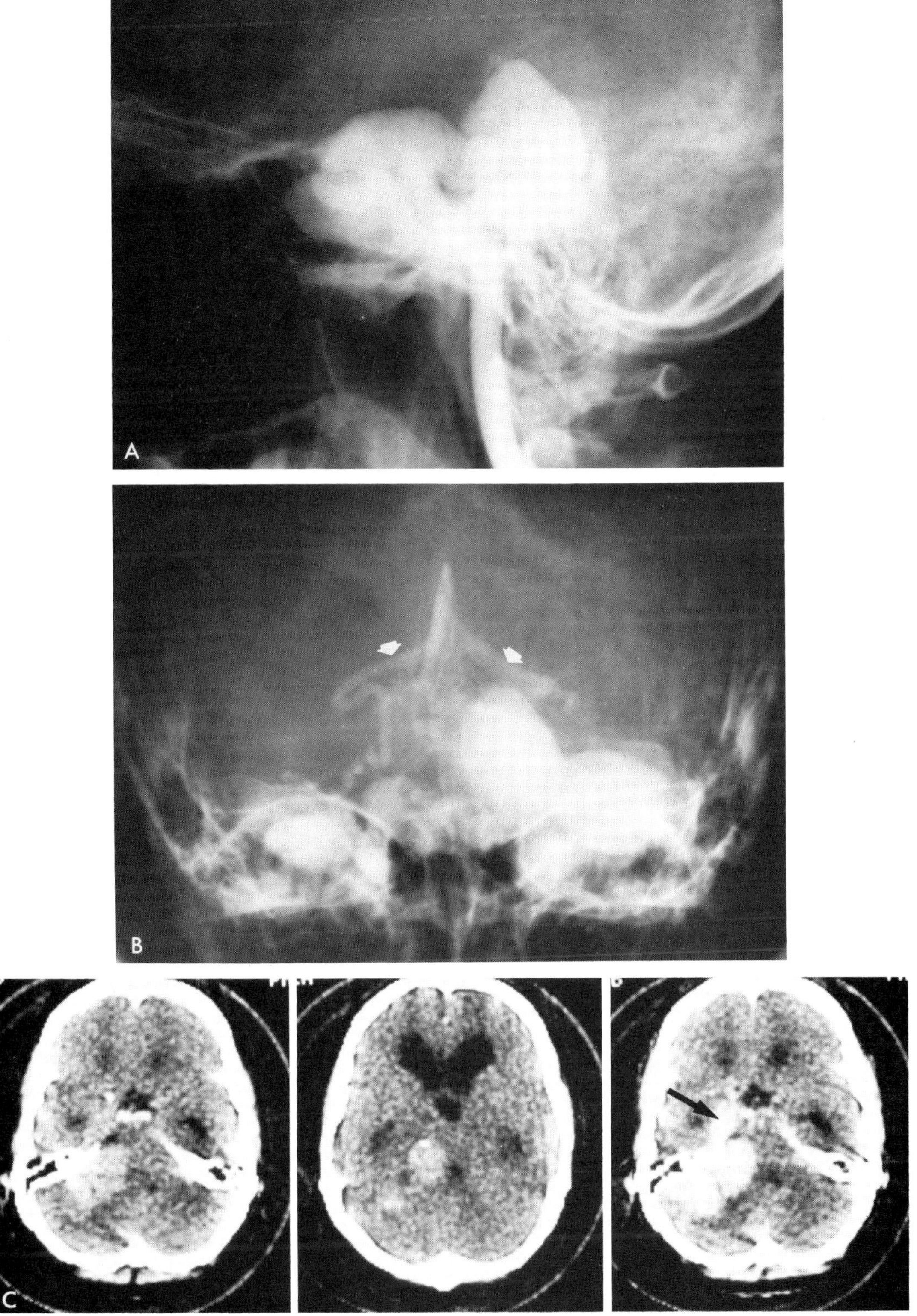

Figure 12–9. *See legend on the opposite page*

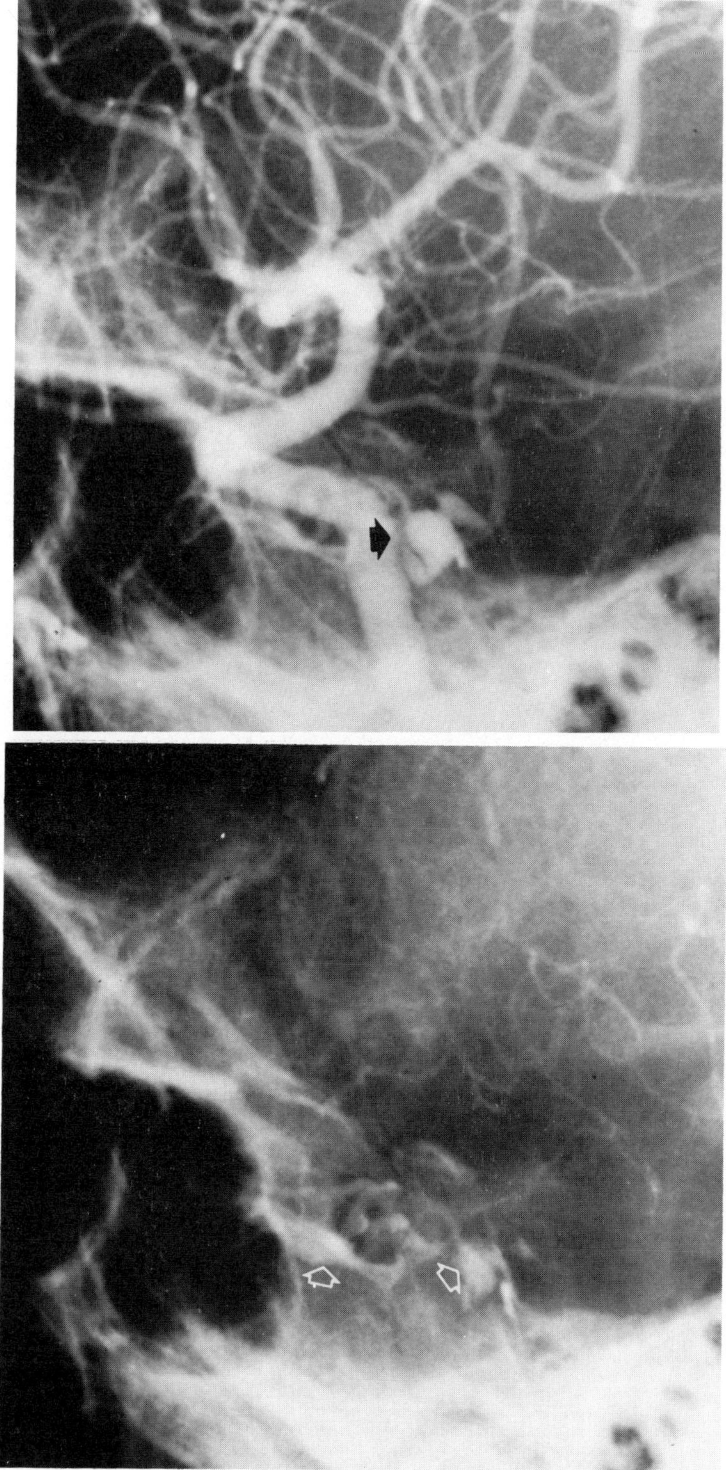

Figure 12–10. CAROTID CAVERNOUS FISTULA: The right carotid arteriogram reveals a tiny fistulous communication (*arrows*) with the veins at the base of the brain. This type of fistula is relatively easy to diagnose but difficult to treat.

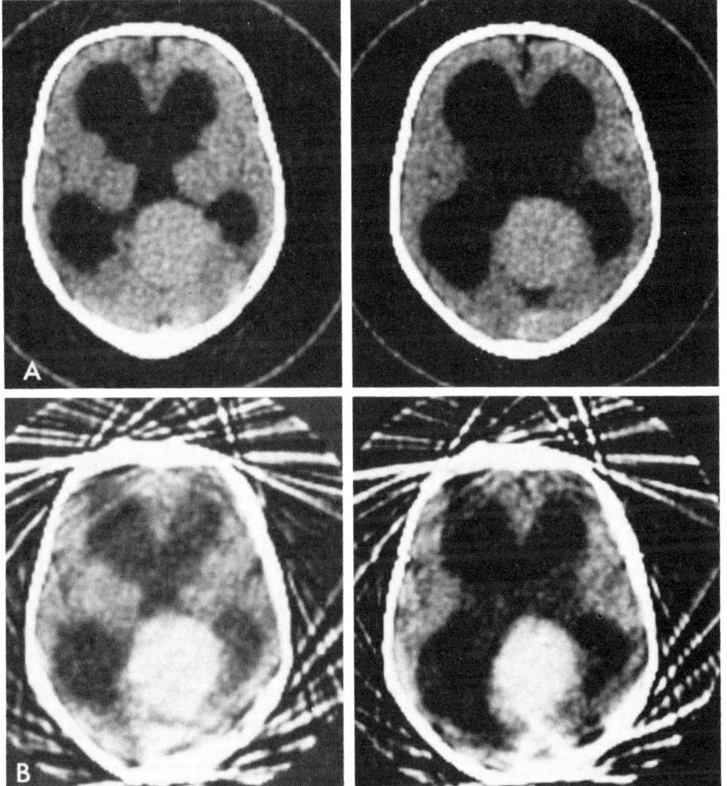

Figure 12–11. VEIN OF GALEN ANEURYSM: *A*, The preinfusion scan reveals a well defined area of increased density in the midline and extending to the right of the midline. There is moderate obstructive hydrocephalus.

B, The postinfusion scan reveals marked homogeneous enhancement of this area.

Illustration continued on the following page

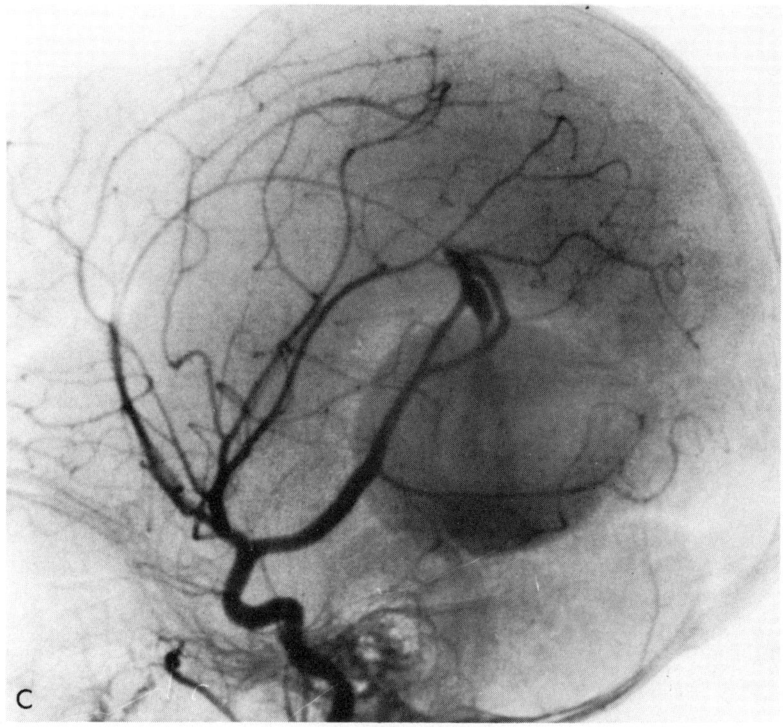

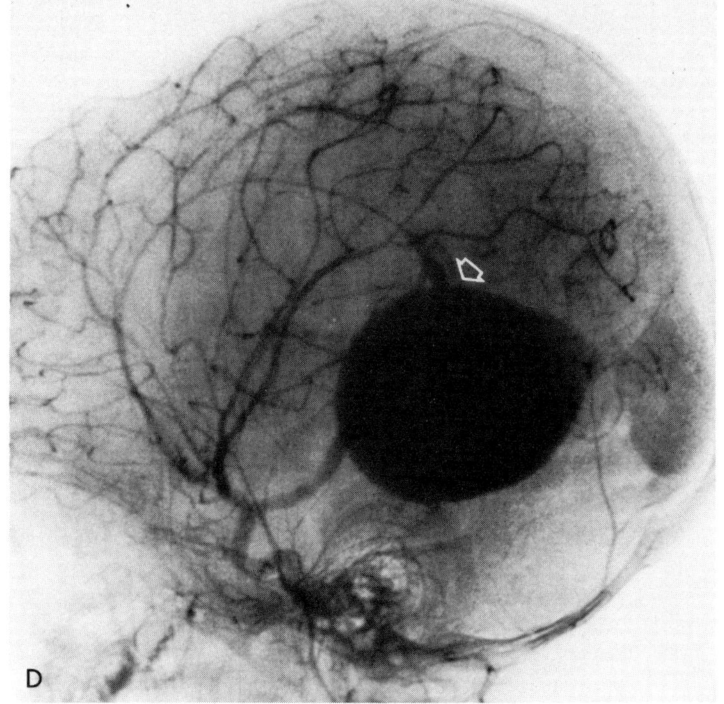

Figure 12–11 *Continued. See legend on the opposite page*

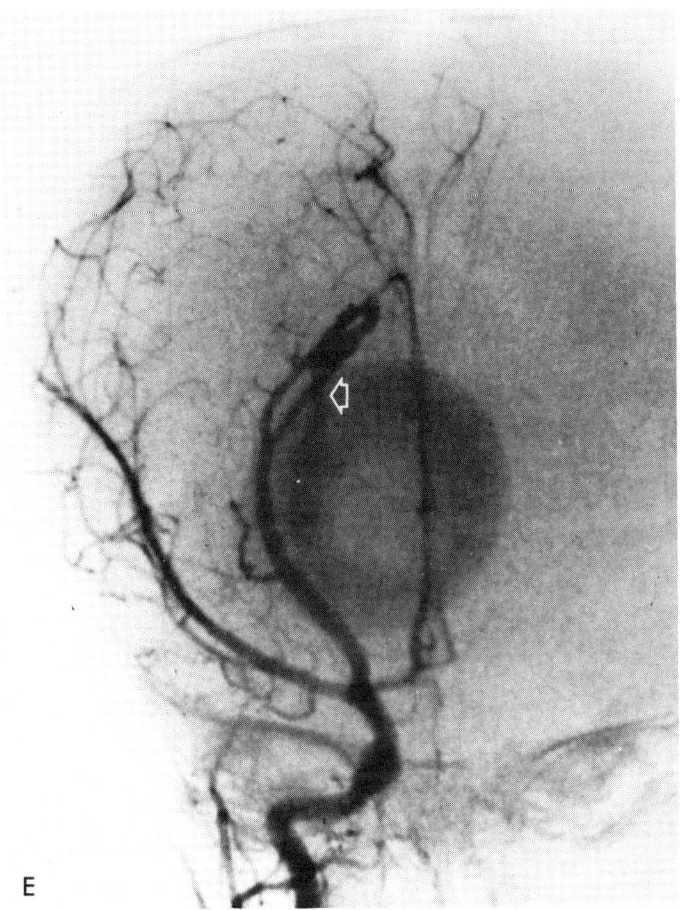

Figure 12–11 *Continued*

C, The right carotid arteriogram demonstrates marked enlargement of the posterior cerebral artery, which communicated directly with the vein of Galen. This is actually an arteriovenous fistula, not a malformation. Note the "jet stream" of contrast material as it enters into the midportion of the vein of Galen. The widened sweep of the pericallosal artery is secondary to the hydrocephalus.

D, The later arterial phase reveals better filling of the vein of Galen *(arrow)* and the region of the torcular Herophili, which are densely opacified while the remainder of the vessels are still in the arterial phase.

E, The AP view again demonstrates the fistulous communication between the deformed and enlarged right posterior cerebral artery and the vein of Galen *(arrow)*, which is asymmetrically enlarged. The "jet stream" of contrast material is again identified.

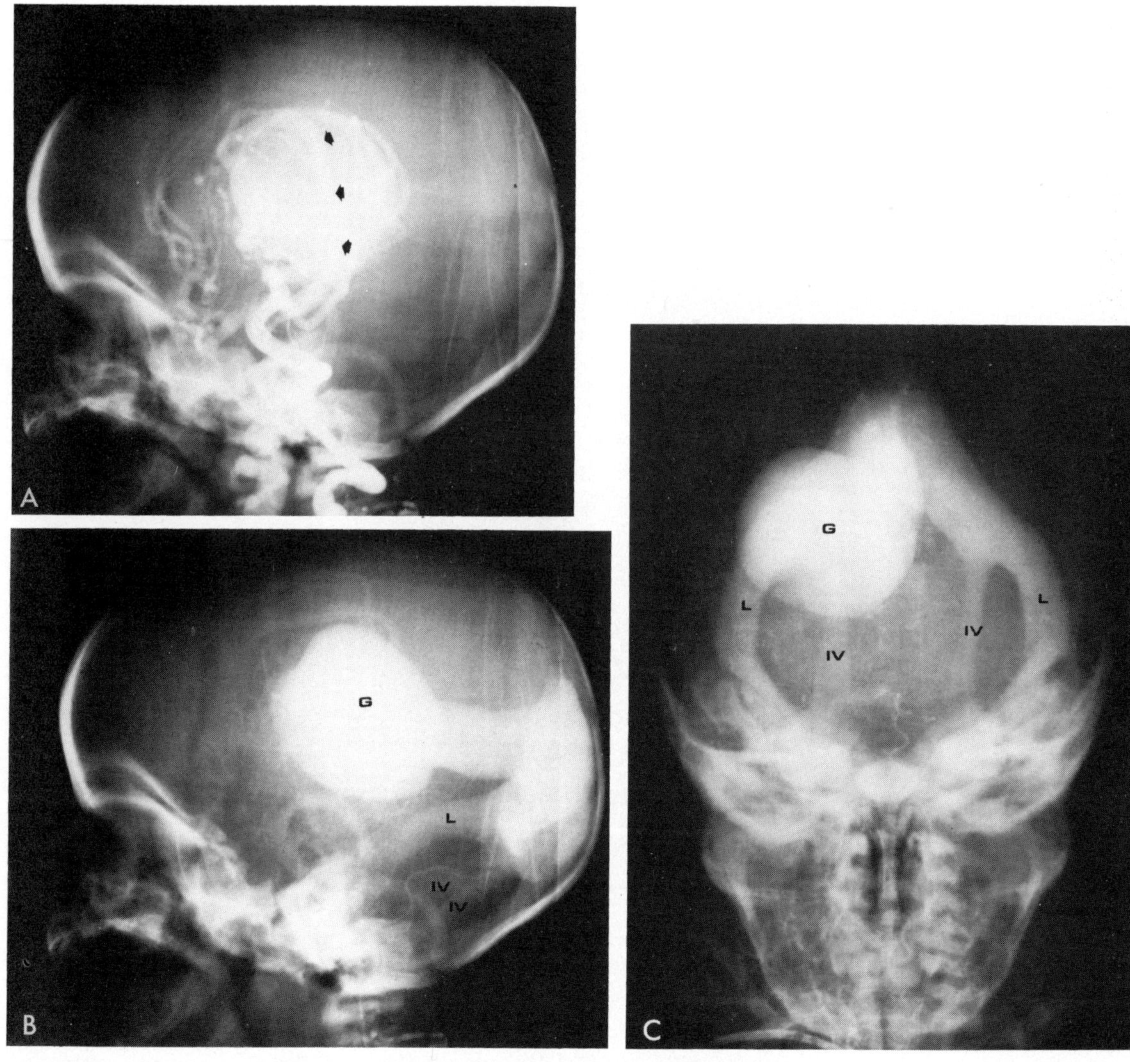

Figure 12–12. VEIN OF GALEN ANEURYSM: *A,* The markedly enlarged posterior cerebral arteries (*arrows*) supply an arteriovenous malformation, resulting in almost instant filling of the vein of Galen. The malformation is never well visualized because it is quite small and is obscured by the enlarged feeding arteries and early draining veins.

B, The vein of Galen (*G*), the straight sinus and the lateral (*L*) and inferior vermian (*IV*) veins are all noted to be densely opacified secondary to rapid shunting of blood through the malformation. There is obstructive hydrocephalus, and the patient presented with congestive heart failure.

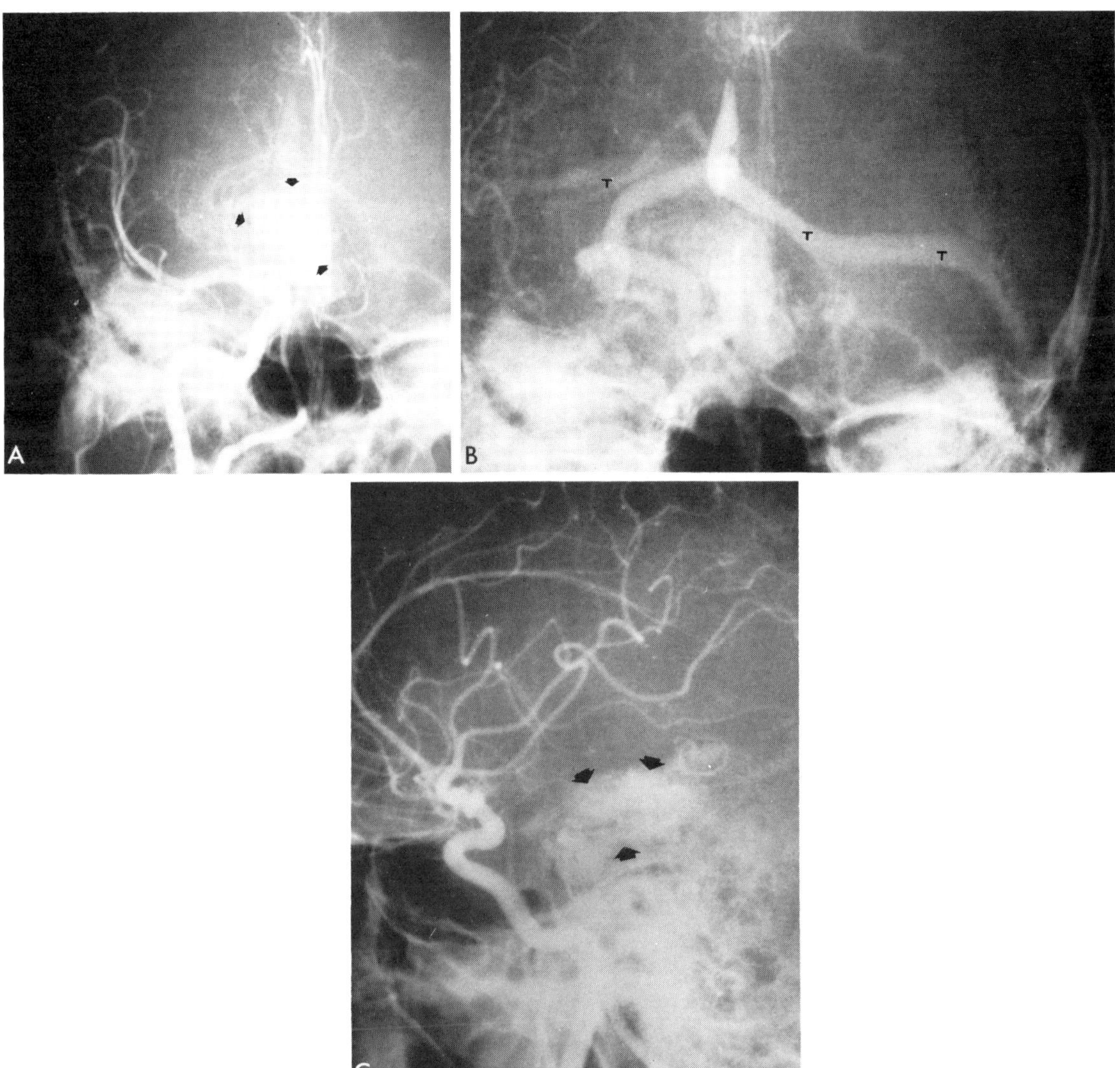

Figure 12–13. ARTERIOVENOUS MALFORMATION OF THE PONS: *A* and *B*, The early and late arterial phases of the right brachial arteriogram reveal an arteriovenous malformation of the right side of the pons. The AVM is supplied by perforating branches to the pons and the posterior cerebral arteries; it drains into the venous plexus at the base and then into the straight sinus and transverse sinuses bilaterally (*T*).

C, This lateral view again demonstrated the malformation (*arrows*) and a widened sweep of the perocallosal artery secondary to obstructive hydrocephalus following a hemorrhage of the malformation. Such a catastrophic event actually is not compatible with life.

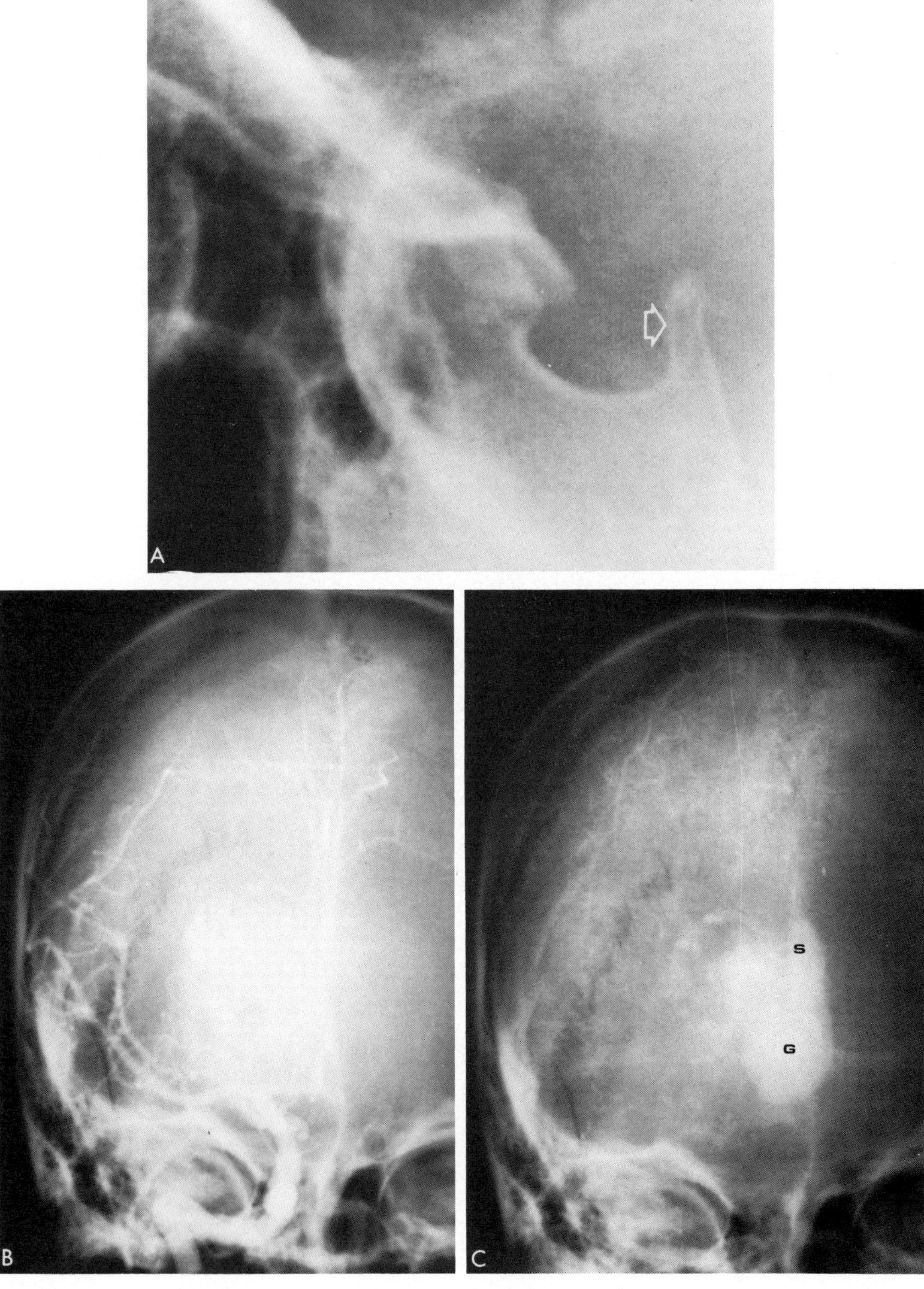

Figure 12–14 *See legend on the opposite page*

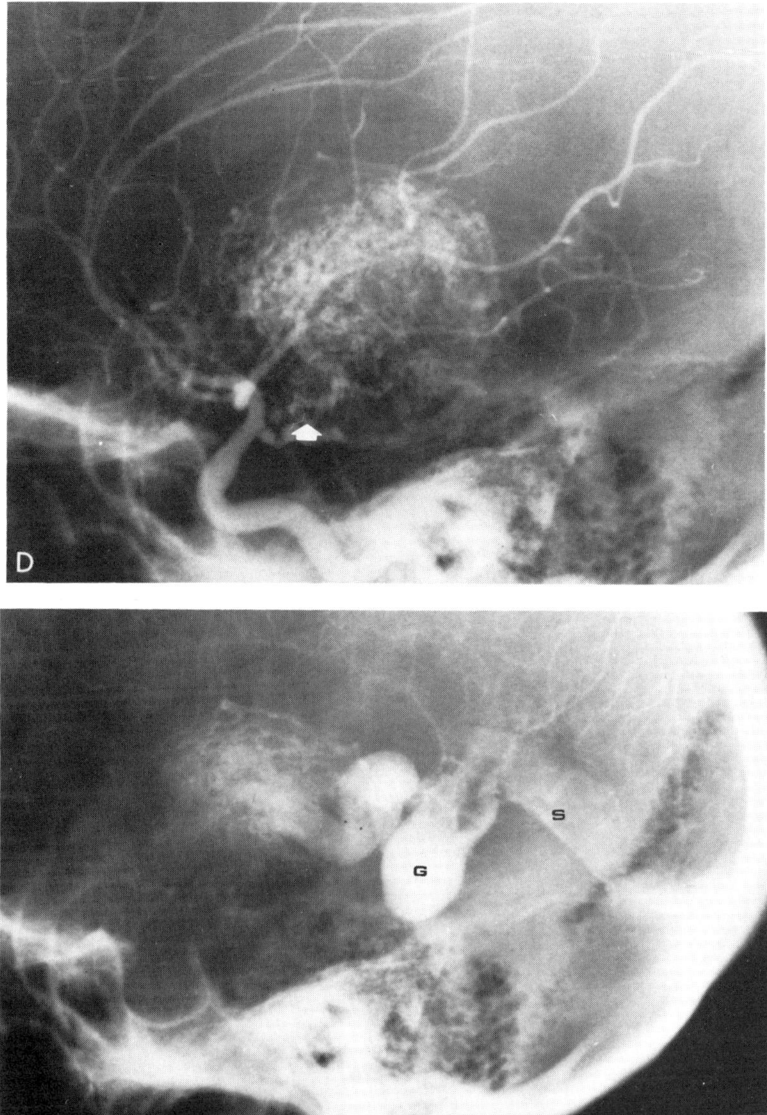

Figure 12–14. BITHALAMIC ARTERIOVENOUS MALFORMATION: *A,* Normal dorsum sella and posterior clinoids (*arrow*); patient aged 13. At age 20 the dorsum sella and posterior clinoids are thinned and the sella is enlarged (see sella in *E*). This change has occurred secondary to obstructive hydrocephalus and continued pounding and transmitted pressure from the third ventricle.

B and *C,* The arterial phase of the right carotid arteriogram reveals a large arteriovenous malformation of the thalamus that is supplied by enlarged thalamoperforating branches from the posterior cerebral arteries that fill from the carotid. *C* shows rapid dense filling of the vein of Galen (*G*) and the straight sinus (*S*).

D, The lateral arterial view shows the enlarged thalamoperforating branches (*arrow*) from the posterior cerebral artery and the mass of abnormal vessels of the malformation outlining the region of the thalamus. There is a widened sweep of the pericallosal artery secondary to obstructive hydrocephalus because of the enlarged vein of Galen.

E, The late arterial view reveals dense opacification of the vein of Galen (*G*) and the straight sinus (*S*).

Illustration continued on the following page

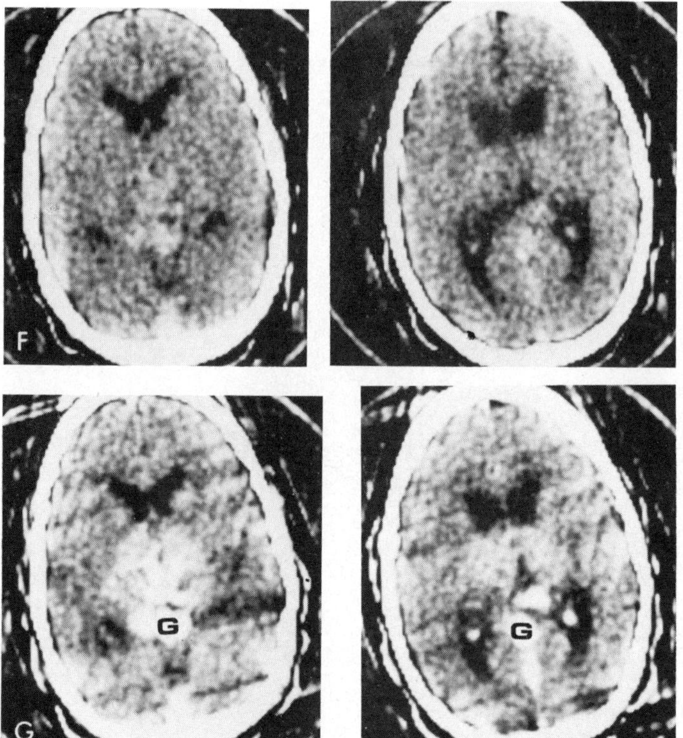

Figure 12–14 *Continued*

F and *G*, The pre- and postinfusion CT scans reveal bithalamic areas of increased density on the preinfusion scan that enhance postinfusion. The dilated vein of Galen is also well demonstrated on the postinfusion scan (*G*). There is moderate obstructive hydrocephalus.

Figure 12–15. RIGHT HEMISPHERE ARTERIOVENOUS MALFORMATION AND LEFT INTRAVENTRICULAR MENINGIOMA: *A*, The preinfusion CT scan reveals a densely calcified meningioma within the left lateral ventricle (*arrow*). In addition, mild asymmetry of the frontal horns of the lateral ventricles is seen.

B, Postinfusion, there is marked homogeneous enhancement of the meningioma. In addition, there is a large area of enhancement in the right hemisphere adjacent to the body of the right lateral ventricle, which has a serpentine pattern. These curvilinear areas of enhancement were shown by arteriography to represent enlarged feeding arteries and early draining veins of a right hemisphere AVM.

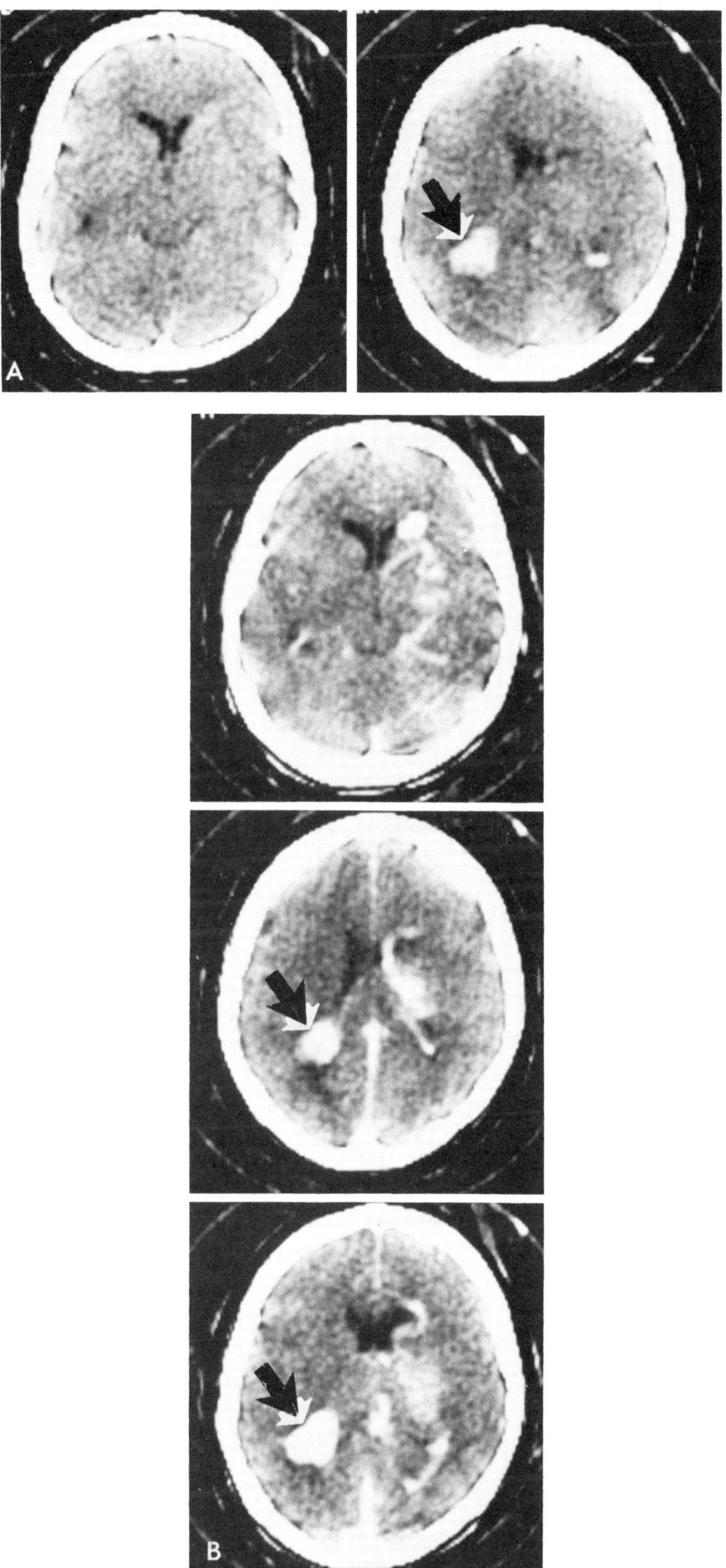

Figure 12–15. *See legend on the opposite page*

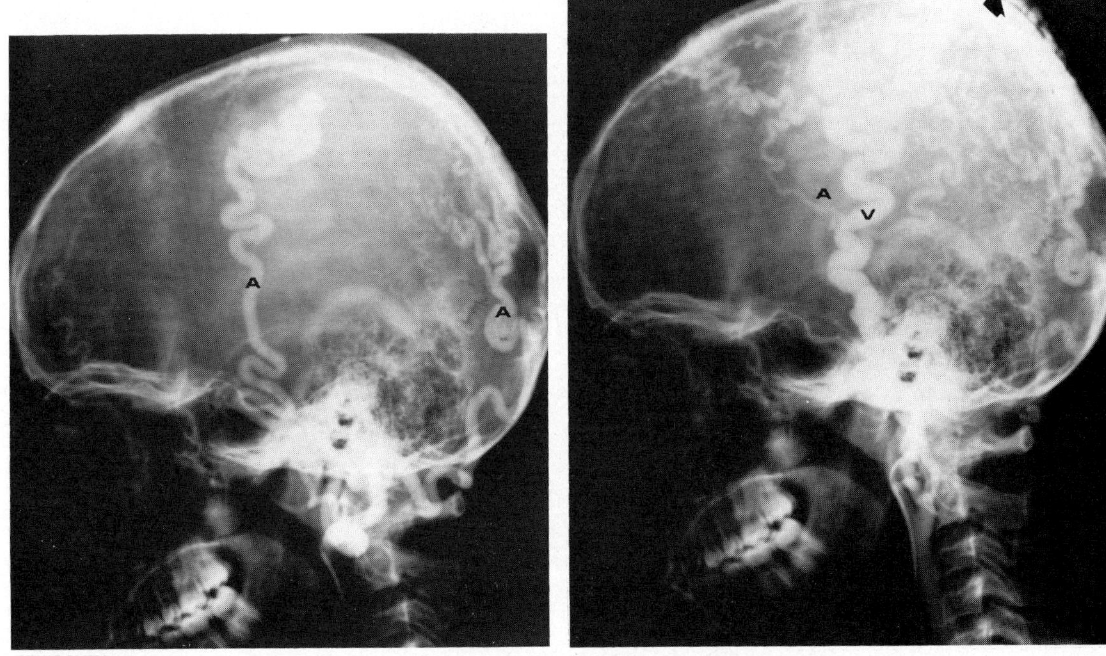

Figure 12–16. SCALP ARTERIOVENOUS MALFORMATION: This patient has a giant scalp arteriovenous malformation that developed following scalp trauma. The selective external carotid arteriogram reveals giant superficial temporal and occipital branches of the external carotid artery (*A*) that supply a large arteriovenous malformation drained by innumerable enlarged draining veins (*V*). The tangential view (*arrow*) reveals that all these vessels lie in the scalp. A similar appearance was seen with arteriography of the opposite external carotid artery.

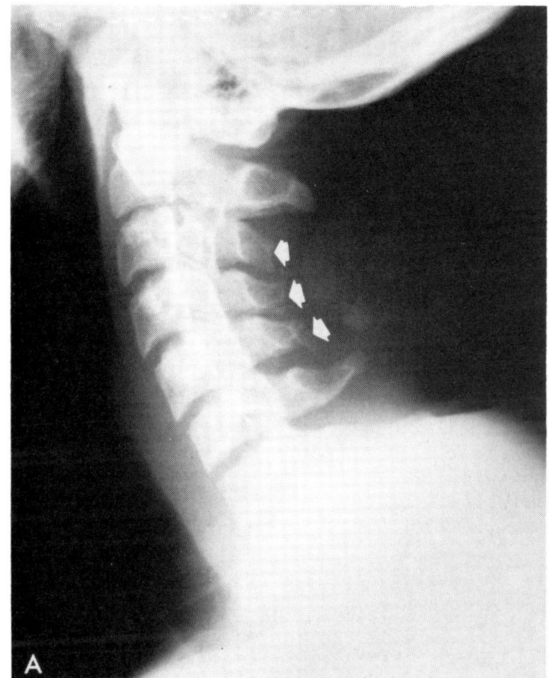

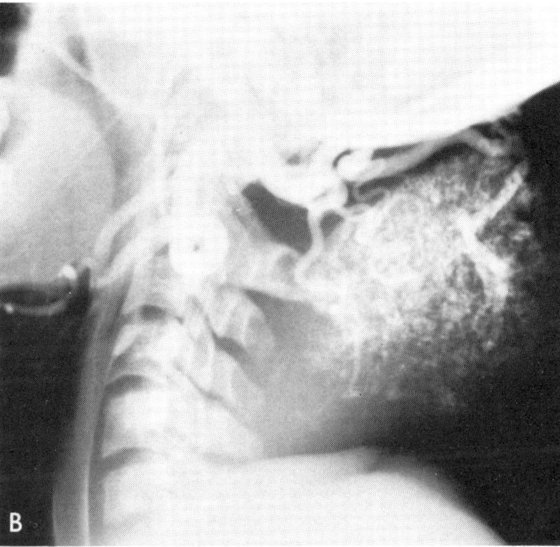

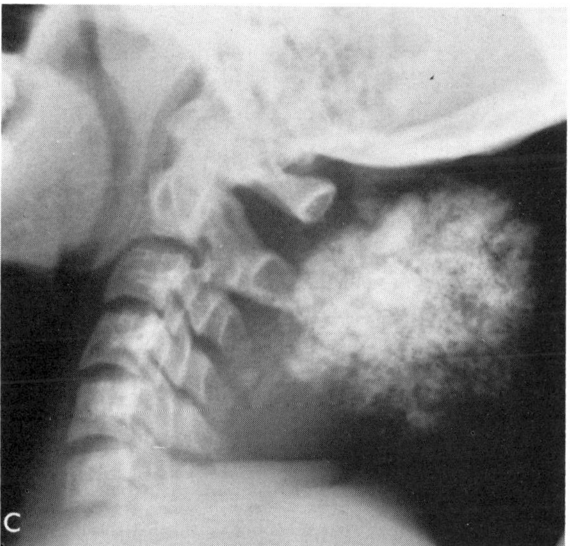

Figure 12–17. ARTERIOVENOUS MALFORMATION OF THE BACK OF THE NECK: *A*, The lateral view of the cervical spine reveals erosion of the spinous processes of the C_3 through C_5 secondary to pressure erosion.

B, Carotid arteriography demonstrates marked enlargement of the common carotid artery and an enlarged occipital branch that supplies the malformation.

C, A later arterial phase shows the large stain of the malformation. Arteriography of the opposite carotid revealed a similar pattern. A portion of the blood supply also arose from the vertebral arteries and from the thyrocervical trunk.

CHAPTER 13

TRAUMA

FRACTURES OF THE SKULL

PLAIN SKULL FILM EXAMINATION

Skull fractures may be classified as linear, comminuted, depressed or compound.

Linear fractures may occur in any area of the calvaria. Fractures involving the base of the skull are particularly difficult to detect. The routine skull series should be inspected closely, with emphasis on the area of interest. It may be necessary for the radiologist to perform a physical examination of the patient to determine the point of injury. If the patient is not present in the department, the films should be "bright lighted" to determine whether there are any areas of soft tissue swelling that might aid in identifying the point of injury.

Linear fractures of the calvaria are radiolucent, with a very well defined border (see Fig. 13–1). A thorough knowledge of the normal anatomy of the skull will help the radiologist avoid mistaking a normal suture line or vascular groove for a linear fracture. This is particularly true in pediatric patients, where sutures and areas of synchondrosis may simulate the appearance of a fracture line. Fractures may be visible on only one view of the skull; therefore, multiple views are obtained for complete evaluation. Simple linear skull fractures extend through both tables of the skull and therefore are more lucent than normal vascular grooves. They do not have the sclerotic border seen with a vascular groove, and they rarely bifurcate — another finding seen with vascular grooves.

The suture line on the outer table of the skull has a serrated appearance, whereas the suture on the inner table of the skull is a straight line. This straight line of the inner table may be mistaken for a fracture.

The posterior branch of the middle meningeal artery courses posterosuperiorly in the squamosal portion of the temporal bone and not uncommonly is mistaken for a fracture — particularly when the history relates to an injury in that region. If the vascular groove is visualized bilaterally, its true nature is more easily established; however, in some cases it may be impossible to differentiate this groove from a fracture.

On the Towne's view of the skull, the occipitomastoid suture frequently is viewed "on-end," and because of its rather straight appearance may easily be mistaken for a fracture. Comparison with the opposite side is helpful for complete evaluation, but may not provide absolute proof of the presence or absence of a fracture. The pediatric skull presents unique problems because of the persistence of normal suture lines and synchondroses in the early years of life (Fig. 13–11). In particular, the mendosal suture of the occipital bone may have the appearance of a fracture. Usually the mendosal suture is bilateral (Fig. 13–11).

Depressed Fractures. The amount of depression of the fracture fragments varies greatly depending on the injury. A depression of 0.5 cm or more is likely to cause damage to the underlying brain and therefore is usually surgically elevated. A tangential view is helpful in determining the amount of depression (see Chapter 2 and Fig. 13–3).

Compound Fractures. External compound fractures result from a communication with the scalp. Internal compound fractures communicate with the paranasal sinuses. Osteomyelitis may occur as a result of compound fractures, and safeguards should be taken to prevent its occurrence (Fig. 13–3).

Base-of-Skull Fractures. Not all fractures of the base of the skull will be identified on the plain films. There may, however, be secondary signs of fractures involving the base of the skull. Clinically, these patients may present with CSF rhinorrhea or CSF otorrhea; if the fracture involves the facial canal, there may be facial nerve palsy. The skull films may reveal an air-fluid level in the sphenoid sinus because CSF has leaked into the sinus or because of the accumulation of blood in the sinus. These air-fluid levels also may be seen in the frontal sinus or in the ethmoid sinus. For these reasons it is strongly recommended that skull films be obtained with the patient in the upright position if at all possible. On the other hand, the air-fluid level can also be demonstrated in cross-table lateral films with the patient in the supine position (see Fig. 13–17).

With tomography, a high percentage of base-of-skull fractures can be identified. To prove the presence of a CSF leak, cotton pledgets are placed in the nose or the ear, and radioactive material is then instilled in the lumbar-subarachnoid space. Later, the pledgets are removed from the nose or ear and scanned. The presence of radioactivity in the pledgets confirms leakage of CSF.

CT scanning of the sinuses after the instillation of Amipaque also may be used to demonstrate a CSF leak. The Amipaque that leaks from the subarachnoid space will be seen to accumulate in a small puddle in the nose.

MEDICOLEGAL ASPECTS OF SKULL FRACTURES

In one study of adult patients with head trauma who were examined with skull radiographs, less than 10 per cent exhibited skull fractures. Most of these were linear and were seen in the cranial vault. No correlation was demonstrated between the physical findings, the patient's symptoms and the radiographic findings. In only two of the 49 patients studied radiologically was the proposed treatment altered.

In one study of a large number of pediatric patients with head trauma, approximately 25 per cent had radiographic evidence of a skull fracture. The skull fracture did not correlate with the clinical seriousness of the patient's symptoms and did not alter the decision for medical care, except in children with depressed or compound fractures. The incidence of serious intracranial sequelae in head injuries, regardless of the presence or absence of a skull fracture, is 9 per cent; the incidence of these sequelae in children without a fracture is 8 per cent. However, because of the need for as thorough an evaluation as possible in patients who have a history of head trauma and possible skull fracture, a routine skull series probably should be obtained in these patients. This is particularly true if there is external evidence of severe head trauma. On the other hand, if one considers cost effectiveness as well as the potential hazards of x-radiation, one might argue that more stringent criteria be applied to patients selected for skull radiography.

Such criteria might include a history of unconsciousness, gunshot wound or skull penetration, previous craniotomy with shunt tube in place. During the physical examination, one should look for:

1. Palpable skull depression or skull fracture.
2. CSF discharge from nose.
3. Battle's sign.
4. CSF discharge from ear.
5. Raccoon's eyes.
6. Blood in the middle ear cavity.
7. Coma or stupor.
8. Focal neurologic signs.

FRACTURE HEALING

Linear fractures may remain apparent for many years after the initial injury. In some cases they may never be completely obliterated. Healing does not occur with callus formation as it does in the long bones; instead, there is gradual bony overgrowth of the fracture site (Fig. 13–5).

TRAUMA — AN OVERVIEW

Specific entities will be discussed later in this chapter. The changes following head trauma are related to the type and severity of the injury and also to the point of injury. Because these changes may or may not be visible on the plain film examination of the skull, a thorough knowledge of normal anatomy is needed in order to evaluate the plain skull examination and any areas of suspicion.

Soft tissue injury (Fig. 13–15) will appear radiographically as an area of soft tissue prominence that becomes visible when the skull films are examined under a bright light. This examination for swelling of soft tissues is of particular importance when the history does not indicate the area or point of interest. Skull fractures may appear as small, thin linear areas of radiolucency to the shattered skull seen with severe head injury (Figs. 13–1 and 13–12).

It is important to remember that most patients who have suffered life-threatening head trauma also have severe injuries to other parts of the body. This will, of necessity, limit the patient's ability to cooperate fully during radiographic examination. It may be necessary to re-examine the patient after the other critical injuries have become stabilized to the point where more particular attention can be given to the bony calvaria. In cases of multiple injury, AP and lateral films may be all that can be obtained at the initial examination. An attempt should be made to evaluate these films as completely as possible, noting any abnormalities that could be associated with intracranial problems and any areas of suspicion that need re-examination (Figs. 13–2 and 13–3).

If possible, when there are no other life-threatening problems a routine skull series should be obtained. The series should include right and left lateral views, PA view, Towne's view and the submentovertex, if possible. As noted earlier, a skull fracture may be visible on only one view, therefore, multiple views are necessary for complete evaluation. Particular attention should be paid to the point of soft tissue injury. Linear skull fractures appear as thin, well defined areas of radiolucency. If visible on the lateral view, they will appear finer and more distinct on the film closest to the side of the injury.

Fractures in the frontal and occipital areas may be visible on only one view. Particular care should be taken to visualize the occipital region on the Towne's view. Likewise, a fracture placed far laterally in the frontal bone or an occipital area may be difficult to visualize on both the PA and the lateral views of the skull. If any such area of suspicion cannot be evaluated by the films available, additional studies, such as oblique views, should be made to rule out a fracture.

The presence of a skull fracture does not imply that there is severe or even *any* intracranial injury. However, it does mean that there has been a certain degree of injury beyond soft tissue damage. On the other hand, the absence of a skull fracture does not rule out the presence of severe and even life-threatening intracranial damage. Trauma may result in extracerebral collections of blood in the subdural or epidural space. Contusion of the brain with edema or clot formation also may be seen. An individual patient may have any combination of these processes. It should be mentioned that the plain film examination remains the best method for evaluation of the presence of a linear skull fracture. The CT scan *may* reveal the fracture line — but if the plane of the fracture is in the same plane as the scan slice, the fracture will not visualize. The bony calvaria should be evaluated by examination of each slice of the CT scan on the viewing screen with manipulation of the window widths and window levels.

Late Effects

Leptomeningeal Cyst. If the skull fracture has resulted in a tear in the dural layer of the meninges, the arachnoid membrane may be tethered in the fracture line after protruding through the dural tear. Over a long period — months or years — the continued transmitted pulsations of the heart beat and respirations to the arachnoid caught in the linear fracture result in a smoothing and widening of the margin of the fracture and a palpable cystic mass outside the bony calvaria — a leptomeningeal cyst (see Fig. 13–7 and Chapter 2).

Porencephalic Cysts. Head trauma that

has resulted in significant intracranial damage destroys a portion of the cerebral tissue. This damage may present initially as an area of edema, areas of infarction, hemorrhage or a combination of these processes. Eventually the acute cerebral damage resolves, sometimes leaving an area of porencephaly in the bed of the previous abnormality. The development of such post-traumatic porencephalic cysts can be observed on serial CT scans. The cysts contain cerebrospinal fluid and consequently are of similar density to the ventricular fluid on the CT scan. The porencephalic cyst also may be demonstrated by pneumoencephalography (Fig. 13–7).

Extracerebral Hematomas

If a fracture extends across the meningeal artery grooves, there is a possibility of shearing the vessel lying in the groove. Damage to the middle meningeal artery may result in an epidural hematoma; therefore, any fracture with this appearance should alert one to the real possibility of intracranial hemorrhage (see Fig. 13–46). Typically, an epidural hematoma is of arterial origin from the middle meningeal artery, but venous bleeding into the epidural space also may occur. Without proper care, this injury may lead rapidly to death.

Head injuries also may result in a subdural hematoma. The amount of trauma necessary to create a subdural or epidural hematoma varies from individual to individual and in different age groups. Very young and very old persons develop subdural hematomas more readily than individuals in other age groups.

Intracerebral Hematomas

In addition to extracerebral accumulations of blood, there may be evidence of intracerebral hematoma formation. The intracerebral hematoma may be remote from the point of skull trauma and may be secondary to "contra-coup" injury to the brain — brain injury opposite the point of skull trauma. This results when there is rapid deceleration of the brain — as from a high-speed motor vehicle accident — and the brain opposite the initial point of injury is stopped suddenly by hitting the cranial vault. This occurs because there is a certain amount of mobility of the brain within the bony calvaria.

The development of intracerebral hematoma may, of course, be at the site of direct trauma. There may be an associated subdural hematoma, an epidural hematoma or a combination of these. The contra-coup damage may occur in any portion of the brain. Commonly affected areas are the anterior temporal lobes, as they are limited by the greater wings of the sphenoid bone, which is a firm bony margin; the frontal lobes and the occipital lobes of the brain. In addition to hematoma formation or in its absence, there may be contusion of the cerebrum, which results in small petechial hemorrhages or edema. Any of these cerebral changes may produce a similar clinical picture, and, in many cases, arteriography will assist in defining the problem but not the true pathologic nature of the intracranial lesion. Only since the development of CT scanning has it become possible to differentiate with certainty between cerebral edema and hemorrhage.

Computed Tomography

The development of computed tomography has brought an entirely new approach to the evaluation of patients with head trauma. When these facilities are available, the CT scan should be the first diagnostic procedure performed on a patient with significant head trauma. *The CT scan provides a more accurate picture of intracranial injury than any other type of diagnostic procedure.* A CT scan of adequate diagnostic quality offers a highly accurate evaluation of intracranial anatomy, and comparison with anatomic sections shows excellent correlation between the scans and the pathologic anatomy.

CT scanning provides a totally new approach to the problems of head injury. Although plain radiography may reveal a skull fracture, the *absence* of a skull fracture does not rule out any of the complications of head trauma discussed earlier. Therefore, any patient who has sustained significant head trauma and in whom there are clinical signs or suspicion of intracranial damage should have an emergency CT scan. It may be necessary to sedate these patients in order to obtain a good quality study. If sedation is used, careful monitoring is necessary. In some cases general anesthesia is needed — especially in the combative or intoxicated patient when immobilization by any other method proves impossible. Indeed, it is these patients who not uncommonly are sent from the emergency room to the scanning room and then directly to the operating room.

In any patient who has suffered severe central nervous system damage, consultation with the neurosurgical service should be obtained as quickly as possible. This is essential because occasional emergency room patients will require bur holes before a diagnosis is made if there is such rapid deterioration that further delay will lead to certain death.

SPECIFIC CT SCAN APPEARANCE IN TRAUMA

With diffuse *cerebral edema* the lateral ventricles will be very small or even invisible, although the CT scan may not reveal a detectable alteration in the density of the brain. Accumulation of blood in the subarachnoid space may make the falx cerebri more readily visible than would be expected because it is outlined by blood on either side. With intraventricular hemorrhage the blood may accumulate in the dependent portions of the lateral ventricles when the patient lies in the supine position. Localized areas of edema may be revealed as areas of radiolucency, with shift of the midline structures to the contralateral side — or merely as shift of the midline structures without definite detectable changes of density in the cerebral tissues. Even small areas of intracerebral hemorrhage are readily demonstrated by the CT scan.

If the scan reveals a subdural hematoma, epidural hematoma or a large intracerebral hematoma the patient can be taken directly to the operating room for surgical correction. Further diagnostic procedures might only delay appropriate treatment. In *selected* cases it may be appropriate to obtain only one midsection cut through the brain. If a large epidural or subdural hematoma is demonstrated, appropriate therapeutic measures may be taken without further delay.

Following acute head trauma there may be dilatation of the lateral ventricles without any other abnormalities. This ventricular dilatation may be caused by a communicating hydrocephalus secondary to subarachnoid hemorrhage, although the etiology in some cases is unknown. The lateral ventricles may then remain unchanged in size, return to normal size or continue to increase in size. Ventricular enlargement not present acutely may later be seen on a follow-up scan. It is believed that this communicating hydrocephalus develops because blood in the subarachnoid space interferes with the absorption of cerebrospinal fluid by the arachnoid villi. CT scans are the ideal method to follow this alteration in ventricular size.

SUBDURAL HEMATOMAS

Subdural hematomas develop between the inner layer of the dura and the arachnoid membrane — hence, the name "subdural hematoma." An acute subdural hematoma is a life-threatening event that results in death in many individuals and in significant morbidity in others.

PLAIN FILM EXAMINATION

Plain film radiography may or may not reveal a skull fracture. A shift of the pineal gland contralateral to the side of the subdural hematoma may be noted. However, the absence of shift does not rule out a subdural hematoma because the subdural accumulations may be bilateral. Also, there may be significant edema on the contralateral side secondary to a contra-coup lesion, preventing a shift of the midline structures even when there is significant intracranial damage. In addition, the pineal gland may not be calcified — and thus of no help in diagnosis. Subdural hematomas also may develop in the posterior fossa. Indeed, posterior fossa subdural hematomas can cause compression of vital structures and the very rapid demise of the patient.

COMPUTED TOMOGRAPHY

In acute subdural hematoma a crescentic extracerebral collection of clotted blood is seen over the affected hemisphere. There will be shift of the midline structures to the contralateral side (see Figs. 13–21 and 13–22). These accumulations vary from small to very large amounts of blood. Sometimes the extracerebral accumulation of blood may be so small that it is barely appreciable (Fig. 13–28). In these cases there is a varying amount of shift of the midline structures to the contralateral side. It is important and often necessary to manipulate the density control system on varying window widths and window levels to better outline the abnormality. Clotted blood measures from 50 to 90 Hounsfield units.

Density manipulation of the CT scanning unit should also be performed so that the bony calvaria also can be viewed and examined for evidence of skull fracture. Both linear and depressed skull fractures can be identified by CT scan. Linear fractures may not be identified if they are not in a plane visualized by the cuts. Failure to visualize a skull fracture on the CT scan therefore does not rule out its presence.

Large acute subdural hematomas may develop the appearance of a hematocrit level (Figs. 13–21 – 13–24). This occurs because the blood components settle when the patient remains in the supine position for a prolonged period. It is unclear exactly what substance it is that produces this level; at the time of surgery, there is no difference in the appearance of the clotted blood — unlike a hematocrit determination.

Acute subdural hematomas are readily identified by CT scanning, whether uni- or bilateral. In addition, the scan may show edema surrounding these extracerebral accumulations and/or evidence of contusion of the brain.

Subacute Subdural Hematomas

A gradual decrease in density of the extracerebral accumulatons of blood takes place post-injury. This results in a mottled appearance of the subdural blood, rather than the white density seen in acute hematomas. It is not known how much time is required before this change in density occurs, because it is often impossible to determine when the patients initially sustained their head trauma. However, early density changes probably occur in the first week post-injury. These patients are frequently alcoholic or demented, and may even give a history of multiple instances of head trauma. Not uncommonly these unfortunate individuals are brought to the emergency room without any useful history.

An associated shift of the midline to the contralateral side is seen in the subacute stage. The subdural accumulation will be less crescentic and more lentiform.

Chronic Subdural Hematomas

CT Scan. During the progression of a subdural hematoma from the acute to the chronic stages, the density of the blood accumulation may be similar (isodense) to the normal brain substance (Fig. 13–36). If this is the case, there may be a shift of the midline but no evidence of a mass lesion or extracerebral accumulation. There may even be an appearance of hemiatrophy on the contralateral side, the shift of the midline appearing to be toward the atrophic side. The greatest danger in these fortunately uncommon cases is that isodense subdural accumulations may be bilateral (Fig. 13–27), thus producing no shift of the midline. It is helpful for diagnosis if the index of suspicion for a subdural hematoma is high in these cases. In patients with isodense bilateral subdural hematomas, the lateral ventricles appear to be elongated and compressed toward the midline.

The lateral ventricles may appear to be smaller than one would normally anticipate for a patient in the older age group because of compression by bilateral subdural hematomas (Fig. 13–37). As these lesions occur frequently in older patients, the absence of cortical sulci provides further evidence of an abnormal scan. The sulci may be obliterated unilaterally or bilaterally, depending on the nature of the lesions.

If bilateral isodense subdural hematomas are a consideration, arteriography may be necessary for more definitive evaluation. A membrane develops around a subdural hematoma 10 to 14 days post-injury. Chronic subdural hematomas may cause enhancement of this membrane on the postinfusion study. This enhancement may be quite subtle (Fig. 13–35) and should be looked for by using varying window widths and window levels; all the cuts should be reviewed, with particular attention given to the very highest cuts. Displacement of the cortical veins away from the inner table on the postinfusion study also may be seen.

Following evacuation of bilateral subdural accumulations, the follow-up CT scan reveals that the lateral ventricles have returned to a more normal size for the patient's age group; also, there may be visualization of the cortical sulci that had not been visible pre-evacuation.

In pediatric patients, *chronic* bilateral subdural hematomas may be associated with dilatation of the lateral ventricles. The appearance on the pneumoencephalogram is of a communicating hydrocephalus, and a similar appearance occurs on the CT scan. The lateral ventricles are dilated and there is evidence of bilateral low density extracerebral accumulations of fluid. The enlargement of the lateral ventricles is thought to be a result of interference with absorption of CSF by the arachnoid villi because of the presence of the bilateral subdural hematomas; however, the exact pathophysiology is not understood.

The author has cases where evacuation of subdural accumulations has resulted in collapse of the cerebrum and accumulation of air in the cranial cavity. It appears that in these cases there is a pre-existing decrease in the normal amount of brain substance. Following removal of the subdural accumulation, the brain is unable to expand and refill the intracranial space.

ARTERIOGRAPHY OF SUBDURAL HEMATOMAS

The AP view is usually most helpful. With a subdural hematoma in the parietal convexity area, the AP view will demonstrate that the branches of the middle cerebral artery group will not reach the inner table of the skull; instead, they are displaced away from the inner table, revealing an avascular crescentic mass outside the cerebral substance. The midline structures will be shifted to the contralateral side.

In the venous phase the cortical veins also will be displaced away from the inner table of the skull in a fashion similar to that noted for the arteries. Both the arteries and the cortical veins run in the subarachnoid space and therefore will be displaced by a subdural accumulation of blood. In addition, there will be a shift of the internal cerebral vein to the contralateral side. Note that subdural accumulations do not cross the midline because they are limited by the reflection of the dura that forms the falx cerebri. Inspection of the films reveals that the cortical veins at the level of the subdural hematoma curve superiorly as they approach the parasagittal region (Fig. 13–41) in order that they may drain into the superior sagittal sinus in normal anatomic fashion. It is because of the falx and superior sagittal sinus and its attachment to the cortical veins that subdural hematomas do not cross the midline.

Subdural hematomas also may develop in the interhemispheric fissure on either side of the falx. This is more readily demonstrated on the CT scan.

When a subdural hematoma is demonstrated by arteriography and there is no shift of the midline structures, one should strongly suspect the presence of a contralateral subdural hematoma or contusion. A study of the contralateral side should be performed in such patients. This may be done by using the cross-compression technique or, if this is unsuccessful in visualizing the opposite side, by subsequent arteriography of that side. The position of the internal cerebral vein should be determined by linear measurement — not by the use of the "eye-ball" technique.

Pitfalls in Diagnosis. If the subdural accumulation is positioned anteriorly, the branches of the middle cerebral artery — which are at the widest biparietal diameter of the skull — will appear to reach the inner table, whereas in reality there is displacement of the branches *away* from the inner table more anteriorly, where the bony calvaria is narrower. This results in failure to visualize the extracerebral accumulation. Although there will be shift of the pericallosal artery to the contralateral side and a less marked shift of the internal cerebral vein, an oblique view of the AP projection toward the side of the suspected subdural will be required. This allows a tangential view of the vessels where they fail to reach the inner table of the skull (Fig. 13–42).

If the subdural accumulation is positioned posteriorly, a similar arteriographic appearance is noted. Again, the branches of the middle cerebral artery will reach the inner table, while the more posterior branches that are displaced away from the inner table will not be seen because of the narrowing of the skull posteriorly. If this is the case a distal shift of the pericallosal artery under the falx and a more marked shift of the internal cerebral vein will be seen. Again, an oblique view away from the side of the hematoma will allow a tangential view of these vessels posteriorly (Fig. 13–42). In fact, when CT scanning is unavailable and an emergency arteriogram is done for a suspected subdural hematoma, a practical and expeditious method of arteriographic study is a standard AP and lateral projection followed immediately by AP runs (arterial phase only), turning the patient obliquely, first toward the ipsilateral side and then toward the contralateral side. This way, either an anteriorly or posteriorly placed subdural hematoma will not be overlooked. The technique is especially helpful if the hematoma happens to be bilateral and is not associated with a shift of the anterior cerebral artery or internal cerebral vein.

It the supratentorial circulation is normal, the infratentorial circulation may require additional study. This is particularly true if hydrocephalus is demonstrated in the supratentorial circulation.

The Lateral View. The lateral view not uncommonly gives a normal or nearly normal appearance in a large percentage of cases. This occurs because the structures are simply displaced out of the plane of view toward the side opposite the hematoma and are frequently not distorted. In other words, the vessel relationships are not changed, but simply moved from their normal positions. This relatively normal appearance is more likely to be seen when the hematoma is over the low convexity and covers a large area. It must be remembered that this is true only when the subdural hematoma is not complicated with other findings, such as an intracerebral hematoma, a cerebral contusion or focal areas of cerebral edema.

On the other hand, if the hematoma is situated in the high convexity or parasagittal area there will be downward displacement of the sylvian triangle. If a subdural hematoma is anterior in its location, the sylvian triangle will be displaced posteriorly, and it will be noted that the vessels in the frontal area do not reach the inner table of the skull (Fig. 13–43). Although absence of vessels adjacent to the inner table of the skull also may be seen with atrophy of the frontal lobes of the brain, if atrophy is present there will be no shift to the contralateral side. This, of course, is true only in the absence of bilateral subdural accumulations. Because the cortical veins must join with the superior sagittal sinus high in the convexity region, these veins will not *appear* to be displaced from the inner table on the lateral view (Fig. 13–43). However, they will be displaced away from the inner table on the AP view obtained in the oblique projection with the patient's head turned toward the side of the hematoma. This is not to say that displacement has not occurred — only that it cannot be appreciated on the lateral view. The sylvian triangle may be displaced posteriorly as well as inferiorly. With a subdural accumulation in the occipital region, the sylvian triangle may be telescoped anteriorly if the mass is retrosylvian—and/or displaced inferiorly if the mass is superior to the sylvian triangle. Obviously, any combination of these changes may be seen, depending on the location of the hematoma.

Other Associated Changes. If there has been *contusion* of the brain, or even an element of subarachnoid hemorrhage, spasm of the vessels may be seen that is similar to that which occurs with a subarachnoid hemorrhage secondary to an aneurysm (Fig. 13–25). If this is the case, the CT scan will demonstrate very small areas of high density secondary to the intracerebral hematoma or petechial hemorrhage, together with some associated edema that appears as areas of radiolucency surrounding the areas of hemorrhage. There may be no evidence of hemorrhage on the CT scan — only areas of lucency secondary to infarction because of spasm or to the edema that follows contusion. This will be associated with shift of the midline structures to the contralateral side. If this is the case, the arteriogram may show a mass effect that is confined to a localized area of edema, or it may reveal diffuse splaying of the vessels if there is massive cerebral edema. With diffuse edema there is no evidence of any specific mass; rather, diffuse changes secondary to the edema are evident.

Most often, trauma results in involvement of the frontal and occipital poles as well as the anterior temporal tips of the brain. In rapid deceleration injuries, primary injury to the brain may occur at the initial point of impact, with secondary edema and contusion at the pole opposite the initial injury — the so-called "contra-coup" lesion. On the other hand, most of the damage may occur at the point of initial injury. Contra-coup lesions develop because the cerebrum is somewhat mobile as it floats in the CSF. Consequently, in rapid deceleration injuries the brian may slide either forward or backward and then be halted by the inner table of the frontal or occipital regions; or, very commonly, the anterior temporal lobes may be injured as they abut the greater wings of the sphenoid that form the anatomic limit of the middle cranial fossa.

Frontal lobe injuries can cause posterior displacement of the anterior cerebral arteries and diffuse splaying of the vascular branches in the frontal poles. If the injury to both frontal poles has been of equal severity, there will be no shift of the midline structures. With an asymmetric injury, the arteriogram will show asymmetric changes that correspond to the extent of damage. Frontal lobe damage will cause posterior displacement of the sylvian triangle. If the damage was severe enough to affect both frontal lobes, frequently there is damage to both anterior temporal lobes as well. The insult to the temporal lobes results in upward displacement of the sylvian triangle secondary to hematoma, contusion or edema of the lobes (Fig. 13–45).

The author has seen two cases in which severe trauma to the back of the skull resulted in a linear fracture of the occipital bone, apparent forward motion of the cerebrum and resulting total anosmia — apparently from shearing of all the olfactory nerves where they pass through the cribriform plate — without any other evidence of damage to the cerebral structures.

Diffuse damage to all the cranial contents from severe head trauma will result in "tetrapolar trauma." In these cases the arteriogram may not reveal very marked alteration, even though very marked cerebral damage actually is present. The CT scan in these cases may show diffuse scattered areas of radiolucency and hemorrhage or only very small lateral ventricles secondary to diffuse cerebral edema. Care must be taken in interpreting small lateral ventricles, depending on the patient's age. If a very old individual has small ventricles, this is more suggestive of diffuse cerebral edema than when small lateral ventricles are seen in a younger patient, in whom it is a normal finding. The CT numbers in diffuse cerebral edema may not accurately reflect the true amount of cerebral damage present. In other words, to show a numerical difference on the CT scans would require such marked alteration in the cerebral fluid content that it is unlikely that the patient could survive.

SUBARACHNOID HEMORRHAGE SECONDARY TO TRAUMA

If an element of subarachnoid hemorrhage is associated with trauma, accumulation of blood in the dependent portions of the lateral ventricles may be evident (Fig. 13–30). A more subtle manifestation is a diffuse increase in density of the falx cerebri that occurs because blood in the subarachnoid space accumulates along the falx and is then apparent on the CT scan. In the older patient, however, the falx may be diffusely calcified even when there is no blood in the subarachnoid space; therefore, this sign must be evaluated on an individual basis. If an old scan is available that did not show this increased density of the falx, or if the increased density resolves on follow-up, the diagnosis of subarachnoid hemorrhage is substantiated.

EPIDURAL HEMATOMAS

An epidural hematoma, as its name implies, is situated outside the dura. It is an extracerebral accumulation of blood in the space between the outer layer of the dura and the inner table of the skull. Generally speaking, epidural hematomas result from arterial bleeding — most frequently from the middle meningeal artery branches. They are frequently, but not always, associated with a fracture that crosses the groove of the meningeal artery branches. Classically, they have a lentiform configuration that is readily demonstrated on both the arteriogram and the CT scan.

Patients with an epidural hematoma may experience a so-called "lucid interval." If this occurs, the patient may have a history of unconsciousness immediately following the injury followed by an interval of total lucidity and a subsequent episode of coma. If the patient is examined during the lucid period, the presence of an epidural hematoma may not be appreciated, and care must be taken not to discharge such a patient from care before a satisfactory period of observation has passed. In our experience this "lucid interval" occurs rarely.

Plain Skull. The plain skull film may be normal. One should look for a fracture that extends across a groove that carries one of the meningeal artery branches. In older patients, the meningeal artery becomes grooved into the inner table of the skull and is more or less fixed in this groove. Therefore, if a fracture extends across the meningeal artery groove, the fixed meningeal artery is very likely to be severed — resulting in hemorrhage into the epidural space.

Epidural hematomas also occur in the posterior fossa; these are frequently associated with a fracture of the occipital bone. Posterior fossa epidural hematomas compress the vital brain stem structures, leading to rapid demise of the patient. They also produce an obstructive hydrocephalus. Thus, if this diagnosis is suspected, appropriate steps should be taken to confirm the diagnosis as rapidly as possible so that appropriate treatment may be undertaken without delay.

Computed Tomography. The CT scan is the diagnostic procedure of choice. The epidural accumulation appears as a lentiform area of blood density in the extracerebral space and is associated with shift of the lateral ventricles to the contralateral side. On occasion, epidural hematomas may resemble a subdural hematoma. Both supratentorial and infratentorial epidural hematomas have a lentiform configuration.

Occasional cases of subfrontal epidural hematoma have a unique and typical configuration in which the classic lentiform configuration is seen in the frontal lobe region but there is only *minimal* shift of the midline structures in spite of the rather large appearing mass (Figs. 13–52 and 13–53). The blood accumulates in the subfrontal region and displaces the brain upward and posteriorly; consequently, the anterior cerebral artery is displaced upward and posteriorly in much the same way as with a subfrontal meningioma. CT scans done in the coronal section are very helpful in confirming the diagnosis of a subfrontal epidural hematoma (Fig. 13–52) but are not necessary for diagnosis when the axial CT scan demonstrates the typical appearance of this disorder. The use of high window widths and window levels may help in the identification of small skull fractures.

Arteriography. The arteriographic changes seen with an epidural hematoma are much the same as those seen with subdural hematomas, and the same diagnostic principles apply. In general, it is nearly impossible to make an absolute differential diagnosis between the two types of abnormalities. Only *rarely* will one be able to demonstrate that the middle meningeal artery is displaced away from the inner table of the skull. This finding, in association with an extracerebral accumulation of blood, will enable one to make the diagnosis of epidural hematoma.

Since the epidural hematoma is outside the dura, one may also see separation of the superior sagittal sinus away from the inner table of the skull by an epidural accumulation of blood that extends across the midline. This is in contradistinction to subdural hematomas, which do not cross the midline but are limited by the falx cerebri.

In the posterior fossa, the torcular and lateral sinuses also may be displaced away from the inner table (Fig. 13–55). Subtraction films may be helpful and sometimes necessary to evaluate these subtle posterior fossa changes.

BIRTH TRAUMA

Trauma to the head at the time of birth may result in subarachnoid hemorrhage and subsequent enlargement of the lateral ventricles secondary to communicating hydrocephalus. There may be actual post-traumatic intracerebral hematoma formation. In addition, other post-traumatic abnormalities such as subdural hematomas also may be evaluated by the CT scan.

Figure 13–60 illustrates a caput succedaneum along the left side of the cranial vault *(arrows)* — in this case associated with large ventricles secondary to subarachnoid hemorrhage and a resulting communicating hydrocephalus.

POSTOPERATIVE TRAUMA

It is not uncommon to observe subdural extracerebral accumulations on CT scans performed following shunting procedures in patients with markedly or even moderately dilated ventricles. Generally speaking, these subdural accumulations do not cause clinically significant changes in the patients' condition;

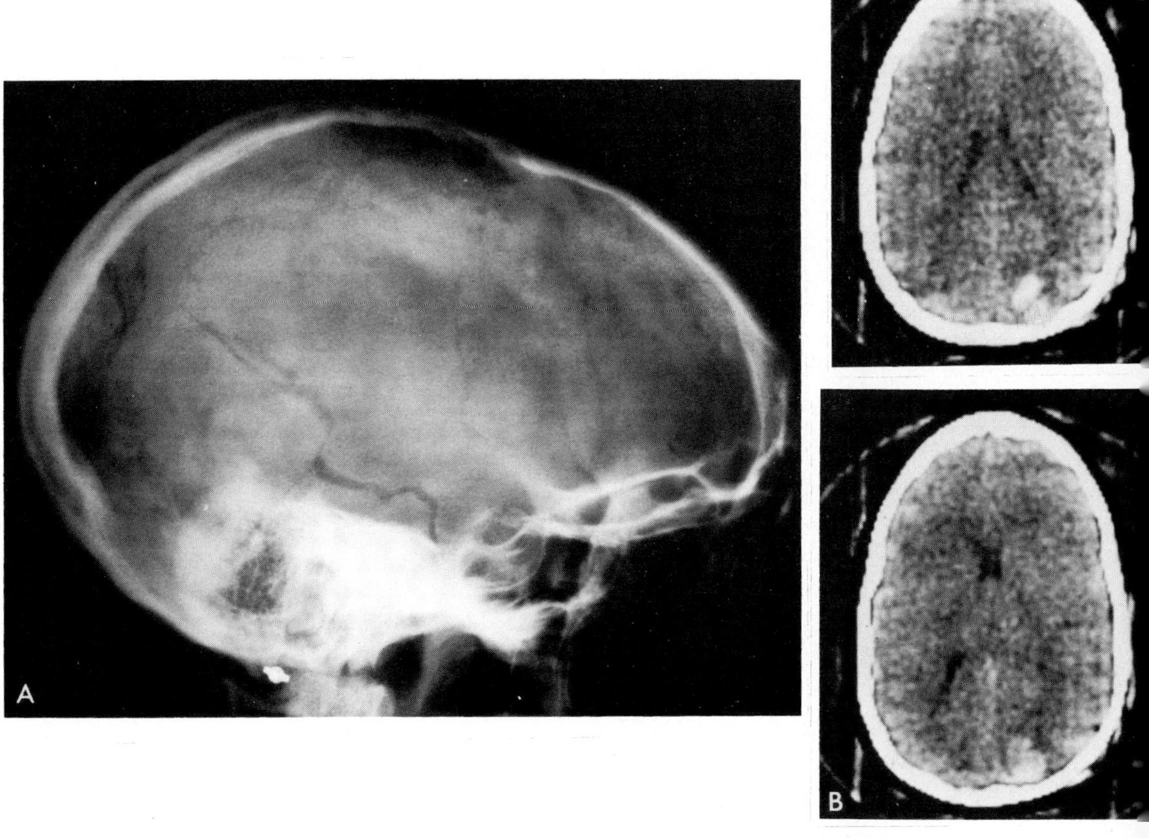

Figure 13–1. LINEAR SKULL FRACTURE: *A*, The linear skull fracture extends from the squamous portion of the temporal bone posteriorly to the posterior parietal bone. There is diastasis of the fracture fragments, and the fracture line has a wavy configuration. There is a second fracture high in the posterior parietal region just above the lambdoid suture.

B, The CT scan reveals a small intracerebral hematoma in the right occipital pole just beneath the inner table of the skull. There is a small amount of surrounding edema and slight compression of the right lateral ventricle.

indeed, the clinical condition is so improved by the shunt procedure that small changes in condition probably are not appreciated. These subdural accumulations are not uncommon, but their incidence was not appreciated until the development of CT scanning and, with it, the ability to follow these patients without the need for invasive procedures. On rare occasions these extracerebral accumulations have been treated with moderate success with subdural shunt tubes. In other cases, this treatment has resulted in re-expansion of the lateral ventricles (Fig. 13–61).

If a craniotomy has been performed, the CT scan will reflect the type of procedure done. The CT scan will reflect these changes following removal of cerebral tissues for decompression or tumor removal.

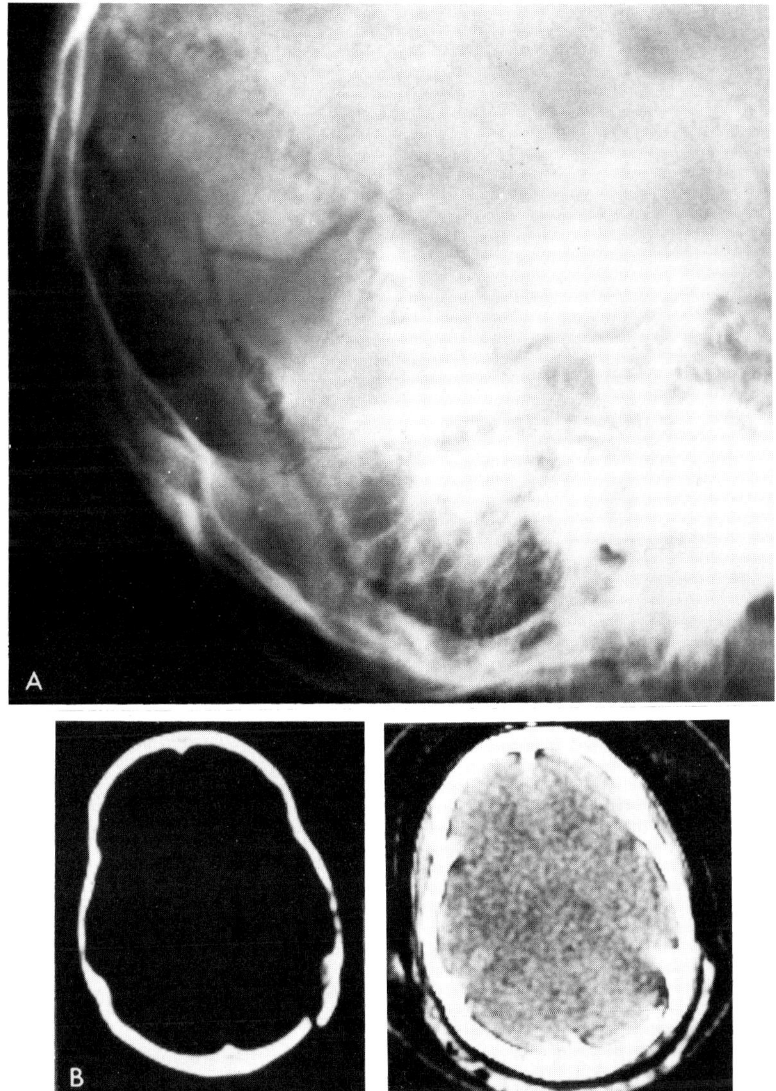

Figure 13–2. DEPRESSED FRACTURE, RIGHT OCCIPITAL: *A*, The plain skull film reveals an irregular fracture line extending from above the mastoid air cells posteriorly and then superiorly through the lambdoid suture and into the occipital bone.

B, The CT scan reveals diastasis of the fracture and depression of the occipital bone at the point of the fracture. There is no evidence of intracerebral hematoma.

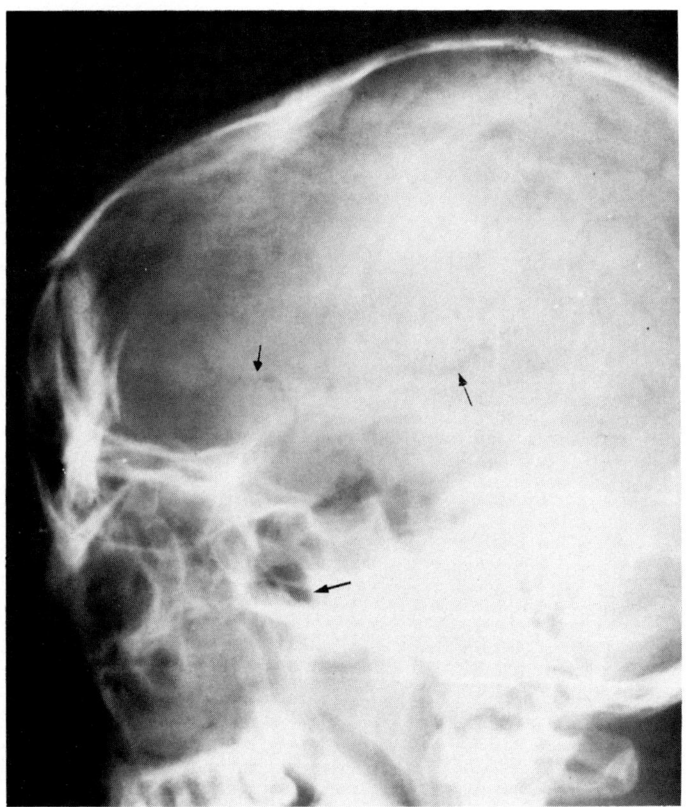

Figure 13–3. COMMINUTED DEPRESSED SKULL FRACTURE AND TRAUMATIC PNEUMOCEPHALUS: There is a large comminuted and depressed fracture in the frontal region. Air is noted in the suprasellar cisterns, and a small amount of air outlines the cerebral gyri *(small arrows)*. The horizontal beam lateral view reveals an air-fluid level in the sphenoid sinus *(large arrowhead)* secondary to CSF or blood in the sphenoid sinus. Note the complete opacification of the paranasal sinuses secondary to hemorrhage and multiple associated facial bone fractures.

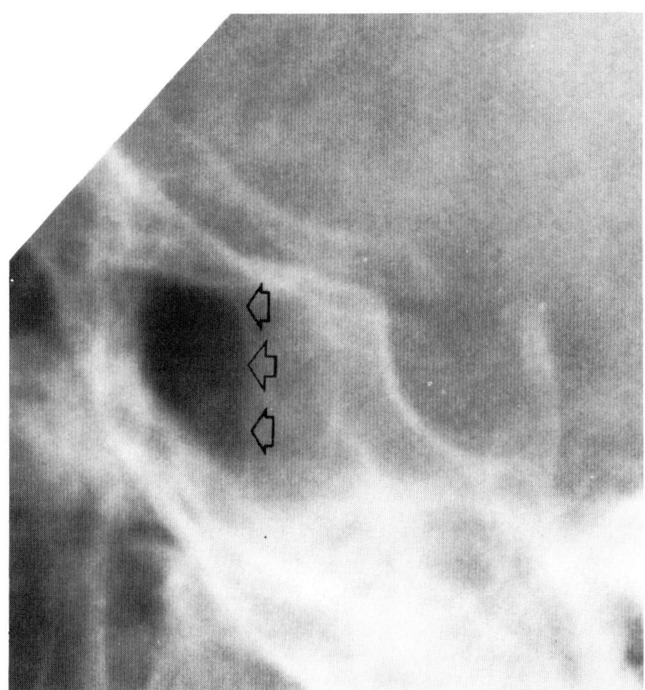

Figure 13–4. AIR-FLUID LEVEL SPHENOID SINUS SECONDARY TO TRAUMA: Films are obtained with the patients in the supine position; thus, air-fluid levels are demonstrated on the horizontal beam "shoot-through" lateral views. The arrows outline an air-fluid level in the sphenoid sinus secondary to either CSF or blood in the sinus following a base-of-the-skull fracture.

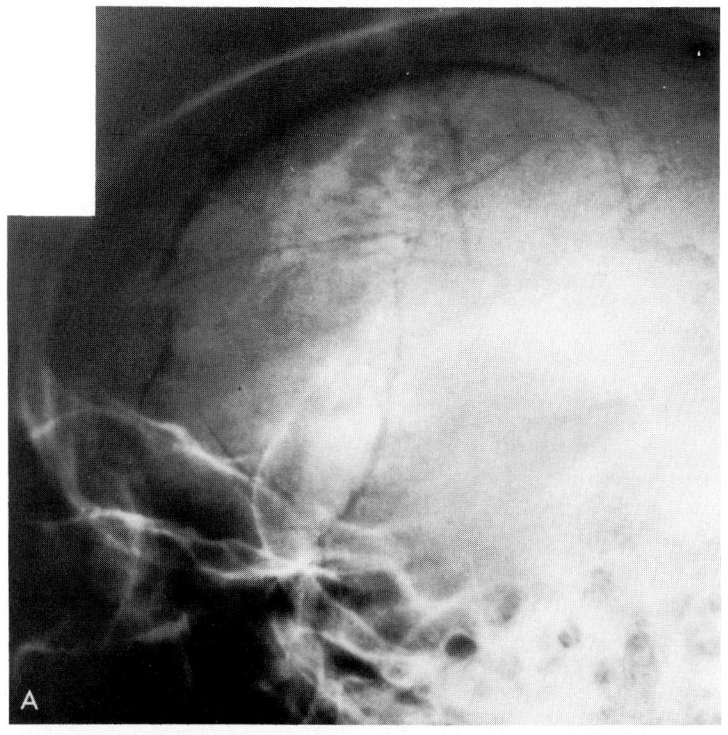

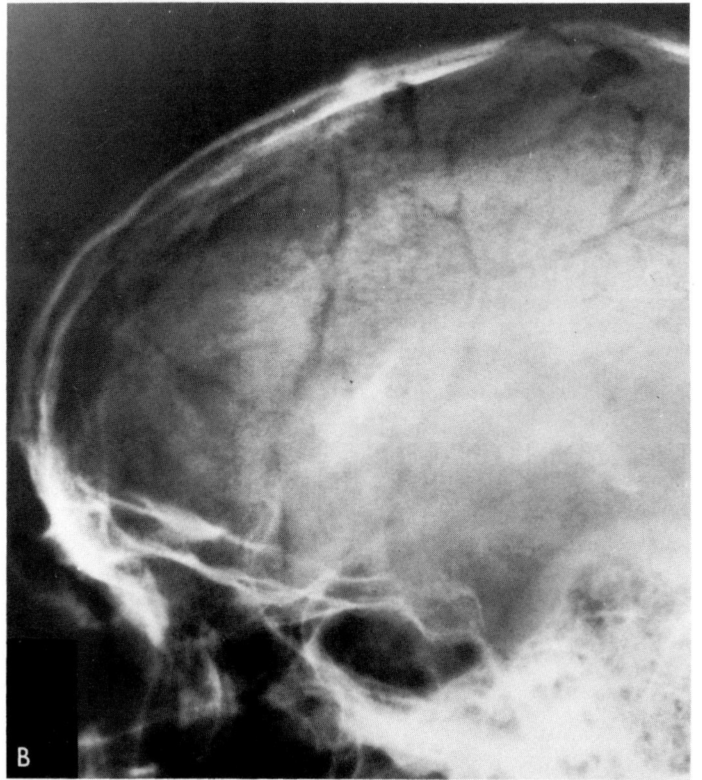

Figure 13–5. COMMINUTED SKULL FRACTURE WITH HEALING: *A*, The initial plain skull films show a comminuted skull fracture involving the frontal and anterior parietal regions.

B, Follow-up examination six months later reveals that the fracture lines have become indistinct owing to secondary bony overgrowth at the fracture sites. Bony union does not occur with callus formation.

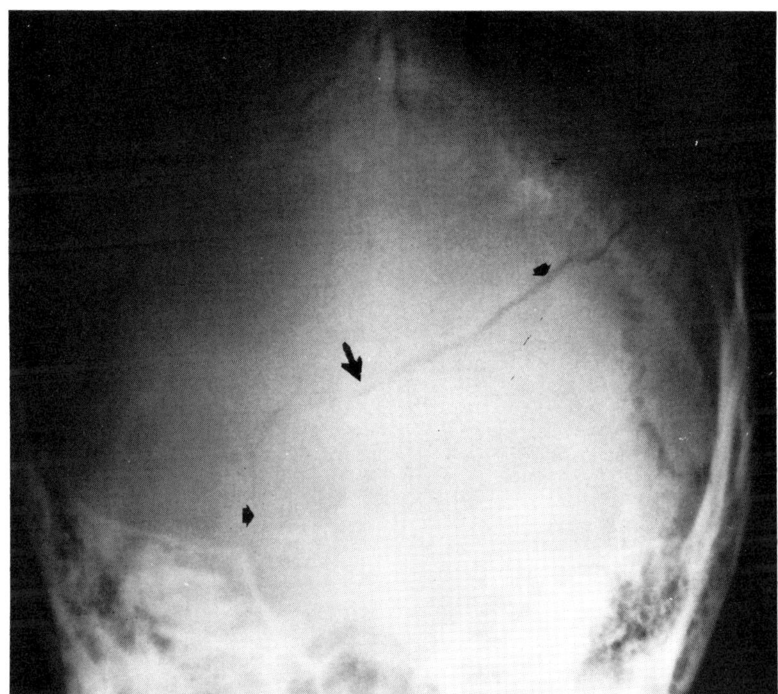

Figure 13–6. LINEAR FRACTURE OF THE OCCIPITAL BONE: The plain film examination reveals a long, diastatic fracture that extends from the left posterior parietal region inferiorly and obliquely across the occipital bone, through the torcular (*large arrow*) and into the foramen magnum (*small arrows*). See also Figure 13–55. This fracture was associated with a posterior fossa epidural hematoma and a contra-coup contusion of the right frontal and parietal lobes.

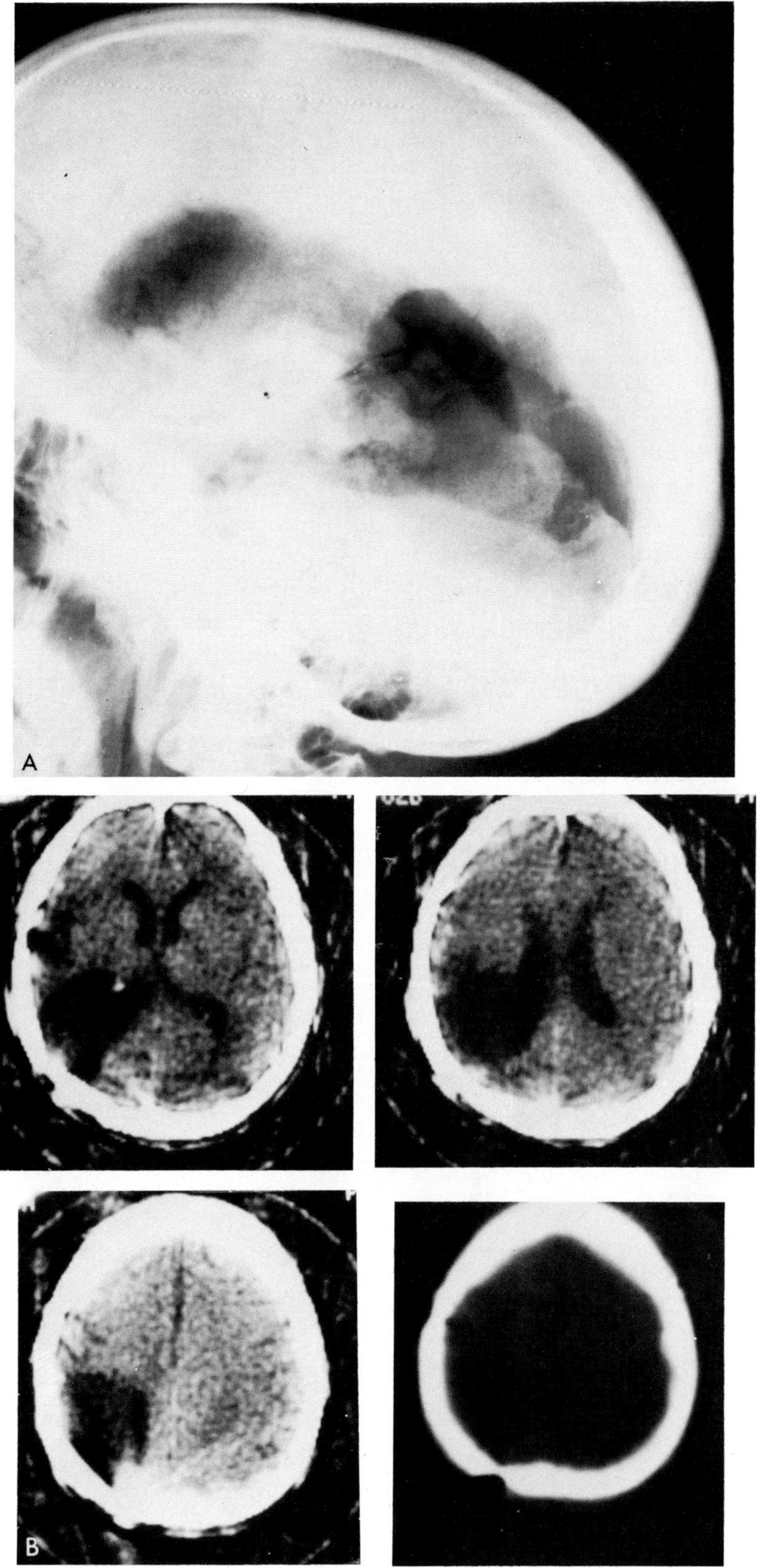

Figure 13–7 *See legend on the opposite page*

Figure 13–7. POST-TRAUMATIC PORENCEPHALIC CYST ASSOCIATED WITH A LEPTOMENINGEAL CYST: *A*, This leptomeningeal cyst is associated with a large porencephalic cyst that fills with air following pneumoencephalography. This right lateral decubitus view also demonstrated the enlarged lateral ventricle secondary to cerebral hemiatrophy.

B, The CT scan of a similar case reveals a porencephalic cyst in the left posterior parietal region that appears to communicate with the occipital horn of the left lateral ventricle. Postoperative changes are also present in the parietal region on the left side. (See also Chapter 2.)

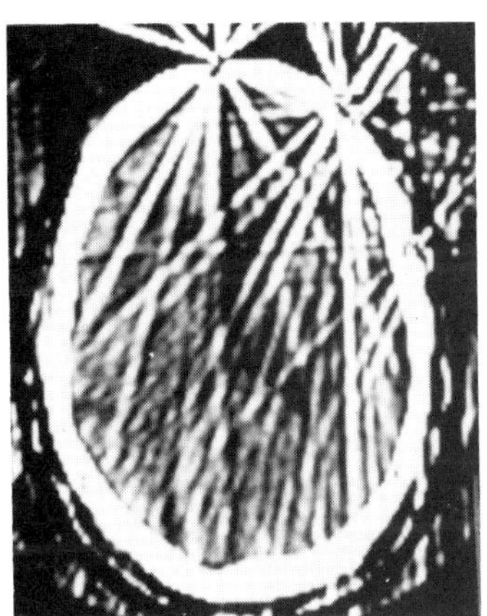
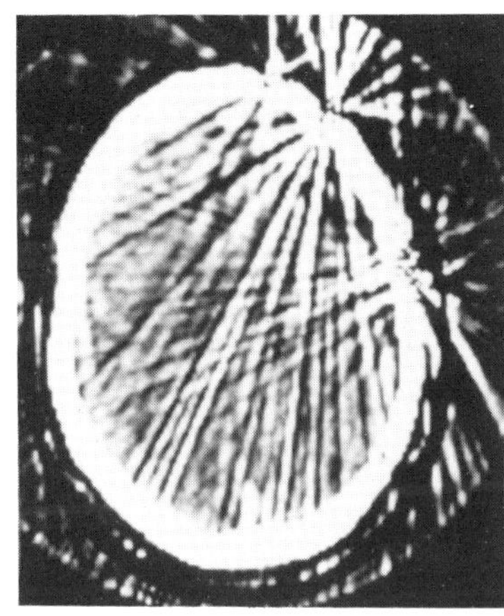
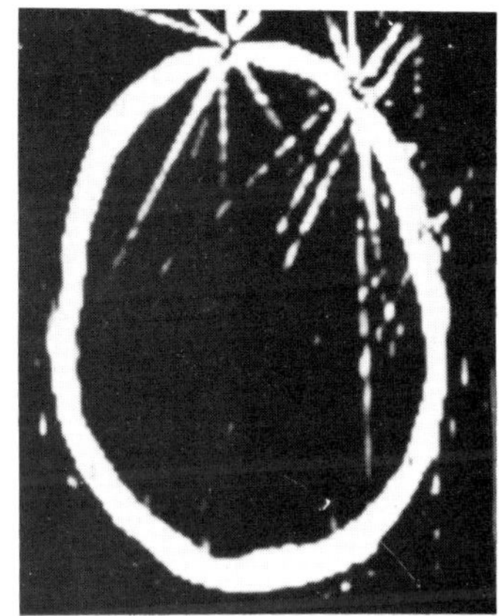

Figure 13–8. GUNSHOT WOUNDS TO SCALP: Multiple shotgun pellets are scattered throughout the scalp. No bullet fragments are inside the bony calvaria: note the computer artifact from the metallic bullets. These pieces of metal may degrade the image to such an extent that the scan is virtually unreadable.

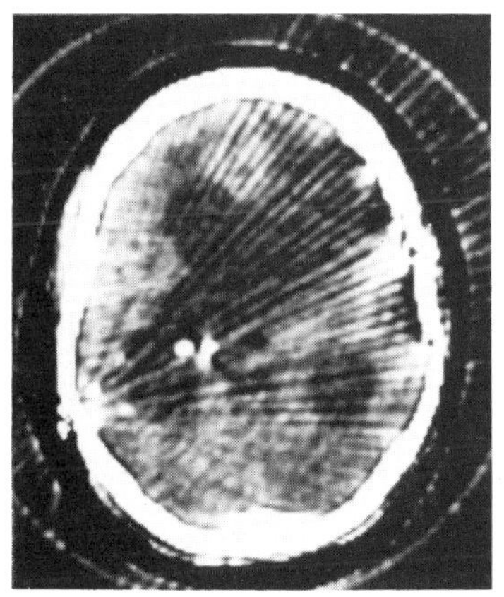
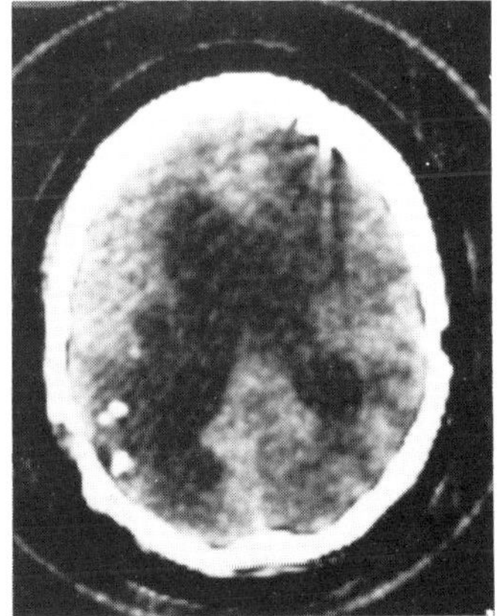

Figure 13–9. GUNSHOT WOUND TO HEAD: The irregularities in the right anterior parietal and left posterior parietal regions represent both the entrance and exit wounds of gunshots. In addition, there are multiple retained bullet fragments within the brain. Note the hydrocephalus — probably the result of a communicating hydrocephalus secondary to subarachnoid hemorrhage — and the multiple scattered areas of radiolucency secondary to brain damage from the gunshots.

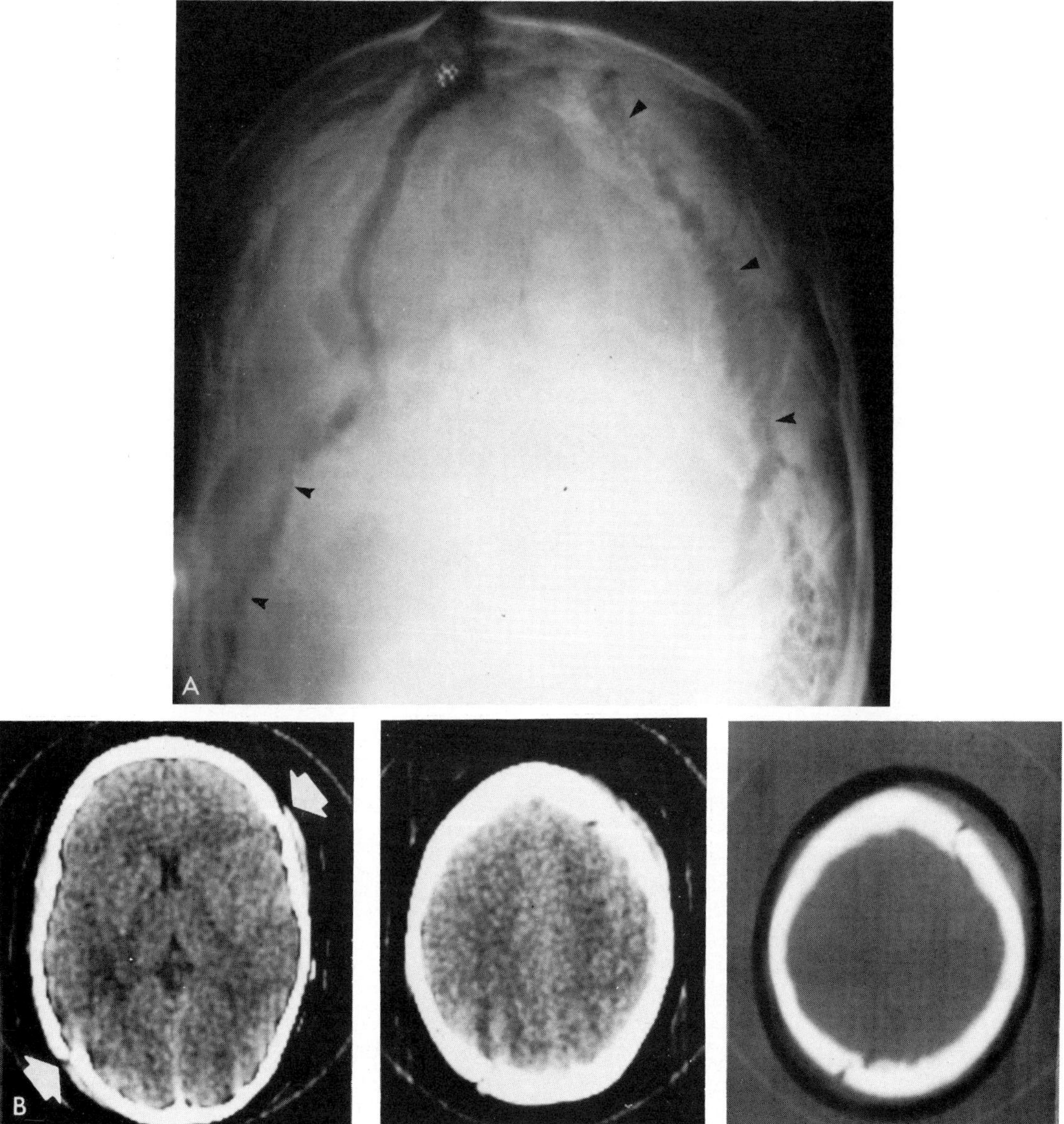

Figure 13–10. LONG LINEAR FRACTURE: *A,* A long linear fracture is noted to extend from the right posterior frontal to the left posterior parietal region. There is some diastasis of the fracture line. Extracranial soft tissue swelling is noted, but the cranial contents appear to be within normal limits.

B, The fracture and its true extent are readily demonstrated on the CT scan viewed at high window width.

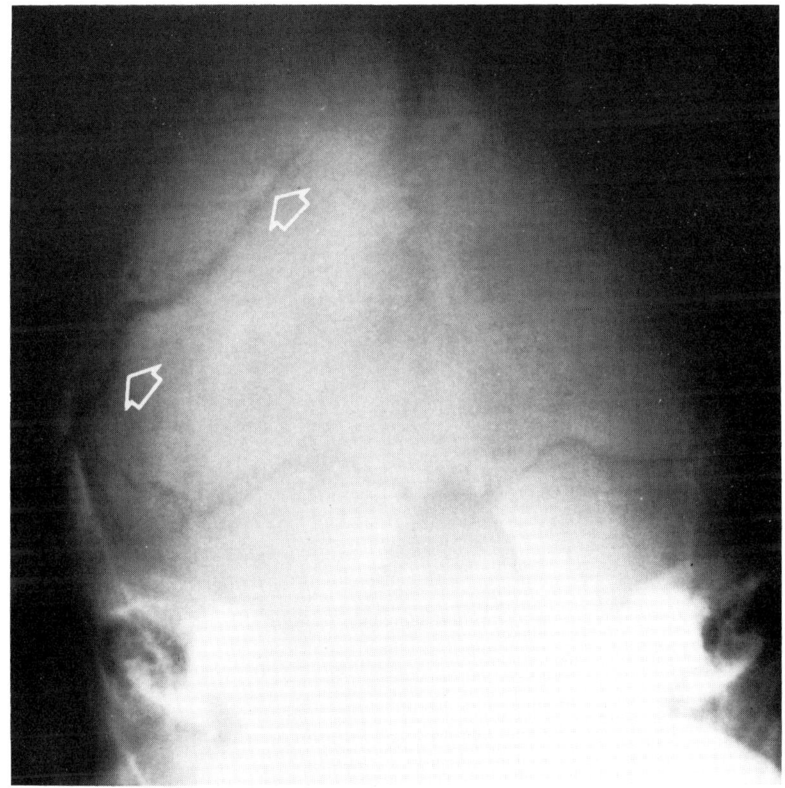

Figure 13–11. OCCIPITAL FRACTURE SIMULATING MENDOSAL SUTURE IN A CHILD: A linear fracture extends across the occipital bone on one side *(arrows)*. The normal mendosal suture is usually bilateral and originates at the posterolateral fontanelle. The mendosal suture is frequently mistaken for a fracture. (See Chapter 2.)

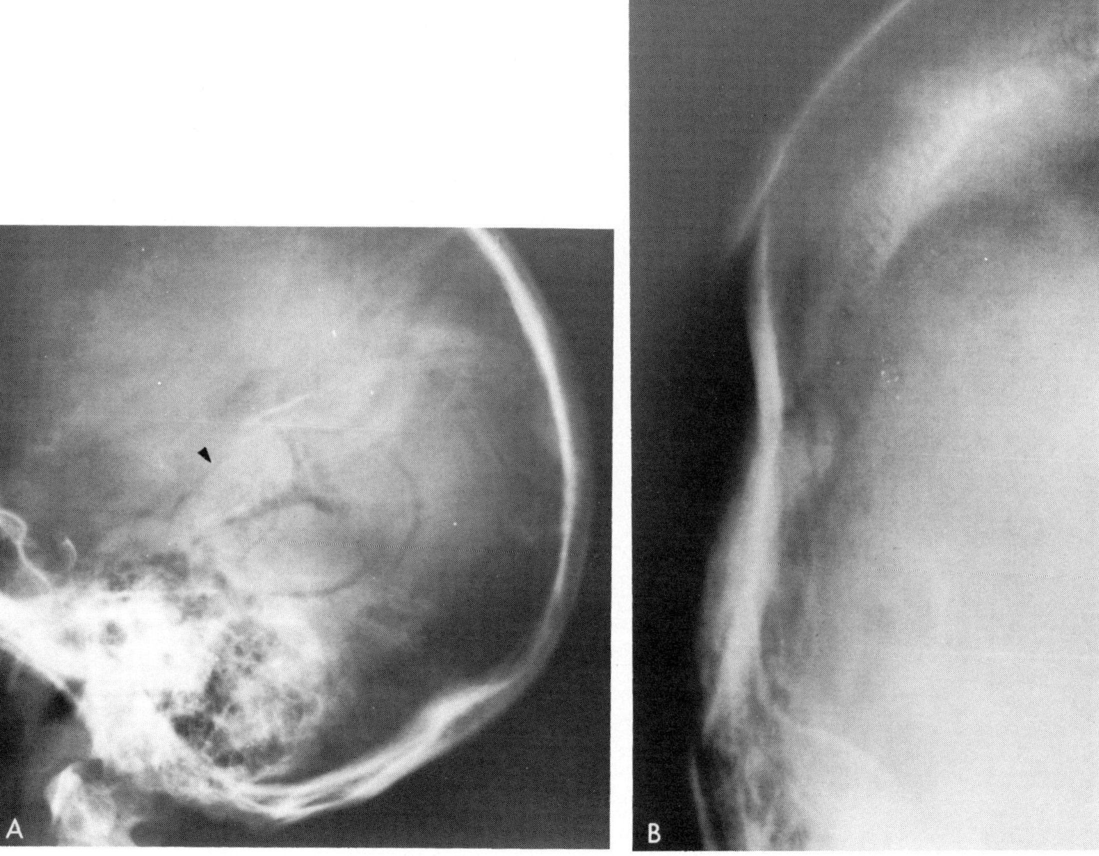

Figure 13–12. DEPRESSED FRACTURE: *A,* The patient has sustained a sharp blow to the calvaria that has resulted in a round and stellate fracture that is depressed in the center portion.

B, The tangential view affords the best method to evaluate the amount of depression of the bony fragments. If the depression of the fracture is greater than 5 mm, it is elevated surgically.

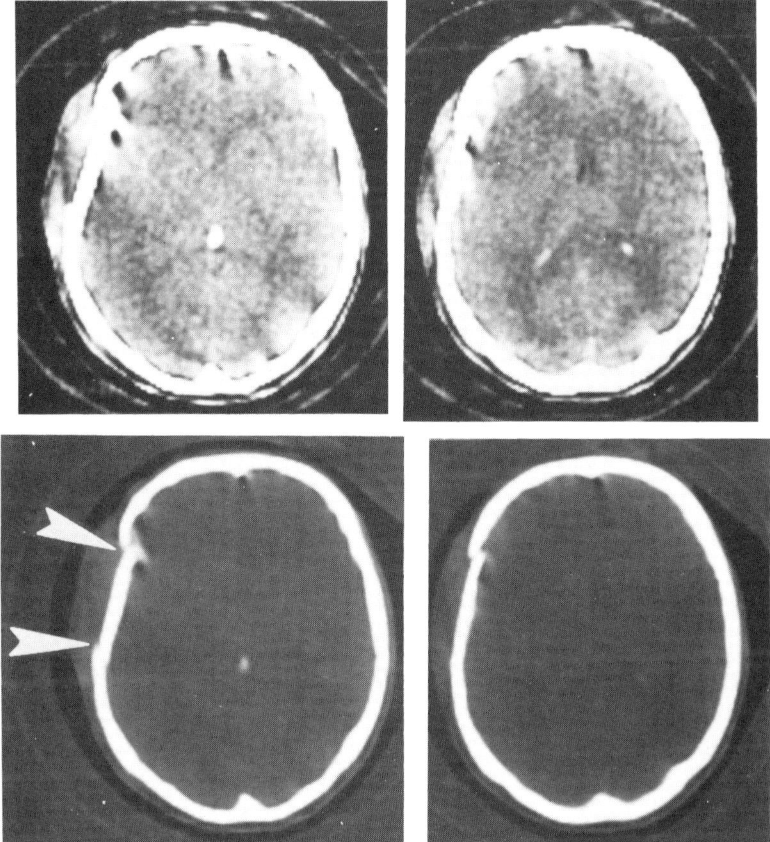

Figure 13–13. DEPRESSED SKULL FRACTURE: There is a large depressed skull fracture in the left posterior frontal region. Note the large extracranial hematoma and swelling of the left hemisphere with very slight shift of the frontal horns to the right side.

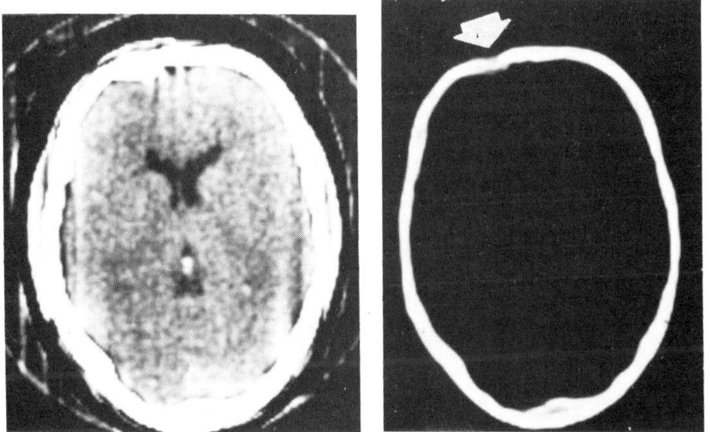

Figure 13–14. SMALL DEPRESSED FRACTURE: A very small depressed fracture in the left parasagittal frontal region is associated with minimal soft tissue swelling. The cranial contents are normal.

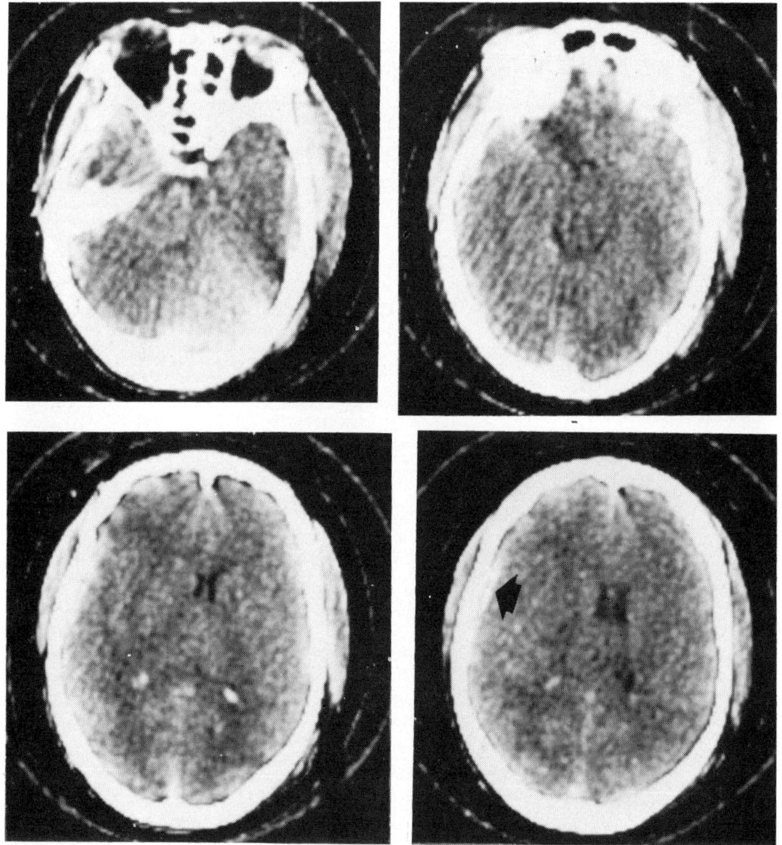

Figure 13–15. ACUTE HEAD TRAUMA: There are bilateral extracranial hematomas and a small left acute subdural hematoma with slight shift to the contralateral side.

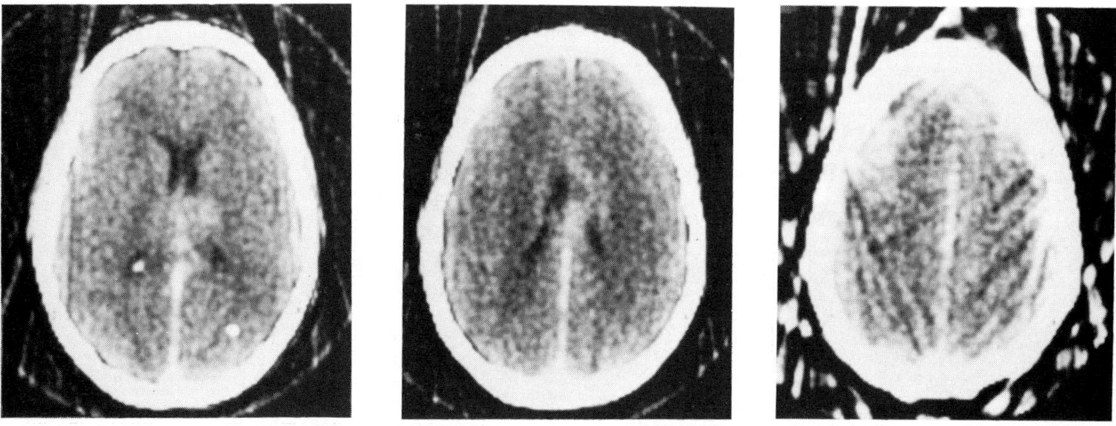

Figure 13–16. DIFFUSE INTRACRANIAL SWELLING: Following a motor vehicle accident this patient developed decerebrate rigidity. The frontal horns and bodies of the lateral ventricles are slightly distorted and compressed to the midline secondary to diffuse intracranial swelling. There is evidence of hemorrhage into the cerebrum deep in the right hemisphere and extending to the right of the midline. This compressed the midportion of the body of the right lateral ventricle. In addition, blood in the subarachnoid space outlines the falx cerebri. (The appearance is similar to that of a postinfusion scan, although the patient has not received an injection of contrast material.)

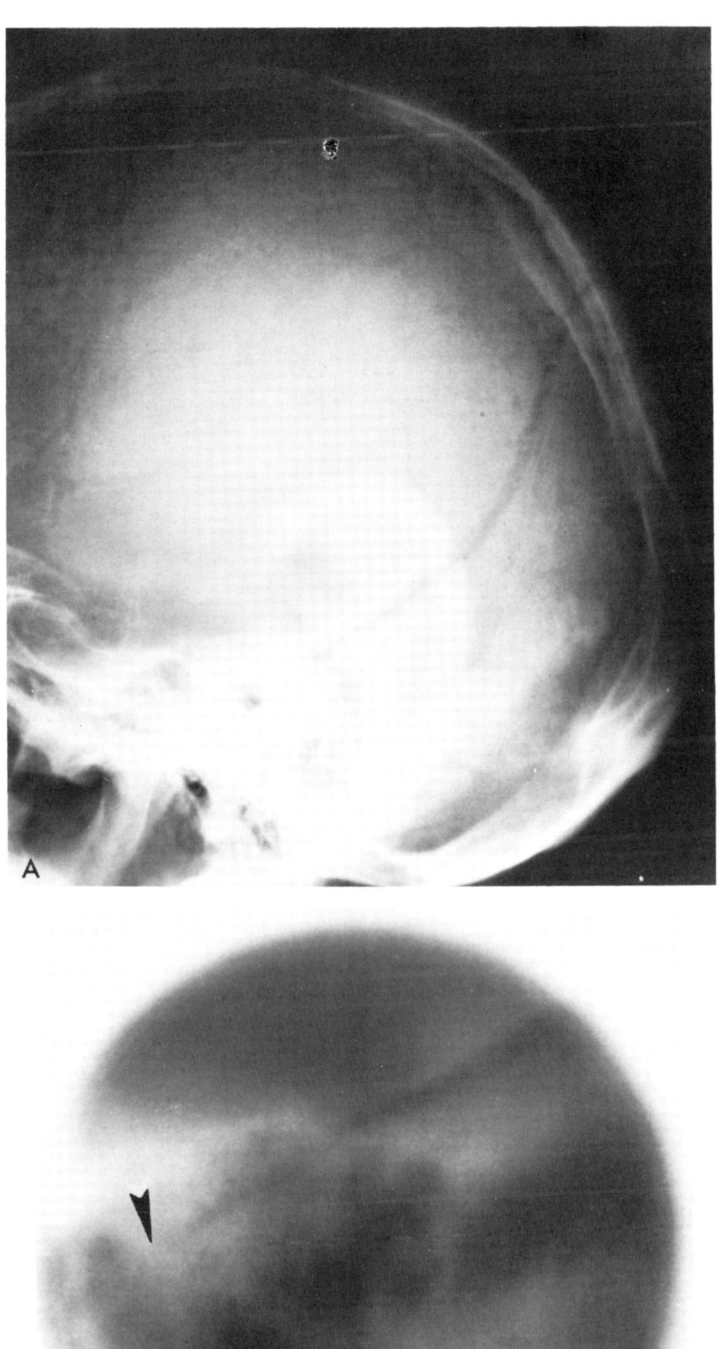

Figure 13–17. SKULL FRACTURE ASSOCIATED WITH A FRACTURE OF THE BASE OF THE SKULL: *A*, This patient presented with CSF otorrhea following severe head trauma. A long linear fracture extends into the petrous bone.

B, The tomogram of the petrous bone best demonstrates the fracture extending into the base of the skull.

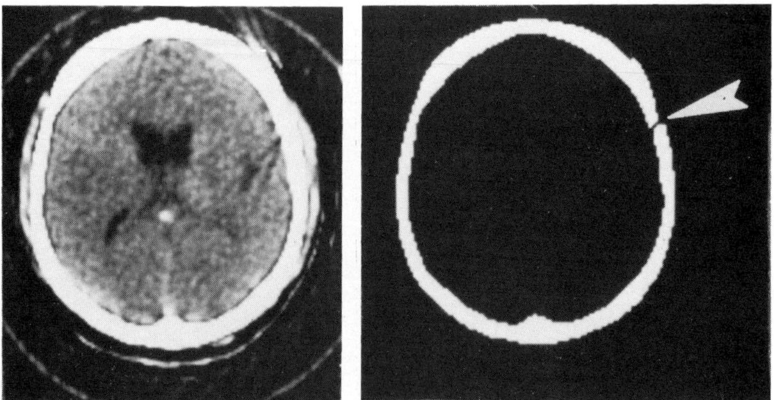

Figure 13–18. LINEAR SKULL FRACTURE: The standard CT appears normal, but the linear fracture is visible by using a high window width and window level.

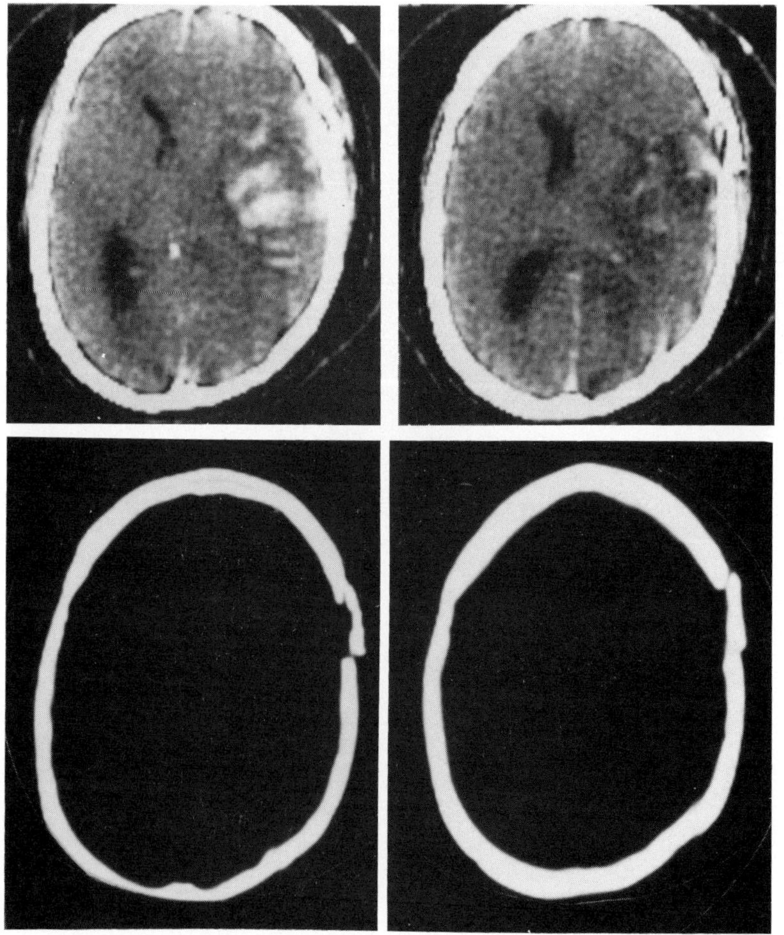

Figure 13–19. COMMINUTED SKULL FRACTURE WITH INTRACRANIAL HEMATOMA: The CT on standard viewing reveals intracerebral hemorrhage and edema and some irregularity of the bony calvaria. On the measure mode the comminuted skull fracture is readily identified.

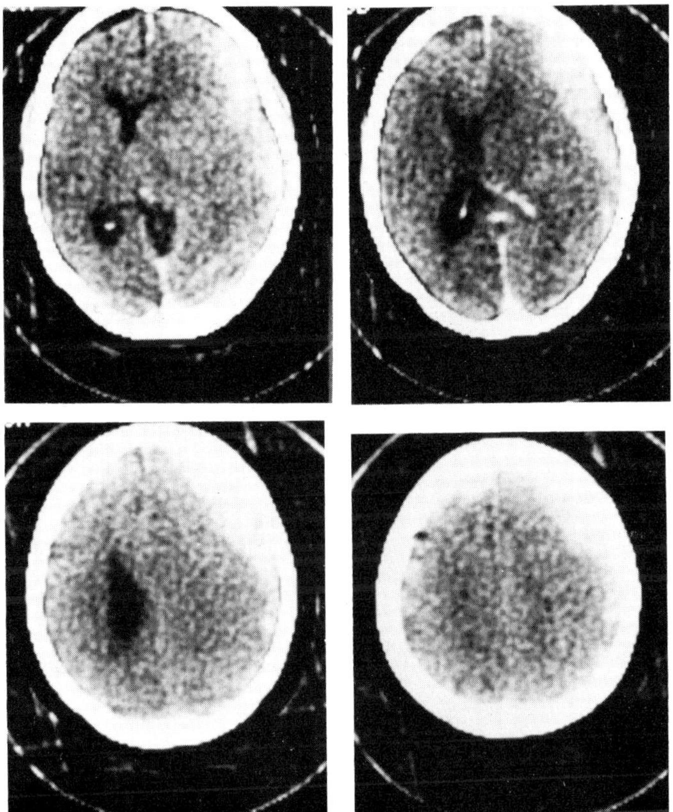

Figure 13–20. ACUTE SUBDURAL HEMATOMA: An area of blood density is seen outside the cerebrum on the right side. It has a crescentic configuration. There is shift to the contralateral side and compression of the right lateral ventricle.

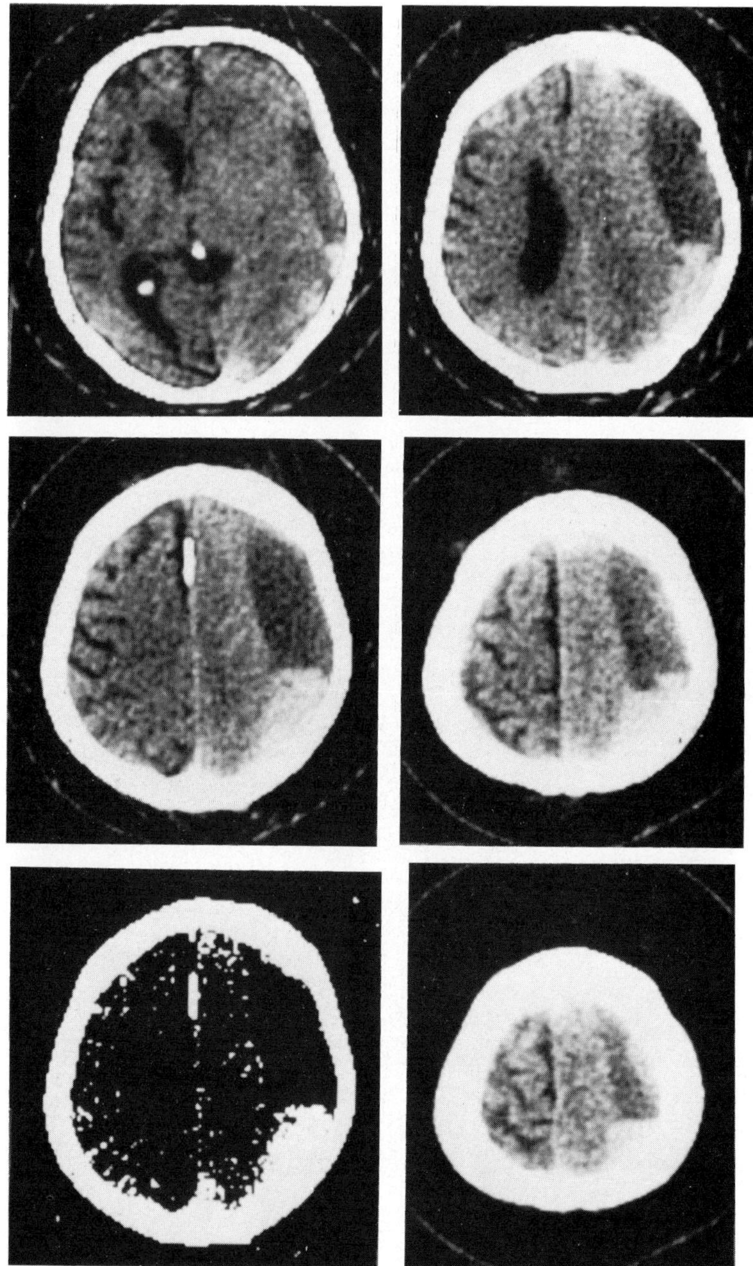

Figure 13–21. ACUTE SUBDURAL HEMATOMA WITH "HEMATOCRIT" LEVELS: The CT scan reveals a large right subdural hematoma, which, because the patient had been placed in the supine position for prolonged periods, has settled, giving a "hematocrit" to the blood in the hematoma. There is shift to the contralateral side and obliteration of the cortical sulci on the side of the hematoma.

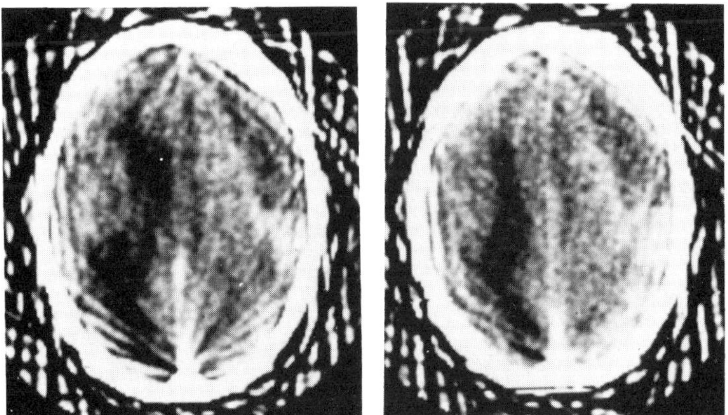

Figure 13–22. ACUTE SUBDURAL HEMATOMA WITH "HEMATOCRIT" LEVEL: There is a large right subdural accumulation of blood with a hematocrit level and shift to the contralateral side. The falx is also well outlined — probably secondary to blood in the subarachnoid space. The scan is degraded by patient motion artifact.

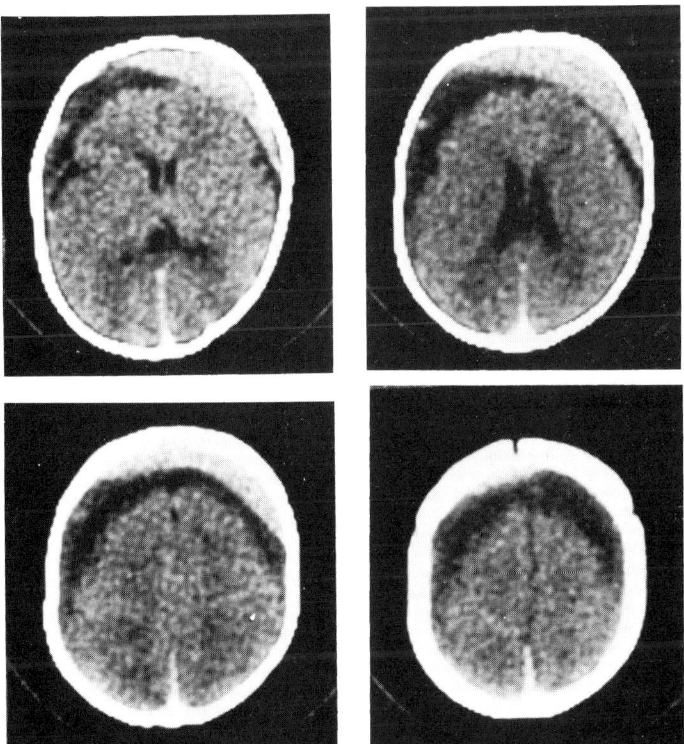

Figure 13–23. BIFRONTAL SUBDURAL HEMATOMA WITH "HEMATOCRIT" LEVELS: Bifrontal subdural hematomas demonstrate the "hematocrit levels" in the frontal region because the baby slept on its stomach and right frontal region.

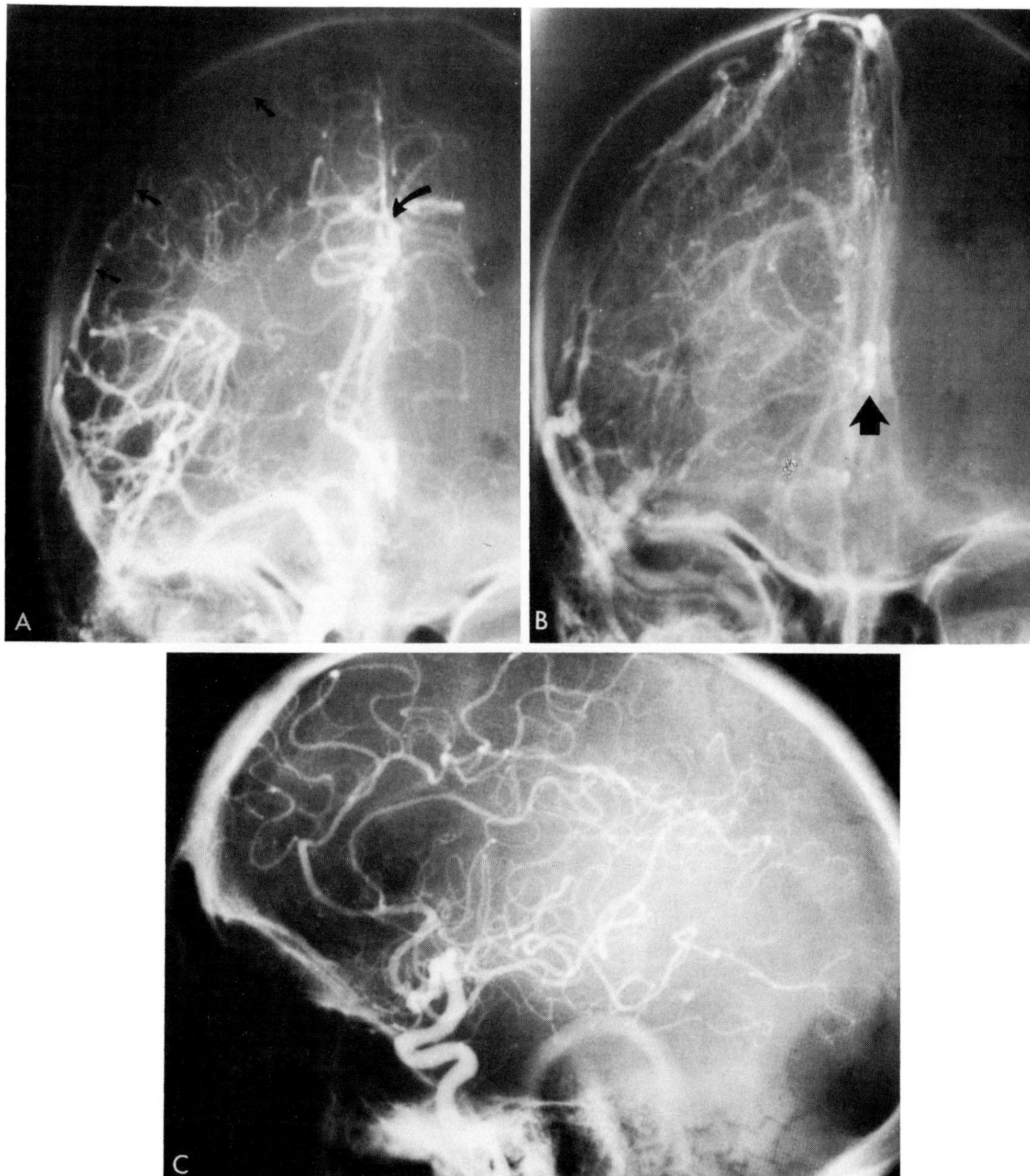

Figure 13–24. ACUTE BILATERAL SUBDURAL HEMATOMAS: *A*, The right carotid arteriogram reveals a crescentic extracerebral accumulation of blood *(small arrows)*. The branches of the middle cerebral artery are displaced by blood away from the inner table of the skull. There is slight shift of the anterior cerebral artery under the falx to the contralateral side *(curved arrow)*.

B, The venous phase also shows displacement of the veins away from the inner table by the blood in the subdural space, but it does not reveal shift of the internal cerebral veins.

C, The lateral view appears essentially normal.

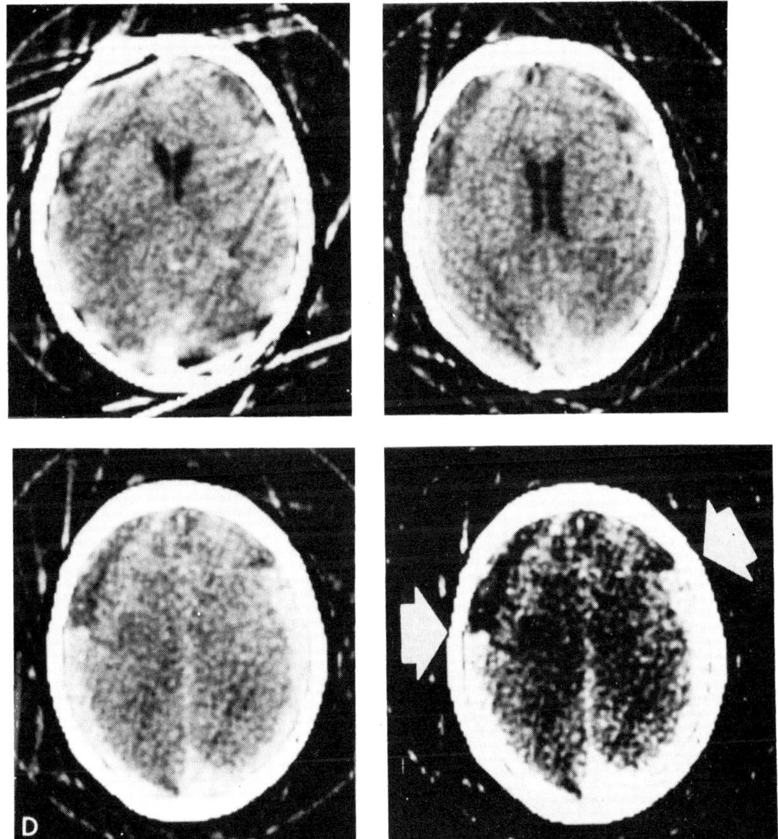

Figure 13–24 *Continued.*

D, The CT scan reveals bilateral crescentic subdural hematomas with "hematocrit" levels, and compression of the lateral ventricles and elongation secondary to the acute hematomas. Because of the bilateral nature of the abnormality, there is no shift of the internal cerebral vein on the arteriogram.

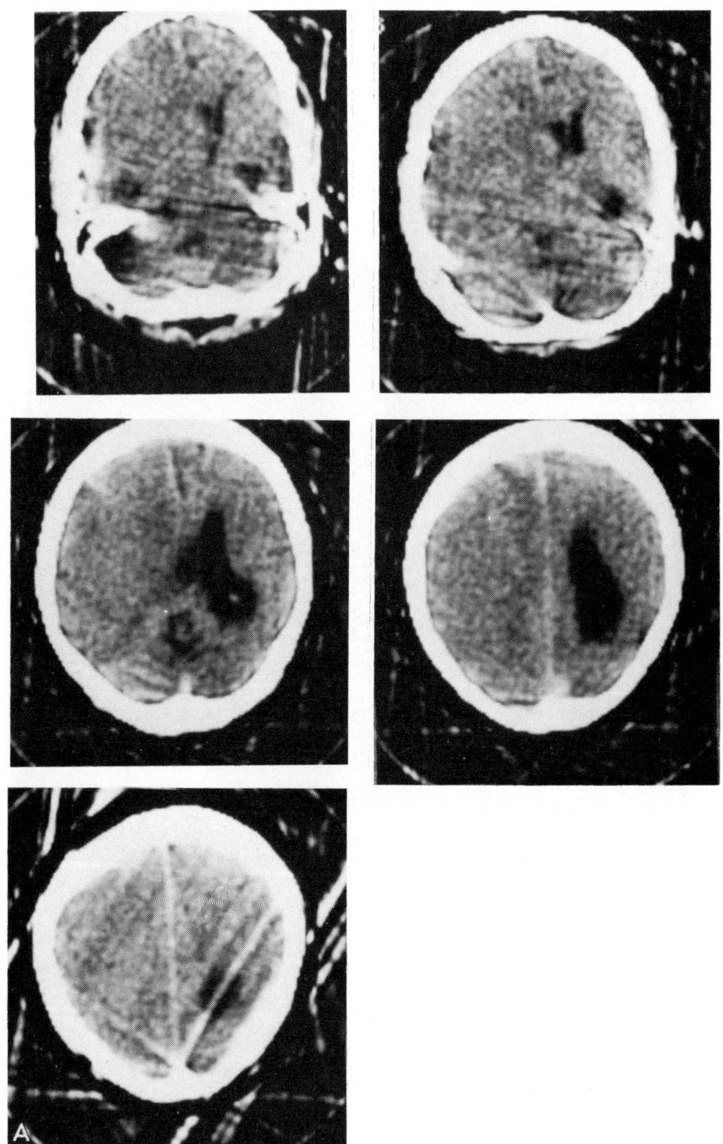

Figure 13–25. ISODENSE SUBDURAL HEMATOMA: *A,* The CT scan reveals marked shift from left to right. There is compression of the body of the left lateral ventricle, but no definite masses or extracerebral accumulations of blood can be identified. There is minimal evidence of edema just to the left of the midline on the 2A and 2B cuts.

The AP arterial *(B)* and venous *(C)* phases of the left carotid arteriogram reveal a crescentic extracerebral accumulation of blood in the high convexity parietal region on the left side *(arrows)*. There is downward displacement of the sylvian point, and proximal and distal shift of the anterior cerebral artery to the contralateral side can be seen.

D and *E,* The right brachial arteriogram reveals shift toward the right side *(arrow)*, and the lateral view shows marked stretching of the anterior cerebral artery and spasm of multiple vessels — probably from blood in the subarachnoid space.

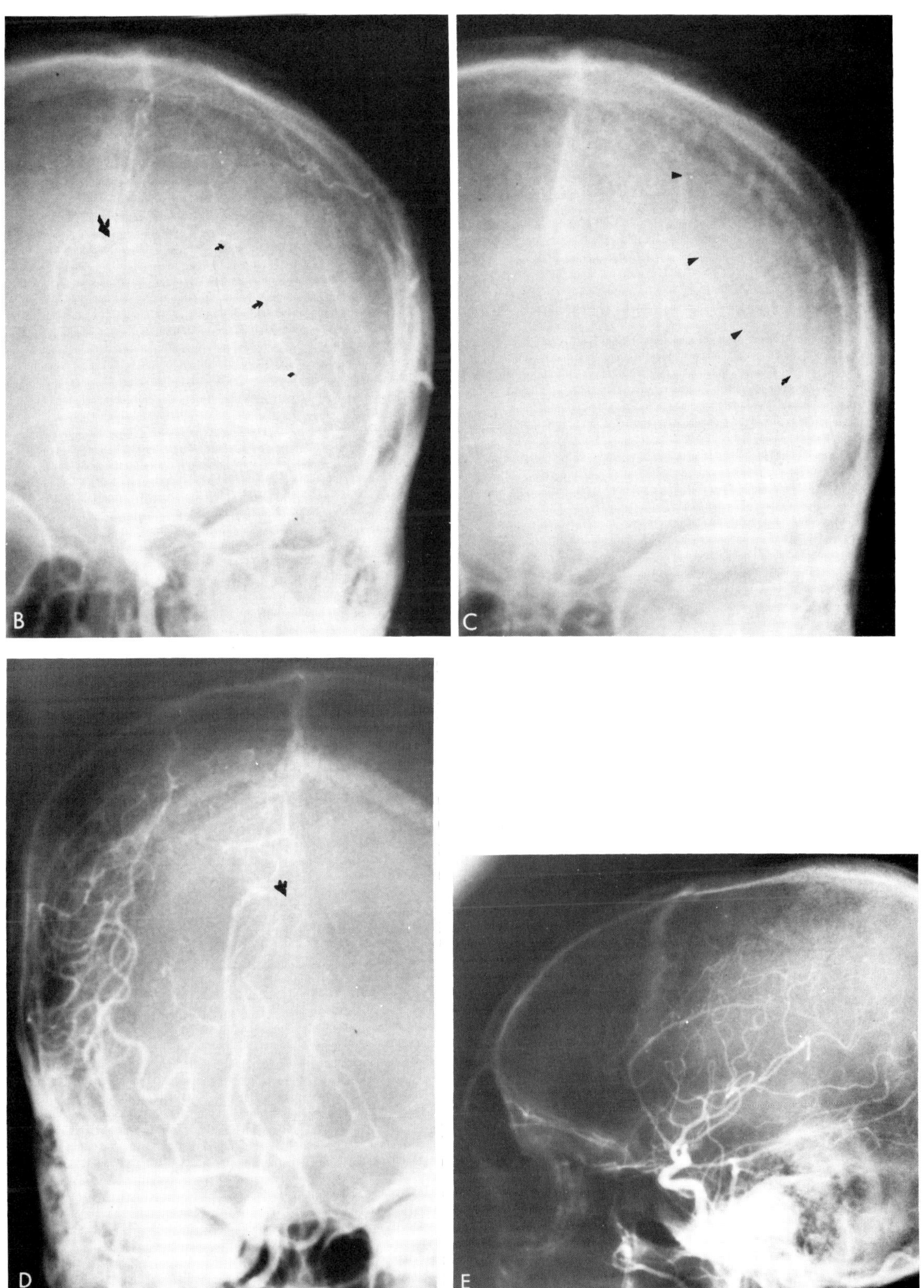

Figure 13–25 *Continued*

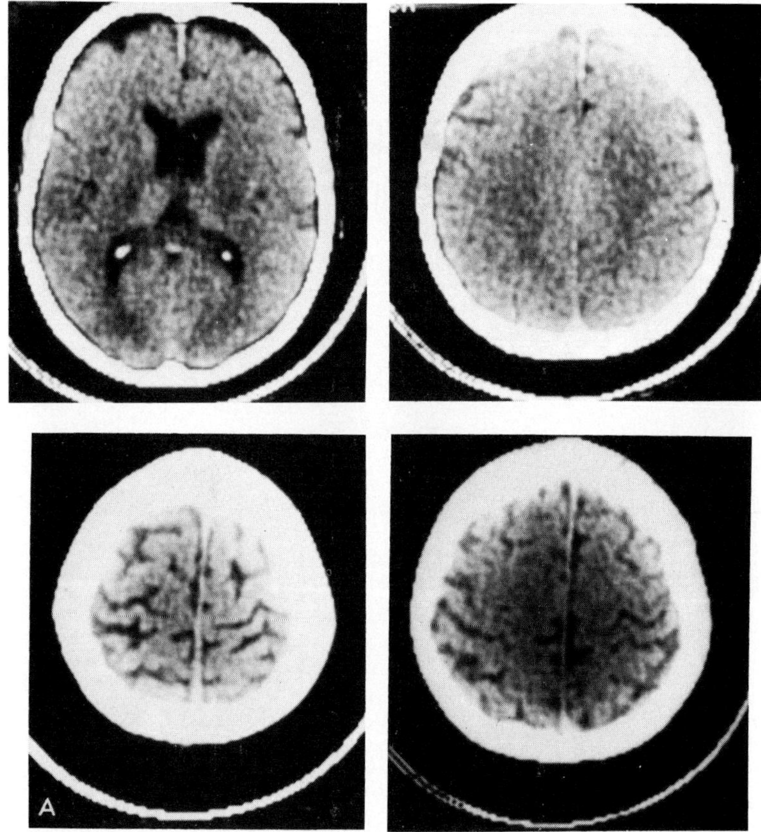

Figure 13–26. CT SHOWING DEVELOPMENT OF A SUBDURAL HEMATOMA: *A*, The initial CT scan was performed because of symptoms of dizziness and right arm tingling. The scan shows mild atrophy with enlargement of the lateral ventricles and the cortical sulci.

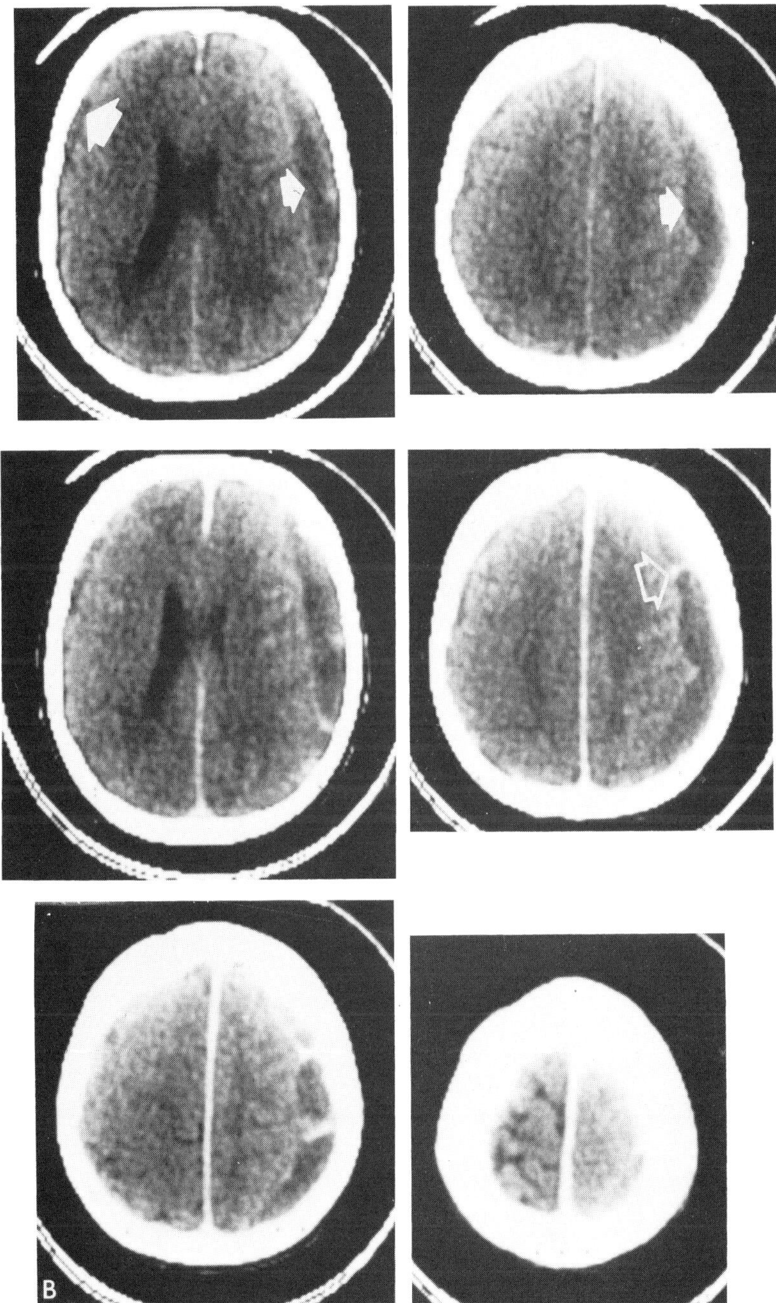

Figure 13–26 *Continued*

B, The follow-up scan two months later reveals a large, chronic right subdural hematoma *(small arrowheads)* and a small, chronic left subdural hematoma *(large arrowhead)* in the left frontal region. Postinfusion, there is enhancement of a membrane around the hematoma and displacement of the cortical vein away from the inner table of the skull *(open arrow)* on the right side. Note also the obliteration of the cortical sulci on the right side as compared to the left — and compared to the initial scan performed two months earlier.

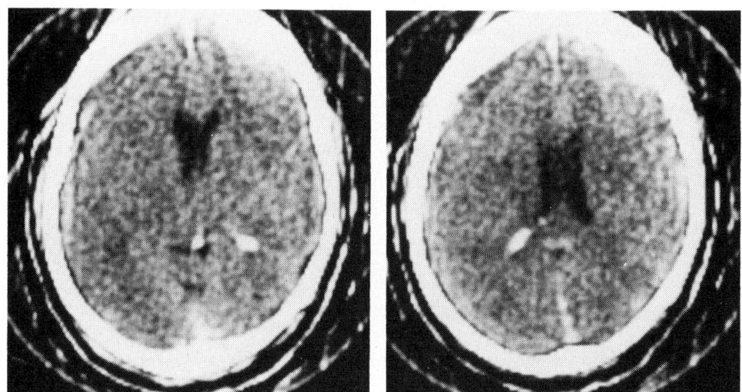

Figure 13–27. BILATERAL ISODENSE SUBDURAL HEMATOMAS: The lateral ventricles are compressed toward the midline and appear elongated secondary to pressure from the bilateral subdural hematomas. There is no real shift of the midline because the accumulations are approximately equal in size. Bilateral, isodense subdural accumulations are easily overlooked on the routine CT scan.

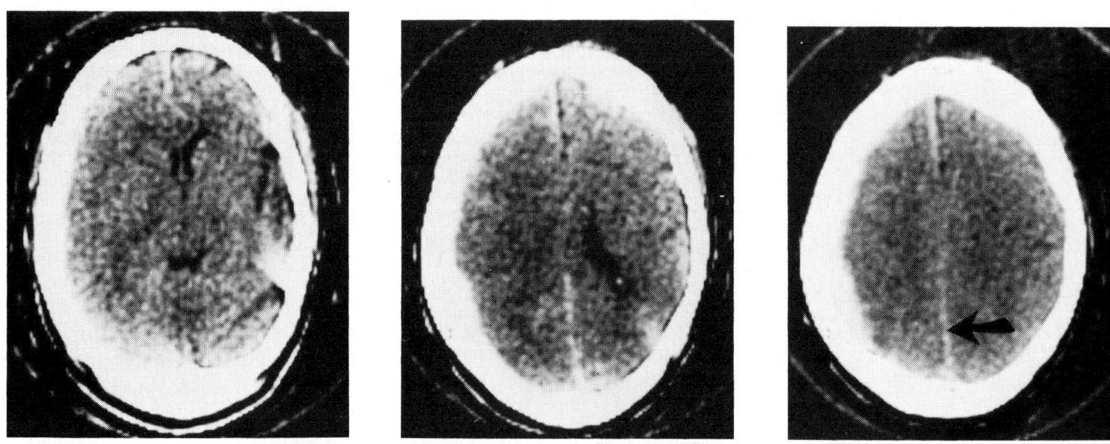

Figure 13–28. SMALL ACUTE LEFT SUBDURAL HEMATOMA: There is a slim acute subdural hematoma on the left side. On standard viewing densities the CT scan gives the appearance of a thickened calvaria on the left side. Manipulating the window width and window level allows for better visualization of the blood accumulation. There is compression of the body of the left lateral ventricle. The falx is dense because of blood in the subarachnoid space *(arrow)*.

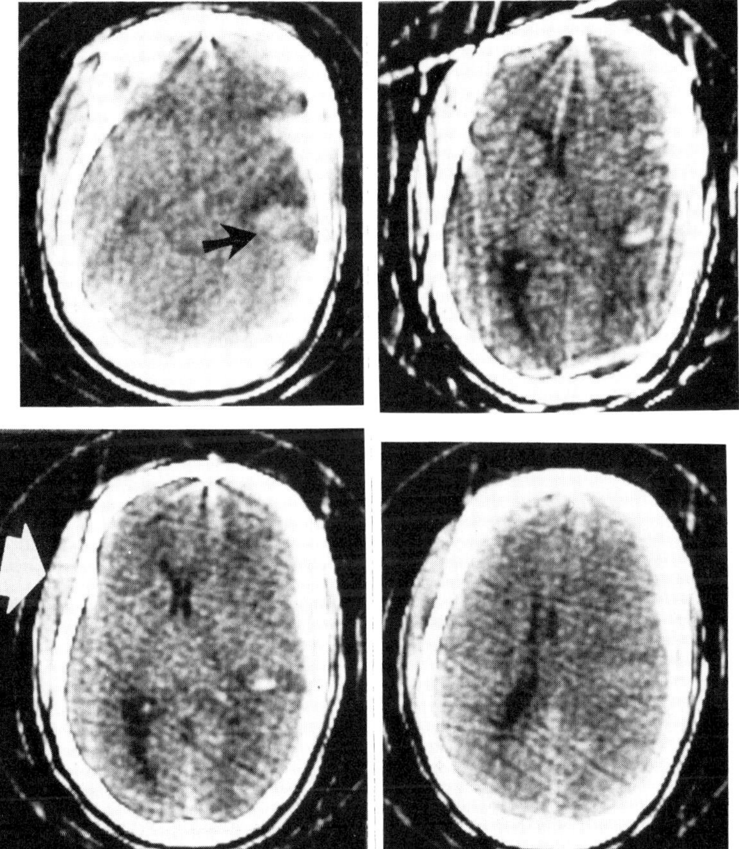

Figure 13–29. SUBDURAL HEMATOMA AND CONTUSION: A large extracranial hematoma is seen on the left side. The "contra-coup" injury has resulted in a small acute subdural hematoma on the contralateral side. In addition, a right temporal hematoma (*arrow*) and areas of contusion with small areas of hemorrhage appear on the higher cuts. There is shift of the midline to the contralateral side — more than would be present with the hematoma alone.

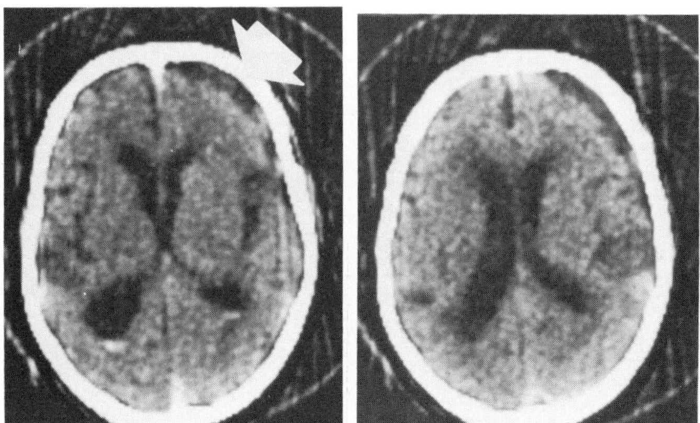

Figure 13–30. SUBACUTE SUBDURAL AND SUBARACHNOID HEMORRHAGE: A small extracerebral collection of fluid is seen in the right frontal area with slight compression of the body of the right lateral ventricle. In addition, there is a small amount of blood with CSF-blood fluid levels present in the dependent portions of the lateral ventricles. These appear as areas of high density on the lowest cut.

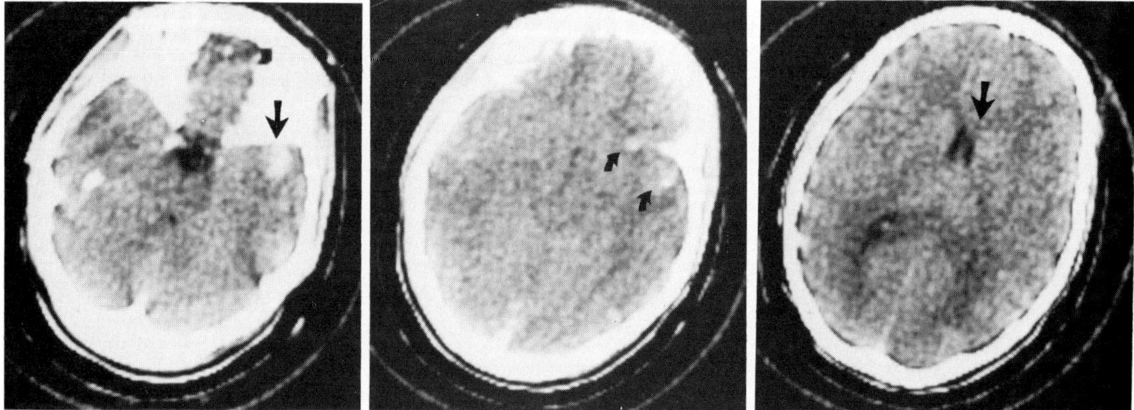

Figure 13–31. TEMPORAL LOBE CONTUSION: A small right temporal lobe hematoma with surrounding edema is noted in the right anterior temporal lobe. There is surrounding edema *(arrows)*. Small areas of edema also are present in the frontal regions bilaterally, and there is a slight shift of the midline to the left.

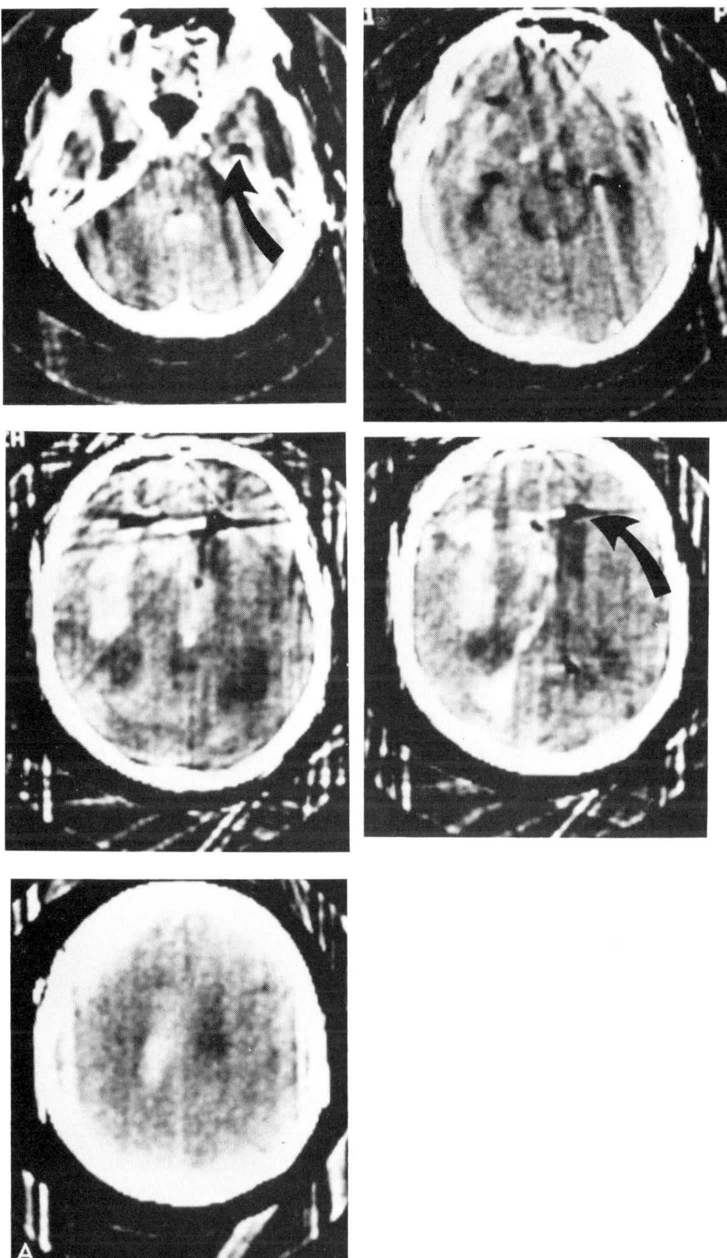

Figure 13–32. SEVERE INTRACRANIAL TRAUMA: *A*, The CT scan shows evidence of intracerebral hemorrhage in the left hemisphere as well as a large intraventricular hemorrhage with blood forming a cast of the left lateral ventricle. In addition, there are multiple scattered accumulations of air in the substance of the brain and within the ventricular system *(arrows)*. These appear as very low density areas. The lowest cut reveals an accumulation of blood in the fourth ventricle that leads to an obstructive hydrocephalus. There is some shift to the contralateral side.

Illustration continued on the following page

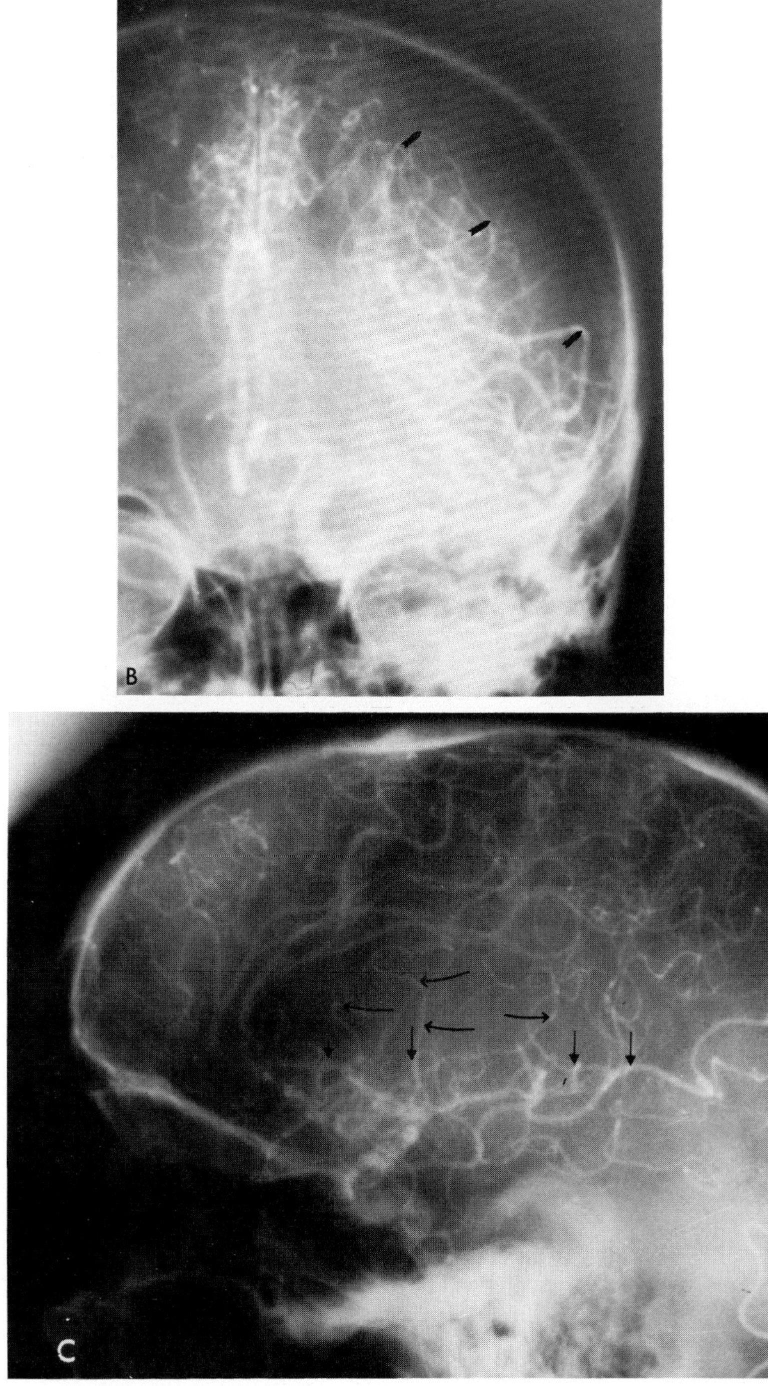

Figure 13–32 *Continued. See legend on the opposite page*

Figure 13–32 *Continued*

B, The AP arterial view reveals shift of the anterior cerebral artery to the contralateral side and downward. There is medial displacement of the sylvian point and an extracerebral accumulation of fluid that displaces the middle cerebral artery branches away from the inner table of the skull *(arrows)*. This subdural hematoma was not seen on the CT scan.

C, The lateral view reveals the downward displacement of the sylvian triangle *(straight arrows)* and the stretching of the branches of the middle cerebral artery group *(curved arrows)*. The changes are secondary to the subdural hematoma and the intracerebral hematoma. Note that the CT scan and arteriograms are complementary for diagnosis of the extent of trauma in this case.

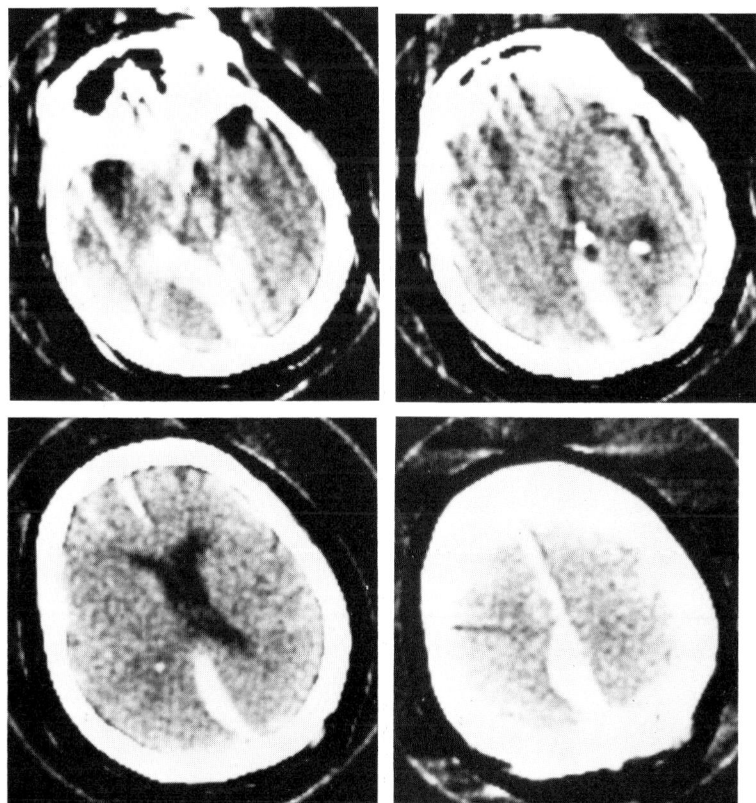

Figure 13–33. INTERHEMISPHERIC SUBDURAL HEMATOMA: The CT scan reveals a well defined area of blood density that lies adjacent to the left side of the falx cerebri and extends down to the tentorium on the left, where blood outlines the free edge of the tentorium. The subdural accumulation expands slightly in the high convexity region. There is a slight shift to the right side.

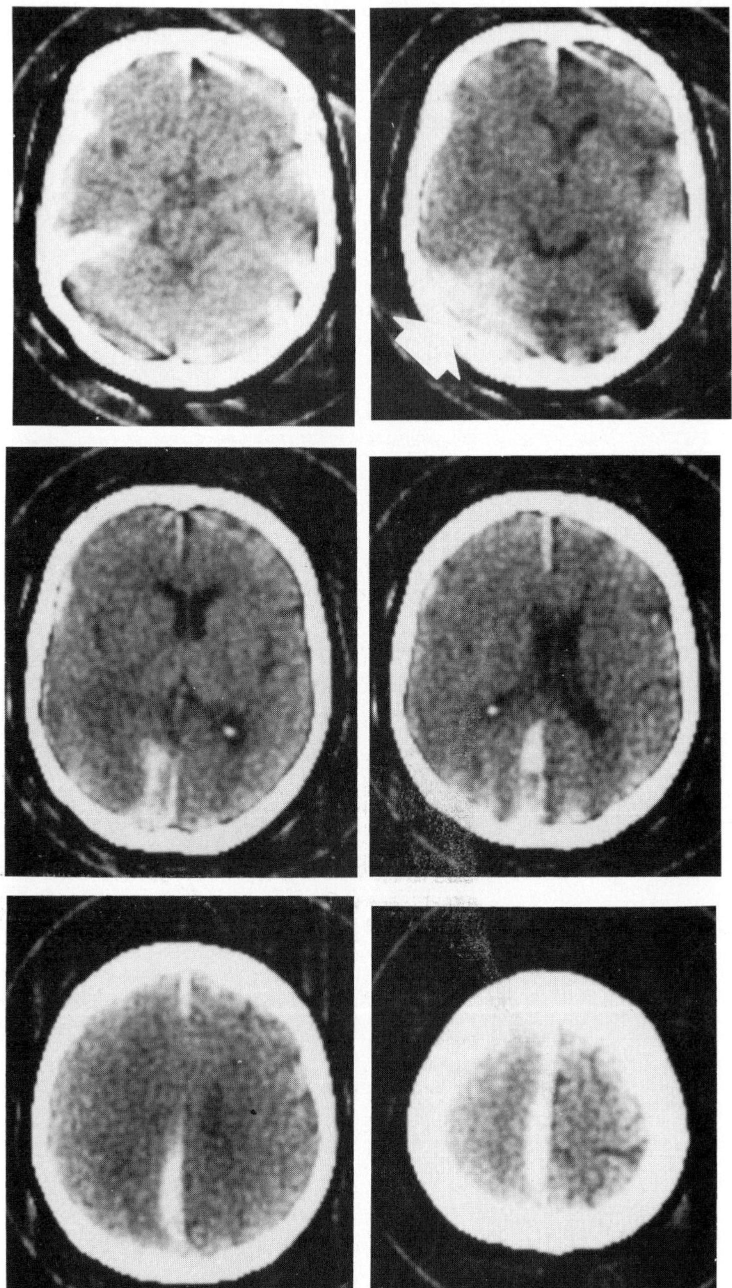

Figure 13–34. INTERHEMISPHERIC SUBDURAL HEMATOMA: There is an interhemispheric subdural hematoma and an accumulation of blood along the supratentorial side of the tentorium *(white arrowhead)*. A very small acute subdural hematoma over the left cerebral hemisphere and a slight shift to the right side can be seen. There is obliteration of the cortical sulci of the left hemisphere.

Figure 13–35. SUBACUTE SUBDURAL HEMATOMA WITH ENHANCING MEMBRANE: The preinfusion scans *(left column)* reveal an extracerebral accumulation of fluid that has a mottled density. There is shift to the contralateral side. After the infusion of contrast material *(right column)*, there is enhancement of the membrane of the subdural hematoma *(arrows)*. The demonstration of a membrane may be especially helpful when a subdural hematoma is chronic and isodense with normal brain tissue. The sign is especially helpful when there are bilateral isodense subdural hematomas and the diagnosis is obscure.

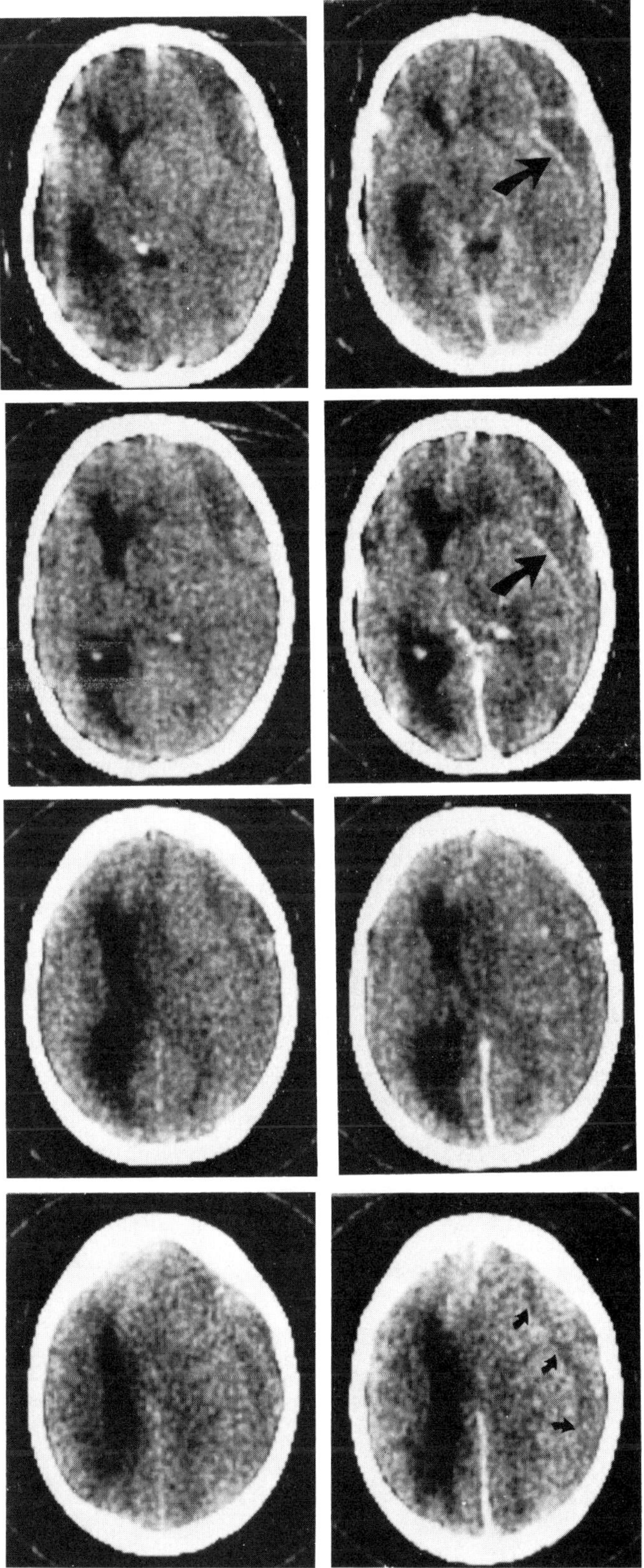

Figure 13–35 *See legend on the opposite page*

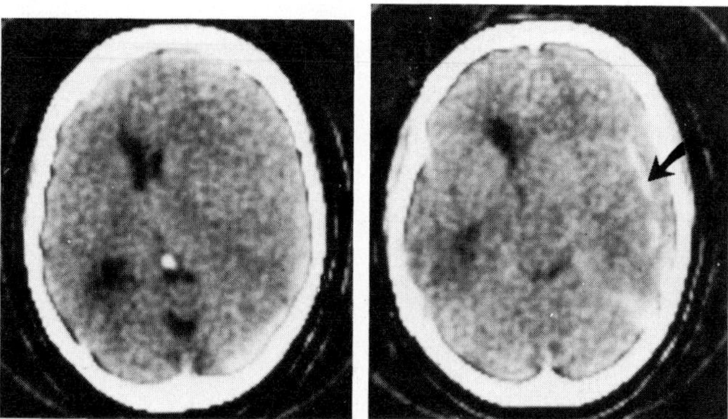

Figure 13–36. ISODENSE SUBDURAL HEMATOMA WITH ENHANCING MEMBRANE: The preinfusion scan *(left)* reveals only shift to the left side. This appearance may be mistaken for left hemiatrophy. The postinfusion scan *(right)* reveals the enhancing membrane of the chronic subdural hematoma *(arrow)*.

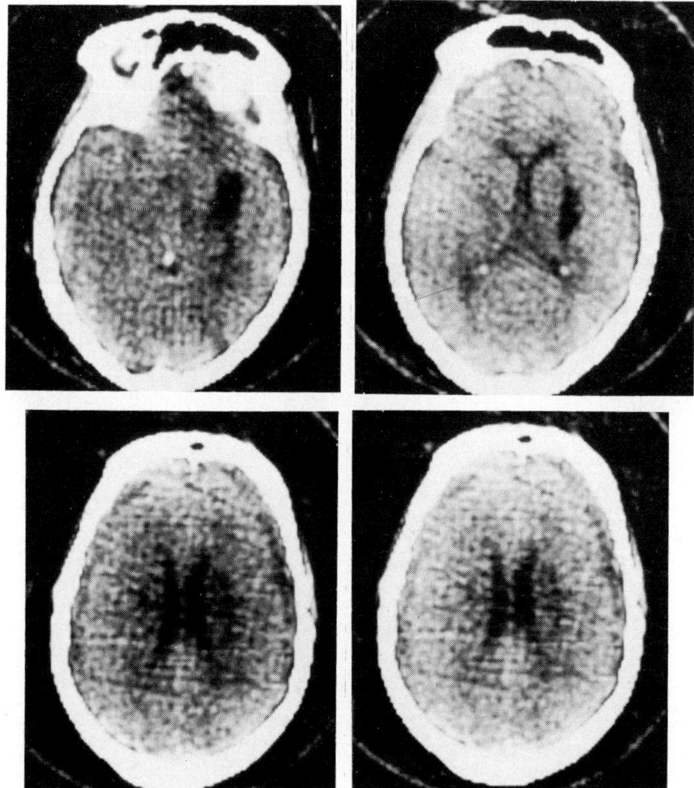

Figure 13–37. BILATERAL CHRONIC SUBDURAL HEMATOMAS: The chronic bilateral subdural hematomas are less dense than normal brain tissue. The lateral ventricles are displaced toward the midline and appear to be elongated. If the subdural accumulations had been isodense, their presence would be difficult to appreciate. In addition, there is an area of porencephaly deep in the right basal ganglia region — probably secondary to an old infarct or basal ganglia hemorrhage.

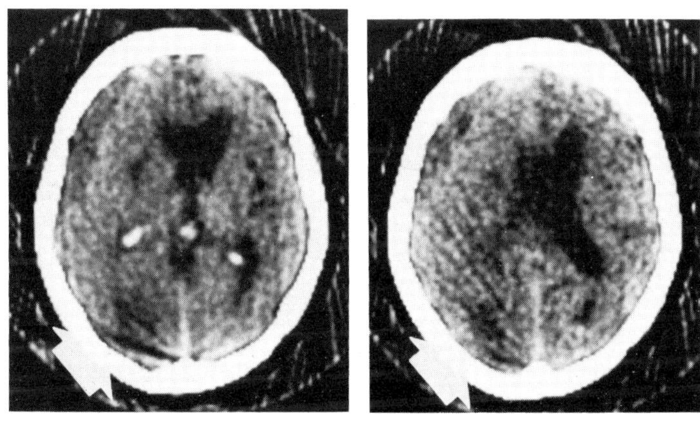

Figure 13–38. CHRONIC SUBDURAL HEMATOMA: A chronic subdural hematoma is seen over the left frontoparietal region. There is shift to the contralateral side. In addition, there is an irregular area of lucency in the left occipital pole (*arrows*) secondary to transtentorial herniation and compromise of the posterior cerebral artery blood supply to the occipital pole on the left side.

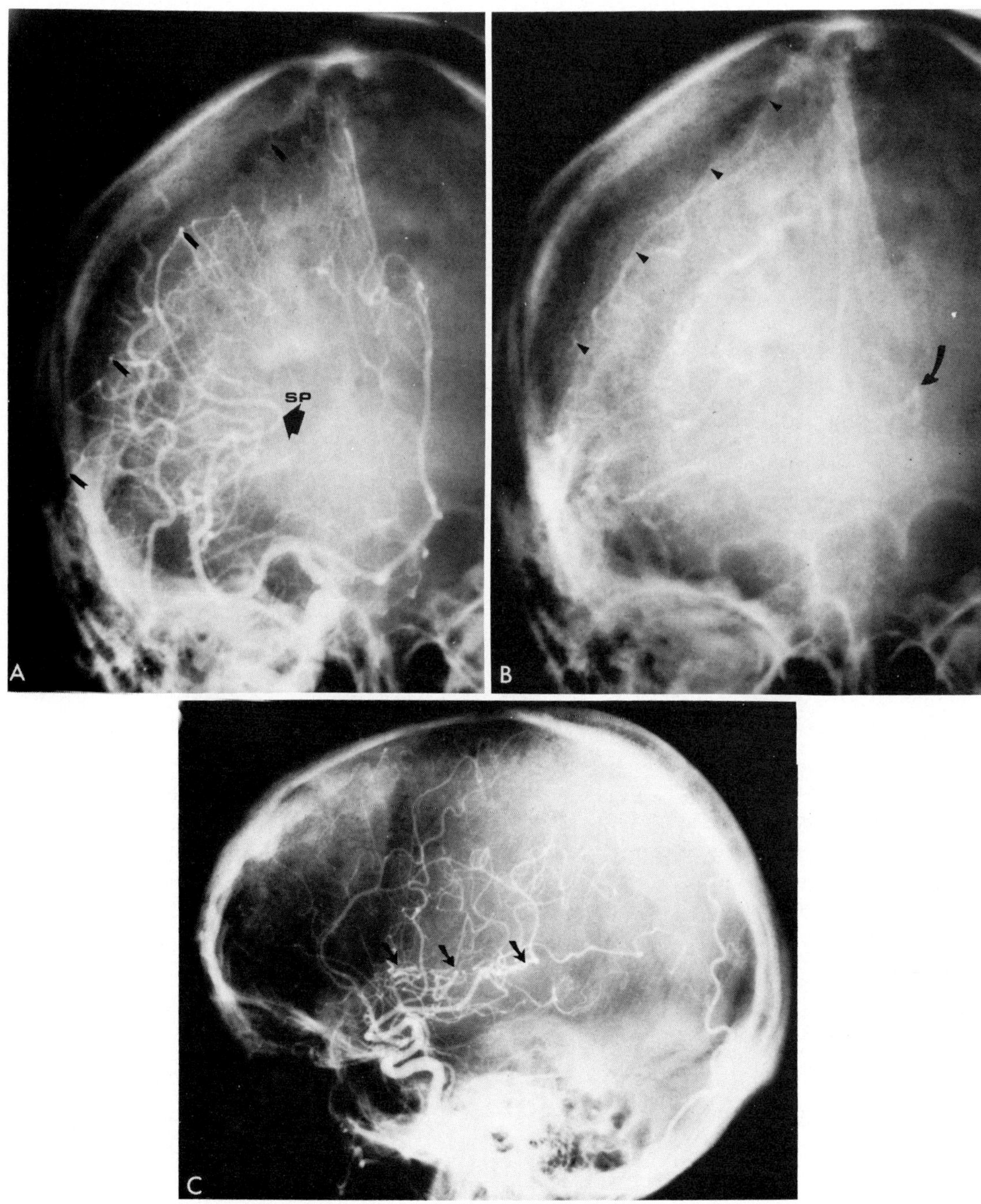

Figure 13–39. *See legend on the opposite page*

Figure 13–39. CHRONIC SUBDURAL HEMATOMA: *A* and *B*, The AP arterial and venous films reveal that the branches of the middle cerebral artery are displaced away from the inner table of the skull (*arrows* in *A*), and there is a distal shift of the anterior cerebral artery under the falx cerebri and downward and medial displacement of the sylvian point (*SP*). The cortical veins are also displaced away from the inner table of the skull (*small arrows*) and there is a marked shift of the internal cerebral vein (*large arrow*). The hematoma has taken on the lentiform configuration typically seen with a chronic subdural hematoma.

C, The lateral view reveals downward displacement of the sylvian triangle by the subdural hematoma, which is suprasylvian in location.

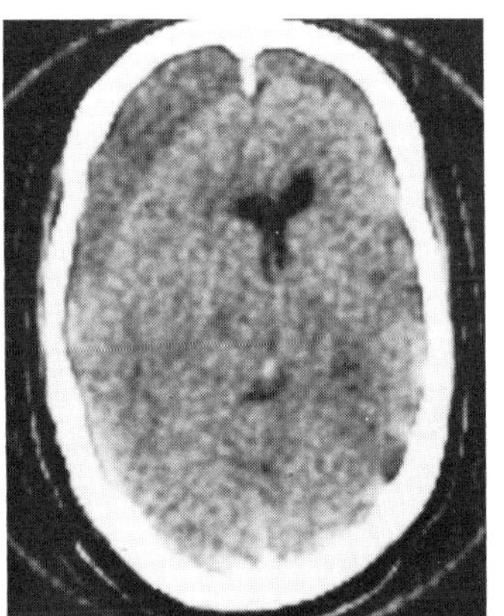

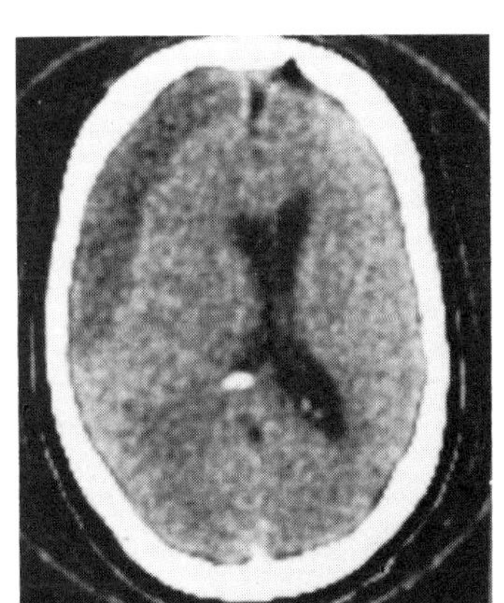

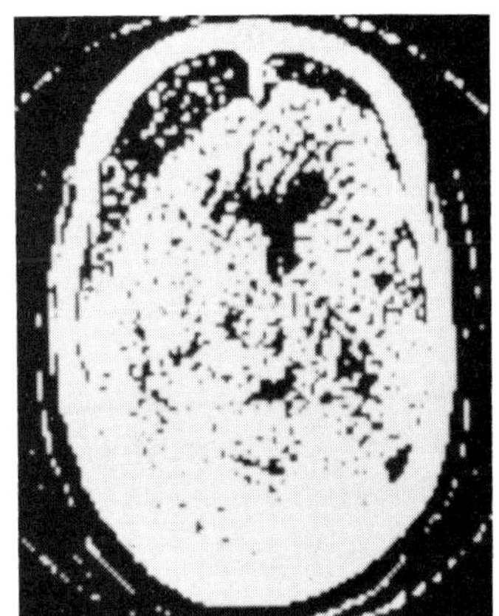

Figure 13–40. CHRONIC SUBDURAL HEMATOMA: A large low density extracerebral accumulation of blood is seen over the left hemisphere anteriorly. Note also a small low density accumulation over the right frontal region and a shift to the right side. The picture taken on the "measure" mode allows ready identification of the chronic subdural accumulation.

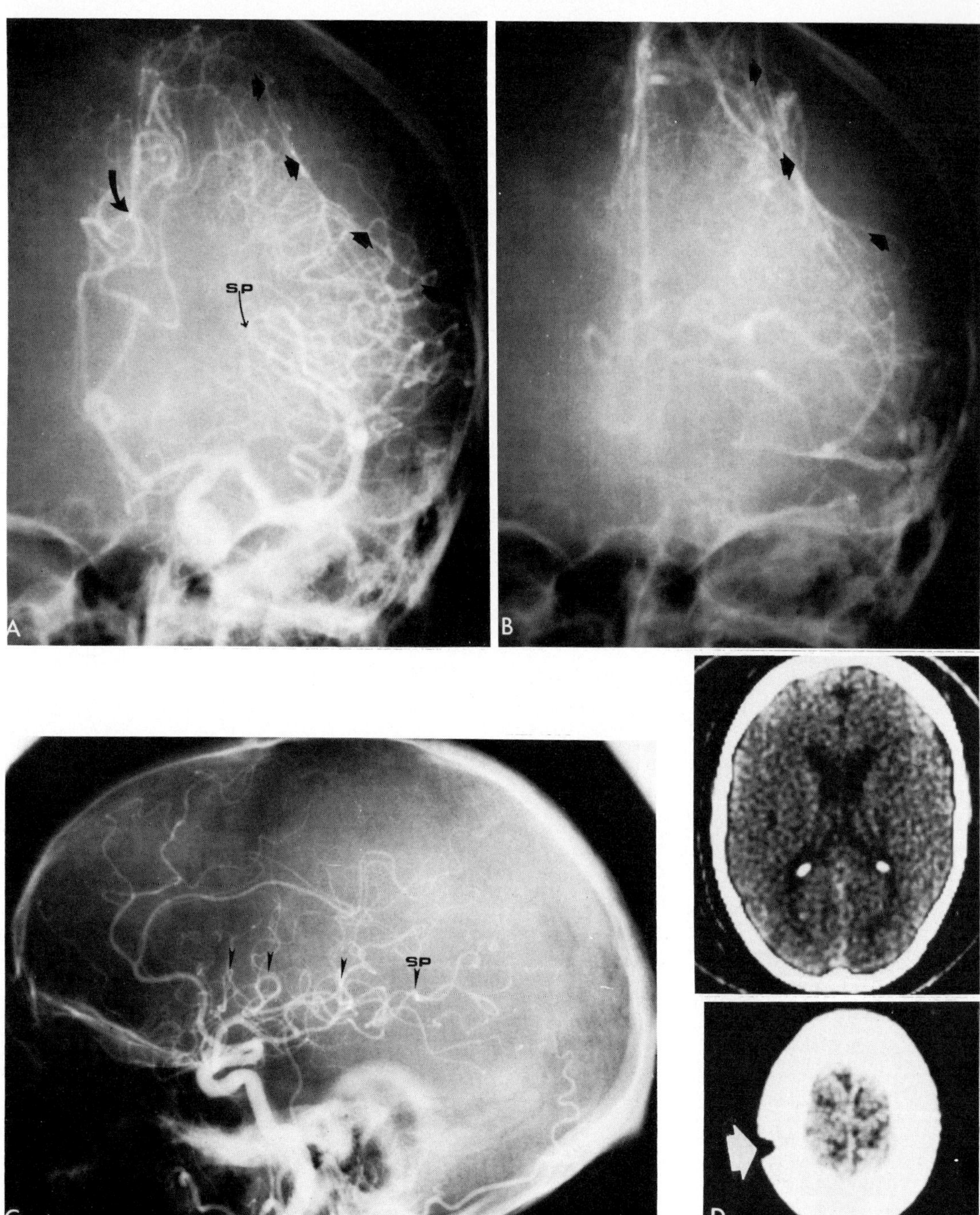

Figure 13–41. CHRONIC SUBDURAL HEMATOMA: *A,* The AP arterial phase reveals a lentiform collection of extracerebral fluid *(arrowheads)* associated with downward and medial displacement of the sylvian point *(SP)*. There is a distal shift of the anterior cerebral artery under the falx cerebri *(large arrow)*.

B, The AP venous phase again demonstrates the lentiform configuration of the chronic subdural hematoma.

C, The lateral arterial view shows downward displacement of the entire sylvian triangle *(arrowheads)*. The sharp angulation of the distal portion of the anterior cerebral artery represents the point where the artery shifts under the falx cerebri.

D, A CT scan obtained postoperatively reveals that the lateral ventricles are in normal position, and the bur hole used for evacuation of the hematoma *(arrow)* is visible on the high cuts. The scan is otherwise unremarkable.

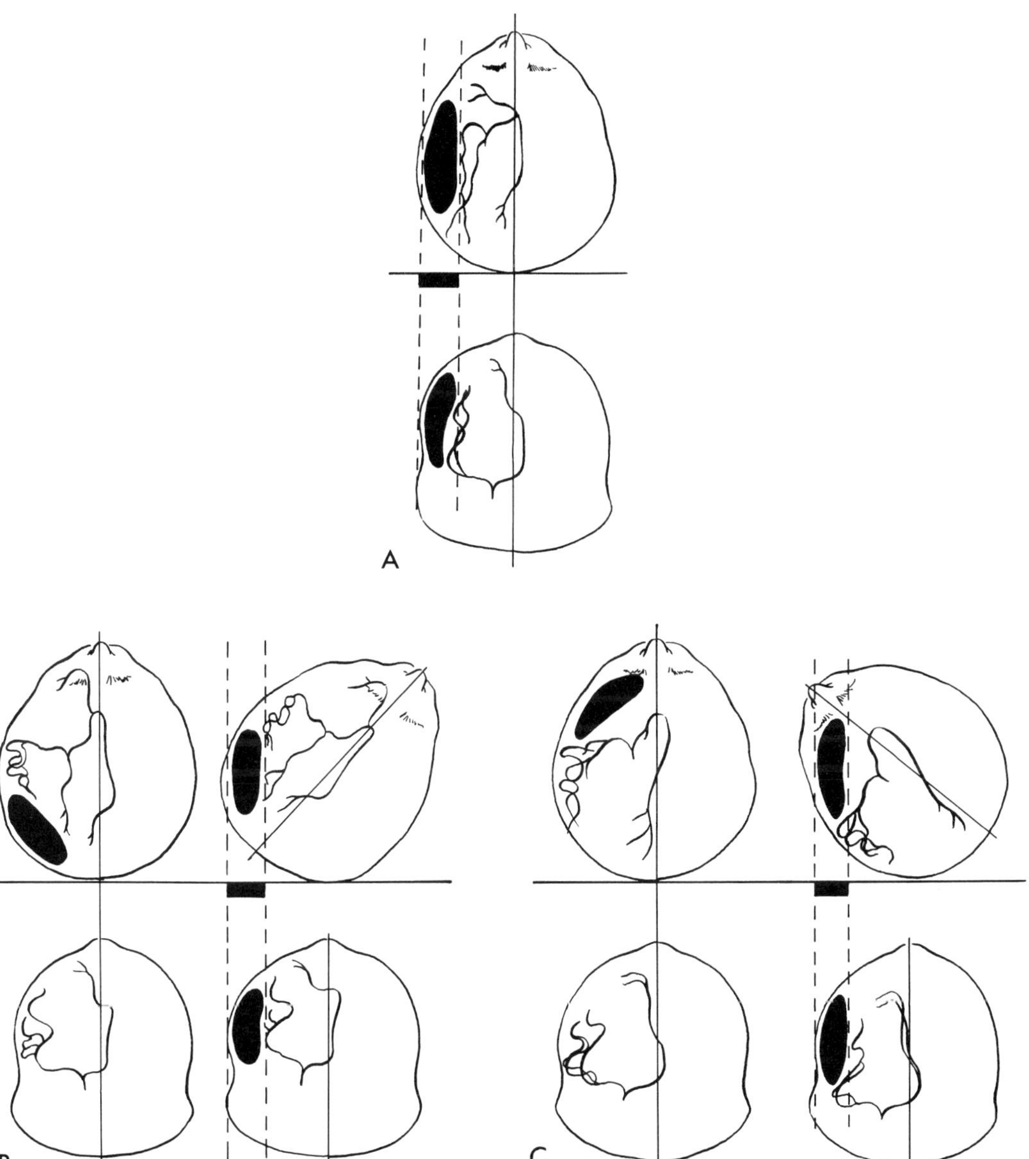

Figure 13–42. ADVANTAGES OF THE OBLIQUE VIEW IN EVALUATING A SUBDURAL HEMATOMA. *A*, A subdural hematoma in the temporal and/or parietal area is readily visible in the standard angiographic projections.

B and *C*, Frontal and occipital subdural hematomas may not be visible in the standard projections, but are better visualized using appropriate oblique projections. (Modified with permission from Radcliffe WB, Quinto FC Jr: Semin Roentgenol *6*:103–110, 1971.)

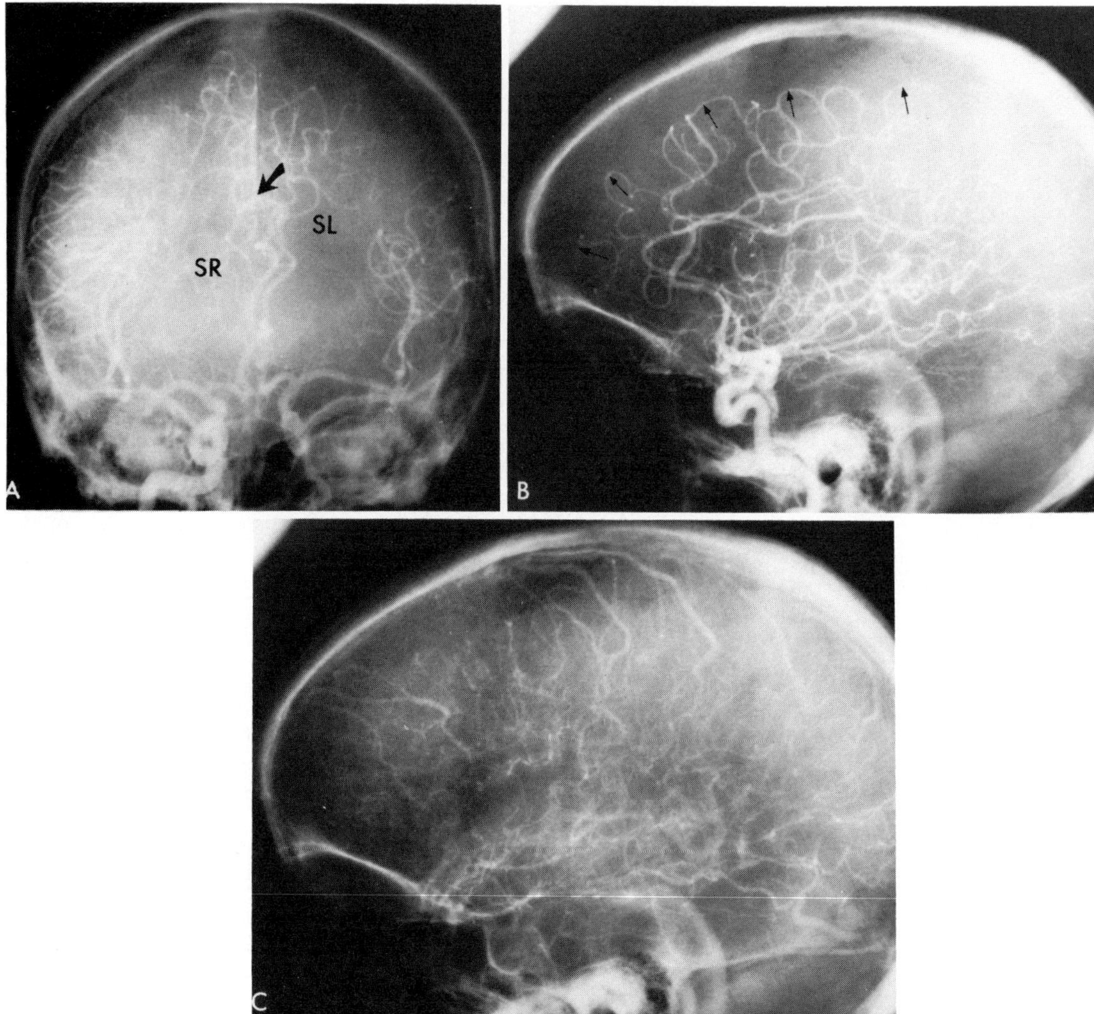

Figure 13–43. FRONTAL SUBDURAL HEMATOMA: *A,* The AP arterial view reveals a distal shift of the anterior cerebral artery (*arrow*). This study, done with cross compression, shows that the sylvian point on the right side (SR) is displaced medially compared with the sylvian point on the normal left side (SL).

B, The lateral view reveals that the distal branch vessels of the anterior cerebral artery are displaced away from the inner table of the skull anteriorly (*arrows*). The pericallosal artery is depressed.

C, The lateral venous phase appears normal. Because the superficial cortical veins must enter the superior sagittal sinus, their actual displacement away from the inner table in the convexity region cannot be appreciated and their entrance into the superior sagittal sinus appears to be normal.

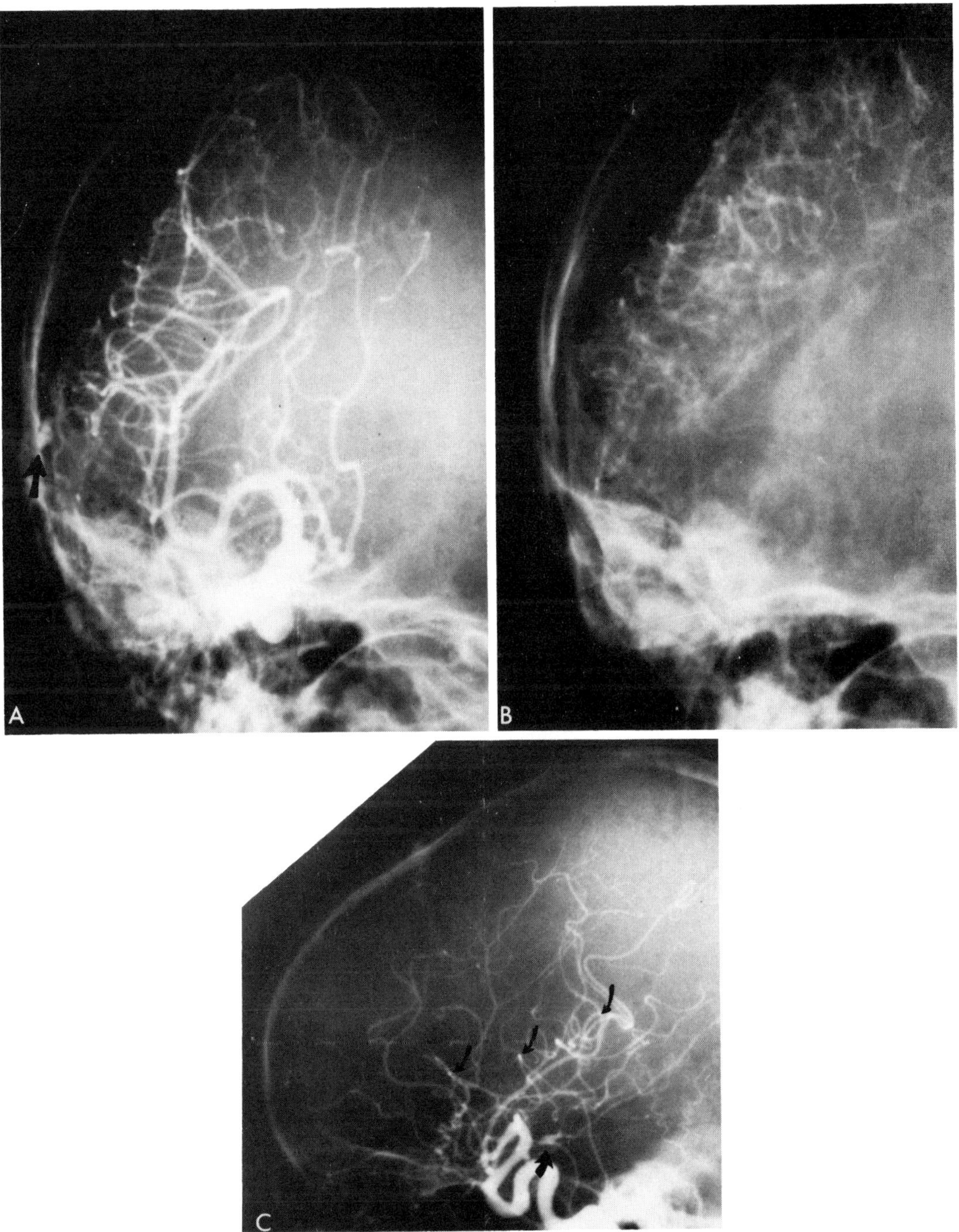

Figure 13–44. CHRONIC POSTERIOR SUBDURAL HEMATOMA: *A* and *B*, The AP arterial and capillary phases of the arteriogram obtained in the left posterior oblique projection reveal the lentiform configuration of a chronic subdural hematoma. The full extent is best appreciated on the oblique view. The arrowhead demonstrates an aneurysm of the middle meningeal artery — possibly post-traumatic.

C, The lateral arterial view demonstrates downward and anterior displacement of the sylvian triangle *(small arrows)* because of the posterior position of the subdural hematoma. The aneurysm of the middle meningeal artery is again demonstrated *(large arrow)*.

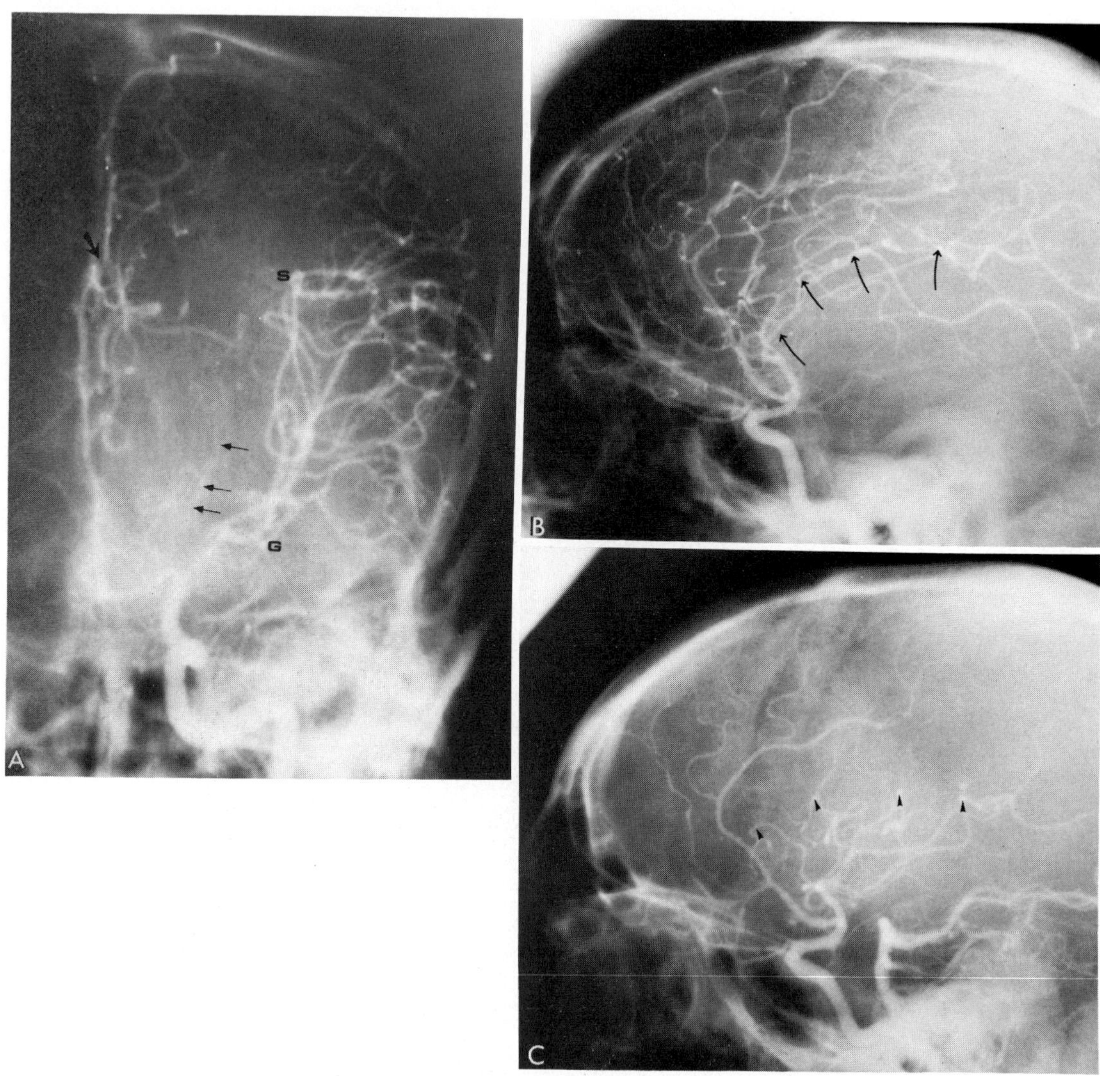

Figure 13–45. BITEMPORAL CONTUSION: *A,* The AP arterial view reveals a distal shift of the anterior cerebral artery under the falx cerebri *(large arrow)*, medial and upward displacement of the sylvian points *(S)*, medial displacement of the lenticulostriate vessels and medial displacement of the genu *(G)*, of the middle cerebral artery and its branches.

B, The lateral artery view shows marked upward displacement of the branches of the left middle cerebral artery *(arrows)*.

C, The lateral view of the right carotid arteriogram reveals upward bowing of the branches that form the roof of the sylvian triangle *(arrows)*, with more marked changes in the midportion of the triangle.

D, The AP arterial view using cross compression demonstrates that the displacements of the middle cerebral artery branches are more marked on the left side and again confirms the shift of the anterior cerebral artery to the right *(arrow)*.

E, The CT scan demonstrates bitemporal radiolucencies consistent with contusion in the temporal lobes. The edema is more marked on the left side.

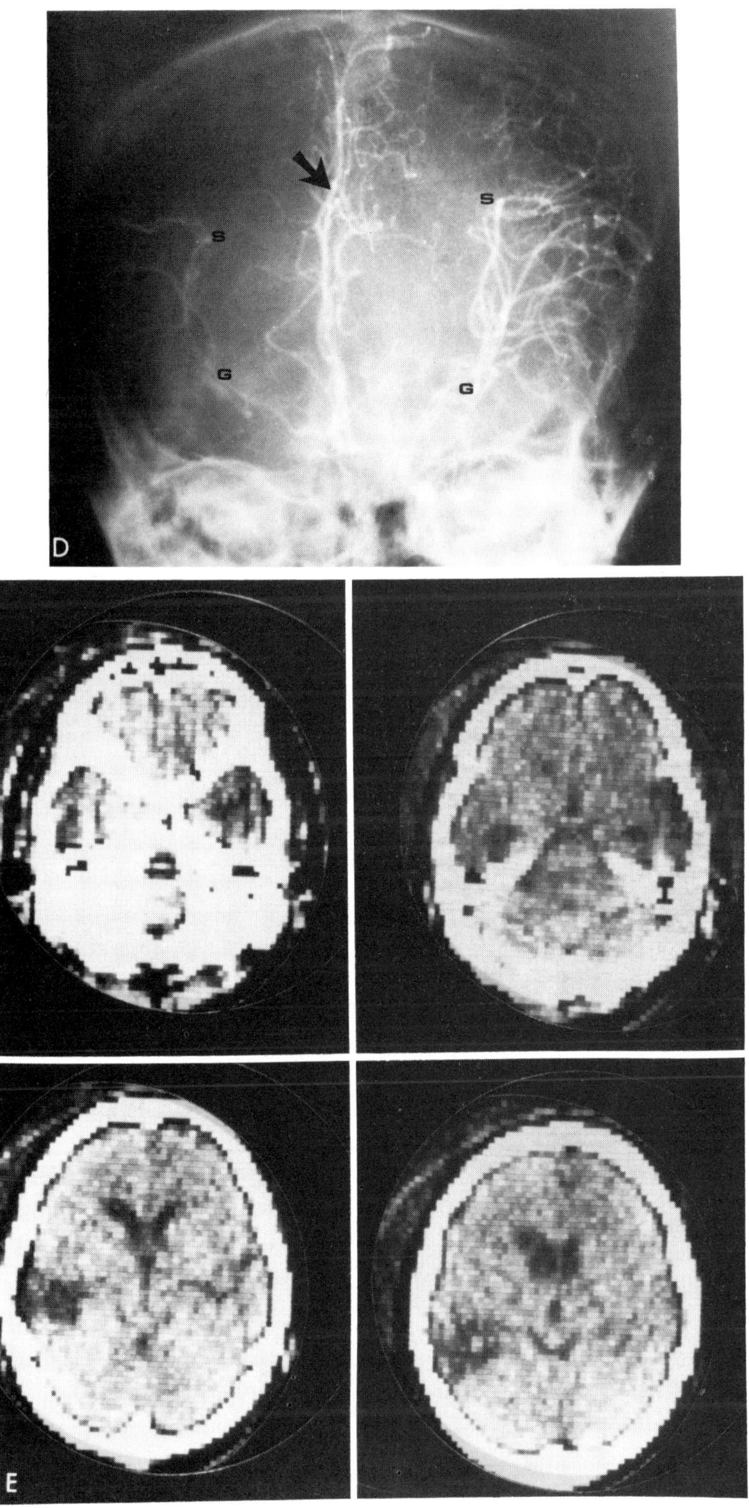

Figure 13–45 *Continued*

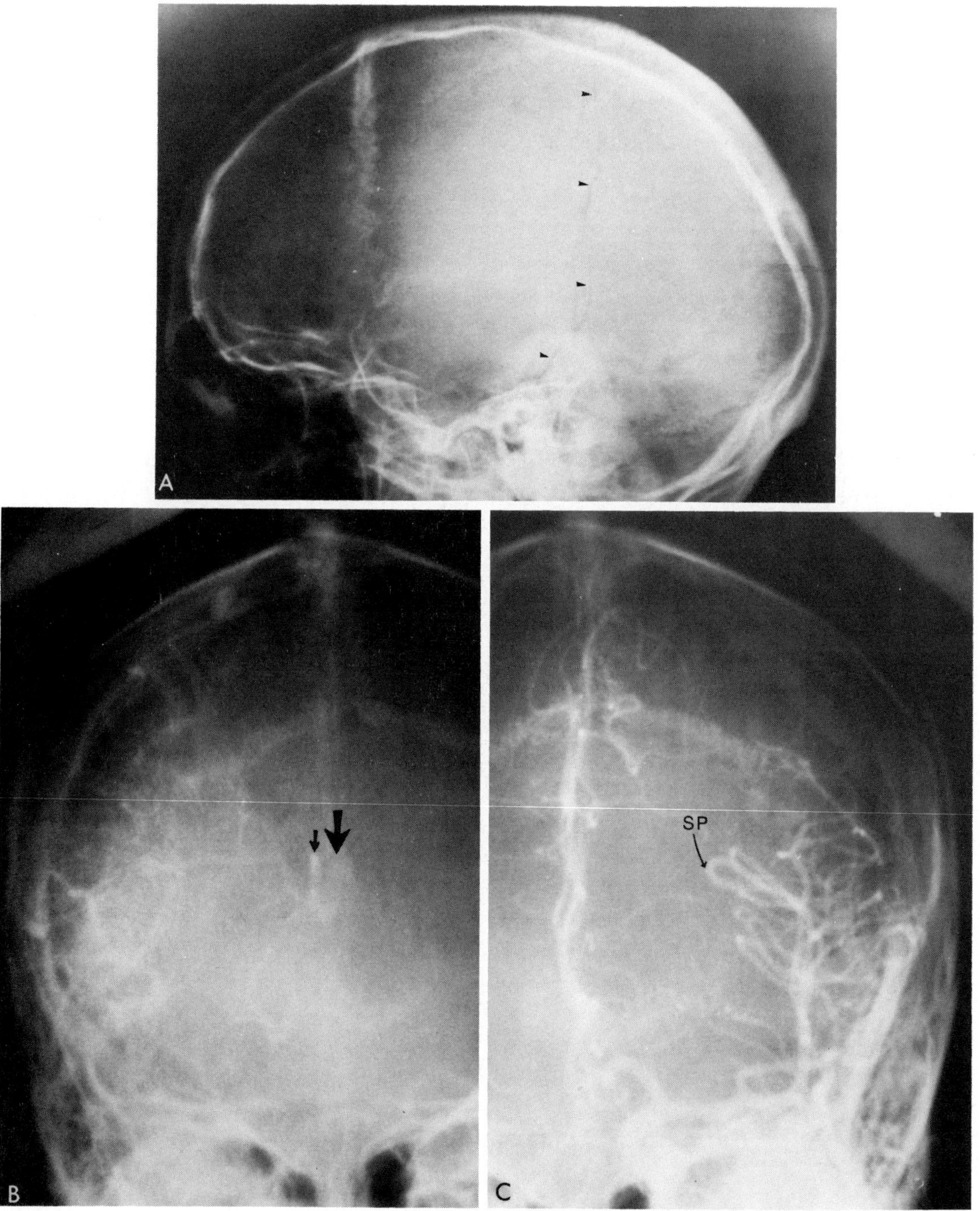

Figure 13–46 *See legend on the opposite page*

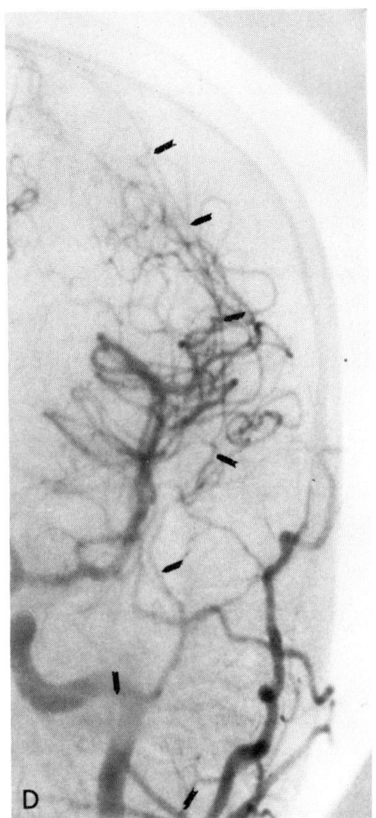

Figure 13–46. EPIDURAL HEMATOMA: *A*, The skull film reveals a long linear skull fracture that extends from one parietal region to the other through the bregma.

B, Because of false localizing signs, a right carotid arteriogram was performed initially. The venous phase reveals shift of the internal cerebral vein *(small arrow)* to the ipsilateral side of the midline *(large arrow)*.

C, The AP arterial phase of the left carotid arteriogram shows slight distal shift of the anterior cerebral artery under the falx cerebri *(arrow)* and medial and downward displacement of the sylvian point *(SP)*.

D, The right posterior oblique projection of the left carotid arteriogram reveals the lentiform extracerebral accumulation of blood and, in addition, shows that the middle meningeal artery is displaced away from the inner table of the skull — confirming the presence of an *epidural* hematoma. The arrowheads trace the origin of the middle meningeal artery from the internal maxillary artery and follow its intracranial course.

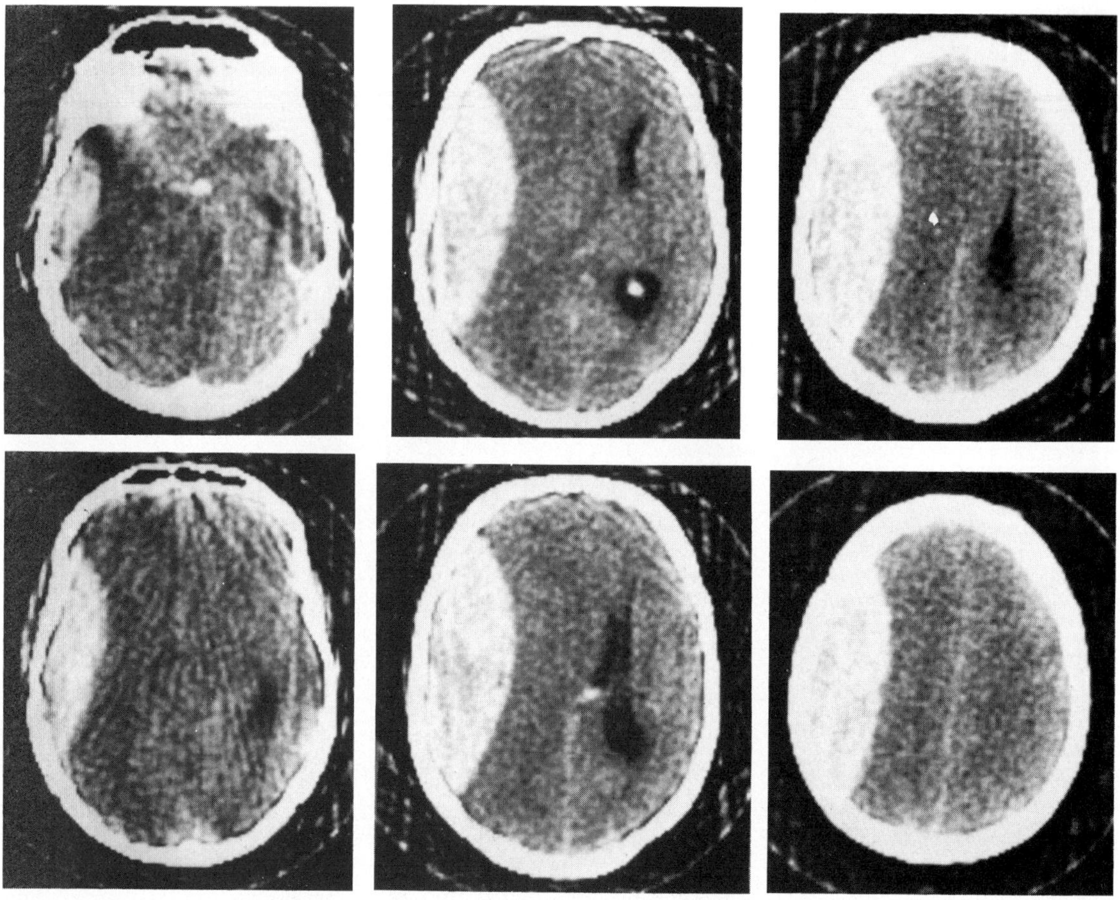

Figure 13–47. EPIDURAL HEMATOMA: The CT scan reveals the typical lentiform accumulation of blood density over the left hemisphere of an acute epidural hematoma. There is marked shift to the contralateral side.

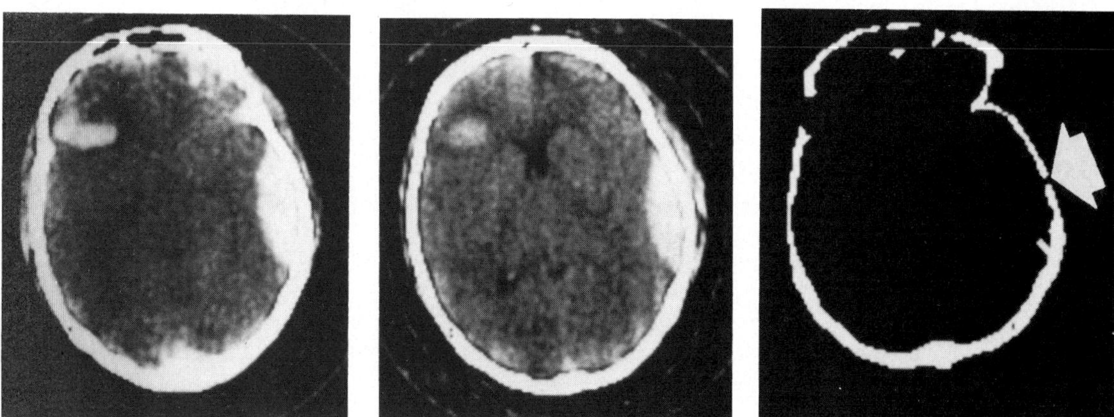

Figure 13–48. EPIDURAL HEMATOMA AND CONTRA-COUP INTRACEREBRAL HEMATOMA: There is a biconcave epidural accumulation of blood over the right hemisphere and an intracerebral hematoma in the left posterior frontal region associated with surrounding edema. The right-sided lesion represents the coup; the left-sided lesion represents the contra-coup. Viewed on the measure mode at high window level, the linear skull fracture is demonstrated *(arrowhead)*.

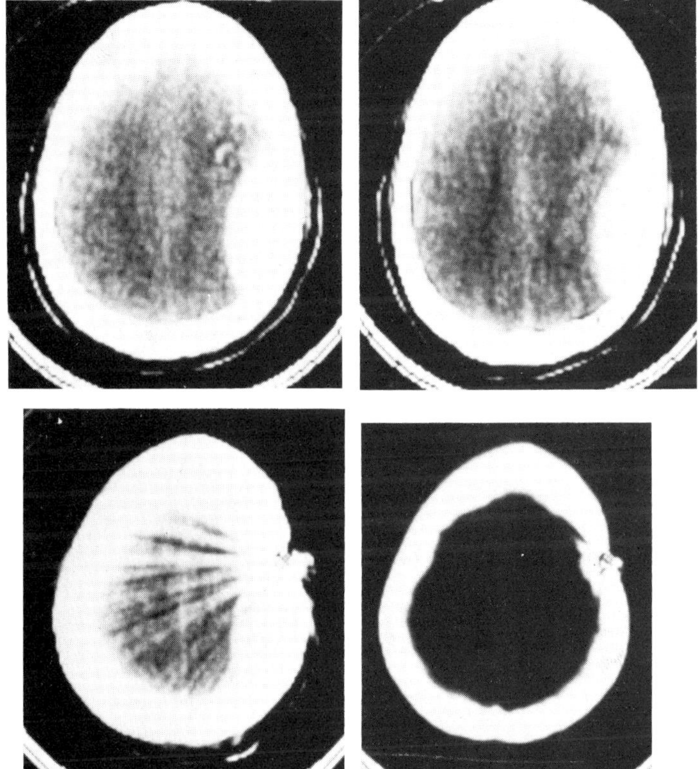

Figure 13–49. EPIDURAL HEMATOMA: A metallic bullet embedded in the outer table of the skull creates computer artifacts on the upper cuts. The bullet did not enter the cranial vault, but created an epidural hematoma high in the right parietal convexity region. An additional small area of contusion can be seen just anterior to the epidural hematoma.

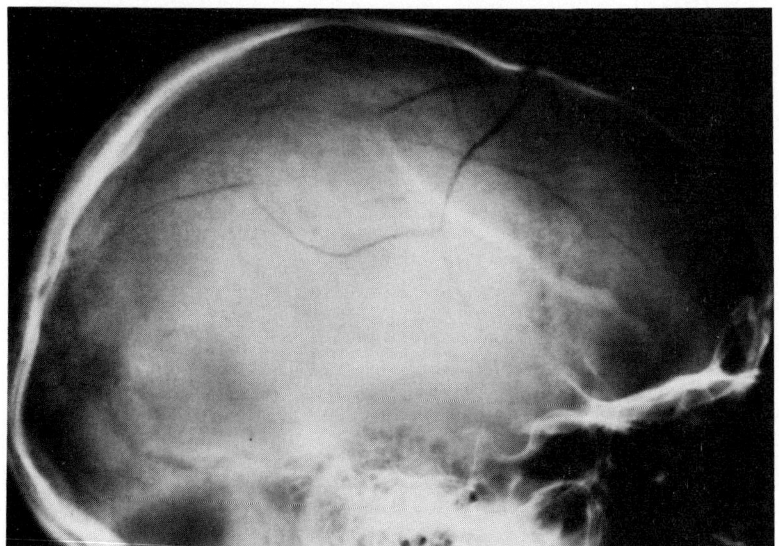

Figure 13–50. COMMINUTED SKULL FRACTURE: The fracture line of this comminuted skull fracture extends across the superior sagittal sinus. This type of fracture is associated with an epidural hematoma.

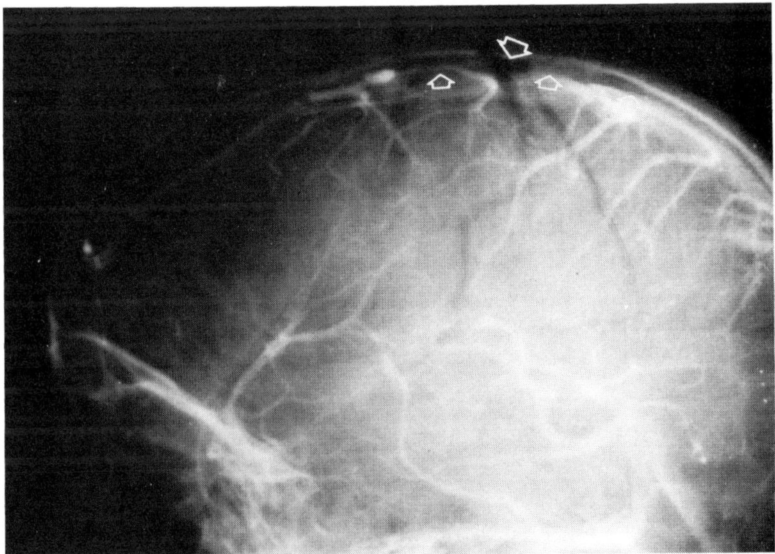

Figure 13–51. EPIDURAL HEMATOMA: The comminuted fracture extends across the superior sagittal sinus, and the later venous phase of the arteriogram reveals that the superior sagittal sinus is displaced away from the inner table of the skull. In this case the epidural accumulation of blood may be venous and secondary to hemorrhage from the superior sagittal sinus.

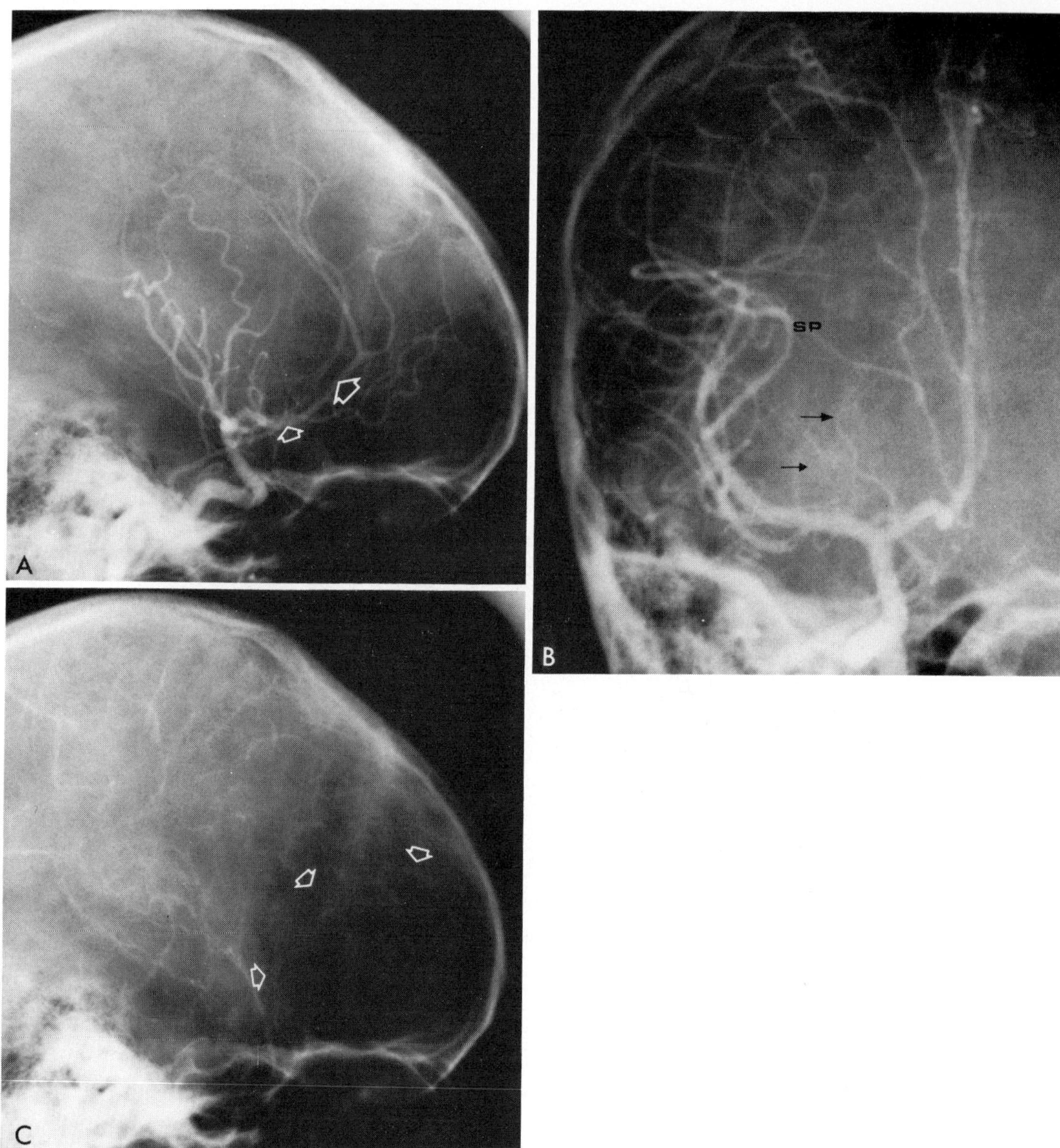

Figure 13–52. SUBFRONTAL EPIDURAL HEMATOMA: *A,* The lateral view of the right carotid arteriogram reveals posterior and upward displacement of the proximal portion of the anterior cerebral artery *(open arrows).* There is a relative paucity of vessels in the frontal pole region.

B, The AP arterial view of the right carotid arteriogram shows medial displacement of the sylvian point *(SP)* and lenticulostriate vessels *(arrows).* There is straightening of the anterior cerebral artery with *minimal* shift to the contralateral side.

C, In the late venous phase, an avascular region *(open arrows)* is seen in the frontal pole. The arteriographic findings are reminiscent of those seen with a subfrontal meningioma.

D, The CT scan reveals a well defined lentiform accumulation of blood density in the right frontal region with *minimal* shift of the midline structures considering the size of the mass. There is some distortion of the frontal horns of the lateral ventricles. The higher cuts reveal a large extracranial hematoma (*arrow*) in the frontal region. The appearance is very typical of a *subfrontal-epidural hematoma.*

E, The CT scan in the coronal section reveals the hematoma located just superior to the orbital roof on the right side. The extracranial hematoma is again identified *(arrow).*

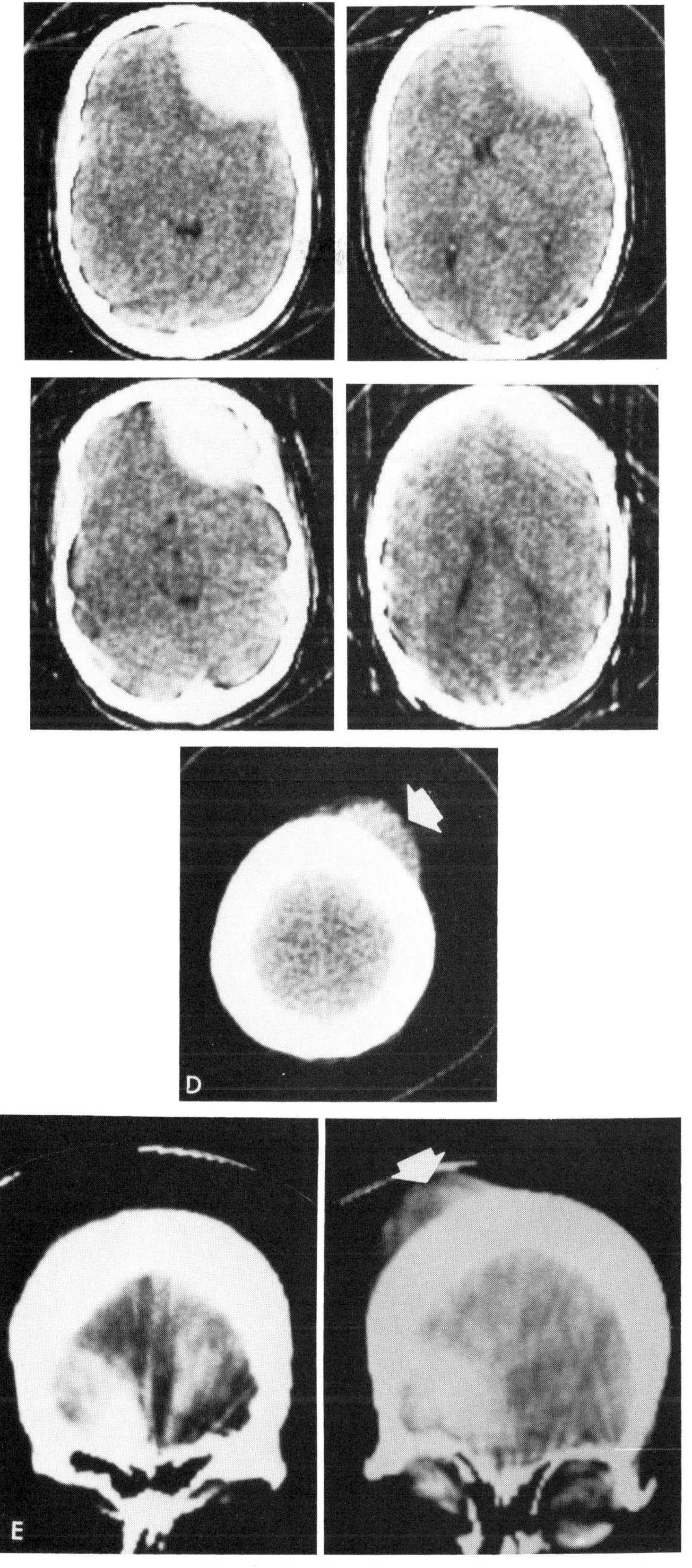

Figure 13–52 *Continued*

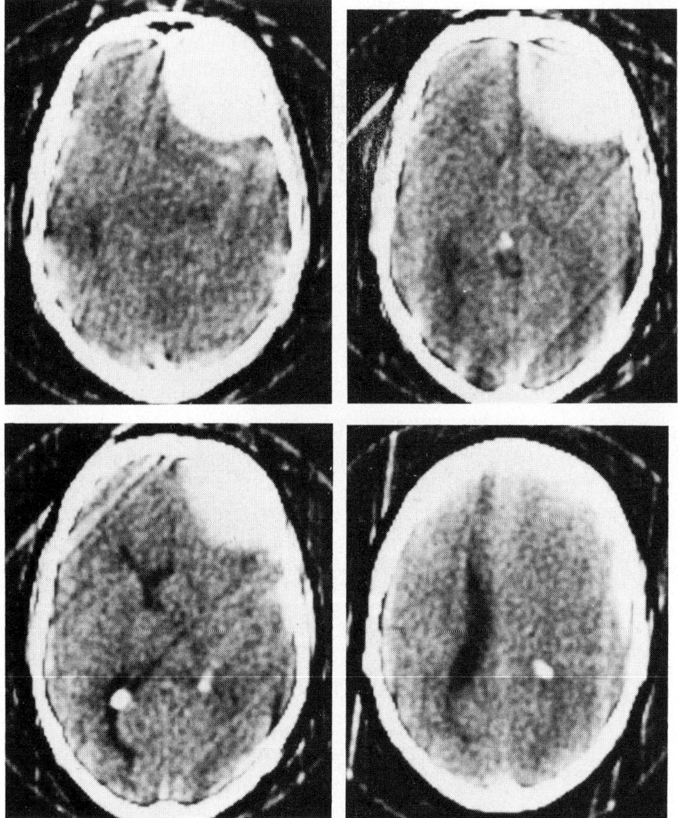

Figure 13–53. SUBFRONTAL EPIDURAL HEMATOMA: There is a biconvex accumulation of blood density in the right frontal region associated with only minimal shift of the midline relative to the size of the hematoma.

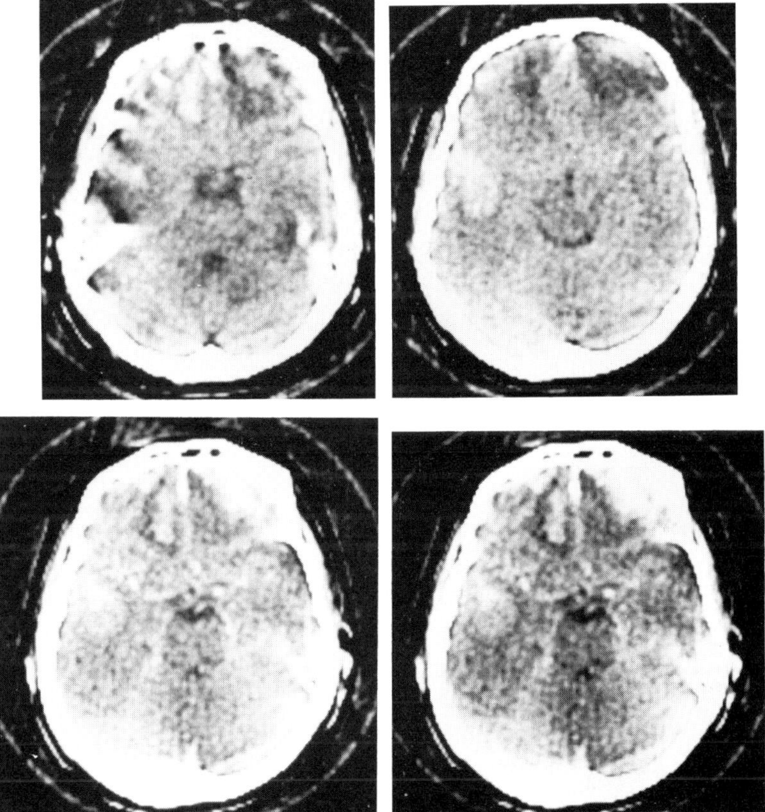

Figure 13–54. MULTIPOLAR TRAUMA: The CT scan shows bifrontal contusions associated with intracerebral hematomas and edema; there is also a left anterior temporal hematoma.

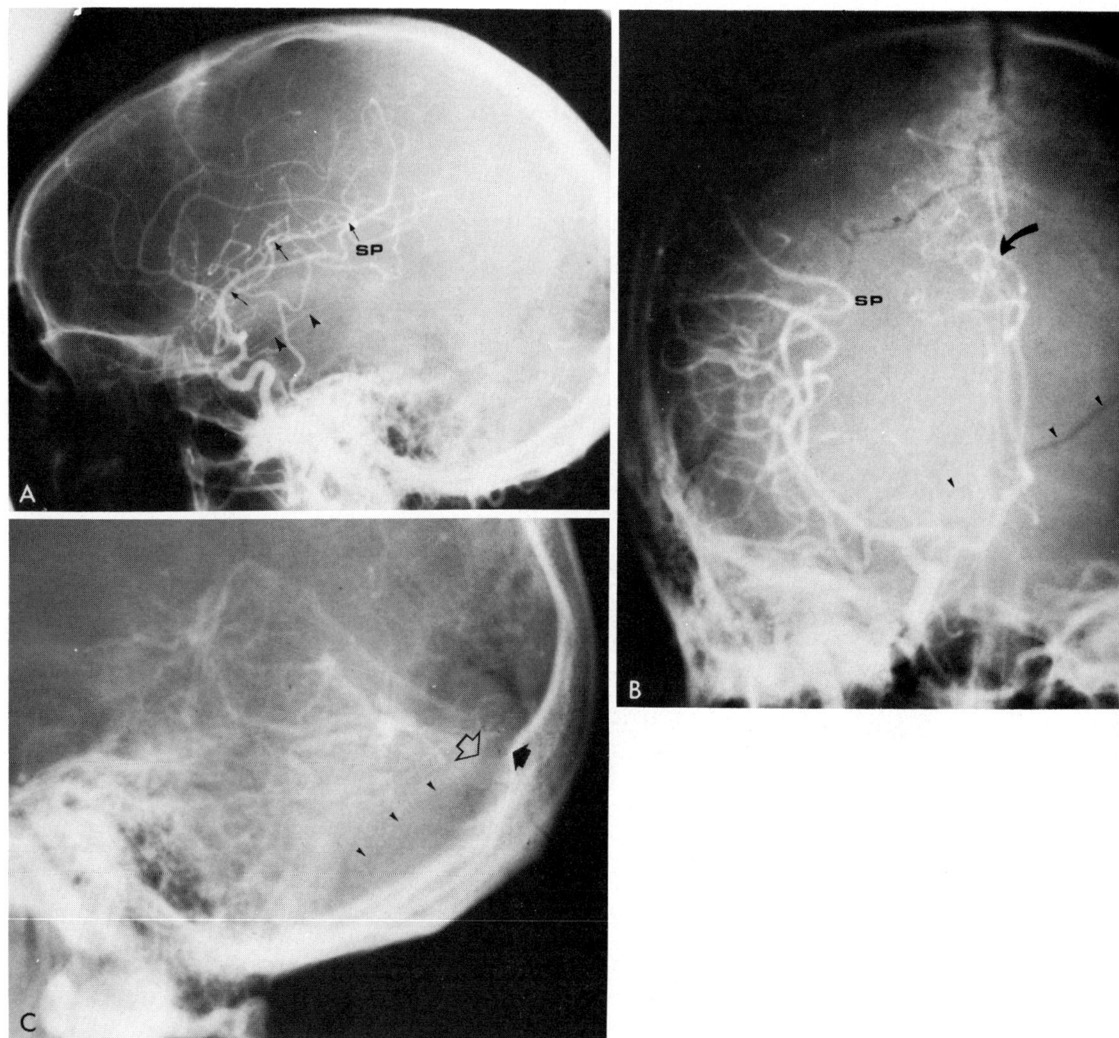

Figure 13–55. HEMISPHERE CONTUSION AND POSTERIOR FOSSA EPIDURAL HEMATOMA: *A,* The lateral view of the right carotid arteriogram reveals upward displacement of the branches of the middle cerebral artery and stretching of the anterior choroidal artery.

B, The AP arterial view demonstrates anterior and posterior shift of the anterior cerebral artery *(large arrow)*. There is medial shift of the sylvian point *(SP)*. The appearance is that of a temporal lobe mass (*arrowheads* demonstrate the occipital fracture.)

C, The late venous phase of the vertebral arteriogram reveals that the torcula *(open arrow)* is displaced anterior to the point of attachment at the internal occipital protuberance *(large black arrow),* and there is anterior displacement of the inferior vermian vein *(small arrowheads).*

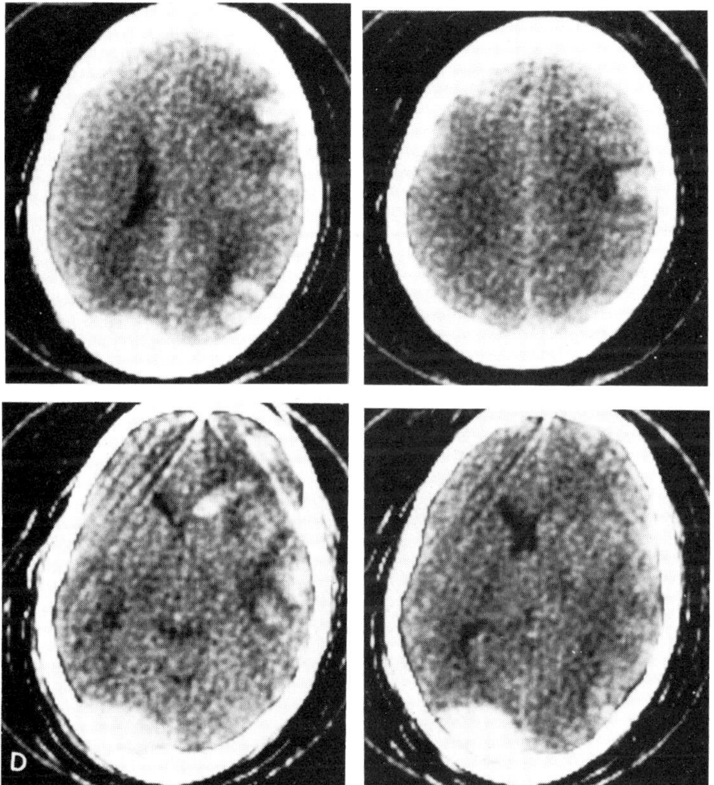

Figure 13–55 *Continued*

D, The CT scan reveals the right temporal contusion and hematoma as well as scattered areas of blood density throughout the right hemisphere in the temporal, frontal and parietal lobes. There is shift to the contralateral side with obliteration of the right lateral ventricle. In addition, a lentiform collection of blood is seen in the posterior fossa and the left occipital region — consistent with an epidural hematoma (surgically proved) (see Fig. 13–6).

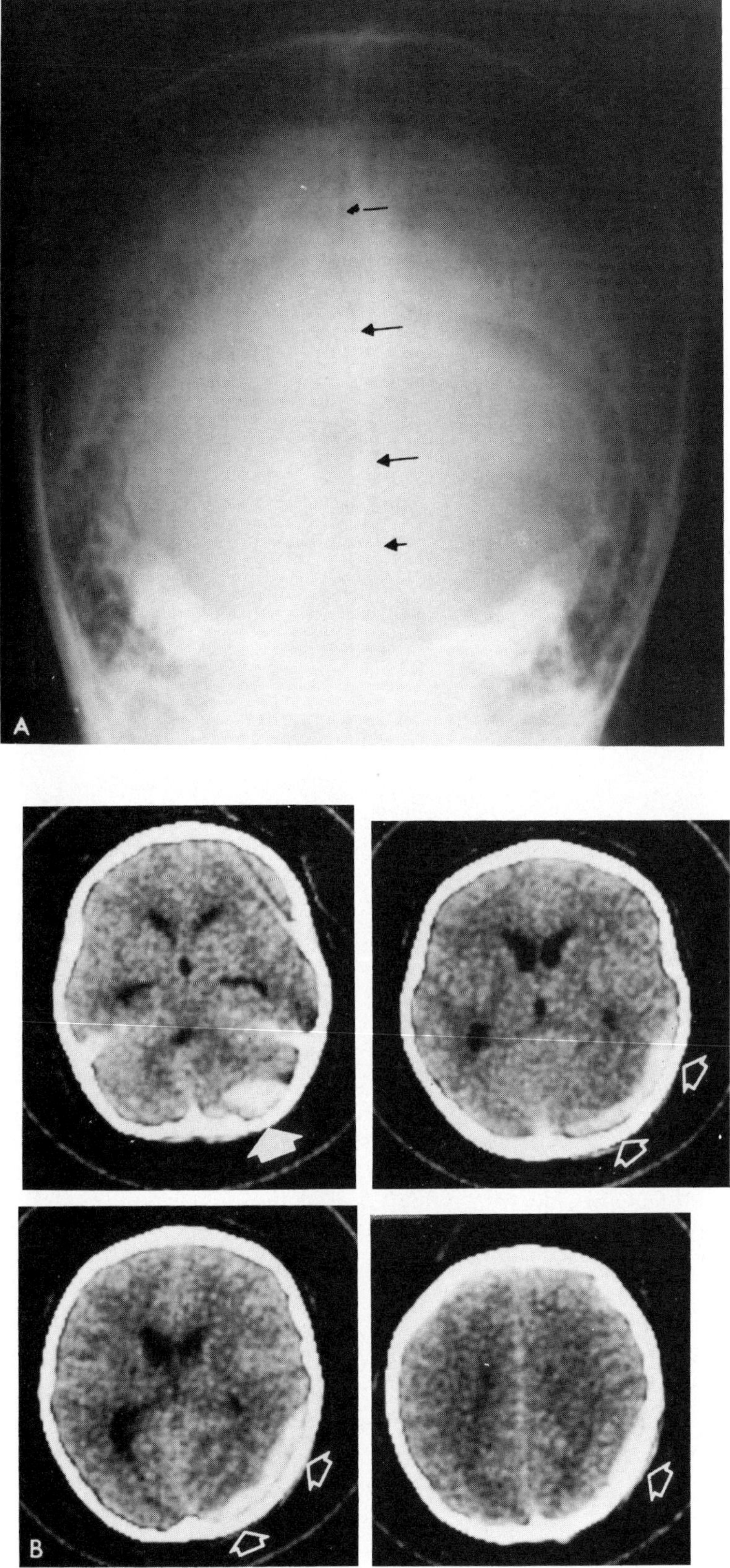

Figure 13–56 *See legend on the opposite page*

Figure 13–56. SUPRATENTORIAL AND INFRATENTORIAL EPIDURAL HEMATOMAS: *A*, The routine skull films revealed a linear skull fracture *(arrows)* extending vertically through the occipital bone and into the foramen magnum.

B, The CT scan shows a lentiform posterior fossa epidural hematoma *(white arrow)* associated with obstructive hydrocephalus. In addition there is a crescentic accumulation of clotted blood in the right supratentorial distribution *(open arrowheads)*, which surgery revealed was in the epidural space.

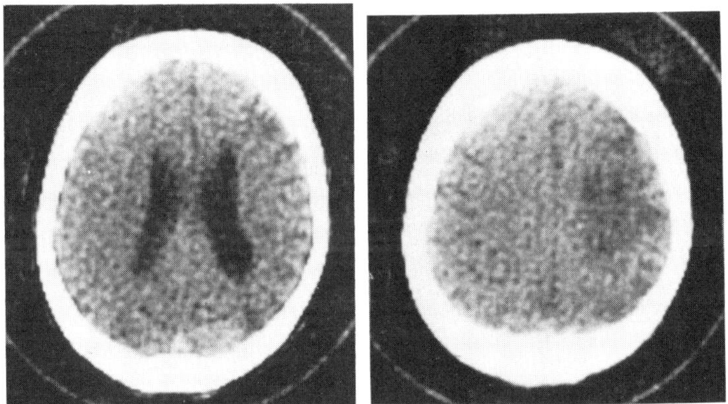

Figure 13–57. OLD ENCEPHALOMALACIA: Remote trauma resulted in a persistent left-sided weakness, and the CT scan revealed an area of low density in the right parietal region secondary to old infarct, hemorrhage or contusion dating from the time of the head trauma.

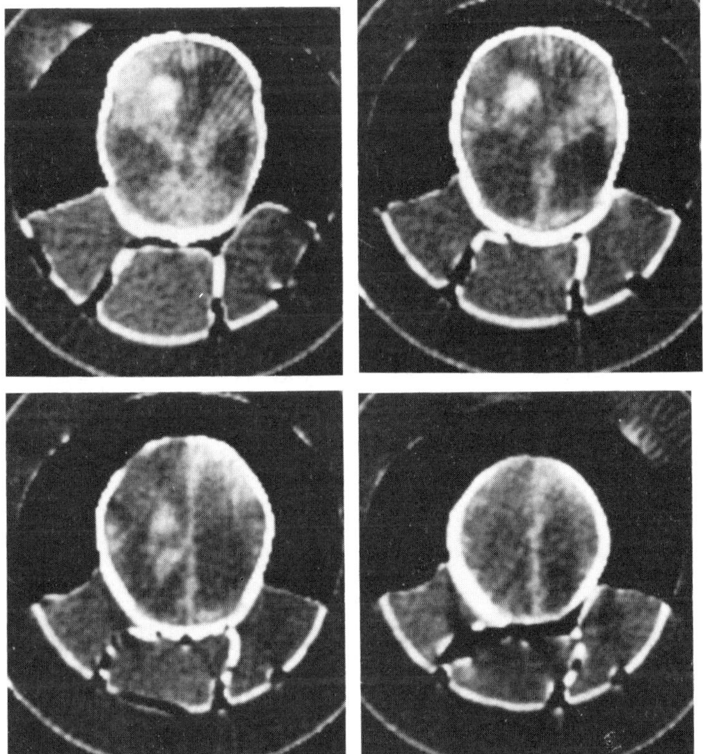

Figure 13–58. BIRTH TRAUMA: The CT scan shows an area of hemorrhage deep in the left hemisphere as well as hydrocephalus presumably secondary to subarachnoid hemorrhage and multiple infarcts following trauma at the time of birth.

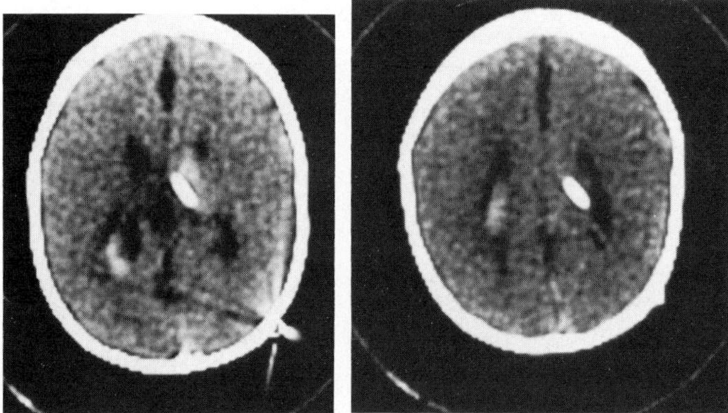

Figure 13–59. POSTOPERATIVE TRAUMA: Shunt tube placement has resulted in intraventricular hemorrhage with clotted blood in the bodies of both lateral ventricles.

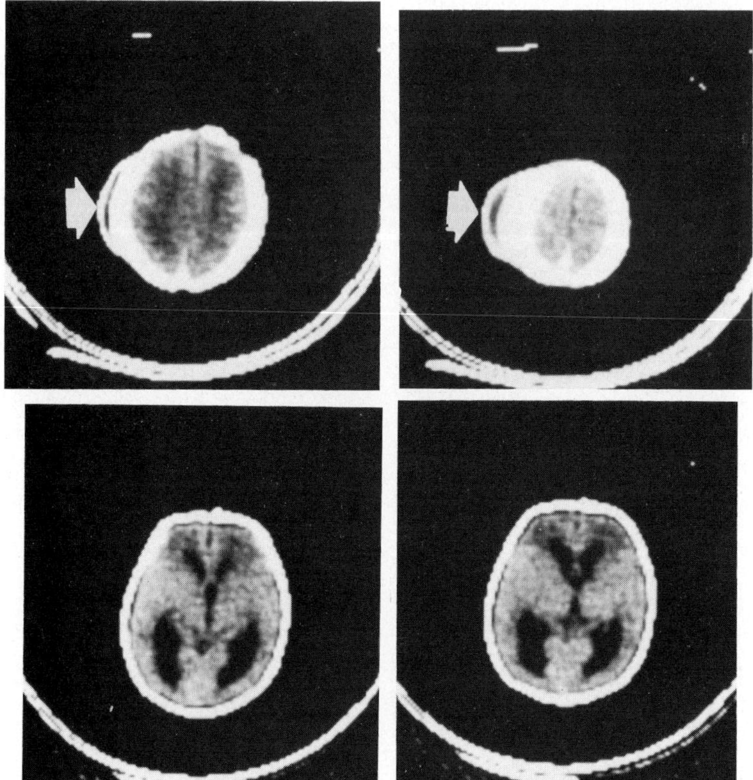

Figure 13–60. CAPUT SUCCEDANEUM: Labor and delivery have resulted in a caput succedaneum in the left parietal extracranial region. In addition, there are large lateral ventricles secondary to a communicating hydrocephalus following subarachnoid hemorrhage and bifrontal radiolucencies secondary to anoxia at the time of birth.

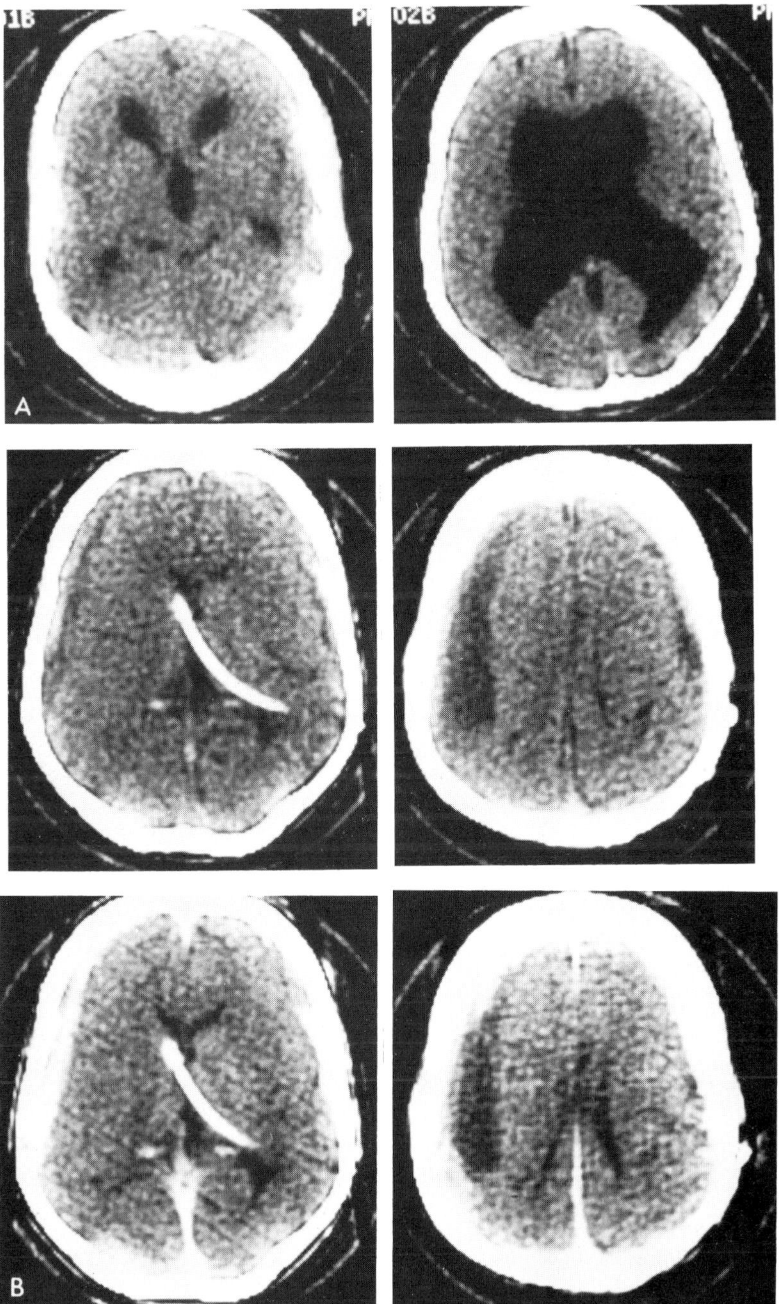

Figure 13–61. AQUEDUCT STENOSIS AND POST-SHUNT SUBDURAL HEMATOMAS: *A*, The initial CT scan showed large lateral ventricles that were found to be secondary to aqueduct stenosis.

B, The post-shunting CT scan reveals the shunt tube in place, bilateral chronic subdural hematomas and enhancing membranes on the postinfusion scan.

Illustration continued on the following page

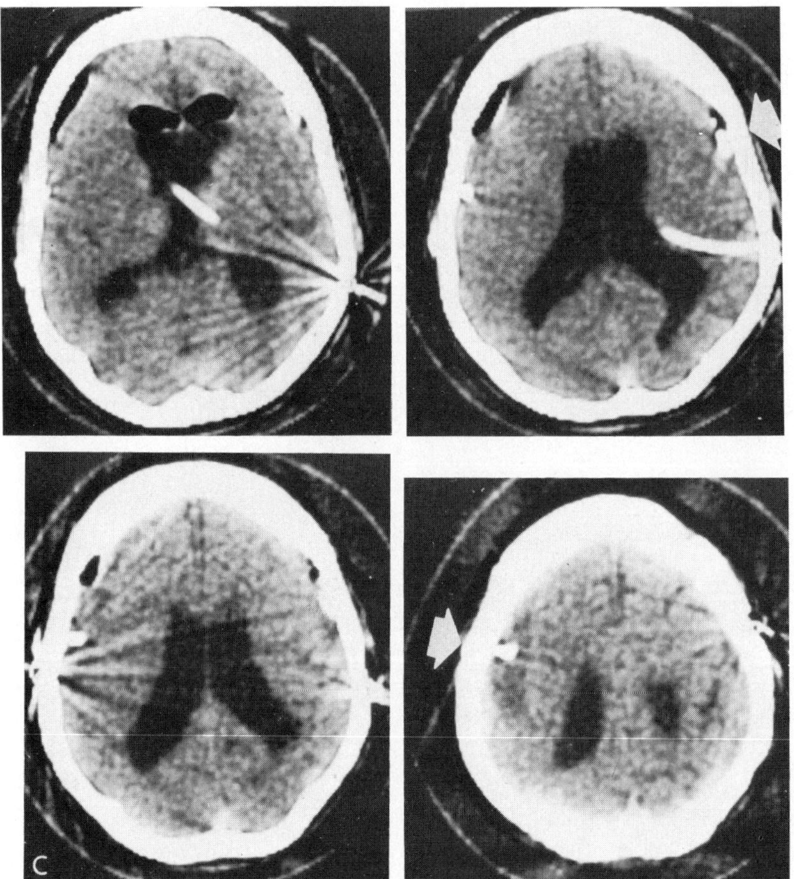

Figure 13–61 *Continued*

C, Shunt tubes were then placed in the subdural spaces bilaterally *(arrowheads)*, and the lateral ventricles were noted to re-expand somewhat. Air is present in the frontal horns of the lateral ventricles secondary to the ventriculogram.

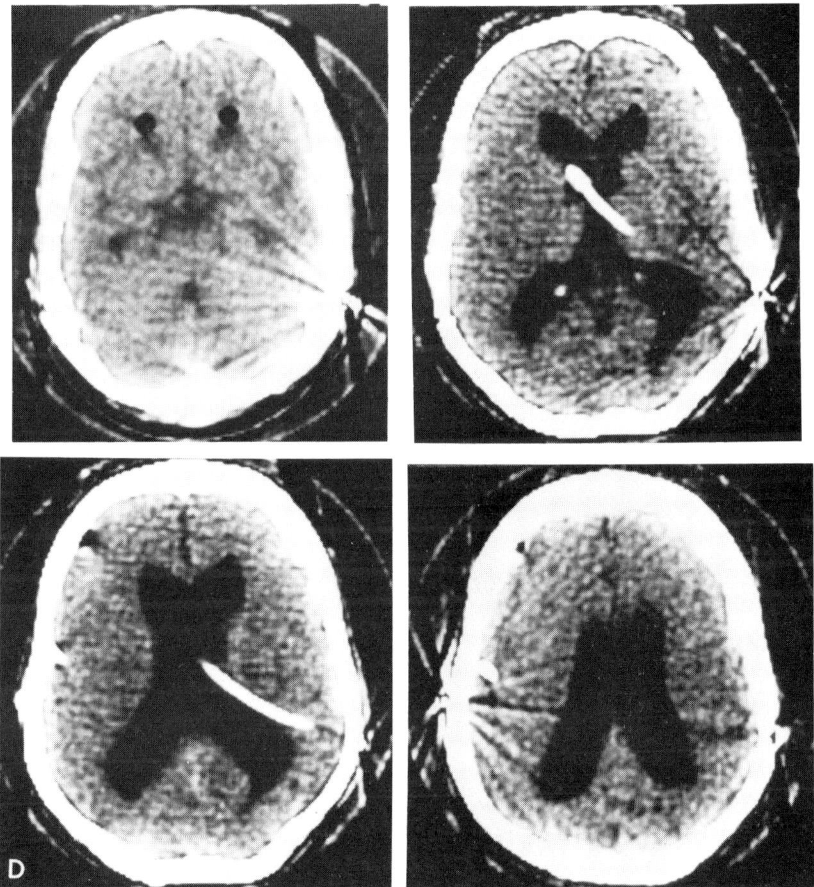

Figure 13–61 *Continued*

D, Subsequent follow-up scans show that the lateral ventricles had remained stable in size and that the subdural accumulations had resolved.

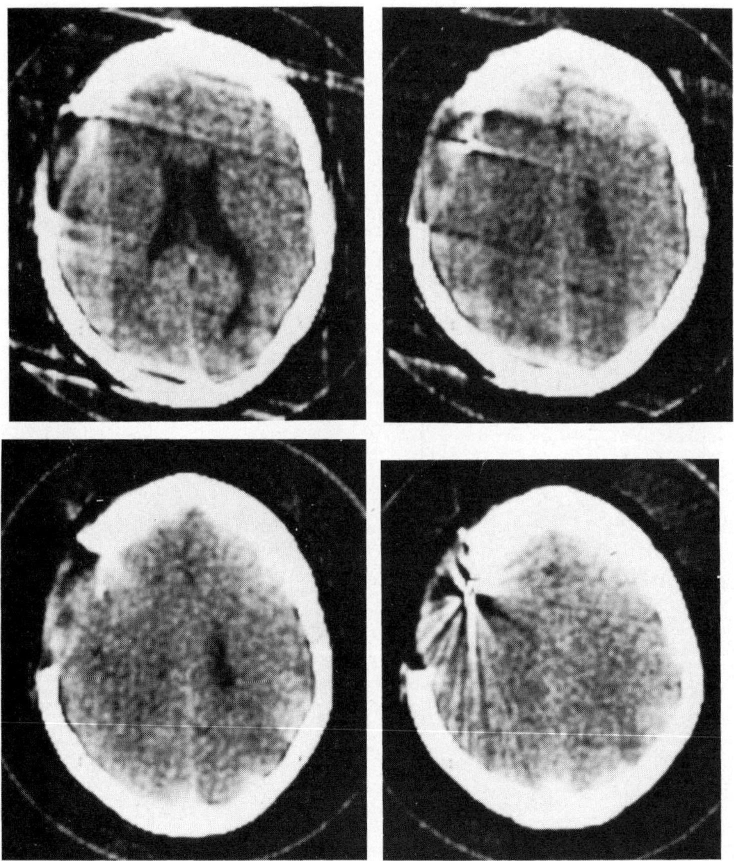

Figure 13–62. POSTOPERATIVE TRAUMA: Following removal of a chronic subdural hematoma, a large craniectomy defect is noted. There is an area of radiolucency beneath the craniectomy site and compression of the body of the left lateral ventricle. Postoperative changes should be correlated with the underlying disease and the surgical procedure.

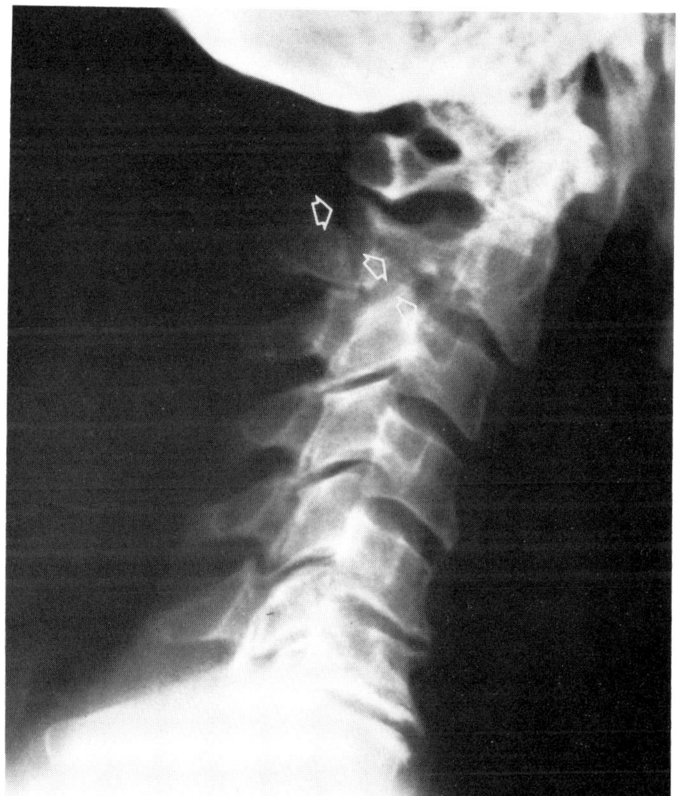

Figure 13–63. HANGMAN'S FRACTURE: This is an extension injury which, by definition, is a fracture dislocation of C_2. The lateral view reveals a fracture through the vertebral body and vertical fractures through the pedicles of C_2 *(arrows)* associated with forward displacement of the body of C_2 relative to C_3. The fracture is unstable because of the bilateral pedicle fractures and disruption of the anterior and posterior longitudinal ligaments and the intervertebral disk.

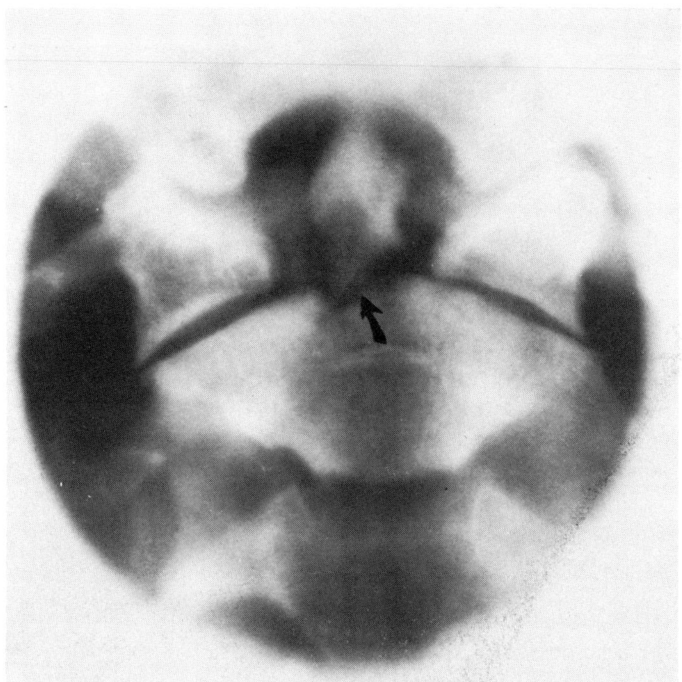

Figure 13–64. ODONTOID FRACTURE: An oblique fracture through the base of the odontoid process is well demonstrated on the tomograms *(arrow)*.

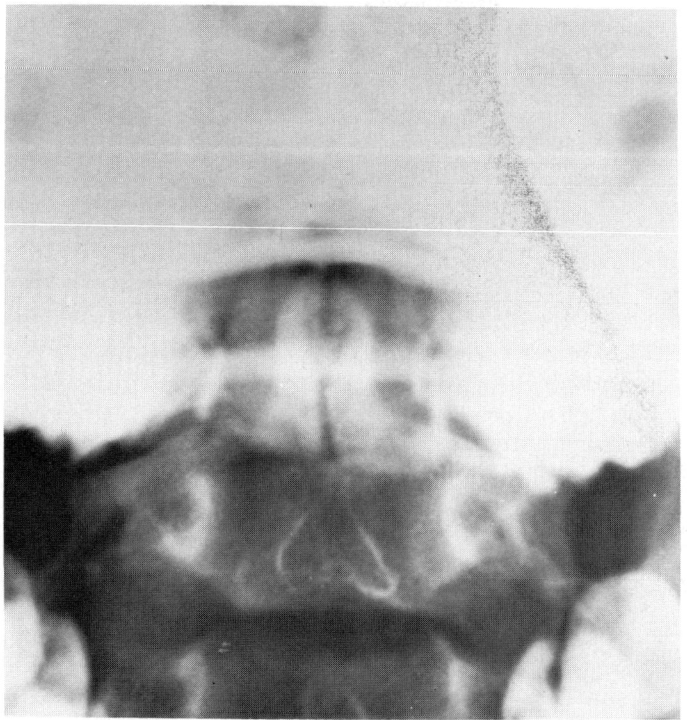

Figure 13–65. FRONTAL INCISORS SIMULATING AN ODONTOID FRACTURE: The incisors may project over the odontoid process and simulate an odontoid fracture or a cleft odontoid. Close inspection of the film reveals that the "cleft" in the odontoid is actually the gap between the incisors as they insert into the maxillary gingivae.

CHAPTER 14

POSTERIOR FOSSA

This discussion of the posterior fossa will focus on the anatomic structures that are in the infratentorial space, with emphasis on the vascular structures. Included in this space are the cerebellum with its right and left hemispheres and the midline cerebellar vermis, which surrounds the fourth ventricle (see Figure 14–1). The pons, medulla, midbrain, quadrigeminal plate and cerebral peduncles will be included in these discussions. The fourth ventricle and the aqueduct of Sylvius are important posterior fossa structures. In addition to these structures, several cisterns are of particular interest in the posterior fossa. Fortunately for us, as students of neuroanatomy, most of the cisterns are named for the particular area with which they are closely related. It should be pointed out that these cisterns are not individual and separate structures; rather, adjacent cisterns are simply extensions or continuations of each other but have been individually named for their related areas.

The cisterna magna is formed by the veil-like arachnoid membrane that extends down from the cerebellar hemispheres. Just anterior and inferior to the cisterna magna are the cerebellar tonsils. The tonsils are situated just off the midline on either side, and are anatomically the lowest point of the cerebellar hemispheres. More inferiorly are the medulla and the junction of the medulla with the spinal cord. Just beneath the medulla bilaterally are the vertebral arteries. These arteries join together in the midline to form the basilar artery below the mid-portion of the medulla. The vertebrobasilar system carries the blood supply to the posterior fossa structures (Fig. 14–1).

Computed Tomography of the Posterior Fossa. Before undertaking a discussion of the various structures of the posterior fossa, a few remarks are in order concerning the angiographic evaluation of posterior fossa lesions. In the supratentorial circulation, because the middle cerebral artery runs in the isle of Reil, which lies deep in the cerebral hemisphere, one is readily able to evaluate vascular displacements. Because of the relatively central location of the sylvian group of vessels, the normal vessel position usually is altered by mass lesions in various locations, whether they are presylvian, retrosylvian, supra- or infrasylvian. However, no such group of vessels runs deep through the central portion of the cerebellum; therefore, one must rely on alterations in the superficial blood vessels, even though they are rather remote from the actual mass lesions. Although some observers have had excellent success with angiographic diagnosis of posterior fossa lesions, I have found it to be less helpful than the CT scan.

The availability of CT scanning has made one appreciate the relative lack of accuracy of angiography in the diagnosis of mass lesions of the cerebellum. In addition, even when vascular alterations are demonstrated on the angiogram, the CT scan gives a more accurate concept of the anatomy of the lesion, whether cystic or solid, and whether it is or is not surrounded by edema. More important, the scan shows whether an

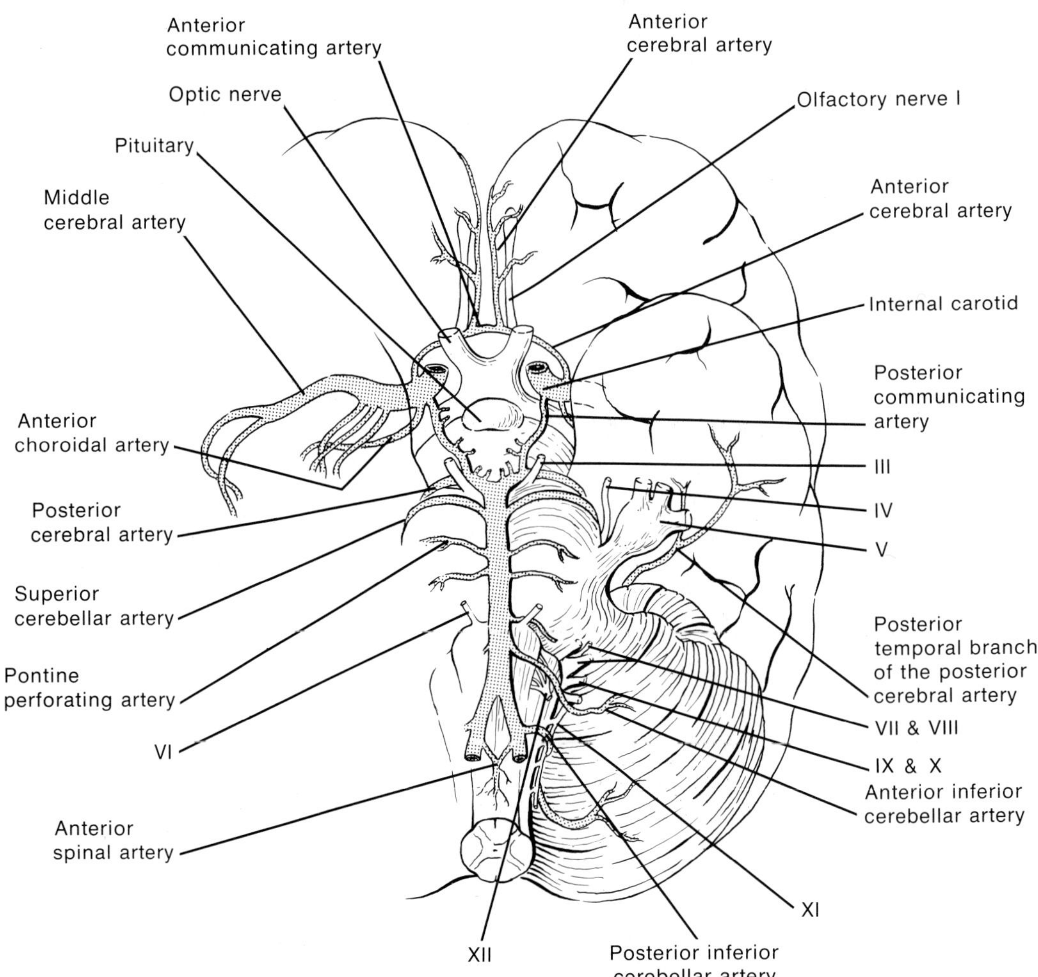

Figure 14–1. CIRCLE OF WILLIS AND POSTERIOR FOSSA VASCULAR SUPPLY: The posterior fossa structures are supplied by the vertebral and basilar arteries. The posterior fossa vessels communicate with the supratentorial circulation via the posterior communicating arteries. The surface anatomy of the base of the brain is also illustrated.

avascular mass represents an acute hematoma. Multiple mass lesions are best demonstrated by CT scanning. The author has seen examples where the CT scan demonstrated a sizable mass lesion and the angiogram was singularly unhelpful — failing, even in retrospect, to demonstrate even the side of the abnormality.

It is becoming apparent that in some cases a definitive operative procedure can be performed on certain posterior fossa lesions without using any invasive studies after evaluation by CT scanning. In addition, the scan can tell us whether there is an associated hydrocephalus, any evidence of supratentorial extension of the mass or an associated supratentorial mass lesion. Although obviously there is no substitute for arteriographic evaluation of such vascular lesions as aneurysms and arteriovenous malformations in the cerebellum or dura, for nearly all other lesions evaluation by CT has greatly enhanced our ability to diagnose both the type and extent of various posterior fossa lesions with far greater accuracy than was ever possible before the development of computed tomography.

It is not unreasonable to expect that in the future angiography will no longer be used for diagnosis; instead, it will serve to demonstrate vessel landmarks and blood supply after the CT scan has revealed a mass lesion. There is, of course, no substitute for the angiogram in defining the position of arterial and venous structures.

Pneumoencephalography. Because arteriographic findings can indicate the presence of tonsillar herniation, arteriography is performed before pneumoencephalography. Pneumoencephalography is dangerous if tonsillar herniation is present. In addition, aneurysms of the vertebral or basilar system also can be ruled out by angiography. This is of more than passing interest, because basilar artery aneurysms can act as mass lesions. Indeed, pneumoencephalography is not indicated if the diagnosis of a basilar artery aneurysm is made by arteriography.

Although pneumoencephalography is an excellent method for the evaluation of posterior fossa mass lesions, the method may be dangerous in the patient with a cerebellar or posterior fossa mass lesion. A lumbar tap may precipitate tonsillar herniation and possibly death, even when proper technique is used.

Ventriculography. Because of these considerations, if tonsillar herniation is demonstrated at arteriography, one may elect not to use pneumoencephalography but rather to perform a ventriculogram.

Ventriculography is performed by instilling air into the ventricular system via a bur hole (or fontanelle tape in young children), usually in the nondominant hemisphere — generally the right side. This is done by the neurosurgeon. A catheter or needle is used, and air or radiopaque contrast material is instilled directly into the ventricular system. By patient manipulation, including posterior somersaulting, the contrast is manipulated into the fourth ventricle and basilar cisterns. If the sylvian aqueduct is occluded, this can also be demonstrated.

Angiography. The posterior fossa circulation may be studied by either right or left brachial arteriography. If studied from the right side, one will also get the "bonus" of seeing the supratentorial circulation on the right side with filling of the right carotid artery. Before other methods such as nuclide brain scanning and computed tomography of the brain were developed, it was helpful to include the supratentorial circulation in order to evaluate the possible presence of hydrocephalus, an abnormal vascular supply arising from the internal carotid system or even evidence of additional mass lesions in the supratentorial compartment. Studies of the carotid circulation are not always needed or desirable and may at times even obscure the visualization of the posterior fossa circulation. Left brachial arteriography will visualize the posterior fossa circulation only. It is beneficial to perform the brachial arteriogram on the side of the suspected mass lesion because the visualization of the position of the PICA and its branches on the involved side is of great diagnostic importance and assists the neurosurgeon in planning a surgical approach. To prevent filling of the carotid circulation at the time of right bra-

Text continued on page 655

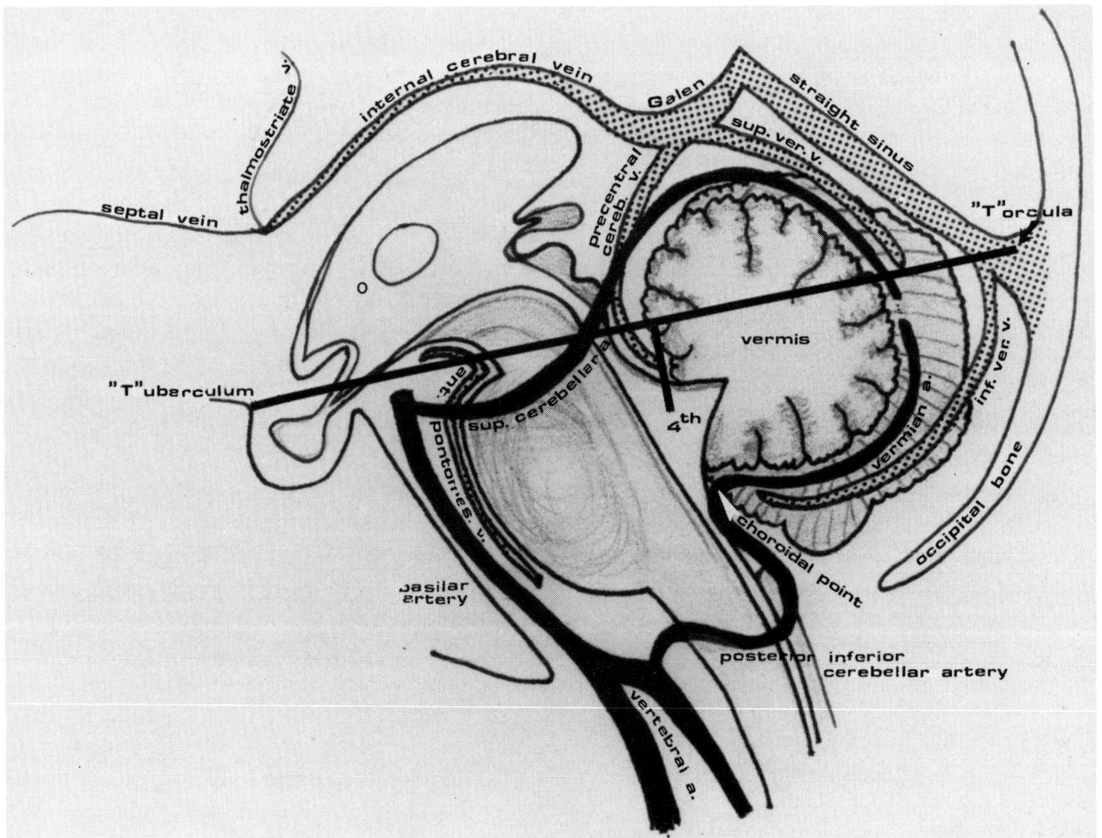

Figure 14–2. TWINING'S LINE: The choroidal point (*white arrow*) lies at approximately the midportion of Twining's line. This line connects the *T*uberculum with the *T*orcula and is also known as the "T-T" line. Most of the important arteries and veins of the posterior fossa are also illustrated in this drawing and should be committed to memory.

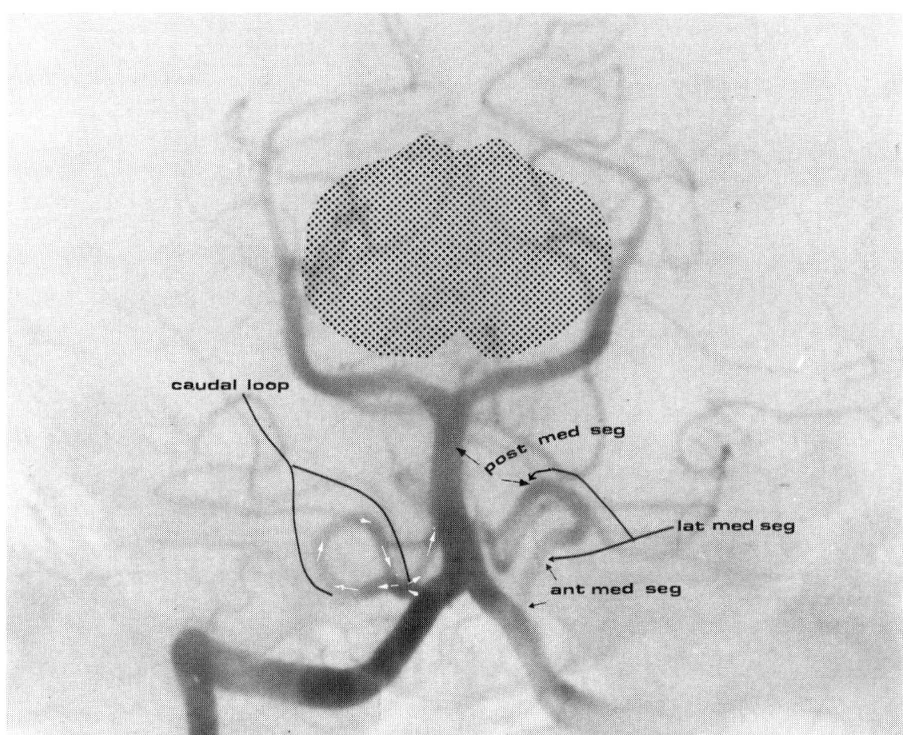

Figure 14–3. NORMAL ANATOMY OF THE POSTERIOR INFERIOR CEREBELLAR ARTERY (PICA): On the left side, the normal segments of the PICA are illustrated; on the right, the course of the PICA is illustrated by the white arrows. The choroidal point is in the midline and is hidden behind the basilar artery, which is filled with contrast material. The posterior cerebral arteries and the superior cerebellar arteries course around the midbrain (shaded area) and nearly meet in the midline in the region of the quadrigeminal plate cistern.

Illustration continued on following page

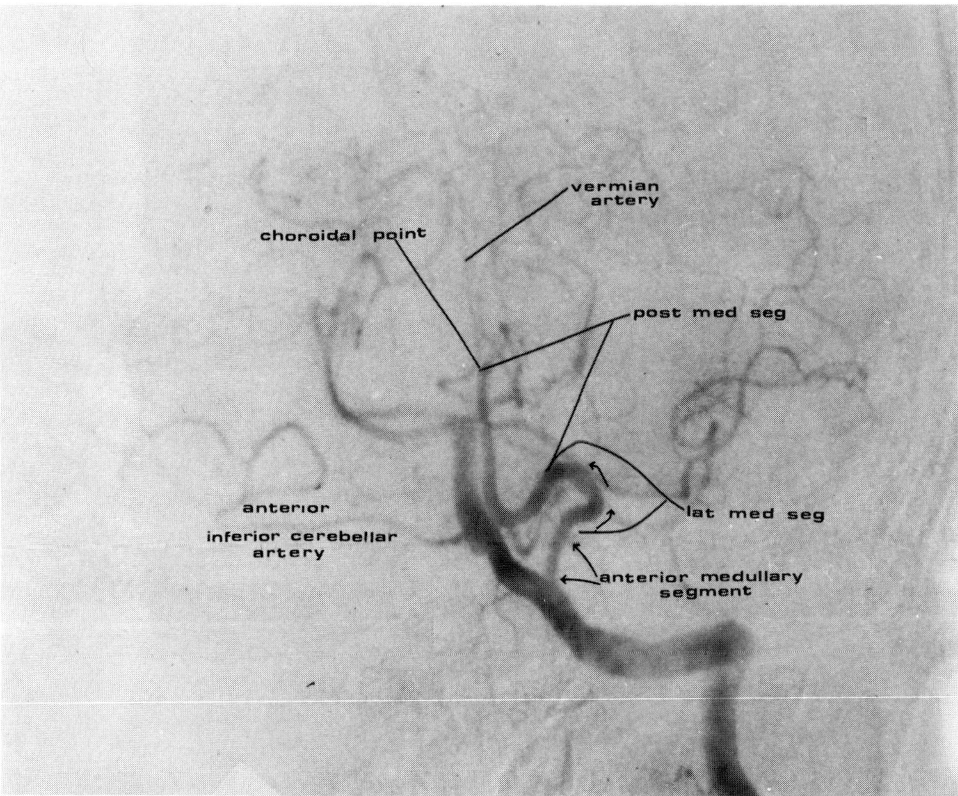

Figure 14–4. CONTINUATION OF FIGURE 14–3: The contrast material has now washed out of the right vertebral artery, and this vessel is now filled with unopacified blood. The anterior inferior cerebellar artery (AICA) is well visualized on the right side, but is obscured by the PICA on the left. The choroidal point is well seen, as are the vermian branches of the PICA. The various segments of the PICA again are demonstrated.

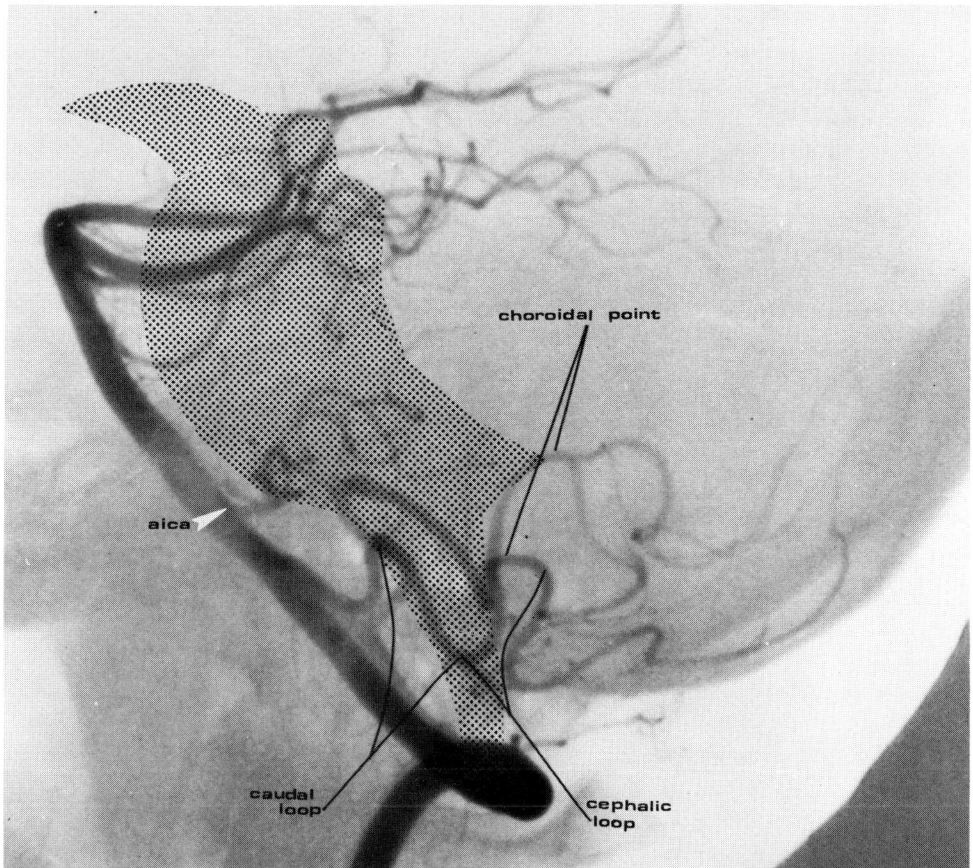

Figure 14–5. LATERAL VIEW: Both the right and the left PICA are filled, and their courses can be traced on the lateral view. The choriodal points are at different levels, but both are normal. The anterior inferior cerebellar arteries (AICA) also can be seen.

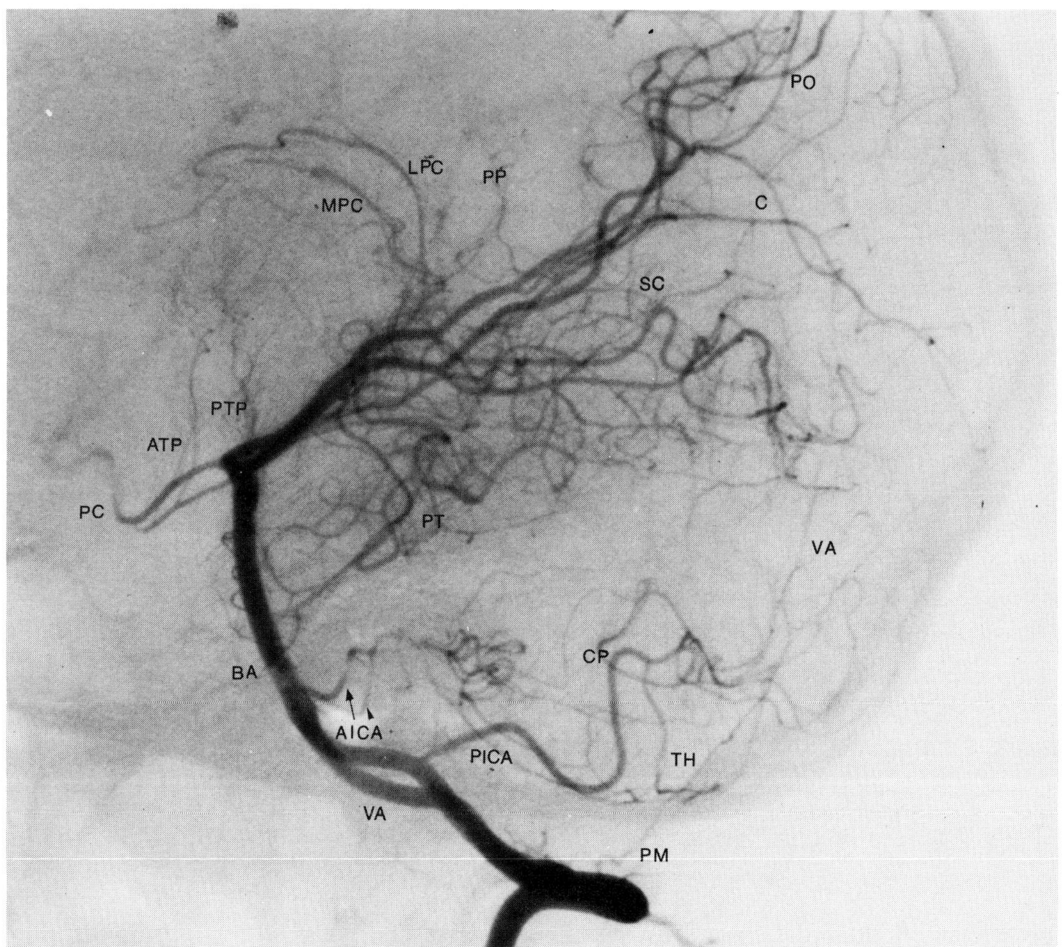

Figure 14–6. The lateral view of the vertebral angiogram in a normal patient using subtraction techniques demonstrates the normal arterial structures in the posterior fossa.

PC Posterior communicating artery; *ATP* Anterior thalamoperforating arteries; *PTP* Posterior thalamoperforating arteries; *BA* Basilar artery; *VA* Vertebral artery; *AICA* Anterior inferior cerebellar artery; *PICA* Posterior inferior cerebellar artery; *CP* Choroidal point; *TH* Tonsillohemispheric branch of *PICA*; *VA* Vermian branch of PICA; *PT* Posterior temporal branch of posterior cerebral artery; *SC* Superior cerebellar arteries; *C* Calcarine branch of posterior cerebral artery; *PO* Parieto-occipital branch of posterior cerebral artery; *MPC* Medial posterior choroidal artery; *LPC* Lateral posterior choroidal artery; *PP* Posterior pericallosal artery; *PM* Posterior meningeal artery.

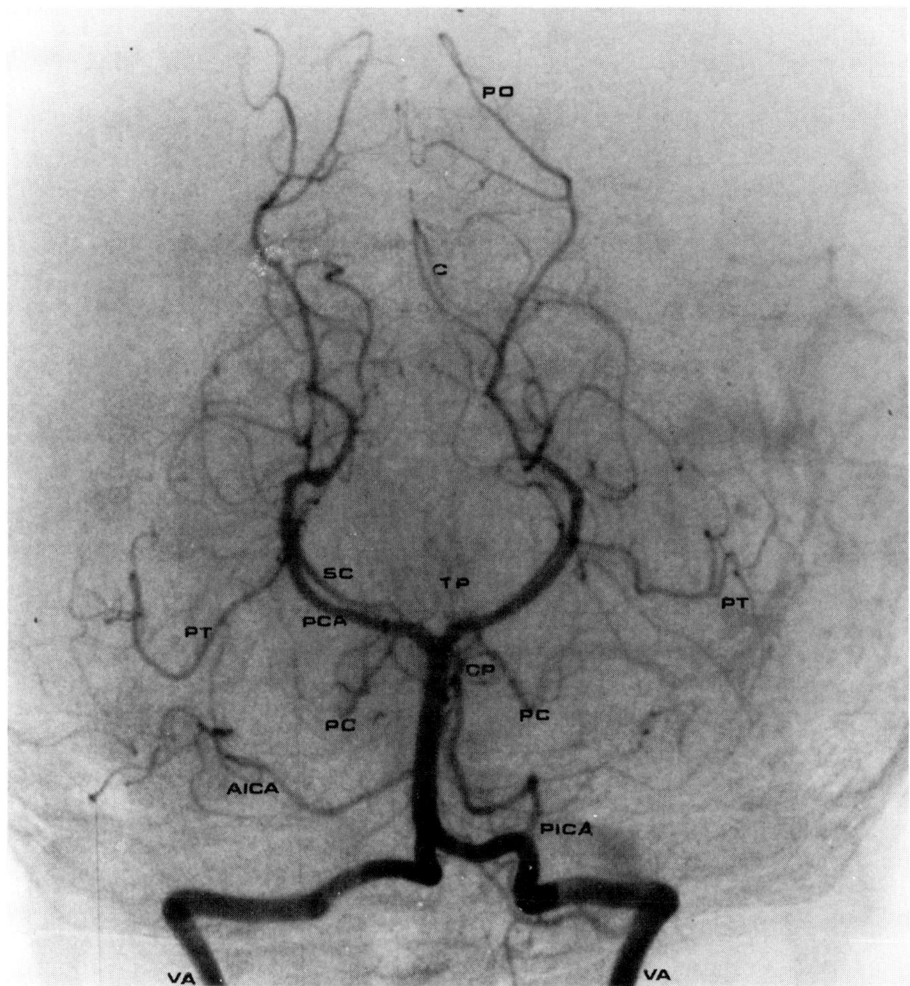

Figure 14–7. The AP view of the vertebral angiogram using subtraction techniques demonstrates the normal arteries in the posterior fossa. The PICA is absent on the right side, a normal anatomic variant.

VA Vertebral artery; *PT* Posterior temporal branch of posterior cerebral artery; *PCA* Posterior cerebral artery; *SC* Superior cerebellar artery; *TP* Thalamoperforating arteries; *C* Calcarine branch of posterior cerebral artery; *AICA* Anterior inferior cerebellar artery; *PO* Parieto-occipital branch of the posterior cerebral artery; *PC* Posterior communicating artery.

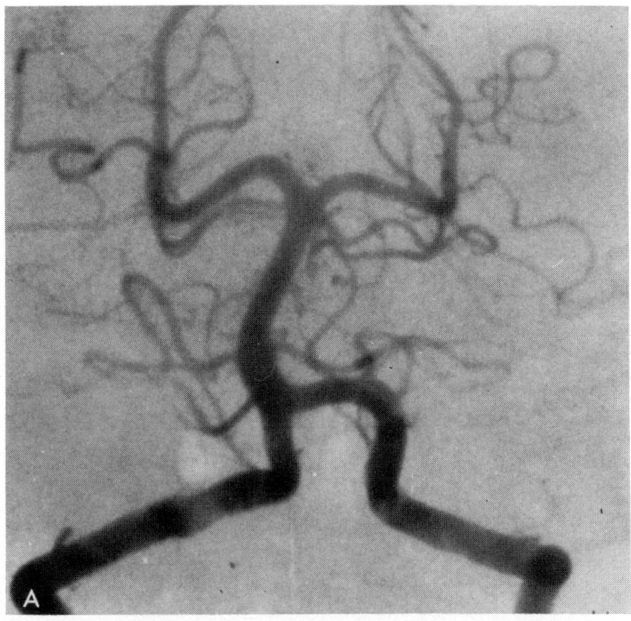

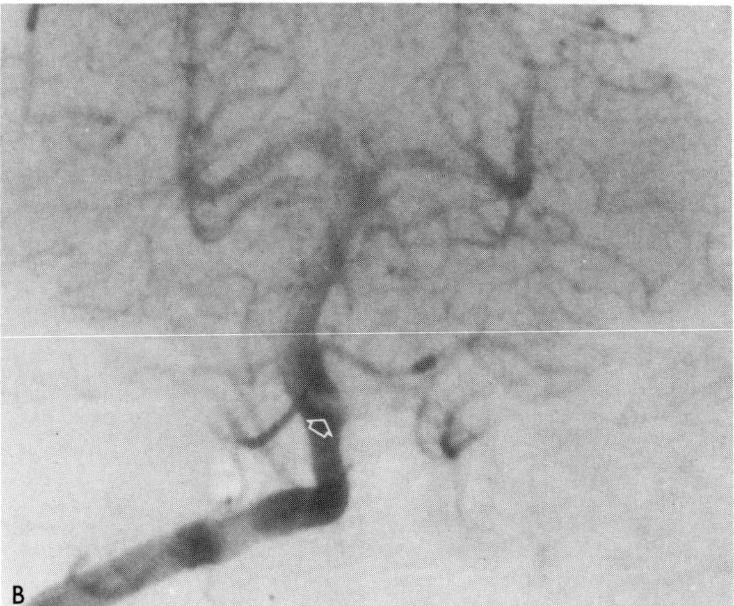

Figure 14–8. NORMAL VERTEBRAL ARTERIOGRAM WITH WASH-OUT: *A* reveals filling of both vertebral arteries from the right vertebral injection. The left vertebral artery is filled by retrograde flow.

B, Later in the arterial phase the contrast material has been washed out of the left vertebral artery; now unopacified blood is flowing up the left vertebral artery, creating a "streaming" effect in the basilar artery. This unopacified blood creates a filling defect in the basilar artery *(white arrowhead)*. This should not be mistaken for an arteriosclerotic plaque or thrombus in the basilar artery.

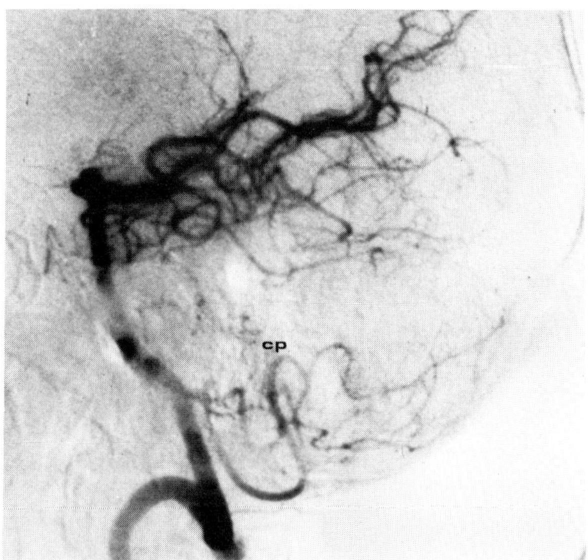

Figure 14–9. NORMAL LOW POSITION OF THE PICA: The PICA originates in a normal position, and the caudal loop extends down below the foramen magnum. There is, however, no evidence of abnormal vascularity or vessel displacement. In addition, note that the choroidal point is in its anticipated normal position *(cp)*. This is not a reflection of tonsillar herniation, but represents a normal variation.

chial arteriography, one can manually compress the right carotid artery in the neck during the time of antegrade flow of the contrast — thus eliminating visualization of the supratentorial circulation.

With the availability of femoral catheterization, selective catheterization of either the right or left vertebral artery can readily be performed in most cases with injection of contrast material directly into the vertebral

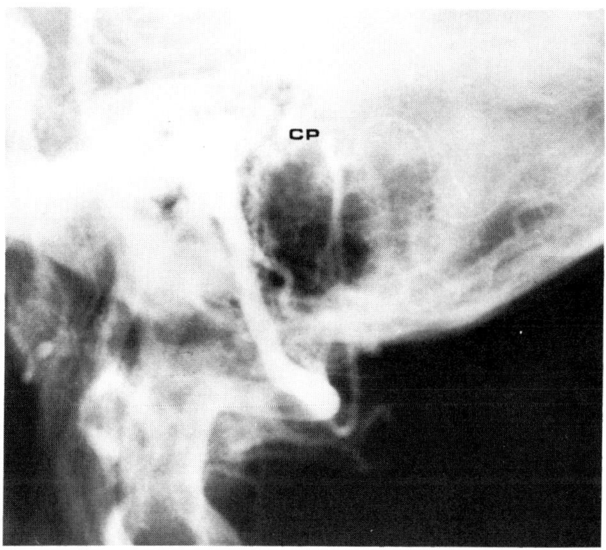

Figure 14–10. NORMAL LOW POSITION OF THE PICA: As in the example in Figure 14–9, the caudal loop of the PICA extends well below the foramen magnum — in this case down to C1 — however, the choroidal point is normal. This is a normal anatomic variation.

artery. Using this method one hopes to fill the vertebrobasilar system; indeed, it may even "wash" the contrast material down the contralateral vertebral artery to a level below the origin of the contralateral PICA. In this fashion one can outline all the posterior fossa structures from one vertebral artery injection and include only the posterior fossa circulation. Depending on the size of the vertebral artery, 3 to 8 cc of contrast material is injected directly into the vertebral artery. With rare exceptions, do not inject more than 8 cc. We use a rate of from 6 to 10 cc per second over a time period necessary to inject the amount desired: e.g., to inject 5 cc we use a rate of 10 cc/sec for 0.5 second. All injections are made with the automatic injector.

As with brachial arteriography, the PICA on the side of the suspected lesion should be visualized if at all possible. If the contrast material does not wash retrograde down the contralateral vertebral artery at the time of injection and evaluation of the opposite side is required, the opposite vertebral artery should be catheterized and injected for full evaluation of the vascular anatomy bilaterally. In some instances, it will be necessary to perform percutaneous brachial angiography if it is technically impossible to catheterize the vertebral arteries selectively — e.g., when there is stenosis of the vessel origin.

NORMAL VASCULAR ANATOMY

The right vertebral artery arises from the right subclavian artery distal to the origin of the right common carotid artery. On the left side, the vertebral artery arises directly from the subclavian artery. In 3 to 6 per cent of cases, the left vertebral artery will be seen to arise directly from the arch of the aorta as a separate vessel (see Chapter 4). In most cases, the vertebral arteries enter into the foramina transversaria of the lateral mass of the cervical vertebrae at the level of C_6. There are anatomic variations, however, and the vertebral artery may enter into the foramina transversaria at any level. The vertebral arteries then course cephalad until they reach the level of C_2. At the C_2 level the artery turns laterally and then superiorly to enter the more laterally placed foramina transversaria of the C_1 vertebral body. Following the exit from the C_1 foramina transversaria, the vertebral artery lies in a groove along the superior margin of the atlas; it then turns anteromedially and passes through the foramina magnum lying anterior to the medulla oblongata. Very shortly thereafter, the vertebral artery joins with its mate from the other side to form the basilar artery (Fig. 14–2). In 5 to 6 per cent of cases, the vertebral artery ends in the PICA.

Three branches of the vertebral artery are of consequence to us as angiographers. In addition to these main branches, a variety of smaller branches feed the musculature of the neck and may be used to supply collateral flow to the vertebral or external carotid system (see Chapter 6). The branches that concern us are the posterior inferior cerebellar artery (PICA), the anterior spinal artery (note that at this point the spinal cord is anatomically positioned dorsal to the vertebral arteries), and the posterior meningeal artery. The posterior spinal artery may arise from the vertebral artery, but more often it arises from the PICA as it courses around the medulla. Note that a posterior spinal artery arising from the vertebral artery would have to course around the medulla to become dorsal or posterior to the cord.

To understand the normal and pathologic anatomy of posterior fossa, one must have a thorough understanding of the anatomy of the normal pathway of the PICA (See Figs. 14–3–14–7). A simple statement, but basic to this understanding, is the fact that the PICA originates from the vertebral artery ventral to the medulla, but ultimately will supply an area that is predominantly dorsal to the medulla. As a consequence, the PICA must follow a course that will allow it to do this.

The PICA has three segments. The initial portion is known as the *anterior medullary segment* because it is still anterior to the medulla at this point. This is best appreciated on the anterior view; on the lateral view, the vessel is directed toward the observer, and its lateral course cannot be recognized because the vessel is foreshortened. This lateral direction is the first step toward this vessel's ultimate position dorsal to the medulla. The PICA then courses inferiorly for a variable distance, forms a loop by reversing its course back upon itself; it proceeds dorsally and cephalad and then courses cephalad toward the fourth ventricle. Most of this loop is lateral to the medulla; it is therefore known as the *lateral medullary segment* (Fig. 14–3). This initial loop, which is convex caudad, is known as the *caudal loop*. When the PICA reaches its position dorsal to the medulla, that portion is known as the *posterior medullary segment* (because it is dorsal or posterior to the medulla). The posterior medullary segment of the PICA then courses cephalad and anteriorly along the posterior margin of the medulla in a near midline position until it reaches the posterior margin of the fourth ventricle. At this point, the PICA gives off a small twiglike branch to the choroid plexus of the fourth ventricle. This point is known as the *choroidal point* (Figs. 14–4 and 14–5). The small branch to the choroid plexus is not usually visible arteriographically, but it may be seen if angiotomography or magnification and subtraction techniques are used (Fig. 14–7).

At the choroidal point, the PICA again reverses its course, turns caudally and bifurcates into the vermian branch and the tonsillohemispheric branches (Fig. 14–6). This loop of the PICA is known as the *cephalic loop* (Fig. 14–5). Note that the caudal loop and the cephalic loop of the PICA share a common limb — that portion just proximal to the choroidal point.

It should also be noted that there is a good deal of normal variation in the position of the PICA. One should be familiar with these normal variations before suggesting a mass lesion or an abnormal course of this vessel. In some cases, the PICA will initially loop upward rather than downward. Again, this is a normal variation and, in most instances, the artery will return to a more "normal" course, and the various loops such as the caudal and cephalic loops will be readily identified.

The normal point of origin of the PICA from the vertebral artery also can vary greatly. The caudal loop of the PICA may extend down to the level of the C_2 vertebral body and still be within normal limits. The fact that the PICA extends this low may suggest a posterior fossa mass lesion. If this is suspected, one should look for other correlating abnormalities. When the caudal loop of the PICA extends very low as a normal anatomic variation, it will be seen that the choroidal point is in normal position and that no other vascular displacements are evident. With true tonsillar herniation secondary to a mass lesion it is the *tonsillar branch* of the PICA that will be displaced below the level of the foramen magnum.

To measure the normal position of the choroidal point, the "T-T" line or "Twining's line" is used as an anatomic measurement (Fig. 14–2). Twining's line extends from the tuberculum sellae (T) to the torcular herophili (T). A line perpendicular to the midpoint of this line should fall approximately in the middle of the fourth ventricle. Therefore, the angiographic choroidal point, which is at the posterior portion of the fourth ventricle, should, in the normal individual, also lie at approximately the midportion of Twining's line.

Distal to the choroidal point, the PICA bifurcates into the tonsillohemispheric and vermian branches (Fig. 14–6). The vermian branches course posteriorly and superiorly just adjacent to the midline and along the posterior margin of the vermis of the cerebellum. The tonsillohemispheric branches of the PICA will be seen to course laterally and then up and over the cerebellar hemispheres. The PICA forms the main blood supply to the lower portion of the cerebellum, and the vermian artery forms anastomotic connections with the superior cerebellar arteries. The tonsillar branch of the PICA *may* course along the inferior border of the tonsil, but it may also loop over or below the tonsil; therefore it is not as reliable a sign as one would like as a reflection of tonsillar herniation. The tonsillar loop *is* displaced inferiorly with tonsillar herniation, however, and this occurs when there is a lesion with enough mass effect to create downward displacement of the tonsil. It is this downward displacement of the tonsillar loop of the PICA that must be looked for when one is concerned about the possibility of a mass lesion in the posterior fossa. One should check also for the position of the choroidal point and other anatomic landmarks that will correlate with or refute the presence of a mass lesion and resulting tonsillar herniation.

Posterior Meningeal Branch of the Vertebral Artery. This vessel arises from the ver-

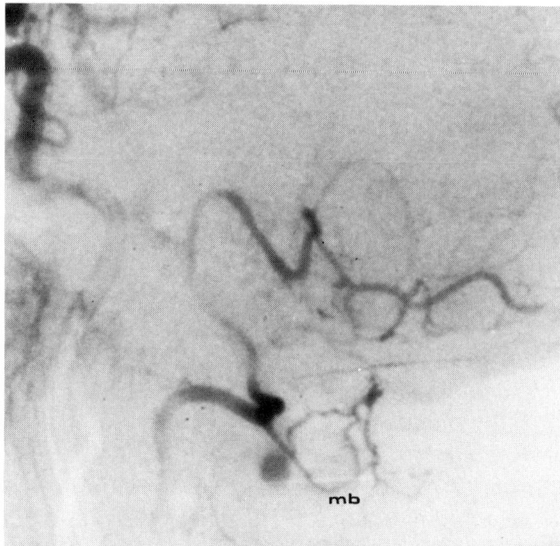

Figure 14–11. VERTEBRAL ARTERY ENDING IN PICA: The vertebral artery ends in the PICA. This normal variation is seen in approximately 25 per cent of individuals. In these patients, the basilar artery and the remainder of the posterior fossa structures will not be filled, and it may be necessary to inject the contralateral vertebral artery. Note muscular branch (mb).

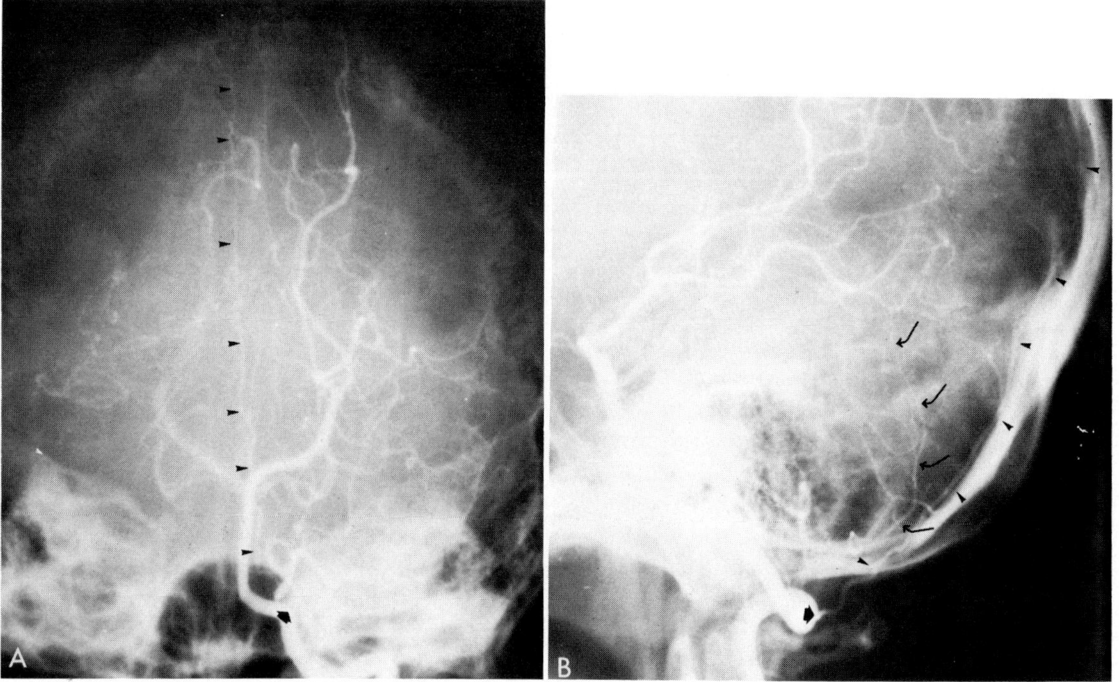

Figure 14–12. NORMAL POSTERIOR MENINGEAL ARTERY: *A* and *B*, The large arrowhead illustrates the origin of the vertebral artery, which is seen to course along the inner table of the skull posteriorly just adjacent to the midline *(small arrowheads)*. The posterior meningeal artery extends past the torcula into the supratentorial circulation. The angled arrows illustrate the vermian branches of the PICA.

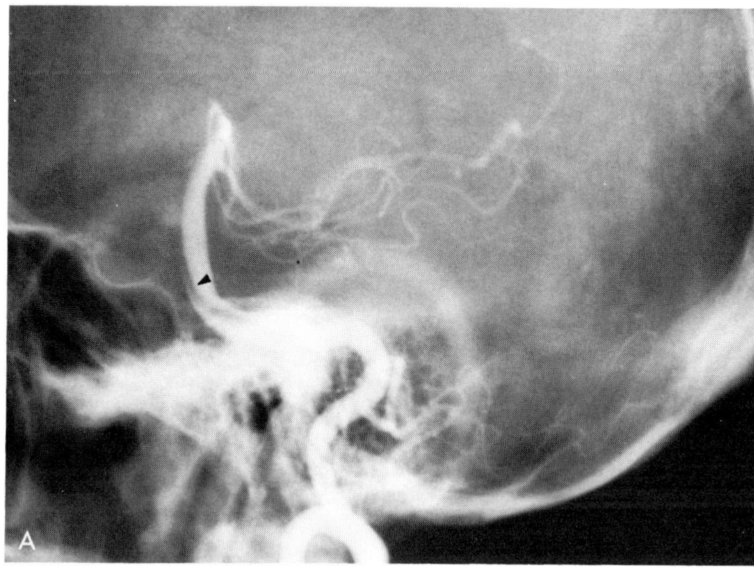

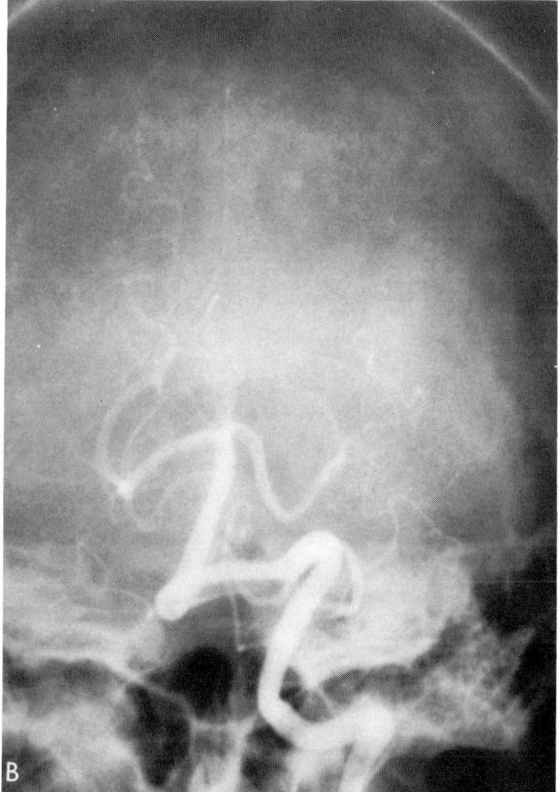

Figure 14–13. TORTUOUS BASILAR ARTERY: *A* and *B*, The basilar artery is seen to be tortuous. A linear filling defect is seen on both the AP and the lateral views; this represents unopacified blood from the opposite vertebral artery *(arrowhead)*. The AP view gives the false appearance that the basilar artery is narrowed because of the stream of unopacified blood. The tortuous artery may simulate a cerebellopontine angle mass, or the patient may complain of hemifacial spasms — apparently from irritation of the nerves in the cerebellopontine angle by the elongated basilar artery.

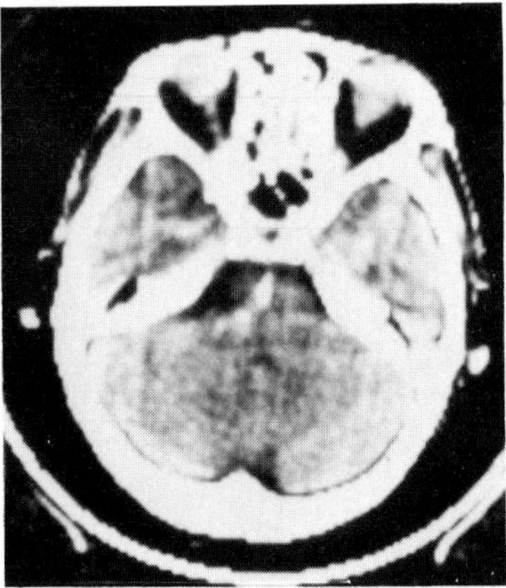
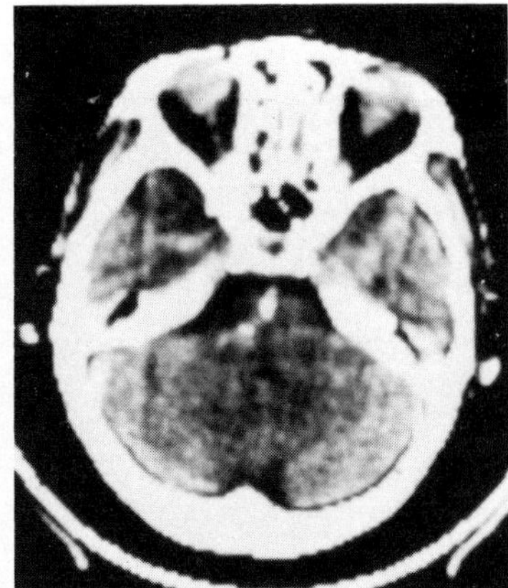
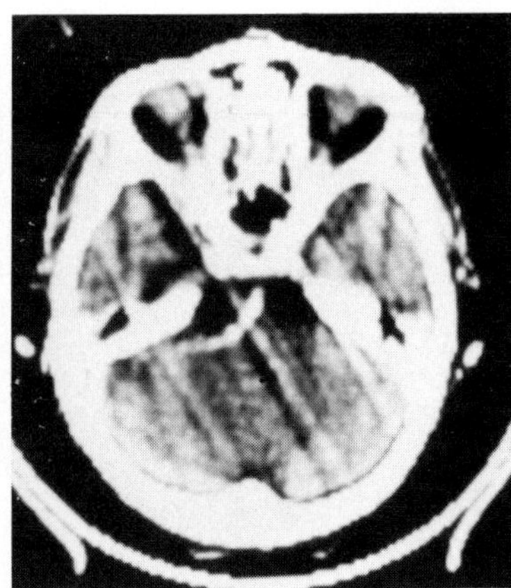

Figure 14–14. CT SCAN OF CALCIFIED TORTUOUS BASILAR ARTERY: The calcified basilar artery is visible on the base cut of the preinfusion scan as it extends obliquely across the pons from left to right in front of the fourth ventricle. Postinfusion, the artery is even better demonstrated.

tebral artery above the arch of the atlas and just below the foramen magnum. The vessel courses superiorly in the midline adjacent to the inner table of the skull. The artery may extend above the tentorium cerebelli and supply the falx cerebri and adjacent tentorium. This vessel may become enlarged with the presence of a meningioma.

Anterior Inferior Cerebellar Arteries. These originate from the basilar artery approximately 1 cm from the origin of the basilar artery. The right and left anterior inferior cerebellar arteries (AICA) are seen and usually can be visualized arteriographically. The AICA will be seen to course laterally; it then enters into and courses out of the internal auditory canal and then around the flocculus of the cerebellum. This unique course of the AICA in the region of the internal auditory canal makes it of particular value when a cerebellopontine angle mass is present. After the AICA exits from the internal auditory canal, it will be seen to course further laterally and supply the cerebellar hemisphere at the level of the great horizontal fissure. The region of the horizontal fissure of the cerebellum is a so-called "watershed" area between the distribution of the superior cerebellar arteries and the posterior inferior cerebellar arteries. There is an inverse relationship between the size of the PICA and the size of the AICA. When the PICA is small — or, in 25 per cent of cases, absent — the AICA is enlarged and supplies the distribution of the PICA.

The basilar artery gives origin to many small pontine perforating vessels; however, these cannot normally be visualized arteriographically except by magnification and subtraction techniques.

Figure 14–15. TORTUOUS VERTEBROBASILAR ARTERY WITH ANEURYSM FORMATION: *A*, The vertebral and basilar arteries are both markedly tortuous and dilated, and the sharp pointed areas of opacification on the arteriogram are accumulations of contrast material in a partially clotted aneurysm.

B, The shaded area outlines the position of the aneursym.

C, The CT scan, postinfusion, reveals the tortuous basilar artery as it courses from right to left along the posterior margin of the right petrous pyramid. The elongated basilar artery protrudes so far superiorly that the outlet of the third ventricle is obstructed, and the dilated occipital horns of the lateral ventricles can be seen (case courtesy of Dr. Martin Bruetman).

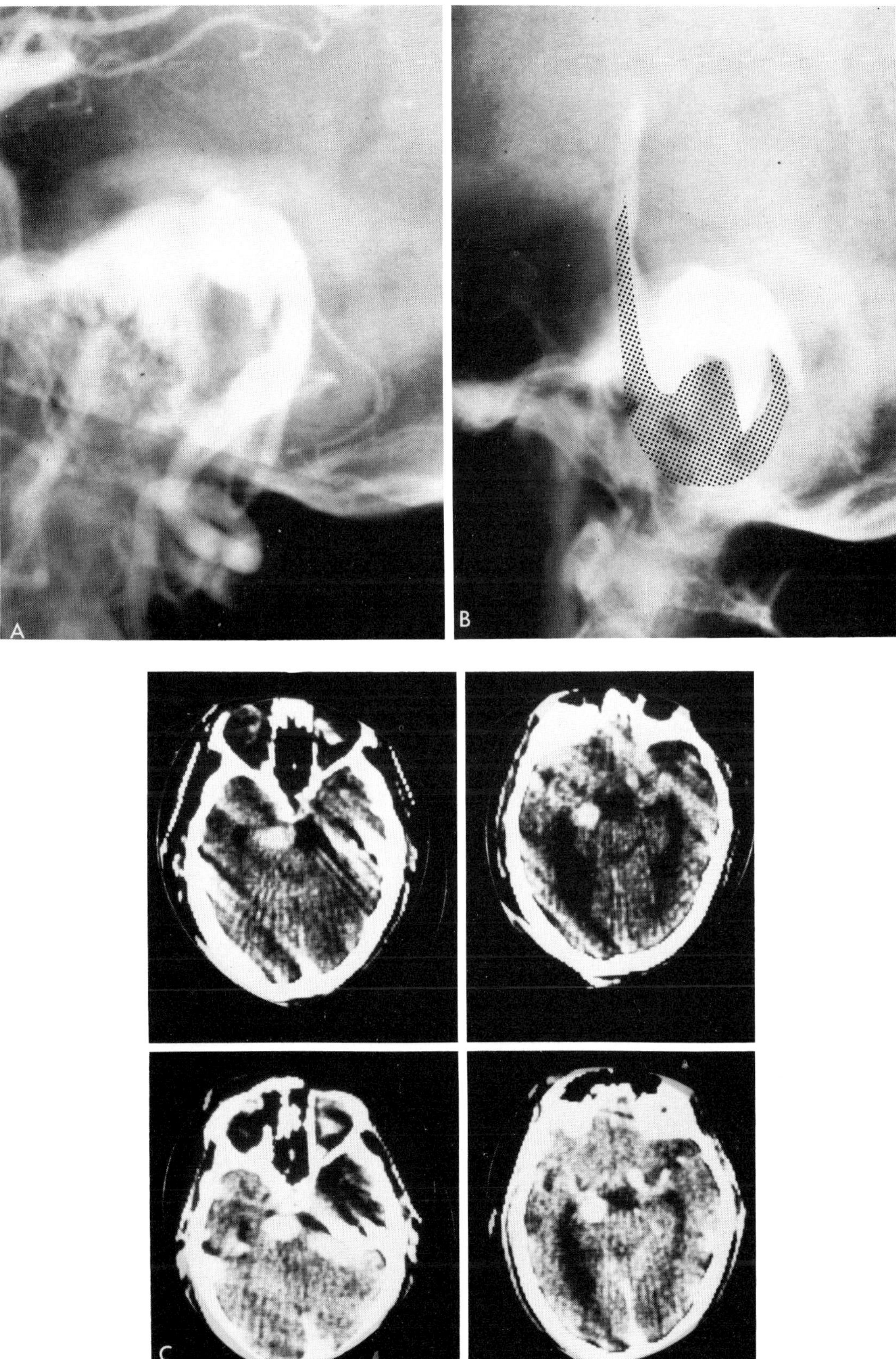

Figure 14–15 *See legend on the opposite page*

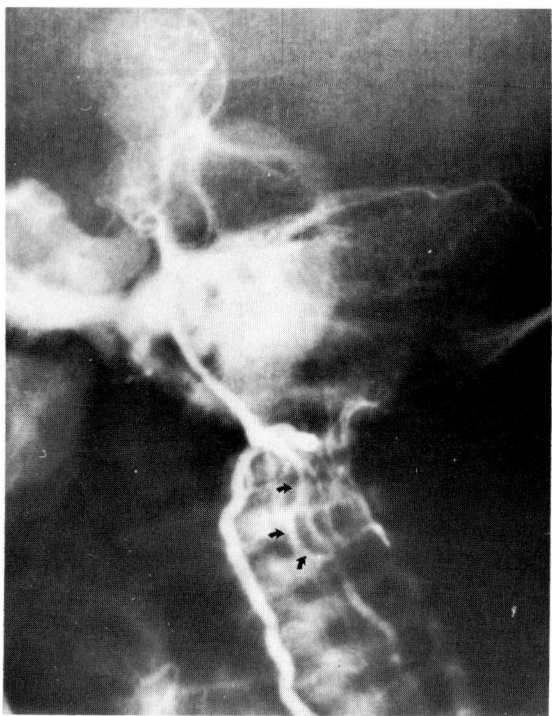

Figure 14–16. ARTERIOGRAM OF THE ARNOLD-CHIARI MALFORMATION: In the Arnold-Chiari malformation the fourth ventricle and the cerebellar tonsils are displaced inferiorly, and the vertebral arteriogram demonstrates that the PICA and the choroidal point and all the branches of the PICA are displaced far below the foramen magnum *(arrows)*. This finding is typical of the Arnold-Chiari malformation.

Superior Cerebellar Arteries. The next branches of the basilar artery that can be visualized arteriographically are the superior cerebellar arteries. They arise from the basilar artery just below the terminal bifurcation into the paired posterior cerebral arteries. If the posterior cerebral arteries arise directly from the carotid system, the superior cerebellar arteries then represent the terminal bifurcation of the basilar artery. This bifurcation is in the interpeduncular fossa. At this level, the superior cerebellar arteries initially course laterally in the perimesencephalic cistern (midbrain portion of the ambient cistern), then posterosuperiorly around the midbrain and then medially until they nearly touch in the midline in the region of the quadrigeminal plate cistern. The superior cerebellar artery branches then course superiorly and posteriorly up and over the vermis of the cerebellum and over the cerebellar hemisphere. Midline branches course posteriorly over the vermis until they anastomose with the vermian branches of the PICA. The superior cerebellar arteries may be either single bilaterally or double bilaterally, or they may be single on one side and double on the opposite side.

The vermian branches of the superior cerebellar artery course quite near the midline just beneath the highest point of the tentorium. The posterior cerebral arteries distribute themselves over the hemispheres more laterally at a lower, more sloping portion of the tentorium. It will be seen, therefore, that even in the normal patient the infratentorial superior cerebellar arteries may project higher than the supratentorial posterior cerebral arteries on the lateral view of a vertebral arteriogram. Review and dissection of a normal preserved anatomic specimen will be very helpful in understanding fully the course of these arteries.

In addition, it should be noted that there can be many normal variations in the course of the posterior cerebral artery. Therefore, caution should be used when interpreting an unusual course as being secondary to mass lesion.

POSTERIOR FOSSA VENOUS ANATOMY

The venous anatomy of the posterior fossa (Figs. 14–17 and 14–18) is as important as the arterial anatomy in the diagnosis of space-occupying lesions in the posterior fossa. The precentral cerebellar vein outlines the anterior margin of the vermis of the cerebellum. This is a single midline vein that is curvilinear and concave posteriorly. This vein originates from below, and drains upward initially, curving first anteriorly and then posteriorly until it joins the posterior portion of the vein of Galen.

Colliculocentral Point. The precentral cerebellar vein originates in the region of the anterior medullary vellum and courses forward until it reaches the inferior colliculi in the region of the quadrigeminal plate. The vein then courses posteriorly and superiorly in a curvilinear line along the anterior margin of the cerebellar vermis; it then proceeds posterosuperiorly where the precentral cerebellar vein joins the vein of Galen. The most anterior point of the curve of the precentral cerebellar is the *colliculocentral point*. Because the vein is situated in the midportion of the posterior fossa, it often is affected if a mass lesion is present.

A line drawn tangent to the precentral cerebellar vein at the level of the colliculocentral point and connected to the choroidal point (see Fig. 14–17) and extending along the limb of the PICA common to both the cephalic and caudal loops falls in the midpoint of the fourth ventricle. This line divides the posterior fossa into the *anterior* and *posterior compartments* (see Figure 14–19). Therefore, abnormalities can be judged by measuring the deviation from the anticipated normal. With masses in the region of the pons or anterior to the fourth ventricle and the aqueduct of sylvius — the anterior compartment — the precentral cerebellar

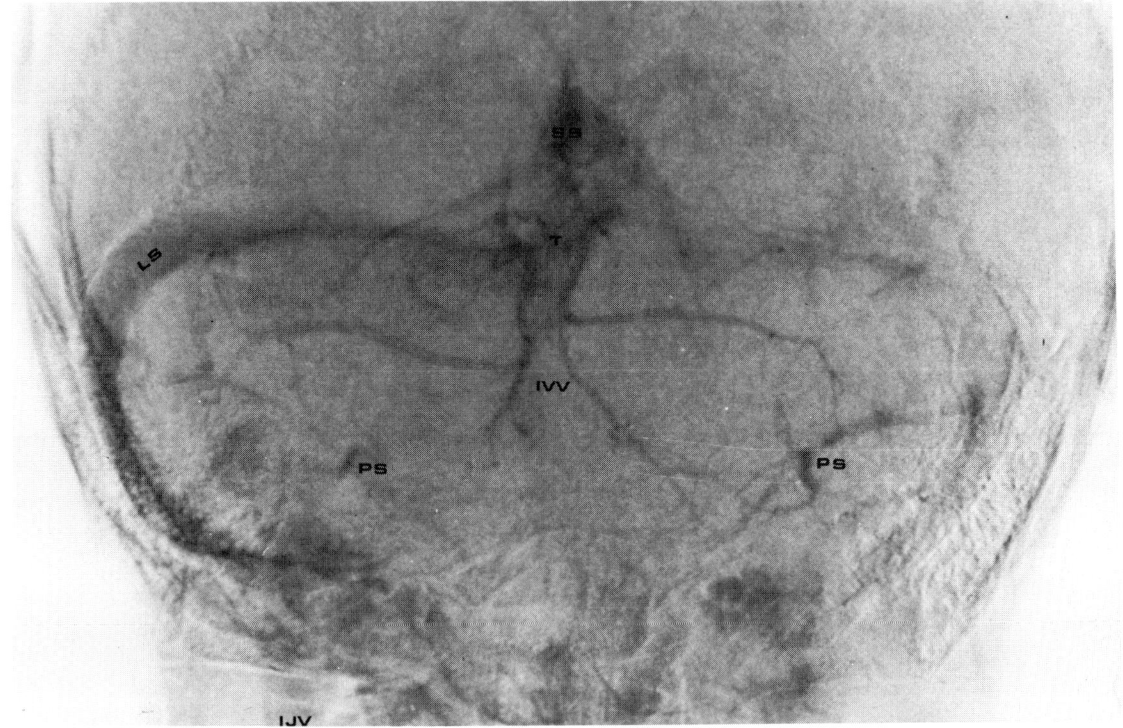

Figure 14–17. The AP view of the venous phase of a vertebral angiogram demonstrates the normal venous structures that one would expect to see using subtraction techniques.

LS Lateral sinus; *PS* Petrosal star; *IVV* Inferior vermian vein; *T* Torcula; *SS* Straight sinus; *IJV* Internal jugular vein.

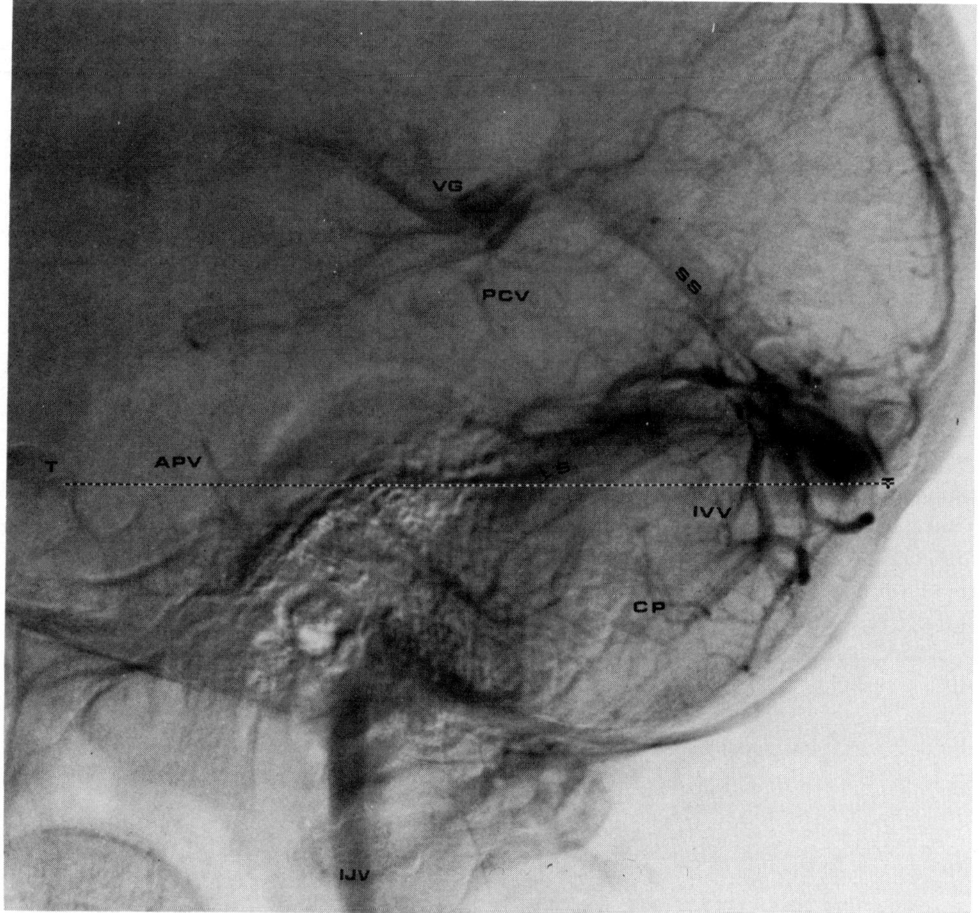

Figure 14–18. The lateral view of the venous phase of a vertebral angiogram demonstrates the normal vascular structures that one would expect to see using subtraction techniques.

VG Vein of Galen; *T-T* Torcula and tuberculum — Twining's line; *PCV* Precentral cerebellar vein; *SS* Straight sinus; *IVV* Inferior vermian vein; *CP* Copular point; *IJV* Internal jugular vein; *APV* Anterior pontomesencephalic vein.

vein is straightened and either loses its normal curvilinear course or is displaced posteriorly. On the other hand, if the mass is in the vermis of the cerebellum or placed more posteriorly in the hemispheres of the cerebellum — the posterior compartment — the precentral vein will be displaced forward. Because of its central position, particular attention should be paid to each angiogram, making special note of the position of this vein. If mass lesions are present in the cerebellar hemispheres, a change in the position of these veins may not be detected because the veins are midline structures. If, however, the lesion is large enough to reach the midline structures, the precentral cerebellar vein will be seen to be displaced anteriorly secondary to this mass lesion. These veins are only rarely visible on the anteroposterior view.

The anterior pontomesencephalic vein lies in intimate association with the anterior inferior margin of the pons, known also as the "belly" of the pons. The origin of this vein is at the level of the posterior perforated substance in the interpeduncular fossa. Because of its intimate association with the pons it is a more accurate representation of the actual position of the pons than is the basilar artery. This is true because the basilar artery may become tortuous secondary to arteriosclerosis and move away from the midline; also, any torsion of the pons may move the basilar artery posteriorly and away from the midline. On the lateral view of the venous phase, the anterior pontomesencephalic vein will be seen to have the shape of a squared hook, with the top of the hook lying in the interpeduncular fossa in the region of the midbrain. The vein then turns caudad to follow along the anterior margin of the pons. The remainder of the course of the vein is obscured by the overlying petrous bones; however, subtraction techniques will allow one to see this vein empty into the basilar venous plexus and ultimately drain via the internal jugular vein.

As in the supratentorial circulation, there are a large number of unnamed veins that course over the surface of the cerebellum. Except for the precentral cerebellar veins, however, there are no deep venous structures that can be used reliably to diagnose the presence or absence of mass lesions.

The *copular point* is just below and behind the fourth ventricle. It marks the beginning of the inferior vermian veins.

The basal vein of Rosenthal will be seen to course along the free edge of the tentorium and around the midbrain in the perimesencephalic cistern until it enters the vein of Galen. This vessel is discussed under the supratentorial venous structures.

The superior vermian veins lie over the upper surface of the vermis of the cerebellum just below the straight sinus. These veins drain anteriorly and superiorly into the vein of Galen. If mass lesions are present, these veins will be seen to be elevated upward and to lie much closer than normal to the straight sinus. This alteration from the normal position with elevation of the superior vermian veins is known as a "closed" or "tight" posterior fossa; it reflects the presence of a space-occupying mass in the posterior fossa.

The inferior vermian veins are paired midline veins that course along the inferior portion of the cerebellar vermis. These veins may be shifted to the contralateral side with cerebellar hemisphere lesions. The position of the patient for filming will affect the position of the vermian veins, since rotation of the head will give the impression that the vein is shifted to one side or the other — even in the absence of a true mass lesion. Therefore, it is of paramount importance that the patient be positioned in a straight anteroposterior projection. In the presence of a mass lesion, there may be poor filling of one or even both vermian veins because of localized increased intracranial pressure. If this is the case, there will usually be other signs of a mass lesion in addition to the finding of poor venous filling. It should be noted that the contralateral vermian vein may not fill well when the injection is made into one vertebral artery, thus giving the impression of a mass lesion in one cerebellar hemisphere, whereas in reality the phenomenon is due to poor filling with contrast of the vessels contralateral to the side injected.

At the base of the skull there is a large venous plexus made up of multiple interconnecting veins. Some of these veins drain into the cavernous sinus, but most of the veins in this plexus drain ultimately into the petrosal sinus and then into the sigmoid sinus and out via the internal jugular vein.

Of particular interest is a group of small tributary veins also known as "brachial veins" (after the Latin word for "arms"). These all join together bilaterally in the shape of a star just above the internal auditory canals. This collection of veins is known as the *petrosal star*. It normally projects just above the internal auditory canal on the AP view. The petrosal star usually will be displaced upward — away from the internal auditory canal — when a mass lesion is present in the region of the cerebellopontine angle. Again, localized increased intracranial pressure may cause poor filling of these veins.

ANTERIOR AND POSTERIOR COMPARTMENTS

The posterior fossa can be divided into two compartments: the anterior compartment and the posterior compartment. These compartments are found by drawing a line connecting the colliculocentral point of the precentral cerebellar vein with the angiographic choroidal point. Examination of the diagram (Fig. 14–19) reveals that this line will course through the fourth ventricle. All masses in front of this line are in the anterior compartment; masses behind the line are in the poste-

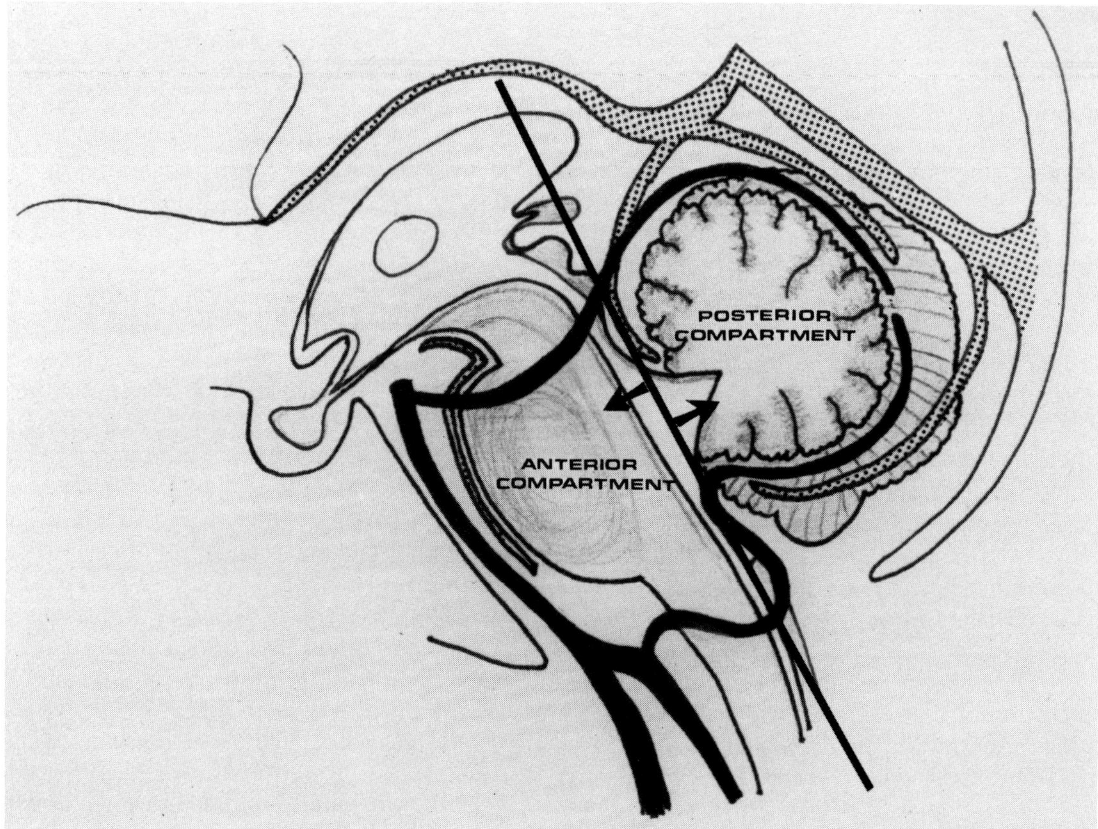

Figure 14–19. ANTERIOR AND POSTERIOR COMPARTMENTS: A line connecting the colliculocentral point of the precentral cerebellar vein with the choroidal point and running along the posterior medullary segment of the PICA divides the posterior fossa into the anterior and posterior compartments.

rior compartment. One anticipates certain angiographic findings with masses in either of these compartments. Therefore, these changes should be looked for when examining a posterior fossa angiogram.

ANGIOGRAPHIC FINDINGS WITH ANTERIOR COMPARTMENT MASSES

1. The basilar artery is closely applied to the clivus.
2. There is *posterior* displacement of the precentral cerebellar vein.
3. The anterior pontomesencephalic vein is closely applied to the clivus.
4. The choroidal point is displaced posteriorly.
5. If the mass is extra-axial — e.g., a clivus meningioma, chordoma or exophytic pontine glioma — the basilar artery is displaced *posteriorly,* as is the anterior pontomesencephalic vein.

Examples of Anterior Compartment Masses

1. Pontine glioma.
2. Acoustic neuroma.
3. Chordoma.
4. Clivus meningioma.
5. Basilar artery aneurysm.
6. Metastases.

ANGIOGRAPHIC FINDINGS OF POSTERIOR COMPARTMENT MASSES

1. The basilar artery is closely applied to the clivus.

2. There is *forward* displacement of the precentral cerebellar vein.
3. The choroidal point and vermian artery are displaced to the contralateral side if the mass is unilateral or if it arises in the midline but extends predominantly to one side.
4. The anterior pontomesencephalic vein is closely applied to the clivus.
5. There is elevation of the superior cerebellar (vermian) veins and arteries.
6. The inferior vermian veins are displaced to the contralateral side.

Examples of Posterior Compartment Masses

1. Medulloblastoma.
2. Cerebellar astrocytoma.
3. Metastases.
4. Hemangioblastoma.
5. Tentorial meningioma.
6. Ependymoma.

In the examples that follow, emphasis has been placed on cases that demonstrate obvious vascular displacements. Particular emphasis is made on masses that give a "classic" appearance, and more esoteric findings have been omitted. Correlation with the CT scan has been made whenever possible. For the most part, cases with normal or nearly normal angiograms have been omitted — even though it is the author's opinion that sizable masses may be present when the angiogram shows only minor or no alterations.

The author recommends the routine use of a Towne's and lateral view, coned down for the posterior fossa, as the initial study in all cases. After review of the films, additional views may be obtained using alterations in the AP positioning — especially with a view centering the internal auditory canals through the center of the orbit. This allows an excellent demonstration of the course of the AICA. The submentovertex view is also very helpful in the diagnosis of mass lesions and aneurysms. Angiotomography is also recommended for the visualization of midline structures. Subtraction views are very helpful and, in many cases, are essential to demonstrate fully the vascular anatomy.

ANTERIOR COMPARTMENT MASSES

CHORDOMA

Chordomas arise from remnants of the notochordal tissues. Intracranially, they arise in the midline, often at the level of the clivus, dorsum sella or region of the spheno-occipital synchondrosis. They may be calcified and result in destructive changes that involve the clivus. The extension and bony destructive properties of these tumors may result in the appearance of a large nasopharyngeal mass. In addition to intracranial tumors, chordomas also occur in the region of the sacrum, where they result in bony destructive changes associated with a large soft tissue mass (no example shown).

CT scans of intracranial chordomas usually reveal a large calcified midline mass.

PONTINE GLIOMA

Pontine gliomas (brain stem gliomas, brain stem astrocytomas) arise in the brain stem and lead to diffuse enlargement of the pons — a finding referred to as "hypertrophy" of the pons. They are more common in boys than in girls, and usually are noted in the first decade of life. The clinical presentation is of multiple cranial nerve palsies. These tumors appear radiographically as anterior compartment masses in the posterior fossa.

CT Scans. The preinfusion scan reveals a mass in the pons that may be radiolucent, isodense or, rarely, of higher density than normal brain tissue. When the tumor is of sufficient size, it is possible to detect an increase in the size of the pons with posterior displacement and compression of the fourth ventricle. There is a varying degree of obstructive hydrocephalus in nearly all cases. Following the infusion of contrast material, there is marked homogeneous enhancement in most cases; however, in some cases no enhancement will be seen. The postinfusion scan also demonstrates the relationship of the mass to the surrounding edema.

Angiography. The basilar artery will be closely applied to the pons except when there is exophytic growth of the tumor. In that case, the basilar artery may actually be displaced posteriorly away from the clivus. There is posterior and downward displacement of the choroidal point and the posterior medullary segment of the PICA. The anterior pontomesencephalic vein will be closely applied to the clivus, and there is posterior displacement of the precentral cerebral vein. The tumors usually are avascular.

Ventriculography and Pneumoencephalography. These studies reveal posterior displacement of the fourth ventricle and compression of the prepontine cistern. The pons measures greater than the maximum of 4 cm in most cases. In the AP view, the fourth ventricle appears to be draped over a mass.

ACOUSTIC NEUROMA

These tumors may originate wherever Schwann cells are found. However, we are interested here in the intracranial tumors and tumors of the eighth cranial nerve in particular. Multiple schwannomas and particularly bilateral acoustic schwannomas (neuromas) are associated with von Recklinghausen's neurofibromatosis.

Histology. There is a surrounding capsule of connective tissue. Microscopic examination reveals either Antoni A or B type cells, the A type demonstrating narrow elongated bipolar cells with little cytoplasm that characteristically are arranged in palisades. In the B type there is less cellular density, and microcysts and vacuolated cells are present. There is a fine honeycombed appearance.

Reticulin fibers are present in both types.

Skull Films. Enlargement and erosion of the internal auditory meatus are evident. In general, the internal auditory canal should not be taller than 8 mm, and there should not be a difference of more than 3 mm between the two sides.

Angiography. Vertebral angiography demonstrates that the anterior inferior cerebellar artery is displaced out of the internal auditory canal by the mass. The basilar artery may be displaced to the contralateral side. The petrosal star is elevated away from the internal auditory canal. Selective external carotid angiography and the use of subtraction techniques may demonstrate a tumor blush. There may or may not be obstructive hydrocephalus.

Computed Tomography. The CT scan without and with the infusion of contrast material is the procedure of choice for the work-up of acoustic neuroma. Most tumors outside of the internal auditory canal that are larger than 1 cm are demonstrated by the postinfusion CT scan. With thin section tomography (1 mm slices), even smaller tumors may be detected. Manipulation of the window width and window level often reveals enlargement of the bony canal. The preinfusion scan frequently is entirely normal. The postinfusion scan demonstrates dense homogeneous enhancement of the tumor. These tumors may exhibit a cystic component, and therefore have a central radiolucency. There may or may not be obstructive hydrocephalus. Even with a fairly sizable tumor, the fourth ventricle may not demonstrate any evidence of shift from its normal position. There may be displacement to the contralateral side or flattening of the anterior margin of the fourth ventricle.

Text continued on page 685

Figure 14–20. TENTORIAL MENINGIOMA: *A* and *B*, The mass lesion is outlined by the dotted gray area. This tentorial meningioma is positioned along the free edge of the tentorium and extends both above and below the tentorium (see Chapter 9). The posterior cerebral artery is displaced on only one side, and the contralateral side is normal. This allows for comparison of the normal with the abnormal side of the lateral view of the arteriogram. The corresponding positions of the posterior cerebral arteries have been labeled on each view (numbers 1, 2 and 3). The PICA is displaced inferiorly and to the contralateral side. The basilar artery is displaced to the contralateral side. The vascular supply is via the tentorial artery, which arises from the internal carotid artery.

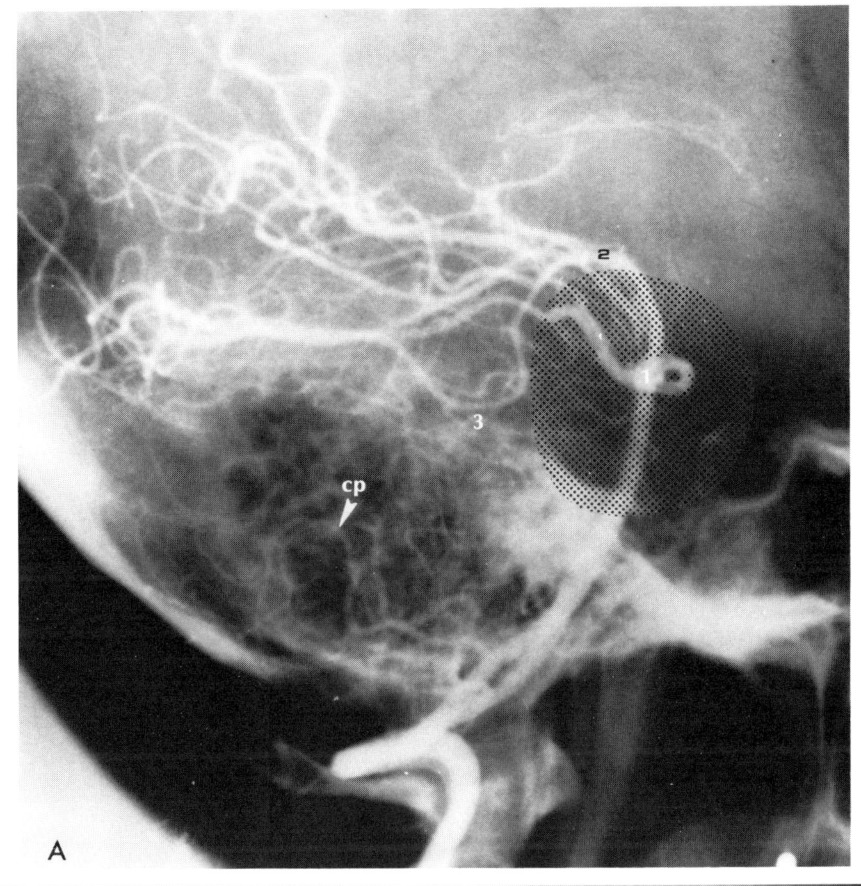

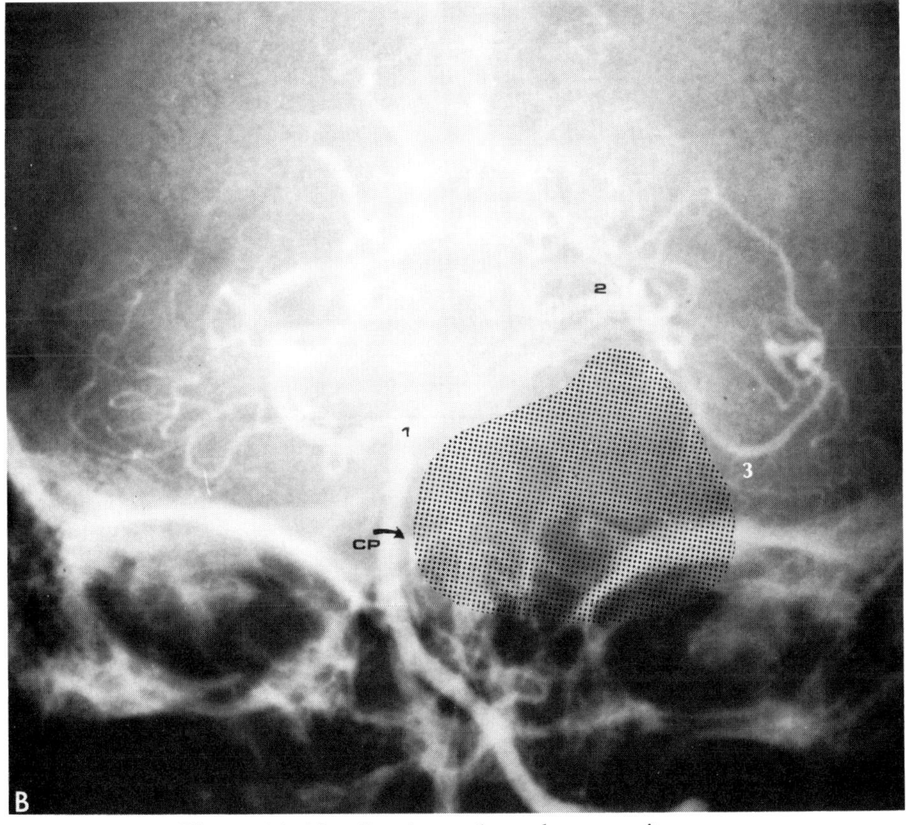

Figure 14–20 *See legend on the opposite page*

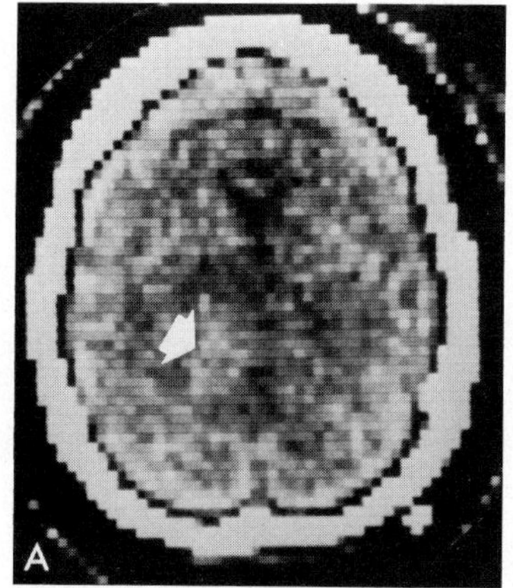

Figure 14–21. TENTORIAL MENINGIOMA: *A,* The CT scan reveals a high density mass lesion along the free edge of the tentorium *(arrowhead).* There is surrounding edema.

B, The AP view of the vertebral arteriogram demonstrates shift of the basilar artery to the contralateral side (*curved arrows*) and elevation of the posterior cerebral and superior cerebellar arteries of the left side.

C, The common carotid arteriogram shows the tentorial artery arising from the internal carotid artery (*open arrowhead*), the blush of the tumor (*closed white arrowhead* on *B* and *C*), and the superficial temporal artery (*black arrowhead*) that does not provide blood supply to the tumor.

Plain film examination approximately three years later (not shown) demonstrated multiple psammomatous calcifications that were not visible on the initial studies.

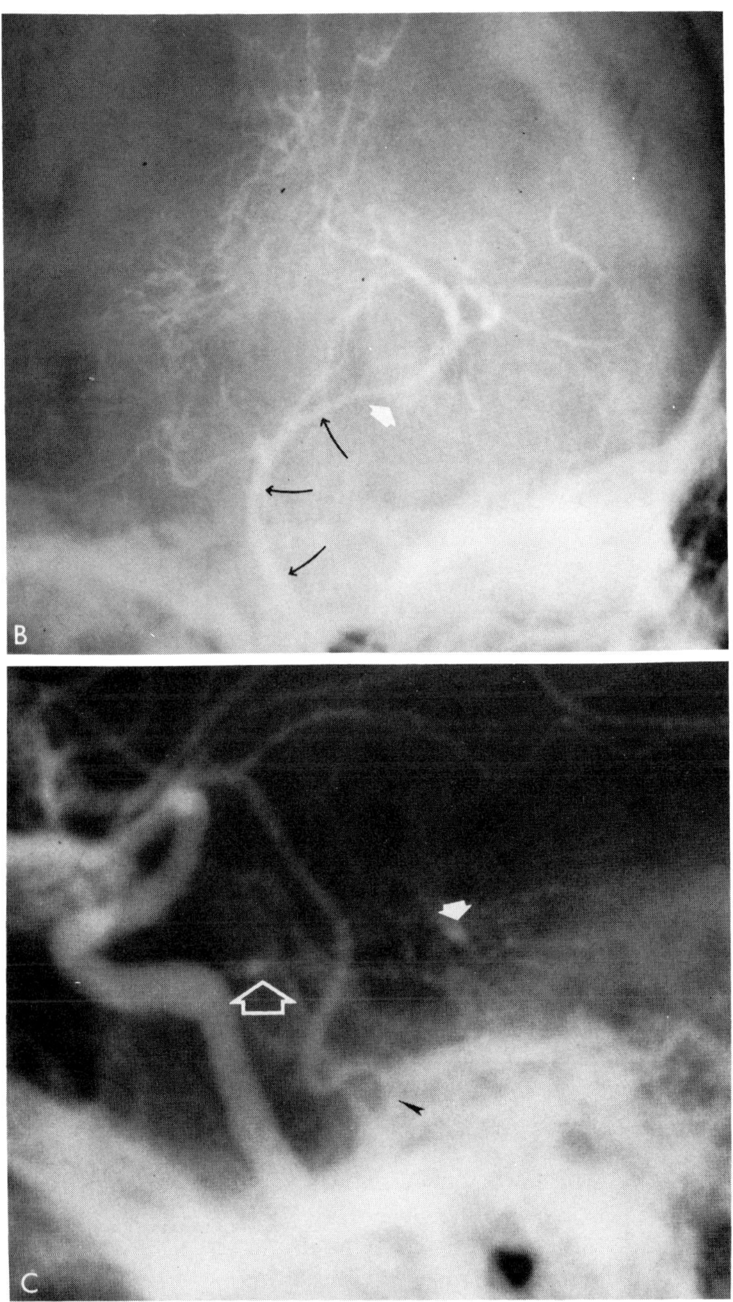

Figure 14–21 *Continued*

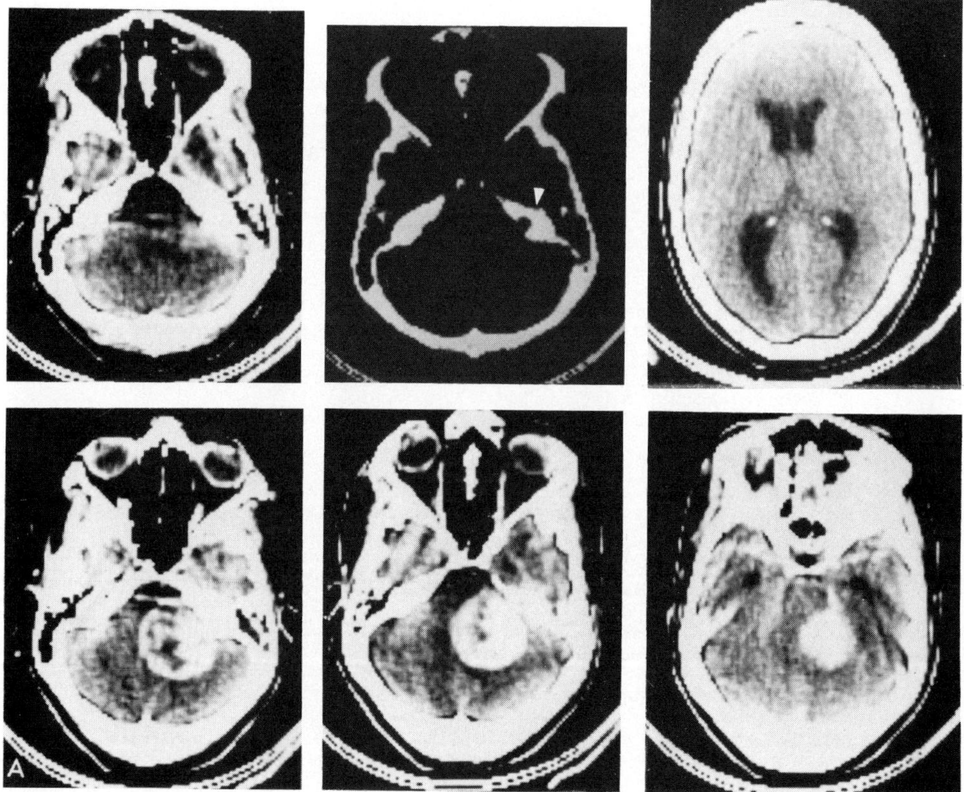

Figure 14–22. RIGHT ACOUSTIC NEUROMA: *A*, The preinfusion scan reveals that the fourth ventricle is displaced to the left of the midline; the tumor is isodense with the normal brain. Viewed at high window width and window level, the right internal auditory canal can be seen to be greatly dilated compared to the left *(arrowhead)*. There is moderate obstructive hydrocephalus. The postinfusion scan shows marked enhancement of the tumor which is closely applied to the right internal auditory canal. There are filling defects in the tumor secondary to cystic change in the tumor or areas of necrosis.

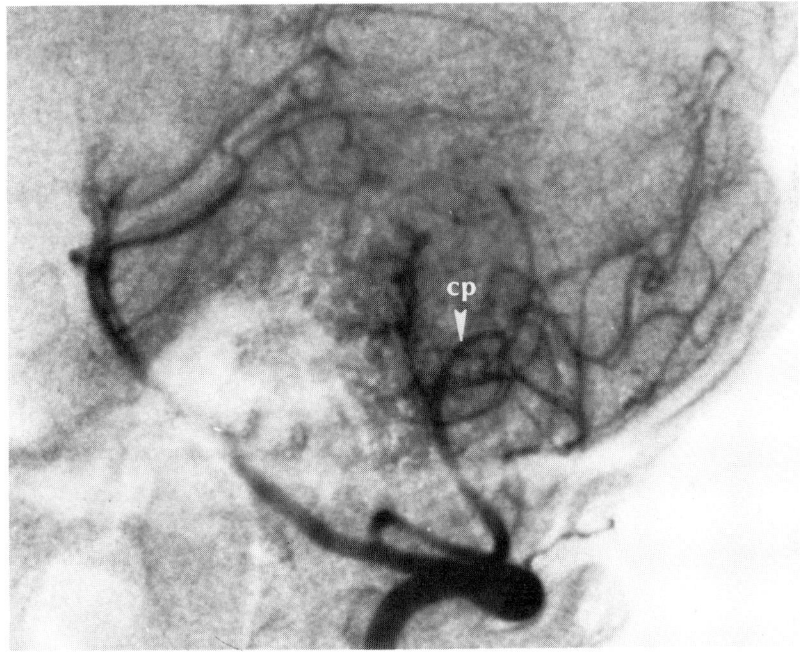

Figure 14–22 *Continued*

B, The lateral view of the right vertebral arteriogram reveals that the choroidal point *(cp)* is displaced inferiorly and there is stretching of some of the branches of the PICA. The basilar artery is closely applied to the clivus.

Illustration continued on the following page

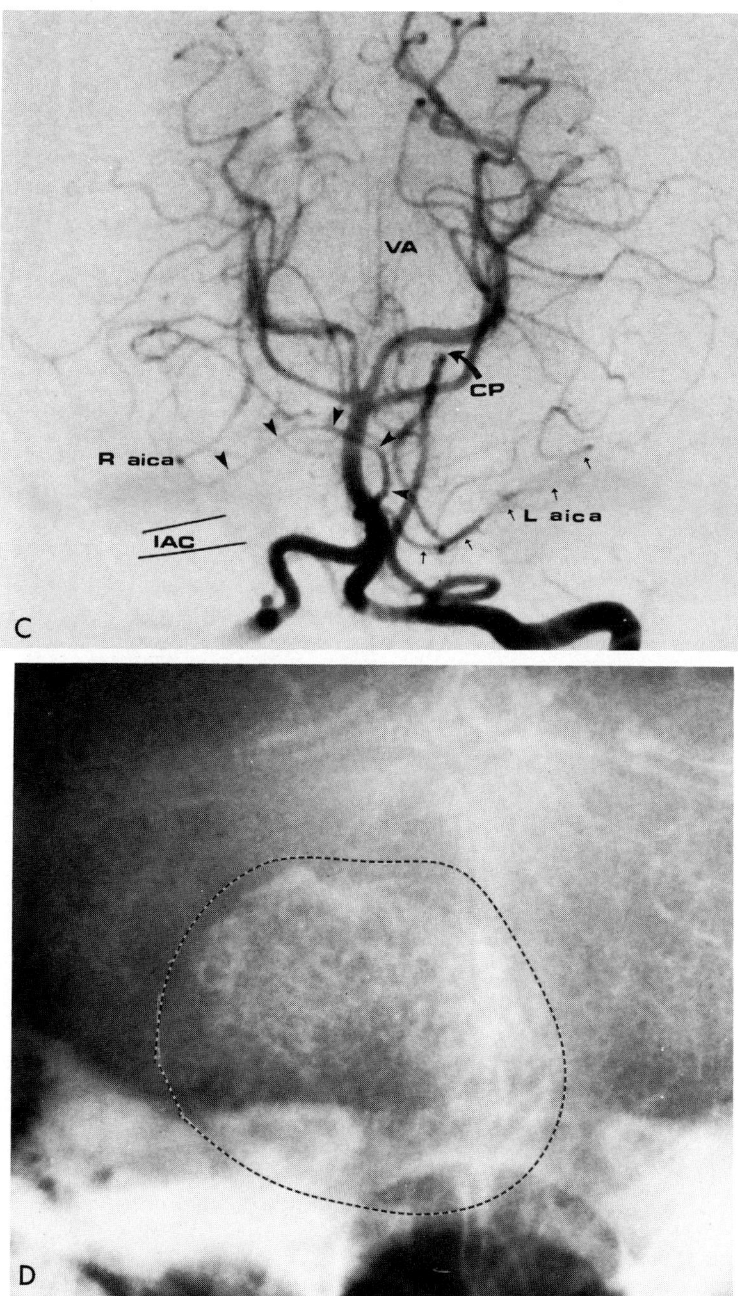

C, The AP view of the right vertebral arteriogram reveals that the left choroidal point (*cp*) is displaced to the left of the midline. The anterior inferior cerebellar artery (*AICA*) is displaced out of the right internal auditory canal (*IAC*) and courses in a curvilinear fashion around a large mass lesion in the right cerebellopontine angle (*arrows*). Left *AICA* (*small arrows*) is normal. The vermian artery (*VA*) is in normal position.

D, The late arterial–early venous phase demonstrates a large area of neovascularity (*dotted line*) and some early draining veins. The abnormal vessels arise from the vertebrobasilar system.

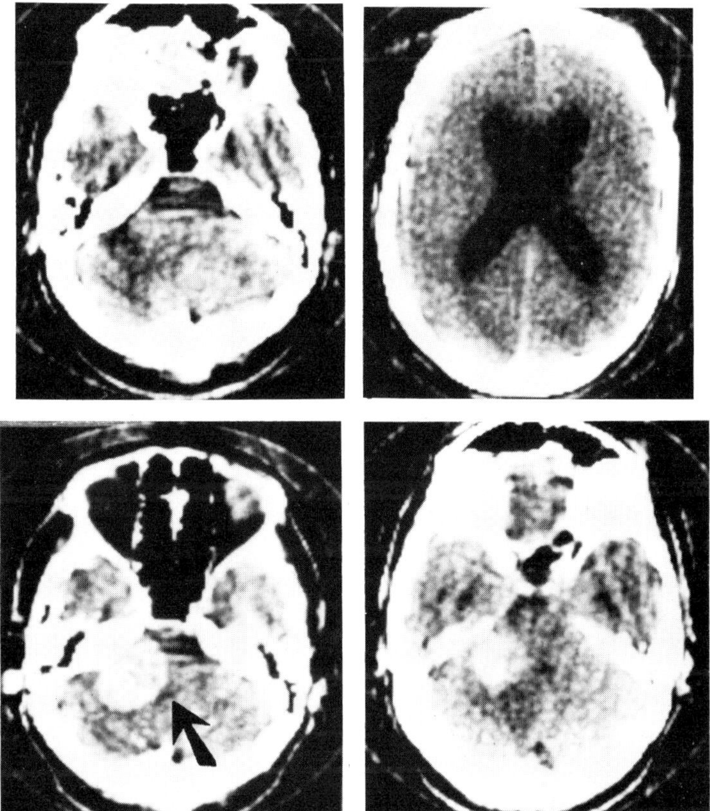

Figure 14–23. LEFT ACOUSTIC NEUROMA: The preinfusion scan reveals a sizable tumor that is isodense with the normal brain substance. The fourth ventricle (arrowhead) is tilted slightly and is displaced to the right of the midline slightly. There is moderately severe obstructive hydrocephalus. The postinfusion scan reveals marked enhancement of the left acoustic neurinoma as it arises from the left porus acusticus.

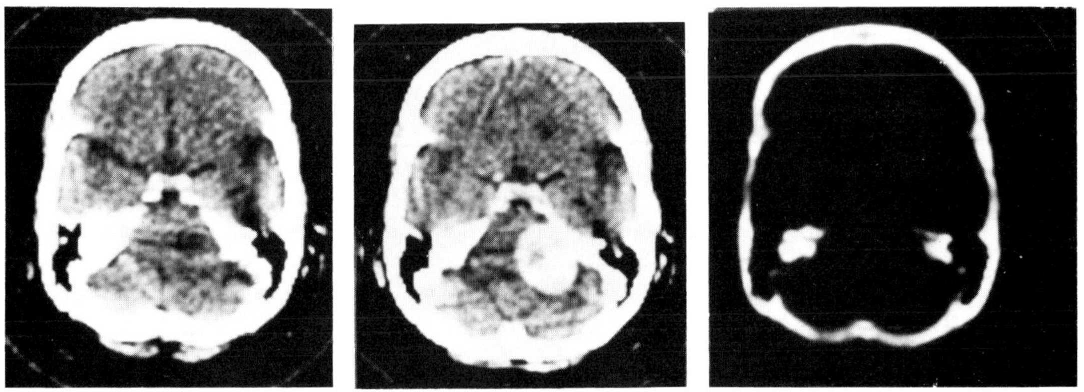

Figure 14–24. CYSTIC ACOUSTIC NEUROMA: The preinfusion scan reveals a well defined low density lesion in the region of the right cerebellopontine angle. The postinfusion scan reveals that this low density area is a cystic portion of the tumor. The fourth ventricle is displaced slightly posteriorly and to the left of the midline. There is slight flaring of the right porus acusticus on the base view.

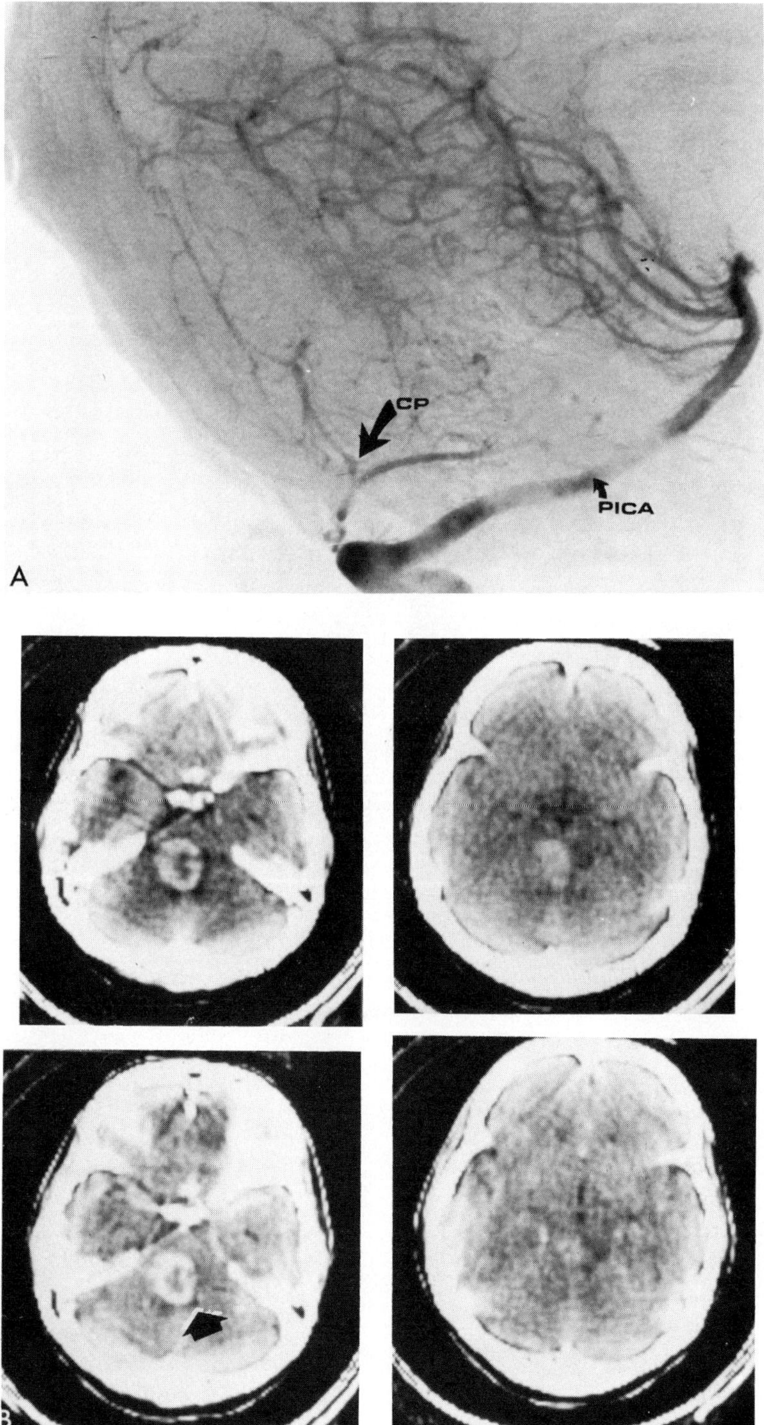

Figure 14–25 *See legend on the opposite page*

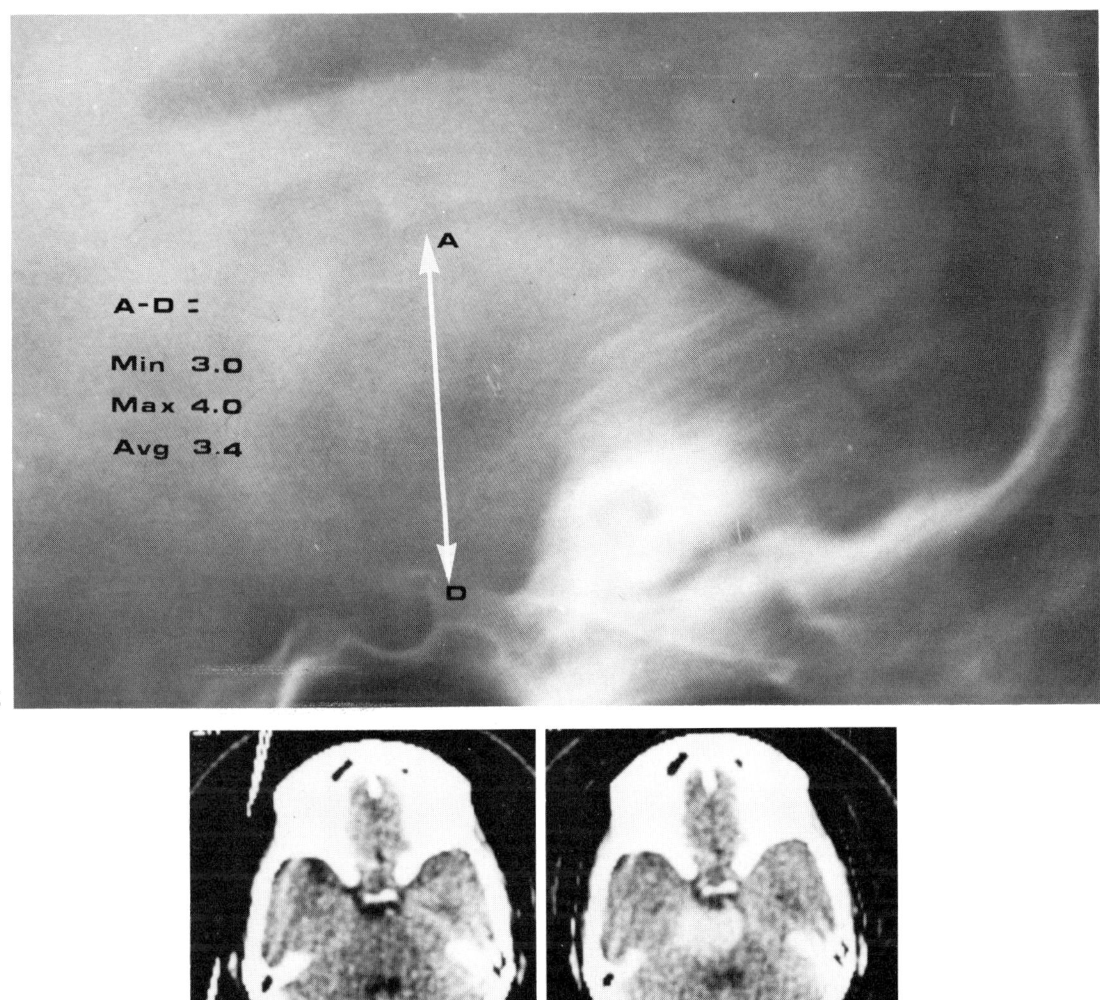

Figure 14–25. PONTINE GLIOMA: *A,* The lateral view of the vertebral arteriogram reveals that the AICA supplies the PICA distribution as an anatomic variation. Its origin is demonstrated by the small arrowhead. The choroidal point *(large arrowhead)* is displaced inferiorly, as are the vermian branches of the PICA, which are closer to the inner table of the skull than one would normally anticipate. The basilar artery is closely applied to the clivus.

B, The CT scan demonstrates a high density cystic lesion on the preinfusion scan. The rim of the tumor is of quite high density and perhaps contains a small amount of calcification. The fourth ventricle is flattened and displaced posteriorly. This is reflected in the arteriogram as the posterior displacement of the choroidal point and the posterior displacement of the vermian branches of the PICA. Postinfusion, there is some enhancement of the rim of the tumor. There is no obstructive hydrocephalus.

C and *D,* In another patient, the pneumoencephalogram *(C)* demonstrates marked widening of the pons secondary to a pontine glioma. The width of the pons from the dorsum sella to the cerebral aqueduct *(A–D)* normally measures an average of 3.4 cm, with a maximum width of 4.0 cm and a minimum width of 3.0 cm.

The CT scan *(D)* also demonstrates widening of the pons, with flattening of the anterior margin of the fourth ventricle. The basilar artery is displaced to the right of the midline. The postinfusion scan demonstrates marked enhancement of the pontine glioma, which in this case is larger on the left side.

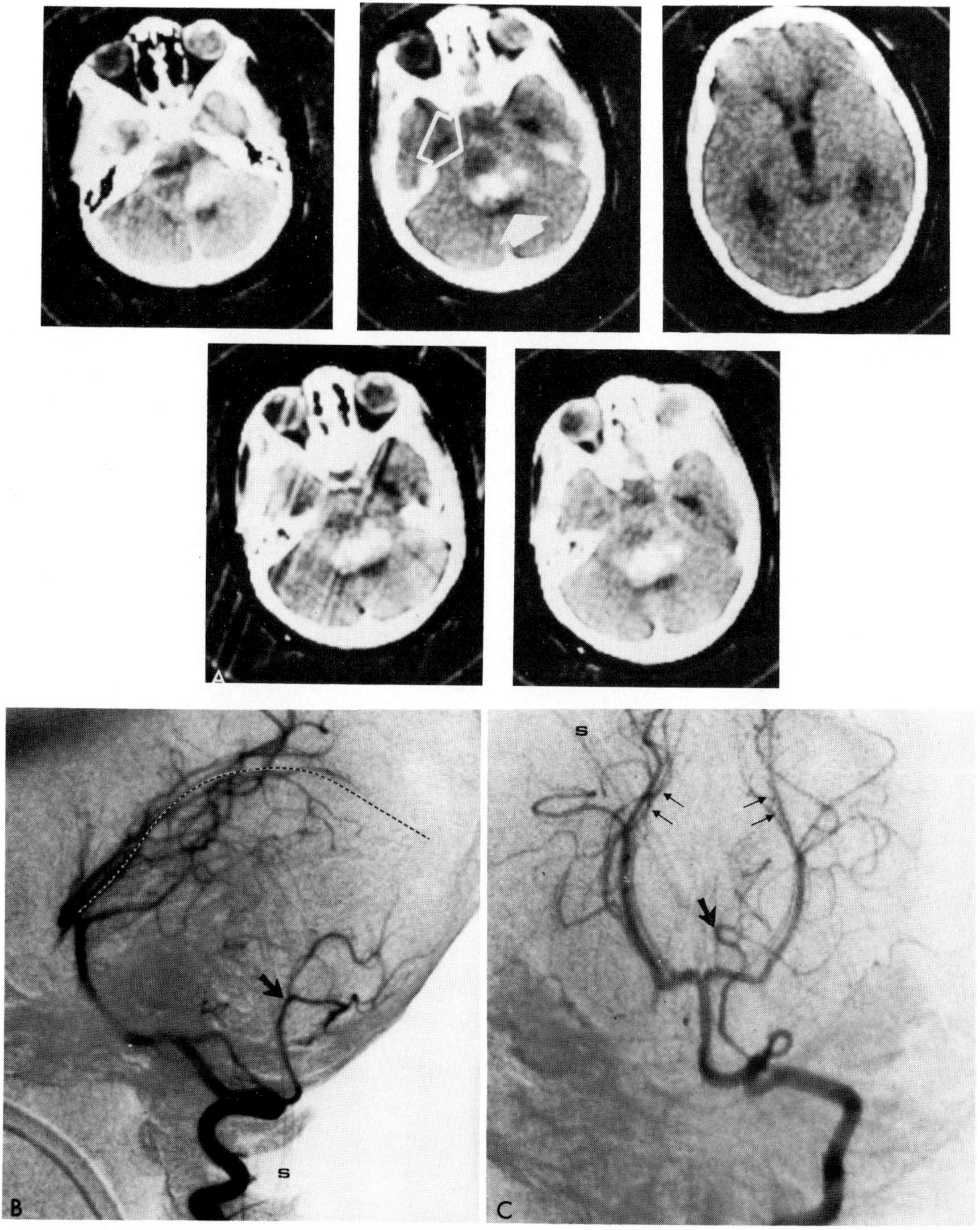

Figure 14–26 *See legend on the opposite page*

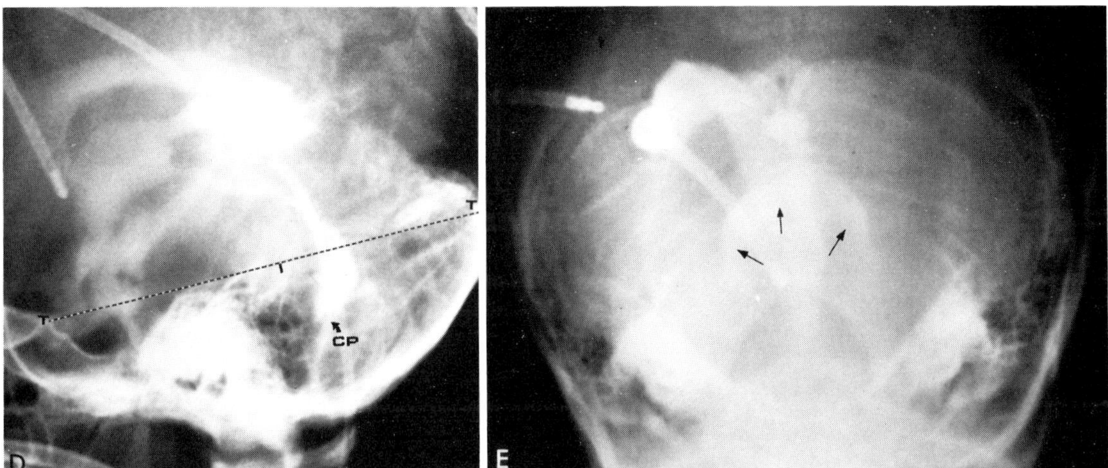

Figure 14–26. LARGE CYSTIC AND CALCIFIED PONTINE GLIOMA: *A*, The CT scan reveals a large cystic *(open arrowhead)* and calcified tumor in the region of the pons which flattens the fourth ventricle and displaces it posteriorly *(white arrowhead)*. There is moderate obstructive hydrocephalus. After the infusion of contrast material there is some enhancement of the tumor.

B, The lateral view of the vertebral arteriogram reveals posterior and inferior displacement of the choroidal point (*arrow*), posterior displacement of the vermian branches of the PICA and stretching of the tonsillohemispheric branches of the PICA. There is superior bowing of the branches of the superior cerebellar arteries *(dotted line)*. A shunt tube *(S)* is now in place.

C, The AP view reveals that the choroidal point *(large arrow)* is displaced slightly to the left of the midline. The branches of the superior cerebellar arteries and the posterior cerebral arteries *(small arrows)* are separated secondary to superior herniation of the posterior fossa contents. The tip of the shunt tube can be seen on the right side (*S*).

D, The Conray-60 per cent ventriculogram demonstrates marked posterior displacement of the fourth ventricle and compromise of the prepontine cistern by a very large, slightly lobulated mass in the region of the pons.

E, The fourth ventricle is flattened and distorted on the AP view by the mass lesion *(arrows)*.

The calcification that was readily apparent on the CT scan could not be identified on the plain films or by other neuroradiologic studies (case courtesy of Dr. Justo Rodriguez).

Figure 14–27. PONTINE GLIOMA WITH POSTERIOR DISPLACEMENT OF THE PRECENTRAL CEREBELLAR VEIN: *A*, The venous phase of the vertebral angiogram reveals reversal of the curve *(dashed line)* of the precentral cerebellar vein *(PCV)* and forward displacement of the anterior pontomesencephalic vein *(APMV)*. These changes reflect the presence of a mass between the two anatomic structures.

B, The pneunoencephalogram reveals marked flattening and posterior displacement of the fourth ventricle and the cerebral aqueduct as well as compromise of the prepontine cistern. The entire pons and medulla are involved with the mass lesion.

C, The CT scan of a different patient demonstrates marked enlargement of the pons by a low density tumor. The fourth ventricle is flattened and displaced posteriorly. The postinfusion scan reveals marked enhancement of the tumor in a homogeneous fashion. The tumor is slightly larger on the left side and displaces the basilar artery to the right of the midline *(arrow)*. The appearance is typical of a pontine glioma.

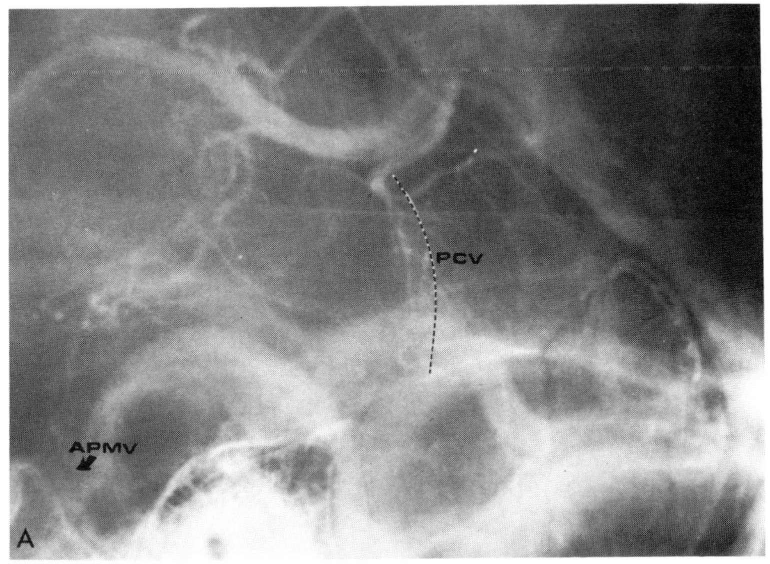

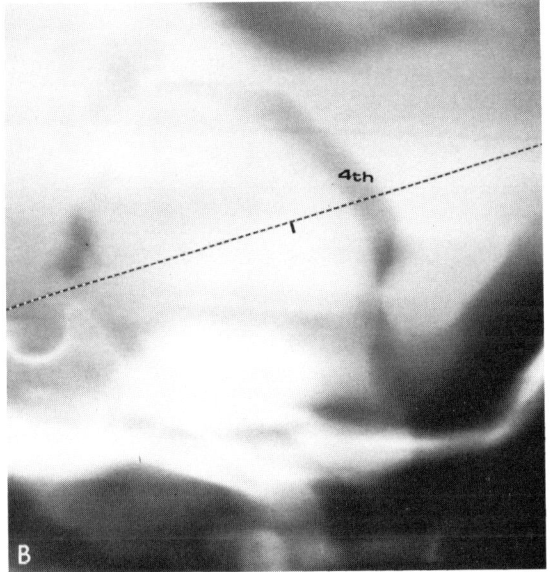

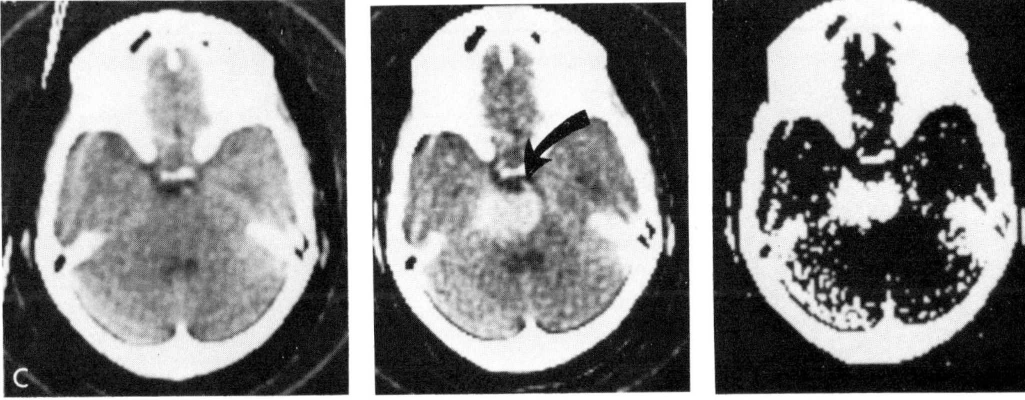

Figure 14–27 *See legend on the opposite page*

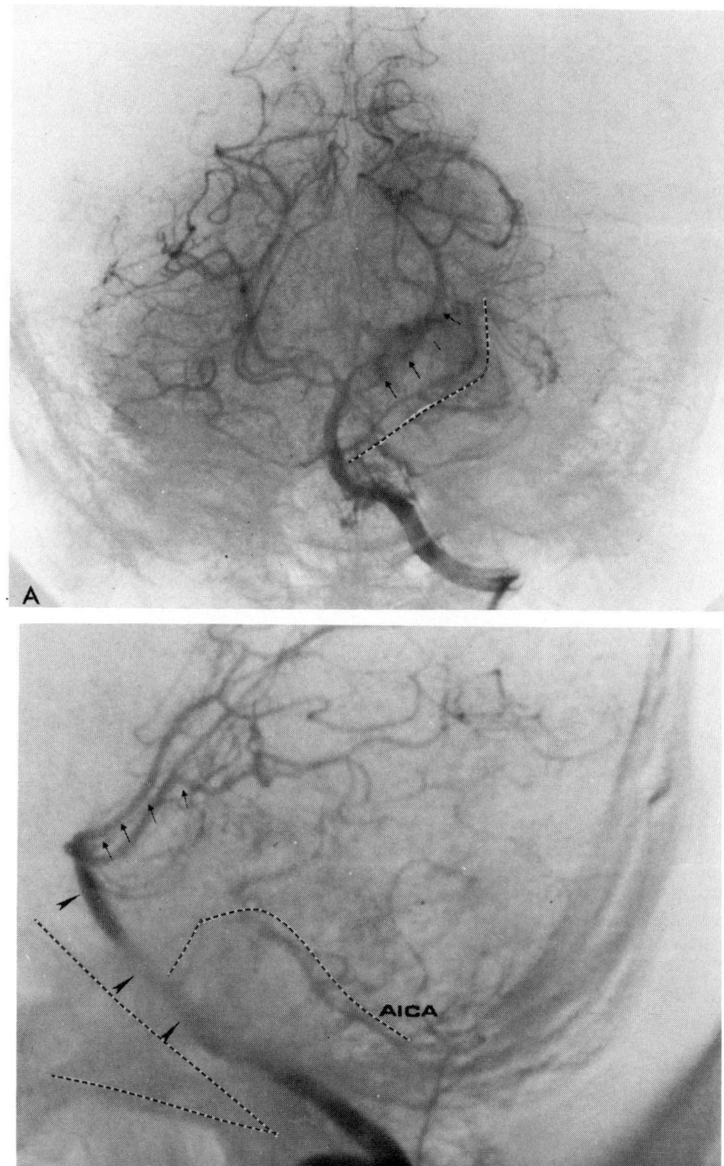

Figure 14–28. EXOPHYTIC PONTINE GLIOMA: *A*, The AP view of the arteriogram demonstrates that the basilar artery is displaced to the right of the midline. The AICA is displaced out of the internal auditory canal (*dashed line*) and there is a large vascular mass in the region of the left cerebellopontine angle. The left superior cerebellar artery is elevated in *A* and *B* (*small arrows*).

B, The lateral view reveals that the basilar artery is displaced posteriorly away from the clivus (*arrows*); the AICA can be seen to be displaced superiorly and posteriorly around a large mass lesion (*dashed line*).

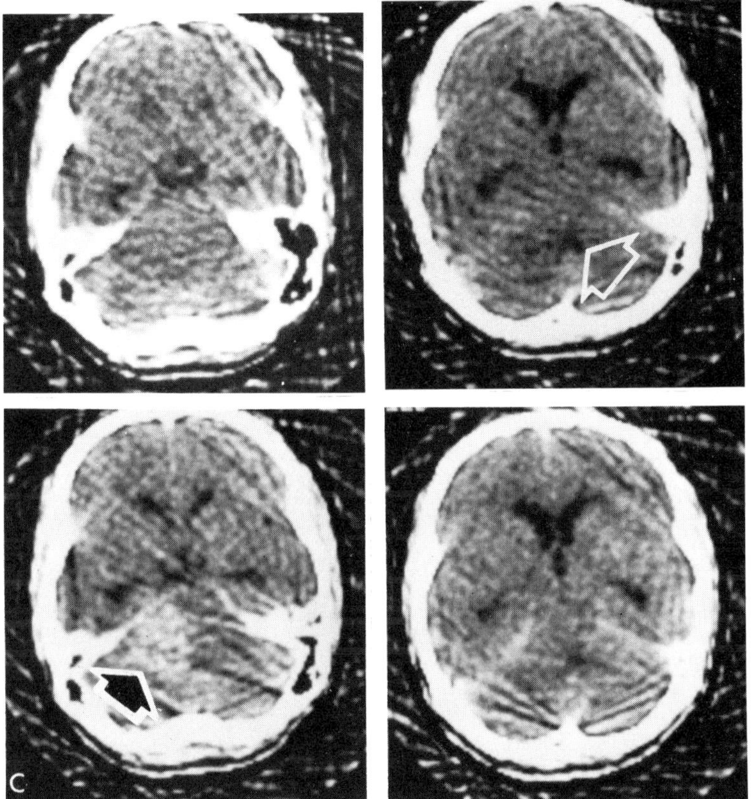

Figure 14–28 *Continued*

C, The preinfusion scan demonstrates an isodense mass displacing the fourth ventricle to the right of the midline, tilting it slightly and displacing the fourth ventricle posteriorly *(open arrowhead)*. The postinfusion scan reveals homogeneous enhancement of the mass (*black arrowhead*). There is moderate obstructive hydrocephalus. (The scan is somewhat degraded by patient motion artifact.)

Although the angiographic appearance suggests an extrinsic mass lesion and the CT scan would seem to support this finding, at operation this proved to be a pontine glioma that had grown in an exophytic fashion — thus simulating an extrinsic mass, but actually being a tumor arising from the pons.

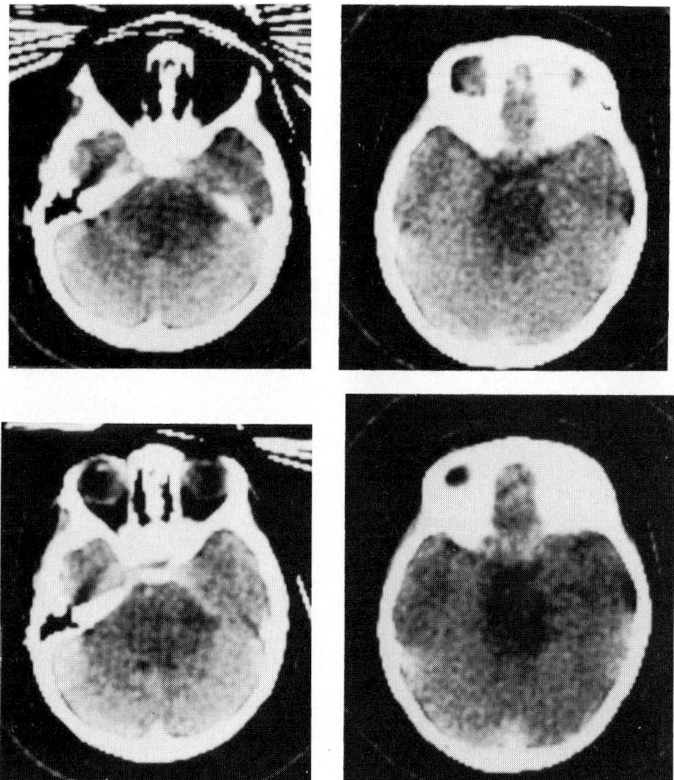

Figure 14–29. LOW DENSITY PONTINE GLIOMA THAT DID NOT DEMONSTRATE CONTRAST ENHANCEMENT: The preinfusion scan shows a large low density mass lesion in the pons that is probably surrounded by edema; it displaces the fourth ventricle posteriorly. There is no change following the infusion of contrast material. This is a large pontine glioma.

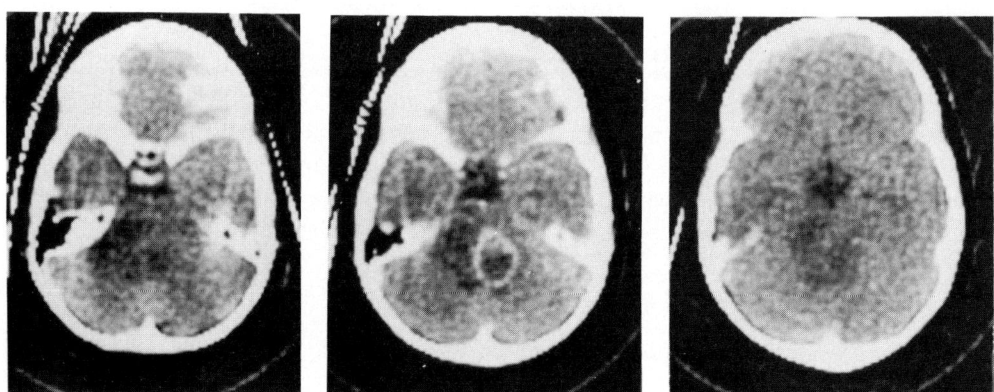

Figure 14–30. PONTINE GLIOMA WITH RING PATTERN OF ENHANCEMENT: The preinfusion scan reveals a large low density lesion in the pons that displaces the fourth ventricle posteriorly. The area of low density appears slightly irregular and appears to spare the anterior portion of the pons on the right side. The postinfusion scan reveals a ringlike oval area of enhancement to the right of the midline and extending to the midline just anterior to the fourth ventricle.

At surgery this was proved to be a pontine glioma.

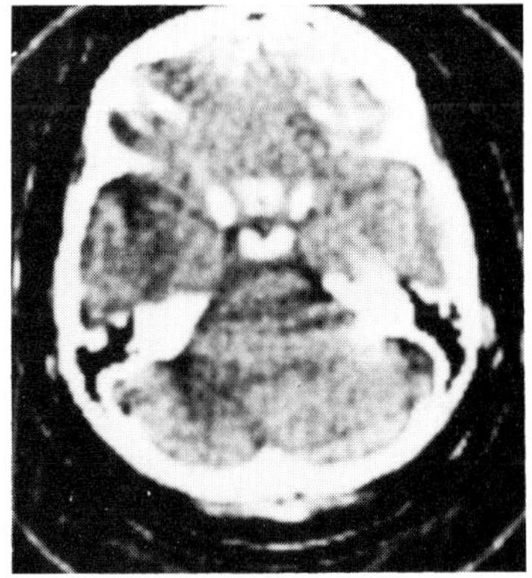

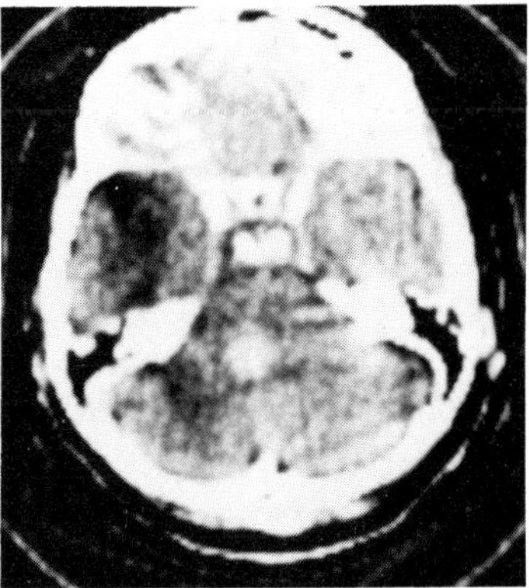

Figure 14–31. METASTASES TO THE REGION OF THE PONS: The preinfusion scan is normal. There is no obstructive hydrocephalus. The postinfusion scan demonstrates a small rounded area of enhancement in the region of the pons and to the left of the midline. The fourth ventricle appears slightly compressed and perhaps displaced slightly to the right of the midline.

This was felt to be a metastatic deposit in a patient with known breast carcinoma and a new onset of a left sixth nerve palsy and right-sided weakness.

POSTERIOR COMPARTMENT MASSES

MEDULLOBLASTOMA

These tumors usually are found in the first decade of life, but may be present in the second or third decade. The lesions arise on the midline in most cases, developing from the primitive cells of the external granular layer of the cerebellum. Occasionally these primitive cells migrate away from the midline; thus, the tumor also may arise off the midline. Although the name might imply a point of origin within the medulla, medulloblastomas most frequently originate from the posterior medullary velum in its inferior portion anatomically at the base of the vermis of the cerebellum. Occasionally, the tumors invade the fourth ventricle. There is a greater than 2:1 male predominance. The medulloblastoma is a posterior compartment mass.

Skull Film. Radiographically visible calcifications are very rare, although calcifications are more frequently identified by CT scan. The skull series most commonly is normal, but it may show evidence of widening of the sutures and other changes secondary to increased intracranial pressure.

CT Scanning. The CT scan with infusion is the procedure of choice for the work-up of a patient with possible medulloblastoma. The scan reveals a varying degree of obstructive hydrocephalus in almost all cases. I have not seen a case that did not demonstrate some degree of hydrocephalus at the time when tumor was visible. The medulloblastoma itself presents as a midline posterior fossa mass. The tumor usually is slightly more dense than normal brain tissue and rarely contains calcification. Frequently there is a variable amount of edema that surrounds the tumor asymmetrically. The fourth ventricle may be obliterated or may be seen to be displaced forward in the midline or slightly to either the right or left.

The mass, at the time of presentation, usually is quite large, commonly occupying half the width of the posterior fossa on those cuts where the tumor is best seen (see Figures 14–32 to 14–36).

Following the infusion of contrast material, there is marked homogeneous enhancement of the tumor. The tumor may seed the subarachnoid space; therefore, metastatic nodules may be seen in the supratentorial region. These are especially demonstrable in the supratentorial distribution on the postinfusion scan. Medulloblastomas also may metastasize to the spinal cord.

Angiography. The angiogram may be normal. These tumors may or may not show evidence of abnormal vascularity, and early draining veins are rare. The vascular displacements vary, depending on the point of origin of the tumors. Although the appearance may be similar to any other mass in the posterior fossa, in general it is that of a posterior compartment mass with anterior displacement of the precentral cerebellar vein. The PICA displacement can be in any direction, depending on the point of origin of the tumor. Because the tumor may grow in the midline or asymmetrically off the midline, the arteries and veins may be either at the midline or displaced to the contralateral side.

The arteriographic findings are not diagnostic. On the other hand, the CT appearance in most cases is very typical, and a diagnosis of medulloblastoma can be made with a high degree of certainty by CT scan.

EPENDYMOMA

These tumors arise from the ciliated ependymoma cells that line the ventricles. In the posterior fossa the tumor arises from the ependymal lining of the fourth ventricle; therefore, it usually presents as a midline tumor in the posterior fossa. Ependymomas are posterior compartment masses.

These tumors are seen in the first two decades of life and are more common in boys than in girls.

Skull Film. Calcifications are not uncommon in ependymomas and present as areas of fine calcification. There may be signs of increased intracranial pressure with split sutures. The skull may be normal.

CT Scanning. These tumors are readily identified on the CT scan. A varying degree of obstructive hydrocephalus is present in nearly all cases. The tumor may be isodense with normal brain tissue, and its presence will be detected by the fact that there is obliteration of the fourth ventricle and obstructive hydrocephalus. Calcifications, if present in the tumor, are readily detected by the CT scan. Following the infusion of contrast material, there is marked homogeneous enhancement of the tumor (see Figure 14–37). (The tumor arises within the fourth ventricle, which is dilated around the mass.) Ependymomas may seed into the supratentorial system or spinal regions via the cerebrospinal fluid pathways.

Angiography. These tumors are vascular with prolonged blush. Vessel displacements vary, depending on the location of the tumor. If the tumor grows inferiorly, the PICA may be splayed apart on either side of the midline. There is nothing specific that will make the angiographic diagnosis absolute.

ASTROCYTOMA

The astrocytoma is the most common posterior fossa tumor in children. In adults, one may also find astrocytomas of the cerebellum that produce similar angiographic changes.

These tumors are typically cystic and lie in the cerebellar hemisphere; therefore, they present as posterior compartment tumors. The lesion may extend to involve the vermis of the cerebellum, or, less commonly, may arise in the midline from the vermis of the cerebellum. These tumors contain a nodule that may be located anywhere in the wall of the cyst. The cyst wall itself is benign, and the nodule is the functioning portion of the astrocytoma (Figs. 14–38 to 14–42).

Skull Film. These tumors may be slow growing and therefore may present as a longstanding process in many children. *Rarely,* there may be bowing of the occipital bone over the cystic tumor. Not infrequently there is splitting of the sutures because of the long standing increased intracranial pressure.

CT Scanning. The CT scan reveals a cystic lesion in the cerebellar hemisphere. The border of the cyst is well defined; there may or may not be surrounding edema. The fluid within the cyst is of higher density than CSF, reflecting its high protein content. There is always a varying degree of obstructive hydrocephalus. Following the infusion of contrast material, there may be enhancement of the nodule of tumor in the wall of the astrocytoma. Not uncommonly, however, the nodule of enhancement reflecting the vascular portion of the tumor is not seen on the CT scan. Even if no enhancing nodule is evident, a cystic lesion in the cerebellar hemisphere that is associated with obstruction hydrocephalus makes the diagnosis of cerebellar astrocytoma possible with a very high degree of certainty in a large proportion of cases.

Angiography. The angiographic findings noted in cerebellar astrocytoma are similar to those seen in any cerebellar mass. The wall of the cyst is benign and does not appear as a vascular structure; however, the nodule of tumor may appear as a vascular mass. In general, the choroidal point of the PICA will be displaced to the contralateral side. The vermian branches of the PICA also will be displaced to the contralateral side, and there is stretching of the hemispheric branches of the PICA. There may be inferior displacement of the tonsillar loops of the PICA, reflecting tonsillar herniation. The vermian branches of the superior cerebellar artery are displaced superiorly.

The superior vermian veins will be displaced close to the straight sinus. The precentral cerebellar vein is displaced anteriorly, and the choroidal point is displaced inferiorly. The basilar artery is closely applied to the clivus and may be displaced across the midline away from the tumor. There is elevation of the superior cerebellar arteries.

In those rare cases where the tumor is particularly long standing, upward bowing of the straight sinus may be seen — an unusual finding because the tentorium and straight sinus are rigid structures.

HEMANGIOBLASTOMA

This is a vascular tumor which arises in the cerebellum from capillary endothelial cells. These tumors vary greatly in size. When the tumors are large and vascular, differentiation from an arteriovenous malformation may be difficult. Typically, the blush of a hemangioblastoma will be noted to persist well into the venous phase. These are posterior compartment masses, although they rarely may involve the brain stem (Figs. 14–46 to 14–48).

Hemangioblastoma associated with retinal hemangiomas and polycythemia is a syndrome known as von Hippel-Lindau's disease; it is one of the phakomatoses. These tumors may be solid or cystic.

Skull Film. Usually normal.

CT Scanning. The CT scan reveals a low density lesion of varying size that may or may not be associated with obstructive hydrocephalus. The postinfusion scan reveals marked homogeneous enhancement of the solid portions of the tumor.

METASTASES TO POSTERIOR FOSSA

Metastatic lesions to the posterior fossa are fairly common. The most common source of metastasis is a primary lung tumor; however, breast carcinoma is another common source. They may be either anterior or posterior compartment masses. Metastases are the most common posterior fossa tumors in adults.

Plain Skull Film. The skull film is usually normal. The progression of the disease is too rapid to allow the changes of increased intracranial pressure to be detected in the sella. Bony metastases may be visible.

CT Scanning. The CT scan performed without and with contrast infusion affords the most accurate assessment of the presence or absence of metastatic deposits in the posterior fossa. Furthermore, the number, position and relationship of the metastatic deposits to other anatomic structures is better defined on the CT scan than by any other diagnostic method now available.

The preinfusion scan may appear normal, or it may reveal radiolucent isodense or high density lesions. There may or may not be displacement or distortion of the fourth ventricle. Obstructive hydrocephalus may or may not be present.

The postinfusion scan reveals a variety of

patterns of enhancement. There may be a ring of enhancement, homogeneous enhancement or any other variety of enhancement imaginable.

Angiography. A variety of abnormal patterns may be seen, depending on the position of the lesions and the multiplicity of lesions.

CEREBELLAR HEMORRHAGE

Hypertensive hemorrhages occur in the cerebellum, but are less frequent in the cerebellum than in the basal ganglia. If of sufficient size, the cerebellar hemorrhage leads to the rapid demise of the patient caused by mass effect with compression of the vital structures in the brain stem. Early diagnosis is therefore important so that the clot can be removed without delay. These are usually posterior compartment hemorrhages. Massive brain stem hemorrhage also may occur.

Plain Skull Film. Normal.

CT Scanning. The preinfusion scan reveals an area of blood density in the cerebellar hemisphere. There may or may not be surrounding edema; the fourth ventricle may be shifted, and there may or may not be obstructive hydrocephalus. A rapid increase in the area of hemorrhage may occur. I have seen one case in which there was a demonstrable increase in the size of the hemorrhage during the time it took to perform the CT scan. Computed tomography is the procedure of choice for diagnosis, and surgery can be undertaken without further work-up. Indeed, delay in diagnosis may lead to the patient's death.

Angiography. Vertebral angiography may demonstrate an avascular mass. The shifts of the various vascular structures will depend on the size and position of the hemorrhage.

Text continued on page 710

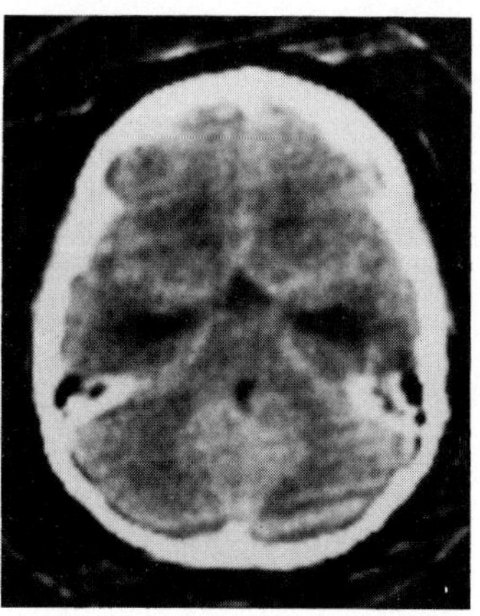

Preinfusion

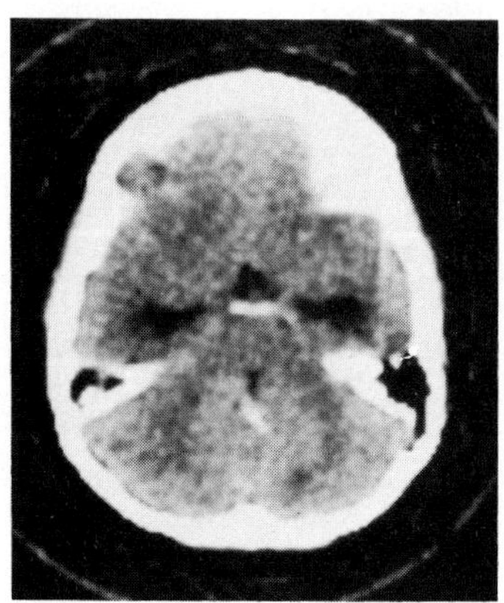

Postinfusion

Figure 14–32. MEDULLOBLASTOMA: The preinfusion scan reveals a posterior fossa mass lesion in the midline that is of higher density than normal brain tissue. There is some surrounding edema that is greater on the right side than on the left. The fourth ventricle is compressed and displaced anteriorly. A curvilinear area of high density can be seen in the midline just behind the fourth ventricle; this probably represents an area of calcification. There is moderate obstructive hydrocephalus, and the dilated temporal horns are visible bilaterally in the middle cranial fossa. Following the infusion of contrast material, there is little or no appreciable enhancement of the tumor mass.

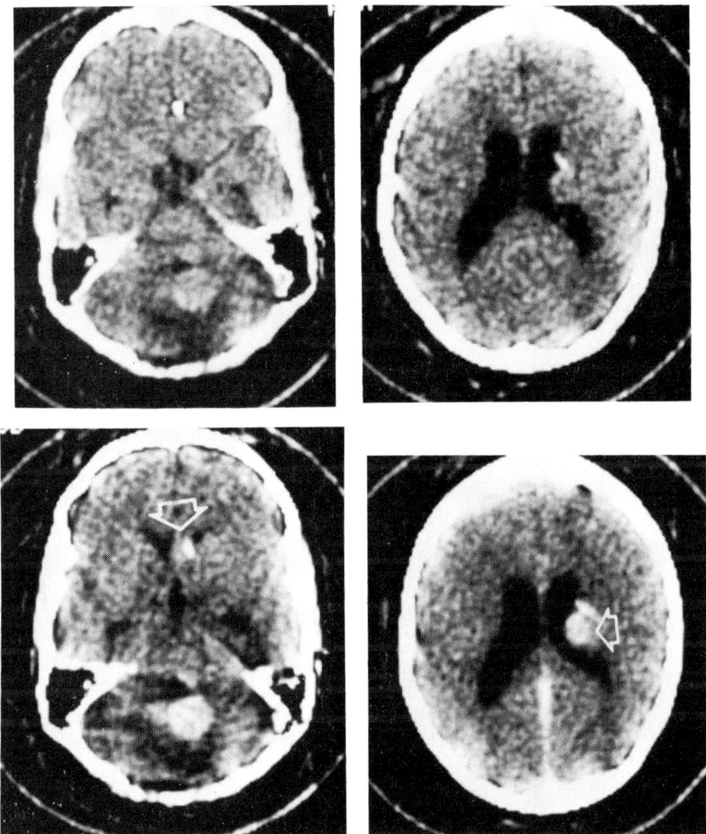

Figure 14–33. MEDULLOBLASTOMA RECURRENT IN THE POSTERIOR FOSSA WITH SUPRATENTORIAL METASTASES: The preinfusion scan reveals a craniectomy defect in the midline in the posterior fossa. Some radiolucency is visible beneath the craniectomy site. In addition, there is a well defined mass lesion behind the fourth ventricle that flattens the fourth ventricle along its right posterior margin. The tip of the shunt tube is visible in the midline at the level of the interhemispheric fissure. There is moderate obstructive hydrocephalus and evidence of a mass lesion that indents the body of the right lateral ventricle.

The postinfusion scan reveals enhancement of the recurrent or remaining tumor in the posterior fossa behind the fourth ventricle. A second deposit of metastatic tumor in the frontal region compresses the right frontal horn. A third metastatic nodule is better seen on the postinfusion scan as it compresses the body of the right lateral ventricle.

This is an example of medulloblastoma that has metastasized to the supratentorial region. This tumor may also spread to involve the spinal cord.

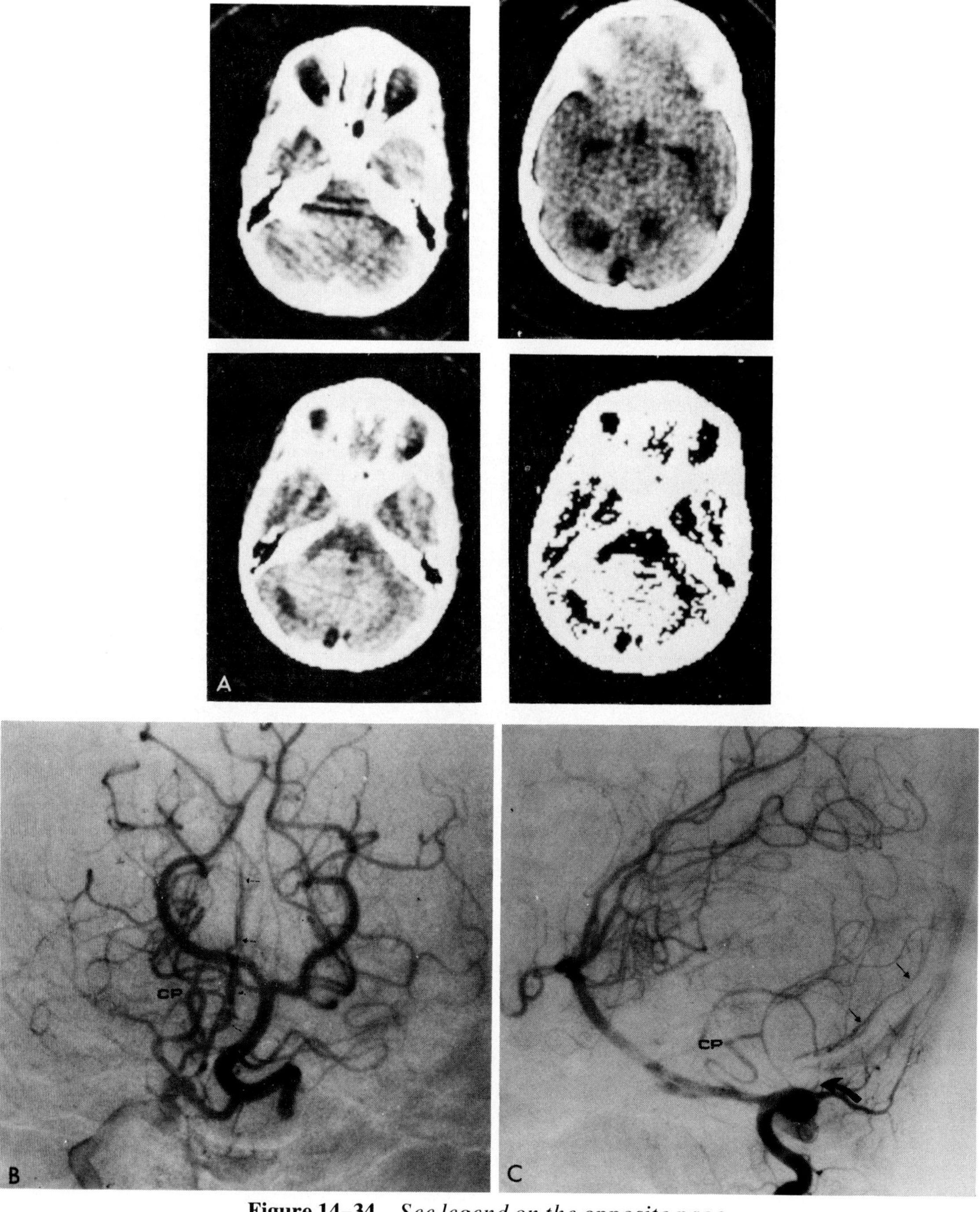

Figure 14–34 *See legend on the opposite page*

Figure 14–34. MEDULLOBLASTOMA: *A*, The preinfusion scan shows a poorly defined mass lesion in the midline in the posterior fossa that has two areas of surrounding edema above it on either side. Following the infusion of contrast material, there is marked homogeneous enhancement of the tumor, which demonstrates some surrounding edema — approximately equal on both the right and the left sides. The tumor appears to be slightly larger on the left than on the right. There is moderate obstructive hydrocephalus in this case.

B, The AP view of the right vertebral arteriogram reveals that both the choroidal point (*CP*) on the right side and the vermian branch of the right PICA are displaced to the right of the midline (*arrows*). This finding is consistent with the CT finding of a tumor slightly larger on the left than on the right side.

C, The lateral view of the right vertebral arteriogram reveals that the choroidal point (*CP*) is displaced inferiorly. There is stretching and splaying apart of the branches of the PICA. The vermian branches are markedly displaced posteriorly (small arrows), and the tonsillohemispheric branches are markedly stretched (*large arrow*). The basilar artery is closely applied to the clivus. No abnormal vessels are seen.

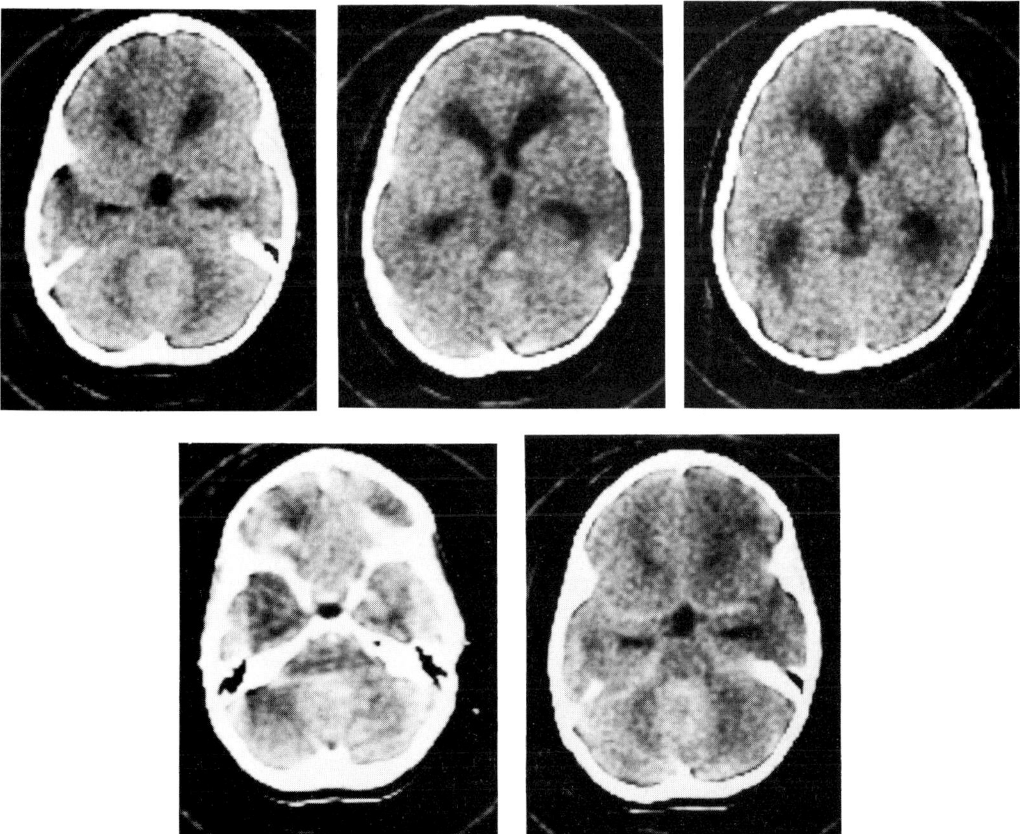

Figure 14–35. MEDULLOBLASTOMA: The preinfusion scan reveals a mass lesion of higher density than the normal brain tissue that is surrounded by edema. The fourth ventricle can be seen to be displaced anteriorly and slightly to the left of the midline. There is moderate obstructive hydrocephalus. The postinfusion scan shows marked homogeneous enhancement of the tumor in the midline. This appearance is very typical of a medulloblastoma.

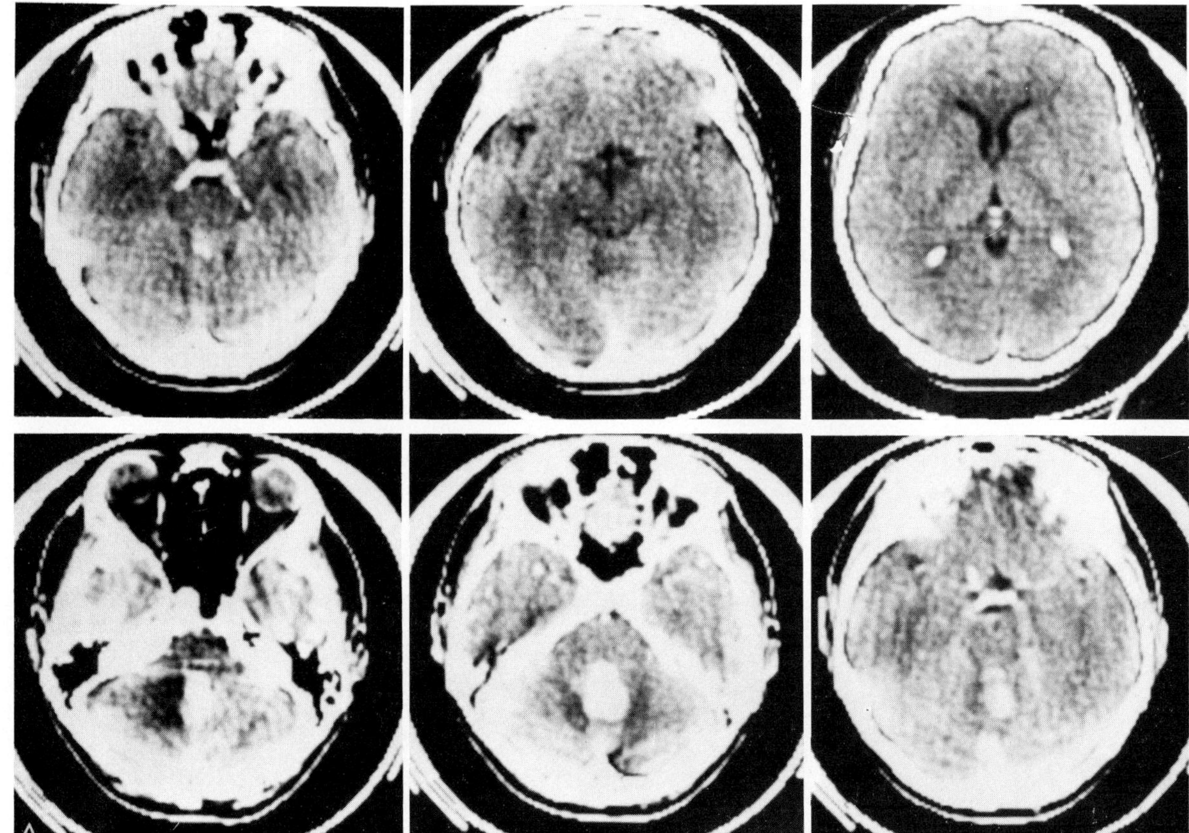

Figure 14–36. MEDULLOBLASTOMA INVADING THE FOURTH VENTRICLE: *A,* The preinfusion scan reveals two small punctate areas of calcification in the midline in the posterior fossa in the anticipated position of the fourth ventricle. The fourth ventricle is never well seen. Otherwise, the scan appears unremarkable, and there is no evidence of obstructive hydrocephalus. After the infusion of contrast material, there is marked homogeneous enhancement of a tumor in the midline in the posterior fossa. It appears to occupy the anticipated position of the fourth ventricle. The appearance is consistent with a medulloblastoma that has invaded the fourth ventricle. However, the appearance is certainly not typical, and the presence of the calcification argues against the diagnosis of a medulloblastoma. Ependymoma of the fourth ventricle appears more likely, and a metastatic lesion to the posterior fossa also should be considered.

B, The lateral view of the right vertebral arteriogram reveals that the choroidal points are displaced anteriorly bilaterally (*CP*). There is stretching of the tonsillohemispheric branches of the PICA anteriorly and marked posterior displacement of the vermian branches of the PICA. No abnormal vessels are seen.

C, The AP view of the arteriogram reveals that the vermian branches of the PICA are splayed apart by the growth of the tumor between the two vessels. The choroidal points *(CP)* also are splayed apart by the tumor in the fourth ventricle. At surgery this proved to be an intraventricular medulloblastoma.

D, The postoperative scan reveals an area of hemorrhage in the midline in the posterior fossa. In addition, there is a large amount of air within the cranial vault and in the suprasellar cisterns.

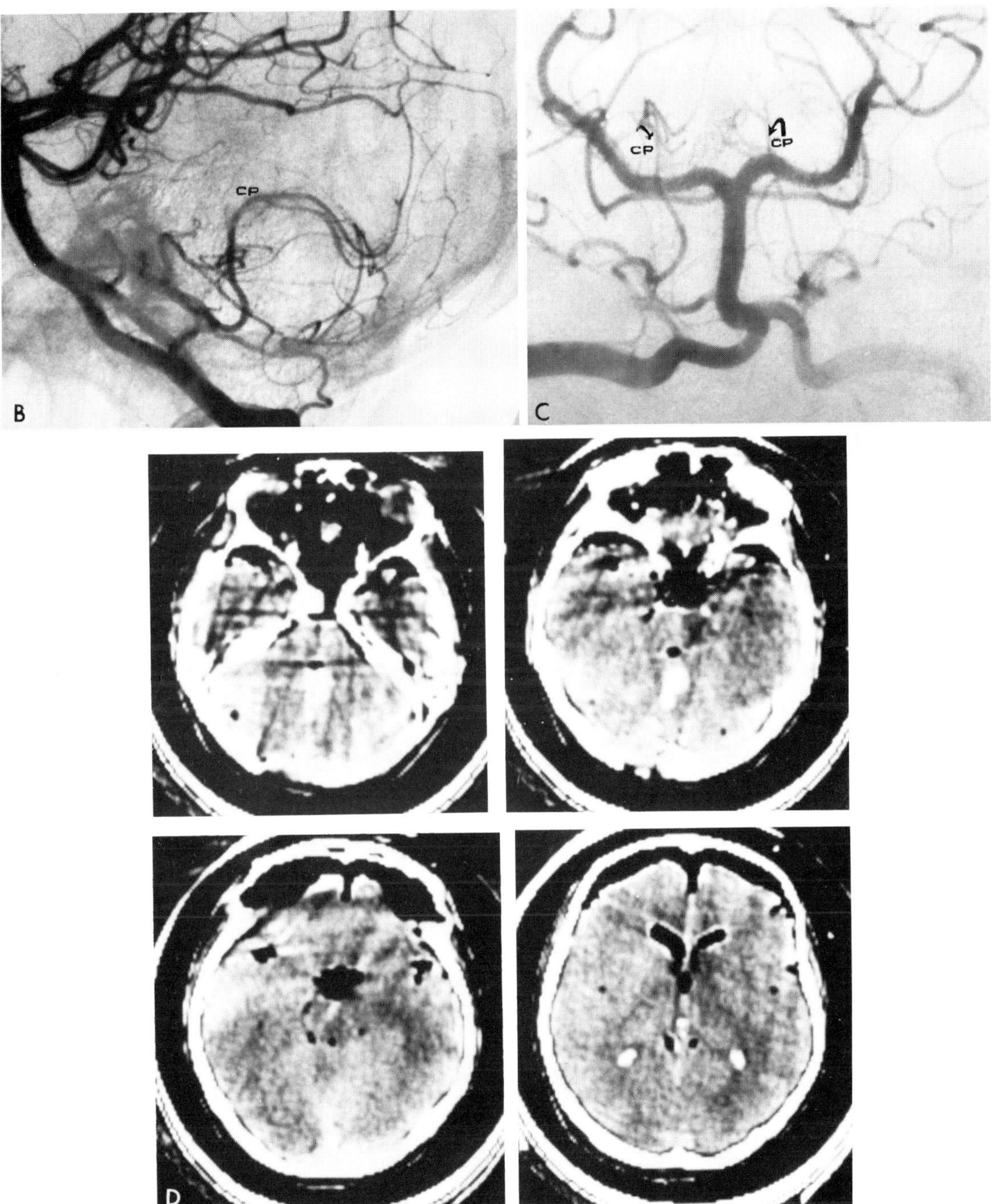

Figure 14–36 *Continued*

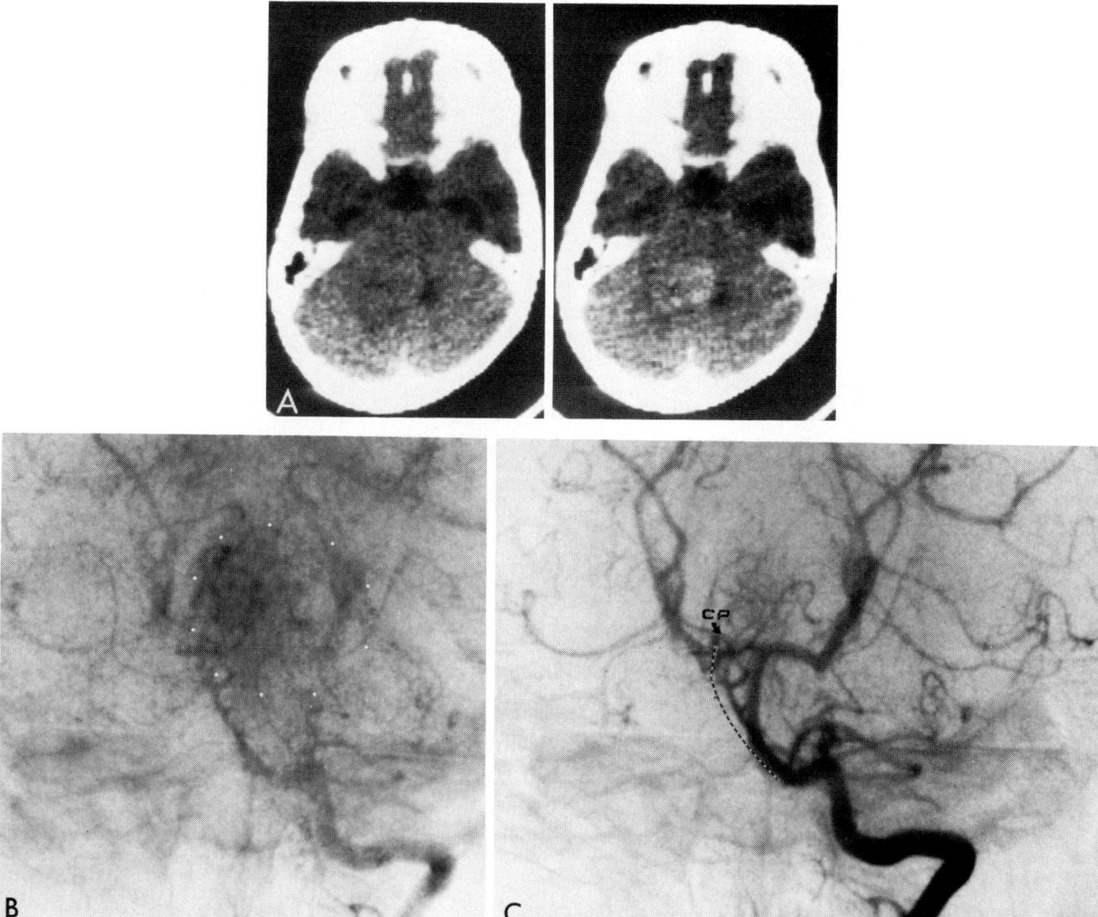

Figure 14–37. EPENDYMOMA: *A*, The preinfusion scan reveals an isodense mass in the midline in the posterior fossa. The fourth ventricle is displaced to the right of the midline around the mass. There is mild to moderate obstructive hydrocephalus. Following the infusion of contrast material, there is moderate enhancement. No calcifications could be detected. The mass is larger on the left than on the right.

The AP view of the left vertebral arteriogram in *B* reveals that the choroidal point (*CP*) is displaced to the right of the midline, and there is curvilinear displacement of the branches of the PICA across the midline to the right side (*dashed line*).

C, There are myriad small tumor vessels arising from the PICA, and the later arterial phase reveals the tumor stain in the midline and extending to the left of the midline (*white dots*).

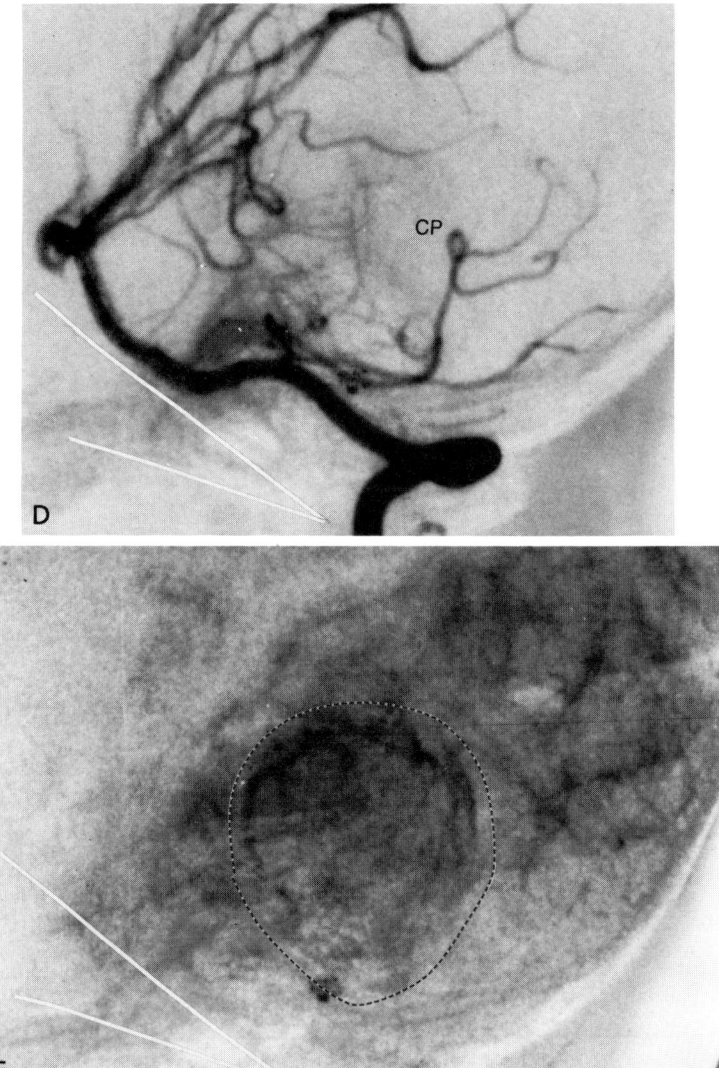

Figure 14–37 *Continued*

D, The lateral view of the vertebral arteriogram reveals marked posterior displacement of the choroidal point *(CP)* and posterior displacement of the vermian branches of the PICA. The white lines outline the clivus.

E, The venous phase reveals a capsular stain of the tumor mass as it is surrounded by draining veins. This lesion was proved at surgery to be an ependymoma.

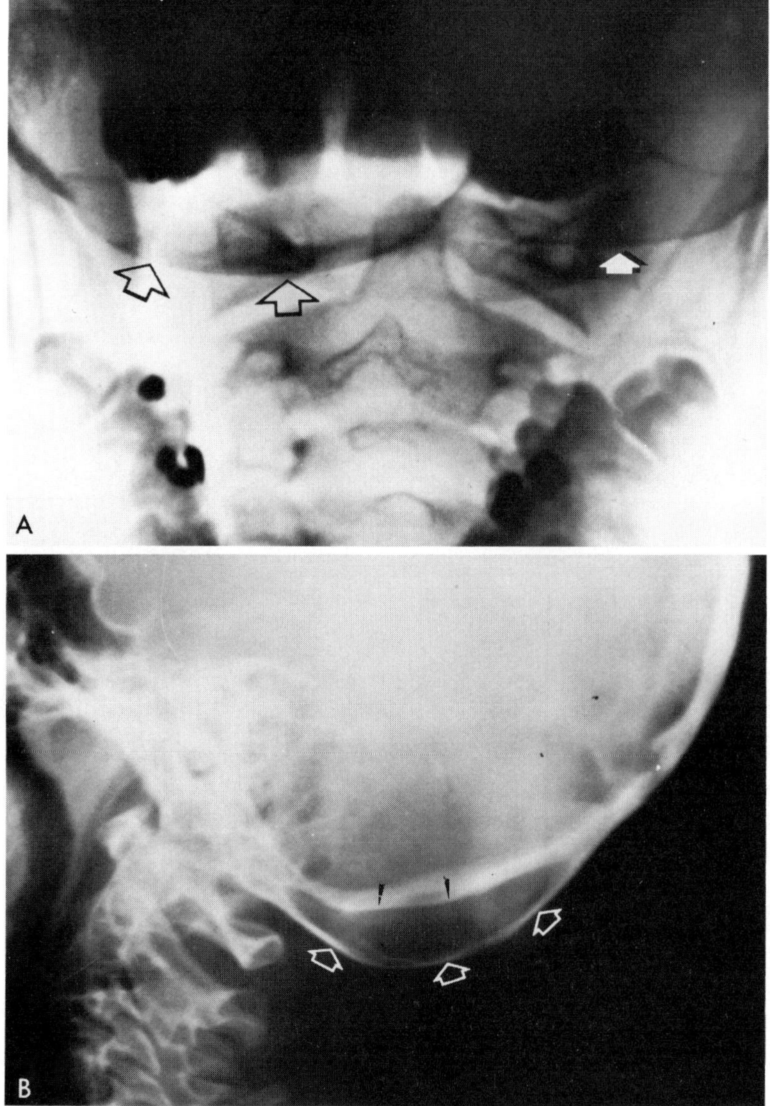

Figure 14–38. CYSTIC CEREBELLAR ASTROCYTOMA: *A,* The open-mouth view of the odontoid process reveals the expansion of the bony margin of the posterior cranial fossa *(open black arrowheads)* on the side of the long standing cystic astrocytoma. The normal left side is demonstrated by the closed white arrowhead.

B, The lateral view of the posterior fossa also demonstrates the expansion of the right side of the posterior cranial fossa *(open white arrowheads)* as compared to the left *(black arrows).* Care must be taken to be sure that this appearance is not due to an "off-lateral" technique of filming rather than to an actual bony expansion.

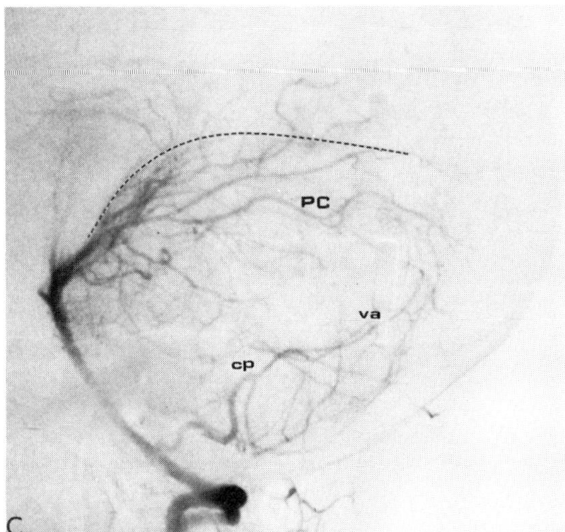

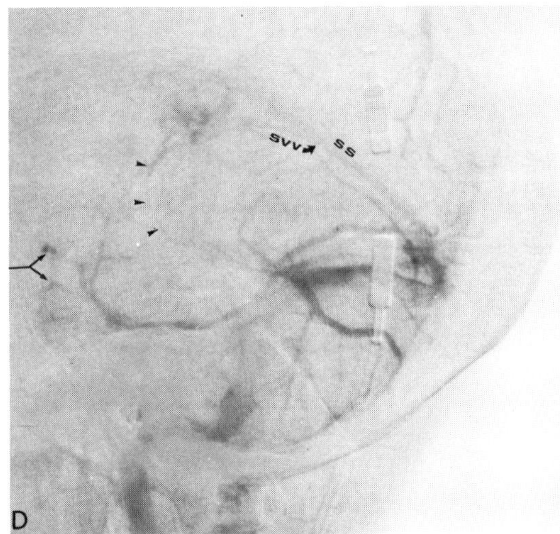

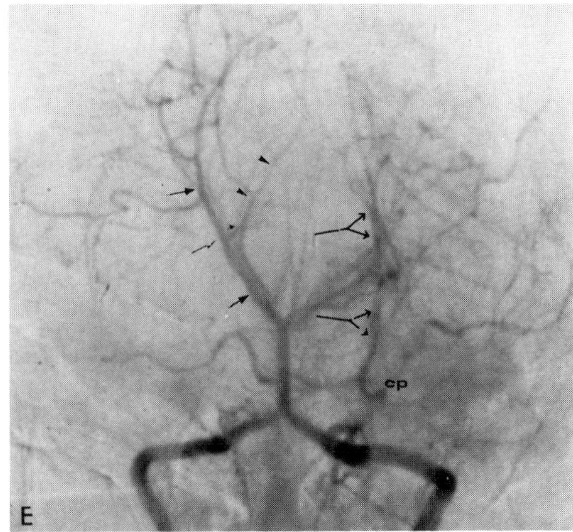

Figure 14–38 *Continued*

C, The lateral view of the arteriogram reveals that the basilar artery is closely applied to the clivus. There is upward displacement of the branches of the superior cerebellar arteries (*dashed line*), which project above the plane of the posterior cerebral arteries *(PC);* there is also posterior displacement of the choroidal point *(cp)* and vermian *(va)* branches of the PICA with marked stretching of the hemispheric branches of the PICA.

D, The lateral venous phase reveals upward bowing of the straight sinus (*ss*) because of the long-standing nature of the problem. The precentral cerebellar vein is displaced anteriorly, indicating involvement of the vermis of the cerebellum (*small arrowheads*). The anterior pontomesencephalic vein is closely applied to the clivus (*double-headed arrow*), the superior vermian veins (*svv*) are displaced close to the straight sinus (*ss*) and there is posterior displacement of the inferior vermian veins. A shunt tubing device is noted in place.

E, The AP view of the vertebral arteriogram demonstrates no filling of the right PICA (anatomic variant); the left PICA and choroidal point (*cp*) are filled and shown to be displaced markedly to the left of the midline, as are all the branches of the PICA (*double-headed arrows*).

In addition there is medial and superior elevation of the posterior cerebral arteries *(long arrows)* and the superior cerebellar arteries *(arrowheads)*. It is unusual for a posterior fossa tumor to affect the supratentorial posterior cerebral arteries; this reflects the long-standing relatively benign nature of the process.

Illustration continued on the following page

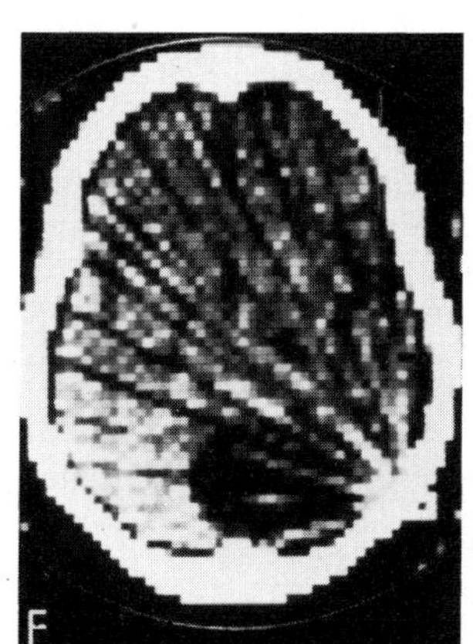

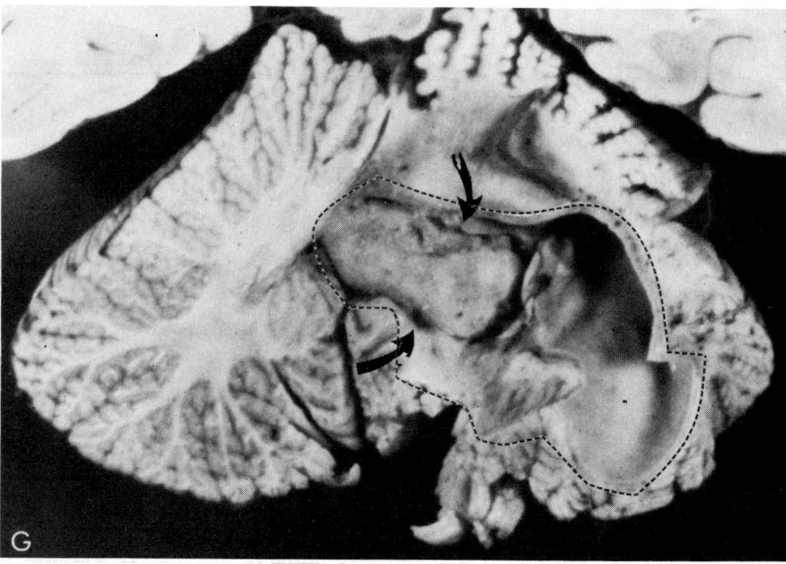

Figure 14–38 *Continued*

F, The CT scan is one of the very earliest scans performed. It readily demonstrates the cystic lesion in the right cerebellar hemisphere. There is some artifact from the metallic shunt tubing device. No postinfusion scan is available.

G, The postmortem pathologic correlation reveals a well-defined, large cystic tumor in the right cerebellar hemisphere with a nodule of tumor that extends into the vermis of the cerebellum *(arrows)*. This correlated with the forward displacement of the precentral cerebellar vein.

This is a classic example of a long-standing, rather benign cystic cerebellar astrocytoma.

Figure 14–39. CYSTIC CEREBELLAR ASTROCYTOMA, RIGHT SIDE: *A*, The AP view of the vertebral arteriogram reveals medial displacement of the right superior cerebellar artery *(dotted line)*. The choroidal point *(CP)* is displaced to the left of the midline, as are the vermian branches of the PICA.

B, The lateral view of the vertebral arteriogram reveals upward bowing of the superior cerebellar arteries *(dotted line)* and a basilar artery that is closely applied to the clivus. The choroidal point *(CP)* is displaced downward, and there is stretching of the branches of the PICA.

C, The lateral venous phase reveals superior displacement of the superior cerebellar veins (*ssv*), which are in very close proximity to the straight sinus. The precentral cerebellar vein (*pcv*) is displaced slightly forward, and the anterior pontomesencephalic (*apmv*) vein is closely applied to the clivus.

D, A CT scan on another patient demonstrates a cystic cerebellar astrocytoma on the right side. The fluid within the cyst measured of higher density than CSF, reflecting the increased protein content of the cyst. The fourth ventricle is displaced forward and tilted slightly by the cystic mass. There is moderate obstructive hydrocephalus. Although these cystic tumors usually have a nubbin of tumor in the wall of the cyst, this area of tumor frequently cannot be demonstrated, even on the postinfusion scan. This is true in this case, and the nodule of tumor is not seen.

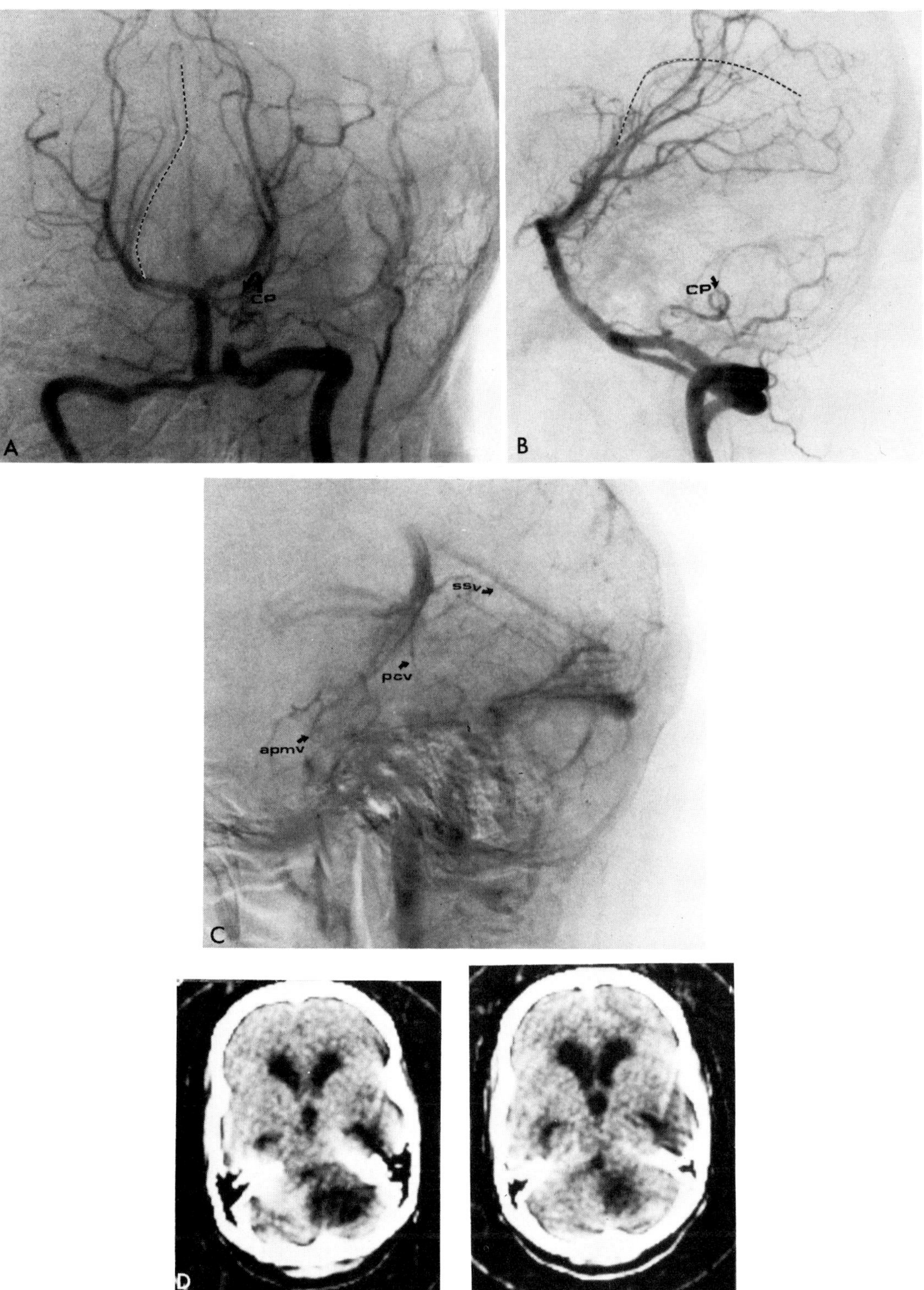

Figure 14–39 *See legend on the opposite page*

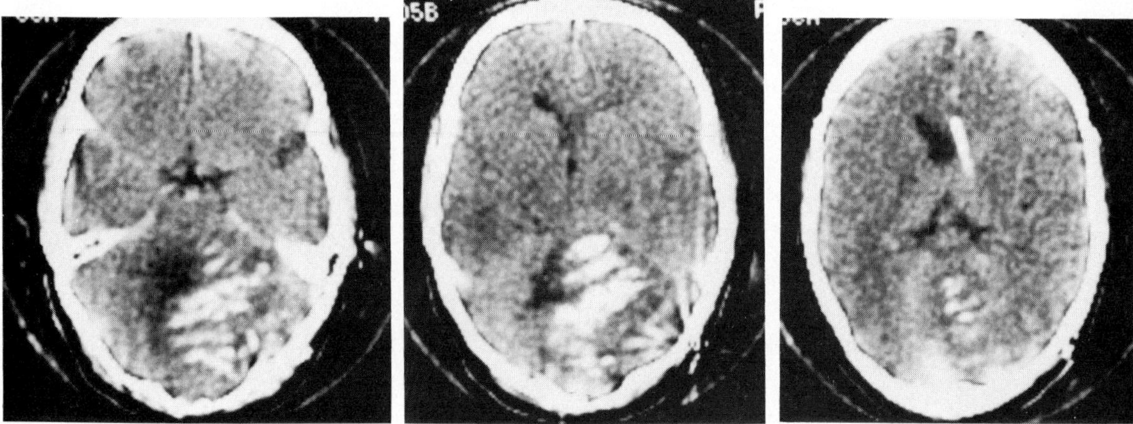

Figure 14–40. CALCIFIED CEREBELLAR ASTROCYTOMA: This patient had had partial removal of a cerebellar astrocytoma in the past, and now has a calcified lesion in the right cerebellar area that is the remnant of the old astrocytoma. The fourth ventricle is slightly compressed and displaced to the left of the midline. A shunt tubing device is in place in the frontal horn of the right lateral ventricle.

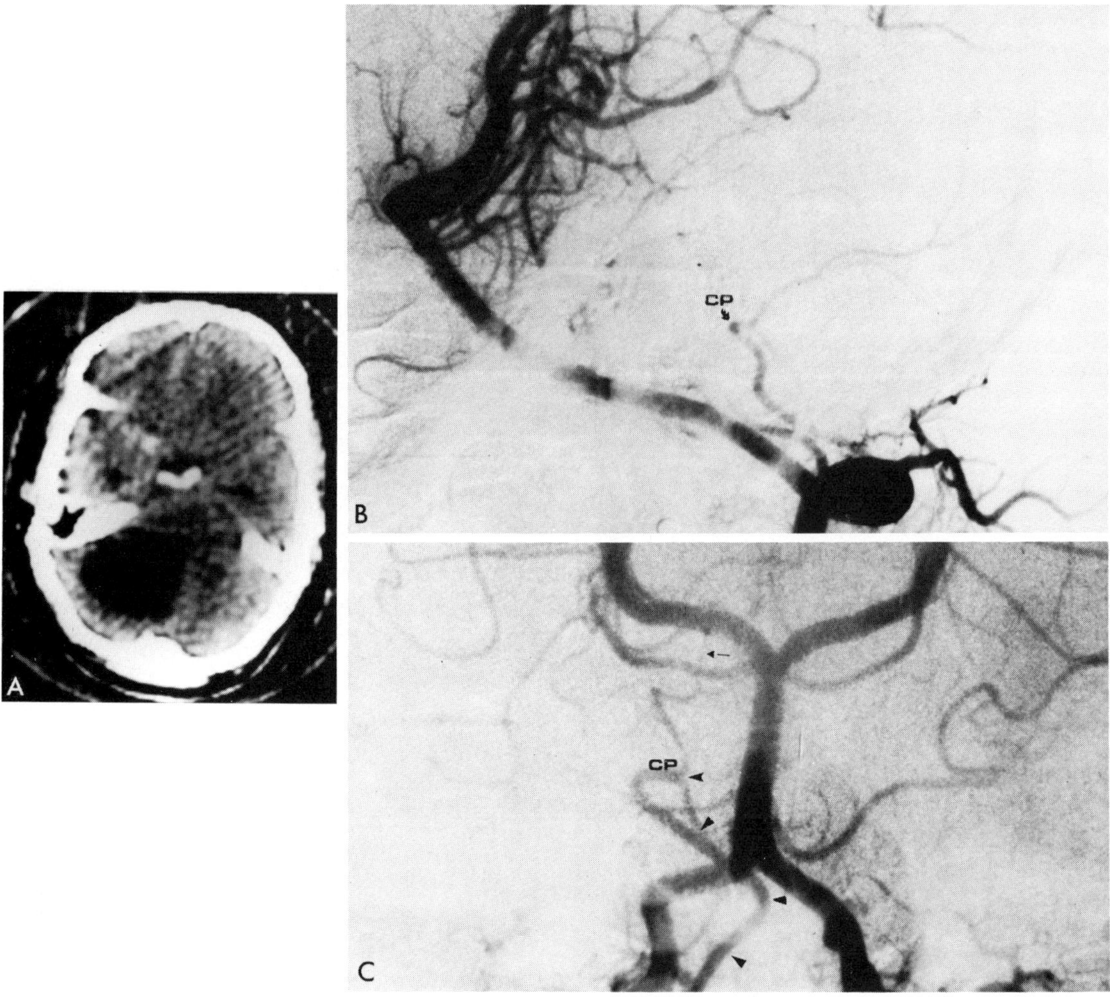

Figure 14–41 *See legend on the opposite page*

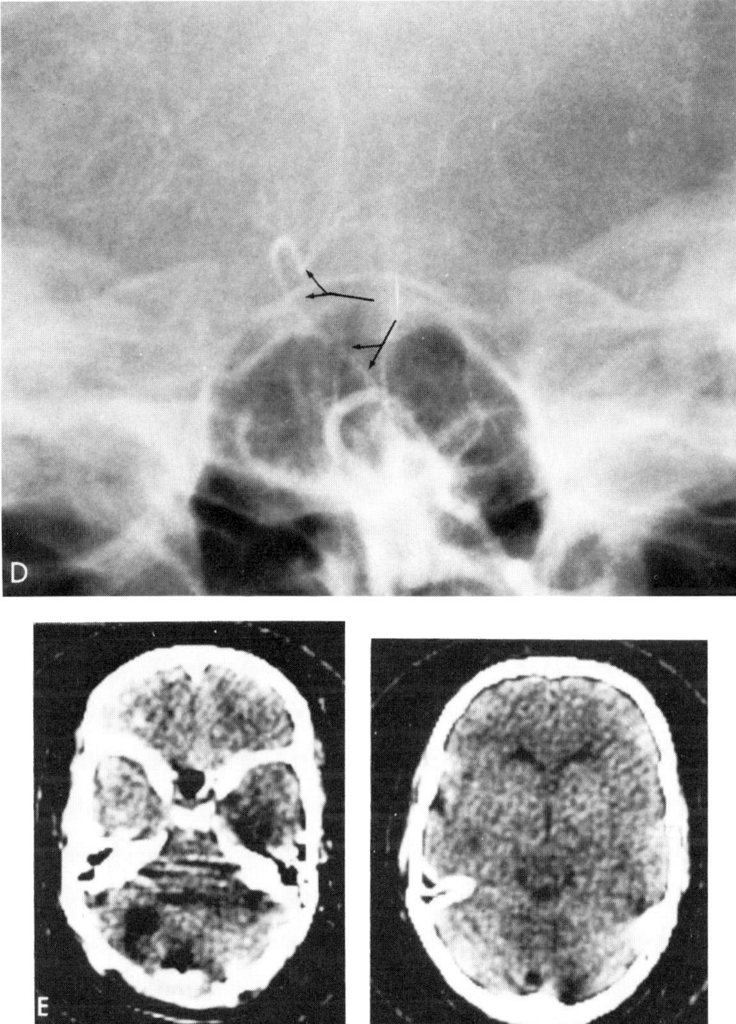

Figure 14–41. CYSTIC CEREBELLAR ASTROCYTOMA, LEFT SIDE: *A*, The CT scan shows a large cystic mass in the left cerebellar hemisphere that has obliterated the fourth ventricle. There was moderate obstructive hydrocephalus. No change could be detected following the infusion of contrast material.

B, The lateral view of the vertebral arteriogram reveals marked downward displacement of the caudal and tonsillar loops of the PICA, reflecting tonsillar herniation. The PICA gives the appearance of being displaced anteriorly; however, the AP view *(C)* discloses that the PICA and the choroidal point *(CP)* actually are displaced far to the right of the midline. The basilar artery is closely applied to the clivus. The black arrowheads follow the course of the PICA; the small arrow demonstrates the vermian branches of the PICA, which are displaced far to the right of the midline.

D, A later film demonstrates that the distal portion of the left PICA is displaced far across the midline to the contralateral side (*double-headed arrows*).

E, A postoperative scan reveals that the tumor has been totally removed. There is only a small cystic area in the bed of the tumor at the site of tumor removal.

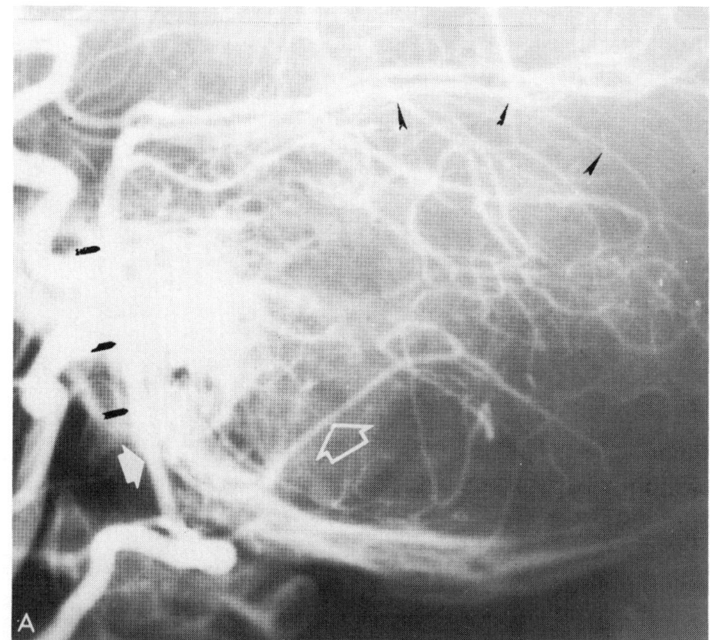

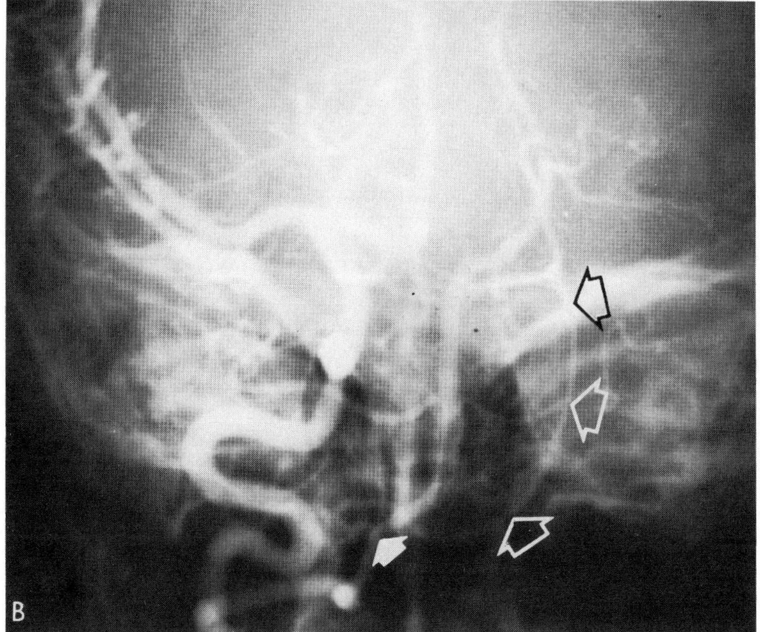

Figure 14–42. CEREBELLAR ASTROCYTOMA, RIGHT SIDE: *A*, The lateral view of the vertebral arteriogram reveals that the basilar artery is closely applied to the clivus *(thick dark arrowheads)*. There is superior displacement of the superior cerebellar arteries *(smaller black arrowheads)*. Marked stretching of the PICA and its branches *(open white arrowhead)* is evident. The origin of the PICA is illustrated by the closed white arrowhead in *A* and *B*.

B, The origin is also well seen on the AP view (*white arrowhead*). In addition, on the AP view one can see that the PICA and its branches are displaced far to the left of the midline (*open arrowheads*).

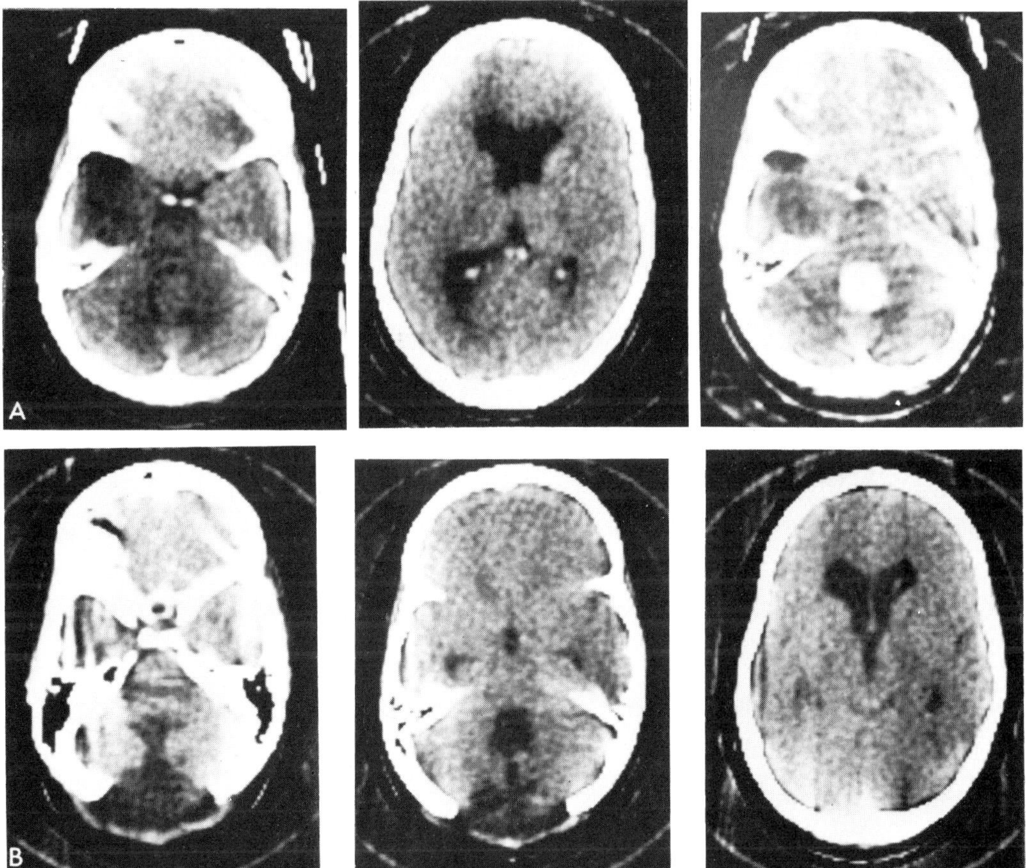

Figure 14–43. CHOROID PLEXUS PAPILLOMA OF THE FOURTH VENTRICLE: *A*, The preinfusion scan demonstrates a mass that is isodense with normal brain tissue but that occupies the anticipated position of the fourth ventricle. There is moderate obstructive hydrocephalus. The postinfusion scan demonstrates homogeneous enhancement of the tumor, which rests in and enlarges the fourth ventricle. At surgery this proved to be a choroid plexus papilloma of the fourth ventricle.

B, Postoperatively, the wide midline craniectomy site can be seen, and the enlarged fourth ventricle is now readily visible. There continues to be enlargement of the lateral ventricles.

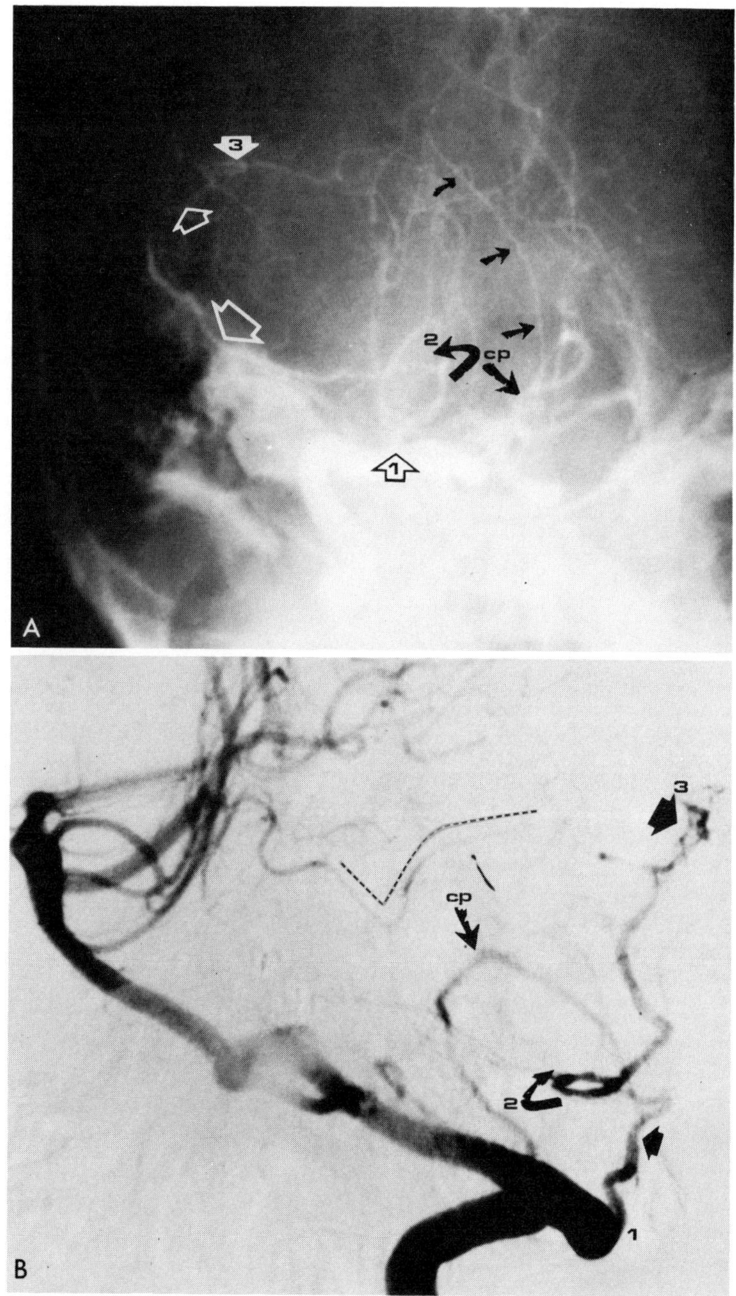

Figure 14–44 *See legend on the opposite page*

Figure 14–44. POSTERIOR FOSSA MENINGIOMA: *A* and *B*, This meningioma is an extra-axial, posterior compartment mass. The AP and lateral views of the right vertebral angiograms demonstrate the origin of the posterior meningeal artery *(1)*, which is greatly enlarged. The meningeal artery takes a sharp turn *(2)* and follows a curvilinear course *(open white arrowheads* on the AP view), where it then supplies the tumor *(3)*. The choroidal point *(cp)* is displaced to the contralateral side, as are the vermian branches *(small black arrowheads)*. The hemispheric branches of the superior cerebellar arteries are displaced in a curvilinear fashion *around* the mass (*open white arrows* in *A* and *dotted line* in *B*). This latter change occurs because the mass is extra-axial; therefore, the branches are not stretched over the mass, but rather are displaced away from it.

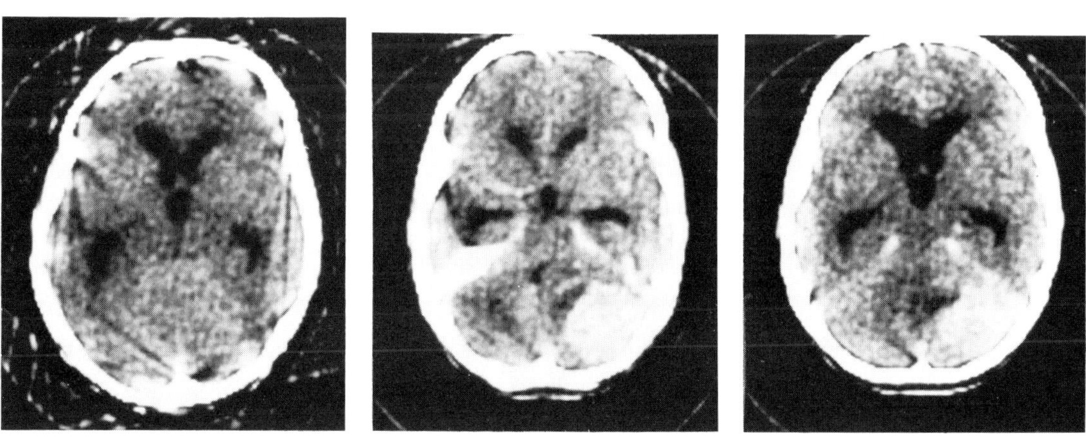

Figure 14–45. CEREBELLAR GLIOBLASTOMA: The preinfusion scan reveals evidence of moderate obstructive hydrocephalus. There appears to be a high density mass in the posterior fossa. The mass is best identified on the postinfusion scan, where there is homogeneous enhancement of a well-defined tumor in the right cerebellar hemisphere. The fourth ventricle is displaced forward and to the left of the midline. A small low density cystic component of the tumor is seen along the anteromedial portion of the mass. Differential diagnosis in this case includes a metastatic tumor or a meningioma. Hemangioblastoma is also a possibility. This lesion was proved surgically to be a glioblastoma.

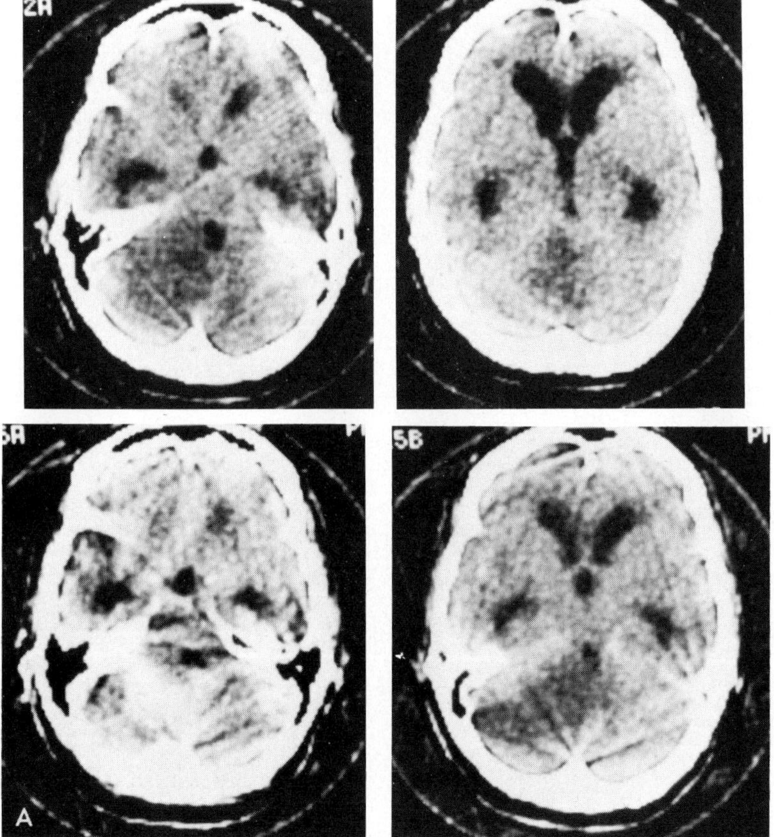

Figure 14–46. HEMANGIOBLASTOMA: *A,* The preinfusion scan reveals a large, poorly defined area of low density in the left cerebellum. The fourth ventricle is displaced forward and to the right of the midline. In addition, there is dilatation of the aqueduct, which also is displaced to the right of the midline. After the infusion of contrast material there is marked homogeneous enhancement of a large tumor mass in the left cerebellum. There is moderate obstructive hydrocephalus.

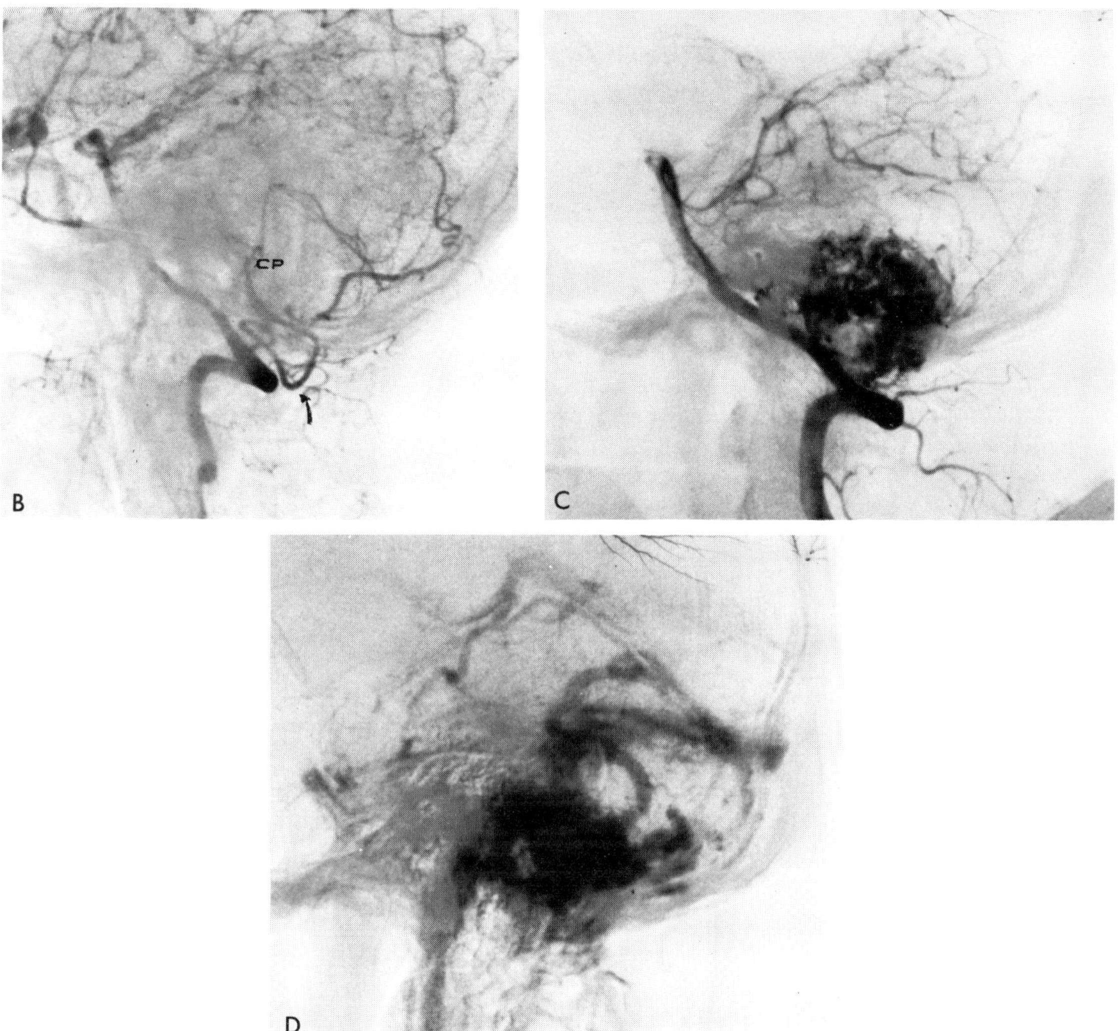

Figure 14–46 *Continued*

B, The early arterial view in the lateral projection of the vertebral arteriogram reveals downward displacement of the PICA and the choroidal point (*CP*), with stretching of the vermian branches of the PICA around a large mass lesion on the posterior fossa.

C, The later arterial view reveals a large, very vascular mass in the cerebellar hemisphere that demonstrates multiple arteries and early draining veins.

D, The later venous phase reveals a prolonged tumor stain, which typically persists well into the venous phase; it again demonstrates the multiple draining veins. In this case, the veins drain predominantly superiorly up to the straight sinus and then to the lateral sinus and internal jugular. This appearance is very typical of a hemangioblastoma of the cerebellum.

This tumor may be part of a syndrome of the Von Hippel-Lindau disease, where the hemangioblastoma of the cerebellum is seen in association with hemangiomas of the retina and renal tumors as well as an elevated hematocrit.

These tumors may be cystic as well as solid. If the tumor is cystic, it may be quite sizeable without creating much mass effect.

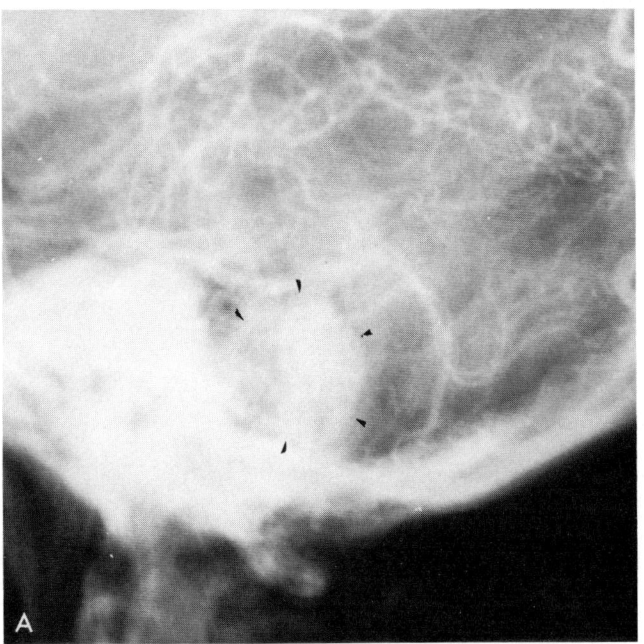

Figure 14–47. HEMANGIOBLASTOMA OF THE CEREBELLAR TONSIL: *A* and *B*, There is a small, nutmeg-sized mass in the region of the cerebellar tonsil very close to the midline. The mass is very vascular, and the stain can be seen persisting well into the venous phase on the AP view (*B*), where the tumor is situated approximately on the midline (*arrows*).

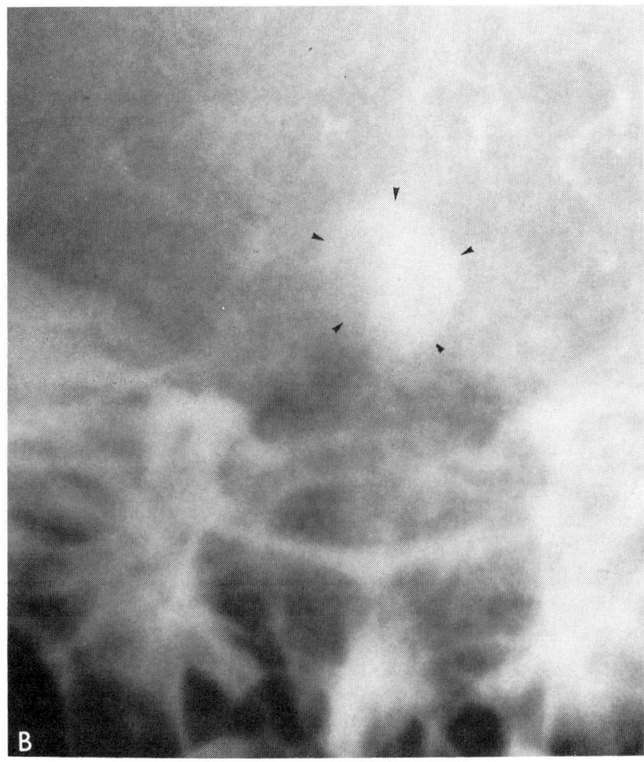

Figure 14–47 *Continued*

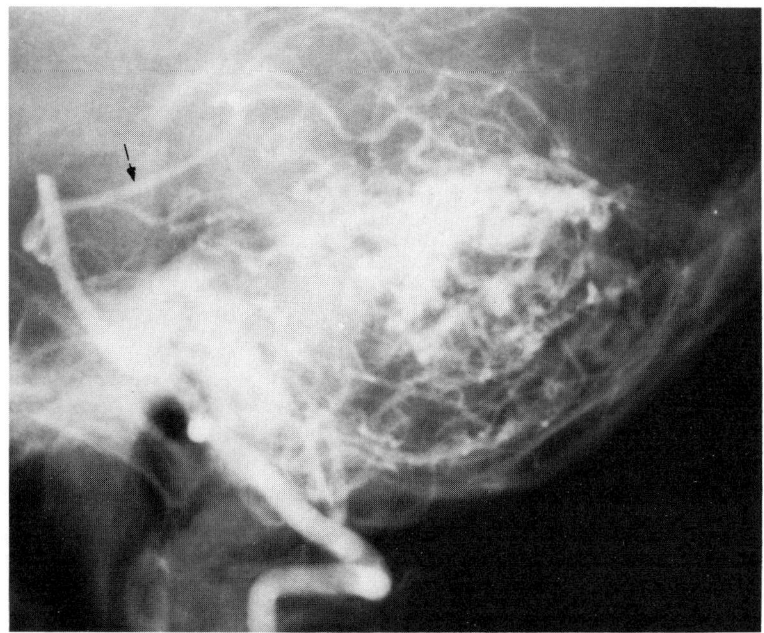

Figure 14–48. HEMANGIOBLASTOMA OF THE ENTIRE CEREBELLAR HEMISPHERE: This surgically proved hemangioblastoma of the cerebellum demonstrates a very vascular tumor of the cerebellum that is fed by enlarged feeding arteries (*arrow*), has a large tangle of abnormal vessels and occupies the entire cerebellar hemisphere. In this case, and in cases similar to this, differentiation from an arteriovenous malformation of the cerebellum is difficult.

MISCELLANEOUS POSTERIOR FOSSA LESIONS

CEREBELLAR HYPOPLASIA

The cerebellum exhibits varying degrees of aplasia and hypoplasia that are congenital and apparently developmental in origin. These variations are readily and beautifully studied by CT scanning.

ARACHNOID CYST OF POSTERIOR FOSSA

Arachnoid cystic lesions of the posterior fossa are seen occasionally and have a fairly typical appearance.

Plain Skull Film. There is thinning of the occipital bone over the cystic abnormality, and there may be a bulging of the bone in the occipital region. The skull may have a dolichocephalic appearance, or that of bathrocephaly.

Angiography. The straight sinus, torcula, lateral sinuses, occipital lobes and cerebellum are displaced anteriorly and away from the inner table of the skull by the cyst.

Pneumoencephalography. The fourth ventricle will be normal in size and configuration. The large arachnoid cyst fills with air.

CT Scanning. The CT scan demonstrates a well defined lesion in the posterior fossa that contains cerebrospinal fluid. The bony calvaria is thinned over the cyst; the fourth ventricle may be visualized and will be normal in size. There is no evidence of obstructive hydrocephalus.

Text continued on page 715

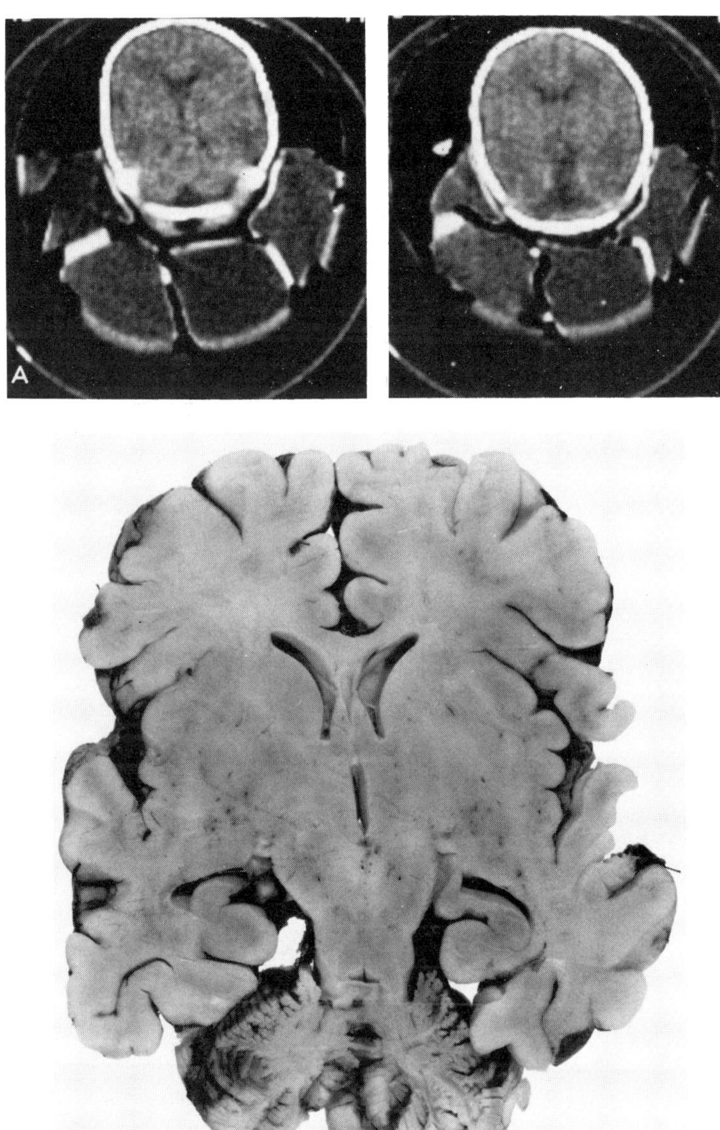

Figure 14–49. CEREBELLAR HYPOPLASIA: The CT scan reveals a large cisterna magna and hypoplasia of the cerebellum with what appears to be a nearly absent vermis of the cerebellum. The pathologic specimen correlates with the CT findings, confirming hypoplasia of the posterior fossa structures.

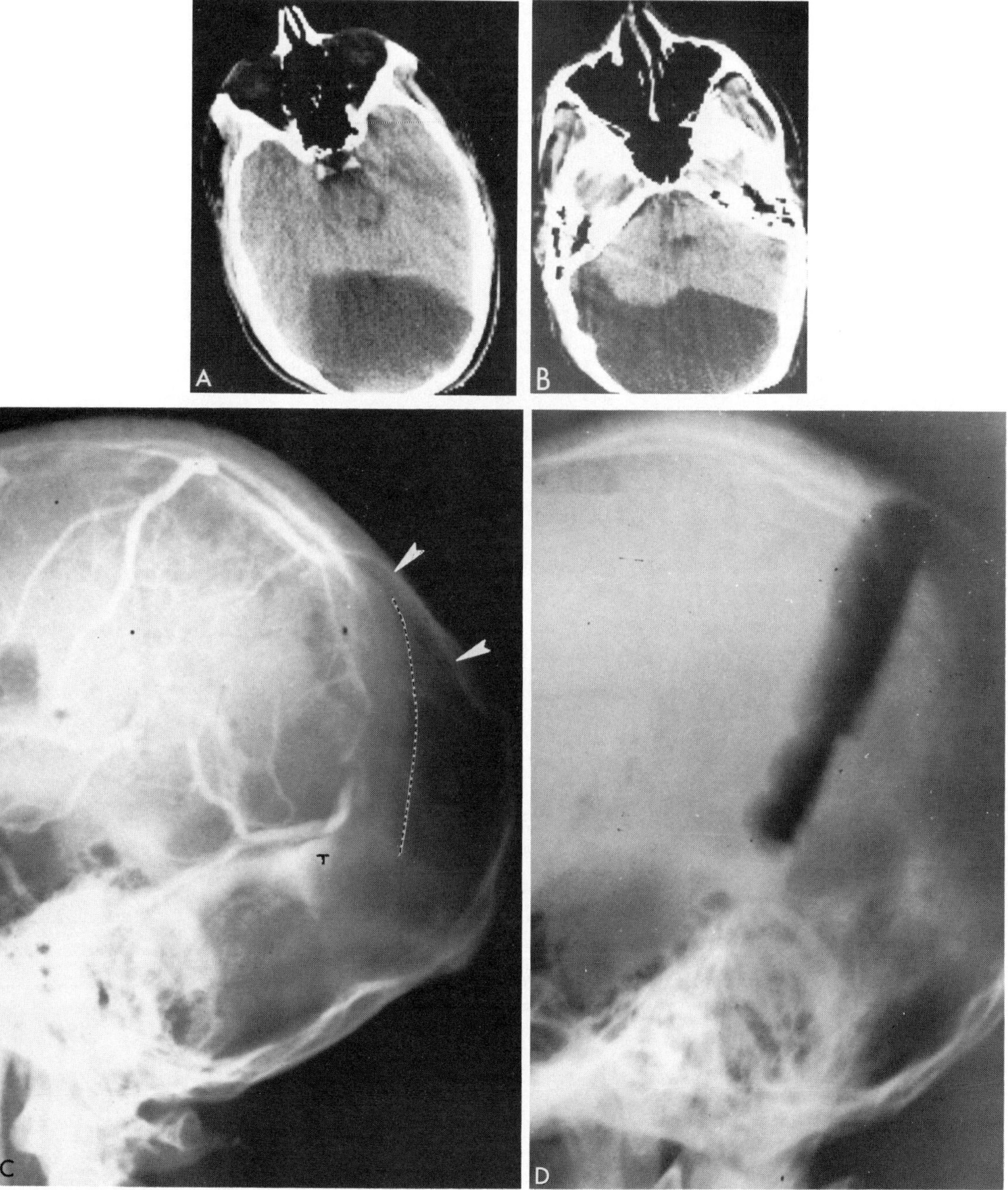

Figure 14–50. POSTERIOR FOSSA ARACHNOID CYST: *A* and *B,* The CT scans reveal a normal appearing fourth ventricle. There is a large CSF-containing structure in the posterior fossa that is positioned behind the lobes of the cerebellum. It thins the inner table of the occipital bone and extends up onto the supratentorial region. The lateral ventricles are within normal limits in size. The plain skull examination (not shown) demonstrated a dolichocephalic appearance of the skull and bathrocephaly.

C, The arteriogram revealed that the torcula *(T)* is displaced far forward from its anticipated position. The straight sinus is also displaced forward, and there is a large vacant area posterior to the torcula.

D, The pneumoencephalogram reveals that this arachnoid cyst fills with air which is freely movable in the cystic cavity. The fourth ventricle could be visualized and appeared to be of normal size and in a relatively normal position.

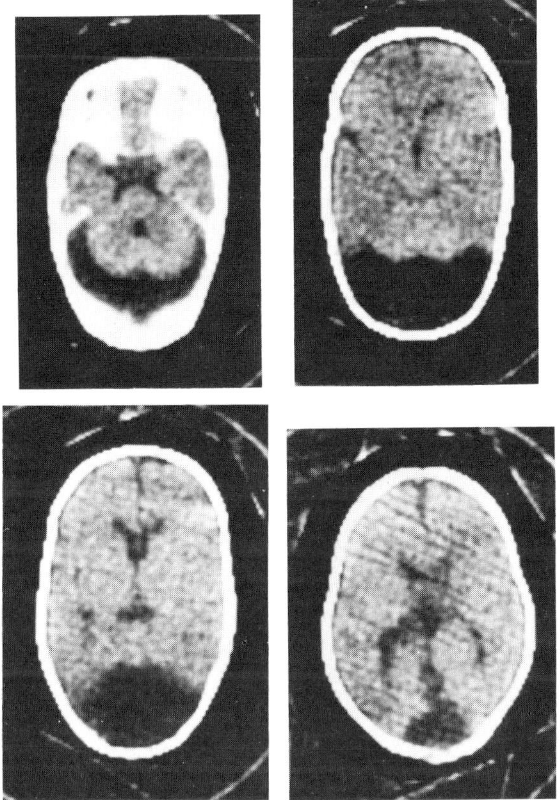

Figure 14–51. ARACHNOID CYST OF THE POSTERIOR FOSSA: There is a dolichocephalic configuration of the skull. The fourth ventricle and the cerebellar hemispheres appear to be normal. There is a large CSF collection posteriorly that produces some thinning of the inner table of the skull.

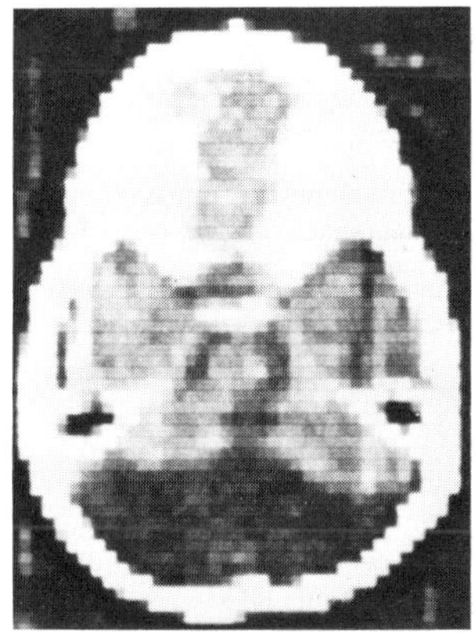

Figure 14–52. POSTERIOR FOSSA HYPOPLASIA AND A GIANT CISTERNA MAGNA: The CT scan demonstrates a markedly hypoplastic cerebellum and a large fourth ventricle that appears to open widely to a large cisterna magna. In this instance, the large cisterna magna is due at least in part to the hypoplasia of the cerebellum.

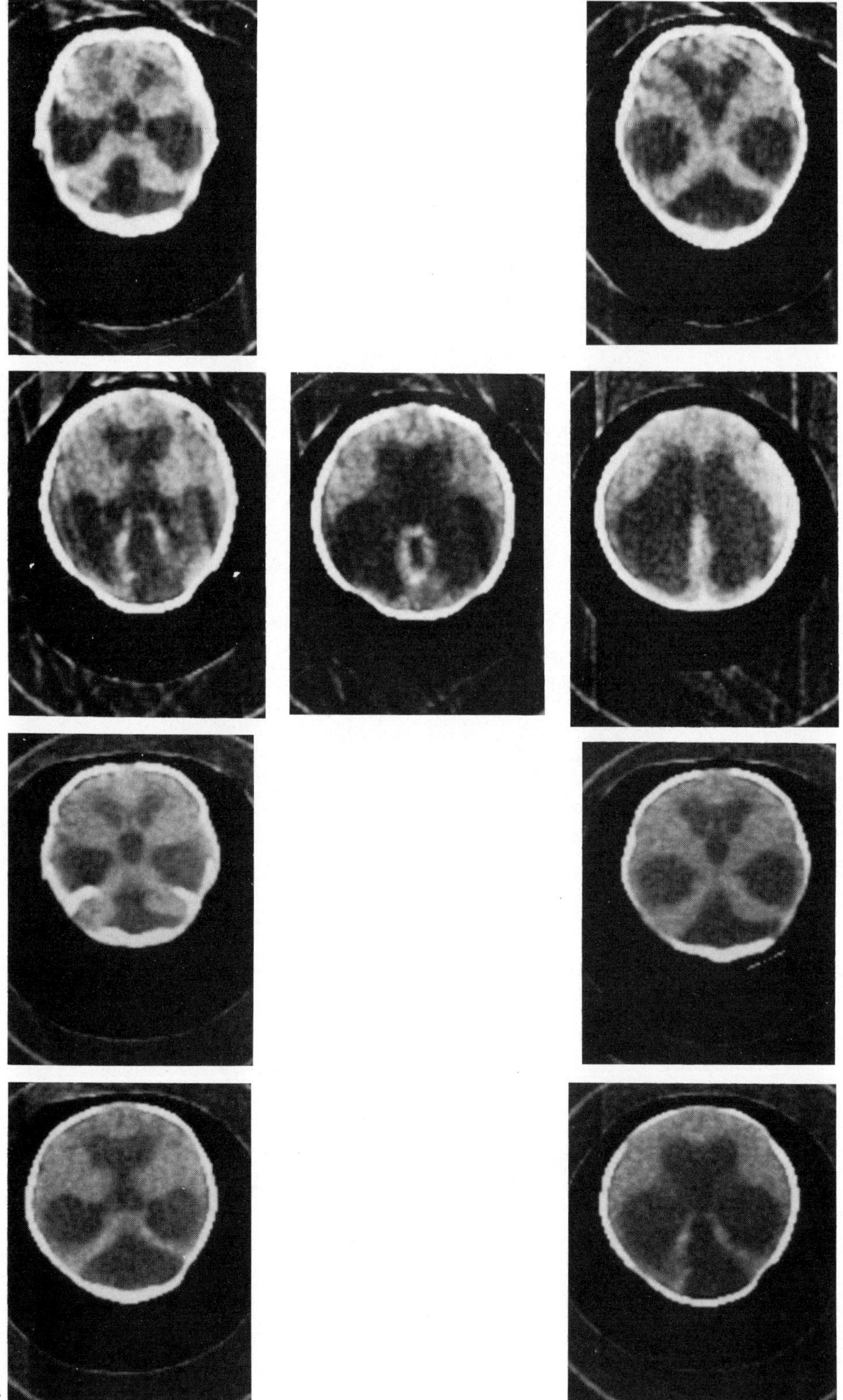

Figure 14–53. DANDY-WALKER CYST: *A,* There is hydrocephalus. The fourth ventricle is large, abnormal in shape and expands and communicates directly to a cystic deformation of the fourth ventricle. The postinfusion scan reveals that the torcula is very high and is positioned above the lambdoid suture. This appearance with torcular-lambdoid inversion is pathognomonic of a Dandy-Walker cyst.

DANDY-WALKER SYNDROME

The pathogenesis is thought to be dilatation of the fourth ventricle secondary to occlusion of the foramen of Magendae and Luschka. There is usually, but not always, dilatation of the lateral and third ventricles.

Angiography. There is upward displacement of the superior cerebellar arteries, downward displacements of the posterior inferior cerebellar artery and a large avascular area in the posterior fossa. The torcula is displaced above the lambdoid suture.

CT Scanning. There is a large CSF-containing cyst in the posterior fossa. A separate fourth ventricle cannot be demonstrated.

The Dandy-Walker cyst (malformation) is to be differentiated from arachnoid cysts of the posterior fossa that may result in enlargement of the bony posterior fossa but are separate from the fourth ventricle. Other varieties of posterior fossa hypoplasias and cerebellar hypoplasias also must be ruled out.

A normally large cisterna magna may give a similar appearance on the CT scan, but in this case the fourth ventricle will be seen as a separate structure that is normal in size and position. This normal anatomic variant is readily demonstrated by CT scanning.

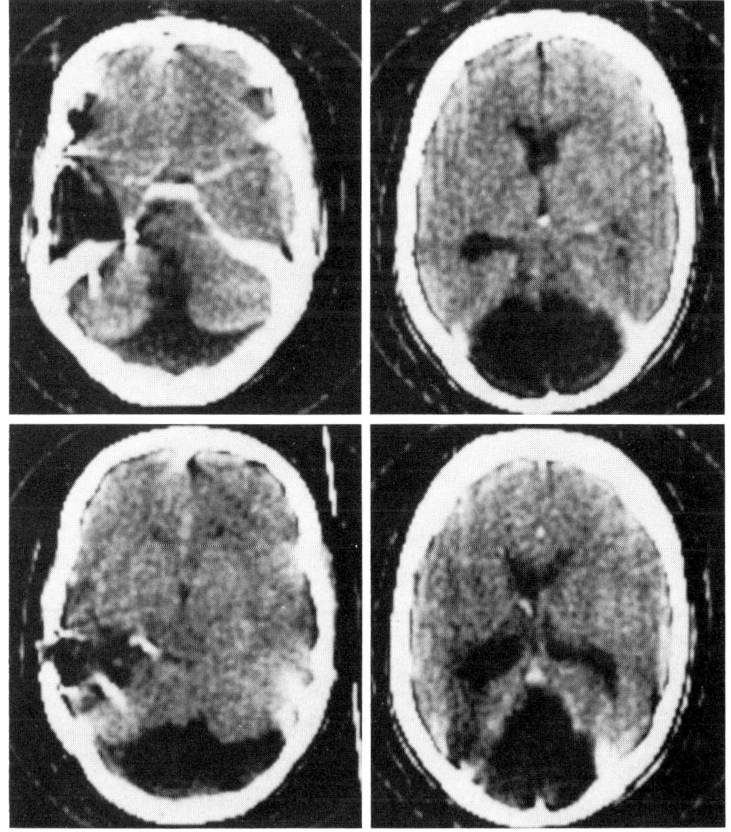

Figure 14–53 *Continued*

B, In another patient, the fourth ventricle demonstrates cystic dilatation — and therefore a normal ventricle is never seen. The CSF-containing structure elevates the torcula-Herophili above the level of the lambdoidal suture. There is mild hydrocephalus. (Postoperative changes are noted in the left temporal region.)

Note that if a normal-appearing fourth ventricle is seen the process is not a Dandy-Walker cyst.

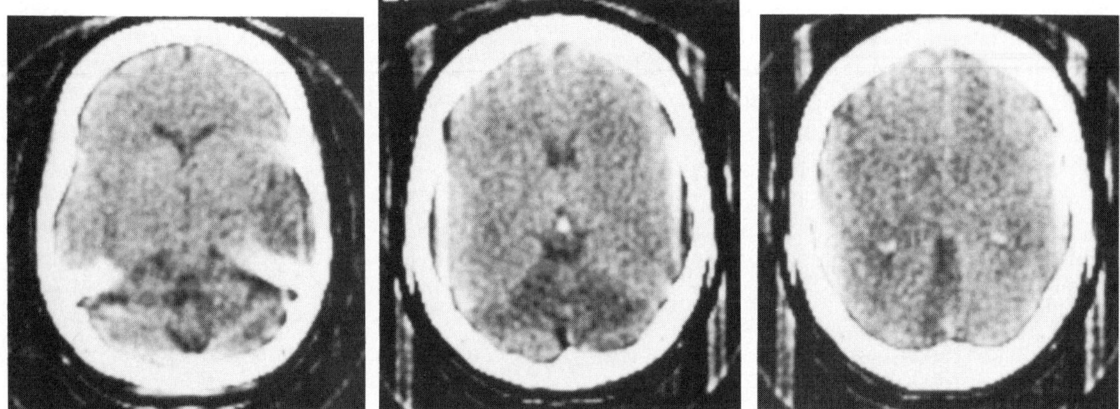

Figure 14–54. POSTERIOR FOSSA ATROPHY: There is diffuse cerebellar atrophy. The fourth ventricle is large, the cerebellopontine angle cisterns are large and the superior cerebellar cistern is large. All these findings reflect cerebellar atrophy.

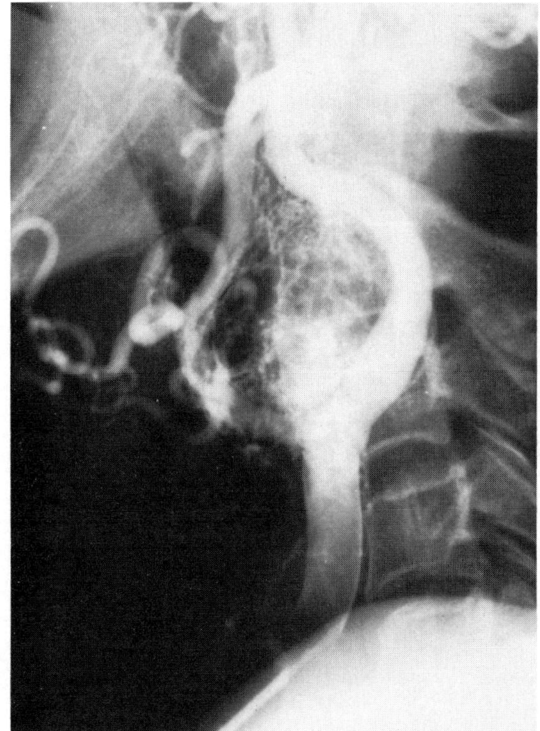

Figure 14–55. CAROTID BODY TUMOR: The common carotid arteriogram reveals a very vascular mass lesion that is fed by branches of the external carotid artery and that splays the internal and external carotid arteries apart. This finding is both classic and consistent with a carotid body tumor. The tumors may occur bilaterally; therefore, the opposite carotid artery should be studied.

GLOMUS JUGULARE, GLOMUS INTRAVAGALE AND CAROTID BODY TUMORS

Glomus jugulare, glomus intravagale and carotid body tumors (chemodectomas) all arise from nonchromaffin paraganglionic tissue. They are very vascular tumors and are supplied by branches of the external carotid artery. The glomus jugulare tumor may also receive blood supply from the vertebral artery. Glomus jugulare tumors may invade the bony margins around the jugular fossa and a mass lesion may be demonstrated in the internal jugular vein by jugular venography.

Glomus intravagale tumors displace the common carotid artery and its branches anteriorly, whereas carotid body tumors arise between the internal and external carotid arteries at the level of the bifurcation and spread them apart.

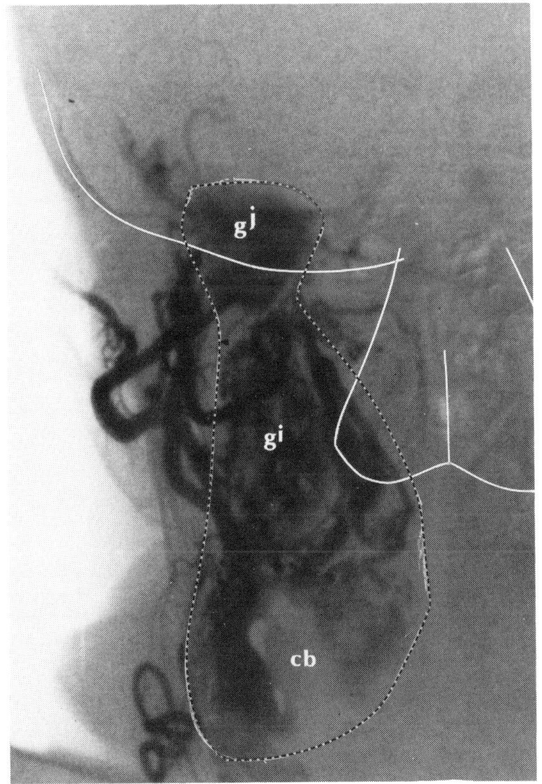

Figure 14–56. GLOMUS JUGULARE, GLOMUS INTRAVAGALE AND CAROTID BODY TUMOR ASSOCIATED WITH A GLOMUS EPITYMPANICUM: The common carotid arteriogram reveals a very vascular multilobulated tumor that is situated at the level of the jugular bulb, the vagus nerve and the carotid bifurcation. The internal carotid artery is occluded secondary to arteriosclerosis. This tumor was discovered after examination revealed a red, pulsating mass behind the tympanic membrane of the ear.

gd glomus jugulare; *gi* glomus intravagale; *cb* carotid body tumor.

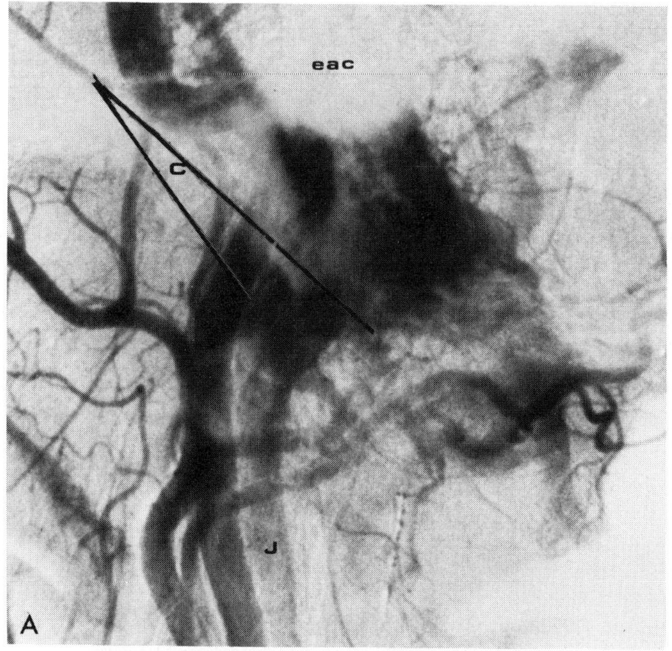

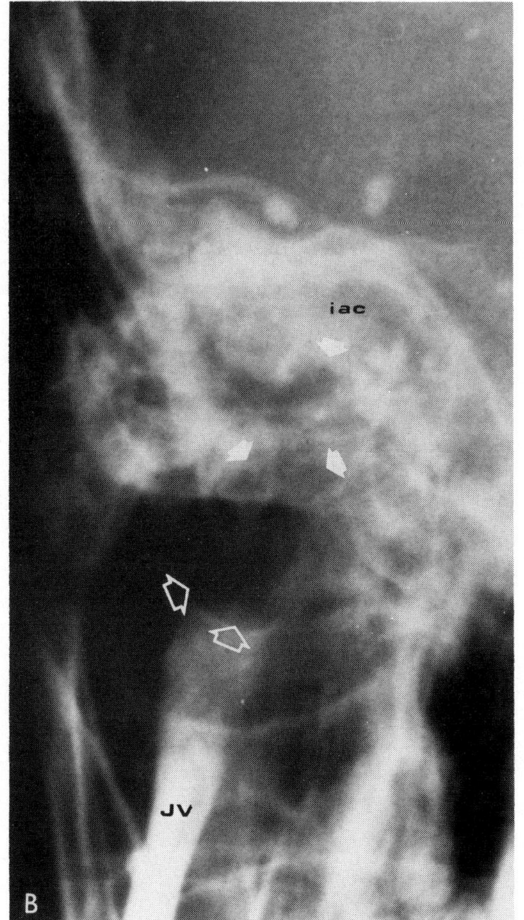

Figure 14–57 *See legend on the opposite page*

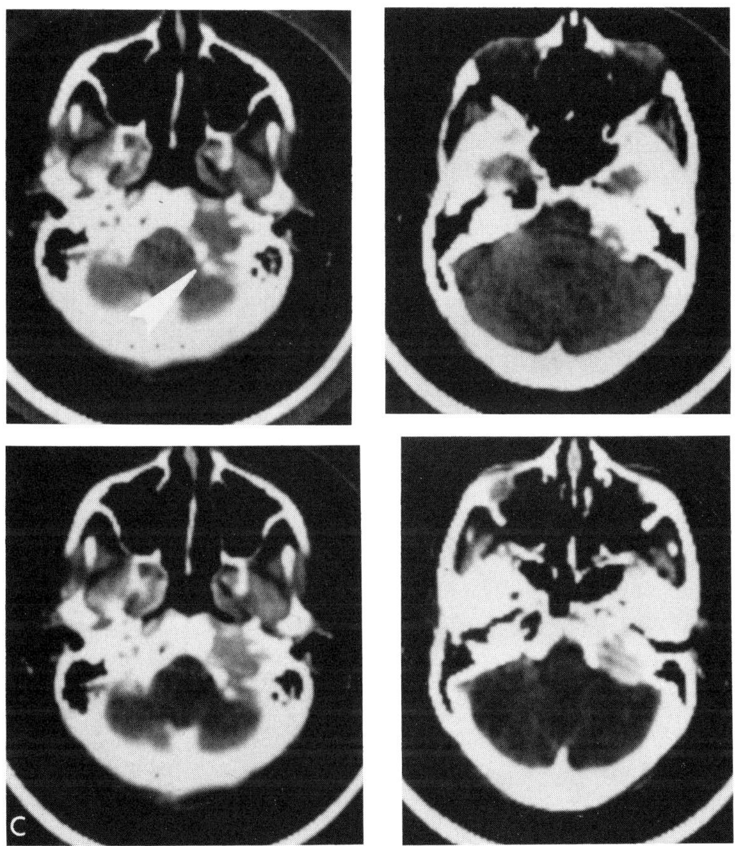

Figure 14–57. GLOMUS JUGULARE TUMOR: *A*, The common carotid arteriogram demonstrates a large vascular mass lesion in the region of the jugular bulb on the left that is supplied by branches of the external carotid artery. The external auditory canal *(eac)* and the clivus *(C)* are labeled, and there is early filling of the internal jugular vein *(J)* because of shunting through the tumor.

B, The jugular venogram demonstrates the tumor mass in the jugular vein *(JV)*, where the tumor obstructs the retrograde flow of contrast material. The lower end of the tumor in the jugular vein is outlined by the open arrowheads; the upper end of the tumor is outlined up to its superior extent in the region of the jugular bulb by the closed arrowheads. This appearance is very typical of a glomus jugulare tumor.

C, The preinfusion scan demonstrates a greatly expanded jugular bulb *(arrow)* with erosion of the bony margin. The area of bony destruction extends to the region of the middle ear. The postinfusion scan demonstrates marked enhancement of this glomus jugulare tumor, which extends posteriorly into the right cerebellar region.

CHAPTER 15

COMPUTED TOMOGRAPHY OF THE ORBIT

Just as computed tomography has assisted in our evaluation of intracranial structures, it has also greatly facilitated the evaluation of patients with orbital pathology. This is generally true of patients with exophthalmos where the CT scan provides a direct view of the orbital contents. Figure 15–1 illustrates the normal anatomic structures visible on the scan.

Orbital scans usually are performed parallel to the base of the skull, and thin or even overlapping cuts can be obtained if desired. The scan also can be performed in the coronal projection; however, the advantage of this projection is not clear. The relationship of the globe to the orbital contents is readily demonstrated. Unilateral exophthalmos is also easily appreciated. Small degrees of bilateral exophthalmos may be difficult to judge because no absolute measurements are yet available. However, the presence of a retro-ocular mass is readily appreciated.

In fact, the ability of the scan to demonstrate the presence or absence of a mass is the greatest asset of CT scanning of the orbit.

The orbital scans should be viewed at a variety of window widths and window levels so that the orbital contents can be viewed to best advantage. The orbit contains a large amount of fat, which can measure as low as −100 h. Special attention also should be directed to the region around the sella turcica, as masses in the sella may present with obscure ocular findings.

The need for orbital venography has decreased since the development of the CT scan, and the indications for this technique are unclear at the present time.

In addition to the abnormalities demonstrated here, a variety of tumors may metastasize to the orbit. If there is bony destructive change this will also be apparent on the scan. If the mass has extended through the orbital roof to involve the cerebral structures, this also can be readily demonstrated on the scan.

Orbital CT, especially in the coronal plane, has also been suggested for use in the diagnosis of facial fractures. The advantages over conventional tomography have not been clearly defined.

Following are multiple examples of entities that can be diagnosed by computed tomography of the orbit. Unfortunately there are, as yet, no absolute criteria available to differentiate between the various retro-ocular masses; therefore, the scans should be viewed in conjunction with other diagnostic tests.

Orbital CT is also very helpful as a follow-up study to evaluate response to treatment.

Text continued on page 729

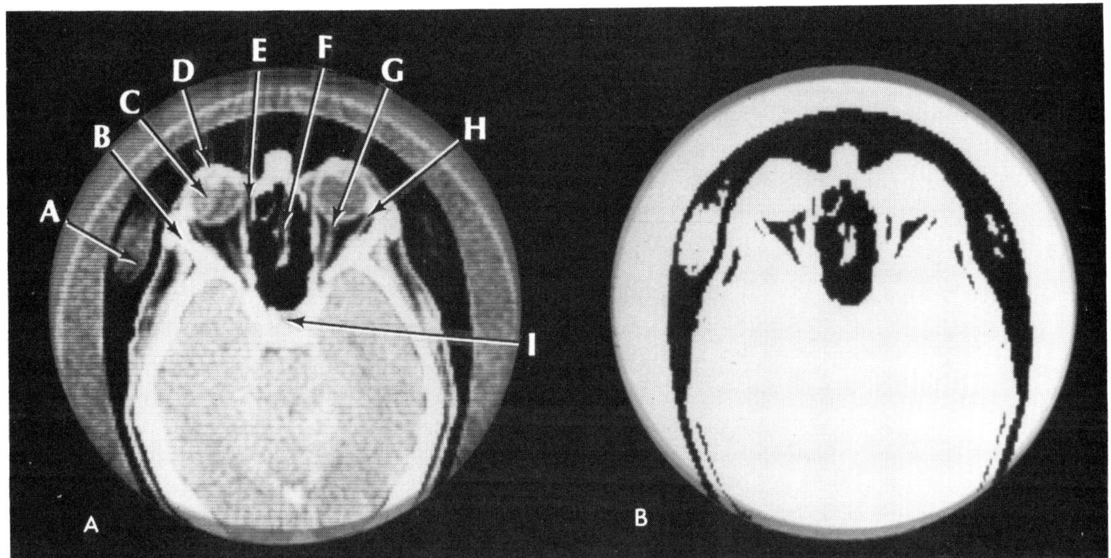

Figure 15–1. *A*, The normal orbits are photographed at a window width of 100; the density is set at a level that best shows the optic nerves. (*A*) The bolus material is also visualized. (*B*) Lateral wall of the orbit. (*C*) Globe. (*D*) Lens. (*E*) Medial wall of the orbit. (*F*) Nasal septum. (*G*) Optic nerve. (*H*) Lateral rectus muscle. (*I*) Region of the sella turcica.

B, Note that the photo on high density setting demonstrates that the optic nerves appear to be asymmetric. This appearance is secondary to the technique of filming and does not imply any abnormality of the optic nerve.

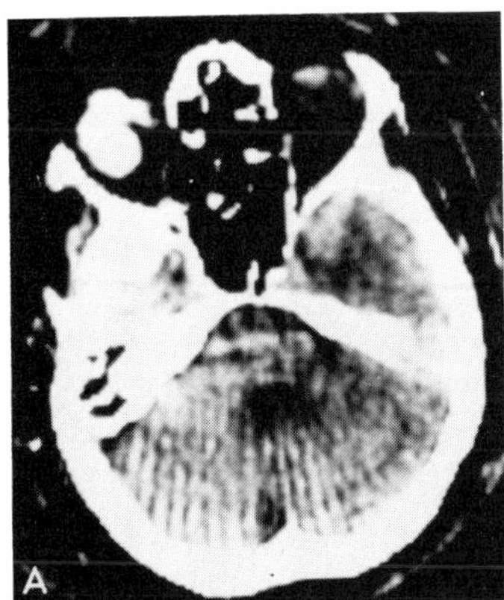

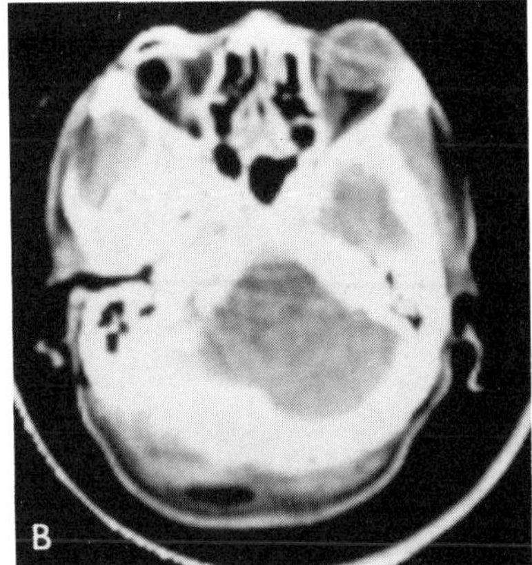

Figure 15–2. ORBITAL PROSTHESIS: *A*, An orbital prosthesis is in place on the left side. The prosthesis is circular and homogeneous in density. A prosthesis also may exhibit a ring configuration with a low density center, as seen in the second example (*B*).

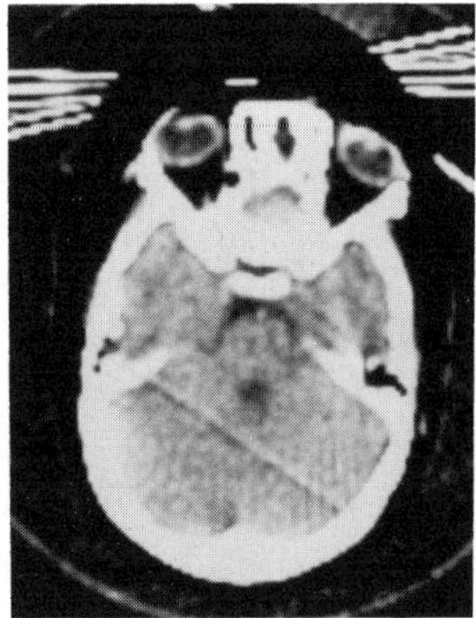

Figure 15–3. HYPERTELORISM: The orbits are wide-set but are otherwise unremarkable.

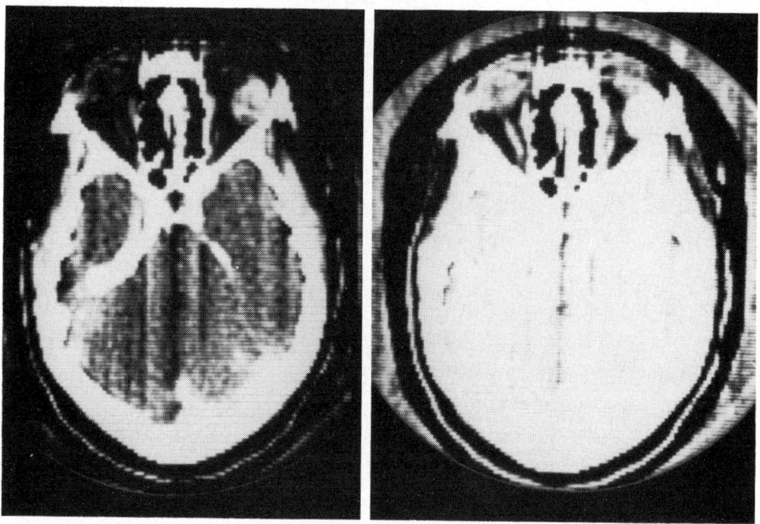

Figure 15–4

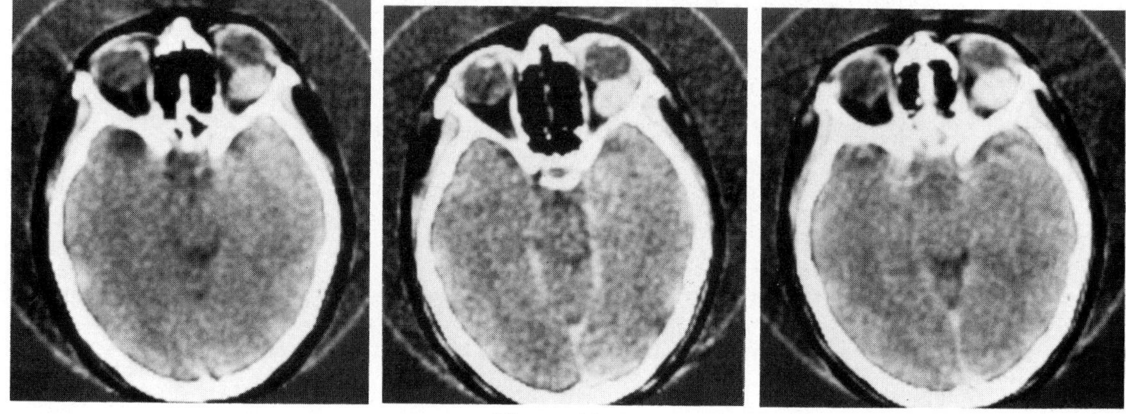

Figure 15–5

Figures 15–4 and 15–5. HEMANGIOMA: These scans demonstrate the typical appearance of orbital hemangioma. The retro-ocular mass is well defined, displaces the globe forward on the affected side, is of relatively high density on the preinfusion scan and enhances homogeneously after the infusion of contrast material.

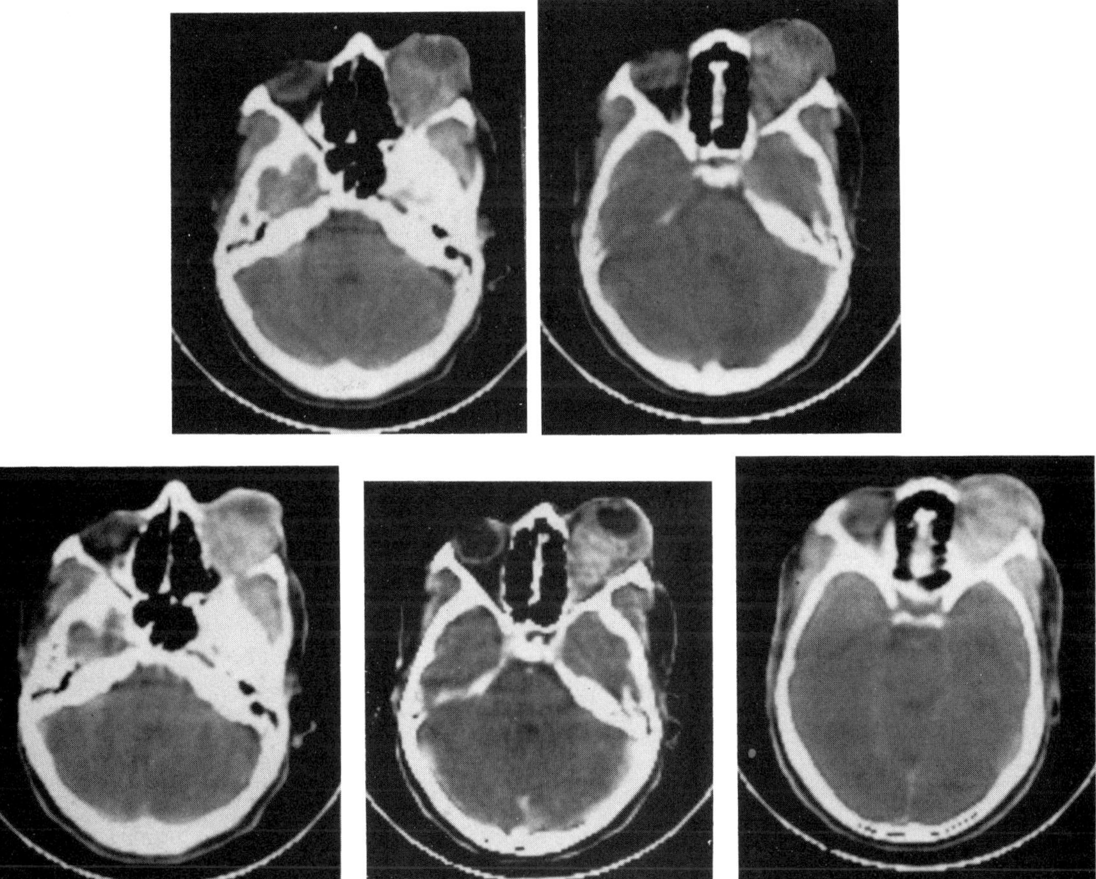

Figure 15–6. HEMANGIOMA: There is a large retro-ocular mass on the right with marked exophthalmos. The mass is so large that the margins are poorly defined and extend around the medial and lateral aspects of the globe. The hemangioma enhances in a homogeneous fashion on the postinfusion scan.

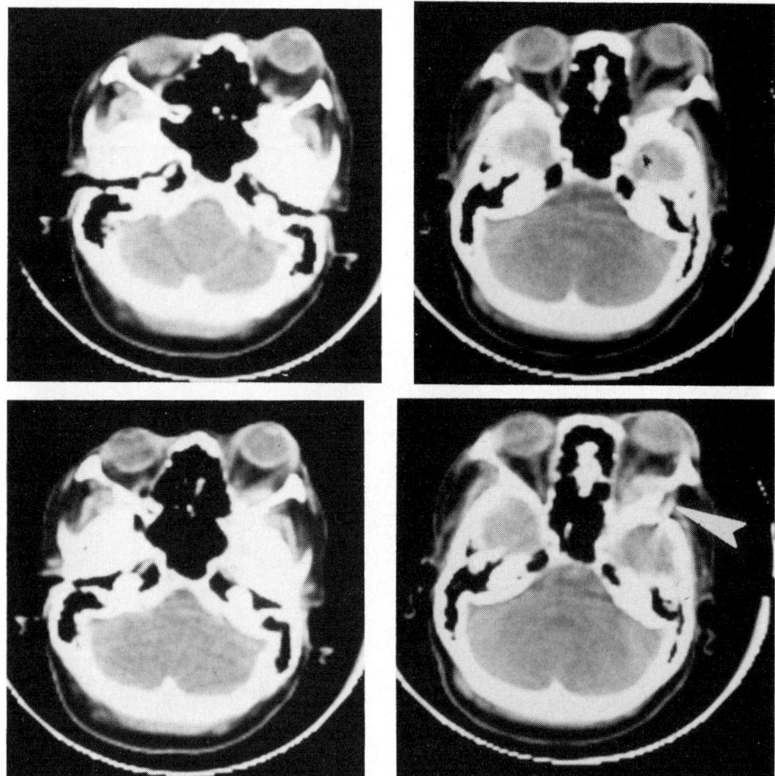

Figure 15–7. ORBITAL MENINGIOMA: Meningiomas may occur in the orbit because the dura and leptomeninges extend along the optic nerve into the orbit. They appear as mass lesions of varying size and are associated with unilateral exophthalmos. The tumors usually are of relatively high density on the preinfusion scan and enhance homogeneously.

In the example shown there is a mass lesion behind the globe on the right that displaces the right globe forward. This is actually a right sphenoid wing meningioma that extends into the globe on the right side. The postinfusion scan reveals the true extent of the tumor outside the orbit (*arrow*). The tumor extends into the right middle cranial fossa and outside the bony calvaria.

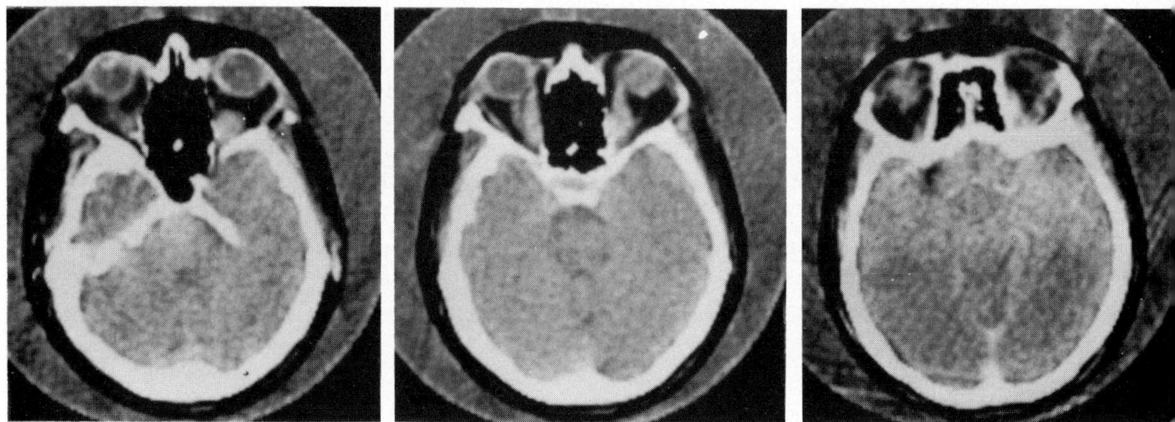

Figure 15–8. HYPERTHYROIDISM: Hyperthyroidism may be associated with unilateral or bilateral exophthalmos. The CT scan in a patient with exophthalmos demonstrates varying degrees of enlargement of the extraocular muscles. At times the muscle enlargement is spectacular. The scan rules out the presence of a mass lesion — a very helpful finding in the case of unilateral exophthalmos, especially in the patient without clinically apparent hyperthyroidism.

The example shown demonstrates marked enlargement of the extraocular muscles. There is marked bilateral exophthalmos.

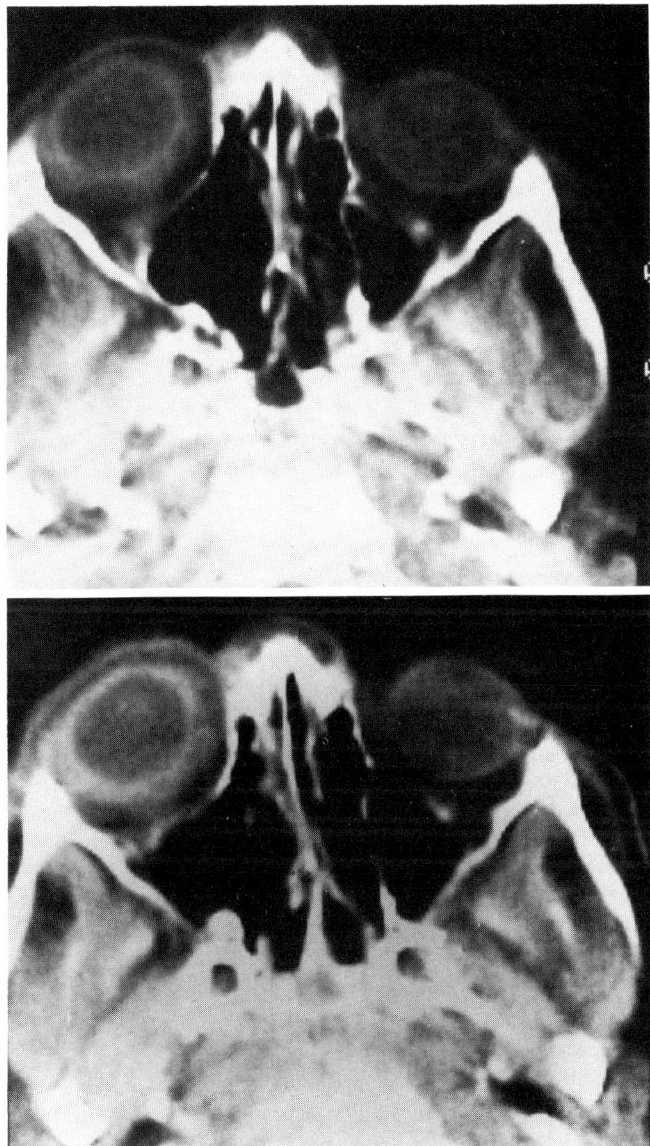

Figure 15–9. ORBITAL PSEUDOTUMOR: The name obviously derives from the fact that, although the abnormality has all the appearances of a tumor, biopsy demonstrates only granulomatous tissue without evidence of a tumor mass. These patients may present with unilateral exophthalmos; thus, the clinical appearance is that of a tumor mass. The CT scan demonstrates an amorphous mass behind the globe and exophthalmos. The mass enhances in a homogeneous fashion on the postinfusion scan, and not infrequently there is also enhancement of the posterior wall of the globe.

Because of the amorphous configuration of the mass and the rimlike enhancement of the posterior margin of globe, the diagnosis of pseudotumor may be suggested. The process may be bilateral.

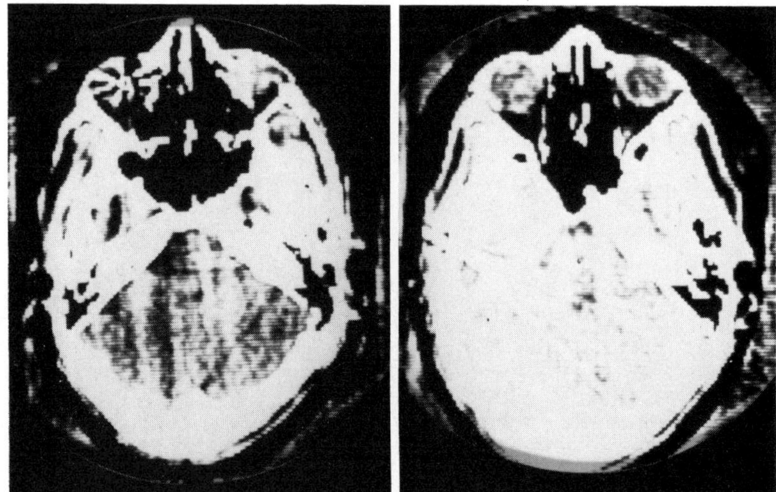

Figure 15–10. FOREIGN BODY IN ORBIT: The orbital scan demonstrates a high density mass directly behind the globe at the level of the optic nerve. The metallic density of the foreign body is readily visualized, and it demonstrates a radiolucent center because of computer artifact. The CT scan has proved to be very helpful for the diagnosis of foreign bodies in the orbit, although exact localization is not always possible.

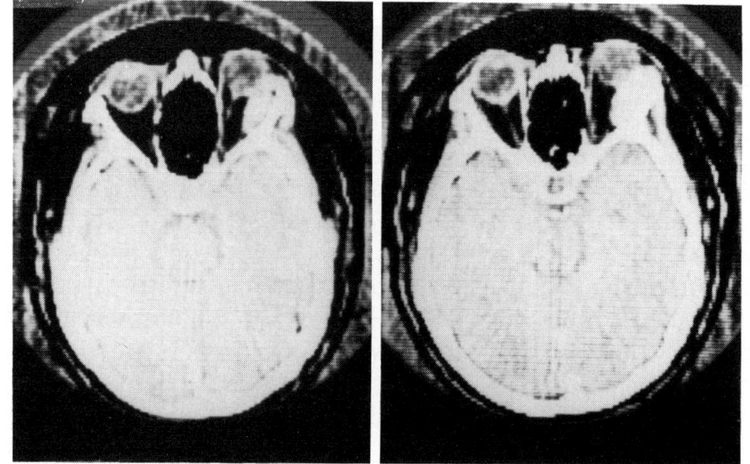

Figure 15–11. RECURRENT HODGKIN'S DISEASE: Hodgkin's lymphoma may present as a retro-ocular mass and progressive unilateral exophthalmos. This potential area of recurrent disease is obviously outside the previous radiation ports. The example shown demonstrates an oval retro-ocular mass that is well defined and that enhances homogeneously on the postinfusion scan.

Unfortunately, the mass has an appearance similar to any retro-orbital mass, and an appropriate history is helpful when suggesting this diagnosis.

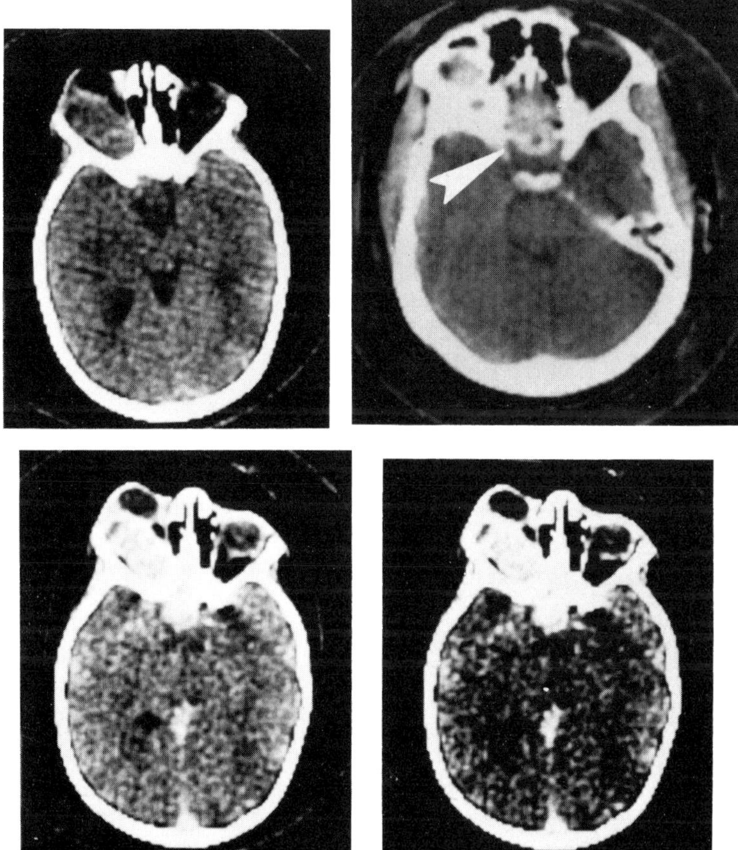

Figure 15–12. OPTIC GLIOMA: The scan demonstrates a mass behind the globe on the left side. There is exophthalmos on the left. Routine views of the optic canal demonstrated enlargement of the canal on the left side. The base cut of the CT scan confirms this finding; it also demonstrates a suprasellar mass, the intracranial extension of the optic glioma. The arrow indicates the left optic canal, which is slightly larger than the right.

There is homogeneous enhancement of the dumbbell-shaped tumor on the postinfusion scan.

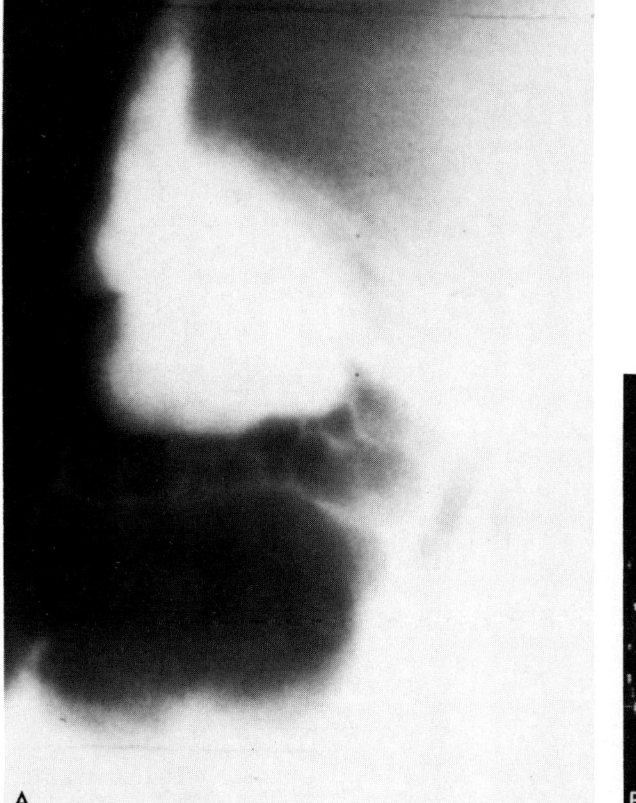

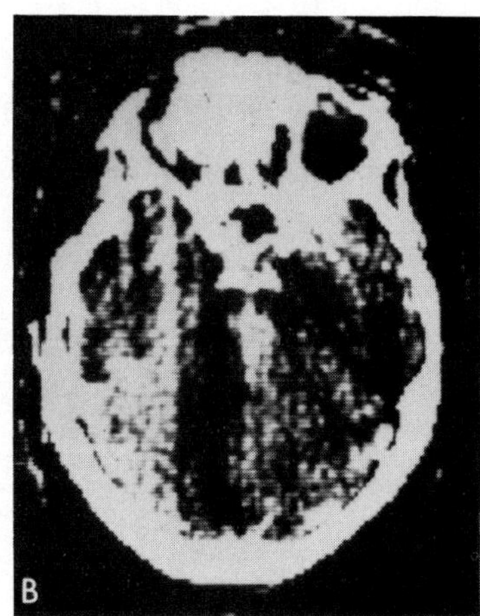

Figure 15–13. OSTEOMA: *A*, The radiographic tomogram (lateral view) demonstrates a well defined, slightly lobulated bony mass in the region of the ethmoid sinus. The finding is consistent with a large osteoma.

B, The CT scan also demonstrates the high density mass. The osteoma is in the region of the ethmoid sinus and extends to either side of the midline. The scan helps to delineate the posterior extent of the mass and rules out the presence of intracranial extension.

ORBITAL VENOGRAM

Although it has been superseded by computed tomography in many centers, orbital venography may be used to demonstrate the cavernous sinus and, consequently, to study the size of intrasellar tumors and their lateral extent, to rule out a cavernous sinus thrombosis and to determine vascular displacements by orbital masses.

Technique. Distention of the frontal vein is achieved by extending the head off the end of the table with the patient supine. A rubber band is then placed circumferentially around the forehead just above the eyebrows. A 19- or 21-gauge "butterfly" (scalp vein) needle is then positioned in the vein. The needle is kept patent by continuous flushing or by connecting the tubing to an intravenous infusion set. The patient is then positioned for filming in the modified Waters' and lateral projections.

The patient is instructed to press his fingers across the zygomatic bone and across the base of the nose in order to compress the facial veins and facilitate retrograde flow of the contrast into the cavernous sinus. Approximately 6 to 8 cc of Contray 60 per cent is then injected slowly to fill the veins of the forehead, the superior ophthalmic veins and the cavernous sinus. A blank film should be obtained at the start of filming so that subtraction films can also be obtained. Magnification technique also may be used.

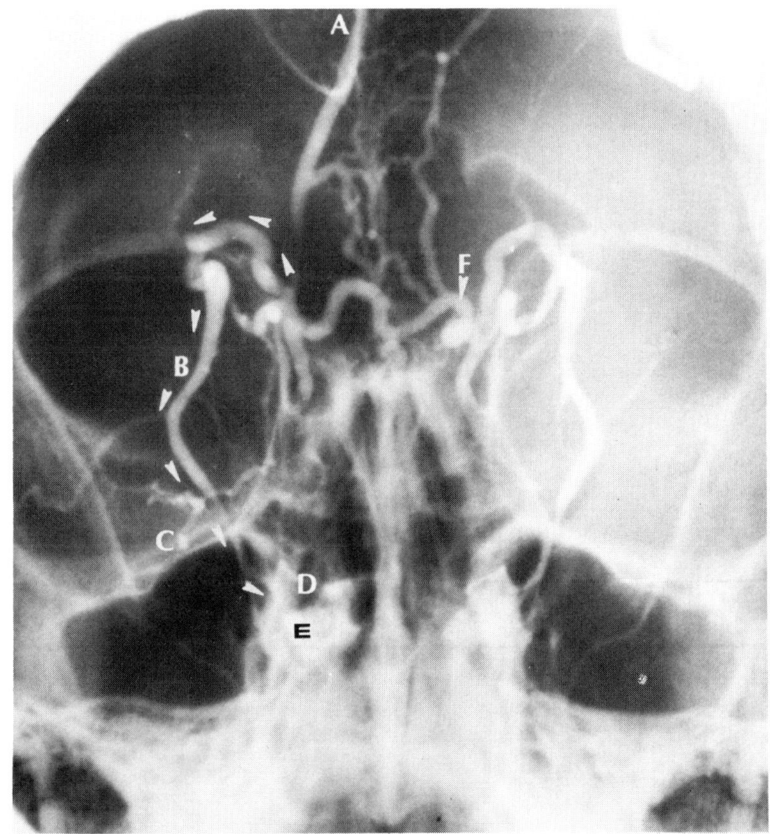

Figure 15–14. ORBITAL VENOGRAPHY: The needle is in place in the frontal vein (not shown), and approximately 6 cc of contrast has been injected. The normal study reveals: A. Frontal vein; B. Superior ophthalmic vein; C. Inferior ophthalmic vein; D. Internal carotid artery filled with unopacified blood and bathed by the contrast; E. Cavernous sinus; F. Angular vein.

At *B* the superior ophthalmic vein courses around the superior rectus muscle medially and downward to the apex of the orbit. The arrows follow the normal blood flow into the cavernous sinus (*E*).

CHAPTER 16

DISORDERS OF THE SPINE AND MYELOGRAPHY

PLAIN FILM EXAMINATION

Before any myelographic procedure is undertaken, routine radiographs of the area of interest should be obtained and reviewed. Any number of disease processes may simulate those that ultimately require a myelogram, and for this reason it is important to be aware of the plain film findings. A thorough understanding of what one should anticipate finding on a plain film provides the basis for interpretation and identification of any variations from normal.

In this chapter, the initial discussion is directed toward the lumbar region; the cervical and dorsal spine will be discussed later. The standard radiographic projections in the lumbar area are the anteroposterior, lateral, oblique, lateral spot of the L_5–S_1 disk space and an additional view of L_5–S_1 obtained in the anteroposterior view with cephalad angulation of the tube for a better view of the disk space.

THE ANTEROPOSTERIOR VIEW

The AP view of the entire lumbar spine (Fig. 16–1) should be examined for alterations in the vertebral body height. Certain conditions will enlarge the vertebral body or bodies; others will lead to loss of vertebral body height. Any alteration in the general contour of the vertebrae also should be noted. Normally there are five lumbar vertebral bodies. Alterations in the number of vertebrae —more or fewer than five — should be noted.

To determine the exact distribution of the vertebral bodies, it is necessary to radiograph and count the vertebral bodies in the various portions of the entire spine. In practice, if there are six lumbar-type vertebral bodies, this is considered "lumbarization" of the S_1 vertebral body; whereas four lumbar vertebral bodies are considered to represent "sacralization" of the L_5 vertebral body.

When unilateral articulation of the lowest vertebral body with the sacrum is found, this vertebra is considered to be a "transitional segment. Also, bilateral articulation of the vertebral body at the lowest lumbar level with the sacrum is considered a more stable situation than unilateral articulation. This is true even when an abnormal increase or decrease in the number of vertebral bodies is seen.

A herniated nucleus pulposus (HNP) may occur at the disks between normally segmented vertebrae and between the sacrum and a

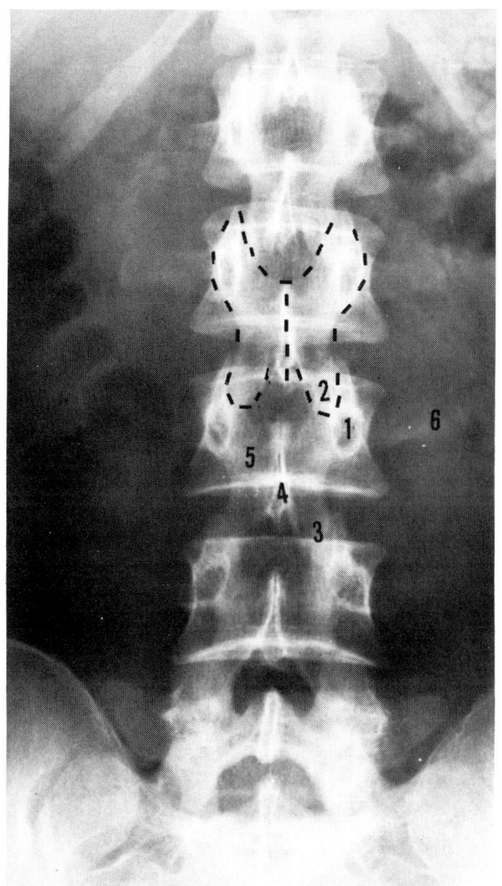

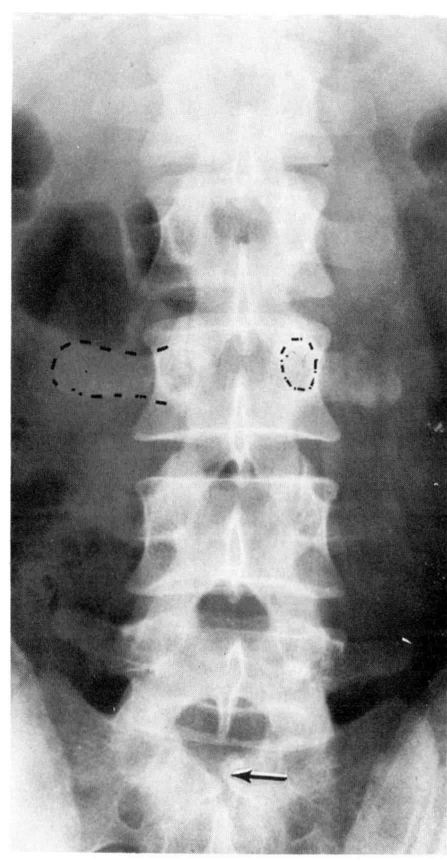

Figure 16–1

Figure 16–2

Figure 16–1. LUMBAR SPINE: On the AP view the pedicles are viewed as oval areas with a dense cortical margin *(1)*. The pedicles project directly posteriorly in the lumbar region and join with the superior and inferior articulating facets *(2 and 3)*. The bone between the superior and inferior facets is the pars interarticularis. The laminae *(5)* then extend medially and posteriorly to join in the midline to form the spinous process *(4)*. The spinous process projects inferiorly in the lumbar region. The transverse process extends laterally *(6)*. The curved dashed lines in the illustration follow the superior and inferior articulating facets. The straight dashed line is on the spinous process.

If a total laminectomy is performed, both laminae are cut and the spinous process is removed. However, more commonly a small portion of the lamina is removed, leaving a small crescentic defect in the lamina. This approach often provides sufficient exposure to a herniated disk.

Figure 16–2. NORMAL ANTEROPOSTERIOR VIEW: The oval dotted line outlines the pedicle. The larger dotted line illustrates the transverse process.

There is also a spina bifida (failure of fusion) of the spinous process of S_1 *(arrow)*.

transitional vertebrae that articulates unilaterally. HNP does not occur between a "sacralized" vertebral body and the sacrum because the disk is hypoplastic and no motion occurs at this level.

Congenital alterations of the vertebral body or spinous processes may be present. Particular note should be made of spina bifida, more marked spinal dysrhaphia or hemivertebrae (Figs. 16–2, 16–3, 16–20).

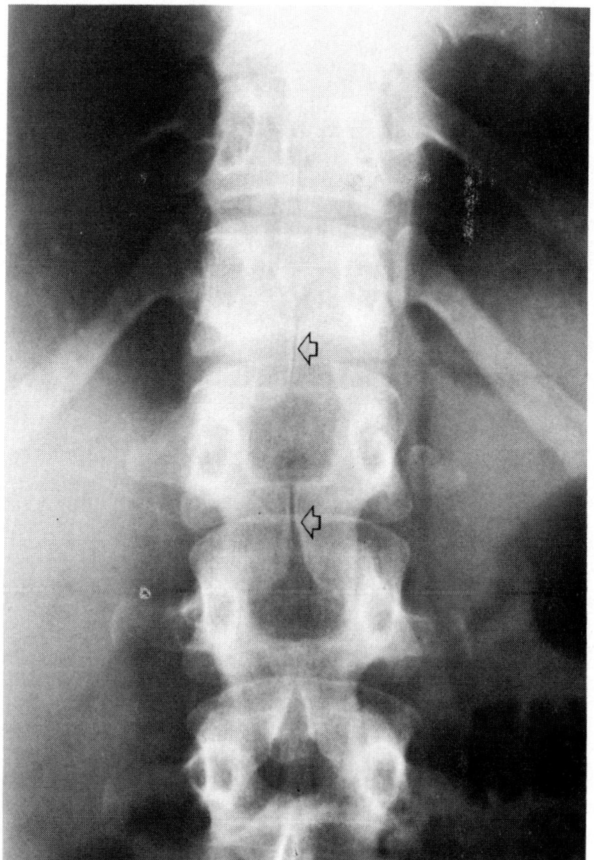

Figure 16–3. SPINA BIFIDA T_{12} AND L_1: There is a failure of fusion of the spinous processes of T_{12} and of L_1 (*arrows*). In this case the finding is of no significance.

THE LATERAL VIEW

The lateral view (Fig. 16–4) also reveals changes in vertebral body height and in the general configuration of the bone. In addition, however, it affords the best view of the height of the disk spaces. Because the mechanics of positioning for radiography in the lateral view create a mild scoliosis of the spine, the lateral spot film of the L_5 disk space is angled to allow for optimal visualization of the disk space at the L_5–S_1 level. There may normally be some narrowing of the posterior aspect of the disk at the L_5–S_1 level (Fig. 16–9).

A spondylolysis, or abnormal break in the pars interarticularis, can be identified on the lateral view, but usually is better seen on the oblique view.

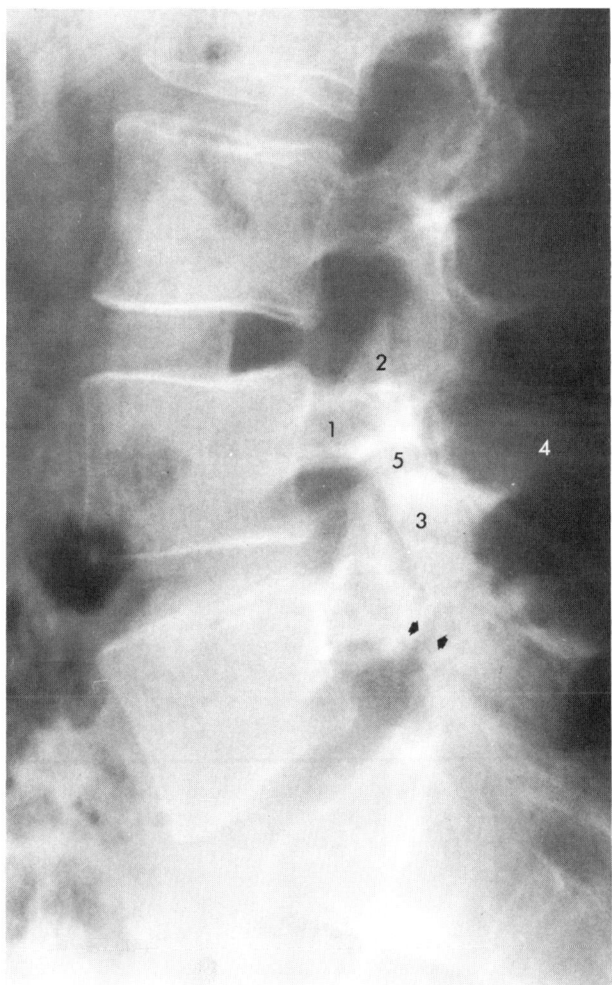

Figure 16–4. LATERAL VIEW OF THE LUMBAR SPINE: This view provides the best evaluation of the heights of the vertebral bodies and the disk spaces. The anatomic structures identified on the AP view also can be seen on the lateral view. *(1)* Pedicle; *(2)* Superior articulating facet; *(3)* Inferior articulating facet; *(4)* Spinous process; *(5)* Pars interarticularis.

The arrows point to a spondylolysis at the L_5 level with a Grade I spondylolisthesis (see text).

THE OBLIQUE VIEWS

Oblique views are obtained with the patient in the prone position. It is easier for the patient to maintain the routine radiographic positions while prone rather than supine. The films are then marked so that when the right side is most dependent (RAO = right anterior oblique) the anatomic right side is marked with an "R." When the left side is most dependent (LAO = left anterior oblique), the anatomic left side is marked with an "L" marker. It is important to understand this because with this positioning the pars interarticularis is viewed through the vertebral body. Consequently, in the RAO position the *left* pars interarticularis is actually displayed. Similarly, in the LAO position the *right* pars interarticularis is viewed. The oblique view best demonstrates the pars interarticularis (Fig. 16–5). This view also allows excellent visualization of the superior and inferior articulating facets and their points of articulation.

The combination of these anatomic parts and the images of the transverse processes and lamina of the spine have the appearance of a "Scottie dog" (Fig. 16–5, *B*). The neck of the dog is the pars interarticularis. A "break" in the pars interarticularis is termed a *spondylolysis* (Figs. 16–6 to 16–8). If spondylosis is present, it appears radiographically as if the "Scottie" were wearing a collar (Fig. 16–6, *B*). Spondylolysis may be congenital or acquired.

Areas of spondylolysis may be identified on both the AP and lateral views of the spine, but are best visualized on the oblique radiograph (Figs. 16–6, 16–7). Spondylolysis commonly leads to instability of the spine at this level and may result in forward displacement of one vertebral body on another. This displacement is termed *spondylolisthesis*. If the upper vertebral body is displaced posterior to the lower vertebral bodies, this is considered a *reverse spondylolisthesis*.

Spondylolisthesis also may occur secondary to degenerative changes and joint space narrowing at the level of the articulation between the superior and the inferior articulating facets. In this case forward displacement of one vertebral body relative to another may occur without spondylolysis.

Text continued on page 739

Figure 16–5. THE OBLIQUE VIEW: *A*, This view provides the best means for evaluation of the pars interarticularis. The oblique view with its combination of structures forms the image of a "Scottie dog" *(B)*. The transverse process is the dog's "nose" and also contributes to the anterior margin of the "eye." The pedicle contributes the posterior margin. The superior articulating facet forms the "ear" and the inferior articulating facet forms the "front leg." The "body" of the dog is formed by the lamina of the vertebral body. *(1)* Transverse process; *(2)* Superior articulating facet; *(3)* Pedicle (the transverse process forms the anterior margin); *(4)* Pars interarticularis; *(5)* Inferior articulating facet; *(6)* Lamina.

The articulation between the superior and inferior articulating facets is well demonstrated. The pars interarticularis forms the neck of the Scottie in the oblique view. Although a pars defect may be visualized on other views, it is best demonstrated on the oblique view.

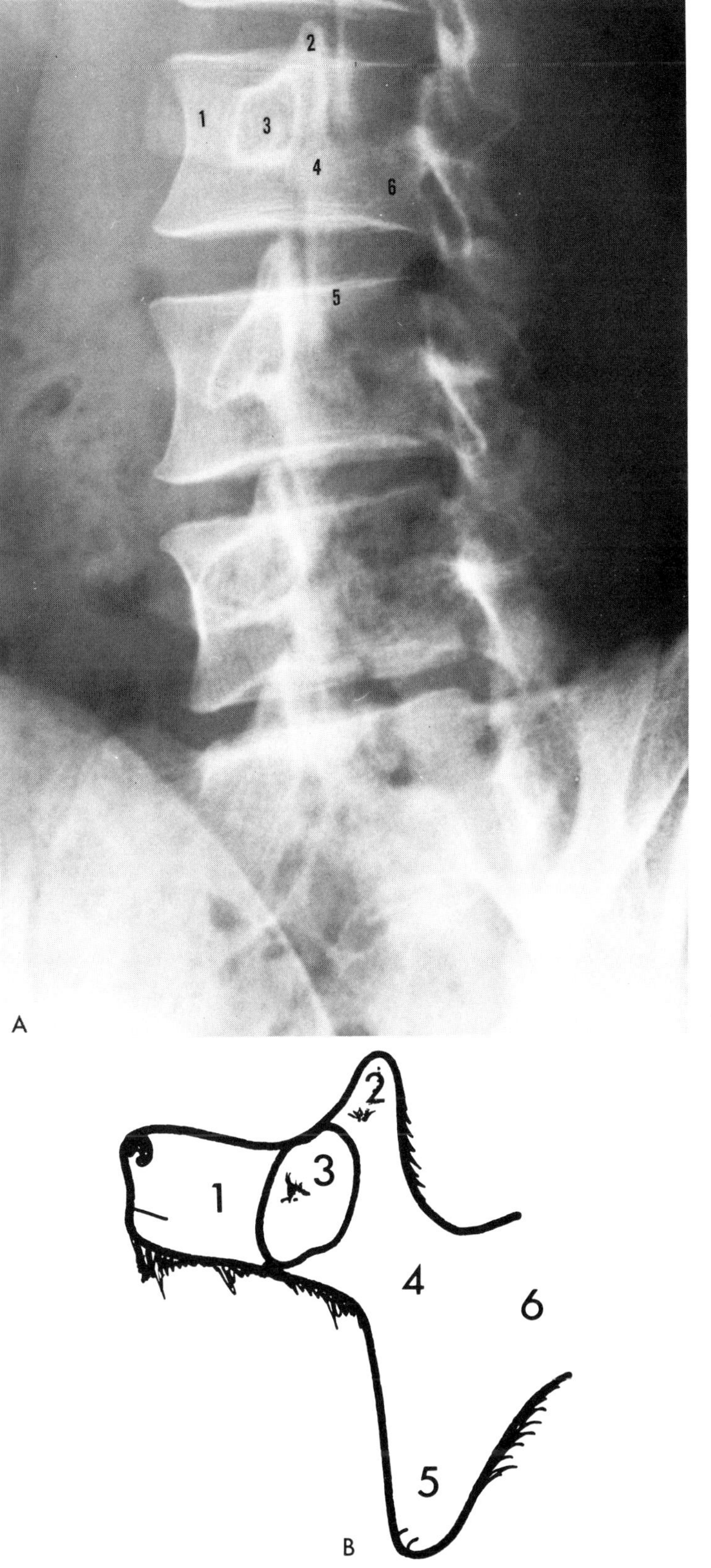

Figure 16–5 *See legend on the opposite page*

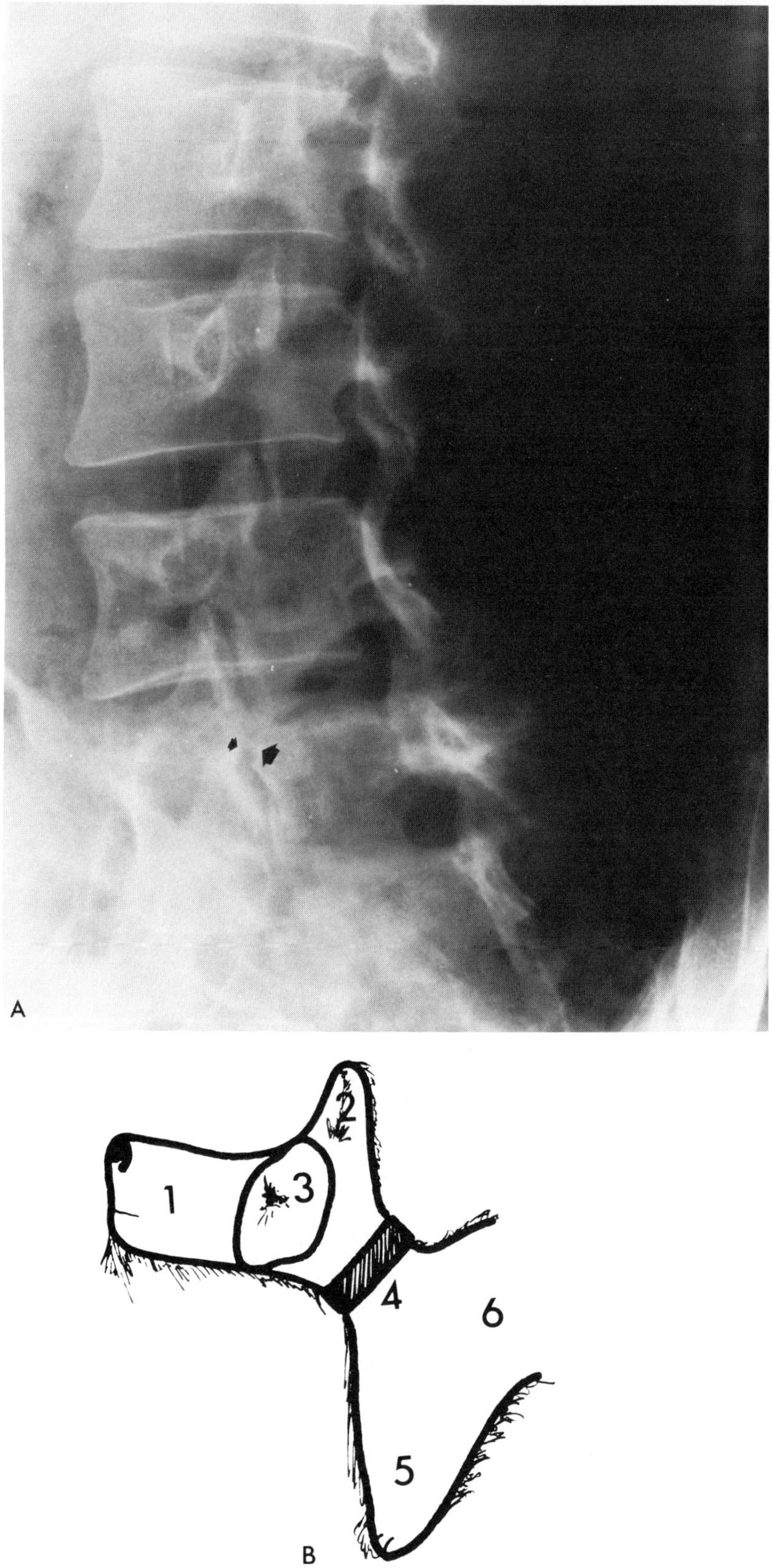

A

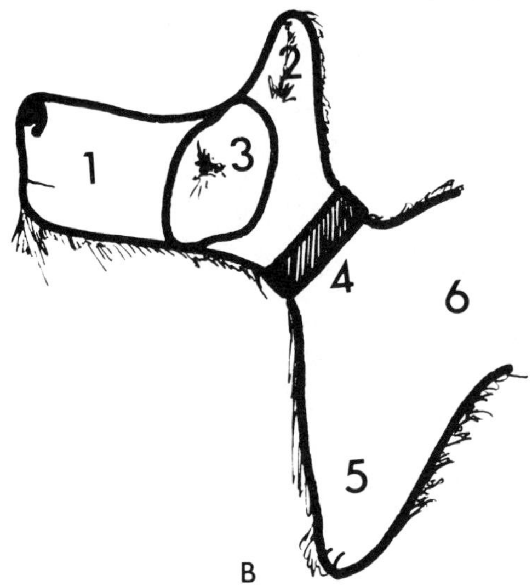

Figure 16–6. OBLIQUE VIEW WITH SPONDYLOLYSIS AT L_5: There is a spondylolysis involving the pars interarticularis at the L_5 level *(arrows)*. This break appears as a radiolucent line — as if the Scottie were wearing a collar.

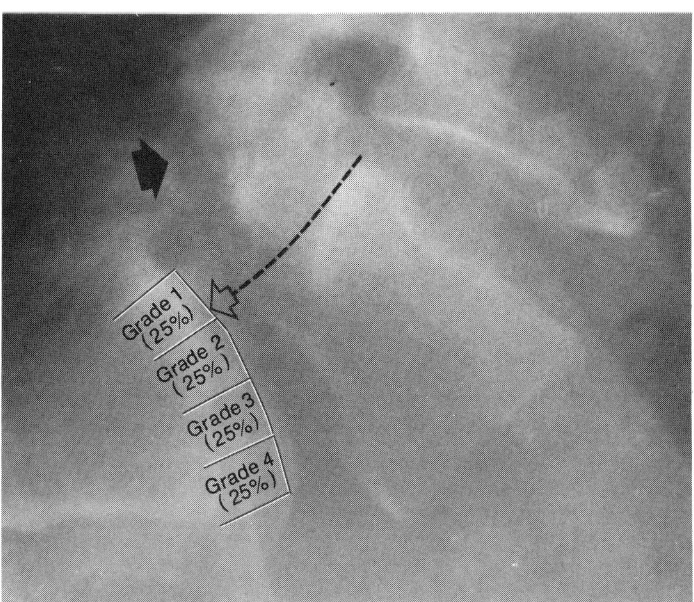

Figure 16–7. SPONDYLOLISTHESIS: One method of grading is pictured above. The superior end-plate of the vertebral bodies is divided into four equal parts. A line is drawn along the posterior margin of the vertebral body above (*dotted line*) and extended down to a point on the end-plate of the reference vertebral body (*open arrowhead*). If displacement of the end-plate is 25 per cent or less, it is a Grade 1 spondylolisthesis; 25 per cent to 50 per cent is Grade 2; 50 to 75 per cent is a Grade 3; 75 per cent or greater is a Grade 4 spondylolisthesis.

The spondylolysis is visible (*closed black arrowhead*) at the L_5 level.

Spondylolisthesis also can occur in the absence of a spondylolysis. In such a case there is interfacet degenerative change and joint space narrowing that allows forward slippage.

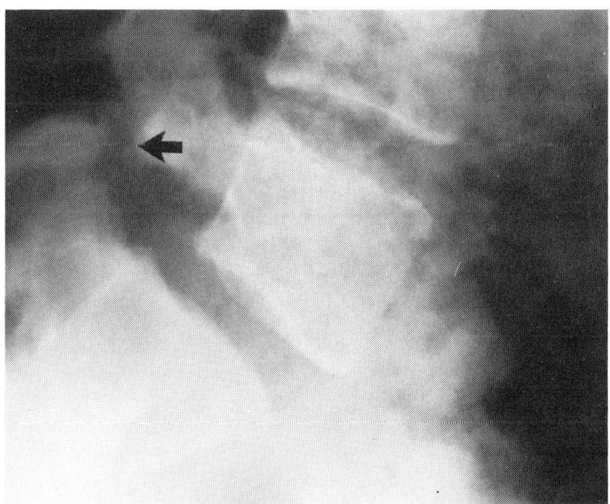

Figure 16–8. LATERAL VIEW OF SPONDYLOLYSIS WITH SPONDYLOLISTHESIS: There is a wide defect in the pars interarticularis in this patient. There is also a Grade I spondylolisthesis with forward displacement of L_5 on S_1.

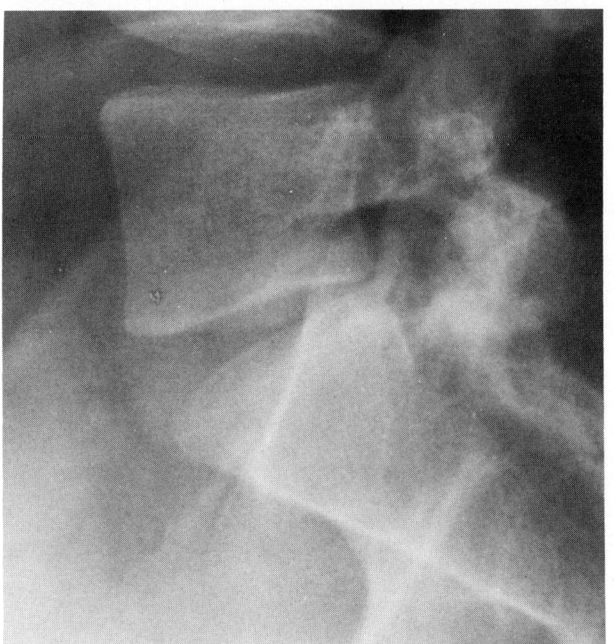

Figure 16–9. NORMAL L_5–S_1: There is narrowing of the L_5–S_1 disk space posteriorly, which probably is normal. In some instances, this may also imply some loss of disk volume and therefore be abnormal.

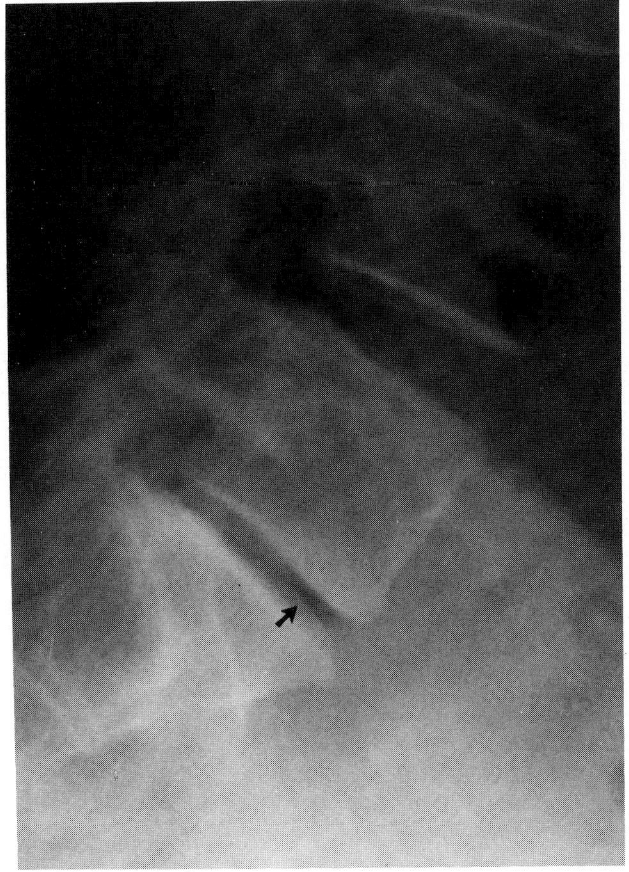

Figure 16–10. "VACUUM DISK": The L_5–S_1 disk is abnormal and has resulted in a vacuum sign. The radiolucent area is not actually a vacuum but reflects the presence of nitrogen in a degenerated disk.

POSTOPERATIVE CHANGES IN THE SPINE

Plain spine radiographs reveal changes that correlate with the surgical procedure. There may be evidence of a partial or complete laminectomy, with or without bony fusion in the lumbar spine.

LUMBAR SPINAL STENOSIS

Patients may have a congenitally small spinal canal. However, the acquired form of spinal stenosis is also of clinical importance. The diagnosis may be suspected on plain spine radiographs or by CT examination of the spine. In the presence of a congenitally small subarachnoid space, superimposed disk disease may cause a patient to become symptomatic, whereas similar changes in a patient with a large subarachnoid space may not cause symptoms. Acquired spinal stenosis may also result from a spondylolisthesis, where the posterior elements are displaced forward and impinge upon the posterior aspect of the subarachnoid space.

The following spine films illustrate a variety of diseases that can be diagnosed by plain film examination.

Paget's Disease. Paget's disease (Figs. 16–12 and 16–13) exhibits an increase in vertical trabeculation that involves the entire vertebral body. Although it may be monostotic, multiple vertebrae usually are involved. The vertebral body in Paget's disease is more dense than in hemangioma and often has a dense outer margin — giving the vertebral body a "picture-window" appearance. The vertebral body usually is enlarged. Paget's disease usually spares the pedicle.

Metastatic carcinoma of the prostate may be considered in the differential diagnosis, but usually does not demonstrate an increased trabecular pattern. Examination of the other bony structures will help to differentiate between the two entities. Metastatic carcinoma of the prostate — of course seen only in men — demonstrates patchy areas of osteoblastic metastatic disease, whereas Paget's

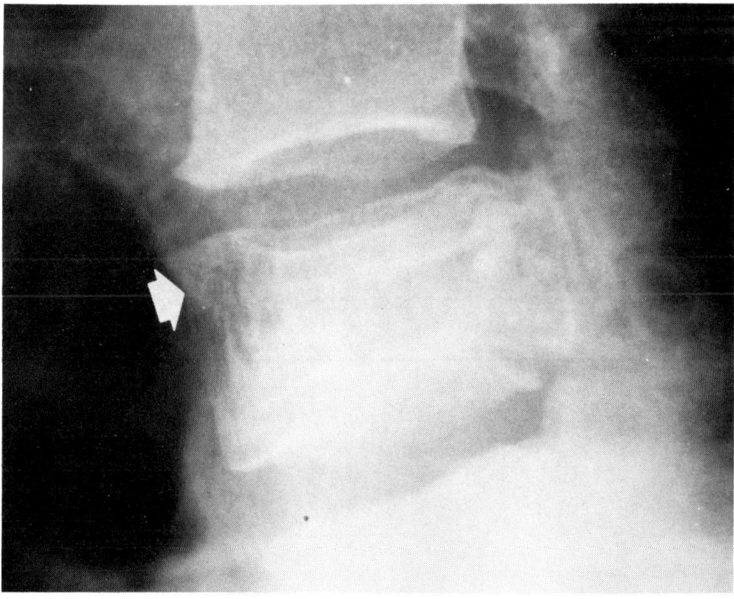

Figure 16–11. HEMANGIOMA: There is a compression fracture of the upper portion of the vertebral body *(arrow)*.

A hemangioma of the spine exhibits increased vertical trabeculae, which form in an attempt to strengthen the vertebral body. These are "stress trabeculae." The affected vertebral body is larger than the remaining vertebral bodies. It should be noted that the hemangioma may involve only a portion of the vertebral body.

disease causes an increase in the bony trabeculae in the other bones. Frequently a sclerosis of the pelvic inlet occurs in Paget's disease, and this often can be seen on routine views of the lumbar spine, helping to differentiate between the two entities.

The enlarged vertebral body of Paget's disease may cause a complete block of the flow of contrast material on myelography. The block has an extradural configuration.

Multiple Myeloma. There may be multiple small osteolytic areas or the multiple myeloma (Fig. 16–14) may present as diffuse osteoporosis of all the visualized bony structures. There may be multiple compression deformities of the vertebral bodies. Multiple myeloma tends to "spare" the pedicles, whereas other types of osteolytic metastatic processes usually involve the pedicles. The actual diagnosis of multiple myeloma depends on confirmatory laboratory data.

Metastatic Disease. Metastatic disease (Figs. 16–14 to 16–17) may be either osteolytic or osteoblastic. It may involve only a single vertebral body, but usually affects multiple vertebral body segments. Because the pedicle is the most vascular portion of the vertebral body, it usually is involved early with blood-borne metastases. Metastatic diseases may lead to compression deformities of the vertebral bodies; not uncommonly, it leads to the clinical syndrome of spinal cord compression. This spinal cord compression may be seen with bony metastases or with soft tissue metastatic deposits in the absence of bony abnormalities.

Osteopetrosis. The bones, including the spine, may exhibit a "bone-within-a-bone" appearance. The increased volume of bone may cause encroachment upon the spinal canal. In addition, the foramina of the base of the skull also may be encroached upon. The

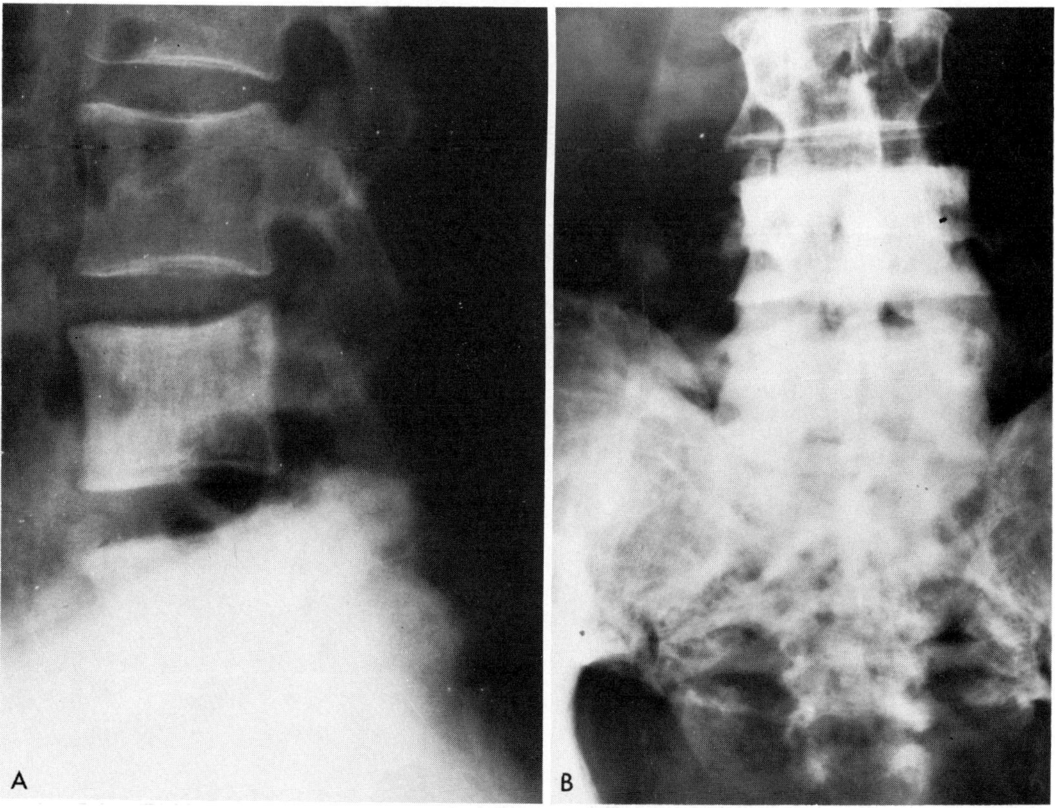

Figure 16–12. PAGET'S DISEASE OF LUMBAR SPINE: *A* and *B*, The lumbar vertebral bodies demonstrate an increase in trabecular markings. In addition, the pelvis also demonstrates a diffuse increase in the trabecular pattern. There is sclerosis of the pelvic inlet.

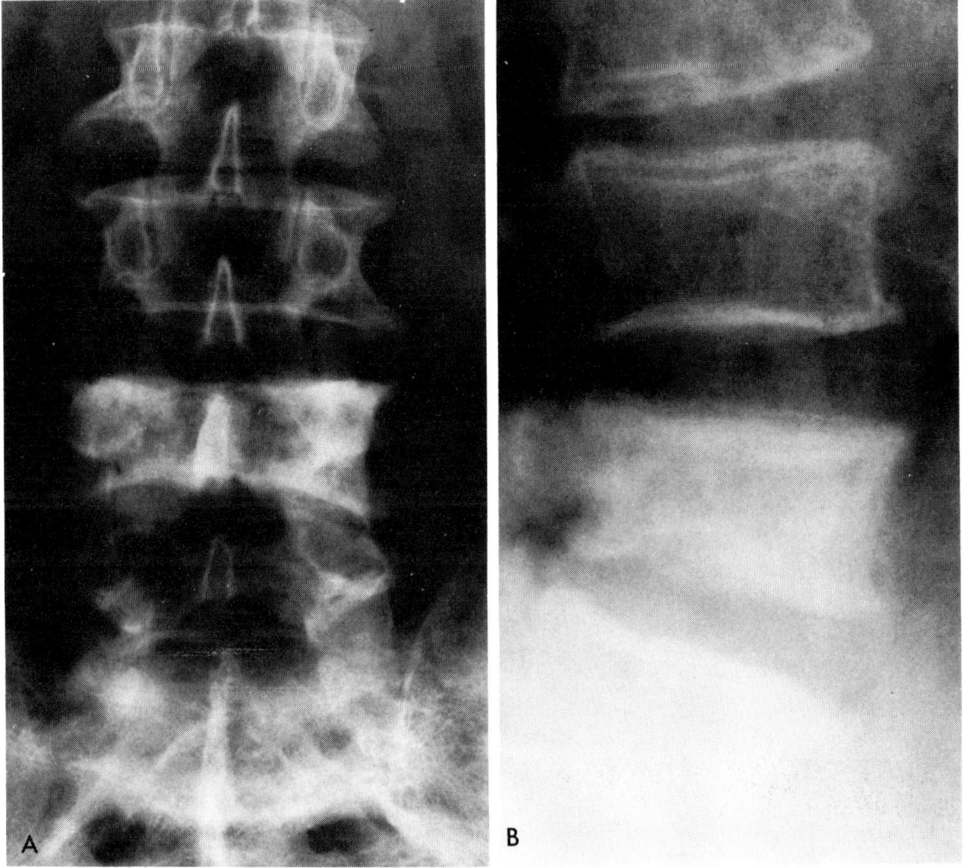

Figure 16–13. PAGET'S DISEASE OF LUMBAR SPINE: *A* and *B*, The L_4 vertebral body is particularly involved. It is larger than the adjacent vertebral bodies, yet has sustained a compression fracture because it is actually weaker than the normal bone. The pelvis also demonstrates an increased trabecular pattern.

optic foramina encroachment may lead to blindness.

Enlarged Spinal Canal. Abnormal scalloping of the backs of the vertebral body may occur in chronic obstructive hydrocephalus (Fig. 16–19) secondary to transmission of increased intracranial pressure down the spinal canal. This is a relatively rare finding, although subtle changes may be found if the plain films of the spine are examined closely. Other processes that may lead to scalloping of the posterior margin of the vertebral bodies and enlargement of the spinal canal are: dural ectasia of neurofibromatosis in the absence of individual neurofibroma; multiple individual neurofibromata; achondroplasia; spinal arachnoid cysts; spinal lipomas; teratomas; astrocytomas; syringohydromyelia or ependymomas.

Hemivertebrae. In this anomaly, a failure of development of one half of the vertebral body occurs because of lack of ossification of one lateral cartilaginous center. An isolated hemivertebra may be present and associated with an acute scoliosis. Most commonly, multiple anomalies are seen, frequently involving multiple vertebral bodies that may have a counterbalancing effect. In addition, there may be other more severe associated problems, such as spinal dysrhaphic states sometimes associated with meningocele or meningomyeloceles.

Text continued on page 746

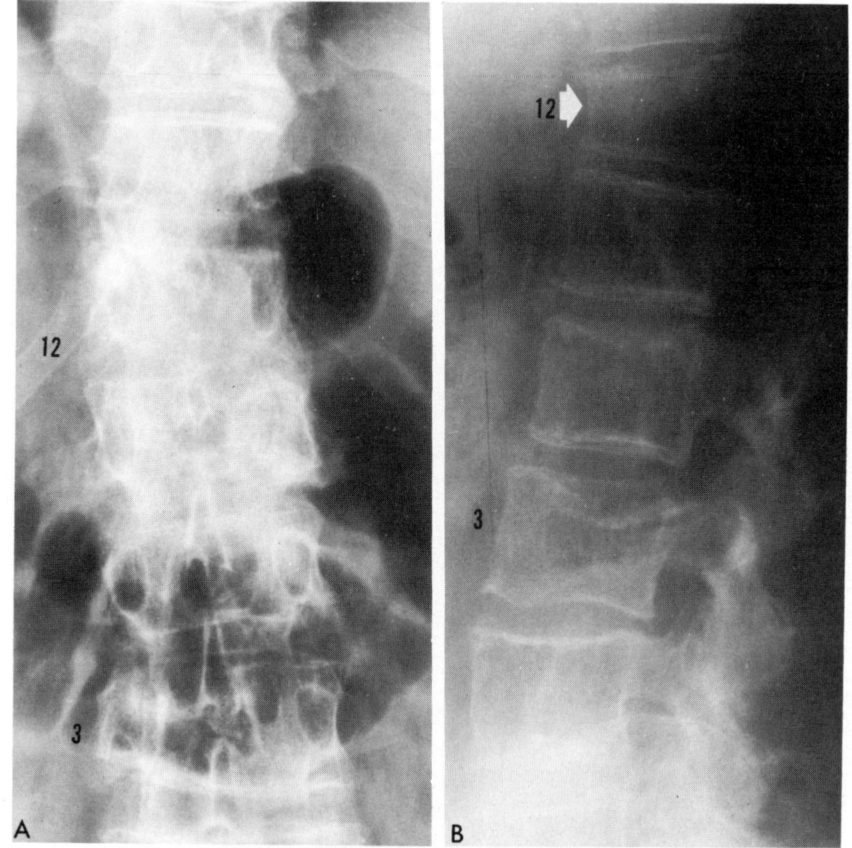

Figure 16–14 *See legend on the opposite page*

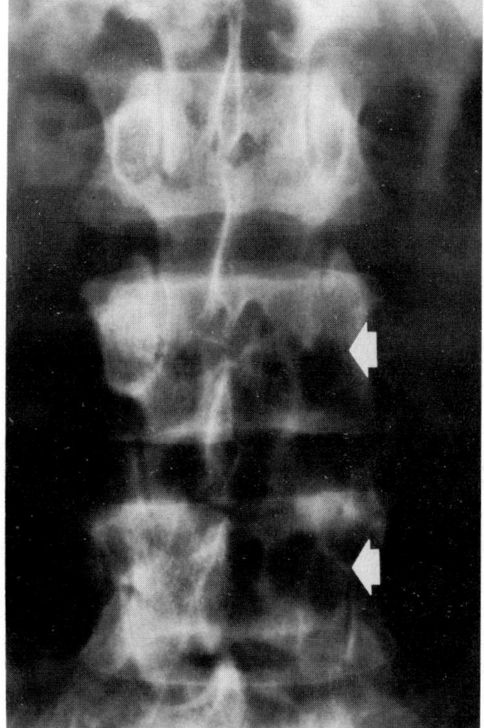

Figure 16–15 *See legend on the opposite page*

Figure 16–14. MULTIPLE MYELOMA: *A* and *B*, There is diffuse deossification of the bony structures. The pedicles are spared. There are compression deformities of the D_{12} and L_3 vertebral bodies.

Figure 16–15. METASTATIC DISEASE: There is lytic destructive metastatic disease involving the left pedicles at L_4 and L_5 (*arrows*). This is the "absent pedicle sign" of metastatic disease.

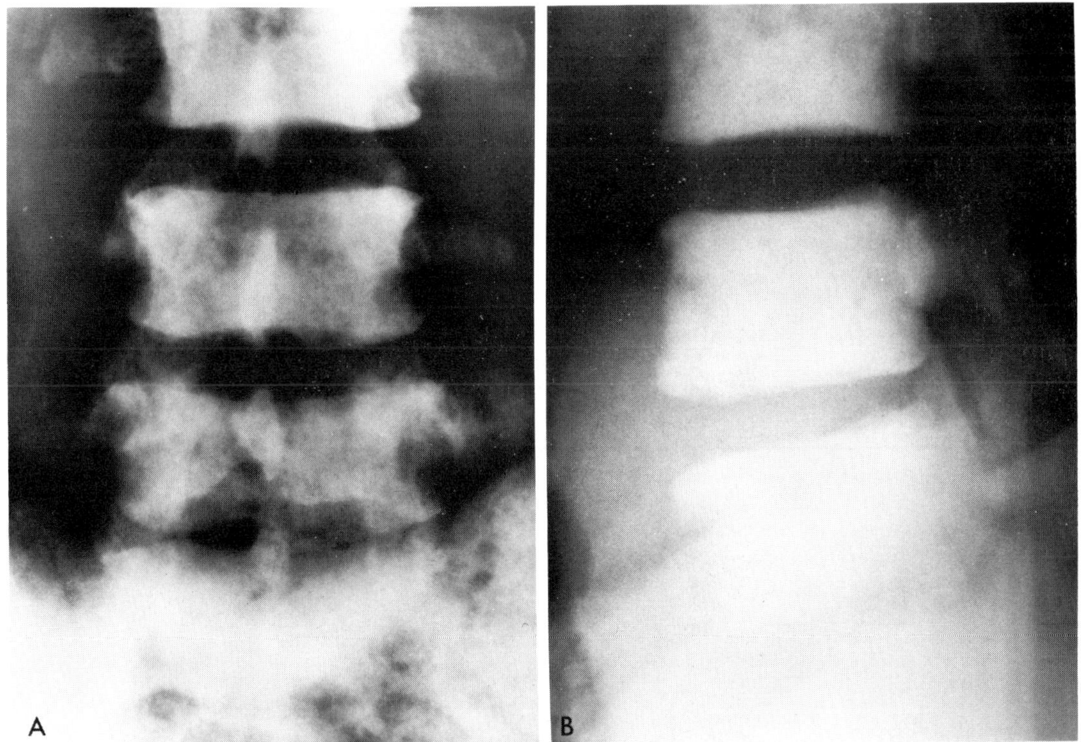

Figure 16–16. OSTEOBLASTIC METASTATIC DISEASE: All of the visualized bony structures demonstrate increased density that is somewhat irregular in its distribution. This is characteristic of osteoblastic metastatic disease. It is differentiated from Paget's disease because of the absence of prominent trabeculae.

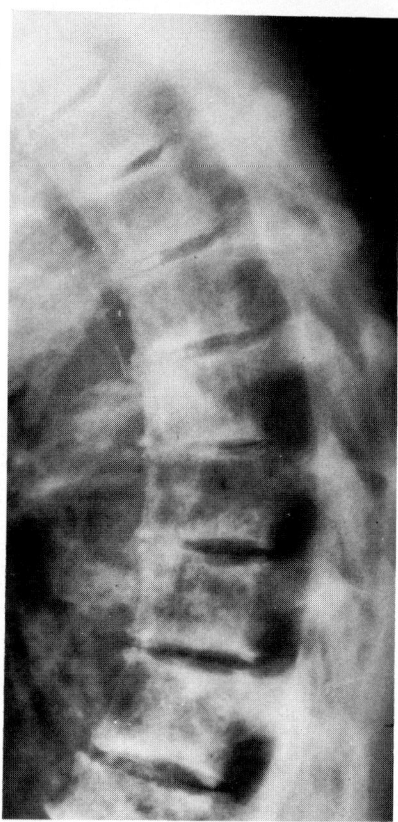

Figure 16–17. MIXED OSTEOLYTIC AND OSTEOBLASTIC DISEASE: The bony structures are diffusely abnormal in appearance. Areas of increased and decreased density occur in a mixed pattern. The pattern is typical of metastatic disease with destructive and reparative bony changes.

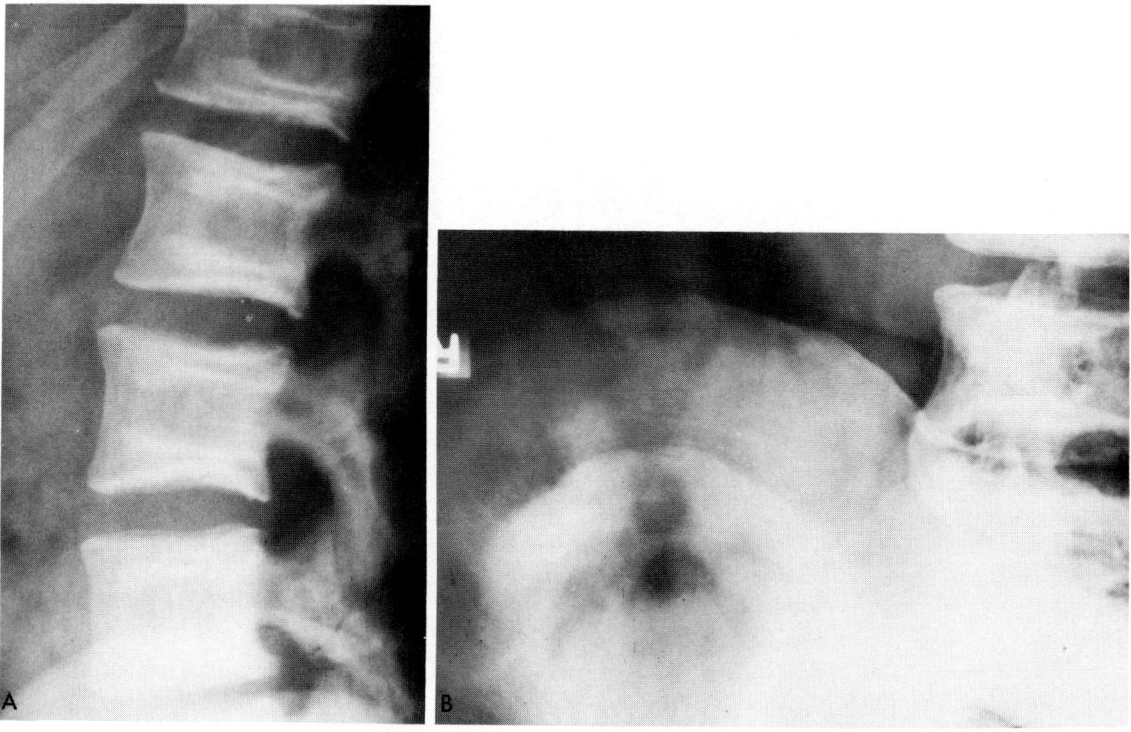

Figure 16–18. OSTEOPETROSIS: *A* and *B*, The bony structures are of diffusely increased density and exhibit a typical "bone-within-a-bone" appearance.

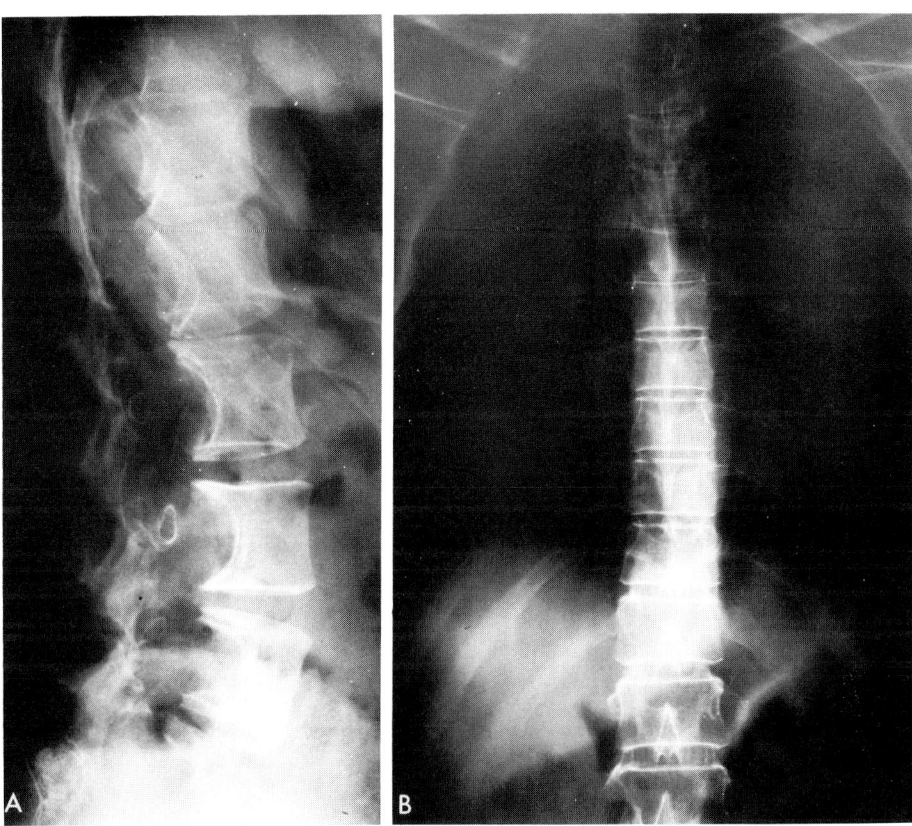

Figure 16–19. CHRONIC INCREASED INTRACRANIAL PRESSURE: The patient had an astrocytoma of the posterior fossa. Because of chronic increased intracranial pressure transmitted to the spine — without tumor actually being present in the spinal canal — there is marked widening of the interpeduncular space in the thoracic region. There is also a marked increase in the AP diameter of the spinal canal in the lumbar region, with marked scalloping of the posterior bodies of all the lumbar vertebrae (case courtesy of Drs. Oscar Sugar and Glen Dobben).

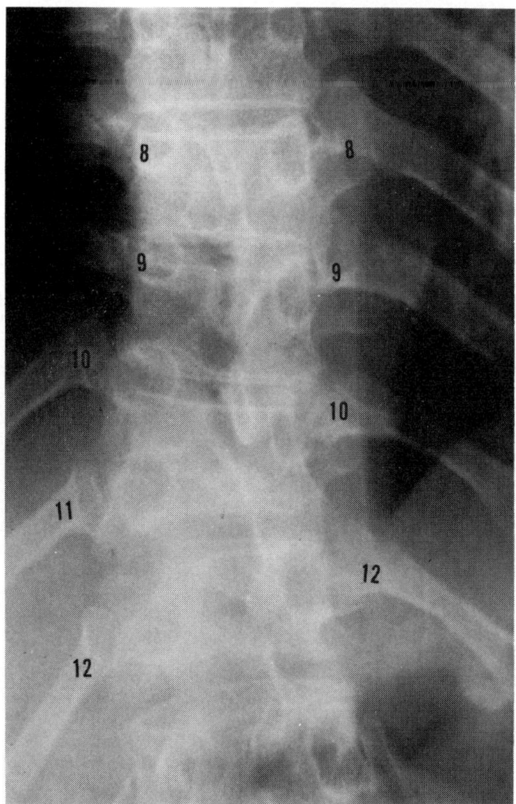

Figure 16–20. HEMIVERTEBRAE: Note that one rib is missing on the left side. There is an absent pedicle at the D_{11} level on the left side with downward displacement of D_{10}. There is only slight distortion of the dorsal vertebral body. More frequently there is a definite wedge-shaped deformity of the vertebral body associated with a scoliosis concave toward the side of the hemivertebrae.

NORMAL ANATOMY OF THE SPINAL CORD

The spinal cord ends, in the majority of cases, at the lower border of the first lumbar vertebrae or at the upper border of the second. The cord is held by the filum terminale, which normally measures no wider than 2 mm and extends caudad from the spinal cord to the lumbar cul-de-sac. The normal cervical enlargement extends from C_3 to D_2 and is widest at C_5–C_6. The lumbar enlargement occurs from D_9–D_{12}, where the cord tapers rapidly in the region of the conus medullaris. The cord then breaks up into multiple nerve roots —the cauda equina — which exit at successive levels. The lumbar cul-de-sac ends at the midbody of S_1 in most cases, but may end higher or lower than this. The spinal cord is sensitive to pressure damage, and compression of a few hours may create irreversible neurologic changes in the cord. Consequently, if spinal cord compression is suspected, rapid diagnosis and treatment are strongly suggested.

MYELOGRAPHY

Myelography (Gr. *myelos,* marrow, medulla and *graphe,* a drawing) is the radiographic visualization or photography of the spinal cord after the injection of a radiopaque substance into the spinal subarachnoid space.

This definition of myelography suggests only a small amount of the information that actually can be gained from a myelogram. In a patient with back pain or progressive neurologic signs, the demonstration of the various disease processes that can affect the spinal cord is necessary for correct diagnosis and proper treatment planning.

The spinal nerves do not originate from the spinal cord at the identical level in the bony spinal column. This is because the cord does not continue to grow with growth of the bony spinal column, but is drawn upward in the canal, leaving the nerves to exit at their proper level even though the actual nerve root level of origin is much higher. One should remember that a spinal cord lesion at the T_{10} level in the bony spinal column corresponds to the clinical neurologic and dermatome level of the umbilicus (see Fig. 16–33). With this in mind, the anatomic location of the lesion causing the patient's signs and symptoms can be roughly ascertained by moving up or down from the level of the umbilicus or T_{10} level.

Because of the possibility of multiple lesions and because of varying biologic responses, the exact anatomic location often cannot be demonstrated by physical examination. Therefore, myelography is necessary for more accurate evaluation. Before myelography is performed, it is essential to obtain and review plain films of the areas to be studied. Review of the plain films is vital because one must be able to correlate and account for possible defects seen on the myelogram with the plain film findings. In addition, after the instillation of contrast material, bony abnormalities may be partially or totally obscured by the contrast medium. This is of particular importance in the cervical area, where one must decide whether a defect is secondary to a bony spur, to a cervical disk or to a combination of the two. In addition, one must always be alert for the possibility of metastatic carcinoma or a congenital abnormality. If evidence for metastatic disease to the bony structures or soft tissues is discovered, this may well alter one's approach to the myelographic study.

CONTRAST MATERIALS

Through the years a variety of contrast materials have been used to outline the spinal cord and subarachnoid space. Among these are:

Air. Dandy reported the use of air for myelography in the 1920s, and air is still in use today as a contrast material for the study of the spinal cord. It is felt to be the medium of choice by many in the field. The use of air causes no long term complications. The patients experience some discomfort at the time of the examination, but otherwise tolerate the procedure well.

Air may be difficult to visualize — even with good patient positioning — and tomography is required in most cases for excellent delineation of the abnormality. In general, air myelography is not now a widely used technique, and the recent introduction of Amipaque may further decrease its use.

Dimeray. This water soluble contrast material was available in the United States for a short time, but subsequently was withdrawn because of complications associated with its use. The material is neurotoxic and could not be used above the level of the conus medullaris. This limitation resulted in an incomplete myelogram because one could not allow the contrast to flow throughout the length of the subarachnoid space — in some cases making it necessary to repeat the myelogram at a later date with another contrast material. Complications with Dimeray are myoclonia, hypotension and grand mal seizures.

Pantopaque (Iodophenylundecanoate). At the present time, Pantopaque, which was originally introduced in 1940, is widely accepted and is the most commonly used myelographic contrast material. It is an ester-based contrast material with firmly bound iodine. Idiosyncratic reactions have been reported, but patients with a history of allergic reactions to intravenous iodinated contrast agents do not develop reactions to subarachnoid Pantopaque. Pantopaque is absorbed from the subarachnoid space at a rate of approximately 1 cc per year. Rarely, Pantopaque may produce arachnoiditis, which may be aggravated by surgery. Arachnoiditis is more likely to occur when the Pantopaque is mixed with blood in the subarachnoid space, and therefore Pantopaque should not be used when the CSF is bloody. When the myelographic procedure is completed, the contrast material should be removed from the subarachnoid space if at all possible.

Conray 60. In the past Conray 60 was used in myelography, but there are certain dangers — the main problem being toxicity to the CNS and the danger of grand mal seizures. In addition, although the contrast is miscible with CSF and usually outlines the individual nerve root sheaths better than Pantopaque, less radiopacity is seen on the radiograph. These studies were frequently performed under general anesthesia. The obvious advantage is that water soluble contrast materials do not require removal at the end of the procedure.

Amipaque (Metrizamide) Myelography

In 1978 a new contrast material, Amipaque, became available for use in myelography. Amipaque is water soluble, but is unique when compared to previously available materials. Earlier water soluble contrast materials were ionic compounds, whereas Amipaque is a molecular solution (see below). This characteristic makes allergic reactions far less likely. Patients who have been allergic to intravenous contrast material do not react to Amipaque. The water soluble compound is resorbed from the CSF and excreted by the kidneys, with approximately 75 per cent removed after 24 hours. Therefore Amipaque need not be removed from the subarachnoid space. At the time of this writing, no *clinically significant* cases of arachnoiditis have been reported following the use of Amipaque. It has low neurotoxicity, but grand mal seizures may develop if the intracranial contents are flooded with Amipaque.

As an added benefit, this contrast is of significant help in diagnosis when used in conjunction with CT scanning of the spine and the intracranial structures.

Amipaque is packaged as a crystalline material and is reconstituted just before the procedure. The solution is mixed in a concentration appropriate to each individual patient (see below). Amipaque is light-sensitive and is stable for 12 hours after reconstitution.

Extracts from the manufacturer's insert (Winthrop Laboratories) describing the chemical structure, reconstitution, dosage and precautions to be followed when using Amipaque are reprinted at the end of this chapter.

INDICATIONS

Myelograms are performed for a variety of reasons. Most often these patients suffer from either acute or chronic back pain and are referred for myelography to rule out the presence of a herniated nucleus pulposus (HNP, ruptured disk). Other patients suffer from multiple sclerosis but have atypical symptoms that require a contrast study to rule out another disease process or possibly a surgically treatable lesion. Metastatic disease often involves both the bony spine and the spinal cord. A syringohydromyelia may involve the lumbar or cervical spine. Meningioma and neurofibroma are other possible causes of back pain. Primary spinal cord tumors, such as ependymomas and astrocytomas, as well as intramedullary metastases are also seen. Arteriovenous malformations that involve the spinal cord also occur. The patient's symptoms may help in differentiating one lesion from another, but in many cases are not helpful.

CLASSES OF LESIONS

Three major classes of lesions are seen at myelography (Fig. 16–21).

The more common types of abnormalities are listed below; however, many other less common lesions may be seen.

1. Extradural lesions:

A. Herniated disc.

B. Metastases.

C. Postoperative change.

D. Neurofibroma (may also be intradural).

E. Hematoma.

F. Spondylosis.

G. Epidural abscess.

H. Paget's disease or other vertebral body processes such as hemangioma, myeloma, chondroma.

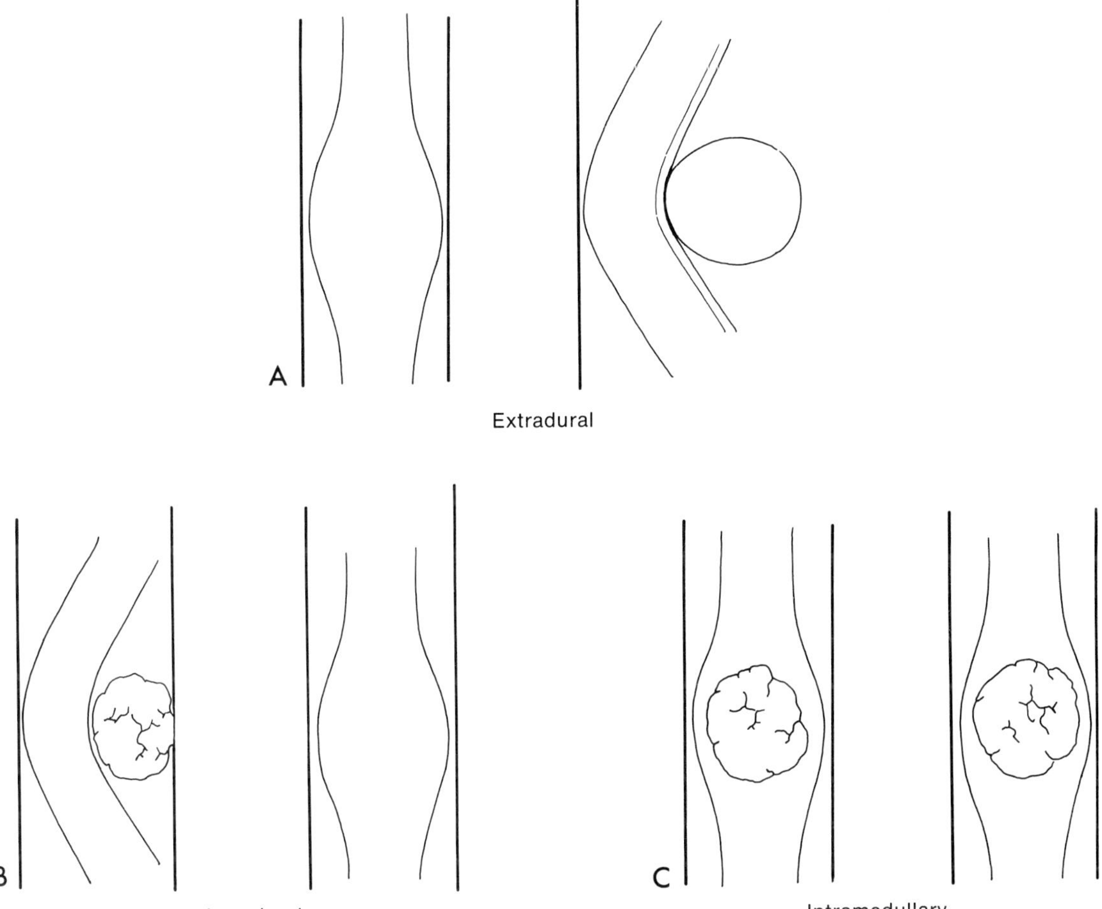

Figure 16–21. These three illustrations demonstrate graphically the roentgen changes seen with the three classes of spine tumors. Note that if only one view is obtained any one of the three varieties may resemble another class: the cord will appear widened and the contrast column will be thinned on either side of the cord. However, it is the view *perpendicular* to this view that more accurately evaluates the true nature of the mass.

A, With an *extradural* mass, such as a herniated disk, both the dura and the subarachnoid space will be pushed, and the contrast will course smoothly over the mass. The cord will be displaced away from the mass and widened by pressure from the mass. The contrast material will be thinned on both sides of the cord.

B, With an *intradural* mass, the contrast will form an acute angle with the tumor at its attachment with the dura. There will be a meniscus going around the mass and a widened contrast column between the mass and the compressed cord. The contrast column on the side of the cord opposite the tumor will be thinned.

C, With an *intramedullary* tumor the cord will appear widened in all views, and the contrast column will be thinned on all sides of the cord in all views.

It is, of course, unusual in radiologic practice to see any of the classic appearances in one standard projection. Therefore, multiple views must be obtained and the patient placed in oblique projection if necessary. All attempts should be made to define the lesion and the class of the abnormality so that proper treatment can be planned. Also, a mass may be of such size as to create a complete block to the flow of contrast material. If this is the case, standard criteria for diagnosis may no longer be helpful. On the other hand, even smaller lesions may take on the characteristics of masses in more than one class, making preoperative diagnosis difficult or impossible.

2. Intradural lesions:
A. Neurofibroma.
B. Meningioma.
C. Metastases — "seeding."
D. Arachnoid cyst.
E. Dermoid.
F. Ependymoma.
G. Lipoma.

3. Intramedullary lesions:
A. Ependymoma (most common).
B. Astrocytoma.
C. Syringohydromyelia.
D. Dermoid.
E. Hematoma or swollen cord.

4. Miscellaneous lesions:
A. Spinal cord arteriovenous malformations.
B. Epidermoid cyst secondary to multiple spinal taps.

Should any of these lesions reach such a size that it completely blocks the flow of contrast, the typical myelographic appearance may be lost. Obviously myelography can no longer be relied upon for exact diagnosis in such patients.

PATIENT PREPARATION

Before the myelographic study, it is helpful if the individual who is to perform it greets the patient at the bedside and discusses the procedure in some detail. Patients are much more cooperative if they understand what the goals of the study will be. In addition, acquaintance with the procedure relieves much of the fear of the unknown, helping the patient to be more relaxed. Not uncommonly, patients have the misconception that a myelogram can lead to lower extremity paralysis. It should be emphasized that patients with neurologic problems often have myelographic procedures — not that the myelographic procedure itself leads to paralysis or neurologic difficulty. In addition, I have found it helpful if the patient is told in some detail about the steps that precede the myelogram.

Patients should be told: (1) whether they will or will not receive premedication before the study; (2) that they will be sent to the radiology department on a cart; (3) that they should empty their bladder before leaving for the study; (4) that they should take nothing by mouth before the study. This is to avoid aspiration of gastric contents should nausea and emesis develop during the procedure. However, patients having Amipaque myelograms should be well hydrated and may be allowed fluids either by mouth or IV.

It is reassuring to the patient to be told that he will be met in the department of radiology by the doctor performing the study. If the patient has been told that the contrast is heavier (or lighter as in the case of air myelography) than cerebrospinal fluid and that manipulation of the radiography table will be done in order to allow the contrast to flow to the areas of interest, this again allows the patient to understand and tolerate better the sometimes uncomfortable positions that must be assumed and held for certain periods of time.

The patient also should be informed that he will be requested to remain flat in bed for 8 hours following a Pantopaque myelogram and to sit up at 30° to 45° for 8 hours following an Amipaque myelogram. Then he must rest in bed, preferably flat, for an additional 16 hours.

Typical Pre-Myelogram Orders

1. Nothing by mouth on day of procedure (except that patients having Amipaque myelograms should be well hydrated either by mouth or IV).
2. 100 mg Nembutal IM on call to radiology.
3. 0.4 mg Atropine IM on call to radiology.
4. Have patient void before coming to radiology.
5. Sign consent.

Typical Post-Myelogram Orders Following Pantopaque Myelogram

1. Flat in bed for 8 hours.
2. Bed rest for 24 hours.
3. Cerebrospinal fluid to be sent for routine and special studies.
4. Push oral fluids.
5. Resume previous orders.
6. Vital signs every 2 hours for 6 hours then per routine.

Typical Post-Myelogram Orders Following Amipaque Myelography

1. Patient to sit up at 30° to 45° angle for 8 hours; then flat in bed for 16 hours.
2. Push oral fluids.
3. Vital signs every 30 minutes for 2 hours, every 60 minutes for 2 hours and every 3 hours for 24 hours.
4. Resume previous diet.
5. Cerebrospinal fluid to be sent for routine and special studies.

These orders can be modified to suit individual needs.

NEEDLES

Many different types of needles are available for myelography (Fig. 16–22). A short beveled needle is desirable. A plain beveled spinal needle can be used, but it is often less than satisfactory when attempting to remove the contrast. When aspiration is attempted, the nerve rootlets may float against the tip of the needle, occluding the outflow. One type of needle has been devised that has a single hole opposite the bevel; this provides two exit pathways for the contrast. There are many variations on this theme; however, the most satisfactory for Pantopaque myelography has been the Cuatico needle (Fig. 16–22), which has an inner stylet with multiple side holes along the distal end of the shaft as well as a distal end-hole. This needle has proved very satisfactory for the removal of contrast material.

One disadvantage of the inner stylet is that while the tip and one or two distal end

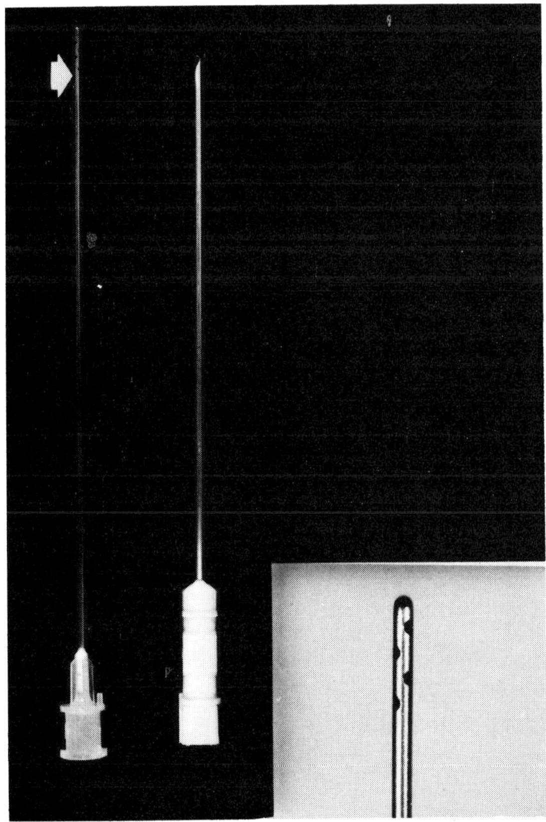

Figure 16–22. MYELOGRAM NEEDLES: The Cuatico needle is a 19-gauge spinal needle with a short beveled point and an inner stylet that is beveled and pointed to fit the hollow needle. In addition, there is a hollow, multi-holed stylet (see inset) that also fits through the needle and projects beyond the bevel of the needle to a point marked by the arrow. This inner core stylet is used to aspirate Pantopaque at the end of the procedure.

holes will be within the contrast material pooled in the ventral subarachnoid space, the rest of the needle's side holes will be in the CSF above the Pantopaque. As a consequence, an excess of CSF may be removed when the Pantopaque is aspirated. This is a disadvantage because in some cases it seems that the occurrence of headache is related to the amount of CSF removed from the subarachnoid space. Indeed, when a large amount of CSF is removed, patients not infrequently complain of headache during the course of the contrast and CSF removal, even though they experienced no discomfort during the course of the examination itself.

In order to avoid excess CSF removal one should check the position of the tip of the needle on the radiographs and advance the tip well into the contrast pool whenever possible. In addition, we have found it helpful to remove as much contrast as possible through the plain beveled needle before using the various types of special inner cannulas. In addition, the author has devised a special needle tip that has only two small, round distal side-holes in addition to the end-hole.

If difficulty is encountered when removing contrast material with the needle at one level, this needle may be removed and the patient retapped at a lower level. This is easily done. The preceding myelogram has demonstrated the appearance of the subarachnoid space at the lower level, and the repeat tap can facilitate contrast removal.

At times a swollen nerve root rests against the tip of the needle, and, in spite of all attempts, the contrast cannot be removed. Again, retapping at another level is strongly suggested. If this is unsuccessful, the contrast should be removed at a later date.

It should be cautioned that if blood is present in the CSF at the time of the initial lumbar puncture, Pantopaque should *not* be instilled in the subarachnoid space because of the possibility of later development of arachnoiditis. Occasionally the initial fluid will be blood-tinged secondary to the tap itself. If this is the case, the obturator should be returned to place and the patient allowed to rest for 10 minutes (by the clock) before proceeding with the study. If the CSF has cleared by that time the examination may be continued. If the fluid remains bloody the procedure should be discontinued and performed 10 to 14 days later. Exceptions to this rule would include a patient with recent cord trauma, where the necessity to evaluate immediately the status of the cord would outweigh considerations of possible future complications. In such a case, air myelography or Amipaque myelography might be desirable.

It should be emphasized that meticulous technique is important when doing myelograms. In addition to precise needle puncture technique, which of course greatly facilitates the performance of the myelogram, rigorous attention to detail is desirable throughout the procedure. Sterile technique should be used throughout. At the time of instillation of contrast material, it is necessary to fill the plastic tubing and syringe full of contrast without allowing any air bubbles to form in the system. If this is not done, small amounts of air will enter the subarachnoid space at the time of contrast instillation. In fact, with fluoroscopic control, one often can seen a small amount of air rise upward while the contrast flows to the dependent portion of the canal. It seems that this air, even though small in amount, may be one reason for the vasovagal response that may develop early in the course of study. (A similar reaction is also seen during pneumoencephalography.) However, even before the procedure is begun, some patients develop a vasovagal reaction with diaphoresis, nausea, hypotension and vomiting. If these reactions occur it is wise to interrupt the procedure, start an IV solution of dextrose and saline and wait until the patient stabilizes before continuing the examination.

TECHNIQUE OF PANTOPAQUE MYELOGRAPHY

In our department, lumbar puncture is performed with the patient in the prone position. A pillow is placed under the abdomen in order to round the back and allow for easier needle placement between the spinous processes. Several types of prepackaged and presterilized myelogram trays are available commercially, or a specific tray set-up can be made.

Needle placement is always performed under fluoroscopic control. If we are interested in the lumbar area, puncture is performed in the midline at the L_2–L_3 or L_3–L_4 interspace (Fig. 16–23), unless, of course, this is the level of interest. In this way, since disk disease is most common in the lower lumbar area, we will avoid the levels most likely to be involved. We use one of two approaches for the initial lumbar tap. If a midline lumbar puncture is to be performed, the L_2–L_3 or L_3–L_4 interspace is identified under fluoroscopic control, and local anesthetic is instilled along the needle tract.

A generous amount of local anesthetic is recommended to make the procedure as painfree as possible. Transitional vertebrae will have been identified by preliminary perusal of the plain films; if there is a variation in the normal number of vertebrae the first non–rib-bearing vertebral body should be considered as the number one lumbar vertebra. The spinous processes angle inferiorly in the lumbar region, and this must be taken into account when performing the puncture. It may be necessary to angle the needle cephalad.

Again, the needle is advanced under fluoroscopic control in the midline until one feels the slight resistance of the ligamenta flavum followed by the slight resistance of the dura. Entrance is then made into the subarachnoid space. It is best to elevate the patient's head before lumbar puncture to allow hydrostatic pressure to expand the subarachnoid space. As the needle is advanced, but before entering the subarachnoid space, it is wise to remove the inner cannula periodically to check for flow of CSF, as it is not always possible to be sure of the exact moment of entrance into the subarachnoid space. After flow has been established, the patient's head is kept elevated to insure flow of CSF, and a sample of fluid is collected and sent to the appropriate laboratories for routine study.

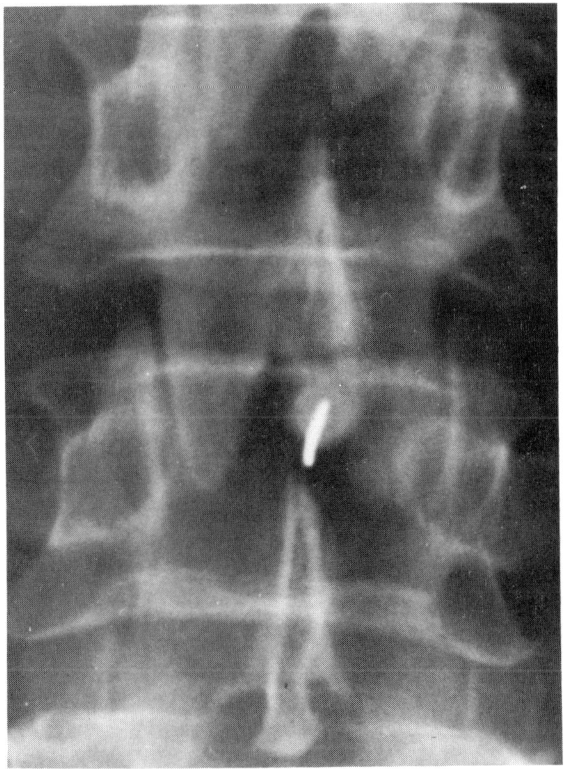

Figure 16–23. MIDLINE NEEDLE PUNCTURE TECHNIQUE: The plastic hubbed needle projects directly in the midline. The tip of the needle is at the mid-portion of the back of the vertebral body. Skin puncture is made just below the spinous process of the superior vertebral body.

For the beginning myelographer it is wise to obtain a cross-table lateral radiograph to check both for radiographic technique and to be certain that the tip of the needle is well centered in the subarachnoid space.

Oblique Puncture Technique. A second — and in many ways preferable — method of lumbar puncture is the oblique approach (Fig. 16–24). When using this method, local anesthetic is placed between the pedicle and the spinous process at the level where lumbar puncture is to be performed. Local anesthetic is then infiltrated along a line directed at the midline and slightly cephalad to the starting point. The puncture needle is then advanced along this oblique line, passing over the lamina of the vertebral body until the "give" of the ligamentum flavum and dura is felt. The needle is then advanced slightly farther until the bevel is well within the subarachnoid space. Again, for the beginning myelographer it is wise to obtain a localization film to check radiographic technique and to confirm the needle position in the lateral projection. This method has the advantage of avoiding any midline scarring that may be present from previous surgery and also of avoiding any calcified longitudinal ligaments that may be present. It is also possible to direct the needle tip easily so that when the subarachnoid space is entered the tip is at the mid- or upper vertebral body level rather than at the disk space. This is important because the needle placement may result in a "needle defect" that occasionally is difficult to differentiate from an organic defect.

When using the midline puncture technique the needle often must be directed cephalad, necessitating entrance into the subarachnoid space at the disk space level. This is suboptimal because entrance at this level, if it has resulted in a needle defect, can mimic the appearance of a defect secondary to a bulging or herniated disk. The needle defect is second-

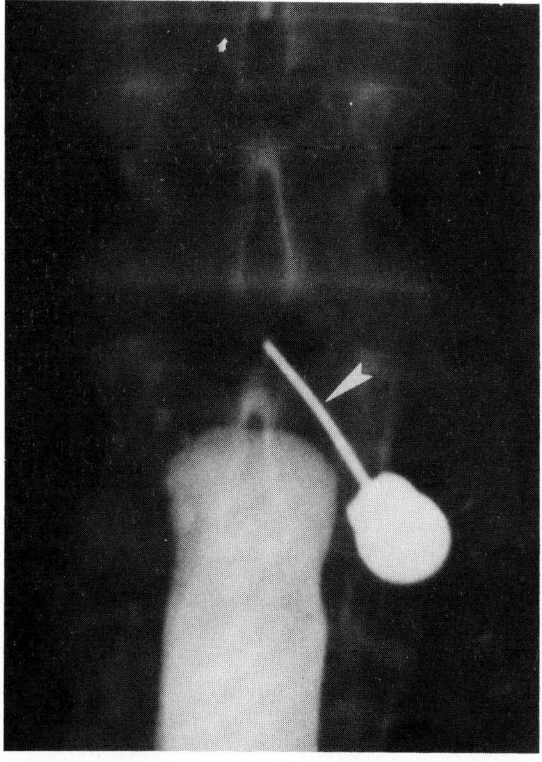

Figure 16–24. OBLIQUE NEEDLE PUNCTURE TECHNIQUE: Skin puncture is made at a level between the vertebral pedicle and the top of the spinous process of the same vertebral body. The needle is then slanted down and forward until lumbar puncture is performed in the midline. The arrowhead marks the skin puncture site.

ary to the puncture — not an anatomic abnormality. When the needle has entered at the vertebral body level, even if a needle defect occurs, confusion with a disk defect is less likely. Furthermore, when using the oblique technique the only bony structure in the direct line to the subarachnoid space is the lamina of the vertebral body. Merely by directing it slightly cephalad, the needle tip will drop over the lamina and into the subarachnoid space. A detailed study of the anatomic skeleton in addition to the radiographs is helpful before undertaking myelographic procedures.

It should be added that when using a sharp small-caliber needle it is less obvious when the tip passes through the dura and into the subarachnoid space. This is particularly true when a 20- or 22-gauge needle is used for instillation of water-soluble contrast material, when needle placement is quite critical (see below under Water-Soluble Contrast Material).

Volume of Pantopaque

The amount of contrast material necessary to perform a myelogram varies from individual to individual, depending on the size of the subarachnoid space and the area of interest. Although this may vary greatly in an individual case, the average amount of contrast is as follow:

AVERAGE RECOMMENDED VOLUMES

Area	*Amount*
Lumbar	9 to 12 cc
Cervical	12 to 15 cc
Thoracic	18 to 24 cc (or more)

Lumbar Myelography

Following removal of a sample of CSF, usually about 5 to 6 cc, Pantopaque is instilled into the subarachnoid space. Varying amounts of contrast material are used, depending on the level of the spine being studied. In the lumbar region, 9 to 12 cc of Pantopaque is usually adequate to cover the areas of interest. A general rule of thumb is to instill enough Pantopaque to outline two disk spaces very well with contrast when the patient is in the upright position. There is a good deal of variation from one patient to the next. Although 6 cc may be all that is needed in one patient, 18 cc or more may be required in another. These recommended amounts should be used only as guidelines, and in any individual case the amount actually used may vary. Each myelogram should be "tailored" to fit the patient.

In addition to the anatomic variations seen from patient to patient, infrequently arachnoid cysts in the lumbar region will hold several cc of contrast material (see Fig. 16–30). Obviously, these must be filled before one can proceed with the myelogram. I have seen one case in which a small occult lumbar meningocele required the instillation of 18 cc of contrast material to reach the L_5—S_1 level.

Both a standard puncture technique and a standard filming technique should be used for each patient. The resulting myelograms are not only more pleasing esthetically, but there is also less likelihood that a particular area will be inadequately evaluated. Parenthetically, at a future date this also will help determine whether any films are missing.

I routinely take:

1. PA vertical beam upright and prone films that cover the lower lumbar area (see Fig. 16–31).
2. Horizontal beam lateral films "cross-table lateral" in the upright and prone positions that cover the lower lumbar area.
3. PA 45° oblique films with the patient in the upright position (vertical beam) and in the prone RAO and LAO positions (if needed) to cover all areas of interest in the lumbar region (see Fig. 16–31).
4. Horizontal beam RAO and LAO "cross-table" projections with the patient upright and prone as needed. These are also done if the myelogram appears normal or to further substantiate findings noted on other views.
5. PA vertical beam spot films in the dorsal and cervical areas are also taken while allowing the contrast material to flow up to the cervical region.

A brief or, if necessary, an extensive examination of the cervical region is suggested in *all* patients with low back pain. A single PA film with the contrast centered in the cervical region may suffice. This dorsal and cervical examination is particularly important if the examination of the lower lumbar region is normal; however, it is also important in others, because the visualized lumbar lesion may not be the actual cause of the patient's clinical problem. I have seen many patients who have had a recent myelogram limited to the lumbar region — only to have a high thoracic or low cervical lesion demonstrated when a re-examination was performed because of persistent or progressive symptoms. After the necessary films are obtained and checked, the contrast material is removed from the subarachnoid space (see below for filming technique with cervical and thoracic myelography).

After the myelographic study, the patient is returned to his room on a cart. He is asked to remain flat in bed for the next eight hours and to remain confined to bed for the next 24 hours. (Following Amipaque myelography the patient should sit up at a 30° to 40° angle for 8 hours. See below.) After this period, a clinical evaluation must be made to determine how much activity each patient is to be allowed. Also, patients are advised to drink additional fluids but are otherwise returned to their previous diet.

If there is any question of total or even high-grade block to the flow of contrast material, it is wisest to be very cautious during the procedure. If a block is suspected and a lumbar puncture performed, only one drop of CSF should be removed from the subarachnoid space — and this only to make certain that the needle is in the subarachnoid space. Then only a small amount of contrast material — 1 to 2 cc — should be instilled. The contrast is then allowed to flow up to the level of the block, where the site is marked with a lead dot or paperclip to facilitate surgery or radiotherapy. If Pantopaque is removed below the level of a block, a "vacuum" effect may result that causes further cord compromise secondary to interruption of vascular supply. Worsening of the patient's symptoms may follow, including paraplegia — a neurosurgical emergency.

If no block is encountered, one may then pool the contrast below the level of the needle, remove the desired amount of fluid for routine study, and proceed with the study without fear of complication. If this lumbar puncture technique is followed closely — even in those patients where suspicion of block is remote — one will not encounter any grave difficulties secondary to excess CSF removal.

The author does not perform myelograms as an outpatient procedure.

Postoperative Changes

The myelogram frequently reveals small indentations on the dorsal or lateral subarachnoid space that are secondary to surgery and of no pathologic significance. However, a ventral defect at the disk space level has the same significance as a ventral defect in a patient who has not had surgery and should be treated accordingly.

Evidence of postoperative arachnoiditis may be seen in patients with recurrent disc disease who do not exhibit a clinical syndrome consistent with arachnoiditis. Therefore, radiographic evidence of arachnoiditis should not deter one from undertaking appropriate treatment.

Subdural Injection (Figs. 16–25 to 16–27)

Because of its bevel, the myelogram needle tip may be only partly in the subarachnoid space and still provide excellent flow of CSF (Fig. 16–25,*A*). However, when one attempts to instill contrast material it will be seen that the contrast enters the subdural and epidural spaces before going into the subarachnoid space (Figs. 16–27, *A* and *B*). These potential spaces allow easy entrance of contrast even under the gentlest of pressure. At times, some of the contrast will simultaneously enter both the subarachnoid and the subdural spaces. This, of course, usually results in an unsatisfactory examination. The study sometimes can be salvaged by advancing the needle deeper into the subarachnoid space and continuing the injection of contrast, or by attempting puncture at another level. If an anterior subdural injection has occurred, the needle should be withdrawn slightly and repositioned in the subarachnoid space.

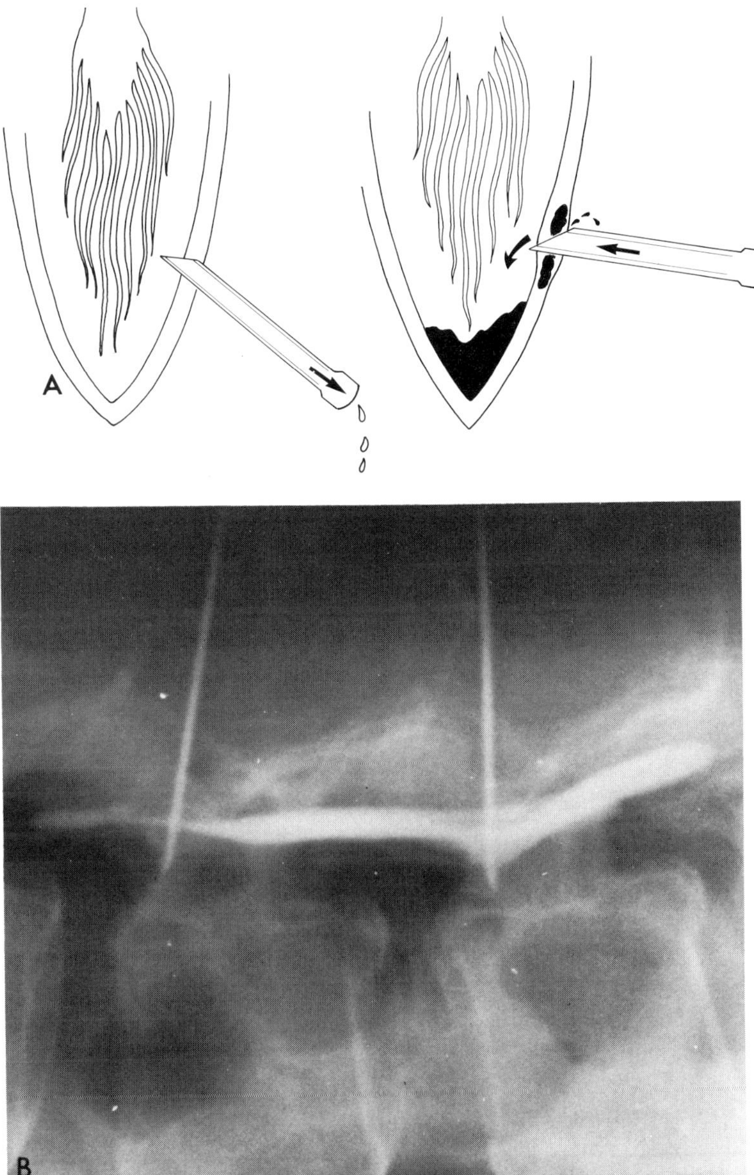

Figure 16–25. SUBDURAL INJECTION OF CONTRAST MATERIAL: *A*, These drawings illustrate the cause of entrance into the subdural space. The use of a long beveled needle should be avoided because of this phenomenon. Note that there will be flow of CSF but that contrast will enter the extradural and subdural spaces.

B, Lumbar puncture was performed without difficulty at the upper level, but there was poor flow of CSF. For this reason a second puncture was performed at the lower level. Flow of CSF was again felt to be adequate; however, after injection of contrast material, it was noted that the contrast had accumulated dorsal to the anticipated position of the subarachnoid space — i.e., in the subdural space. Usually most of this contrast material can be aspirated from the subdural space.

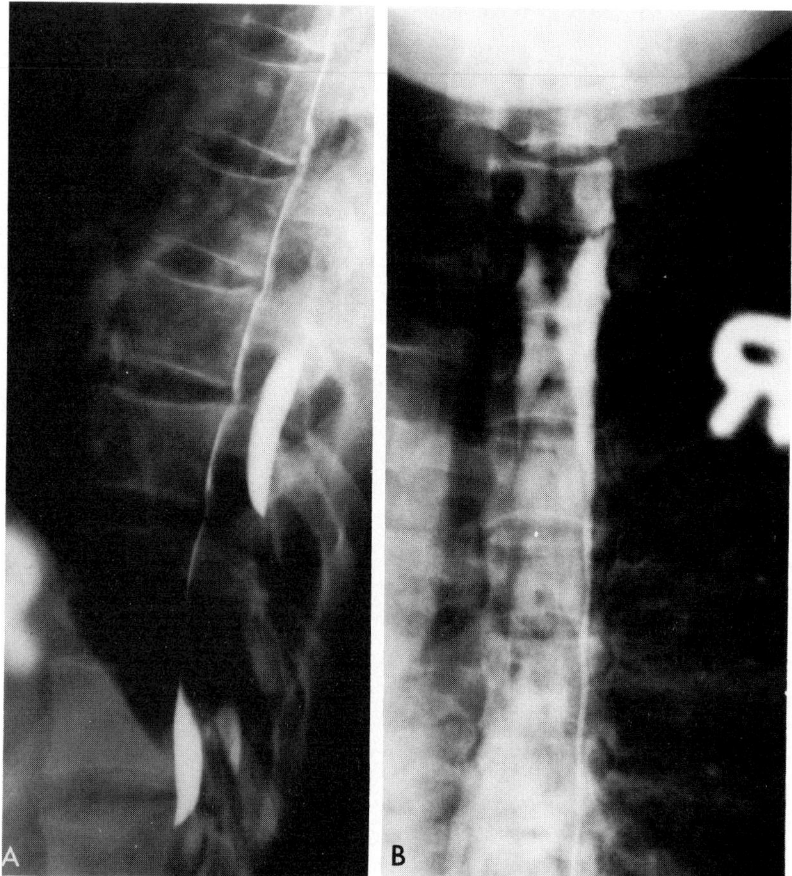

Figure 16–26. SUBDURAL CONTRAST: *A* and *B*, A large amount of contrast material has entered into the ventral subdural space, and a small accumulation of subdural contrast material is present in the dorsal subarachnoid space. Notice that the dorsal spinal cord cannot be visualized. This subdural contrast flowed freely up into the cervical region. Generally speaking, subdural contrast material does not flow readily, but tends to move slowly and over only one or two vertebral body segments.

If contrast is injected into the subdural space, it usually will be noted at fluoroscopy that the material collects under the tip of the needle and does not drop readily into the lumbar cul-de-sac like "lead balls in water" (Fig. 16–25). The contrast may enter the subdural or epidural space even with apparently adequate needle positioning. This may occur because the dura has thickened following previous surgery or an inflammatory process. Another possibility is that the tip of the myelographic needle has been dulled by multiple use, and the dura is carried forward by the needle, not punctured by it.

When contrast material is in the subdural space, the top of the contrast does not oscillate up and down with changes in respiration and the transmitted pulsation of heart beat as it does when the contrast is in the subarachnoid space. Also, if the contrast material is in the subarachnoid space one may ask the patient to cough and note under fluoroscopy that the contrast material "jumps" because of transmitted changes of pressure. When contrast material is in the subdural space, there is usually no or little fluoroscopic evidence of changes with transmitted pressure differences — or they may be less pronounced than when the material is in the subarachnoid space. In addition, any contrast material that is in the subdural space will not flow *readily* up to the cervical subarachnoid space.

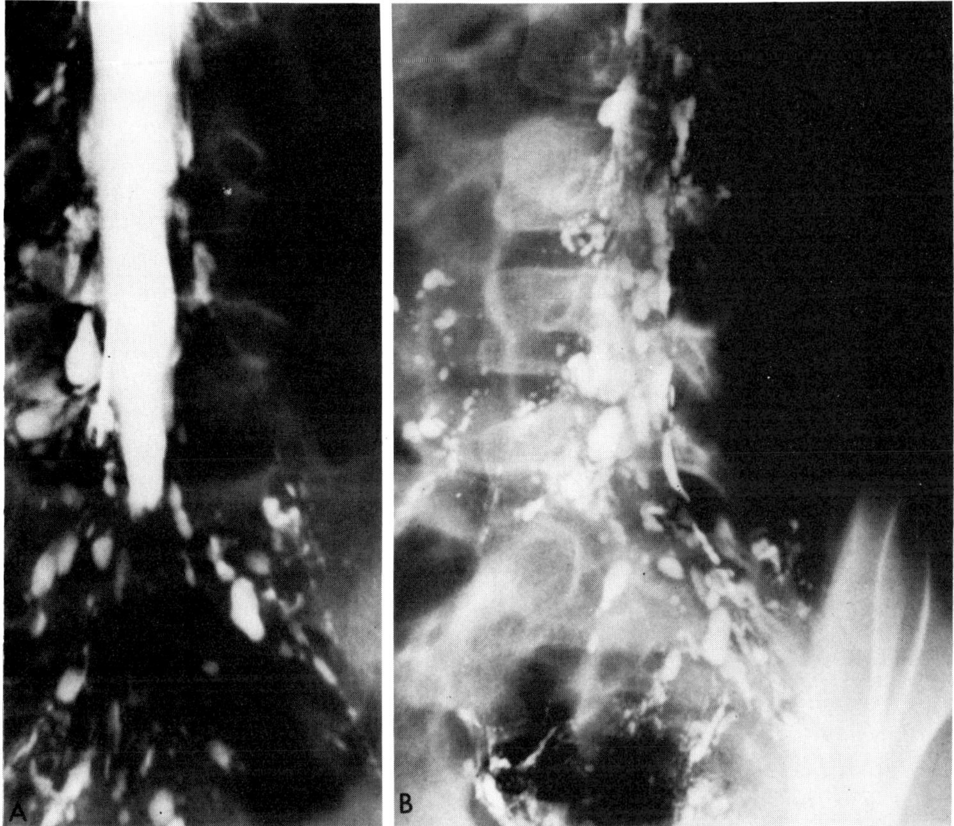

Figure 16–27. EXTRADURAL PANTOPAQUE: *A*, A large amount of Pantopaque is noted in the extradural space. This contrast tracks peripherally along the nerve pathways. There is also a large amount of contrast material in the subarachnoid space. Fluoroscopy should be performed intermittently during the instillation of contrast material to avoid this large accumulation of contrast in the extradural space.

B, Following the aspiration of contrast material from the subarachnoid space a moderate amount of contrast is also noted in the subdural space, forming a linear pattern that outlines the lumbar spinal column.

At times, however, it may be very difficult to identify subdural contrast material. I have witnessed one case where contrast flowed up to the cervical region without difficulty (Fig. 16–26). Lateral views may be helpful for further evaluation and may demonstrate that contrast has accumulated in the subdural space either ventrally or dorsally (Fig. 16–25). With subdural accumulation of the contrast, the spinal cord cannot be visualized.

If an injection of contrast does occur subdurally, removal should be attempted by pooling the material under the tip of the needle and aspirating as much as possible. If the needle cannot be repositioned, the patient may be retapped at another level and the procedure continued. More ideally, the examination should be discontinued and attempted again 10 days to 2 weeks later. In an emergency, the contrast material should be instilled via a C_1–C_2 tap and removed at a later date.

Technique of Cervical Tap

With lateral fluoroscopy with the patient in the supine or prone position, local anesthesia is administered and the needle is positioned in the posterior portion of the cervical subarachnoid space anterior to the posterior limit of the subarachnoid space (Fig. 16–67).

The needle is advanced until the "give" of the dura is felt, and then slightly farther until the tip is well into the cervical subarachnoid space. The needle position can be readily checked by fluoroscopy in the anteroposterior position if desired.

If lateral or biplane fluoroscopy is not available, a C_1–C_2 tap may be performed after the patient is placed in the lateral position with the head level and the chin flexed upon the chest. After instillation of local anesthetic, the spinal needle is again placed in position in the cervical subarachnoid space. When the stylet is removed, CSF will be noted to "well up" into the hub of the needle, even with the patient in a horizontal position. If desired, the patient may be placed in a modified Trendelenburg position to promote flow of CSF. After fluid removal, contrast material may be instilled under fluoroscopic control with the patient in the lateral decubitus position, or the patient may be placed supine by keeping the neck flexed on the chest. The contrast material cannot be removed from the cervical subarachnoid space via cervical tap; therefore only the amount of contrast material needed to complete the study should be used.

If no obstruction is encountered, contrast will accumulate in the lumbar subarachnoid space. It can then be removed via lumbar tap. We have used this method quite frequently in patients where a complete block to flow seems likely. It is especially useful in patients with metastatic disease, where outlining the upper border of the lesion is often all that is necessary before treatment.

TECHNIQUE OF AMIPAQUE MYELOGRAPHY

Lumbar Myelography

Amipaque may be instilled into the lumbar subarachnoid space using the same technique previously described for Pantopaque. The patient may be prone or in the lateral decubitus position. A short beveled 20- or 22-gauge spinal needle is used, and lumbar tap is performed at the L_2–L_3 level.

It is recommended that 6 cc of CSF be removed and the contrast material instilled in the lumbar subarachnoid space. The total amount instilled should not exceed 3 gm of Amipaque. The package insert suggests using the dilutions and amounts of contrast material shown on page 838. The recommended amounts should *not* be exceeded.

For a routine lumbar myelogram the author recommends the use of 11 to 14 cc of Amipaque in the 190 mg I/2 ml concentration. In an individual case, the myelogram may require the full 15 cc of of 190 mg I/2 ml or only 2 to 3 cc for complete evaluation. Each case should be judged separately so that an appropriate but not an excessive amount of contrast material can be used.

Although the contrast material is water-soluble, it is heavier than CSF; therefore, it initially accumulates in the dependent portion of the subarachnoid space. In the lumbar area, filming can be done using the method described for Pantopaque. Alternatively, films can be obtained by using only horizontal beam cross-table lateral radiography. With this technique, the lumbar tap can be performed with the patient in the lateral decubitus position. Films are then obtained with the patient in the right lateral decubitus position, the RAO position, the prone cross-table true lateral position, and in the left anterior oblique and left lateral decubitus positions. Because of the low density of Amipaque, it is preferable to use low kilovoltage technique — approximately 70 kv and high Mas — to increase radiographic contrast. In addition, it is important to collimate the films closely to increase radiographic detail. If the puncture needle is removed, the close collimation of the films may make exact identification of the individual levels difficult; therefore, it is preferable to leave the needle in place until filming has been completed. All patient movements should be done slowly to prevent excess admixing of the Amipaque with CSF. In general, patient movement should be kept to a mimimum.

Because of the possibility of precipitating a grand mal seizure with intracranial contrast material, it is very important that the head of the patient be kept elevated throughout the procedure or that the procedure be closely monitored fluoroscopically to prevent the inadvertent entrance of excessive amounts of the contrast intracranially. However, because thoracic or even cervical lesions can mimic lumbar disk disease, I prefer to allow the contrast material to flow up to the cervical region after films of the lumbar area have been obtained. The Amipaque flows more easily than Pantopaque and is not readily visible fluoroscopically in the thoracic area; therefore, fluoroscopy should be performed intermittently in the cervical region while allowing the contrast to flow cephalad and checking for the accumulation of contrast in the cervical region. *Great* care must be taken so that the contrast does not flood into the intracranial region; in fact, an attempt should be made to *prevent* it from entering the cranial vault. After PA and lateral films and any additional views are obtained in the cervical region, the head is again elevated, the contrast is allowed to return to the lumbar subarachnoid space and the patient is returned to his room in an upright position. As noted earlier, the patient is kept in a 30 to 40° angle upright position for 8 hours. He then lies flat in bed for the next 16 hours. To minimize complications, the patient should be kept well hydrated before and after the procedure. It is advisable to ask the patient to remain quiet during the 24 hours following the procedure in order to lessen the risk of admixing the Amipaque. This precaution may decrease morbidity. The author also suggests aspirating as much of the contrast material as possible at the termination of the procedure, although this has not definitely been shown to decrease morbidity.

Cervical Myelography with Amipaque

Amipaque may be used for cervical myelography using the lumbar approach. With this method, a standard lumbar puncture is performed and 10 cc of 250 to 300 mg I/2 ml is instilled. The contrast is then placed, under fluoroscopic guidance, in the cervical subarachnoid space without further delay. The patient should be kept in the head-down position during the instillation. The contrast material admixes with CSF and becomes more dilute than when it is instilled directly into the cervical region; but, if performed without delay, the procedure allows for adequate visualization of the cervical region. Again, care must be taken to prevent the inadvertent entrance of excess contrast material into the cranial vault.

It is also possible to instill the contrast material directly into the cervical subarachnoid space via a C_1–C_2 lateral cervical tap with the patient in the prone position. With this technique the needle is placed in the cervical subarachnoid space (Fig. 16–67), a CSF sample is collected, and 10 cc of 22 mg I/2 ml contrast is instilled under fluoroscopic guidance. The normal cervical lordosis holds the contrast material in the cervical region. PA and lateral films are obtained; then PA oblique films are obtained by using appropriate film positioning and tube angulation — preferably without moving the patient. The oblique views allow excellent visualization of the nerve rootlets as they exit anterolaterally in the cervical region. If necessary, the patient may be rotated into the oblique position with the right side elevated slightly for viewing the right roots and the left side elevated slightly for viewing the left roots; however, this is less desirable than tube angulation.

If the dorsal aspect of the cervical subarachnoid space does not fill satisfactorily, the patient may be placed supine and the contrast allowed to bathe the posterior margin of the foramen magnum. Do *not* allow the contrast material to flood the intracranial system.

Lateral tomograms may be helpful for complete evaluation, and may be obtained with the patient either prone or supine, depending on the clinical situation.

Thoracic Myelogram with Amipaque

A lumbar puncture is performed, 3 to 5 cc of CSF is removed, and approximately 12 cc of 220 to 250 mg I per ml is instilled. The patient is then placed in the lateral decubitus position with the head cocked toward the ceiling. The head of the table is then tipped slowly down, and the contrast is allowed to flow into the dorsal region. Films are then obtained in the lateral and horizontal beam AP positions. The table is then tilted head-up to reaccumulate the contrast in the lumbar region, and the same procedure is repeated in the opposite lateral decubitus position. All motions should be made slowly to prevent admixing and consequent dilution of the contrast material.

At the end of the procedure the contrast is accumulated in the lumbar subarachnoid space, and the patient is returned to his room in a sitting position. The patient should remain sitting for 8 hours and then lie flat in bed for the next 16 hours, remaining relatively immobile.

Computed Tomography

Computed tomography of the spine can be performed at any level after the instillation of Amipaque.

Tips on Amipaque Myelography

1. Use fluoroscopic control to determine the amount of contrast material necessary.
2. The patient should remain as immobile as possible to minimize the amount of admixing of the contrast with CSF both during and after the myelogram.
3. Do not allow the contrast to flood the intracranial region because a grand mal seizure may result.
4. The presence of blood in the subarachnoid space has *not* been shown to complicate a myelographic procedure performed with Amipaque.
5. Patients should be kept well hydrated before and after the use of Amipaque to decrease morbidity.
6. Amipaque is not yet approved for use in children, although extensive pediatric trials have been performed in other countries.

COMPLICATIONS OF MYELOGRAPHY

Pantopaque.

1. Headache.
2. Coccygodynia.
3. Traumatic herniated intervertebral disk secondary to puncture technique with traumatic perforation of the anulus fibrosus.
4. Transection of nerve filament.
5. Confusion.
6. Iatrogenic intraspinal epidermoid.
7. Arachnoiditis.
8. Intravenous injection of contrast.
9. Vasovagal reaction with hypotension, nausea, vomiting, dizziness, diaphoresis and lightheadedness or even fainting.

Amipaque (added complications).

1. Grand mal seizures if an excessive amount of contrast material enters the intracranial area.
2. Severe nausea and vomiting.
3. Severe headache.

Arachnoiditis (Figs. 16–28 and 16–29)

Arachnoiditis can be seen following trauma and for unknown reasons. However, postsurgical arachnoiditis and the arachnoiditis seen after myelography are far more common and of greater interest and concern to those involved in the diagnosis and treatment of low back pain. The entity appears to be rare, although its exact incidence is unknown.

The myelogram in a patient with arachnoiditis reveals mild radiographic changes consisting of matting of the nerve roots (which appear thickened and clumped), obliteration of the nerve root sleeves and more extensive radiographic changes revealing irregular lacy interruption of filling of the entire lumbar subarachnoid space. In its most severe form, there may be a complete block to the flow of contrast material.

Pantopaque alone has been shown to produce arachnoiditis in some cases. The risk appears to be potentiated by blood in the subarachnoid space; thus, if blood is admixed with CSF at the time of myelography, Pantopaque should not be instilled. In addition, Pantopaque myelography followed by surgery may also aggravate arachnoiditis. The *exact* causes have not yet been identified. No known treatment has been shown to be truly effective with arachnoiditis.

Amipaque has produced microscopic evidence of arachnoiditis in all rats given an injection in the subarachnoid space. However, there have not yet been any proved clinically significant cases of arachnoiditis when Amipaque is used in the recommended doses. This is apparently true even when contrast material is admixed with blood before use, although this has not yet been proved clinically.

Text continued on page 770

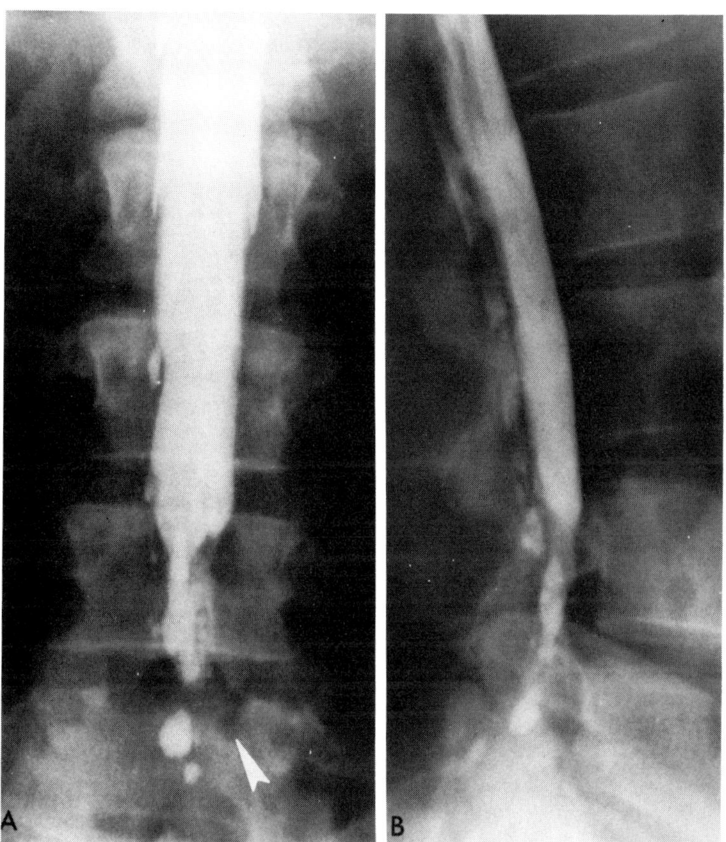

Figure 16–28. POSTOPERATIVE ARACHNOIDITIS: *A*, Instillation of contrast material was performed via a C_1–C_2 tap because there was no flow of CSF following several attempts at lumbar tap. There is failure of filling of the lumbar cul-de-sac below the L_4 level, with irregular globular accumulations of contrast material. There is obliteration of the nerve rootlets at L_2 and L_3. The partial laminectomy site is noted at 15 on the left side *(arrow)*.

B, The lateral view reveals that the nerve rootlets of the cauda equina are matted together to form an almost solid structure, which is placed dorsally in the lumbar subarachnoid space. The appearance is typical of arachnoiditis.

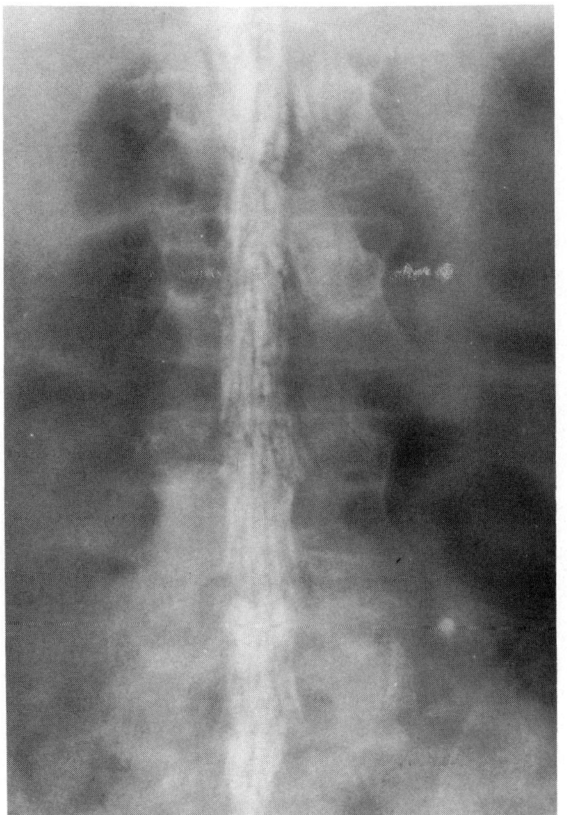

Figure 16–29. SEVERE ARACHNOIDITIS: Multiple attempts at lumbar puncture resulted in failure to obtain CSF. Contrast material was then instilled via a C_1–C_2 tap. The Pantopaque flowed slowly into the lumbar subarachnoid space, where there was demonstrated a diffusely abnormal pattern of accumulation of contrast with a lacelike, reticular pattern. The etiology was unsolved, but was felt to have an inflammatory basis. It is impossible to remove the contrast material in this situation.

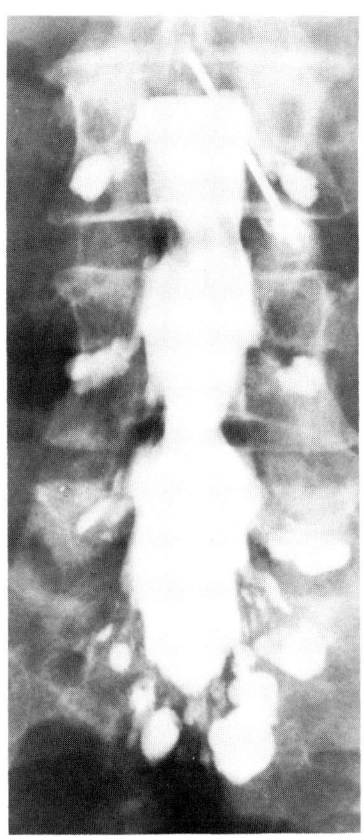

Figure 16–30. NORMAL TARLOV'S CYSTS (PERINEURAL CYSTS): Multiple cystic accumulations of contrast material are noted along the extensions of the nerve root sleeves. These are a normal anatomic variant and occur in different sizes and numbers. It may be impossible to remove contrast material that accumulates in these cystic areas. Indentations upon the contrast material at the L_4–L_5 and L_5–S_1 disk spaces are consistent with lumbar disk disease.

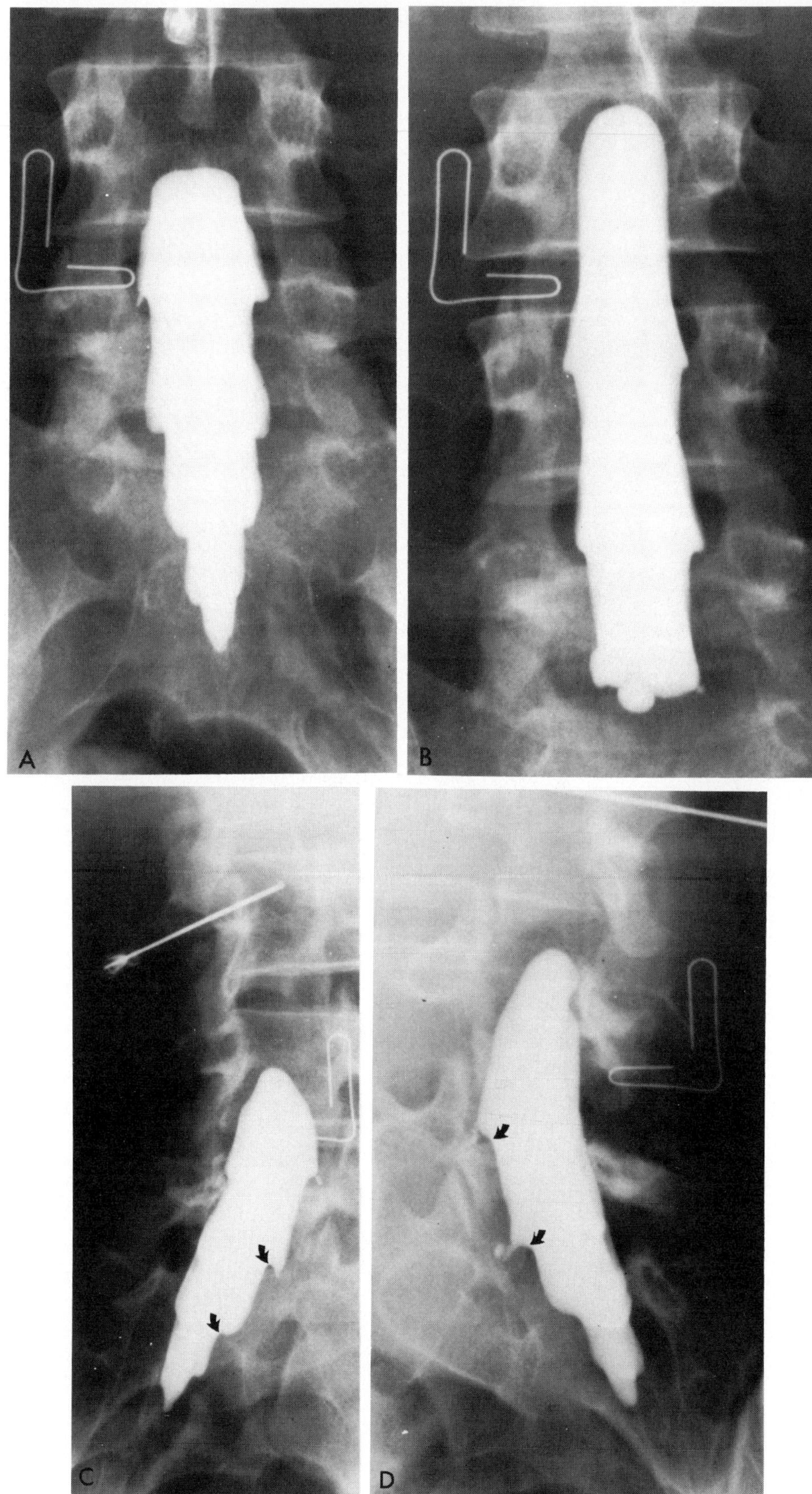

Figure 16–31 *See legend on the opposite page*

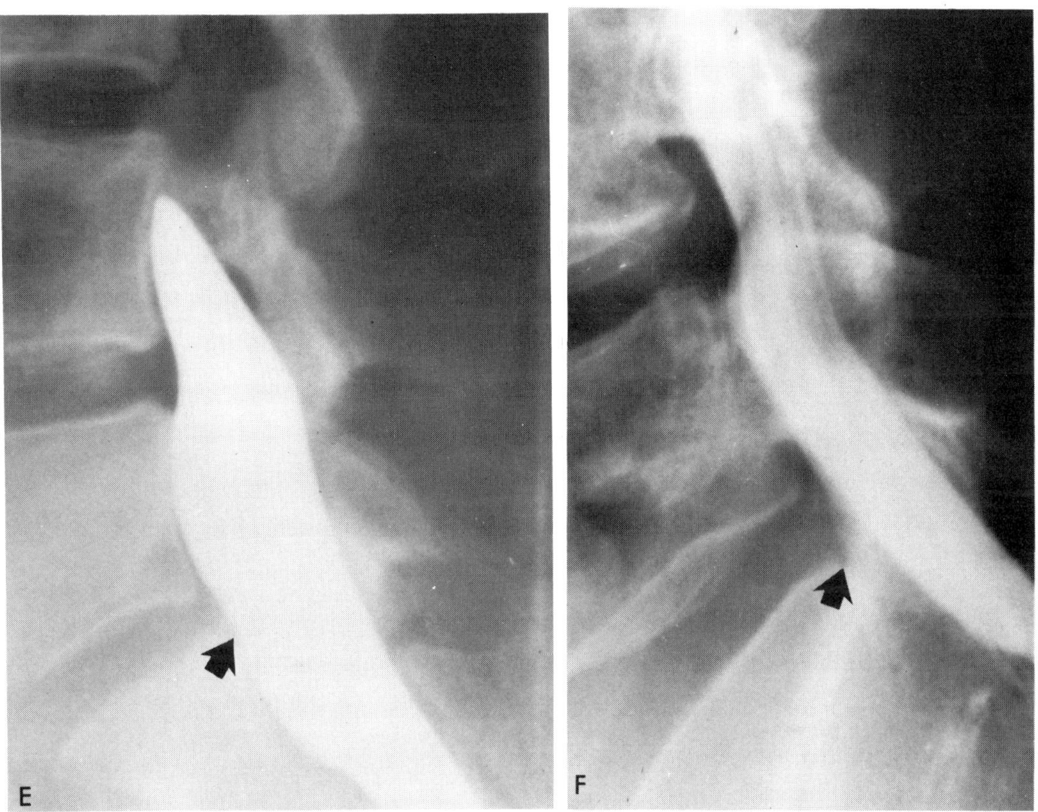

Figure 16–31. NORMAL MYELOGRAM: *A*, The upright PA view reveals side-to-side symmetry of the nerve rootlet sleeves.

B, The prone film continues to show symmetric nerve root filling.

C and *D*, The oblique views again reflect the symmetric filling of the nerve root sleeves, which do not vary by more than 1 mm from one *(arrows)* to the next when one side is compared to the opposite.

E, The lateral view of the normal myelogram demonstrates that the subarachnoid space is closely applied to the posterior margin of the vertebral bodies. (The arrow marks the upper margin of S_1.)

F, At the L_5–S_1 level, there is a large extradural space. The contrast column is posteriorly located away from the posterior margin of the vertebral bodies (the arrow marks the upper margin of S_1). This alteration is present up to the mid-portion of L_5. With a large extradural space the presence of a small- or even moderate-sized abnormal disk would not be appreciated on the myelogram.

A bulging disc is present at L_4–L_5.

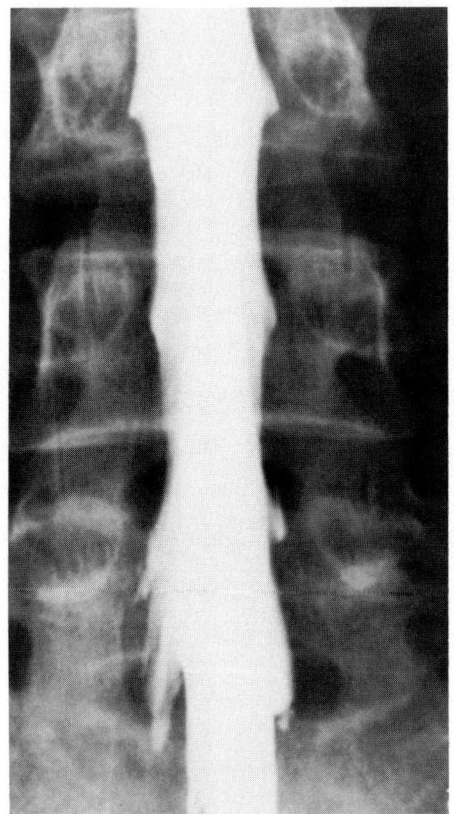

Figure 16–32. NORMAL ANATOMIC VARIATION: Here there is asymmetric filling of the nerve root sleeves. However, close inspection reveals that this is most likely due to an anatomic variation in the pattern of nerve root filling. No changes were seen on the lateral views.

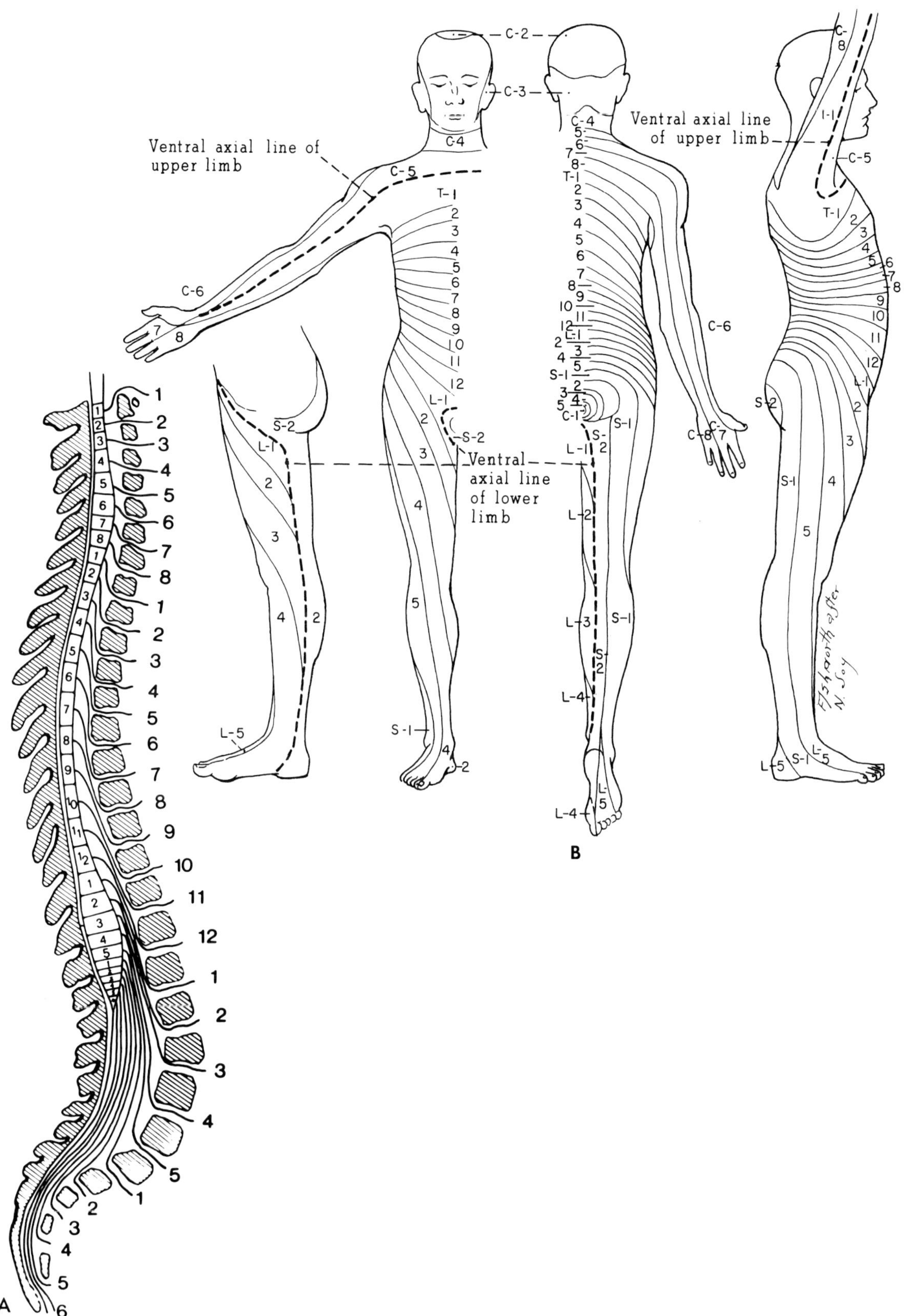

Figure 16–33. *A,* Normal spinal cord nerve exit levels relative to the bony spinal canal. *B,* The dermatome levels of the spinal cord nerves. (From Jacob SW, Francone CA, Lossow WJ: Structure and Function in Man, 4th ed. Philadelphia, WB Saunders, 1978.)

AMIPAQUE (METRIZAMIDE) CISTERNOGRAPHY WITH COMPUTED TOMOGRAPHY

A lumbar puncture is performed, and 4 to 6 cc of 180 mg I/2 ml Amipaque is instilled in the lumbar subarachnoid space. The patient is then placed in the 45° head-down position for five minutes and kept in the 15° head-down position until the completion of the scan. The contrast may be allowed to flow cephalad with the patient either prone or supine; the patient may be rotated 360° several times to facilitate the entrance of Amipaque into the lateral ventricles. Initially, the contrast should be kept below the puncture site and then allowed to flow rapidly cephalad to prevent leakage out of the puncture site.

The CT scan is then performed, either immediately or up to several hours after instillation. The contrast outlines the basilar cisterns, the fourth ventricle, the lateral ventricles and the cortical sulci. The patient should be kept in the 15° head-down position during the scan; this can be accomplished by placing him on a firm board or an emergency room stretcher.

Mass lesions appear as areas of negative contrast bathed by the high density of the Amipaque. This technique is especially helpful for use with mass lesions in the region of the sella turcica. It would appear that the availability of this new contrast material for cisternography may further decrease or eliminate the need for pneumoencephalography.

DISCOGRAPHY (Figure 16–44)

Discography is another method used to evaluate the presence or absence of disk disease. A needle is inserted into the disk, and contrast material (Conray 60) is instilled to demonstrate that the needle is in the disk and to evaluate the quality of the disk. A normal disk will accommodate only 1 to 2 ml of contrast, and the material will remain in a central location within the nucleus pulposus. If there is a break in the fibrous annulus of the disk, the contrast will be noted to run out of the disk at the point of break. In a posteriorly herniated nucleus pulposus, the contrast will run out posteriorly into the spinal canal. Discography can be used to diagnose an abnormal disk when the myelogram is normal or equivocal.

With a large extradural space at the disk space levels, a herniated nucleus pulposus not visualized at myelography may be demonstrated at discography. This is especially true at the L_5–S_1 level. On the other hand, a normal discogram may further substantiate the normal findings of other examinations. Discography can be used in either the lumbar or cervical region. The injection of contrast and disk puncture should be done with care so as not to create a break in the anulus fibrosus and perhaps a herniated nucleus pulposus.

The use of discography alone for diagnosis is to be discouraged. Neoplasms of the cauda equina may present with signs and symptoms similar to those seen with a herniated nucleus pulposus and would be missed if myelography were not performed.

Pitfalls and Accuracy. The procedure usually is performed under general anesthesia because it may be quite painful. At times, it may be technically impossible to position the needle in the disk space. It is theoretically possible to precipitate a herniated nucleus pulposus by puncturing the anulus fibrosus. With increasing age, an intervertebral disk undergoes a normal degeneration; the disk may appear to be abnormal, but this is not clinically significant.

Although discography has its limitations, a normal myelogram and a normal discogram can obviate unnecessary surgery.

RADIOGRAPHIC DIAGNOSIS OF LUMBAR DISK DISEASE

By far the most common type of extradural lesion demonstrated by myelography is the abnormal disk, which usually is seen at the disk space level and which creates a smooth extradural type of indentation on the contrast column. Occasionally the nucleus pulposus may be extruded out of the disk space and displaced either cephalad or caudad, creating an extradural defect not at the disk space level. This results in an appearance more suggestive of metastatic disease than disk disease. The history may help one differentiate between the two entities.

In lumbar disk disease, the symmetry or lack of symmetry of the subarachnoid space is of great importance when one attempts to make a diagnosis of an abnormal lumbar disk. Very small defects at the disk space levels may be considered to be protruding disks; larger defects, bulging disks and the largest defects, or those with a complete block to the flow of contrast material, may be considered to be herniated disks or, more accurately, herniated nucleus pulposus (HNP).

Symmetry or lack of symmetry of the nerve root sleeves as they extend down along the nerve should be noted in particular. If the disk is laterally placed, elevation of the affected nerve root sleeve and an edematous nerve root will be seen. The swelling of the nerve is secondary to irritation and/or mechnical compression. One should compare the appearance of the root sleeves from one side to the other on all views obtained. If the disk is not lateralized, the elevation will be symmetric. There will also be a ventral defect on the contrast column in the lateral films. With a laterally placed disk, there is often a prominent "double density" shadow on the cross-table lateral films (Fig. 16–37). This finding confirms what is seen on the other views. The radiographic appearance is created by the laterally placed disk elevating one side of the subarachnoid space more than the other.

When in doubt about the presence of a disk, the oblique views obtained with the horizontal beam (cross-table) are sometimes helpful in establishing the presence of a small, laterally placed disk. In complete block secondary to a herniated nucleus pulposus, the obstruction usually is at the level of the disk space, arising from the ventral aspect of the subarachnoid space. With this type of complete block, the contrast column will have a "brush border" appearance similar to the end of a paint-brush. This is most prominent in the cauda equina region, where the nerve roots are compressed together. This appearance is quite characteristic — nearly pathognomonic — of an extradural defect (Figs. 16–40 and 16–41). In addition, close inspection of the preliminary films may show the rare finding of a calcified degenerated disk fragment that has been extruded into the spinal canal (Fig. 16–34).

Abnormal disks are most common at the L_4–L_5 and L_5–S_1 levels. They also may occur at higher levels. These changes may be seen at multiple levels, and in 8 to 10 per cent of individuals are present at both L_4–L_5 and L_5–S_1.

Very rarely in adults one will encounter a lipoma or arachnoid cyst in the lumbar canal. While destruction of the vertebral pedicles may provide evidence of metastatic disease, pressure erosion or undercutting of the pedicles may be seen with growing tumors, such as neurofibromas, lipomas or arachnoid cysts. Scalloping of the backs of the vertebral bodies may be seen with long standing increased intracranial pressure (Fig. 16–19), with dural ectasia of neurofibromatosis in the presence of individual neurofibromata or with a lipoma or other spine tumors such as dermoids of the spine.

The subarachnoid space may be closely applied to the posterior aspect of the vertebral bodies (Fig. 16–31). If this is the case, a protruding bulging or herniated disk will produce a ventral indentation on the contrast column. These defects in the contrast column can be readily identified. However, a certain percentage of patients will demonstrate a large extradural space; the contrast column is then displaced away from the posterior aspect of the vertebral bodies. If this is the case, protruding or bulging disks may not produce an indentation on the contrast column. Indeed, if this extradural space is large enough, even the presence of a herniated disk may not be appreciated because the contrast column is displaced so far from the disk. The large extradural space is seen most commonly at the L_5–S_1 level, but sometimes extends up to the L_4 L_5 level.

In patients with a large extradural space and a normal myelogram it is helpful to perform an epidural venogram to evaluate the presence or absence of an abnormal disk. Discography also may aid in diagnosis in these cases.

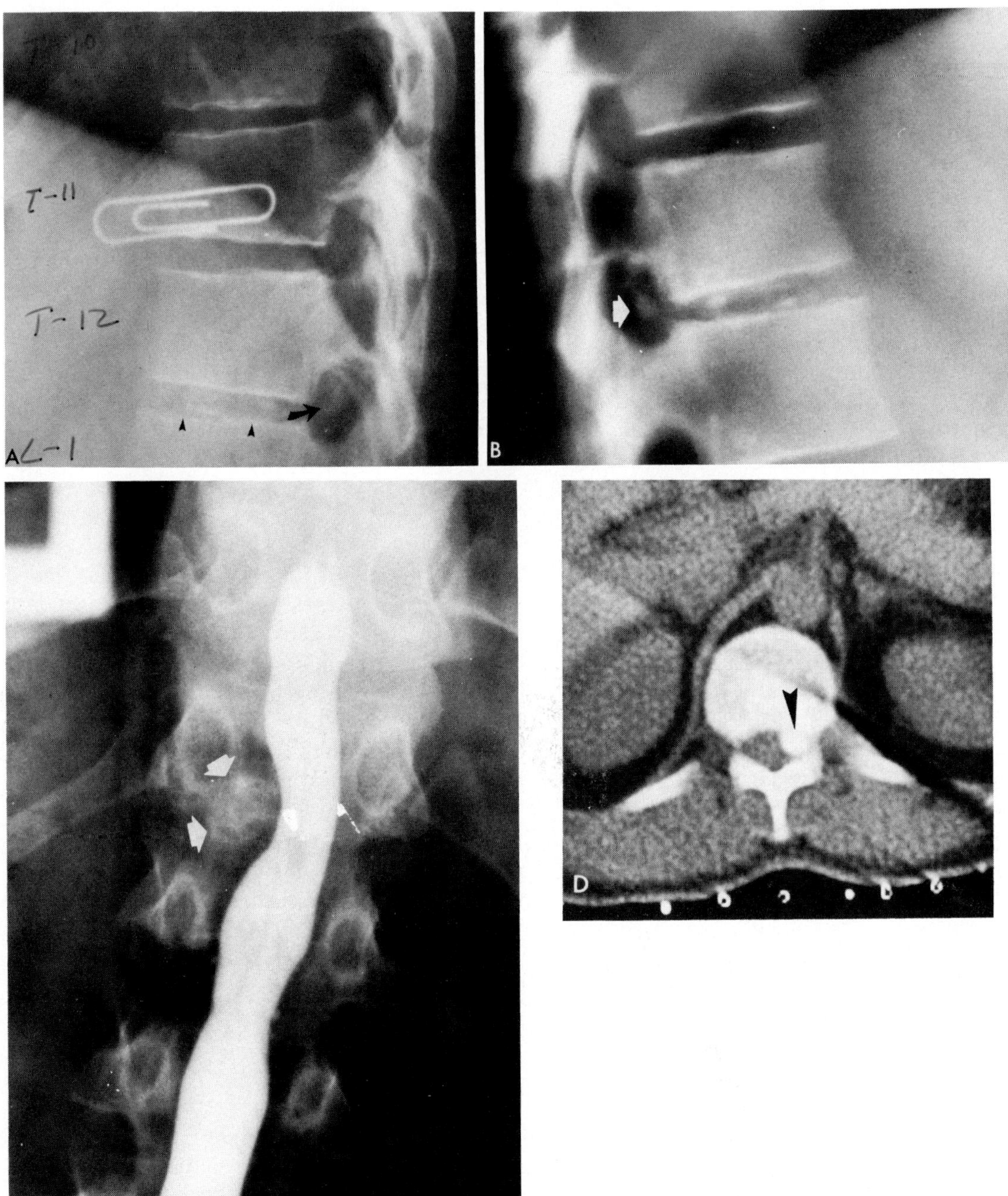

Figure 16–34. CALCIFIED HERNIATED NUCLEUS PULPOSUS: *A,* The lateral view reveals a calcified disk at the D_{12}–L_1 level *(arrowheads)*. In addition, there is an area of calcification posterior to the disk space that represents an extruded fragment of the calcified disk *(large arrow)*.

B, The lateral tomographic view shows the extruded calcified disk, which rests in the spinal canal *(white arrow)*.

C, The myelogram reveals that the column of contrast material flows around the calcified fragment *(arrows),* which rests to the left of the contrast column.

D, Computed tomography of the spine at this level reveals the abnormal area of calcification as it projects into and impinges upon the spinal canal *(arrow)*.

ACCURACY OF THE MYELOGRAM IN LUMBAR DISK DISEASE

Even in the presence of a herniated nucleus pulposus, the myelogram may be normal. The myelogram will be accurate in 80 to 85 per cent of cases. In most patients with normal myelograms, surgery will reveal the herniated disk at L_5–S_1. Far laterally placed disks may not be visualized by myelography, and a large extradural space also may interfere with visualization of an abnormal disk.

Postoperative Myelogram. Dorsal and lateral defects on the contrast column may be secondary to scar formation from a surgical procedure. A ventral defect should, however, be viewed with the same suspicion as a ventral defect noted on the preoperative myelogram.

Text continued on page 781

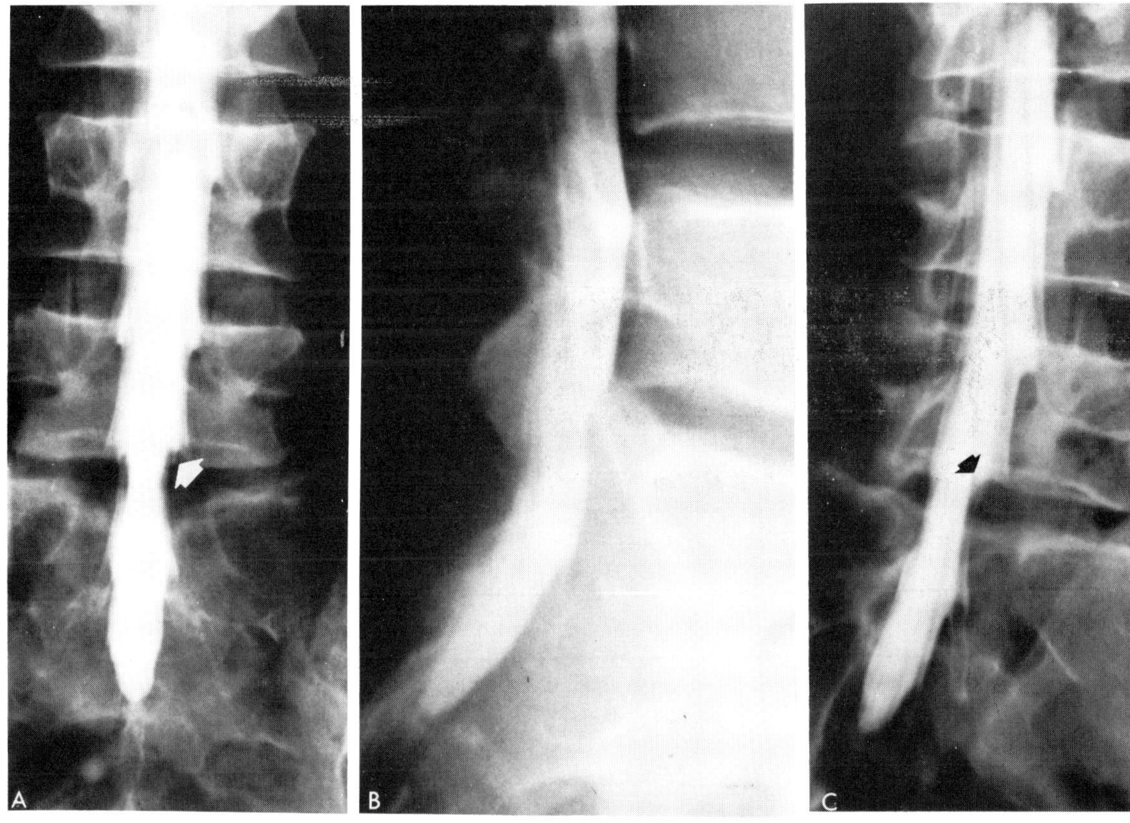

Figure 16–35. HERNIATED NUCLEUS PULPOSUS L_5–S_1, RIGHT SIDE. Myelogram (water-soluble contrast material): Routine views in the (*A*) PA, (*B*) lateral and (*C*) PA oblique views reveal a bulging disk at the L_5–S_1 level. On the PA view there is elevation of the nerve root sleeves bilaterally, but slightly more on the right side. A similar change is noted on the oblique view (*C*), which also reveals a slight indentation in the subarachnoid space (*arrow*). The lateral view (*B*) reveals a ventral defect in the subarachnoid space at the disk space level. Note the excellent visualization of the individual nerves of the cauda equina when the water-soluble contrast is used.

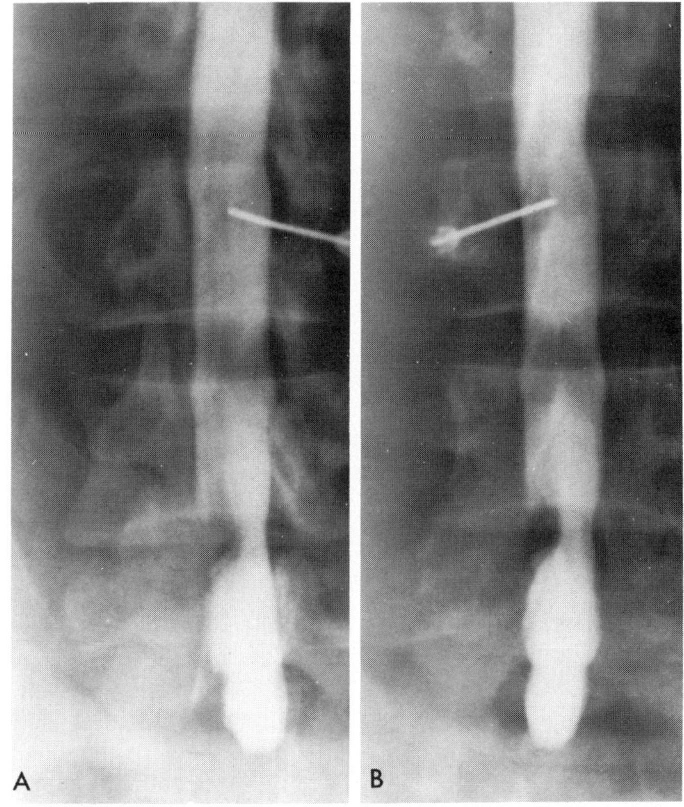

Figure 16–36 *See legend on the opposite page*

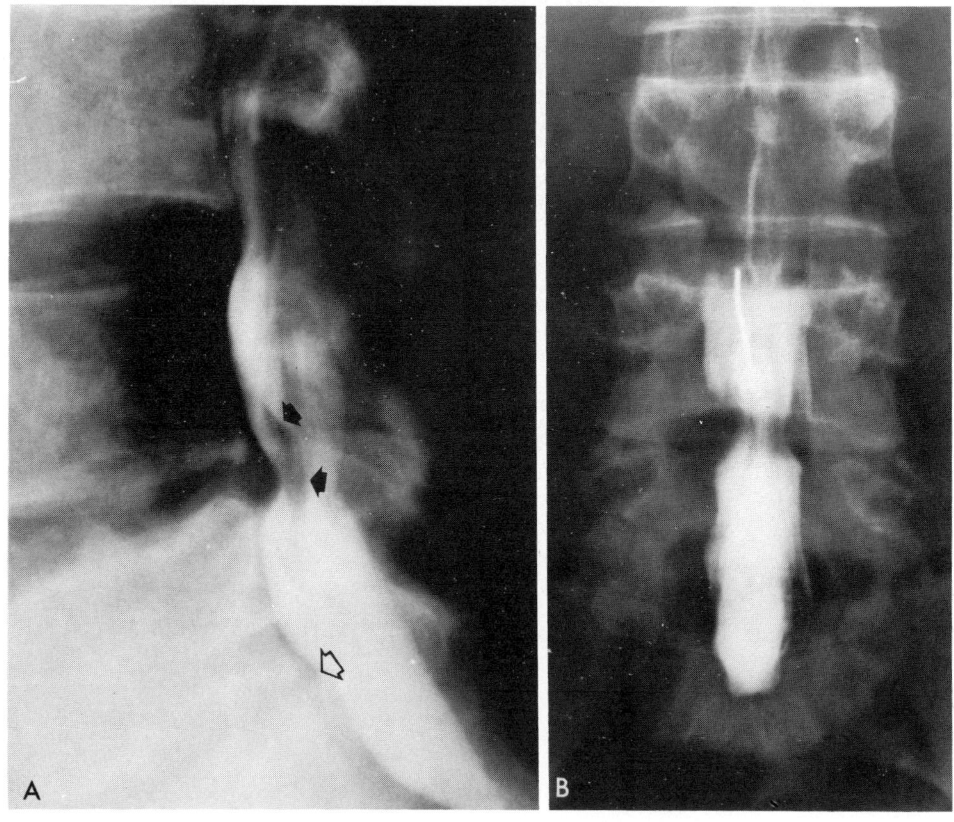

Figure 16–37 *See legend on the opposite page*

Figure 16–36. HERNIATED NUCLEUS PULPOSUS—UNILATERAL: The right anterior oblique *(A)* and PA *(B)* views reveal a large extradural indentation upon the subarachnoid space at the L_4–L_5 level on the left side. This finding is consistent with a herniated nucleus pulposus laterally placed on the left side. The nerve roots are edematous and can be seen just above the defect on the left. Note that there is poor nerve root sleeve filling at all levels, raising the possibility of previous arachnoiditis that has obliterated the sleeves.

Figure 16–37. HERNIATED NUCLEUS PULPOSUS: *A,* The lateral view reveals an indentation upon the ventral aspect of the subarachnoid space at the L_4–L_5 disk space level. In addition there is a double density shadow *(arrows)*. This occurs because the Pantopaque column is displaced further posteriorly on one side than on the other, since the herniation of the disk is larger on one side.

B, The PA view confirms this impression and reveals a bilateral defect, larger on the left side. In addition, there is reversal of the normal lordotic curve (open arrow in *A*) as well as posterior narrowing at the L_5–S_1 disk level—a finding that is very suggestive of a bulging disk at the L_5–S_1 level.

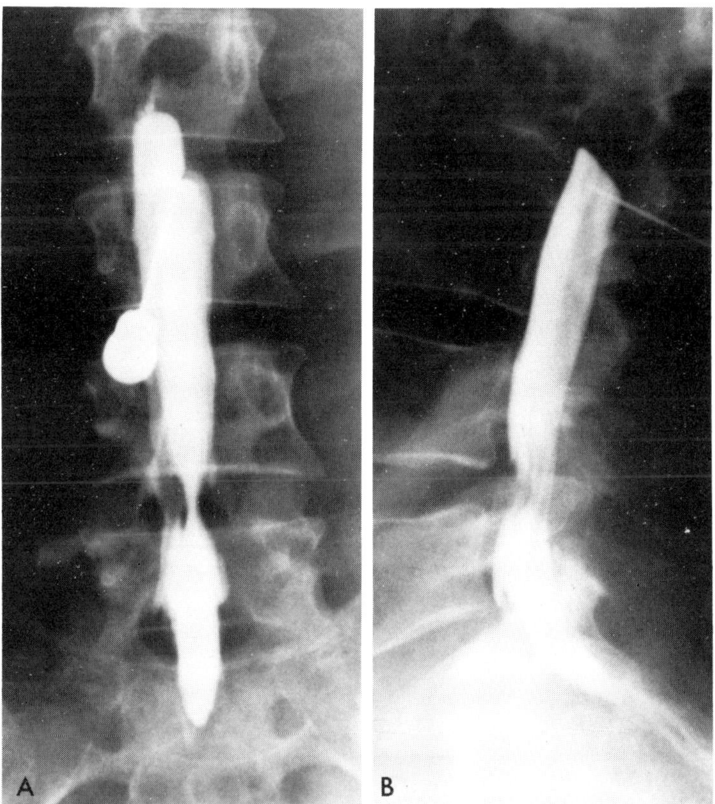

Figure 16–38. HERNIATED NUCLEUS PULPOSUS: *A* and *B,* There is a large disk at the L_4–L_5 level with swollen nerve roots and an "hourglass" deformity of the Pantopaque column. Incidentally, notice the "needle" defect of the site of the lumbar puncture on the PA view *(A)*. A ventral defect is seen in the contrast column at the disk level on the lateral view at L_4–L_5.

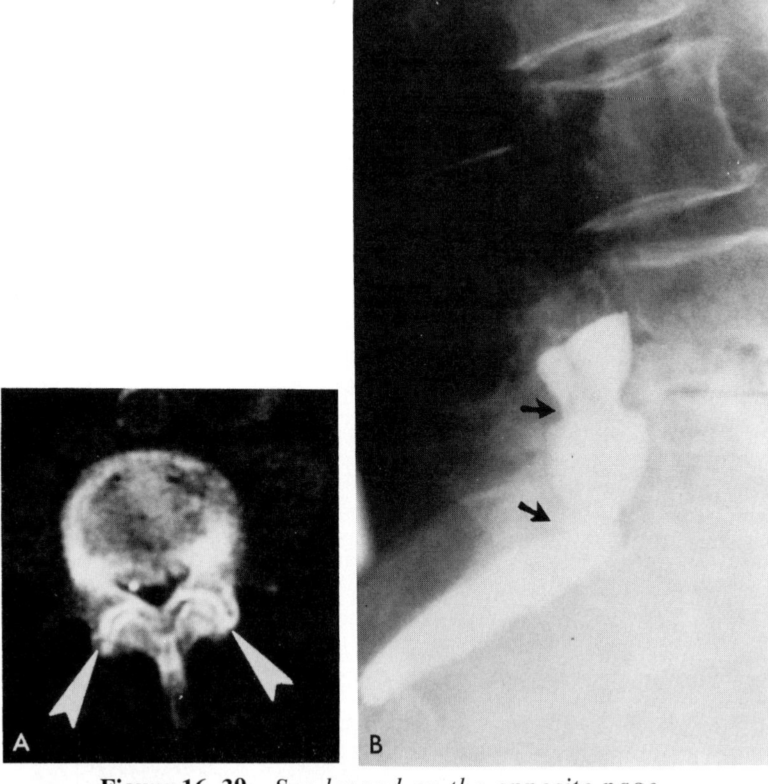

Figure 16–39 *See legend on the opposite page*

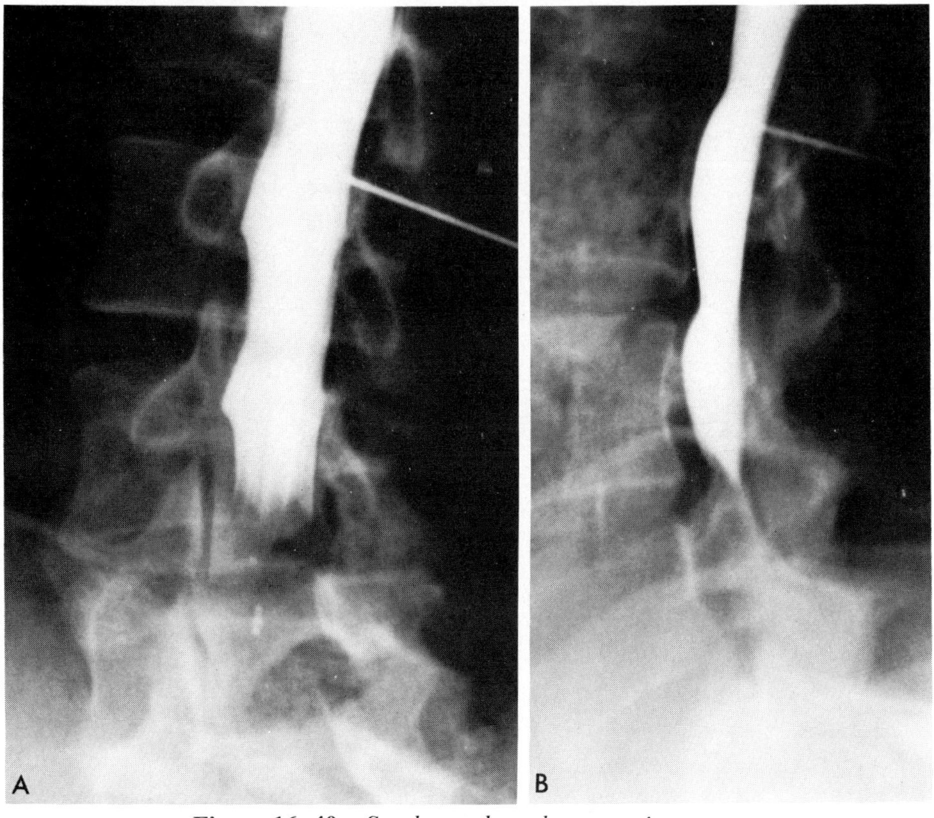

Figure 16–40 *See legend on the opposite page*

Figure 16–39. NARROW SPINAL CANAL: *A*, There is narrowing of the L_4–L_5 disk space and of the L_5–S_1 disk space, with posterior osteophytes that impinge on the ventral aspect of the contrast column. In addition there is hypertrophy of the ligamentum flavum and interfacet degenerative change, with impingement on the dorsal aspect of the Pantopaque column.

B, The CT scan confirms the presence of osteophytes and bony sclerosis about the articulating facets *(arrows)*. A single droplet of Pantopaque is in the subarachnoid space.

These changes have resulted in an acquired spinal stenosis.

Figure 16–40. LARGE HERNIATED NUCLEUS PULPOSUS—PANTOPAQUE: There is a complete block to the flow of contrast at the L_4–L_5 level. The contrast column has the typical "paint-brush" appearance of an extradural defect. The lateral view *(B)* demonstrates that the defect appears to arise from the ventral aspect of the contrast column just at the disk level.

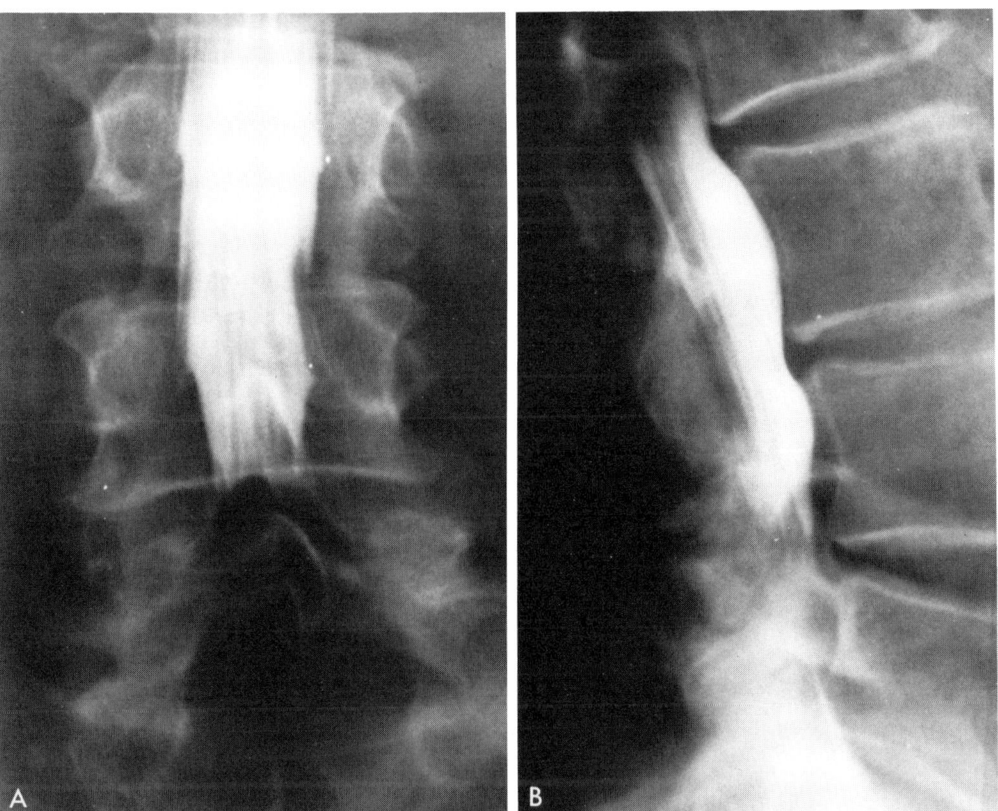

Figure 16–41. LARGE HERNIATED NUCLEUS PULPOSUS, WATER-SOLUBLE CONTRAST: *A* and *B*, There is a complete block to the flow of contrast, which has a "paint-brush" border. The obstruction is at the disk space level. Note the visibility of the individual nerve rootlets of the cauda equina.

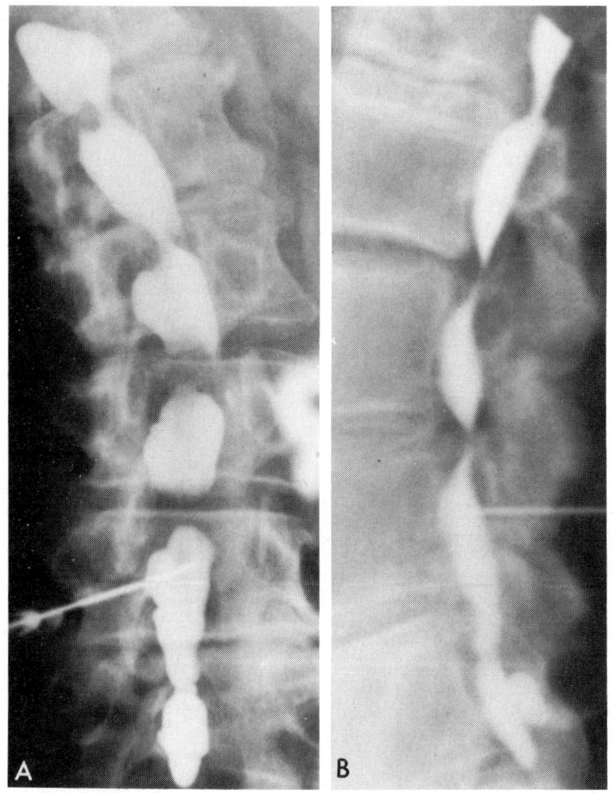

Figure 16–42. MULTIPLE DISKS: *A* and *B*, Defects are noted at all disk space levels. In addition, there is impingement on the posterior aspect of the contrast column, resulting in a narrow spinal canal.

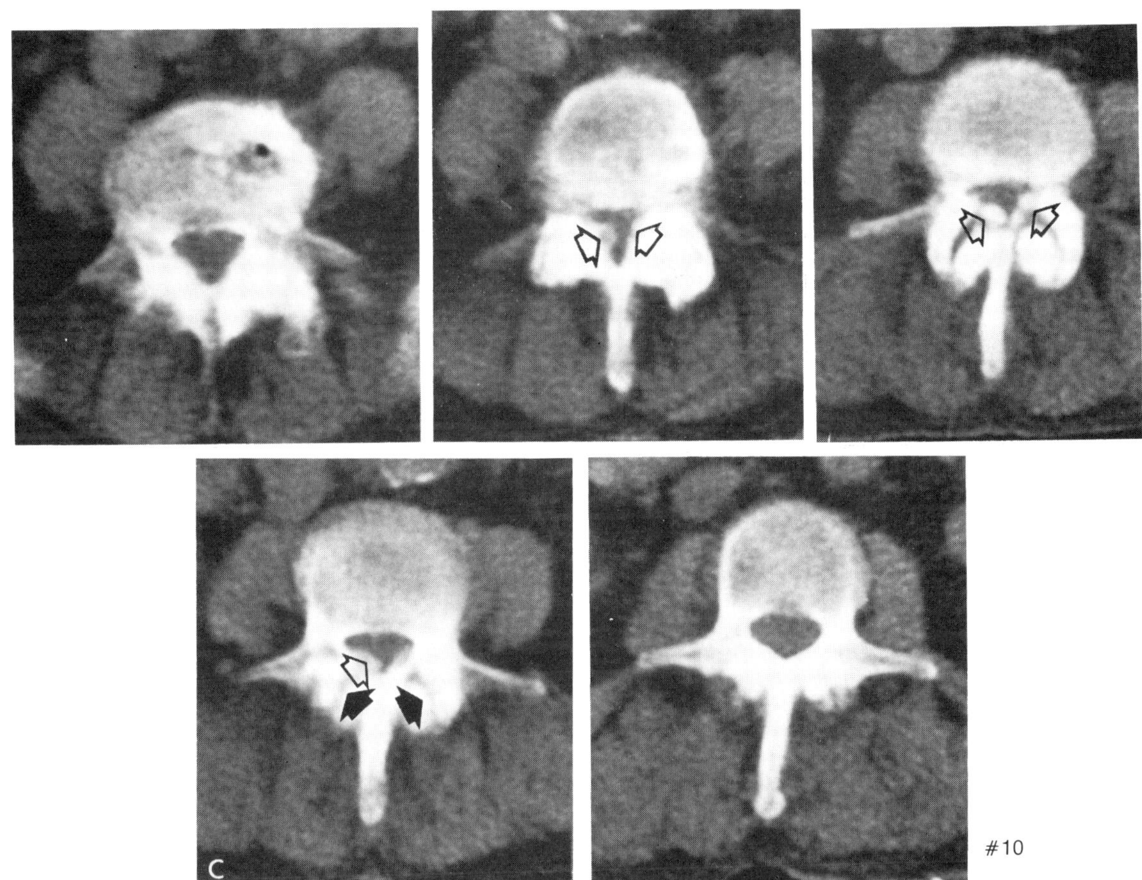

Figure 16–42 *Continued*

C, The CT scan demonstrates a relatively normal spinal canal in the low lumbar region (#16). The higher cuts, however, demonstrate marked hypertrophic degenerative change and encroachment on the spinal canal *(open arrows)*. In addition, there is narrowing of the interfacet joints secondary to degenerative disease *(closed arrows)*. In the upper lumbar region, the spinal canal again takes on a more normal appearance (#10).

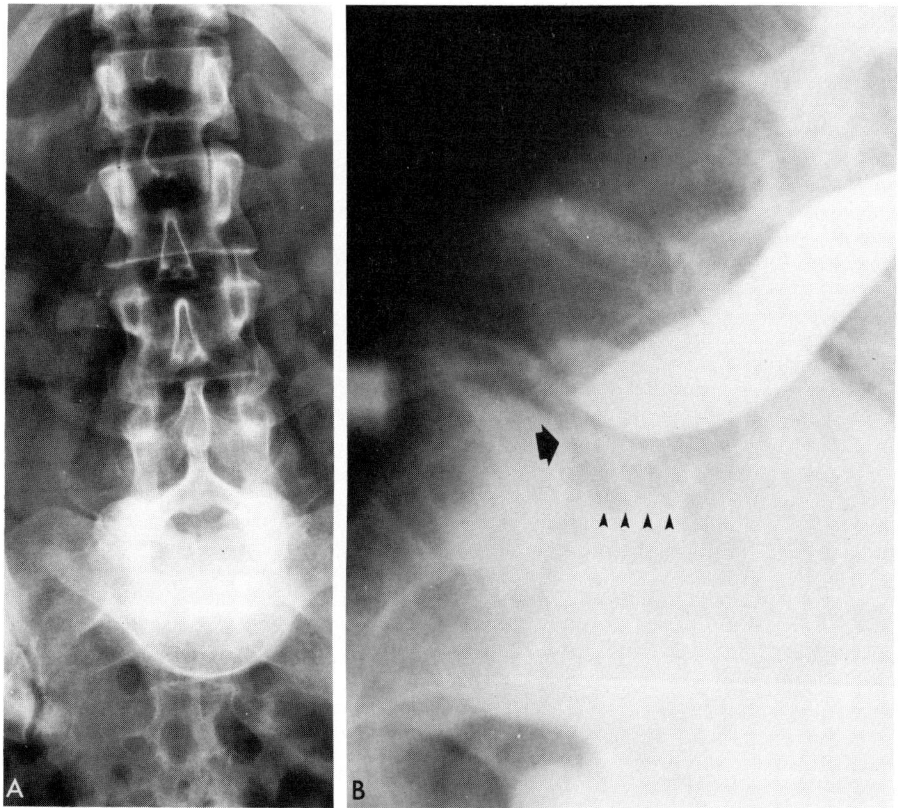

Figure 16–43. CONGENITAL SPONDYLOLISTHESIS: *A*, AP view of the lumbar spine reveals a "Napoleon Hat Deformity" because of marked forward displacement of L_5 on S_1.

B, The lateral view of the myelogram reveals deformity of the sacrum *(large arrowhead)* and marked forward displacement of L_5 on S_1 — Grade 2 spondylolisthesis, secondary to spondylolysis at the L_5 level. There is complete block of the flow of contrast at the upper border of S_1. A large space is seen between the contrast column and the posterior body of L_5 (*four small arrowheads*).

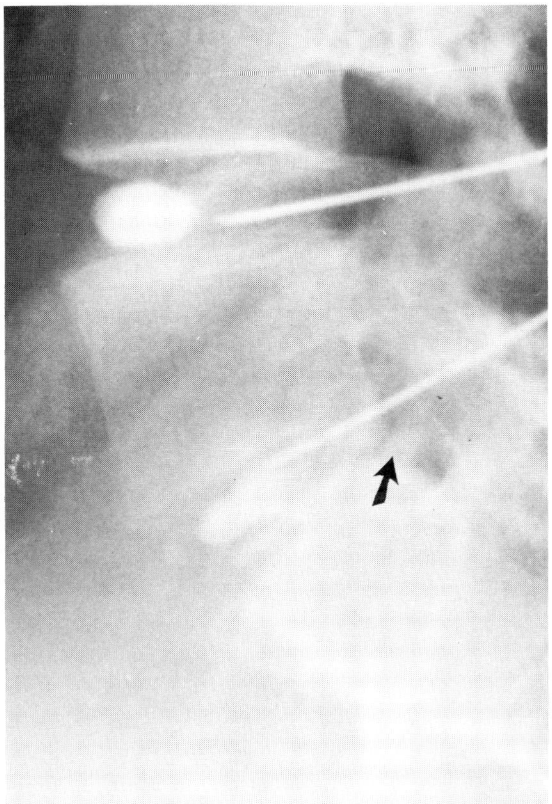

Figure 16–44. NORMAL DISCOGRAM: Via a posterolateral oblique approach, the tips of the needles are placed in the L_4–L_5 and L_5–S_1 disk spaces. Conray 60 is injected. The L_4–L_5 disk is normal and assumes an oval configuration. The L_5–S_1 disk demonstrates an irregular collection of contrast, which exits from the disk space posteriorly into the spinal canal. This is consistent with a herniated nucleus pulposus at this level.

SPINAL CORD TUMORS

EXTRADURAL

Second only to disk disease, metastatic disease is the most common type of extradural defect seen in an active clinical neuroradiology service. The size of the defect depends on the size of the metastatic lesion, which often is associated with abnormalities of the bony structures at the level of involvement (Fig. 16–45). When metastases are suspected, a close inspection of the preliminary films will be rewarding in many cases. If multiple abnormal levels (Fig. 16–46) are found, the patient will more likely be a candidate for radiation therapy than for surgical treatment.

In metastatic disease, the contrast column is compressed at a level other than at the disc space; not infrequently, multiple lesions can be demonstrated (Fig. 16–46). Myelographic abnormalities secondary to metastatic disease may or may not be associated with a detectable bony abnormality. Careful examination of the plain films may reveal a productive or, more commonly, a destructive lesion. Look carefully for a destroyed pedicle, since these often are the first areas involved by metastatic disease.

A complete extradural block to the flow of contrast material will give a "paint-brush border" appearance and may demonstrate what appears to be a circumferential narrowing of the subarachnoid space.

Primary tumors that commonly metastasize to the spine or its soft tissues are: (1)

breast; (2) lung; (3) multiple myeloma; (4) lymphoma.

INTRADURAL-EXTRAMEDULLARY

Neurofibromas (Figs. 16–47 and 16–48) and meningiomas are the most common tumors in this category. In neurofibroma, the patient may be known to have neurofibromatosis, and the plain film of the spine may reveal widening of one or even several of the neural foramina at the level of the neurofibromas. This enlargement is secondary to the dumbbell configuration of the neurofibroma (see Figs. 16–76 to 16–78). In these cases there is frequently a rather small intradural spinal component and a relatively large extradural soft tissue component outside the spinal canal that may be palpable in some cases.

Rarely, meningiomas may demonstrate a similar appearance, with widened neural foramina, because of bilobed development of the tumor. There is a marked predominance of meningiomas in women — about 80 to 85 per cent. Meningiomas occur most often in the thoracic spine.

The myelographic appearance of an intradural lesion is quite typical (see Fig. 16–21). At the point of origin of the tumor the cord will be displaced to the contralateral side — away from the tumor. The contrast column will form an acute angle with the tumor at its point of attachment to the dura and then bathe the tumor, creating a curvilinear line that has the appearance of a meniscus. If the tumor is of sufficient size, the spinal cord will not only be displaced away from the tumor but will also be flattened by the mass. Because the cord is flattened against the dura on the side away from the tumor, the contrast column on that side will be noted to form an acute angle with the spinal cord and with the dura. This appearance is very typical of an intradural extramedullary tumor. If the spinal cord is viewed as one is looking directly at the tumor, it may appear as if the cord is merely widened, with the contrast column thinned on either side. The appearance, because of the widening of the cord, is similar to that seen with a mass that is purely intramedullary. If at all possible, great care must be taken to obtain and examine closely views that are at 90° angles to one another. Failure to do so will result in errors of diagnosis. This is important because intradural lesions may be cured surgically, whereas intramedullary tumors usually cannot.

INTRADURAL-INTRAMEDULLARY

As the name implies, these lesions arise from within the substance of the spinal cord. The most common tumor of the intramedullary type is the ependymoma; the second most common is the astrocytoma — then syringohydromyelia abnormalities and then a variety of less common lesions. The myelographic abnormality demonstrates widening of the spinal cord in all views. This results in narrowing of the contrast column at the point of the mass lesion. If there is a complete block to the flow of contrast material, the contrast column will be widened and the contrast will form an acute angle with the mass at the level of the tumor (see Figs. 16–86, 16–93, 16–94). In all projections the appearance of the contrast column and its relationship to the spinal cord will be the same. If the widening of the cord is secondary to a tumor, this area of cord widening usually will be limited; if the cord widening is secondary to a syringohydromyelia, the cord will appear to be widened over a much longer segment.

Summary. Each of the three classes of spinal cord tumors may mimic the appearance of another if examined in only one view. Therefore, it cannot be overemphasized that views of the abnormality should be obtained in *multiple* projections for a more accurate diagnosis.

In addition, if any of the abnormalities reach sufficient size to cause a complete block to the flow of contrast material, the diagnostic criteria are often obscured or take on an appearance consistent with two different classes of tumors. Thus, an accurate diagnosis cannot be made. In some cases, additional information can be gained by instilling contrast material both above and below the level of the block in order to characterize the abnormality better. With a complete block, surgical decompression is usually performed; therefore, the information to be gained by both myelographic studies must be weighed against the risks involved.

DIASTEMATOMYELIA

This uncommon lesion consists of a fibrous or bony band that extends from front to back in the spinal canal at the lower thoracic level. This structural abnormality sometimes can be seen on the plain radiograph or by tomography, but more commonly it is not detected until the time of the myelogram. In addition to any physical symptoms that the patient may have, this abnormality is often associated with spinal dysraphism. Tomograms of the bony structures reveal a developmental abnormality in all cases. Because of the bony spur that divides the subarachnoid space, the cord is also split or divided in some fashion. This splitting and tethering of the cord by the bony spicule is the cause of the patient's symptoms and may lead to a scoliosis. Myelography reveals that the contrast material flows around the bony defect, creating a double shadow where the dorsal cord is divided. Because this abnormality is often fibrous rather than bony, the myelogram may be the only procedure that outlines the diastematomyelia.

Computed tomographic body scanning of the spinal column is helpful in the diagnosis of diastematomyelia. The technique is of great value, particularly after the instillation of Amipaque, when the CT scan may be the only procedure necessary to outline the abnormal anatomy (Fig. 16–51).

Text continued on page 792

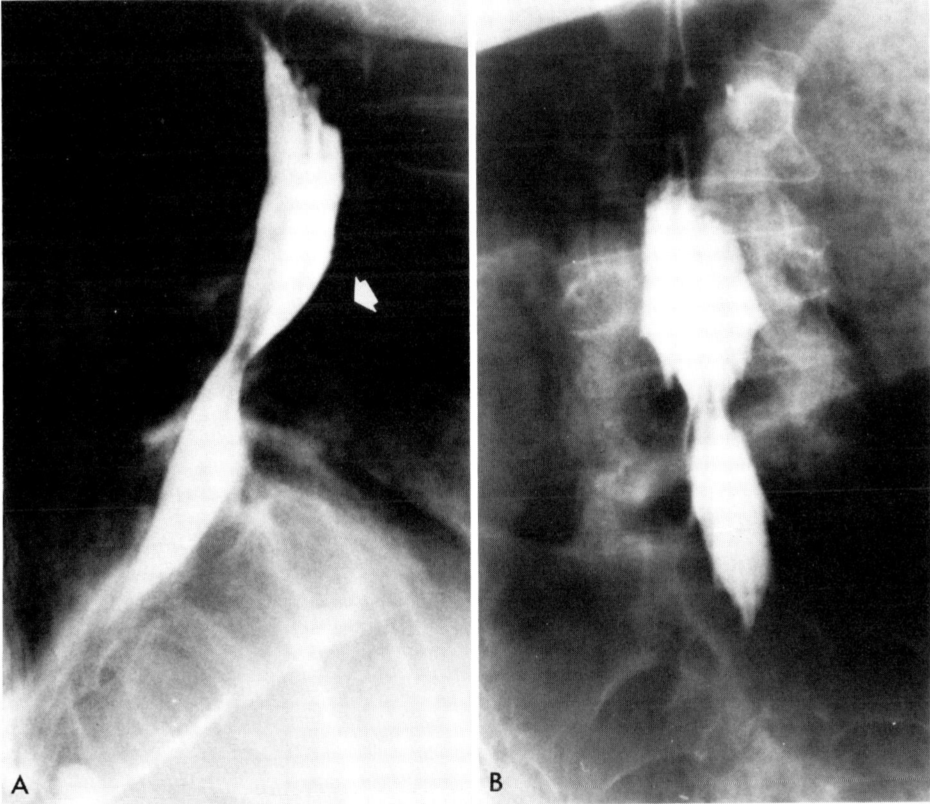

Figure 16–45. METASTATIC DISEASE: *A*, The lateral view reveals a ventral defect on the contrast column that extends over the level of the L_5 vertebral body and the two adjacent disk spaces. The white arrowhead marks the inferior plate of L_4. There is lytic destruction of the L_5 vertebral body, and the large soft tissue component results in the myelographic defect.

B, The PA view reveals irregular indentations on the Pantopaque column that extend over the vertebral body level. Destruction of the pedicles secondary to metastatic disease is again noted at L_5.

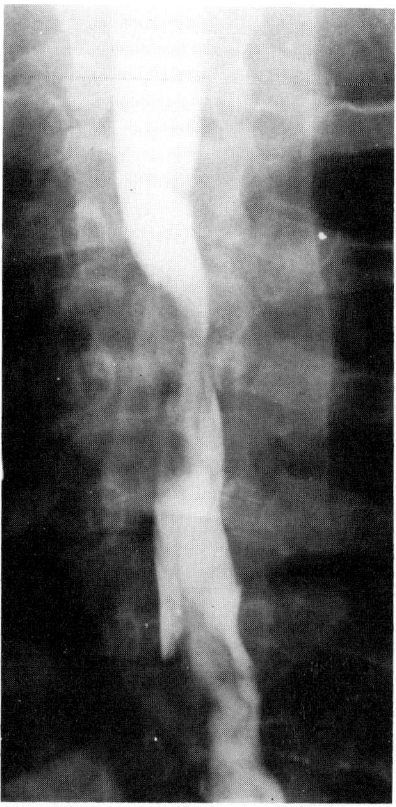

Figure 16–46. METASTASES: There are multiple indentations on the contrast column secondary to multiple metastatic deposits in the extradural space. This patient had a lymphoma.

Figure 16–47. NEUROFIBROMATOSIS: *A*–C, Views in both the lumbar and cervical regions reveal multiple rounded filling defects of the nerve rootlets. In the cervical region the cervical cord is displaced to the left by the large tumor *(white arrowhead),* while higher in the cervical region the cervical cord is compressed *(open white arrows).* These neurofibromas are the so-called "dumbbell tumors," which also have a soft tissue neurofibroma outside the neural foramina. At times the portion of the tumor outside the central canal is palpable in the neck.

D, The CT scan in another patient with neurofibromatosis demonstrates a dumbbell tumor *(T)* present in the soft tissues of the neck. The neurofibroma also extends into the spinal canal and widens the bony neural foramina *(arrow).*

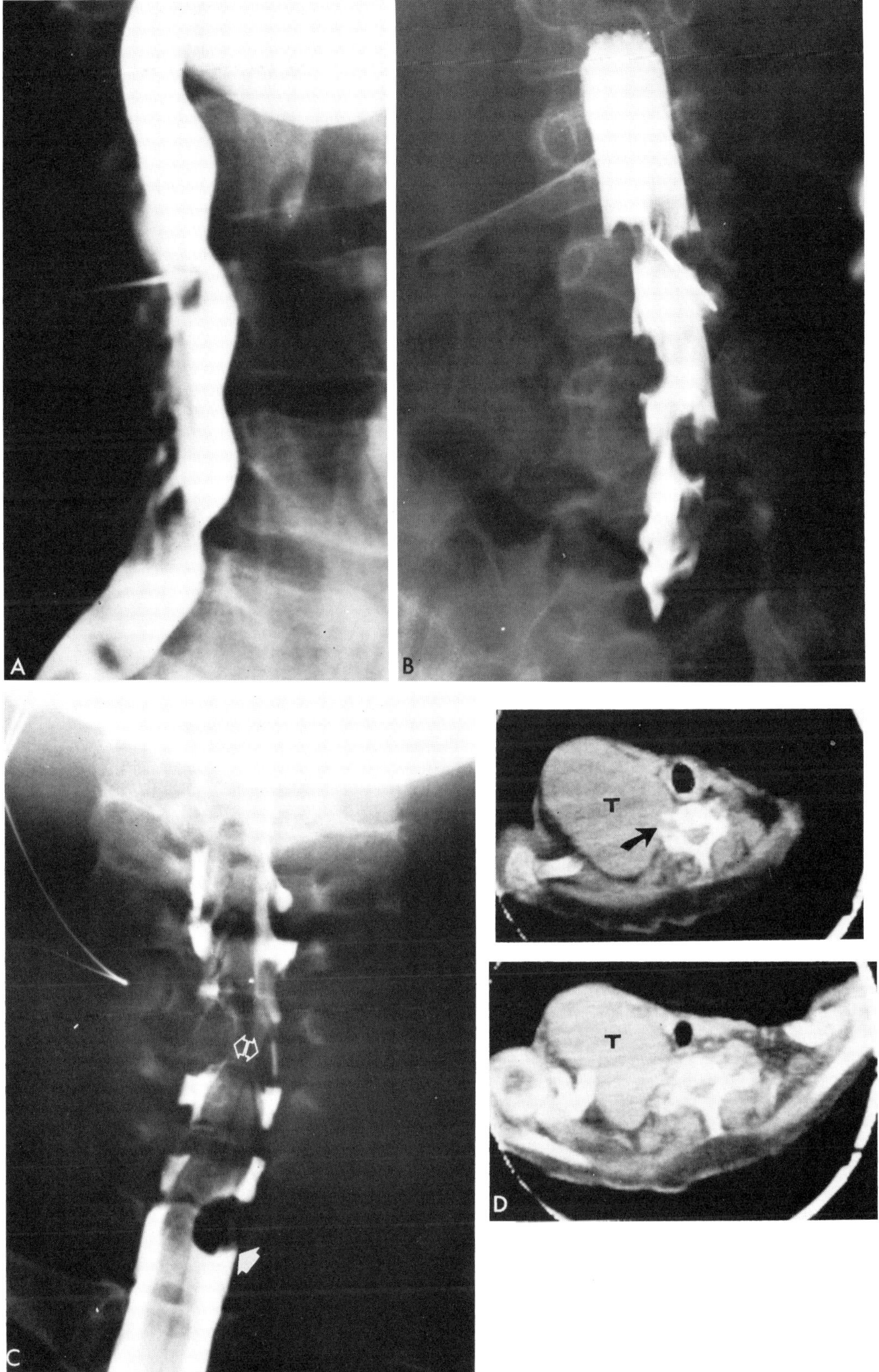

Figure 16–47 *See legend on the opposite page*

Figure 16–48. EPENDYMOMA: *A* and *B,* The lateral and PA views reveal a classic intradural extramedullary mass. The crescentic outline of the tumor by the contrast material can be readily identified on both views. The PA view shows the cord displaced to the left. Also present are large dilated vessels that overlie the cord.

C, Because of suspected disk disease, the lumbar puncture was initially performed in the lower lumbar region. Large dilated blood vessels are noted below the level of the block.

The tumor may actually arise from the nerve roots of the cauda equina and therefore be an intramedullary tumor.

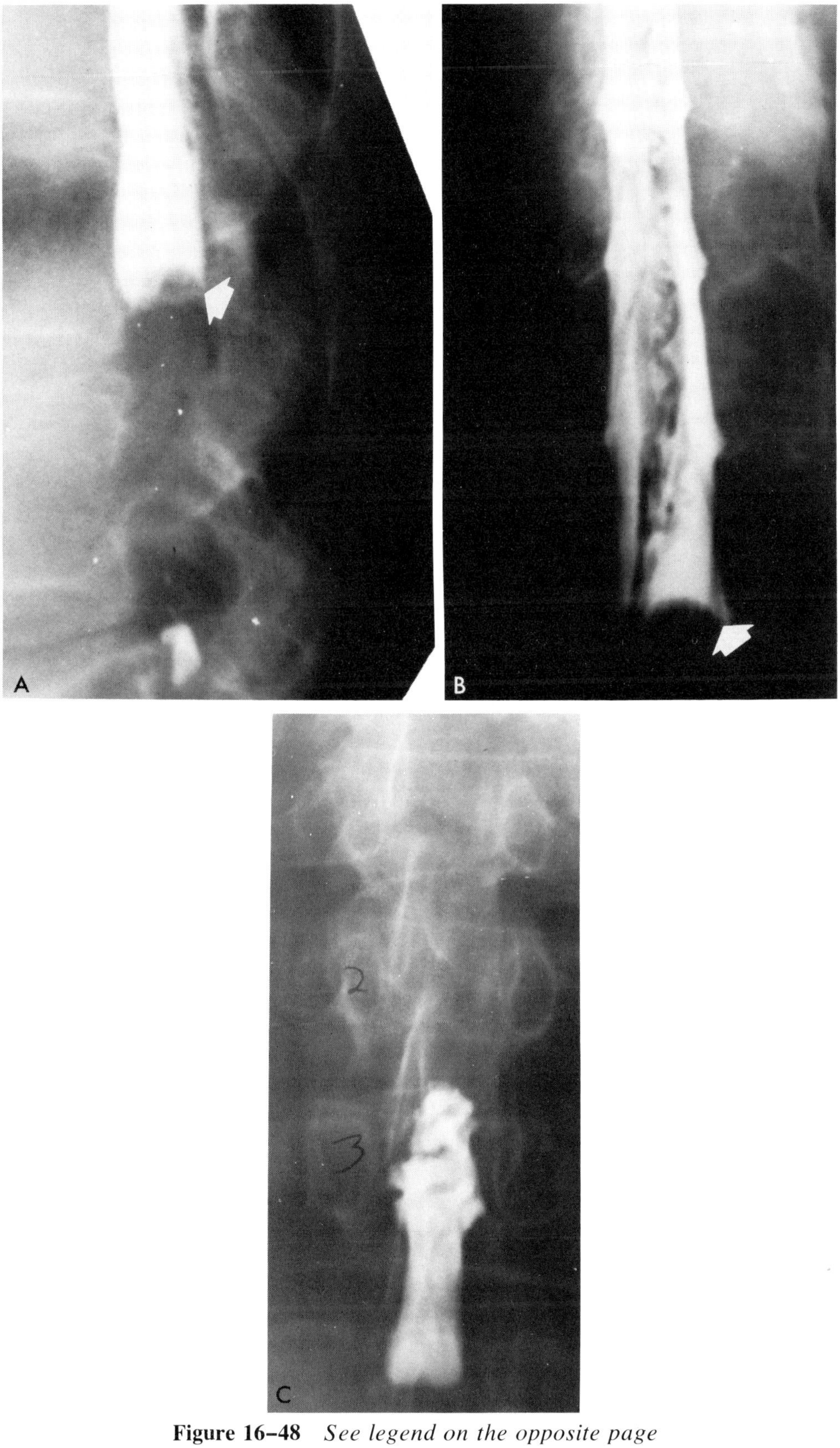

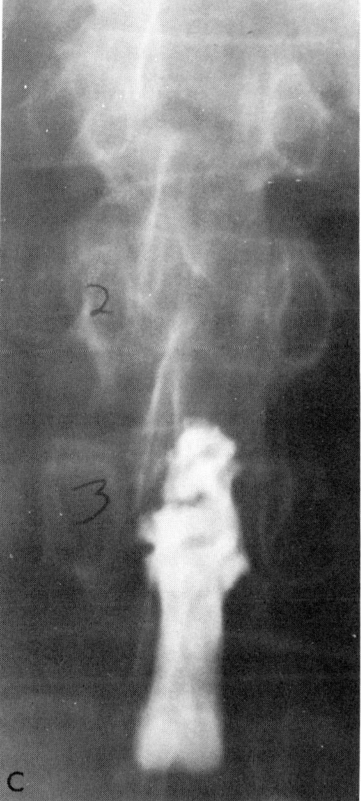

Figure 16–48 *See legend on the opposite page*

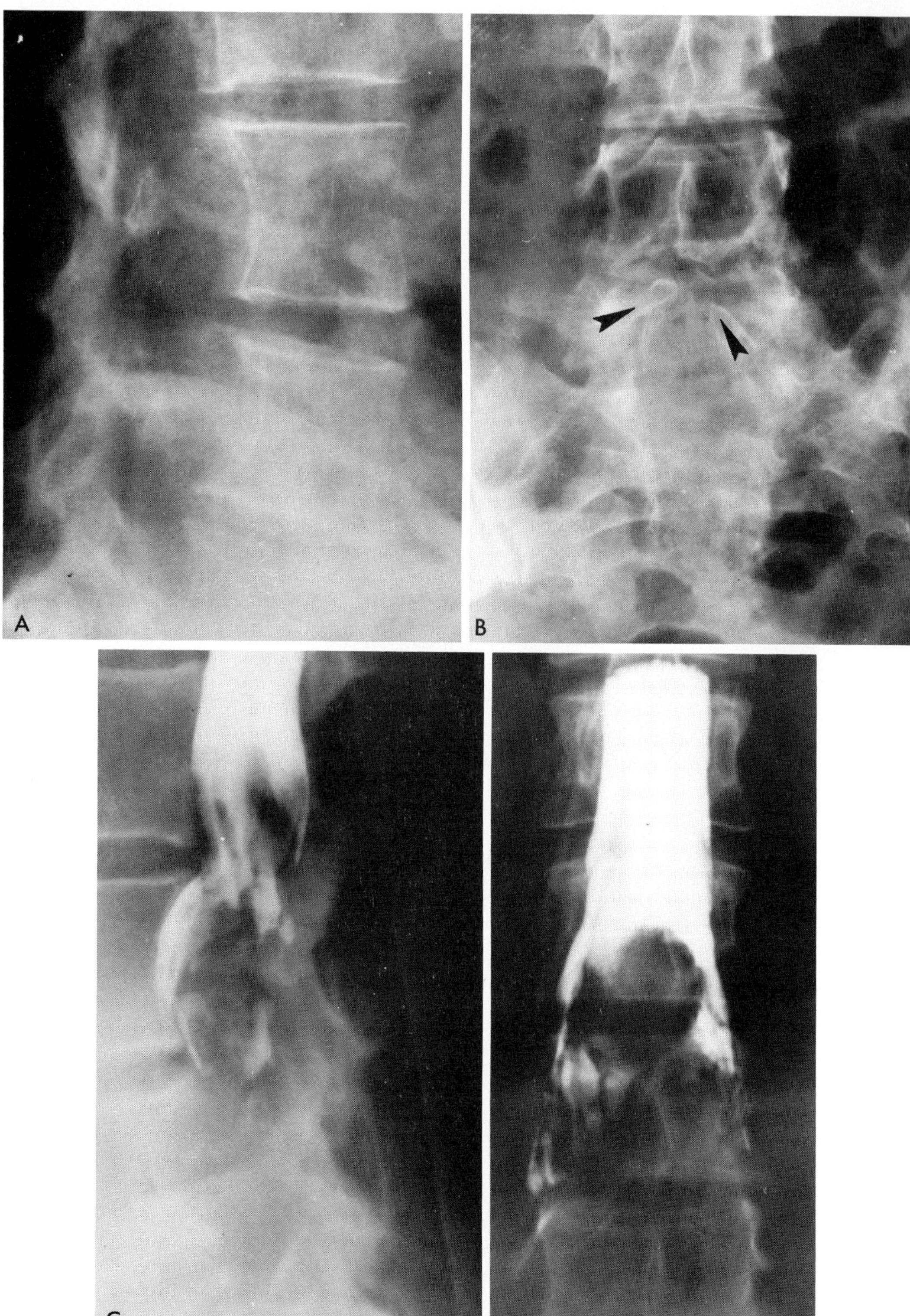

Figure 16–49. DERMOID OF CAUDA EQUINA: *A* and *B,* Plain film examination of the lumbar spine reveals a marked increase in the lateral and AP diameter of the subarachnoid space, with scalloping of the posterior aspects of all the lower vertebral bodies. In addition, there is a spina bifida of the L_5 vertebral bodies *(arrows).*

C and *D,* The myelogram reveals a large lobulated mass lesion that has expanded the lumbar subarachnoid space. The Pantopaque column outlines the upper border of the tumor.

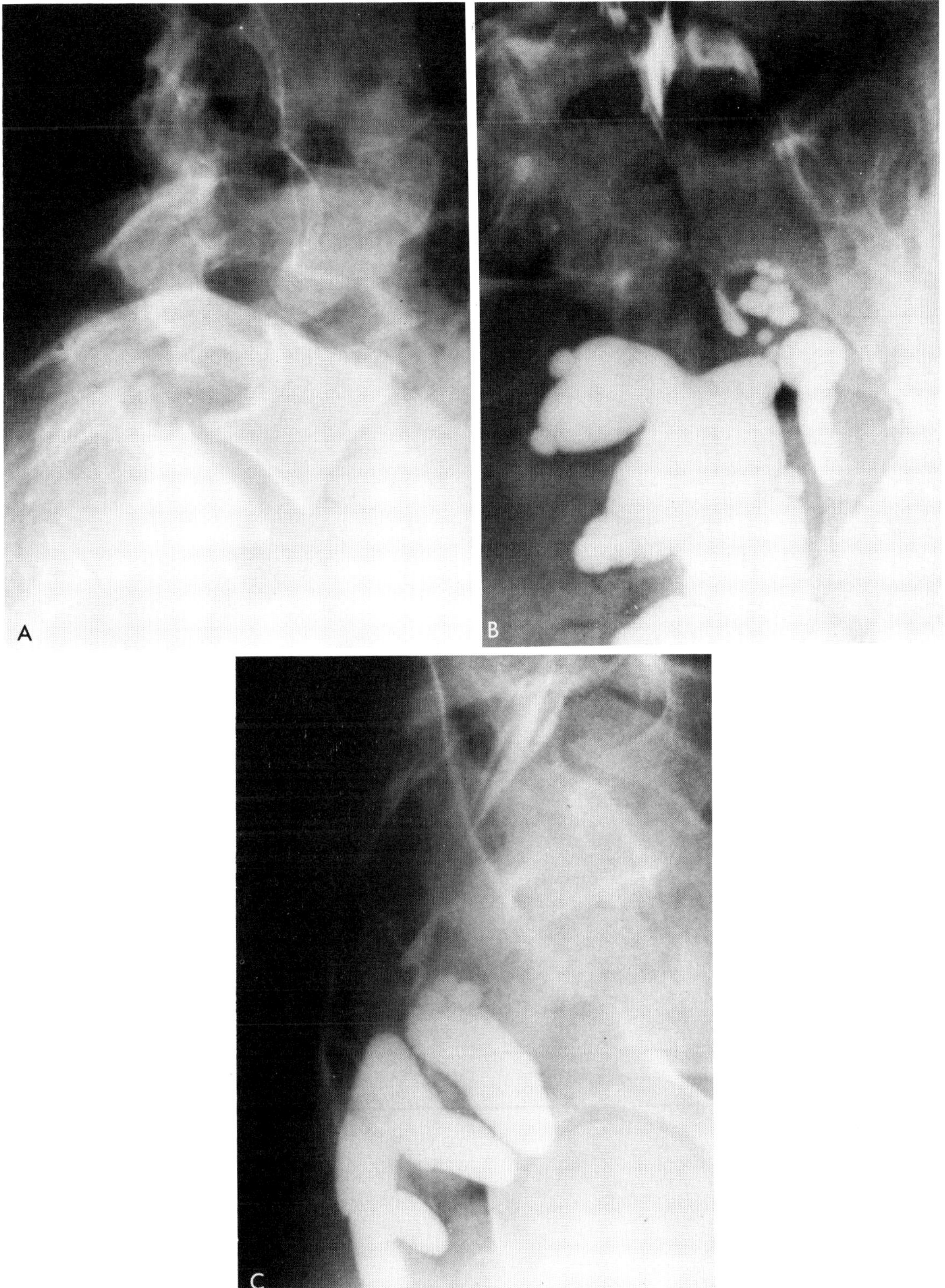

Figure 16–50. ANTERIOR SACRAL MENINGOCELE: *A*, Plain film examination reveals marked scalloping of the posterior aspects of all of the lumbar and sacral vertebral bodies. There is an increase in the AP and lateral diameters of the subarachnoid space.

B and *C*, Following the instillation of Pantopaque, a large anterior sacral meningocele is filled with contrast material. On the lateral view, the meningocele projects into the pelvic canal. This may present as a pelvic mass on physical examination.

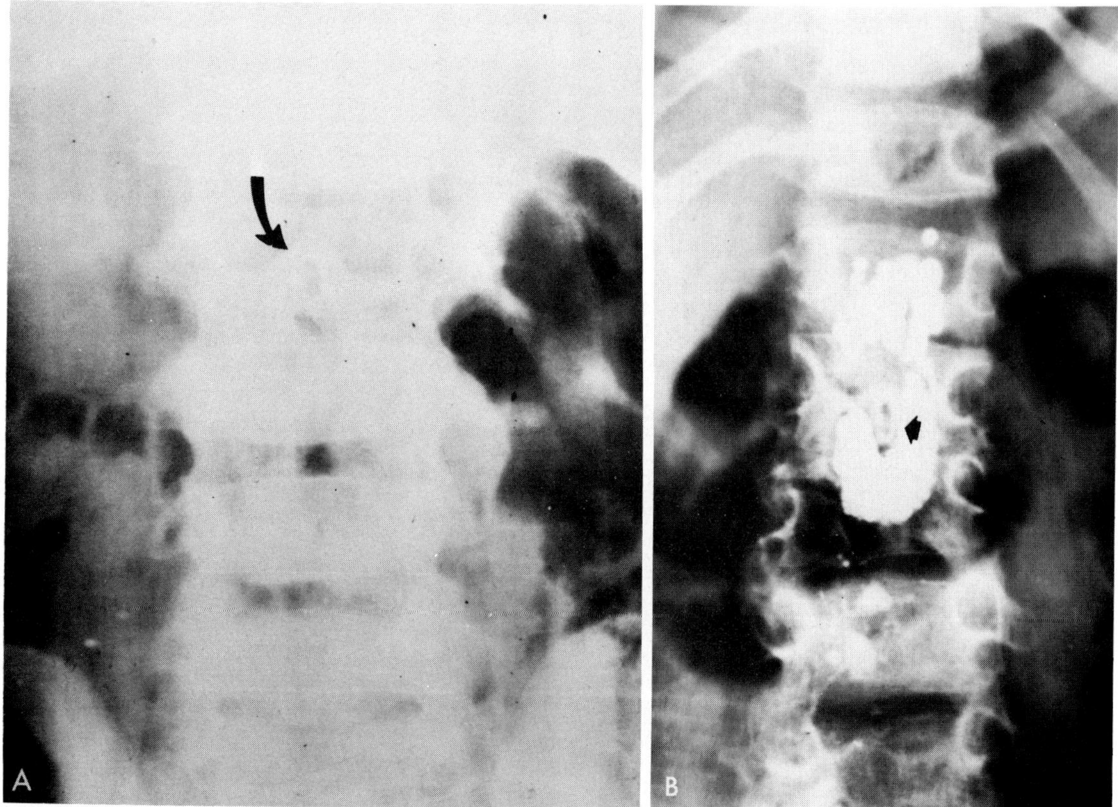

Figure 16–51. DIASTEMATOMYELIA: *A*, Plain film examination reveals a bony spur in the midline of the spinal canal at the L_3 level.

B, Myelographic study in another case of diastematomyelia reveals the bony cleft surrounded by Pantopaque. Note the abnormal vertebral bodies at the level of the bony cleft. Diastematomyelia is always associated with a bony abnormality of the vertebral bodies.

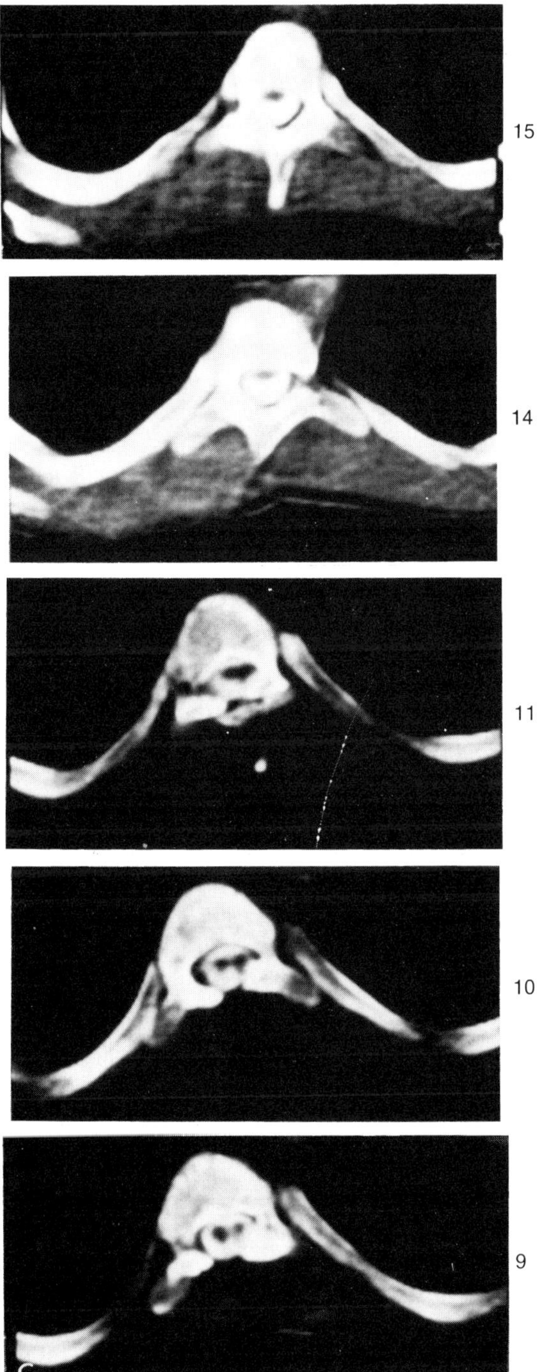

Figure 16–51 *Continued*

C, The CT scan following the instillation of Amipaque demonstrates evidence of spinal dysrhaphia (#11, 10, 9) with absence of the spinous processes. In addition, a diplomyelia (double spinal cord) has developed because of the diastematomyelia. The bony spur had previously been removed surgically. The diplomyelia is best seen on #09, 10 and 11; above this level (#14, 15), a normal cord and bony spinal column are demonstrated.

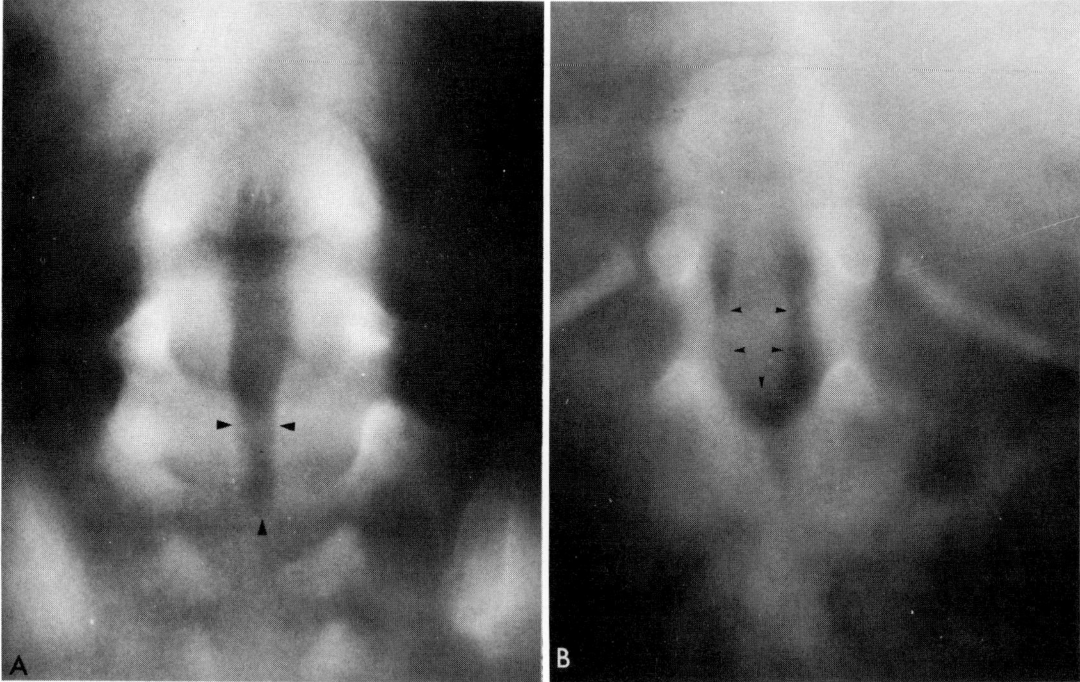

Figure 16–52. AIR MYELOGRAM: *A,* The outline of the lumbar cul-de-sac *(arrowheads).* Higher in the spinal canal *(B),* the air outlines the conus medullaris of the spinal cord *(arrowheads).* These views were obtained with the patient in the supine position with the body in the Trendelenburg position. Tomographic views are necessary.

CERVICAL SPINE RADIOGRAPHIC ANATOMY

Radiography of the cervical spine includes anteroposterior, lateral and oblique views as well as an AP view of the odontoid process (Fig. 16–53). C_2–C_7 will be considered together in this section; C_1 will be considered separately.

The cervical spine vertebrae are unique when compared to those of the remainder of the spine. A well developed "lateral mass" is present on each of the cervical vertebral bodies. The pedicles of the cervical vertebrae project more posterolaterally than elsewhere in the spine and so are less well seen in the AP projection. The lateral mass is made up of: (1) Transverse process; (2) Foramina transversaria; (3) Articulating facets; (4) Apophyseal joints.

The foramina transversaria at the C_1 level are more lateral in position than at other levels of the cervical spine. The vertebral artery normally enters the foramina transversaria at C_6, but may enter at any level. The vertebral artery exists above C_2; it then courses laterally and then superiorly, where it re-enters the foramina transversaria of C_1 and turns 90° posteriorly to lie in a groove along the top of the C_1 vertebral body. It then courses anteromedially to enter the skull through the foramen magnum.

The odontoid process is in close relationship to the anterior arch of C_1, and should not be displaced posteriorly more than 3 mm in the adult (Fig. 16–57). The odontoid is held in position by the transverse and cruciate ligaments. Following soft tissue trauma or in rheumatoid arthritis (which causes relaxation of the ligaments), there may be subluxation of the odontoid from the atlas. Trauma also may result in fractures of the odontoid. A variety of other fractures may occur (Fig. 16–58), but a discussion is beyond the scope of this book.

Unlike studies of the lumbar spine, positioning for oblique views no longer reveals the areas of interest "through" the vertebral bodies. When the patient is in the RAO position, we view the lateral masses and the right neural foramina. The anatomic right marker will indicate the right side, which is the side of interest. Similarly, with the patient in the LAO position we view the left neural foramina and left lateral mass. This radiographic projection in the cervical region occurs because the lateral mass is nearly lateral to the vertebral body. The articulation of each lateral mass with the adjacent lateral mass is the apophyseal joint. This is a synovial joint, and degenerative changes may occur at this level and encroach posteriorly upon the neural foramina.

Each cervical vertebral body contains a small thin piece of bone that projects superiorly along the lateral and superior edge of each vertebra. This is the *uncinate* process. Each higher vertebral body is consequently beveled along its inferior lateral margin in a corresponding fashion so that it articulates with the uncinate process to form the *joints of Luschka* (Fig. 16–53). The joints of Luschka are not true synovial joints, but do develop degenerative osteophytes. The *normal* uncinate process should not be mistaken for osteophytes.

The normal cervical spinal cord itself measures 10 mm in its anteroposterior dimension. The cervical subarachnoid space is limited anteriorly by the back of the vertebral bodies and posteriorly by the level where the laminae of each side fuse together to form the dorsal spinous process. *Where* they fuse appears as a white line — the spinal laminar line — on the lateral view because the point of bony union is viewed tangentially. The average anteroposterior dimension of the bony subarachnoid space normally measures 17 mm. It may normally measure 14 mm at a minimum and 20 mm at a maximum.

In general, the indications for cervical myelography are similar to those for lumbar myelography. If the study is being performed with particular reference to the cervical area, the lumbar tap for contrast instillation can theoretically be performed at any level in the lumbar region. It should be noted that if the study is being done for possible cervical disk disease, there is often symptomatic or asymptomatic lumbar disk disease as well. Thus it is best to perform the puncture at L_3–L_4 — away from the most common levels of lumbar disk disease.

Following instillation, the contrast material is allowed to flow cephalad while the patient extends the neck and elevates the head, assisted by a pillow under the chin. At the same time, the table is tilted with the patient's head down until the contrast reaches the cervical region. The head should be kept straight. Once the contrast is in the cervical region, the patient may be returned to the horizontal position, as the normal cervical lordosis will hold the Pantopaque in the cervical region. Films should be obtained in the PA and lateral projections, with the contrast covering all levels of the cervical spine, including the clivus. (Note that since the advent of computed tomography of the head most of the intracranial portion of the study will be covered by a routine head scan.) In addition, films may be obtained in both the PA prone vertical beam oblique projections as well as in the lateral horizontal (cross-table) oblique projections. Again, the radiographic filming should be altered to aid and facilitate diagnosis in each individual case (Fig. 16–60).

Because of various alterations in radiographic equipment and myelographic filming, it is difficult to speak of cervical cord size in terms of absolutes; rather, it must be discussed in terms of its relationship to the bony cervical spine. The cord can be seen outlined in the pool of Pantopaque (Fig. 16–60) as the gray shadow in the middle of the Pantopaque pool.

The cervical spinal cord normally has an area of widening in its mid-portion that is largest at the C_6 level but that expands from C_3 to T_3. This normal widening should not be mistaken for an intramedullary lesion. The normal thoracic cord is smaller than the cervical cord and is approximately the size of the smallest digit of the hand. This normal localized area of widening of the cord serves to accommodate the increased numbers of nerve cell bodies at these levels that supply the upper extremity.

The cervical cord in its widest dimension should be no wider than two-thirds of the interpeduncular distance. This distance is measured from the medial side of each pedicle as seen on the PA radiograph. Also, the cord should be no wider than three-fourths of the width of the subarachnoid space measured from one side of the contrast column to the other.

The nerve root pouches also can be seen readily as they exit through each neural foramen (Fig. 16–60). Several small nerves can be seen at each level. In addition, the anterior spinal artery often can be readily visualized along the ventral aspect (Fig. 16–61) of the cord as it is outlined by the contrast. Again, any defects detected on the myelogram should be correlated with the routine cervical spine radiographs. With the patient's neck well extended and not rotated, the contrast material can be pooled in such a way that both the ventral and dorsal aspects of the cervical subarachnoid space can be covered by the Pantopaque column (Figs. 16–64 and 16–65). In this way, mass lesions and other filling defects can be ruled out in either the dorsal or ventral aspect of the cord. In some cases, however, it will be necessary to remove the lumbar puncture needle and turn the patient on his back. If Pantopaque is used, it can then be run up to the cervical region to the level of the cisternae magnae and even into the fourth ventricle to evaluate the presence of a mass lesion around the posterior margin of the foramen magnum (Figs. 16–66, 16–81 and 16–82). In this case, lumbar tap can be repeated at the termination of the procedure and the contrast material removed; or the patient may be brought back to the department for contrast removal at a later date. The same procedure can be followed when Amipaque is used.

The cervical nerve roots arise from the cervical cord and course anteroventrally to their point of exit via the neural foramina. Each root will be seen to be made up of several small rootlets (Fig. 16–60). The right cervical nerves are best demonstrated with oblique views with the patient in a gentle LAO position. Likewise, the left cervical nerves are best demonstrated in the RAO projection. An excessive oblique positioning will cause the heavier-than-CSF contrast to flow away from the area of interest. Ideally, and if the equipment allows, the oblique views should be obtained by angulation of the tube and appropriate film positioning without moving the patient. This is particularly true if water-soluble contrast material is used, because patient motion causes dilution of the contrast material.

On the lateral view, there is often a prominent ventral bulge on the subarachnoid space in the upper cervical level behind the odontoid process. This, however, is due to ligaments — not to a tumor (Fig. 16–62, *A*). Care must be taken to avoid calling this normal finding a pathologic process. In addition, the dentate ligament may be seen on the lateral projections as a lucent line in the mid-portion of the contrast column (Fig. 16–63).

A MYELOGRAM IN CERVICAL SPONDYLOLYSIS

Spondylolysis. This all-inclusive term implies a general degenerative process in the cervical spine. The process includes a variety of changes that occur in the cervical spine, including osteophyte formation around the joints of Luschka, bulging or herniated cervical disks (which would not be visible on plain films of the spine), degenerative changes of the facets and disk space narrowing.

Trauma has been implicated as a cause, but spondylolysis appears to be more prevalent with increasing age and unrelated to overt trauma. The changes seen with age may be related to the multiple small "traumas" of daily living. It does appear that trauma may be a factor in some cases, and constitutional factors may be incriminated in others.

The uncovertebral "joints" will be considered to be true joints and therefore susceptible to arthritic changes. Plain films will reveal the formation of bony osteophytes at a single or multiple level. These changes are most common at C_5–C_6 and, next-most-common, at C_6–C_7. These uncovertebral osteophytes may be seen to impinge on the neural foramina in the oblique views and to project posteriorly in the midline, where the osteophytes may reach to the ventral aspect of the spinal cord.

The myelogram will reveal changes reflecting the findings seen on routine plain film examination. Osteophytes around the joints of Luschka and lateral in position will obliterate the nerve roots and produce small triangular defects in the contrast column. Midline osteophytes will indent the contrast column and produce one or more ventral bars in the cervical region. In the absence of a cervical disk, the contrast column will be closely applied to the posterior margin of the osteophyte.

The vast majority of cases with or without herniated disk — 95 per cent — occur at C_5–C_6 or C_6–C_7. Again, review of the preliminary films usually reveals degenerative changes with osteophytes that can be seen to impinge on the neural foramina — particularly in the oblique projections (Figs. 16–70 to 16–74).

If bony osteophytes encroach upon the cervical subarachnoid space and the ventral aspect of the spinal cord, there can be clinical evidence of spinal cord compression and pyramidal tract signs. Symptoms also may result from pressure on the anterior spinal artery, resulting in interference with the blood supply to the cord. By inspection of the lateral view of the cervical spine one can actually measure from the most posterior extent of the osteophyte to the spinal laminar line (Fig. 16–53), which marks the posterior extent of the cervical subarachnoid space, to obtain the *bony* width of the cervical canal. If this measures 11 mm or less, there is definite evidence of bony compromise of the cervical cord. This is true because at least 1 mm must be allowed for accommodation of the posterior spinal ligament connecting the vertebral bodies and the ligamentum flavum dorsally connecting the vertebral laminae in addition to the meningeal coverings of the spinal cord. Therefore, a measurement of 12 mm might be considered suspicious for cord compression by bony encroachment. In a congenitally small or stenotic cervical canal, these osteophytes will produce symptoms sooner than in a patient with a large anteroposterior spinal canal diameter.

In cases of cervical disk disease, there is thinning of the contrast column at the levels of the disk in the PA views; interruption of nerve root filling at the abnormal levels is best shown on the oblique views. These findings should always be confirmed by cross-table lateral projections of the mid- and upper cervical spine and a swimmer's view to include the lower cervical and upper thoracic spine levels. In addition, cross-table oblique views may be used to better define the side of involvement.

At myelography, there may be complete obstruction to the flow of contrast material at the level of the large cervical osteophytes and/or disks. This obstruction to flow (Fig. 16–74) is most commonly seen with the patient in the extended position. Indeed, when the neck is flexed and the chin is placed on the chest, contrast will often flow beyond the level of block. This maneuver should certainly be attempted in order to evaluate the abnormal levels fully and accurately. It may become necessary to instill contrast above the block via a C_1–C_2 in order to outline the upper border of the block more accurately. With impingement on the cord from a ventral disk, one can at times actually see widening of the cord (Figs. 16–67, 16–73 and 16–74). This widening is due to a flattening of the cord in the anteroposterior dimension, and this finding will be confirmed on the lateral views. It should not be mistaken for an intramedullary tumor. All abnormal levels should be studied, using at least two projections — ideally obtained at 90° angles to one another.

If there is herniation of the nucleus pulposus in the cervical region in addition to bony osteophytes, there may be compromise of the cord by soft tissue abnormalities not visible on plain film radiographs of the spine. These disk defects will be identified on the myelographic study when the contrast column is displaced farther than can be accounted for by the bony osteophyte alone (Figs. 16–72 to 16–74).

It is not always possible to be certain whether myelographic changes are secondary to a cervical disk or to bony osteophytes. Patients with myelographic changes secondary to spondylolysis are a common problem in an active clinical practice. Their management can be challenging and difficult.

MENINGIOMAS AND NEUROFIBROMAS
(Figs. 16–76–16–82)

Neurofibromas of the cervical region may be associated with widening of the neural foramina secondary to pressure erosion. Neurofibromas and meningiomas represent most of the intradural extramedullary tumors seen in the cervical region. With intradural lesions, there will be a sharp angle made with the contrast column, a rounded defect of the tumor itself and displacement of the cord away from the mass. Again, it is advisable to obtain views of the abnormal levels in two projections. If only one view is obtained, it may appear that there is cord displacement similar to that seen with an extradural lesion. In the upper cervical level, the low-lying cerebellar tonsils should not be mistaken for a mass lesion along the dorsal aspect of the cord (Fig. 16–67). Similarly, the dura and ligamentum flavum may be noted to form a corrugated pattern with the patient's head in the extended position—a normal finding (Fig. 16–64).

SYRINGOHYDROMYELIA

Syringohydromyelia is seen most commonly in the cervical cord region (Fig. 16–86). In these cases the patient may have minimal symptoms, but usually will have a history of long duration and may have Charcot joints involving the upper extremity (Fig. 16–86). Plain films of the cervical spine usually reveal a widened AP and lateral diameter of the spinal canal.

In syringomyelia, the cord will be noted to be widened over multiple vertebral body segments. The widened cord usually extends into the region of the thoracic cord. The wide cervical cord associated with a syrinx and demonstrated with standard myelography usually will collapse with air myelography. This use of air myelography also rules out the presence of a spinal cord tumor. The syrinx collapses when an air myelogram is performed because the air flows cephalad when the head is raised, while the fluid within the syringohydromyelia sac flows caudally in the enlarged canal by the force of gravity.

It is helpful to perform lateral tomography at the time of air myelography. At times it may be impossible to differentiate a noncollapsing syrinx from an intramedullary primary cord tumor. Direct puncture of the syrinx has been performed, followed by instillation of contrast material or air.

It is hoped that with improved resolution of CT units the diagnosis of this type of spinal cord abnormality will be possible without the use of contrast material. At present, the use of Amipaque with CT scanning has been shown to be helpful in the diagnosis of cord abnormalities.

Text continued on page 824

Figure 16–53. NORMAL LATERAL VIEW OF THE CERVICAL SPINE: *A, 1.* Pedicle; *2.* Spinous process; *3.* Lateral mass. The small arrows indicate the uncinate process. The large arrow points to the posterior limitation of the subarachnoid space, the point where the laminae join to form the spinous process. A white line (the spinolaminar line) is visible radiographically.

B, Normal AP view of the cervical spine: 1. Pedicle; *2.* Spinous process; *3.* Lateral mass. The small arrows outline the tracheal air shadow. The large arrow demonstrates the uncinate process at the level of the joint of Luschka.

C, Normal oblique view of the cervical spine, LAO position: 1. Pedicle; *3.* Lateral mass, viewed obliquely. The large arrowhead demonstrates the joint of Luschka, where osteophytes develop and may be noted to encroach upon the neural foramina. The black arrow: the right pedicle viewed on end; small arrows; the neural foramina at the C_6–C_7 level.

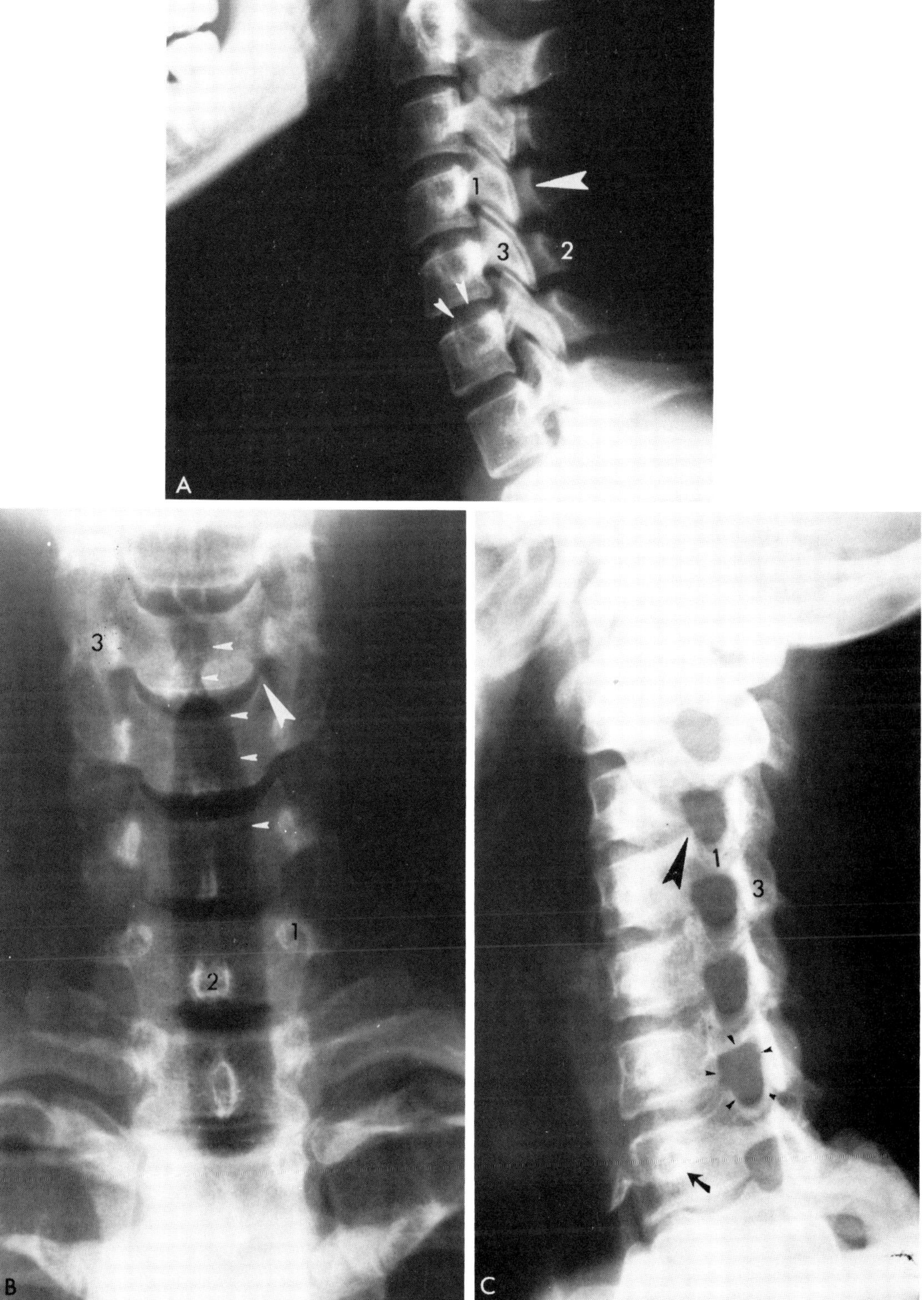

Figure 16–53 *See legend on the opposite page*

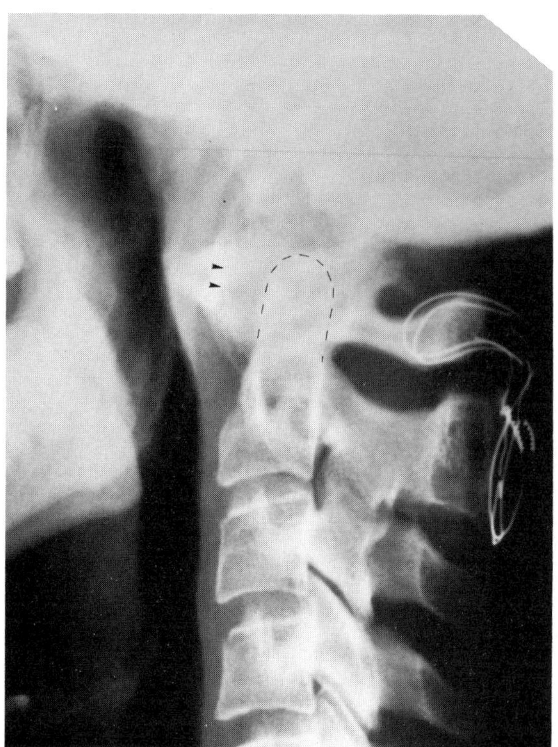

Figure 16–54. RHEUMATOID ARTHRITIS: There is atlantoaxial dislocation secondary to laxity of the ligaments. The arrowheads mark the posterior margin of the anterior arch of C_1. Stabilization had been attempted by the use of wires surrounding the posterior elements of C_1 and C_2, but the wires subsequently broke.

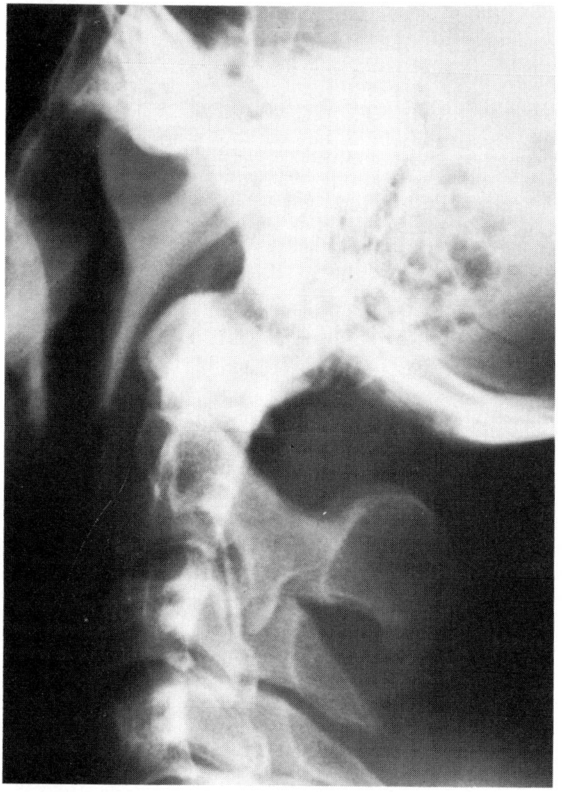

Figure 16–55. Congenital absence of the posterior arch of C_1.

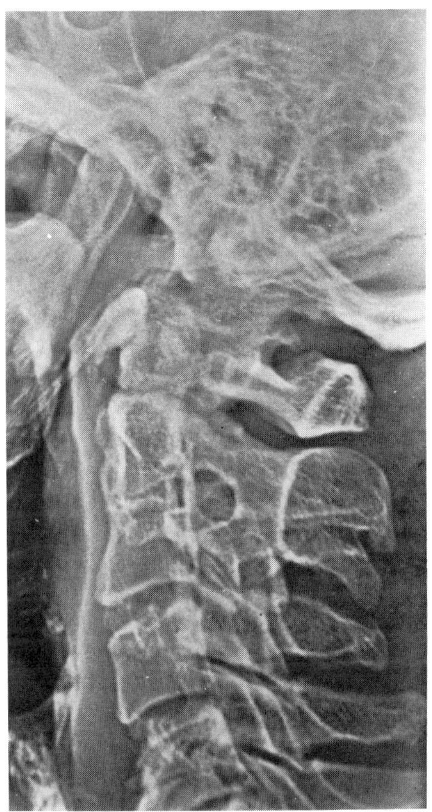

Figure 16–56. KLIPPEL-FEIL: This congenital anomaly may occur alone or with other anomalies. The Klippel-Feil anomaly is fusion (failure of segmentation) of two or more cervical vertebral bodies. This fusion results in a decrease in the normal motility of the spine. There may be an associated Arnold-Chiari malformation.

"Block vertebrae": A lateral xeroradiogram of the neck reveals fusion of the vertebral bodies and the spinous processes of the C_2 and C_3 vertebral bodies. The problem is really one of failure to segment, not one of fusion.

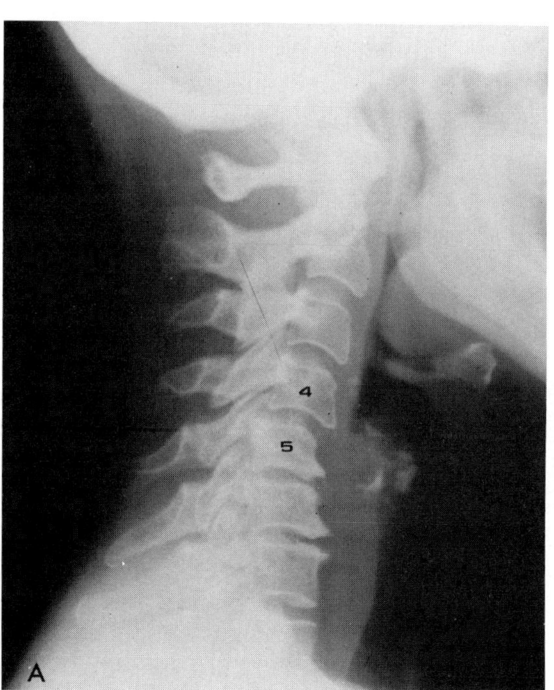

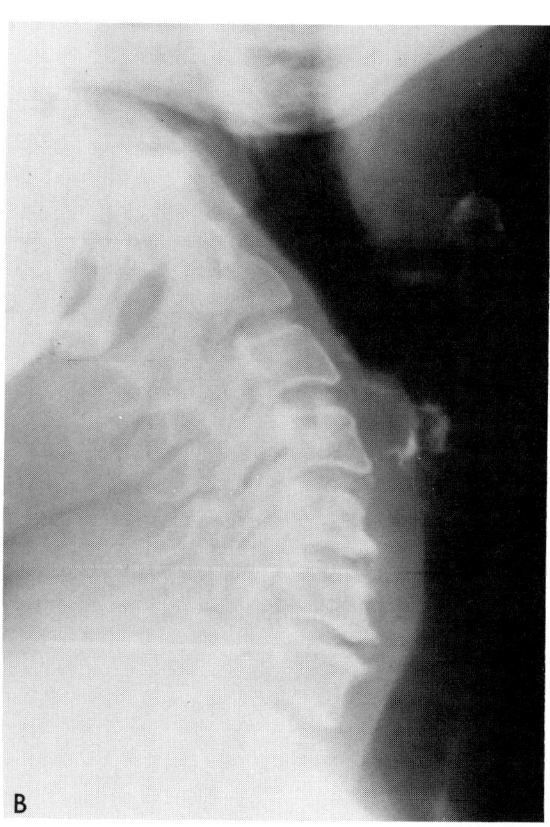

Figure 16–57. POST-TRAUMATIC SUBLUXATION: In flexion *(A)* there is forward displacement of C_4 on C_5; in extension *(B)* the vertebral bodies return to normal alignment.

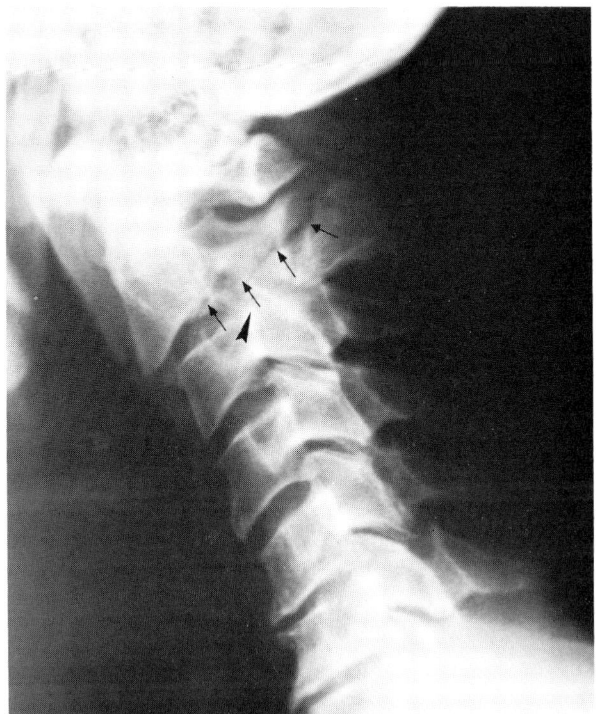

Figure 16–58. HANGMAN'S FRACTURE: A fracture extends through the lateral masses and laminae as well as the spinous process of the C_2 vertebral body (*arrows*). There is forward subluxation of C_2 on C_3. (*Arrowhead* illustrates back of C_3.)

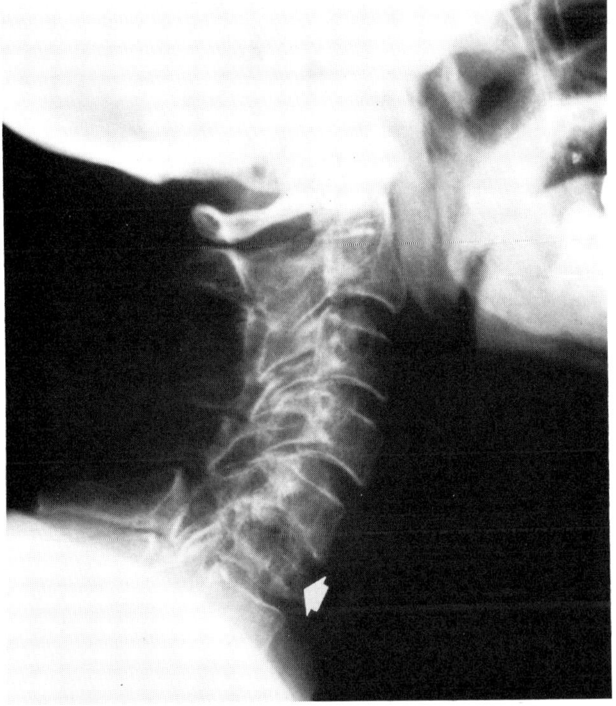

Figure 16–59. METASTATIC DISEASE TO THE CERVICAL SPINE: Osteolytic bony destructive change involves the C_6 vertebral body. There is collapse of the vertebral body. The bony and soft tissue components may result in cord compression and paraplegia.

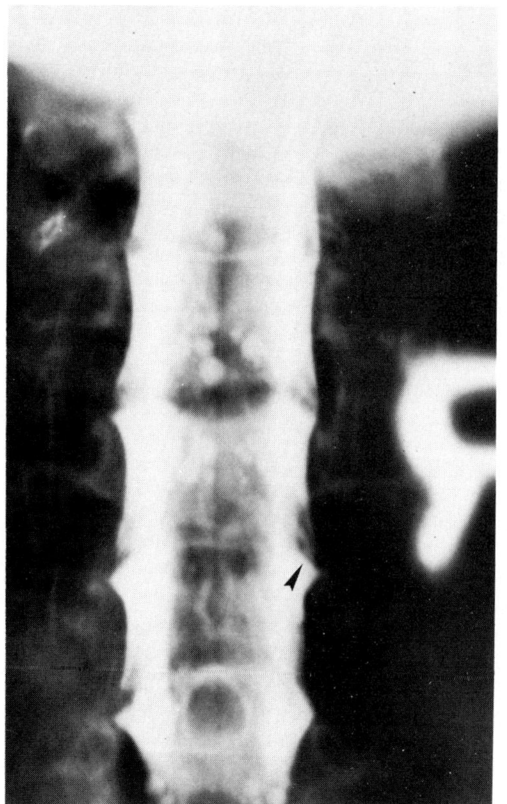

Figure 16–60

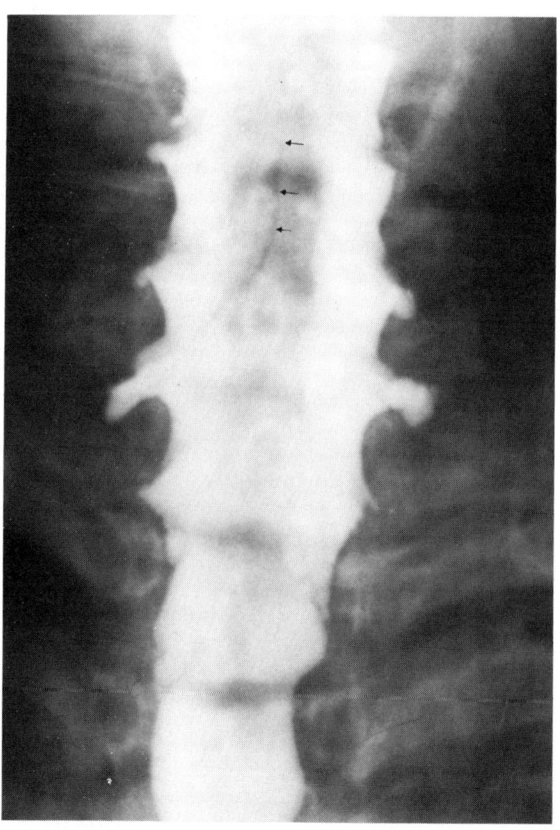

Figure 16–61

Figure 16–60. NORMAL CERVICAL MYELOGRAM: The PA view reveals good filling of all the nerve rootlets *(black arrowhead)* as they exit through the neural foramina. At each level the nerves appear as multiple threadlike shadows in the Pantopaque. The cervical spinal cord is a gray shadow in the center of the column of contrast. There is normally a widening of the cervical cord, with the widest point at the level of C_5–C_6. The anterior spinal artery is a radiolucent shadow in the midline; this lies at the anterior aspect of the cervical cord.

Figure 16–61. The lateral extensions of the subarachnoid space result in the appearance of multiple cystlike deformities. These should not be mistaken for a nerve root avulsion. The anterior spinal artery *(small arrows)* also can be seen.

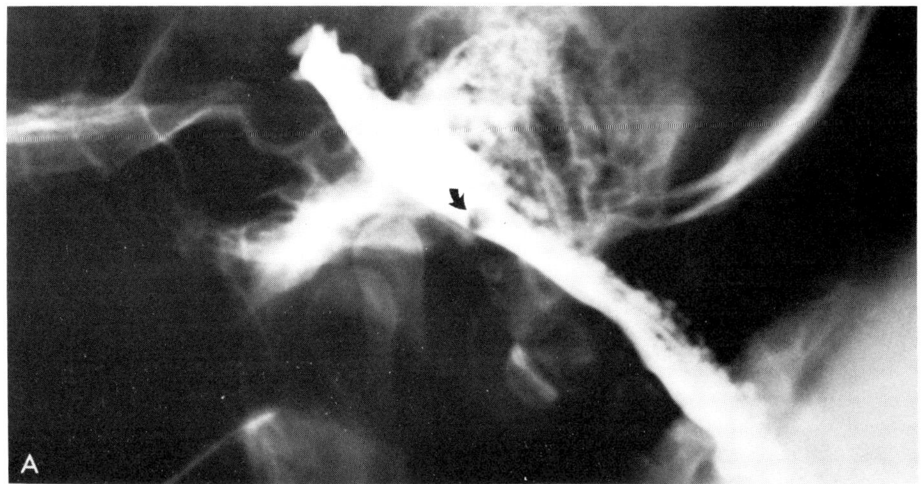

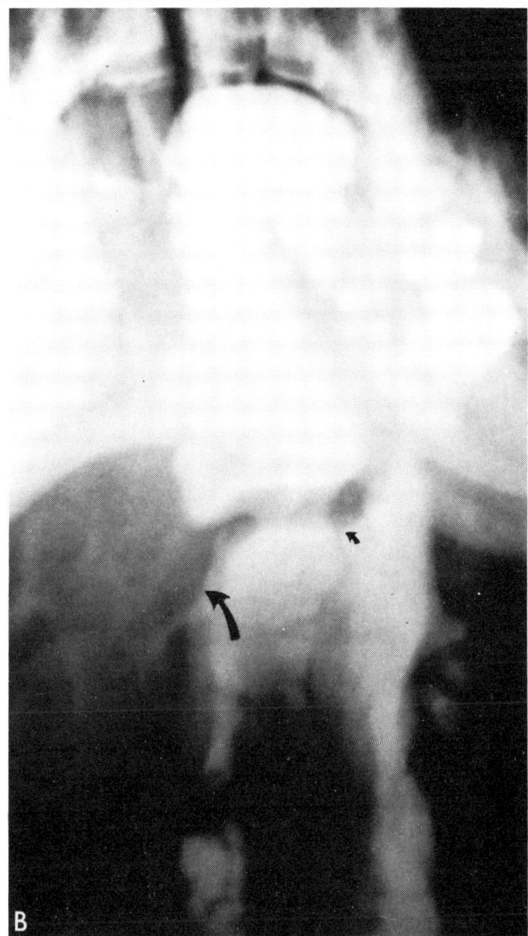

Figure 16–62. *A*, The lateral view, with the Pantopaque column on the clivus, outlines the negative shadow of the vertebral artery *(arrow)*. The Pantopaque column is held at the level of the dorsum sella and posterior clinoids by the membrane of Liliequist ("the radiologists' friend"). This membrane prevents entrance of Pantopaque into the middle cranial fossa. The normal odontoid reveals that there may be a large separation between the odontoid and the contrast column. This separation is caused by ligaments and is a normal finding that should not be mistaken for a tumor.

B, The corresponding PA view reveals the tortuous vertebral artery *(large arrow)* and its point of junction with the opposite vertebral artery (*small arrow*) to form the basilar artery. The upper margin of the contrast material is outlined by the curvilinear membrane of Liliequist.

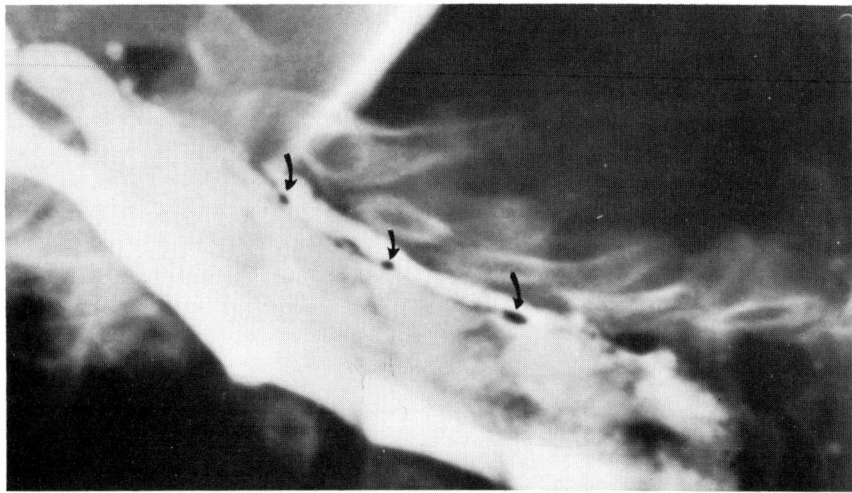

Figure 16–63. DENTATE LIGAMENTS: The oblique view may reveal the points of attachment of the dentate ligaments. These are fan-shaped structures that extend from the cord to the dura laterally. The small radiolucency is the lateral point of attachment *(arrows);* these serve to stabilize the spinal cord. There are 21 points of attachment of the spinal cord by the dentate ligament.

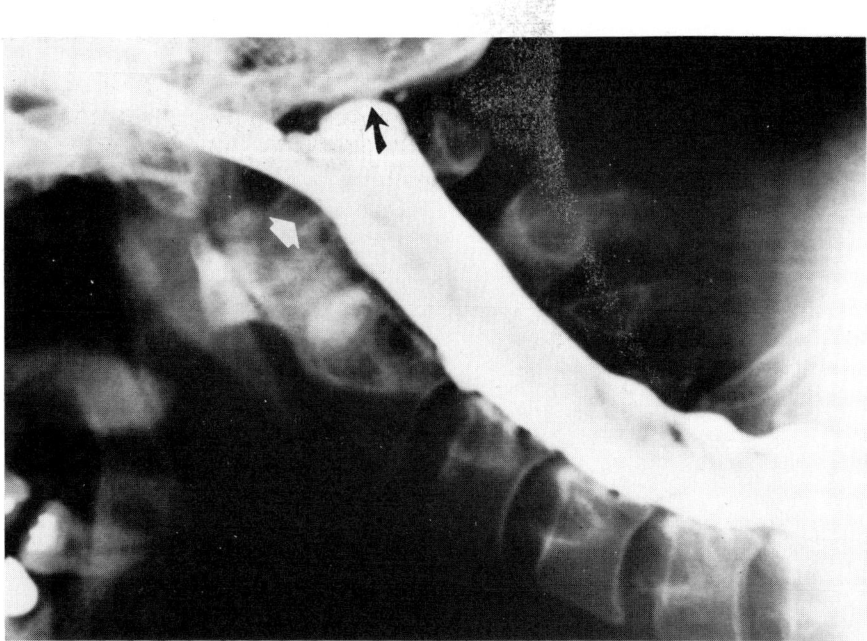

Figure 16–64. DURAL FOLDS: The entire cervical subarachnoid space is outlined by contrast up to and including the posterior margin of the foramen magnum *(black arrow).* The posterior margin of the odontoid process *(white arrow)* demonstrates a normal separation from the contrast column. The dura and ligamentum flavum indent the contrast column posteriorly in a corrugated fashion.

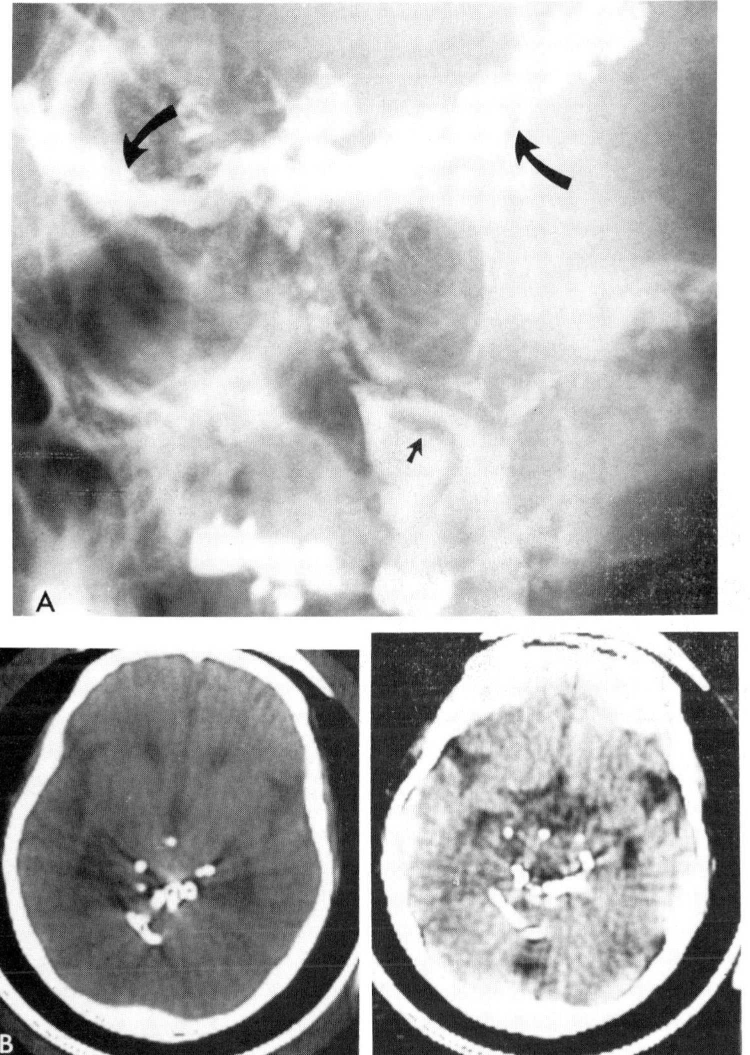

Figure 16–65. INTRACRANIAL PANTOPAQUE: *A*, A large amount of contrast material has entered into the cranial vault and outlines the sylvian fissures bilaterally *(large arrows)*. The vertebral arteries are also well outlined *(small arrow)*.

B, The CT scan demonstrates droplets of retained Pantopaque in the subarachnoid space. A large amount of Pantopaque can degrade the image and make the scan uninterpretable.

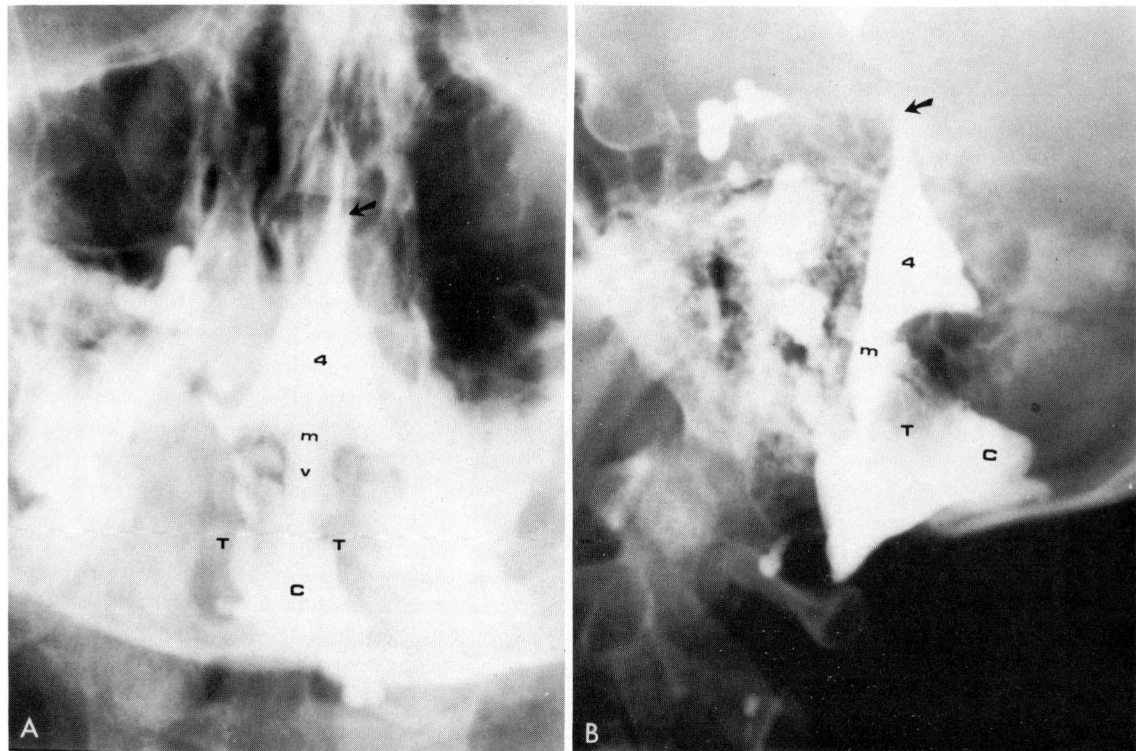

Figure 16–66. SUPINE MYELOGRAPHY OF THE POSTERIOR FOSSA: *A* and *B*, The contrast material flows readily up into the cisternae magnae and the fourth ventricle. It may be necessary at times to place the patient in this position to rule out a tumor of the region of the foramen magnum. *4,* Fourth ventricle; *m,* Foramen of Magendie; *v,* Vallecula; *T,* Cerebellar tonsils; *C,* Cisternae magnae; *arrow,* Aqueduct of Sylvius.

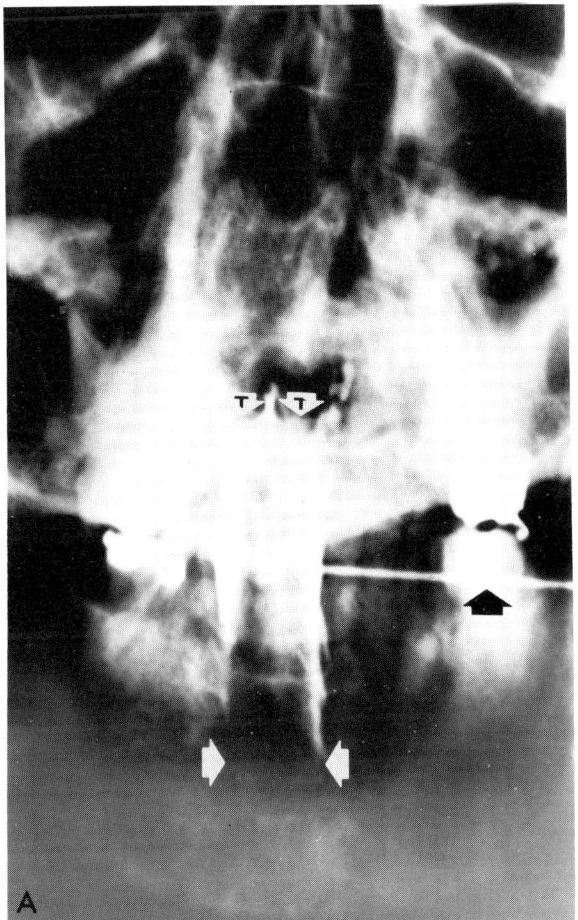

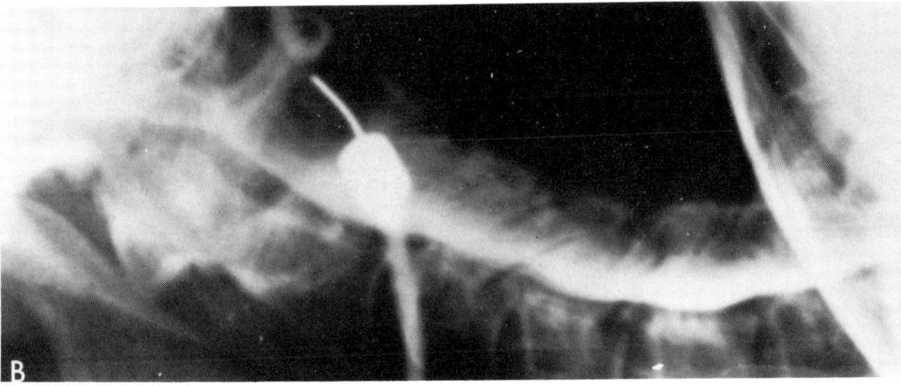

Figure 16–67. CEREBELLAR TONSILS: *A*, Myelogram performed via C_1–C_2 tap reveals a complete block to the flow of contrast material in the lower cervical region secondary to a herniated cervical disk *(white arrowheads)*. The needle is in place *(black arrowhead)*. The contrast material outlines the cerebellar tonsils with the patient in the supine position *(T)*.

B, The lateral view demonstrates the correct needle position for a lateral cervical tap. The needle is at the C_1–C_2 level and is far enough dorsal in position to avoid the spinal cord.

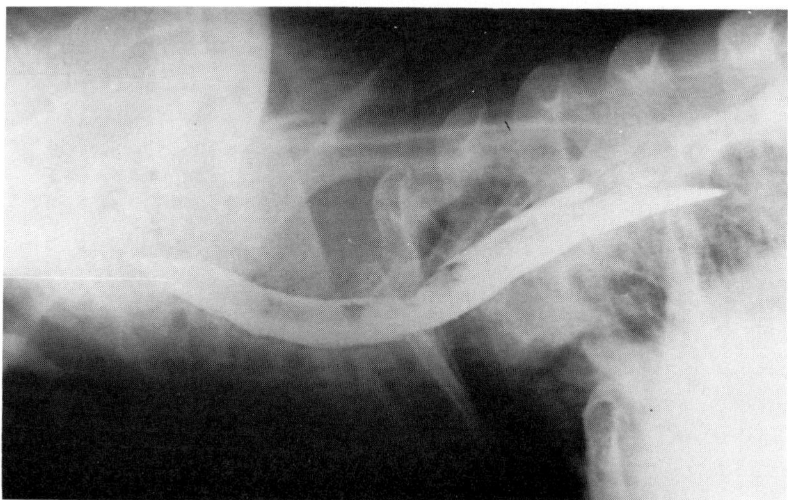

Figure 16–68. NORMAL MYELOGRAM — SWIMMER'S VIEW: The swimmer's view allows excellent visualization of the lower cervical and upper thoracic region without the overlying shoulders.

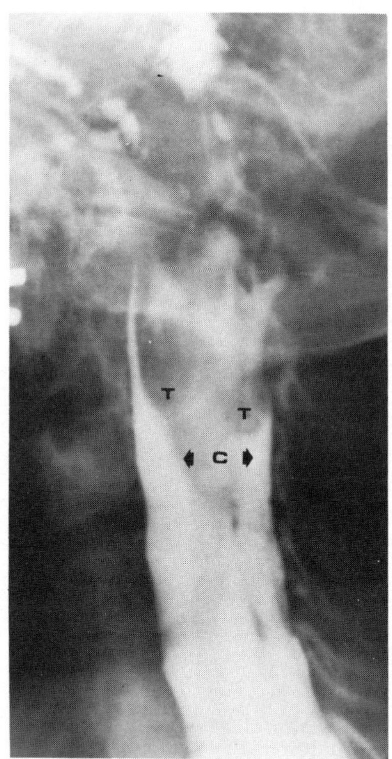

Figure 16–69. ARNOLD–CHIARI MALFORMATION: The cervical myelogram outlines the low lying cervical tonsils, which extend down to the C_3 level *(T)*. The cervical cord is outlined *(C)* below the cerebellar tonsils. There is a high degree of obstruction to the flow of contrast material at the level of the foramen magnum. The cervical cord is wide in the mid- and lower cervical regions because of a hydromyelia associated with the Arnold-Chiari malformation (courtesy of Drs. Oscar Sugar and Glen Dobben). Because of the downward displacement of the cord with the Arnold-Chiari malformation, the cervical nerve rootlets often will be seen to slant upward, whereas in the normal patient they slant inferiorly.

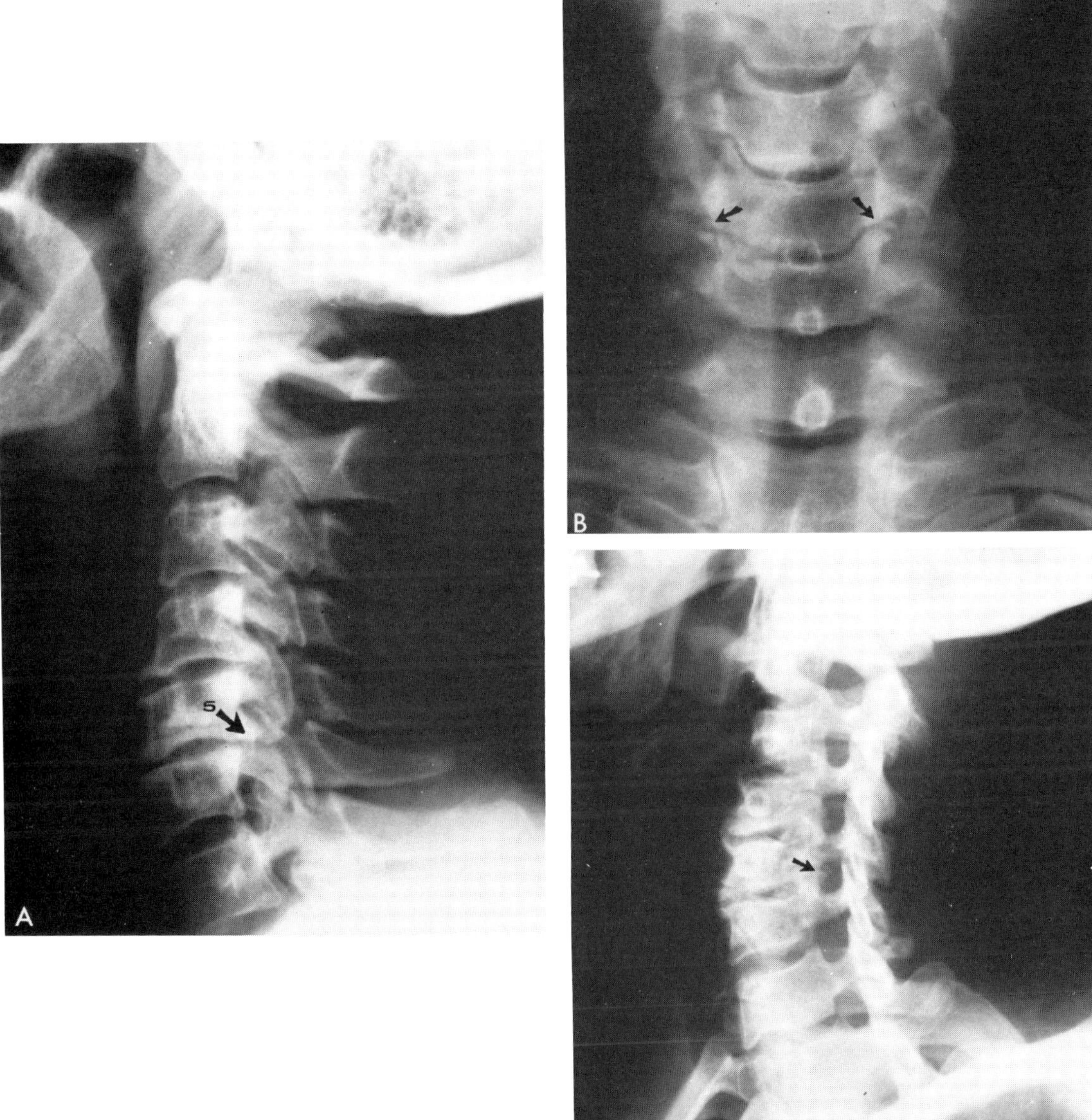

Figure 16–70. CERVICAL ARTHRITIS: *A,* The lateral view reveals degenerative changes, with narrowing of the C_4–C_5 and C_5–C_6 disk spaces. There is anterior spur formation and large posterior osteophytes at these levels. The posterior osteophytes are marked at the C_5 level on all views, but are readily visible at the C_4–C_5 level also.

B, The AP view demonstrates the bony overgrowth about the uncinate processes bilaterally. This extends posteriorly into the spurs, which impinge upon the neural foramina.

C, The oblique view allows visualization of the neural foramina and demonstrates the encroachment by the bony osteophytes *(arrow).* Note that the level above also demonstrates the osteophytes, while the remainder of the neural foramina are oval and without evidence of impingement by spur formation.

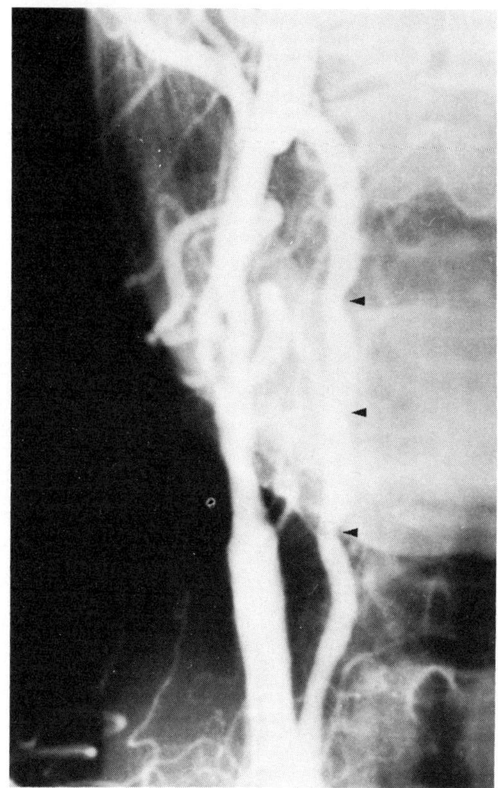

Figure 16–71. These osteophytes about the uncinate processes may also indent the vertebral artery *(arrows)* as it courses in the foramina transversaria.

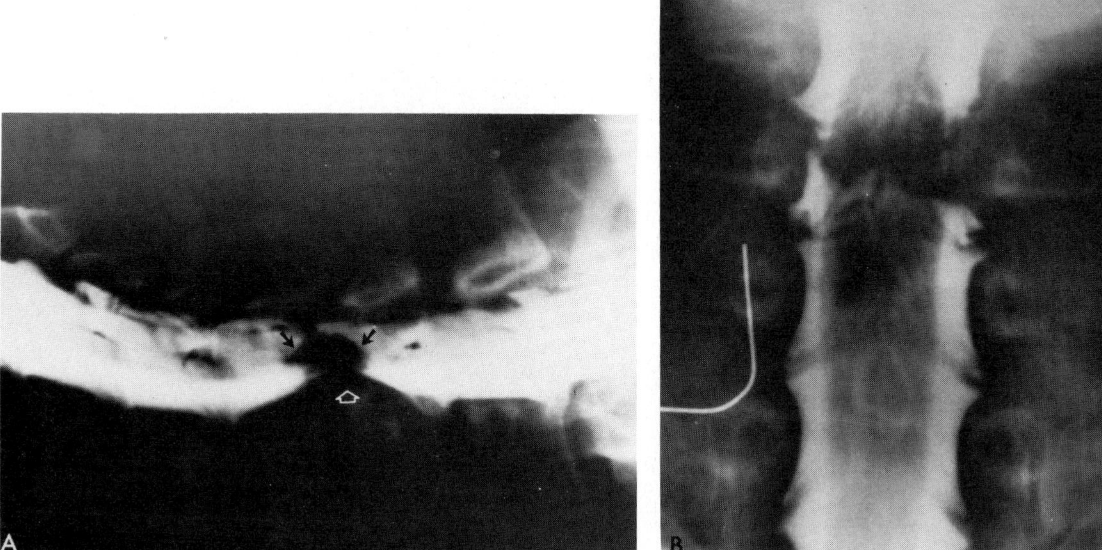

Figure 16–72. BONY OSTEOPHYTES AND HERNIATED CERVICAL DISK: *A,* The lateral view reveals a ventral indentation on the contrast column that extends beyond the bony spur *(open arrowhead)*. This is a finding when a herniated cervical disk is present. In addition, there is a double density shadow (*black arrows*) because the disk is larger on one side than on the other.

B, The PA view confirms this finding and demonstrates poor nerve root filling and a lateral defect in the contrast column. This filling defect frequently takes on a wedge-shaped appearance with a herniated disk. There is mild widening of the cord at this level secondary to compression by the osteophytes and the cervical disk.

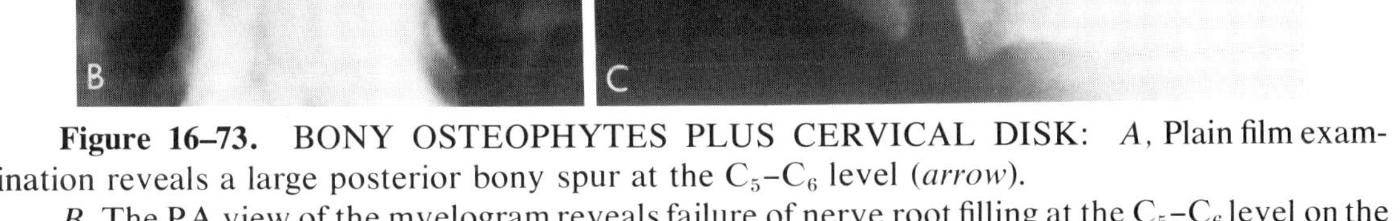

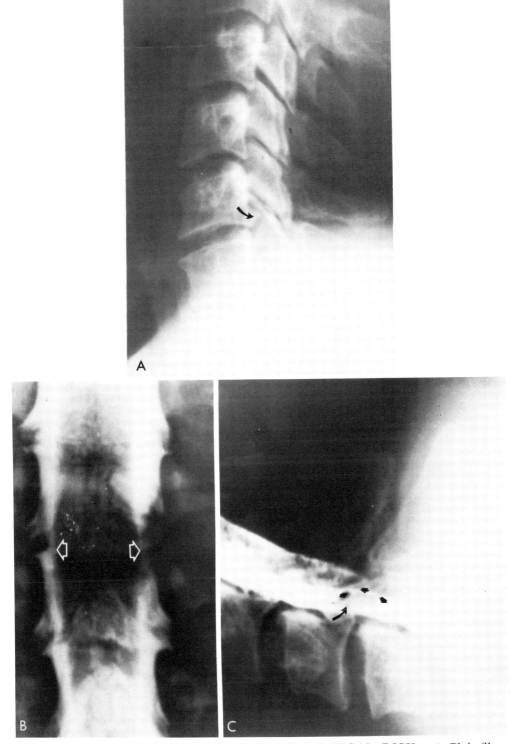

Figure 16–73. BONY OSTEOPHYTES PLUS CERVICAL DISK: *A*, Plain film examination reveals a large posterior bony spur at the C_5–C_6 level (*arrow*).

B, The PA view of the myelogram reveals failure of nerve root filling at the C_5–C_6 level on the right side (at the side of the osteophyte). There is localized widening of the cord *(arrows)* at this level because of compression.

C, The lateral view reveals that the bony spur *(long arrow)* is associated with a large cervical disk that displaces the contrast material and creates a double density shadow *(small arrows)*.

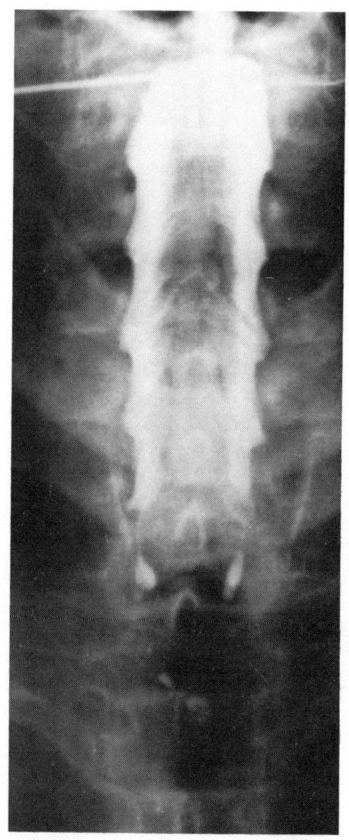

Figure 16–74. CERVICAL DISK WITH NEAR COMPLETE BLOCK TO THE FLOW OF CONTRAST: Through a C_1–C_2 tap with the patient in the supine position, contrast material is placed in the cervical subarachnoid space. There is a near complete block to the flow of contrast at the C_6–C_7 level that is associated with widening of the cord. A large ventral defect was present on the lateral view.

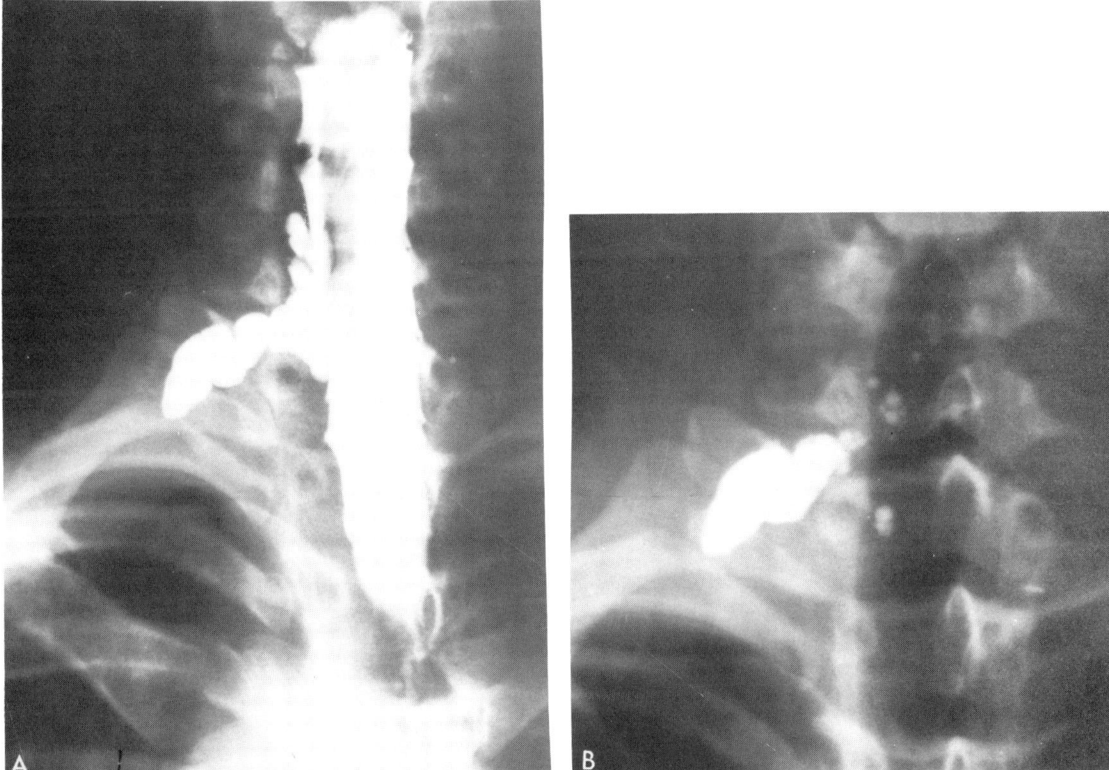

Figure 16–75. NERVE ROOT AVULSION: *A*, The Pantopaque collects in a sac made up of the arachnoid protruding through a dural tear. The end of the avulsed nerve, which is pulled from the cord, retracts distally in the arachnoid sac. In addition to the marked change at the C_7–T_1 level, there has also been a less marked avulsion at the C_6–C_7 level.

B, When the contrast material is drained from the cervical subarachnoid space, the rest of the contrast is still present in the sac (courtesy of the Carle Clinic Radiologists, Urbana, Illinois).

Figure 16–76. NEUROFIBROMA, DUMBBELL TUMOR: *A* and *B*, Plain film examination reveals a marked difference in the size of the neural foramina at the C_2–C_3 level bilaterally *(arrows)*.

C, Myelography reveals an intradural tumor at the C_2–C_3 level on the right side. The cervical cord is displaced to the contralateral side. Associated with this is a second portion of the tumor, which extends into the soft tissues of the neck (not seen). The "waist" of the tumor is created by the compression of the bony neural foramina—thus resulting in the "dumbbell" appearance.

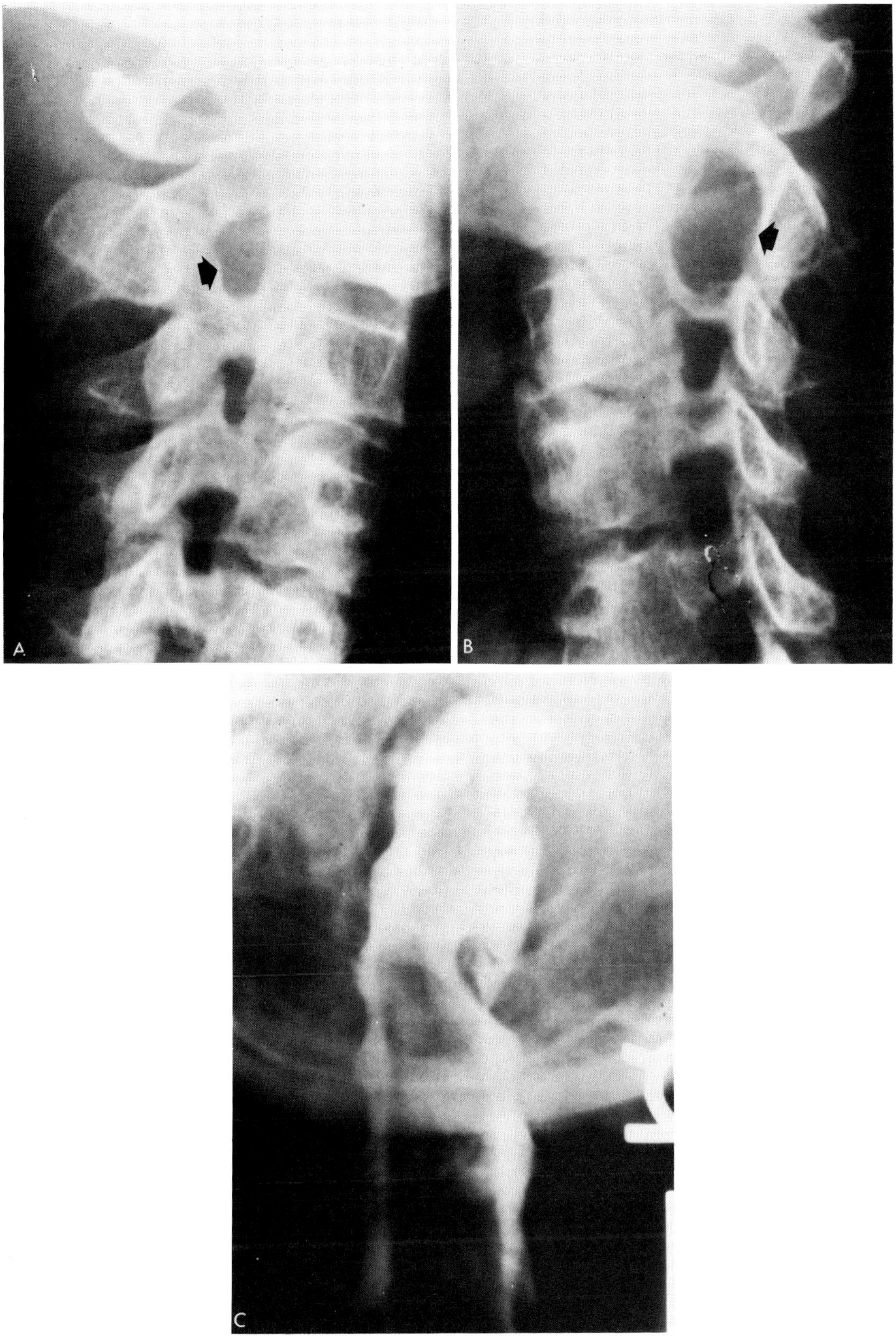

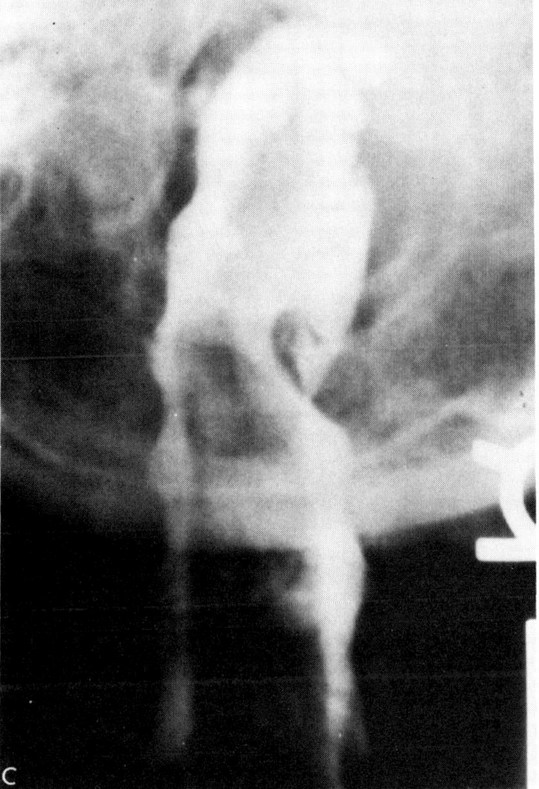

Figure 16–76 *See legend on the opposite page*

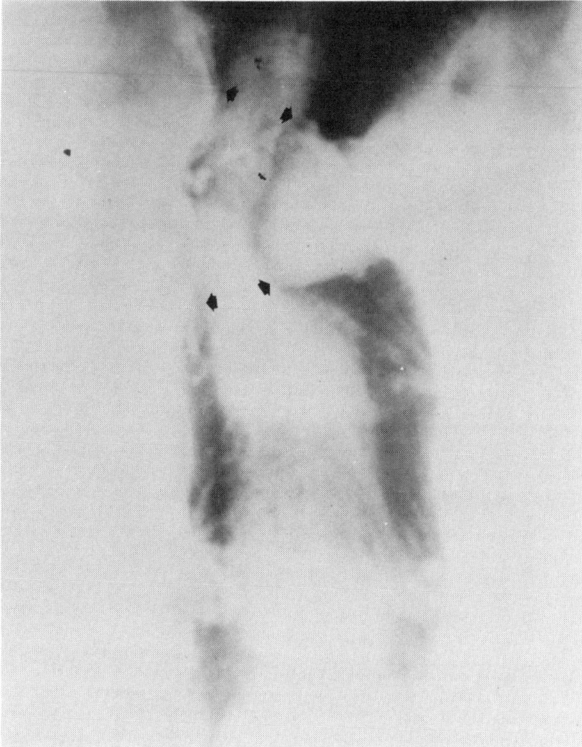

Figure 16–77 *See legend on the opposite page*

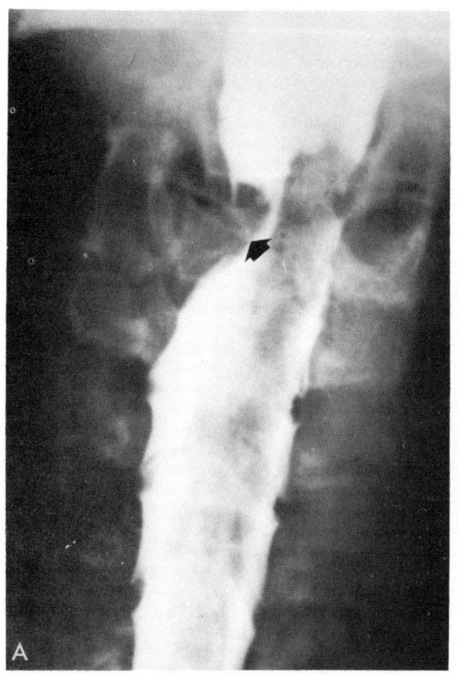

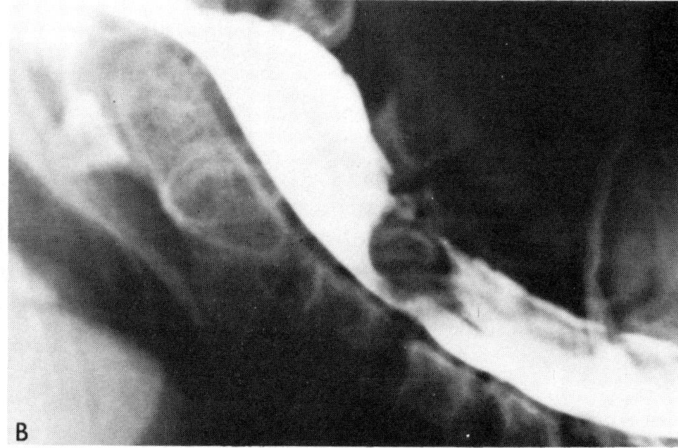

Figure 16–78 *See legend on the opposite page*

Figure 16–77. NEUROFIBROMA: A rather angulated neurofibroma is present at the C_2–C_3 level. The tumor is intradural and displaces the cord to the contralateral side, resulting in a marked compression of the cord localized to the area of the tumor *(arrowheads)*. There were no plain film changes in this case.

Figure 16–78. NEUROFIBROMA; DUMBBELL TUMOR: *A*, This patient was diagnosed as having multiple sclerosis; however, the myelogram reveals an intradural, slightly angulated neurofibroma *(arrow)* at the C_3–C_4 level on the left side. The cervical cord is displaced to the contralateral side and compressed by the neurofibroma.

B, The lateral view reveals the tumor as seen end-on, where it appears as a rounded filling defect. There was no alteration of the neural foramina on plain film examination, but the patient had a palpable mass in the soft tissues of the neck at this level which subsequently proved to be the extradural portion of this dumbbell neurofibroma.

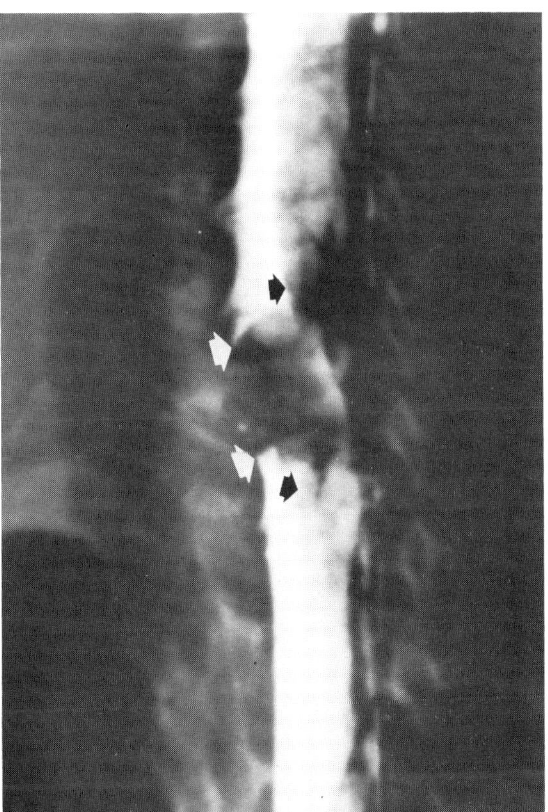

Figure 16–79. MENINGIOMA: There is a well rounded intradural tumor on the left side in the low cervical region. The sharp angle of the contrast material at the point of attachment of the tumor to the dura is well demonstrated *(white arrowheads)*. The cervical cord is displaced to the contralateral side *(black arrowheads)* and compressed.

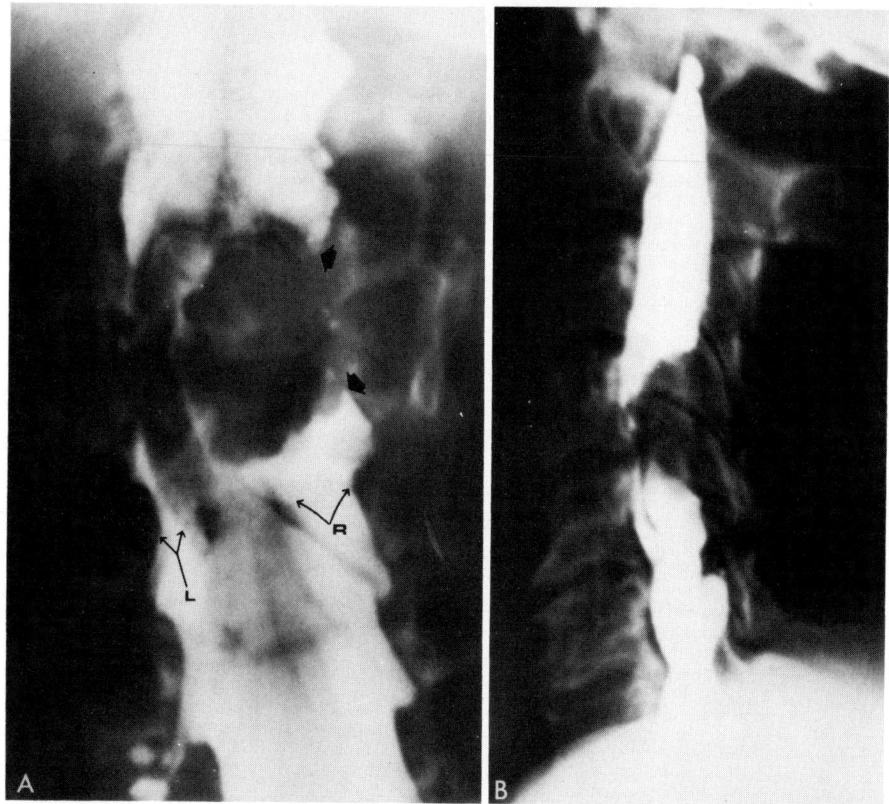

Figure 16–80. MENINGIOMA: *A,* A well rounded but slightly lobulated tumor is seen on the right side in the midcervical region. The point of attachment to the tumor is well demonstrated by an acute angle of Pantopaque (*black arrowheads*). The cord is displaced to the contralateral side at the level of the tumor and is markedly compressed by the mass. The subarachnoid space on the right side (*R*) is much larger than the subarachnoid space on the left side of the cord (*L*).

B, This lateral view demonstrates that the semicircular tumor arises from the dorsal aspect of the cervical subarachnoid space.

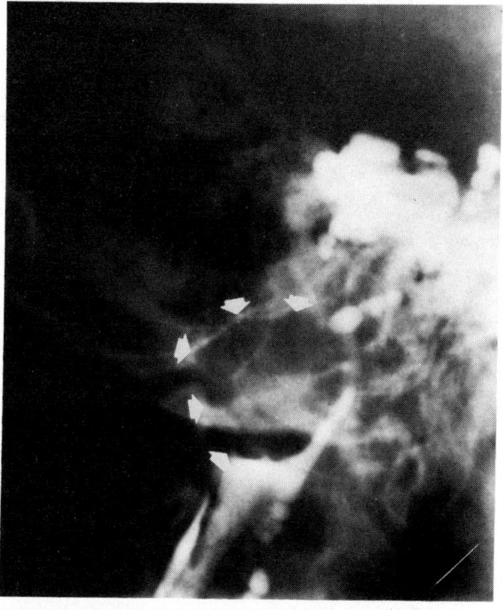

Figure 16–81. FORAMEN MAGNUM MENINGIOMA: The contrast material bathes the posterior aspect of the foramen magnum and demonstrates a meningioma *(white arrows)* of the dorsal aspect of the foramen magnum.

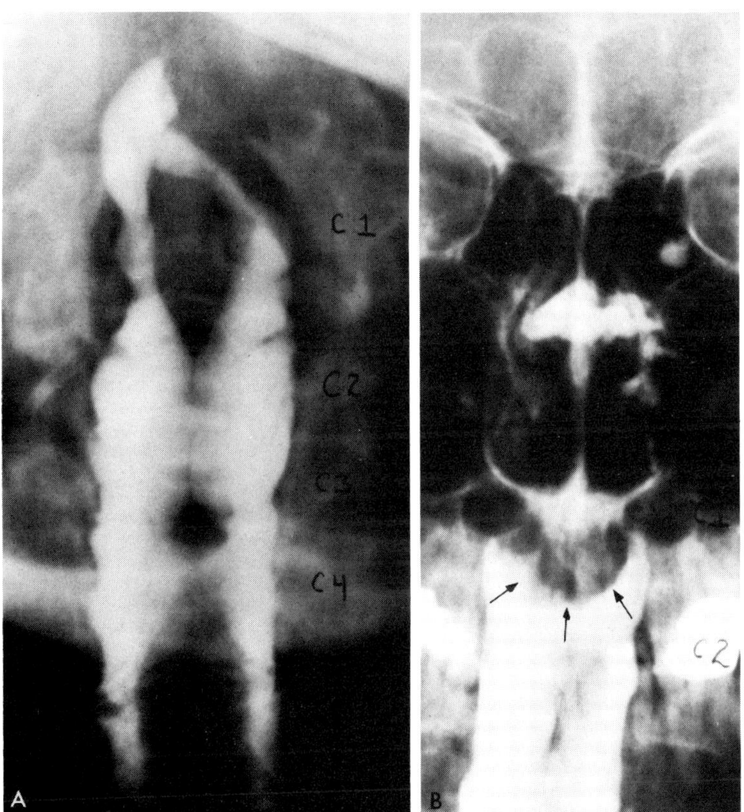

Figure 16–82. FORAMEN MAGNUM MENINGIOMA: *A*, Myelography performed in the routine prone position reveals no definite abnormalities; however, when the patient is placed in the supine position after removal of the needle *(B)*, the AP view demonstrates a filling defect in the upper cervical magnum region *(black arrows)*.

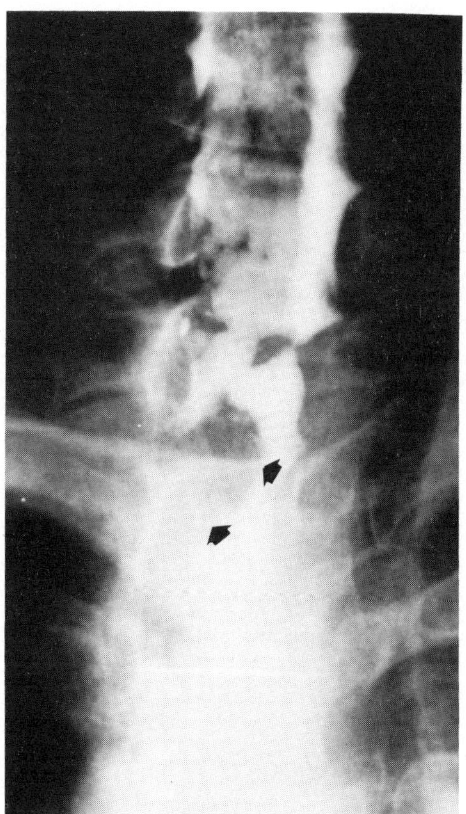

Figure 16–83. HEMATOMA SIMULATING AN INTRADURAL TUMOR: Myelography demonstrates a tumor in the upper thoracic region that has the appearance of an intradural mass lesion *(arrows)*. At fluoroscopy there was a high degree of obstruction to the flow of contrast material. This was proved at surgery to be a hematoma in the subarachnoid space secondary to anticoagulants.

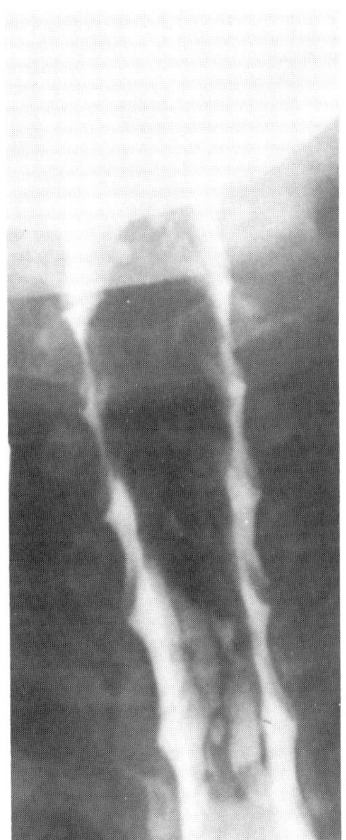

Figure 16–84

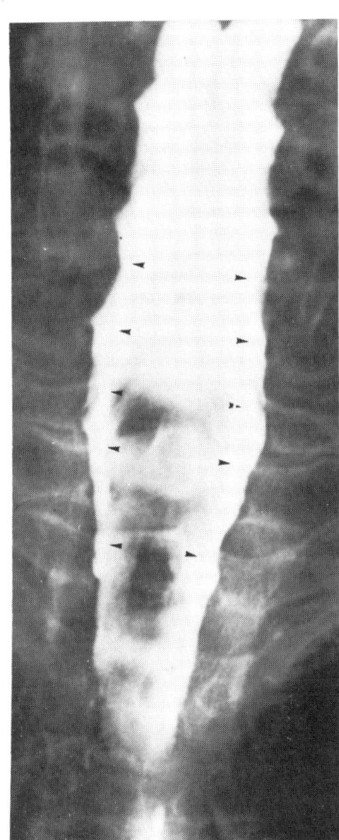

Figure 16–85

Figure 16–84. INTRAMEDULLARY TUMOR: The cervical cord is widened and there is bilateral thinning of the contrast material in the subarachnoid space. There was a similar appearance on the lateral view. Surgery revealed an astrocytoma (courtesy of Drs. Oscar Sugar and Glen Dobben, University of Illinois).

Figure 16–85. INTRAMEDULLARY TUMOR: There is widening of the lower cervical and upper thoracic cord *(arrowheads)*. Surgery revealed an astrocytoma.

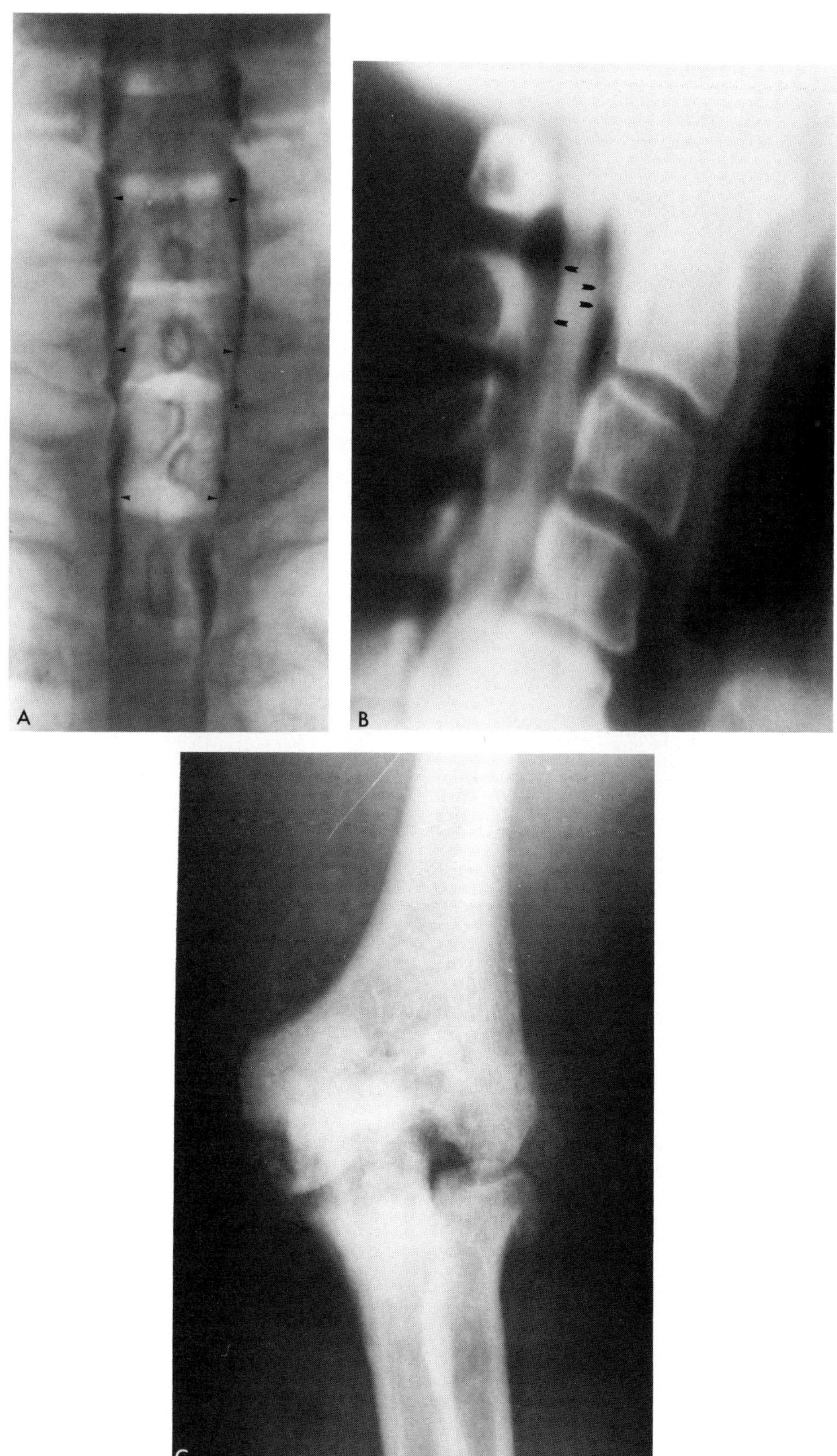

Figure 16–86 *See legend on the opposite page*

Figure 16–86. SYRINGOHYDROMYELIA: *A*, There is diffuse widening of the cord that extends throughout the entire cervical region and well down into the thorax. The cervical cord has almost obliterated the subarachnoid space bilaterally *(arrowheads)*. Incidentally, there is a spina bifida of the T_1 spinous process.

B, Air myelography reveals that the cervical cord collapses and becomes very narrow *(arrowheads)*. The cord is surrounded by the radiolucent shadow of the surrounding air. The collapse of the cervical cord occurs when the patient's head is elevated and the fluid in the hydromyelic sac flows by gravity to a more distal position in the cord.

C, Charcot Joint: The elbow demonstrates a marked amount of soft tissue calcification and degenerative changes surrounding the elbow. The bony structures continue to be well ossified. The appearance is typical of a Charcot joint.

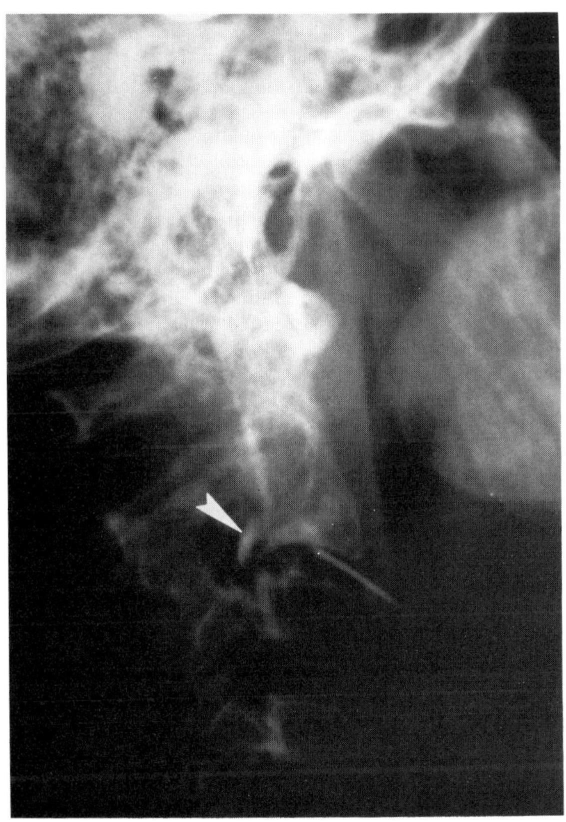

Figure 16–87. CERVICAL DISCOGRAM: The needle is placed in the C_1–C_2 disk space, and Conray 60 is injected. Although a small amount of the contrast material is noted to remain in the disk space, most exits out of the disk space posteriorly *(arrowhead)*. This is an abnormal finding seen with a herniated nucleus pulposus in the cervical region.

THORACIC (DORSAL) SPINE

Anteroposterior and lateral views of the dorsal spine are obtained routinely. Inspection of the vertebrae should be performed in a manner similar to that described for the corresponding views of the lumbar spine. Diastematomyelia (Fig. 16–51), if present, is associated with congenitally abnormal vertebral body and is usually found in the lower dorsal or upper lumbar region. Herniated disks are uncommon in the thoracic region.

IVORY VERTEBRA

The single white vertebra or "ivory vertebra" (Fig. 16–88) is seen most commonly with Hodgkin's disease or the non-Hodgkin's lymphomas. The ivory vertebra also may be seen with osteoblastic metastatic disease, myeloid metaplasia, Paget's disease, fluorosis or osteopetrosis.

MYELOGRAPHY OF THE DORSAL CORD

The dorsal spinal cord may be studied by filling the entire column with contrast material. More commonly, approximately 18 to 24 cc of Pantopaque is used. After removal of 10 to 12 cc of CSF, the contrast is instilled very slowly into the lumbar subarachnoid space. The patient is then placed in the lateral decubitus position, and the contrast is allowed to flow cephalad by tilting the table in the Trendelenburg position until the entire dependent side of the dorsal spine is outlined by contrast (Fig. 16–89). With the patient in the true lateral position, films are then obtained in the lateral and AP projections.

Care should be taken to make sure that the patient holds his head tipped upward with his ear resting on his upper shoulder. This will insure that contrast material is held in the cervical region and does not flow into the cranial vault. After the necessary films have been obtained, the patient is returned to a prone, head-up position. The contrast is again pooled in the lumbar subarachnoid space and then allowed to flow cephalad, with the patient positioned in the opposite lateral decubitus position. A similar technique is used with water-soluble contrast material and is described under the discussion on Amipaque myelography.

SPINAL CORD ARTERIOVENOUS MALFORMATIONS

Spinal cord arteriovenous malformations (Fig. 16–95) are seen infrequently. They do, however, have a rather characteristic appearance on myelography. Most commonly, they appear as wormlike accumulations of dilated vascular channels upon the dorsal aspect of the cord. If this diagnosis is suspected, it is necessary to remove the needle and place the patient in the supine position, allowing the contrast to flow into the dorsal region of the cord. A large amount of contrast may be necessary, and reports of using up to 100 cc of Pantopaque have been published. In addition, it may become necessary to study these abnormalities by spinal arteriography. Arteriovenous malformations of the cord may be suspected in patients who have had subarachnoid hemorrhage and when no intracranial source of bleeding has been identified in spite of multiple arteriographic examinations.

Spinal cord arteriography is a lengthy procedure, requiring selective catheterization of the artery of Adamkiewicz and as many lumbar arteries as possible, with serial filming after injection of contrast. The use of magnification and subtraction techniques allows better visualization of any vascular malformations of the cord (see Chapter 12). There are dangers inherent in spinal cord arteriography, including the possibility of paralysis of the lower extremities because of occlusion of the blood supply to the cord and because of a direct toxic reaction of the cord to the contrast material. Therefore, caution should be used when performing the procedure. Because of its meticulous nature, this procedure is of necessity quite prolonged and physically taxing for the patient and the individuals performing the study.

NERVE ROOT AVULSION

A severe injury to either the brachial plexus or more rarely the lumbar plexus may result in an avulsion of the nerve root at its attachment to the spinal cord (Fig. 16–75). This injury appears to be secondary to a stretching of the nerve beyond its endurance, as when the patient suffers a harsh traction injury on an arm or leg. This type of damage to the brachial plexus is irreversible and generally results in a partially or totally frail upper extremity.

The myelographic appearance is very characteristic. The cord appears intrinsically normal, but the contrast material readily enters a sac of the arachnoid layer of the meninges that formed when the cervical nerve was pulled from the spinal cord at its point of attachment. The severed end of the nerve will be found at the distal end of the sac, where it retracts after being pulled from the cord. Although the contrast material readily *enters* this sac, its egress is often not seen — even after returning the patient to the upright position. Attempts have been made surgically to anastomose this avulsed nerve to the cord, but have not met with success. Similar damage to the lumbar plexus is rare and is associated with extensive soft tissue and bone damage.

EPIDURAL ABSCESS

Abscesses in the epidural space are not common but may be seen — particularly in drug addicts with a history of intravenous drug abuse. They also may develop following dental procedures. Epidural abscesses (not illustrated) may or may not be associated with a bony abnormality. The patient often experiences severe pain, and the extradural block to the flow of contrast material typically extends over a long length of the spinal column.

Text continued on page 832

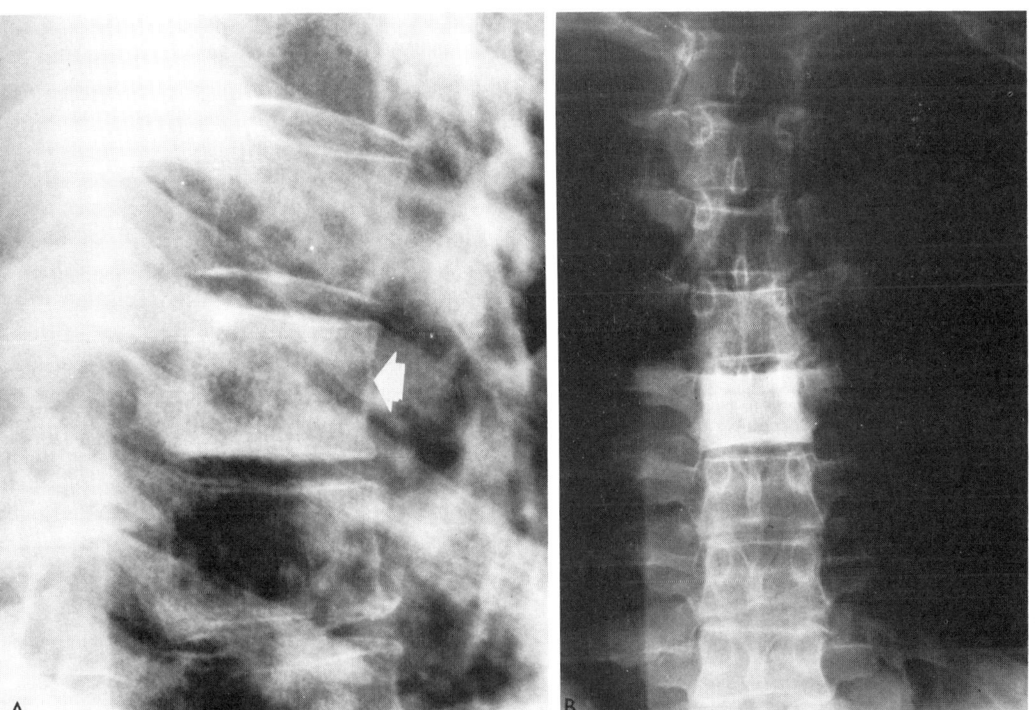

Figure 16–88. "IVORY VERTEBRAE": There is marked sclerosis of the D_7 vertebral body. This is an ivory vertebra secondary to involvement with Hodgkin's disease.

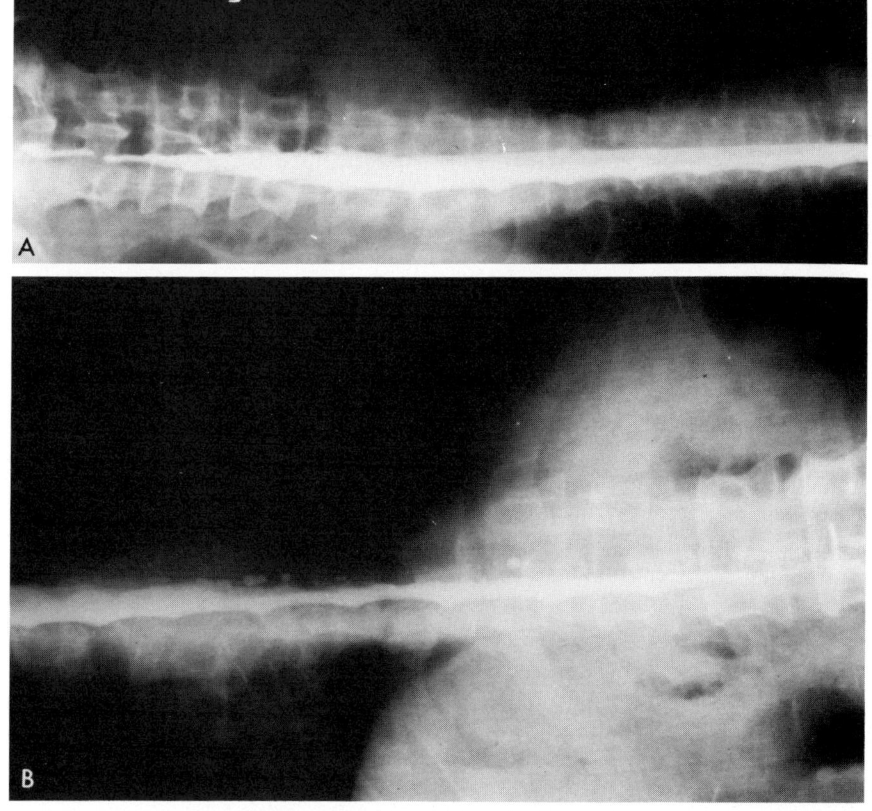

Figure 16–89 *See legend on the opposite page*

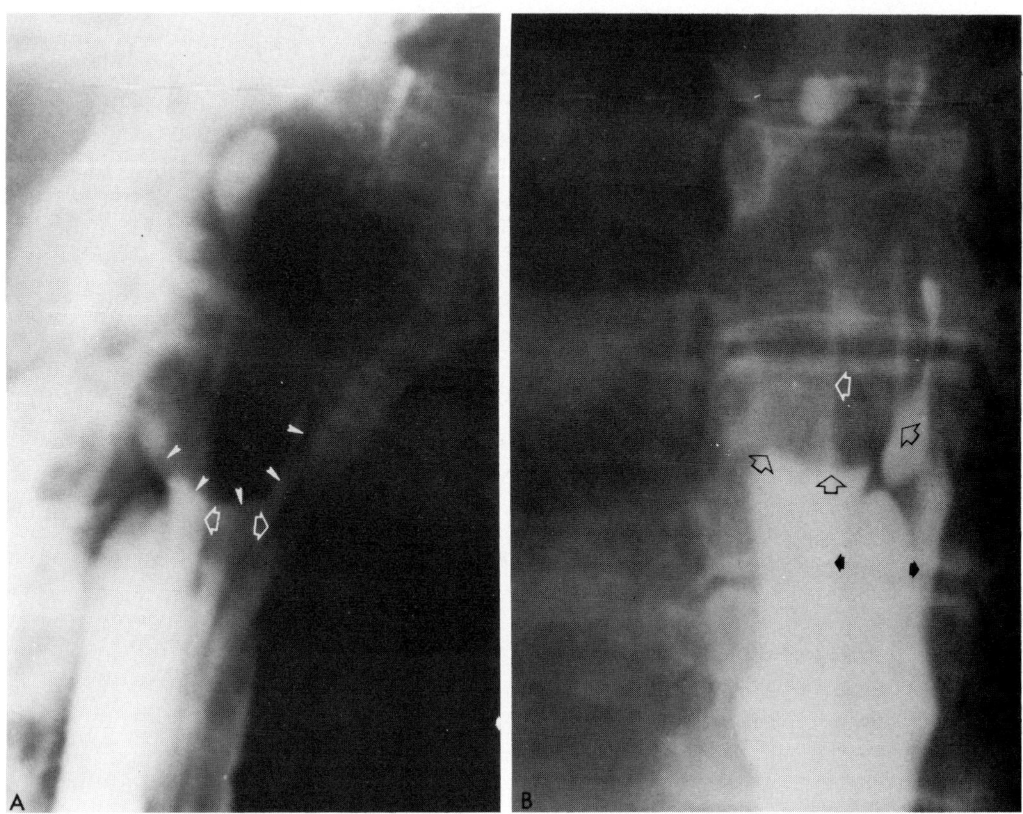

Figure 16–90 *See legend on the opposite page*

Figure 16–89. NORMAL THORACIC MYELOGRAM: *A* and *B*, The patient is placed first in one lateral decubitus position and then in the opposite lateral decubitus position, and films are obtained in the PA and true lateral positions. The lateral decubitus positions are illustrated here.

Figure 16–90. THORACIC MENINGIOMA: *A*, The oblique view reveals a well rounded tumor *(arrowheads)* that is intradural in configuration. The thoracic cord is displaced ventrally *(open arrowheads)*.

B, The PA view reveals that the cord is displaced to the right *(black arrowheads)*. The tumor is again well demonstrated *(open black arrowheads)*, and a small amount of the contrast has outlined the thoracic cord behind the tumor *(open white arrowhead)*, demonstrating its position to the right of the midline.

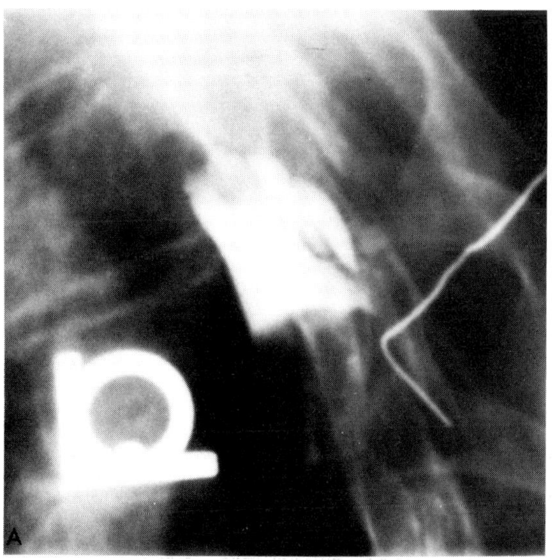

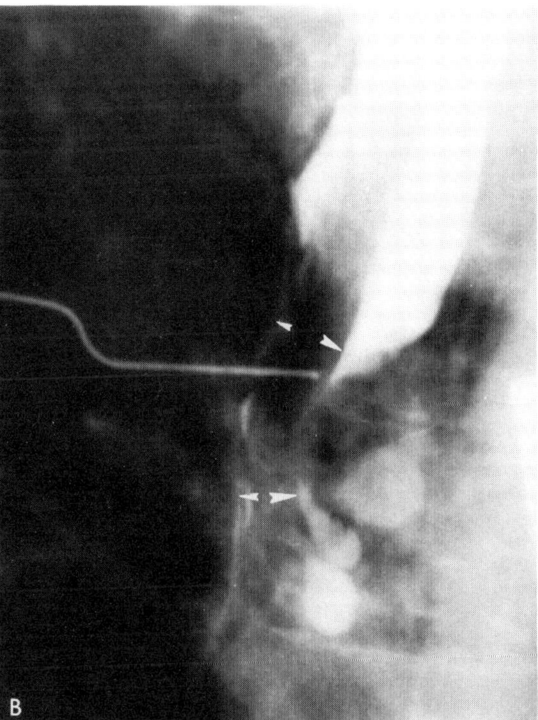

Figure 16–91. THORACIC MENINGIOMA: *A*, The lateral view reveals that the meningioma has the typical intradural configuration. The cord is not seen on this view. The open paper clip is taped to the patient's back as a marker to aid in the surgical approach.

B, The oblique view reveals that the cord is displaced and compressed *(arrowheads)* by the tumor. In this view the tumor has almost an extradural configuration. This patient was originally thought to have multiple sclerosis.

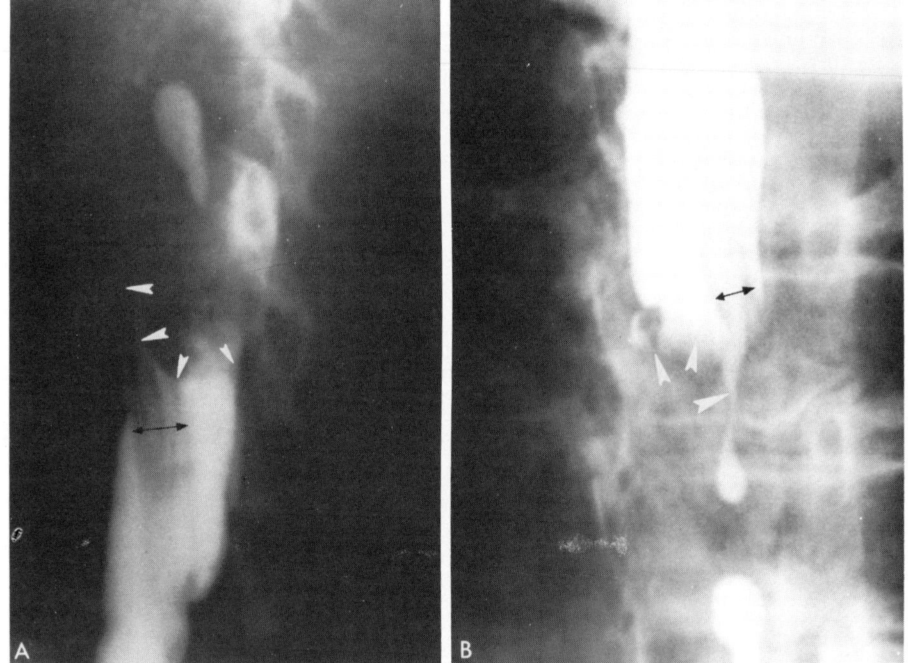

Figure 16–92 *See legend on the opposite page*

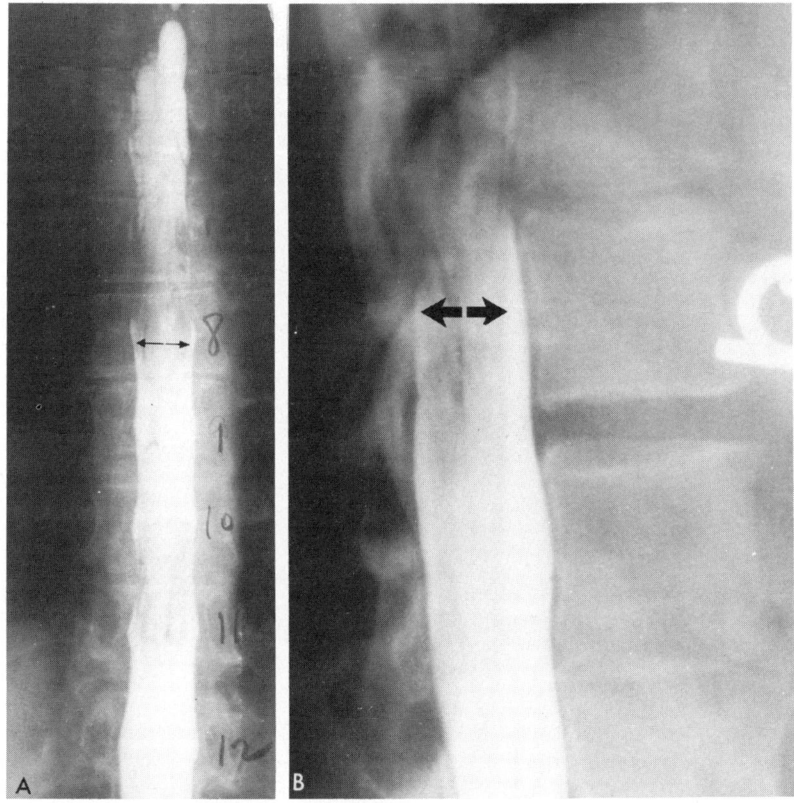

Figure 16–93 *See legend on the opposite page*

Figure 16–92. THORACIC MENINGIOMA: *A*, The lateral view reveals the meniscus sign seen with an intradural lesion *(white arrowheads)* and demonstrates the displacement of the dorsal cord *(black double-headed arrow)* and the compression of the cord at the level of the meningioma.

B, The PA view reconfirms these findings. The meningioma (*white arrows*) is dorsal and to the left of the thoracic cord (*double-headed black arrow*).

Figure 16–93. THORACIC ASTROCYTOMA: The PA *(A)* and lateral *(B)* views demonstrate diffuse widening of the entire visualized portion of the cord (*double-headed arrows*). There is marked compromise of the thoracic subarachnoid space. Surgery confirmed the presence of an astrocytoma of the thoracic cord.

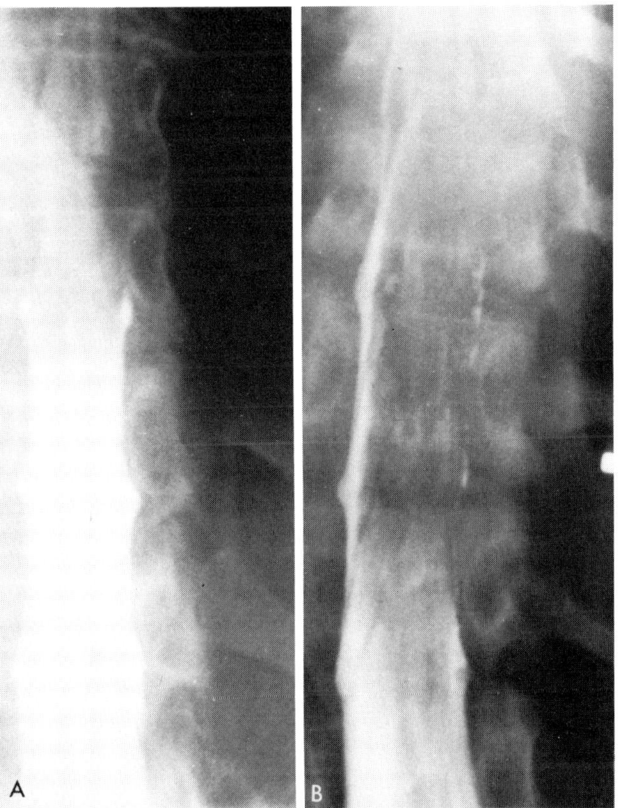

Figure 16–94. THORACIC GLIOMA: *A* and *B*, Diffuse widening of the entire visualized thoracic spinal cord is present, with near-complete obliteration of the thoracic subarachnoid space. There is a complete block to the flow of contrast material. Surgery confirmed the presence of a glioma of the thoracic spinal cord.

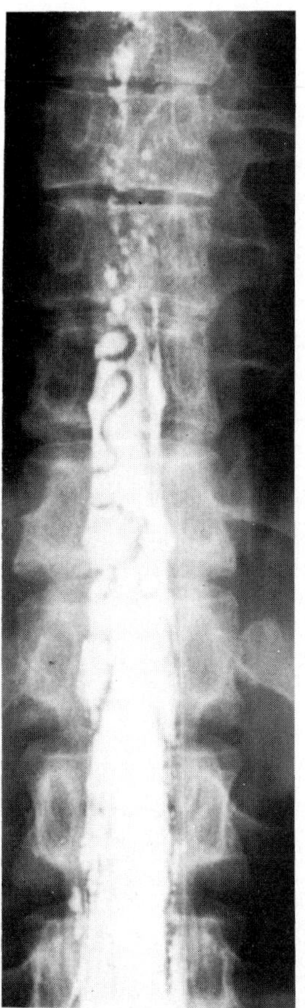

Figure 16–95. ARTERIOVENOUS MALFORMATION OF THE THORACIC SPINAL CORD: With the patient in the supine position, multiple, enlarged tortuous vessels can be readily demonstrated over the thoracic spinal cord. This appearance is very typical for the enlarged arteries and draining vessels associated with an arteriovenous malformation of the cord (see Chapter 12).

Figure 16–96. A SPINAL DYSRHAPHIA AND MENINGOMYELOCELE: *A* and *B*, Plain film examination demonstrates marked widening of the spinal canal with marked deformity of the spinous processes in the lower thoracic and lumbar region *(large white arrowheads)* and bony clefts in the spinous processes *(black arrow)*. This bony deformity is associated with a soft tissue mass that contained both the meninges and the neural tissues — a meningomyelocele.

C, Myelography demonstrates an ectatic spinal canal extending from the midthoracic through the entire lumbar region (courtesy of Drs. Oscar Sugar and Glen Dobben, University of Illinois).

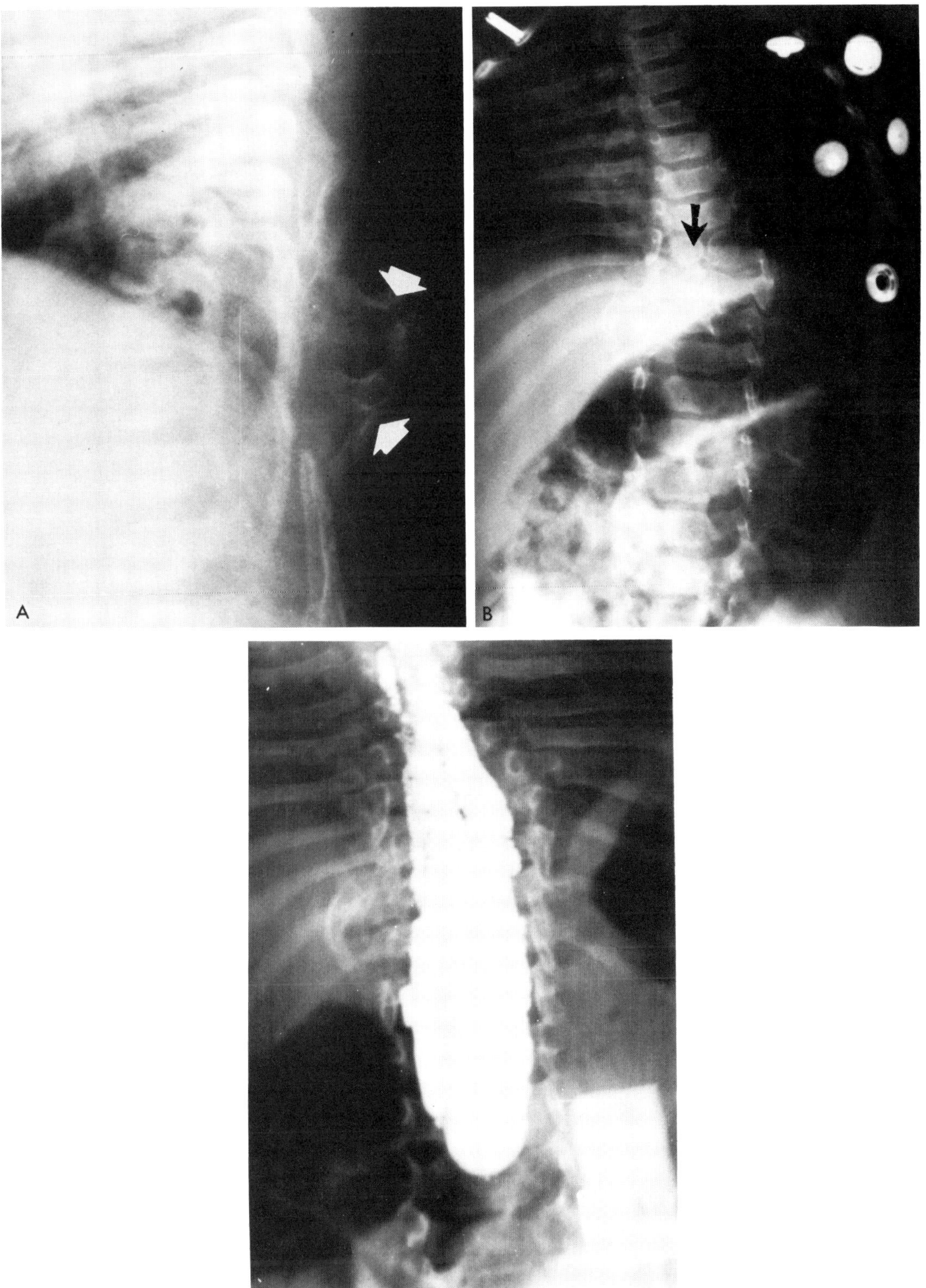

Figure 16–96 *See legend on the opposite page*

EPIDURAL VENOGRAPHY

Selective catheterization of the ascending lumbar veins is performed, using the Seldinger technique. Failure to fill the anterior internal vertebral veins is significant, as is posterior displacement of these veins. Venography is of no help in the postoperative patient, and should not be performed in the patient allergic to contrast material.

Epidural venography is helpful in patients with a normal myelogram and in those with a wide epidural space.

Because of anatomic variations in the venous system, some feel that venography is not helpful. Others find the accuracy similar to that of myelography. The author has not been impressed with the value of epidural venography.

CEREBELLOPONTINE ANGLE CISTERNOGRAPHY

Cerebellopontine angle cisternography (Fig. 16–97) was and is a popular procedure for the diagnosis of space-occupying lesions in the cerebellopontine angle. One begins by following the identical procedures used for myelography. Lumbar tap under fluoroscopic control is performed with the patient in the prone position. When studying the cerebellopontine angle, one needs to use only a small amount of contrast material; in fact, a large amount of contrast may tend to flood the cistern and obliterate the areas of interest.

After the insertion of contrast, the patient is placed in the head-down prone position until the material is noted to accumulate on the clivus. The patient's head is then turned to either the right or left until the Pantopaque is seen to flow into the internal auditory canal. With this maneuver, in the absence of a mass lesion the contrast should readily enter the internal auditory canal. At times, small droplets of contrast will reach even the most lateral portion of the canal. If a mass lesion is present, the contrast will flow around the space-occupying lesion at the porus acusticus. After radiographs have been obtained in this position, the patient's head is then turned to the opposite direction, and the maneuver is repeated.

The eighth and seventh cranial nerves exit from the internal auditory canal, and the usual clinical history is that of involvement of these two nerves. Involvement of the fifth cranial nerve suggests that the tumor has reached a certain size. The fifth cranial nerve and its trigeminal ganglion rest in Meckel's cavity, which is an outpouching of the dura along the top of the petrous bone 1.5 cm from the internal auditory canal. Therefore, if the fifth as well as the seventh and eighth cranial nerves are involved, this implies that the tumor is at least 1.5 cm in size. This can be readily appreciated at myelography. In the normal study, the shadow of the trigeminal ganglion occasionally can be seen along the top of the petrous ridge. At the termination of the procedure, the contrast is returned to the lumbar subarachnoid space and removed through the puncture needle.

The use of biplane fluoroscopy in conjunction with a 90° tilt table will simplify the procedure greatly. After the contrast is centered in the cervical region, the patient is placed in the lateral decubitus position, with the head in the true lateral position. Fluoroscopy is then performed in the anteroposterior horizontal projection and the table is tilted slowly down until the Pantopaque is seen to drop into the dependent internal auditory

Figure 16–97. NORMAL CEREBELLOPONTINE ANGLE MYELOGRAM: *A* and *B*, On the right side *(A)* the contrast material flows readily into the internal auditory canal *(I)*. The oval window is well demonstrated *(O)*. On the left *(B)*, an excessive amount of contrast obscures visualization of the internal auditory canal *(arrow)*. Further manipulation of the contrast material allows better visualization of the canal. The CT scan demonstrated excellent visualization of the normal-appearing internal auditory canals.

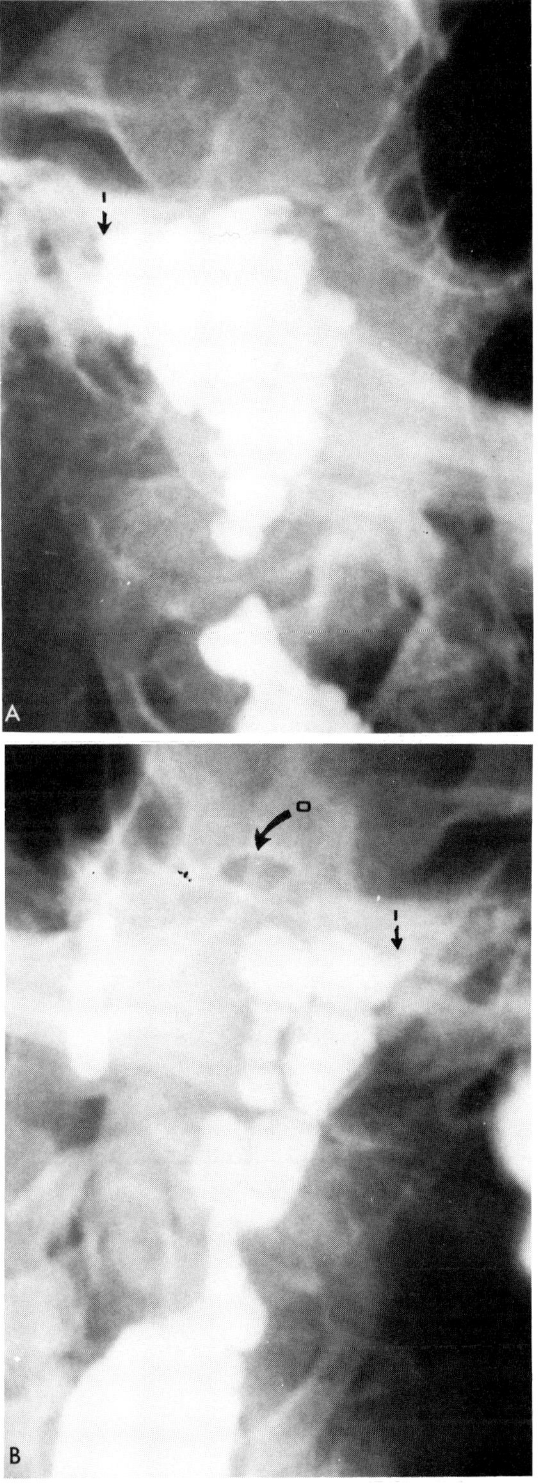

Figure 16–97 *See legend on the opposite page*

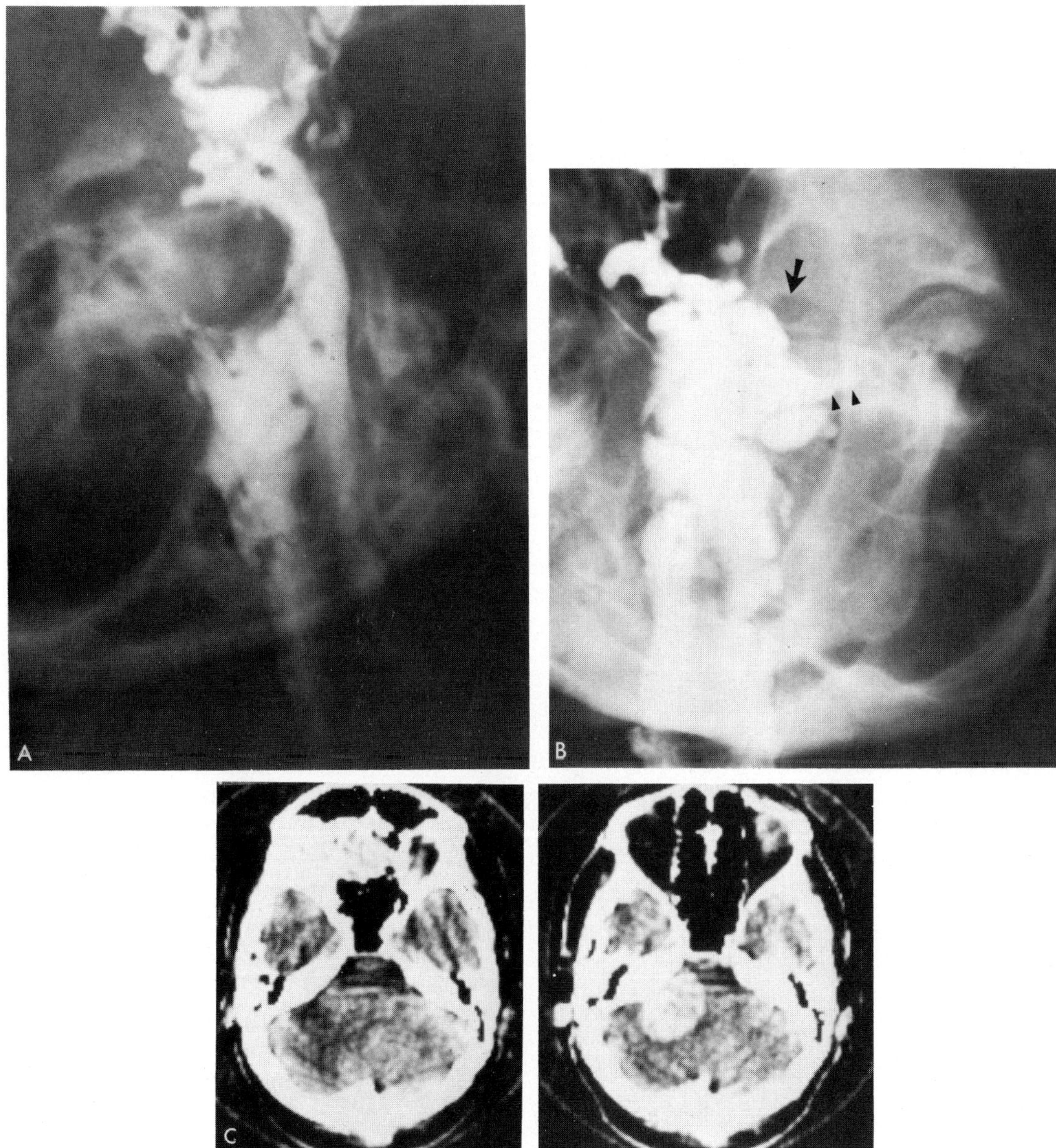

Figure 16–98. ACOUSTIC NEURINOMA: *A,* On the left side the acoustic neurinoma is demonstrated as a rounded radiolucent filling defect in the Pantopaque column. *B,* On the right side the Pantopaque flows readily into the internal auditory canal *(arrowheads).* The foramen ovale *(large arrow)* is well demonstrated. *C,* CT scan with and without the infusion of contrast material reveals an isodense tumor in the region of the left internal auditory canal with marked homogeneous enhancement of the tumor after the infusion of contrast material. This appearance is typical of an acoustic neurinoma.

canal. In the presence of a tumor the contrast will be seen to flow around the mass in the cerebellopontine angle. The radiographic tubes then can be manipulated to allow views in the lateral as well as the anteroposterior projections. When one side is completed, the patient is then placed in the prone position, and the maneuver is repeated. At the end of the study, the contrast material is returned to the lumbar subarachnoid space and removed.

The upper limits of normal in size of the internal auditory canal is 8 mm in the mid- or tallest area, with no more than a 3 mm difference between the two sizes. Occasionally greater differences are seen, however, and even larger internal auditory canals can be normal. The most common tumors of the cerebellopontine angle are acoustic neurinomas, meningiomas (which rarely present with deafness) and the epidermoids (cholesteatomas). Fifth and seventh nerve neurinomas also can be seen, but are rare. Arachnoid cysts also may occur in the cerebellopontine angle and can lead to enlargement of the internal auditory canal.

Amipaque and/or air cisternography used with computed tomography or radiographic tomography probably will replace Pantopaque cisternography.

AIR MYELOGRAPHY

In addition to positive contrast materials, it is also possible to use air as a myelographic contrast agent (see Fig. 16–52). This method is useful in the acutely injured patient to rule out the presence of cord edema resulting in complete block to the flow of contrast. When the diagnosis of syringomyelia is suspected, the procedure is performed using the C_1–C_2 approach with the patient in the supine Trendelenburg position. Initially, a large amount of CSF is removed from the cervical subarachnoid space, and then air is instilled. The patient is placed in the Trendelenburg position to allow the air to rise into the lumbar region. Then further CSF is removed, and the procedure is continued until the CSF has been replaced by air in the subarachnoid space. Radiographs are then obtained. It is vital that tomographic studies be available for complete evaluation. Without tomography it is impossible to evaluate thoroughly the relationship between the cord and the subarachnoid space.

Air myelography is particularly useful in trauma patients with subarachnoid hemorrhage when it is undesirable to use Pantopaque in the presence of blood in the CSF. With a complete block, air may be instilled from below and Amipaque from above, or vice versa, with the patient placed in the appropriate head-down or head-up position for films and tomograms if appropriate.

SPINAL TRAUMA AND COMPUTED TOMOGRAPHY

We have found that computed tomography enhances our ability to diagnose the anatomic deformities seen with spinal trauma. In fact, in most cases this method is preferable to radiographic tomography — especially because in most cases these patients cannot be moved into the lateral position because of the possibility of aggravating their deficit. The instillation of Amipaque into the subarachnoid space also facilitates study of these patients. In Figure 16–99 the fractures of the posterior elements are well demonstrated, and the level of the complete block is also readily demonstrated by the fact that the Amipaque does not accumulate in the lower subarachnoid space.

The anatomy of the bony abnormalities and the interruption of the flow of CSF are well demonstrated by this method; in fact, they are better demonstrated than by any other method.

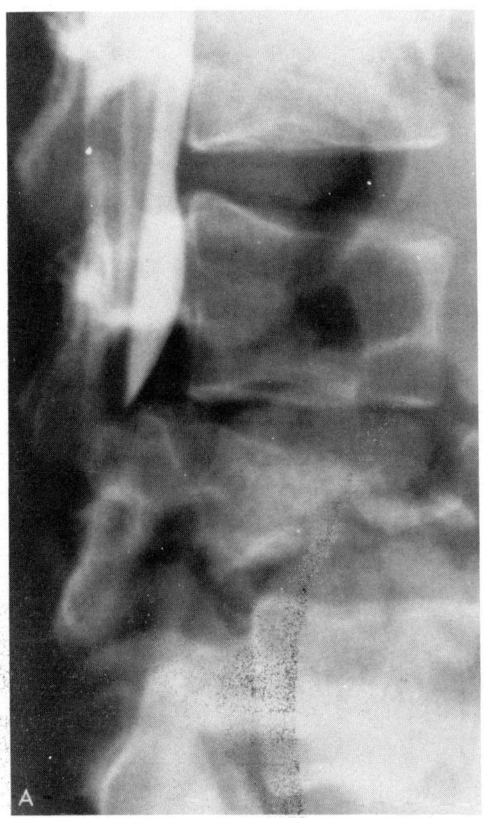

Figure 16–99. LUMBAR SPINE FRACTURE WITH AMIPAQUE MYELOGRAM AND CT SCAN: After the instillation of contrast material at the C_1–C_2 level, a complete block to the flow is encountered at the level of the fracture. The L_3 vertebral body is noted to be compressed and deformed. There is posterior displacement of the posterior aspect of L_3. The contrast column is displaced posteriorly, and the nerves of the cauda equina are compressed.

B, The true extent of the fracture is better appreciated on the CT scan:

#16: The thoracic cord is normal *(arrow)*. Note the anterior and posterior roots as they enter and exit from the spinal cord. The subarachnoid space is filled with Amipaque.

#15: The transverse process demonstrates a comminuted fracture *(arrow)*.

#12: The nerves of the cauda equina are distributed in the lumbar subarachnoid space and bathed by Amipaque.

#07: The comminuted fracture of L_3 can now be seen. Note that the Amipaque is no longer seen because there is a complete block to flow.

#06: A fracture is seen through the spinous process and articulating facet *(arrow)*. Note the comminuted pieces of the L_3 vertebral body. A portion of the vertebral body has been displaced posteriorly into the spinal canal.

#05: There is diastasis of the interfacet articulation *(arrow)*.

#04: There is a fracture through the lamina of the vertebral body and bilateral distraction of the interfacet joints.

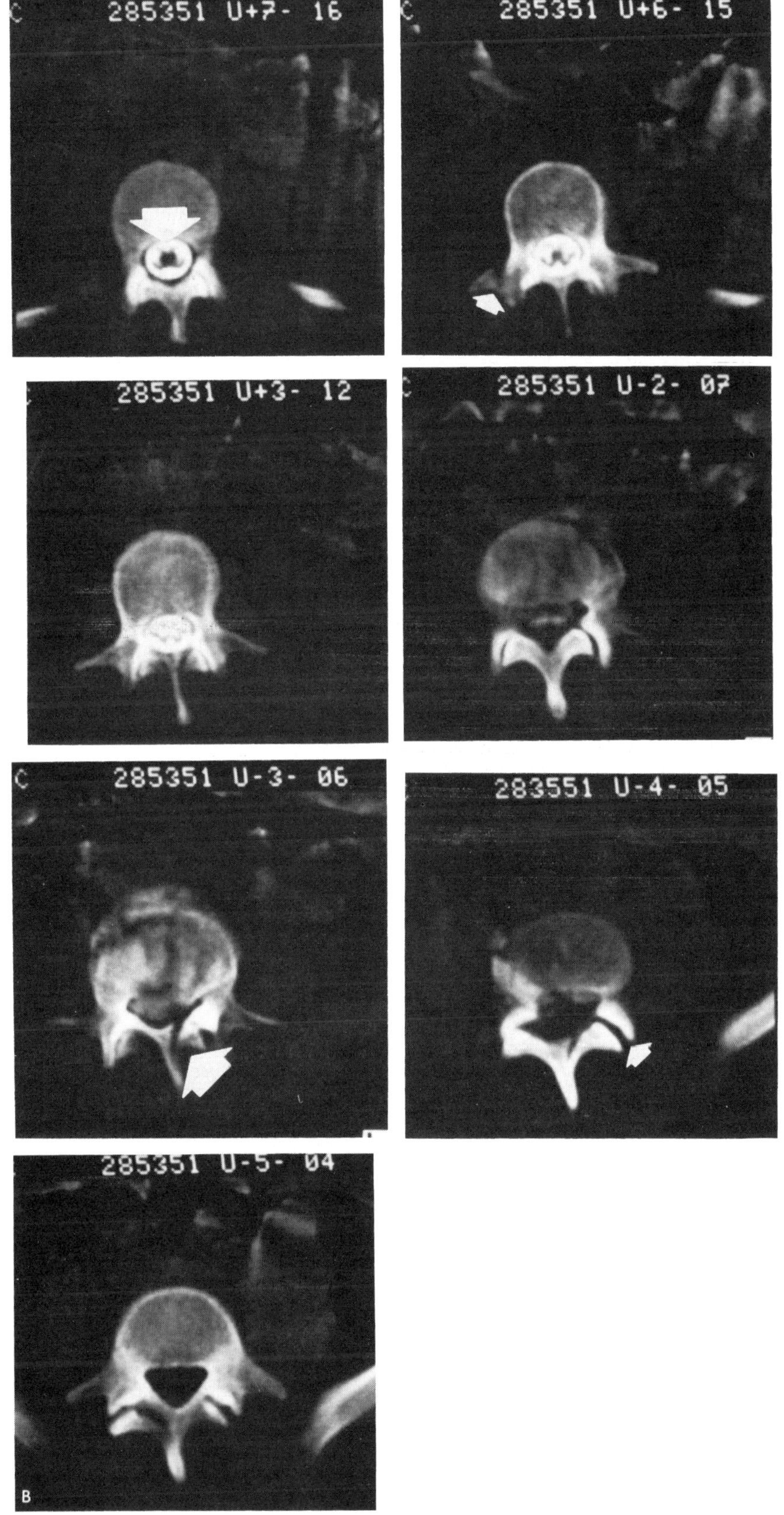

Figure 16–99 *Continued*

AMIPAQUE: DOSAGE, RECONSTITUTION AND MANUFACTURER'S WARNINGS*

The recommended usual and maximum doses of AMIPAQUE are summarized in the following table:

DOSAGE TABLE

Procedure	*Conc. of Solution (mgI/ml)*	*Usual Recommended Dose* (ml)*	*Max. Dose Total (mgI)*
Lumbar myelogram	170–190	10–15	2850
Thoracic myelogram	220	12	2640
Cervical myelogram (via lumbar injection)	250–300	10	3000
Cervical myelogram (via lat. cervical inj.)	220	10	2200
Total columnar myelography	250–280	10	2800
CT cisternography (via lumbar inj.)	170–190	4–6	1140

*Refer to RECONSTITUTION TABLE for preparation of Solution.

RECONSTITUTION TABLE

Conc. of Solution (mgI/ml)	*Volume of Diluent to be Added* 3.75 g Vial (ml)	6.75 g Vial (ml)
170	8.9	16.1
180	8.3	15.0
190	7.8	14.0
220	6.5	11.7
250	5.5	10.0
260	5.2	9.4
270	5.0	9.0
280	4.7	8.5
290	4.5	8.1
300	4.3	7.8
	The volume of the final solution will equal the volume of the diluent + 1.7 ml	The volume of the final solution will equal the volume of the diluent + 3.1 ml

The volume of the final solution will exceed the amount required to achieve the recommended dosage. For precise volume for injection refer to DOSAGE TABLE.

WARNINGS

If grossly bloody CSF is encountered, the possible benefits of a myelographic procedure should be considered in terms of the risk to the patient.

Fatal reactions have been associated with the administration of water-soluble contrast media. Although no fatal reactions have been associated with AMIPAQUE, it is of utmost importance that a course of action be carefully planned in advance for the immediate treatment of serious reactions; and that adequate and appropriate facilities and personnel be readily available in case of a severe reaction.

Caution is advised in patients with a history of epilepsy, severe cardiovascular disease, chronic alcoholism or multiple sclerosis. *Elderly patients* may present a greater risk following myelography. The need for the procedure in these patients should be evaluated carefully. Special attention must be paid to dose and concentration of the medium, hydration, and technique used.

Patients who are receiving anticonvulsants should be maintained on this therapy. Should a seizure occur, intravenous diazepam or phenobarbital sodium is recommended.

Care is required in patient management to prevent inadvertent intracranial entry of a large dose or concentrated bolus of the medium. Direct intracisternal or ventricular administration for standard radiography (not CT) is not recommended.

Prophylactic anticonvulsant treatment with barbiturates or diazepam orally for 24 to 48 hours should be considered in patients with evidence of inadvertent intracranial entry of a large or concentrated bolus of the contrast medium since there is an increased risk of seizures in such cases.

Drugs which lower the seizure threshold, especially phenothiazine derivatives, including those used for their antihistamine properties should not be used with AMIPAQUE. Others include MAO inhibitors, tricyclic antidepressants, CNS stimulants, psychoactive drugs described as analeptics, major tranquilizers, or antipsychotic drugs. Such medication should be discontinued at least 48 hours before myelography, should not be used for the control of nausea and vomiting, and should not be resumed for at least 24 hours postprocedure.

*Reprinted, with permission, from the package insert provided by the distributors, Winthrop Laboratories, Division of Sterling Drug Inc., New York, N.Y. For further details, see current package insert.

BIBLIOGRAPHY

Plain Skull Films

Albright F, Reifenstein EC Jr: The Parathyroid Glands and Metabolic Bone Disease. Baltimore, Williams & Wilkins, 1948.

Barnett DJ: Radiologic aspects of craniopharyngiomas. Radiology *72*:14, 1959.

Bentson JR et al: Computed tomography in intracranial cysticercosis. J Comput Assist Tomography *1*(4):464, 1977.

Bull JWD, Nixon WLB, Pratt RTC: The radiological criteria and familial occurrence of primary basilar impression. Brain *78*:Part 2, 229, 1955.

Bull JWD, Nixon WLB, Pratt RTC, Robinson PK: Paget's disease of the skull and secondary basilar impression. Brain *82*:10, 1959.

Camp JD: II. The normal and pathologic anatomy of the sella turcica as revealed by roentgenograms. Am J Roentgenol *12*:143, 1924.

Camp JD: Symmetrical calcification of cerebral basal ganglia; its roentgenologic significance in diagnosis of parathyroid insufficiency. Radiology *49*:568, 1947.

Camp JD: Significance of intracranial calcification in the roentgenologic diagnosis of intracranial neoplasms. Radiology *55*:659, 1950.

Camp JD, Nash LA: Developmental thinness of the parietal bones. Radiology *42*:42, 1944.

Carbajal JR et al: Radiology of cysticercosis of the central nervous system, including computed tomography. Radiology *125*(1):127, 1977.

Childe AE: Localized thinning and enlargement of the cranium with special reference to the middle fossa. Am J Roentgenol *70*:1, 1953.

Cushing, H: Experiences with orbito-ethmoidal osteomata having intracranial complications. With the report of four cases. Surg Gynecol Obstet *44*:721, 1927.

DiChiro G: The width (third dimension) of the sella turcica. Am J Roentgenol *84*:26, 1960.

Dyke CG: Indirect signs of brain tumor as noted in routine roentgen examinations; displacement of pineal shadow. A survey of 3000 consecutive skull examinations. Am J Roentgenol *23*:598, 1930.

Dyke CG, Davidoff LM, Masson CB: Cerebral hemiatrophy with homolateral hypertrophy of the skull and sinuses. Surg Gynecol Obstet *57*:588, 1933.

Etter LE: Atlas of Roentgen Anatomy of the Skull. Springfield IL, Charles C Thomas, 1955.

Gouliamos AD et al: Computed tomography and skull radiography in the diagnosis of calcified brain tumor. Am J Roentgenol *130*(4):761, 1978.

Hobaek A: Fibrous dysplasia — fibro-osteoma —Osteoma of the facial bones and skull. Acta Radiol *36*:97, 1951.

Holt, JF, Dickerson WW: The osseous lesions of tuberous sclerosis. Radiology *58*:1, 1952.

Kasabach HH, Dyke CG: Osteoporosis circumscripta of the skull as a form of osteitis deformans. Am J Roentgenol *28*:192, 1932.

Kido DK et al: Comparative sensitivity of CT scans, radiographs and radionuclide bone scans in detecting metastatic calvarial lesions. Radiology *128*(2):371, 1978.

King AB, Gould DM: Symmetrical calcification in the cerebellum. Am J Roentgenol *67*:562, 1952.

Klotz O: Studies on calcareous degeneration. I. The process of pathological calcification. J Exp Med *7*:633, 1905.

Leeds NE, Seaman WB: Fibrous dysplasia of the skull and its differential diagnosis. A clinical and roentgenographic study of 46 cases. Radiology *78*:570, 1962.

List CF, Holt JF, Everett M: Lipoma of the corpus callosum. A clinicopathologic study. Am J Roentgenol *55*:125, 1946.

McGregor M: The significance of certain measurements of the skull in diagnosis of basilar impression. Br J Radiol *27*:171, 1948.

McRae DL: Occipitalization of the atlas. Am J Roentgenol *70*:23, 1953.

McRae DL: Observations on craniolacunia. Acta Radiol (Diag) *5*:55, 1966.

Martin GI et al: Computer-assisted cranial tomography in early diagnosis of tuberous sclerosis. JAMA *235*(21):2323, 1976.

Merrill V: Atlas of Roentgenographic Positions, 2d ed. St. Louis, CV Mosby, 1959.

Moss ML: The pathogenesis of premature cranial synostosis in man. Acta Anat *37*:351, 1959.

Norman D, Diamond C, Boyd D: Relative detectability of intracranial calcifications on computed tomography and skull radiography. J Comput Assist Tomography *2*:61, 1978.

Obrador S: Clinical aspects of cerebral cysticercosis. Arch Neurol Psychiatr *50*:457, 1948.

Osborn AG, Saville T: The basal ganglia on cranial computed tomography; normal anatomy and pathology. Comp Axial Tomography *1*:245, 1977.

Pepper OHP, Pendergrass EP: Hereditary occurrence of enlarged parietal foramina; their diagnostic importance. Am J Roentgenol *35*:1, 1936.

Poppel MH, Jacobson HG, Duff BK, Gottlieb C: Basilar impression and platybasia in Paget's disease. Radiology *61*:639, 1953.

Rhodes BA, Greyson ND, Hamilton CR Jr et al: Absence of anatomic arteriovenous shunts in Paget's disease of bone. N Engl J Med *287*:686, 1971.

Rothner AD et al: Agenesis of the corpus callosum revealed by computerized tomography. Dev Med Child Neurol *18*(2):160, 1976.

Schunk H, Maryuama Y: Two vascular grooves of the external table of the skull which simulate fractures. Acta Radiol *54*:186, 1960.

Seur NH et al: Arachnoid cyst of the middle fossa with paradoxical changes of the bony structures. Neuroradiology *12*(3):177, 1976.

Simmons DR, Peyton WT: Premature closure of the cranial sutures. J Pediatr *31*:528, 1947.

Sprague RG, Haines SF, Power MH: Metabolic effects of parathyroid hormone, dihydrotachysterol and calciferol in case of pseudohypoparathyroidism. Proc Central Soc Clin Res *17*:16, 1944; J Lab Clin Med *30*:363, 1945.

Stauffer HM, Snow LB, Adams AB: Roentgenologic recognition of habenular calcification as distinct from calcification in the pineal body. Its application in cerebral localization. Am J Roentgenol *70*:83, 1953.

Vogt BC, Deck MDF: The clivus deformity of the Arnold Chiari malformation. Radiology *36*:147, 1941.

Weed LH: A note on calcification in cerebral neoplasms. Arch Neurol Psychiatr *6*:190, 1914.

Weinstein MA et al: Diagnosis of juvenile angiofibroma by computed tomography. Radiology *126*(3):703, 1978.

Wood EH Jr: Some roentgenological and pathological aspects of calcification of the choroid plexus. Am J Roentgenol *52*:388, 1944.

Yakovlev PI, Guthrie RH: Congenital ectodermoses (neurocutaneous syndromes) in epileptic patients. Arch Neurol Psychiatr *26*:1145, 1931.

Yu HC, Deck MDF: The clivus deformity of the Arnold-Chiari malformation. Radiology *10*:613, 1971.

Computed Tomography

Abrams HL et al: Computed tomography: cost and efficacy implications. Am J Roentgenol *131*(1):81, 1978.

Alderson PO et al: Computerized cranial tomography and radionuclide imaging in the detection of intracranial mass lesions. Semin Nucl Med 7(2):161, 1977.

Ambrose JA: Computerized transverse axial tomography. Br J Radiol *46*:401, 1973.

Ambrose JA: The usefulness of computerized transverse axial scanning in problems arising from cerebral haemorrhage, infarction or oedema. Br J Radiol *46*:736, 1973.

Ambrose JA: Computerized transverse axial scanning (tomography): II. Clinical application. Br J Radiol *46*:1023, 1973.

Ambrose JA: Computerized x-ray scanning of the brain. J Neurosurg *40*(6):679, 1974.

Ambrose JA, Hounsfield GN: Computerized transverse axial tomography, abstracted. Br J Radiol *46*:148, 1973.

Ambrose JA, Gooding MB, Richardson AE: An assessment of the accuracy of computerized transverse axial scanning (EMI scanners) in the diagnosis of intracranial tumor. A review of 366 patients. Brain *98*:569, 1975.

Bardfield PA, Passalaqua AM, Braunstein P, Raghavendra BN, Leeds NE, Kricheff I: A comparison of radionuclide scanning and computed tomography in metastatic lesions of the brain. J Comput Assist Tomography *1*:315, 1977.

Barrington NA et al: Indications for contrast medium enhancement in computed tomography of the brain. Clin Radiol *28*(5):535, 1977.

Becker H et al: The base of the skull: a comparison of computed and conventional tomography. J Comput Assist Tomography *2*(1):113, 1978.

Berg B et al: Nonsurgical care of brain abscess: early diagnosis and follow-up with computerized tomography. Ann Neurol *3*(6):474, 1978.

Bergström M et al: Variation with time of the attenuation values of intracranial hematomas. J Comput Assist Tomography *1*(1):57, 1977.

Bhave DG et al: Scattered radiation doses to infants and children during EMI head scans. Radiology *124*(2):379, 1977.

Braun IF et al: Dense intracranial epidermoid tumors. Computed tomographic observations. Radiology *122*(2):717, 1977.

Butler AR, Horii SC, Kricheff II, Shannon MB, Budzilovich GN: Computed tomography in astrocytomas: a statistical analysis of the parameters of malignancy and the positive contrast-enhanced CT scan. Radiology *129*:433, 1978.

Byrd SE et al: Coronal computed tomography of the skull and brain in infants and children. I. Technique and results. Radiology *124*:705, 1977; II. Clinical value. Radiology *124*:710, 1977.

Byrd SE et al: Computed tomography in the evaluation of encephaloceles in infants and children. J Comput Assist Tomography *2*(1):81, 1978.

Byrd SE et al: Two projection computed tomography: the axial and Towne projections. Radiology *128*:512, 1978.

Claveria L, Sutton D, Tress BM: The radiological diagnoses of meningioma. The impact of EMI scanning. Br J Radiol *50*:15, 1977.

Clifford JR et al: Comparison of radionuclide scans with computer-assisted tomography in diagnosis of intracranial disease. Neurology (Minneap) *26*:(12):119, 1976.

Constant P et al: CT appearances of the normal tentorial hiatus and expanding lesions of the incisura. J Neuroradiol *5*(1):27, 1978.

Cornell SH et al: Individualized computer tomography of the skull with the EMI scanner using the 160 × 160 matrix. Am J Roentgenol *126*(4):779, 1976.

Crocker EF et al: The effect of steroids on the extravascular distribution of radiographic contrast material and technetium pertechnetate in brain tumors as determined by computed tomography. Radiology *119*:471, 1976.

Davis JM et al: Expanded high iodine dose in computed cranial tomography: a preliminary report. Radiology *131*:373, 1979.

Davis KR et al: Some limitations of computed tomography in the diagnosis of neurological diseases. Am J Roentgenol *127*(1):111, 1976.

Drayer BP, Rosenbaum AE, Higman HB: Cerebrospinal fluid imaging using serial metrizamide CT cisternography. Neuroradiology *13*:7, 1977.

Dublin AB et al: Computed tomography in the evaluation of herpes simplex encephalitis. Radiology *125*(1):133, 1977.

Enzmann DR et al: Computed tomography of granulomatous basal arachnoiditis. Radiology *120*(2):341, 1976.

Evens RG et al: Economic analysis of body computed tomography units including data on utilization. Radiology *127*(1):151, 1978.

Forssell A et al: Computed tomography of the paranasal sinuses. Adv Otorhinolaryngol *24*:42, 1978.

Gado MH, Phelps ME, Coleman RE: An extravascular component of contrast enhancement in cranial computed tomography. Radiology *117*:589, 1975.

Gado MH, Hanaway J, Frank R: Functional anatomy of the cerebral cortex by computed tomography. J Comput Assist Tomography *3*(1):1, 1979.

Glyndensted C: Measurements of the normal ventricular system and hemispheric sulci of 100 adults with computed tomography. Neuroradiology *14*:183, 1977.

Hahn FJY, Rim K: Frontal ventricular dimensions on normal computed tomography. Am J Roentgenol *126*:593, 1976.

Hammerschlag SB et al: Computed tomography of the skull base. J Comput Assist Tomography *1*(1):75, 1977.

Handa J et al: Computerized tomography in Moyamoya syndrome. Surg Neurol *7*(5):315, 1977.

Haymen LA, Evans RA, Hinck VC: Rapid high dose (RHD) contrast cranial computed tomography: a concise review of normal anatomy. J Comput Assist Tomography *3*(2):147, 1979.

Horsley RJ et al: Radiation exposure from EMI scanner-multiple scans. Br J Radiol *49*(585):810, 1976.

How many CT scanners? (letter). N Engl J Med *297*(13):731, 1977.

Hounsfield GN: Computerized transverse axial scanning (tomography). I. Description of system. Br J Radiol *46*(552):1016, 1973.

Huckman MS, Grainer LS, Clasen RC: The normal computed tomogram. Semin Roentgenol *12*(1):25, 1977.

Jacoby CG et al: Computed tomography in cerebral hemiatrophy. Am J Roentgenol *129*(1):5, 1977.

Kazner E et al: Computer assisted tomography in primary malignant lymphomas of the brain. J Comput Assist Tomography *2*:125, 1978.

Kinkel WR: Right is right. Orientation of CT images of the head. Neurology (Minneap) *27*(1):98, 1977.

Kramer RA: Vermian pseudotumor: a potential pitfall of CT brain scanning with contrast enhancement. Neuroradiology *13*:229, 1977.

Kramer RA, Janetos GP, Perlstein G: An approach to contrast enhancement in computed tomography of the brain. Radiology *16*:641, 1975.

Krishnamoorthy KS et al: Evaluation of neonatal intracranial hemorrhage by computed tomography. Pediatrics *59*(2):165, 1977.

Laster DW, Moody DM, Ball MR: Resolving intracerebral hematoma: alteration of the "ring sign" with steroids. Am J Roentgenol *130*:935, 1978.

Lee KF et al: CT evidence of grey matter calcification secondary to radiation therapy. Comput Tomography *1*(1):103, 1977.

LeMay M, Kido DK: Asymmetries of the cerebral hemispheres on computed tomograms. J Comput Assist Tomography *2*:471, 1978.

McCullough EC et al: An evaluation of the quantitative and radiation features of a scanning x-ray transverse axial tomography: the EMI scanner. Radiology *111*(3):709, 1974.

McGeachie RE, Gold LHA, Latchaw RE: Periventricular spread of tumor demonstrated by computed tomography. Radiology *125*:407, 1977.

Mandybur TI: Intracranial hemorrhage caused by metastatic tumors. Neurology *27*:650, 1977.

Messina AV: Computed tomography: contrast enhancement in resolving intracerebral hemorrhage. Am J Roentgenol *127*(6):1050, 1976.

Messina AV, Chernik NL: Computed tomography: the "resolving" intracerebral hemorrhage. Radiology *118*:609, 1975.

Mikhael MA: Case report. Diminished density surrounding a meningioma verified to be an overlying cystic astrocytoma. J Comput Assist Tomography *1*:349, 1977.

Naidich TP et al: Computed tomography in the diagnosis of extra-axial posterior fossa masses. Radiology *120*(2):333, 1976.

Naidich TP et al: The tentorium in axial section. I. Normal CT appearance and non-neoplastic pathology. Radiology *123*:631, 1977.

Naidich TP et al: The normal contrast-enhanced computed tomogram of the brain. J Comput Assist Tomography *3*(2):16, 1977.

New PFJ et al: Computed tomography with the EMI scanner in the diagnosis of primary and metastatic intracranial neoplasms. Radiology *114*:75, 1975.

New PFJ, Aranow S: Attenuation measurements of whole blood and blood fractions in computed tomography. Radiology *121*:635, 1976.

Norman D et al: Computed tomography in the evaluation of malignant glioma before and after therapy. Radiology *121*:85, 1976.

Osborn AG: The medical tentorium and incisura: normal and pathological anatomy. Neuroradiology *13*(2):109, 1977.

Osborn AG: Diagnosis of descending transtentorial herniation by cranial computed tomography. Radiology *123*(1):93, 1977.

Osborn AG et al: The evaluation of ependymal and subependymal lesions by cranial computed tomography. Radiology *127*(2):397, 1978.

Paxton CR, Ambrose JA: The EMI scanner. A brief review of the first 650 patients. Br J Radiol *47*(561):530, 1974.

Perry BJ, Bridges C: Computerized transverse axial scanning (tomography): III. Radiation dose considerations. Br. J. Radiol *46*(552):1048, 1973.

Ramsey, RG: Computed Tomography of the Brain. Philadelphia, WB Saunders, 1977.

Scott WR et al: Computerized axial tomography of intracerebral and intraventricular hemorrhage. Radiology *112*:73, 1974.

Swartz R et al: Computed tomography: the cost-benefit dilemma. Radiology *125*(1):251, 1977.

Tadmor R et al: Computed tomography in primary malignant lymphoma of the brain. J Comput Assist Tomography *2*:135, 1978.

Tamaki N et al: Dynamics of cerebrospinal fluid circulation evaluated by metrizamide CT cisternography. J Comput Assist Tomography *3*(2):209, 1979.

Thomson JL: The computed axial tomograph in acute herpes simplex encephalitis. Br J Radiol *49*(577):86, 1976.

Vassilouthis J, Ambrose JA: Computerized tomography scanning appearance of intracranial meningiomas. J Neurosurg *50*:320, 1979.

von Holst H et al: Titanium clips in neurosurgery for elimination of artefacts in computer tomography (ct) a technical note. Acta Neurochir (Wien) *38*(1–2):101, 1977.

Weinstein MA et al: White and gray matter of the brain

differentiated by computed tomography. Radiology *122*(2 Suppl):699, 1977.

Wendling LR: Intracranial venous sinus thrombosis: diagnosis suggested by computed tomography. Am J Roentgenol *130*(5):978, 1978.

Wiggli U et al: Normal computed tomography anatomy of the suprasellar subarachnoid space. Radiology *128*(1):65, 1978.

Wortzman G et al: Cranial computed tomography: an evaluation of cost effectiveness. Radiology *117*(1):75, 1975.

Yock DH, Marshall WH: Recent ischemic brain infarcts at computed tomography: appearance pre and post contrast infusion. Radiology *117*:599, 1975.

Zimmerman RD, Leeds NE, Naidich TP: Ring blush associated with intracerebral hematoma. Radiology *122*:707, 1977.

Angiographic Technique and Applied Cerebrovascular Embryology and Normal Anatomy

Amundsen P et al: Cerebral angiography by catheterization — complications and side effects. Acta Radiol *1*:164, 1963.

Andersen PE: The lenticulo-striate arteries and their diagnostic value. A preliminary report. Acta Radiol *50*:84, 1958.

Azambuja N, Lindgren E, Sjögren SE: Tentorial herniations. I. Anatomy. Acta Radiol *46*:215, 1956; III. Angiography. Acta Radiol *46*:232, 1956.

Baker HL Jr: A new approach to percutaneous subclavian angiography. Proc Staff Meet Mayo Clin *35*:169, 1960.

Baker HL Jr: Cerebral angiography: technics and results. Proc Staff Meet Mayo Clin *35*:482, 1960.

Barbieri PL, Verdecchia GC: Vertebral arteriography by percutaneous puncture of the subclavian artery. Acta Radiol *48*:444, 1957.

Begg AC: Radiographic demonstration of the "hypoglossal artery." A rare type of persistent anomalous carotid-basilar anastomosis. Clin Radiol *12*:187, 1961.

Bierman HR: On the intravascular knotting of catheters. Vasc Surg *6*:155, 1972.

Broman T, Forssman B, Olsson O: Further experimental investigations of injuries from contrast media in cerebral angiography. Summation of various injurious factors. Acta Radiol *34*:135, 1950.

Broadridge AT, Leslie EV: Cerebral angiographic contrast media. A comparison of Hypaque 45% and Urografin 60% and an assessment of the relative clinical toxicity of Urografin 60%, Hypaque 45%, Diaginol 25%, and Diodone 35% in carotid arteriography. Br J Radiol *31*:556, 1958.

Carpenter MB, Noback CR, Moss ML: The anterior choroidal artery. Its origins, course, distribution, and variations. Arch Neurol Psychiatr *71*:714, 1954.

Chase NE, Kricheff II: The comparison of the complication rates of meglumine iothalamate and sodium diatrizoate in cerebral angiography. Am J Roentgenol *95*:852, 1965.

Chinichian A et al: Knitting of an 8-French "headhunter" catheter and its successful removal. Radiology *104*:282, 1972.

Chou SN et al: Some angiographic features of brain abscess. J Neurosurg *24*:693, 1966.

Coddon DR, Krieger HP: Circumstances surrounding complications of cerebral angiography. Analysis of 546 consecutive cerebral angiograms. Am J Med *25*:580, 1958.

Crawford T: The pathological effects of cerebral arteriography. J Neurol Neurosurg Psychiatr *19*:217, 1956.

Ecker AD: The Normal Cerebral Angiogram. Springfield, IL, Charles C Thomas, 1951.

Ecker AD, Riemenschneider PA: Angiographic Localization of Intracranial Masses. Springfield, IL, Charles C Thomas, 1955.

Elias WS: Intracranial fibromuscular hyperplasia. JAMA *218*:254, 1971.

Epstein N: Acute reactions to urographic contrast media. Ann Allergy *39*:139, 1977.

Feild JR, Robertson JT, DeSaussure RL Jr: Complications of cerebral angiography in 2,000 consecutive cases. J Neurosurg *19*:775, 1962.

Feild JR, Lee L, McBurney RF: Complications of 1,000 brachial arteriograms. J Neurosurg *36*:324, 1972.

Fischer HW, Doust VL: An evaluation of pretesting in the problem of serious and fatal reactions to excretory urography. Radiology *103*:497, 1972.

Gabrielsen TO, Heinz ER: Spontaneous aseptic thrombosis of the superior sagittal sinus and cerebral veins. Am J Roentgenol *107*:579, 1969.

Galloway JR, Greitz T: The medial and lateral choroid arteries: an anatomic roentgenographic study. Acta Radiol *53*:353, 1960.

Greitz T: A radiologic study of the brain circulation by rapid serial angiography of the carotid artery. Acta Radiol (Suppl) 140, 1956.

Hanafee W, Stout P: Subtraction technic. Radiology *79*:658, 1962.

Hassler O, Saltzman GF: Angiographic and histologic changes in infundibular widening of the posterior communicating artery. Acta Radiol *1*:321, 1963.

Hawkins IF, Tonkin A: Deflector method for nonsurgical removal of knotted catheters. Radiology *106*:705, 1973.

Hilal SK: Hemodynamic changes associated with the intra-arterial injection of contrast media. New toxicity tests and a new experimental contrast medium. Radiology *86*:615, 1966.

Hodes PJ et al: Cerebral angiography. Fundamentals in anatomy and physiology. Am J Roentgenol *70*:61, 1953.

Holder JC, Cherry JF: The use of a tip deflecting guide in untying a knotted arterial catheter. Radiology *128*:808, 1978.

Holman CB: The application of closed-circuit television in diagnostic roentgenology. Proc Mayo Clin *38*:67, 1963.

Horwitz NH, Dunsmore RH: Some factors influencing the nonvisualization of the internal carotid artery by angiography. J Neurosurg *13*:155, 1956.

Huang Y, Wolf B: Angiographic features of the pericallosal cistern. Radiology *82*:14, 1964.

Kaplan HA: The transcerebral venous system. Arch Neurol *1*:148, 1959.

Kaplan AD, Walker AE: Complications of cerebral angiography. Neurology *4*:643, 1954.

Kuhn RA: Brachial cerebral angiography. J Neurosurg *17*:955, 1960.

Laine E et al: Phlebography in tumors of hemispheres and central grey matter. Acta Radiol *46*:203, 1956.

Lasser BC: Basic mechanisms of contrast media reactions. Theoretical and experimental considerations. Radiology *91*:63, 1968.

Lasser EC, Walters AJ, Lang JH: An experimental basis for histamine release in contrast material reactions. Radiology *110*:49, 1974.

Lasser EC et al: Steroids: theoretical and experimental basis for utilization in prevention of contrast media reactions. Radiology *125*:1, 1977.

Leeds NE et al: Serial magnification cerebral angiography. Radiology *90*:1171, 1968.

Lima PM de A: Cerebral Angiography. New York, Oxford University Press, 1950.

Lin PM et al: Importance of the deep cerebral veins in cerebral angiography, with special emphasis on the orientation of the foramen of Monro through visualization of the "venous angle" of the brain. J Neurosurg *12*:256, 1955.

Lindgren E: Percutaneous angiography of the vertebral artery. Acta Radiol *33*:389, 1950.

LoZito JC: Convulsions: a complication of contrast enhancement in computerized tomography (letter). Arch Neurol *34*:649, 1977.

Mani RL, Eisenberg RL: Complications of catheter cerebral arteriography: analysis of 5,000 procedures. III. Assessment of arteries injected, contrast medium used, duration of procedure, and age of patient. Am J Roentgenol *131*:871, 1978.

Maslowski HA: Vertebral angiography. Percutaneous lateral atlanto-occipital method. Br J Surg *43*:1, 1955.

Mokrohisky JF et al: The diagnostic importance of normal variants in deep cerebral phlebography. With special emphasis on the true and false "venous angles of the brain" and evaluation of venous angle measurements. Radiology *67*:34, 1956.

Morello A, Cooper IS: Arteriographic anatomy of the anterior choroidal artery. Am J Roentgenol *73*:748, 1955.

Naidich TP et al: The tentorium in axial section. II. Lesion localization. Radiology *123*:639, 1977.

Newton TH, Kramer RA: Clinical uses of selective external carotid arteriography. Am J Roentgenol *97*:458, 1966.

Olivecrona H: Complications of cerebral angiography. Neuroradiology *14*:175, 1977.

Padget DH: The circle of Willis, its embryology and anatomy. In: WE Dandy: Intracranial Arterial Aneurysms. Ithaca, NY, Comstock, 1944.

Patterson RH Jr, Goodell H, Dunning HS: Complications of carotid arteriography. Arch Neurol *10*:513, 1964.

Pygott F, Hutton CF: Vertebral arteriography by percutaneous brachial artery catheterization. Br J Radiol *32*:114, 1959

Radner S: Vertebral angiography by catheterization. A new method employed in 221 cases. Acta Radiol (Suppl) 87, 1951.

Rapoport SI, Levitan H: Neurotoxicity of x-ray contrast media. Am J Roentgenol *122*:186, 1974.

Raynor RB, Ross G: Arteriography and vasospasm. The effects of intracarotid contrast media on vasospasm. J Neurosurg *17*:1055, 1960.

Saltzman GF: Patent primitive trigeminal artery studied by cerebral angiography. Acta Radiol *51*:329, 1959.

Saltzman GF: Angiographic demonstration of the posterior communicating and posterior cerebral arteries. I. Normal angiography. Acta Radiol *51*:1, 1959; II. Pathologic angiography. Acta Radiol *52*:114, 1959.

Scheinberg P, Zunker E: Complications of direct percutaneous carotid arteriography. Arch Neurol *8*:676, 1963.

Seldinger SI: Catheter replacement of the needle in percutaneous arteriography. A new technique. Acta Radiol *39*:368, 1953.

Stanley RJ, Pfister RC: Bradycardia and hypotension following use of intravenous contrast media. Radiology *121*:5, 1976.

Stauffer HM et al: Biplane stereoscopic cerebral angiography. Acta Radiol *46*:262, 1956.

Stein HL: Successful nonsurgical removal of a knotted preshaped coronary artery catheter. Radiology *109*:469, 1973.

Sugar O: Discussion of "use and limitations of angiography." Proceedings of International Conference on Vascular Diseases of the Brain. Neurology *11*:91, 1961.

Takahashi M, Kawanami H: Complications of catheter cerebral angiography: an analysis of 500 examinations. Acta Radiol (Diag) *13*:248, 1972.

Tuohimaa PJ, Melartin E: Neurotoxicity of iothalamates and diatrizoates. II. Historadioautographic study of rat brains with 131-Iodine tagged contrast media. Invest Radiol *5*:22, 1970.

Vitek JJ: Femoro-cerebral angiography: analysis of 2,000 consecutive examinations, special emphasis on carotid arteries catheterization in older patients. Am J Roentgenol *118*:633, 1973.

Weiner IH, Azzato NM, Mendelsohn RA: Cerebral angiography. A new technique; catheterization of the common carotid artery via the superficial temporal artery. J Neurosurg *15*:618, 1958.

Wolf BS, Newman CM, Schlesinger B: The diagnostic value of the deep cerebral veins in cerebral angiography. Radiology *64*:161, 1955.

Wood EH, Bream CA: Enlargement radiography without special apparatus other than a very fine focal spot tube. North Carolina Med J *15*:69, 1954.

Young DA, Maurer RM: Successful manipulation of a knotted intravascular catheter allowing nonsurgical removal. Radiology *94*:155, 1970.

Ziedses des Plantes BG: Planigraphie en subtractie. Röntgenographische Differentiatiemethoden. Thesis, 1934.

Ziedses des Plantes BG: Subtraktion. Eine röntgenographische Methode zur separaten Abbildung bestimmter Teile des Objekts. Fortschr Geb Röntgenstrahlen *52*:69, 1935.

Ziedses des Plantes BG: Application of the roentgenographic subtraction method in neuroradiology. Acta Radiol (Diag) *1*:961, 1963.

The Abnormal Angiogram

Baker HL Jr: Intracerebral hemorrhage masquerading as a neoplasm. A difficult neuroradiologic problem. Radiology *78*:914, 1962.

Brant-Zawadski M, Enzmann DR: Computed tomographic brain scanning in patients with lymphoma. Radiology *129*:67, 1978.

Cairns H, Russell DS: Intracranial and spinal metastases in gliomas of the brain. Brain *54*:377, 1931.

Chase NE, Taveras JM: Temporal tumors studied by serial angiography — review of 150 cases. Acta Radiol (Diag) *1*:225, 1963.

Crocker EF et al: The effect of dexamethasone upon the accumulation of meglumine iothalamate and technetium pertechnetate in cerebral tumors as determined by computed tomography. J Nucl Med *17*:528, 1976.

Deck MD et al: Computed tomography in metastatic disease of the brain. Radiology *119*(1):115, 1976.

Ethelberg S, Vaernet K: The angiographic configuration of intracerebral metastatic tumors. Radiology *61*:39, 1953.

Feiring EH, Shapiro JH: Evaluation of angiography in the diagnosis of suprasellar tumors. Am J Roentgenol *92*:811, 1964.

Goree JA, Dukes HT: The angiographic differential diagnosis between the vascularized malignant glioma and the intracranial arteriovenous malformation. Am J Roentgenol *90*:512, 1963.

Hardman J: The angioarchitecture of the glioblastoma multiforme type of tumor and its bearing on angiography. Lisboa méd *15*:329, 1938.

Heinz ER, Cooper RD: Several early angiographic findings in brain abscess including "the ripple sign." Radiology *90*:735, 1968.

Huang YP, Wolf BS: Veins of the white matter of the cerebral hemispheres (the medullary veins): diagnostic importance in carotid angiography. Am J Roentgenol *92*:739, 1964.

Huckman MS et al: Angiographic clinico-pathologic correlates in basal ganglionic hemorrhage. Radiology *95*:79, 1970.

Jefferson A, Sheldon P: Transtentorial herniation of the brain as revealed by the displacement of arteries. Acta Radiol *46*:480, 1956.

Johnson RT, Yates PO: Clinico-pathological aspects of pressure changes at the tentorium. Acta Radiol *46*:242, 1956.

Kricheff II, Taveras JM: The angiographic localization of suprasylvian space-occupying lesions. Radiology *82*:602, 1964.

Leeds NE, Taveras JM: Diagnostic value of changes in local circulation time in frontal and parietal tumors. Acta Radiol *1*:332, 1963.

List CF, Hodges FJ: Differential diagnosis of intracranial neoplasms by cerebral angiography. Radiology *48*:493, 1947.

Mandybur TI: Intracranial hemorrhage caused by metastatic tumors. Neurology *27*:650, 1977.

Margolis MT, Newton TH: Methamphetamine ("speed") arteritis. Neuroradiology *2*:179, 1971.

Pollock JA, Newton TH: The anterior falx artery; normal and pathologic anatomy. Radiology *91*:1089, 1968.

Potts DG, Taveras JM: Differential diagnosis of space-occupying lesions in the region on the thalamus by cerebral angiography. Acta Radiol (Diag) *1*:373, 1963.

Rumbaugh CL et al: Cerebral vascular changes secondary to amphetamine abuse in the experimental animal. Radiology *101*:345, 1971.

Russell DS, Rubinstein LJ: Pathology of Tumors of the Nervous System, 2d ed. Baltimore, Williams and Wilkins, 1963.

Scatliff JH et al: Vascular structures of glioblastomas. Am J Roentgenol *105*:795, 1969.

Torkildsen A: Carotid angiography. With special reference to the diagnosis of cerebral gliomas. Acta Psychiatr Neurol Scandinav (Suppl) 55, 1949.

Wood EH Jr, Himadi GM: Chordomas: a roentgenologic study of sixteen cases previously unreported. Radiology *54*:706, 1950.

Zimmerman HM: Introduction to tumors of the central nervous system. In: J Mincker (ed): Pathology of the Nervous System, Vol II. New York, McGraw-Hill, 1971.

Zimmerman HM: The ten most common types of brain tumor. Semin Roentgenol *6*:48, 1971.

Arteriosclerosis

Alcala H, Gado M, Torack RM: The effect of size, histologic elements and water content on the visualization of cerebral infarcts. Arch Neurol *35*:1, 1978.

Alvarez WC: Little Strokes. Philadelphia, JB Lippincott, 1966.

Bergstrom M et al: Variation with time of the attenuation values of intracranial hematomas. J Comput Assist Tomography *1*(1):57, 1977.

Campbell JK et al: Computed tomography and radionuclide imaging in the evaluation of ischemic stroke. Radiology *126*:695, 1978.

Crawford ES et al: Surgical treatment of atherosclerotic occlusive lesions in patients with cerebral arterial insufficiency. Circulation *20*:168, 1959.

Davis KR et al: Cerebral infarction diagnosis by computerized tomography. Am J Roentgenol *124*:643, 1975.

Davis KR et al: Computed tomography of cerebral infarction: hemorrhagic, contrast enhancement, and time of appearance. Comput Tomogr *1*:71, 1977.

Denny-Brown D, Meyer JS: The cerebral collateral circulation. II. Production of cerebral infarction by ischemic anoxia and its reversibility in early stages. Neurology *7*:567, 1957.

Drayer BP et al: Physiologic changes in regional cerebral blood flow defined by Xenon-enhanced CT scanning. Neuroradiology *16*:220, 1978.

Ehrenfeld WK, Hoyt WF, Wylie EJ: Embolization and transient blindness from carotid atheroma: surgical considerations. Arch Surg *93*:787, 1966.

Garcia JH, Kamijyo Y: Cerebral infarction. Evaluation of histopathological changes after occlusion of a middle cerebral artery in primates. J Neuropathol Exper Neurol *33*:408, 1974.

Ghoshhajra K et al: CT detection of intracranial aneurysm in subarachnoid hemorrhage. Am J Roentgenol *132*:613, 1979.

Gonzalez LL, Wiot JF, Boyd AD: Retrograde flow in the vertebral artery. Arch Surg *91*:185, 1965.

Julian OC et al: Ulcerative lesions of the carotid artery bifurcation. Arch Surg *86*:803, 1963.

Kendall BE, Radue EW: Computed tomography in spontaneous intracerebral haematomas. Br J Radiol *51*:563, 1978.

Kinkel WR, Jacobs L: Computerized axial transverse tomography in cerebrovascular disease. Neuroradiology *26*:924, 1976.

Kishore PRS, Lin JP, Kricheff II: Fibromuscular hyperplasia of internal carotid artery and stationary waves. Acta Radiol (Diag) (in press).

Kuhn RA: The revolution produced by cerebral angiography in management of the patient with "stroke." J Med Soc New Jersey *56*:68, 1959.

Larson EB, Omenn GS, Loop JW: Computed tomography in patients with cerebrovascular disease: impact of a new technology on patient care. Am J Roentgenol *131*:35, 1978.

Margolis MT, Newton TH: Collateral pathways between cavernous portion of the internal carotid and external carotid arteries. Radiology *93*:834, 1969.

Mount LA, Taveras JM: Further observations of the significance of the collateral circulation of the brain as demonstrated arteriographically. Tr Am Neurol Ass, 109, 1960.

Mueller RL, Hinck V: Thyrocervical steal. Am J Roentgenol *101*:128, 1967.

Norton GA, Kishore PRS, Lin J: CT contrast enhancement in cerebral infarction. Am J Roentgenol *131*:881, 1978.

Patel A, Toole JF: Subclavian steal syndrome — reversal of cephalic blood flow. Medicine *44*:289, 1965.

Ring BA: Angiographic recognition of occlusion of isolated branches of the middle cerebral artery. Am J Roentgenol *89*:391, 1963.

Shaw C, Alvord EC, Berry RG: Swelling of the brain following ischemic infarction with arterial occlusion. Arch Neurol *1*:161, 1959.

Siekert RG: Diagnosis and classification of focal ischemic cerebrovascular disease. Proc Staff Meet Mayo Clin *35*:473, 1960.

Taveras JM: Angiographic observations in occlusive cerebrovascular disease. Neurology *11*:86, 1961.

Taveras JM: Multiple progressive intracranial arterial occlusions: a syndrome of children and young adults. Am J Roentgenol *106*:235, 1969.

Taveras JM, Mount LA, Friedenberg RM: Arteriographic demonstration of external-internal carotid anastomosis through the ophthalmic arteries. Radiology *63*:525, 1954.

Vander Eecken HM: Discussion of "collateral circulation of the brain." Proceedings of International Conference on Vascular Diseases of the Brain. Neurology *11*:16, 1961.

Vander Eecken HM, Adams RD: The anatomy and functional significance of the meningeal arterial anastomoses of the human brain. J Neuropathol Exper Neurol *12*:132, 1953.

Walshe TM, Hier DB, Davis KR: The diagnosis of hypertensive intracerebral hemorrhage: the contribution of computed tomography. Comput Tomogr *1*:63, 1977.

Weisberg LA, Nice CM: Intracranial tumors simulating the presentation of cerebrovascular syndromes: early detection by cerebral computed tomography (CCT). Am J Med *63*:517, 1977.

Wiggis WS et al: Clinical and computerized tomographic study of hypertensive intracerebral hemorrhage. Arch Neurol *35*:832, 1978.

Wing SD et al: Contrast enhancement of cerebral infarcts in computed tomography. Radiology *121*:89, 1976.

Wood EH, Farmer TW: Cerebral infarction simulating brain tumor. Radiology *69*:693, 1957.

Aneurysms

Allcock JM, Drake CG: Postoperative angiography in cases of ruptured intracranial aneurysm. J Neurosurg *20*:752, 1963.

Allcock JM, Drake CG: Ruptured intracranial aneurysms. The role of arterial spasm. J Neurosurg *22*:21, 1965.

Chase NE et al: Brachial angiography for the evaluation of carotid artery occlusion in the treatment of "posterior communicating" aneurysm. Radiology *91*: 1140, 1968.

Crompton MR: Mechanisms of growth and rupture in cerebral berry aneurysms. Br Med J *1*:1138, 1966.

Dandy WE: Intracranial Arterial Aneurysms. Ithaca, NY, Comstock, 1944.

Davis KR et al: Computed tomographic evaluation of hemorrhage secondary to intracranial aneurysm. Am J Roentgenol *127*:143, 1976.

Fisher CM, Roberson GH, Ojemann RG: Cerebral vasospasm with ruptured saccular aneurysm—the clinical manifestations. Neurosurgery *1*(3):245, 1977.

Fletcher TM, Taveras JM, Pool JL: Cerebral vasospasm in angiography for intracranial aneurysms. Incidence and significance in one hundred consecutive angiograms. Arch Neurol *1*:38, 1959.

Fox JL, Boez TC, Jakoby RH: Differentiation of aneurysm from infundibulum of the posterior communicating artery. J Neurosurg *21*:135, 1964.

Griffith HBM, Cummins BH, Thomson JLG: Cerebral arterial spasm and hydrocephalus in leaking arterial aneurysms. Neuroradiology *4*:212, 1972.

Hayward RD, O'Reilly GVA: Intracerebral haemorrhage. Lancet *1*:4, 1977.

Hunter CR, Mayfield FH: The oblique view in cerebral angiography. J Neurosurg *12*:79, 1955.

Kricheff II, Chase NE, Ransohoff JR: The angiographic investigation of ruptured intracranial aneurysms. Radiology *83*:1016, 1964.

Liliequist B, Lindqvist M, Valdimarsson E: Computed tomography and subarachnoid hemorrhage. Neuroradiology *14*:21, 1977.

Lin JP, Kricheff II: Angiographic investigation of cerebral aneurysm (technical aspects). Radiology *105*:69, 1972.

Locksley HB: Report on the cooperative study of intracranial aneurysms and subarachnoid hemorrhage. Natural history of subarachnoid hemorrhage, intracranial aneurysms and arteriovenous malformations: based on 6368 cases in the cooperative study. J Neurosurg *25*:219, 1966.

Martland HS: Spontaneous subarachnoid hemorrhage and congenital "berry" aneurysms of the circle of Willis. Am J Surg *43*:10, 1939.

Mount LA, Taveras JM: Cerebral angiographic studies following surgical treatment of intracranial aneurysms. Angiographic evaluation of results. Acta Radiol *46*:333, 1956.

Ojemann RG, New PFJ, Fleming TC: Intracranial aneurysms associated with bacterial meningitis. JAMA *198*:1222, 1966.

Potts DG: Variations of the circle of Willis associated with intracranial aneurysms. Thesis for the Degree of Doctor of Medicine, New Zealand, 1960.

Russell DS: The pathology of spontaneous intracranial haemorrhage. Proc. Roy Soc Med *47*:689, 1954.

Sahs AL: Intracranial aneurysms and polycystic kidney. Arch Neurol Psychiatr *63*:524, 1950.

Schneck SA, Kricheff II: Intracranial aneurysm rupture, vasospasm and infarction. Arch Neurol *11*:668, 1964.

Scotti G et al: Computed tomography in the evaluation of intracranial aneurysms and subarachnoid hemorrhage. Radiology *123*:85, 1977.

Wood EH: Angiographic identification of the ruptured lesion in patients with multiple cerebral aneurysms. J Neurosurg *21*:182, 1964.

Inflammatory and Degenerative Diseases

Allen JH, Martin JT, McClain LW: Computed tomography in cerebellar atrophic processes. Radiology *130*:379, 1979.

Arimitsu T et al: White-gray matter differentiation in computed tomography. J Comput Assist Tomography *1*:437, 1977.

Banna M: The ventriculo-cephalic ratio on computed tomography. J Canad Assoc Radiol *28*:208, 1977.

Barr AN et al: Bicaudate index in computerized tomography of Huntington disease and cerebral atrophy. Neurology *238*:1196, 1978.

Bentson J et al: Steroids and apparent cerebral atrophy on computed tomography scans. J Comput Assist Tomography *2*:16, 1978.

Bjoergen JE, Gold LHA: Computed tomographic appearance of methotrexate-induced necrotizing leukoencephalopathy. Radiology *122*:377, 1977.

Bosch EP, Cancilla PA, Cornell SH: Computerized tomography in progressive multifocal leukoencephalopathy. Arch Neurol *33*:216, 1976.

Brennan RE, Stratt BK, Lee KF: Computed tomographic findings in cerebral hemiatrophy. Neuroradiology *17*:17, 1978.

Campbell AMG et al: Cerebral atrophy in young cannabis smokers. Lancet *2*:1219, 1971.

Carlen PL et al: Reversible cerebral atrophy in recently abstinent chronic alcoholics measured by computed tomography scans. Science *200*:1076, 1978.

Carroll BA et al: Diagnosis of progressive multifocal leukoencephalopathy by computed tomography. Radiology *122*:137, 1977.

Duda EE, Huttenlocher PR: Computed tomography in adrenoleukodystrophy. Radiology *120*:349, 1976.

Enzmann DR, Lane B: Cranial computed tomography findings in anorexia nervosa. J Comput Assist Tomography *1*:410, 1977.

Fox JH et al: Cerebral vascular enlargement: chronic alcoholics examined by computerized tomography. JAMA *236*:365, 1976.

Gawler J: Computerized tomography (the Emi scanner): a comparison with pneumoencephalography and ventriculography. J Neurol Neurosurg Psychiatr *39*:203, 1976.

Gonzales CF, Lantieri RL, Nathan RJ: CT scan appearance of the brain in the normal elderly population. Neuroradiology *16*:120, 1978.

Gosling RH: The association of dementia with radiologically demonstrated cerebral atrophy. J Neurol Neurosurg Psychiatr *18*:129, 1955.

Greenberg HS, Halverson D, Lane B: CT scanning and diagnosis of adrenoleukodystrophy. Neurology *27*:884, 1977.

Gyldensted C: Measurements of the normal ventricular system and hemispheric sulci of 100 adults with computed tomography. Neuroradiology *14*:183, 1977.

Haug C: Age and sex dependence of the size of normal ventricles on computed tomography. Neuroradiology *14*:201, 1977.

Haughton VM et al: CT detection of demyelinated plaques in multiple sclerosis. Am J Roentgenol *132*:213, 1979.

Heinz ER, Martinez J, Haenggeli A: Reversibility of cerebral atrophy in anorexia nervosa and Cushing's syndrome. J Comput Assist Tomography *1*:415, 1977.

Heinz ER et al: Computed tomography in white-matter disease. Radiology *130*:371, 1979.

Hershey LA, Gado MH, Trotter JL: Computerized tomography in the diagnostic evaluation of multiple sclerosis. Ann Neurol *5*:32, 1979.

Huckman MS, Fox J, Topel J: The validity of criteria for evaluation of cerebral atrophy by computed tomography. Radiology *116*:85, 1975.

Huckman MS, Fox J, Ramsey RG: Computed tomography in the diagnosis of degenerative diseases of the brain. Semin Roentgenol *12*:63, 1977.

Huckman MS, Ramsey RG, Shenk GI: CT scanning in patients with suspected cerebral metastases. J Comput Assist Tomography *2*:511, 1978.

Kaszniak AW et al: Predictors of mortality in pre-senile and senile dementia. Ann Neurol *3*:246, 1978.

Kuehnle J et al: Computed tomographic examination of heavy marijuana smokers. JAMA *237*:1231, 1977.

Lane B, Carroll RA, Pedley TA: Computerized cranial tomography in cerebral diseases of white matter. Neurology *28*:534, 1978.

McGeachie RE et al: Diagnosis of Pick's disease by computed tomography. J Comput Assist Tomography *3*:113, 1979.

Nardizzi LR: Computerized tomographic correlation of carbon monoxide poisoning. Arch Neurol *36*:38, 1979.

Ramsey RG, Huckman MS: Computed tomography of porencephaly and other cerebrospinal fluid-containing lesions. Radiology *123*:73, 1977.

Robertson WC et al: Computerized tomography in demyelinating disease of the young. Neurology *27*:838, 1977.

Shapiro WR, Chernik NL, Posner JB: Necrotizing encephalopathy following intraventricular instillation of methotrexate. Arch Neurol *28*:96, 1973.

Terrence CF, Delaney JF, Alberts MC: Computed tomography for Huntingdon's disease. Neuroradiology *13*:173, 1977.

Victor M, Adams RD, Mancall EL: A restricted form of cerebellar cortical degeneration occurring in alcoholic patients. Arch Neurol *1*:579, 1959.

Weinstein MA, Ducheseneau PM, MacIntyre WJ: White and gray matter of the brain differentiated by computed tomography. Radiology *122*:699, 1977.

Weinstein MA et al: Interval computed tomography in multiple sclerosis. Radiology *129*:689, 1978.

Wendling LR et al: Transient, severe periventricular hypodensity after leukemic prophylaxis with cranial irradiation and intrathecal methotrexate. J Comput Assist Tomography *2*:502, 1978.

Wolpert SM: The ventricular size on computed tomography. J Comput Assist Tomography *1*:222, 1977.

Meningiomas

Ambrose J, Gooding MR, Richardson AE: An assessment of the accuracy of computerized transverse axial scanning (EMI scanner) in the diagnosis of intracranial tumor. A review of 366 patients. Brain *98*(4): 569, 1975.

Banna M, Appleby A: Some observations on the angiography of supratentorial meningiomas. Clin Radiol *20*:375, 1969.

Bernasconi V, Casinari V: Caratteritische angiografiche dei meningiomi del tentorio. Radiol Med *43*:1015, 1957.

Claveria L, Sutton D, Tress BM: The radiological diagnosis of meningioma. The impact of EMI scanning. Br J Radiol *50*(589):15, 1977.

Cooper M, Dohn DF: Intracranial meningiomas in childhood. Cleveland Clin *241*(4):197, 1974.

Cushing H, Bailey P: Tumors Arising from the Blood-Vessels of the Brain. Springfield, IL, Charles C Thomas, 1928.

Cushing H, Eisenhardt L: Meningiomas. Springfield, IL, Charles C Thomas, 1938.

Felson B (ed): A primer on cerebral angiography. Semin Roentgenol *6*(1), 1971.

Felson B (ed): Computerized cranial tomography I. Semin Roentgenol *12*(1), 1977.

Felson B (ed): Computerized cranial tomography II. Semin Roentgenol *12*(2), 1977.

Frugoni P et al: A particular angiographic sign in meningiomas of the tentorium: the artery of Bernasconi and Cassinari. Neurochirugia *2*:142, 1960.

Gammal TE et al: Further causes of hypertrophied tentorial arteries. Br J Radiol *40*:350, 1967.

Hirsch LP, Mancall EL: Giant meningiomas of the posterior fossa. JAMA *240*:1626, 1978.

Hoessly GF, Olivecrona H: Report on 280 cases of verified parasagittal meningioma. J Neurosurg *12*:614, 1955.

Lin JP et al: Brain tumors studied by computerized tomography. Adv Neurol *15*:175, 1976.

Mikhael MA: Case report: diminished density surrounding a meningioma. Verified to be an overlying cystic astrocytoma. J Comput Assist Tomography *1*(3):349, 1977.

Newton TH, Potts DG (eds): Radiology of the Skull and Brain. Angiography, Vol 1, Books 1-2. St Louis, CV Mosby, 1971.

Quest DO: Meningiomas: an update. Neurosurgery *3*(2):221, 1978.

Salamon GM et al: An angiographic study of meningiomas of the posterior fossa. J Neurosurg *35*(6):731, 1971.

Scatliff JH, Guinto FC Jr, Radcliffe WB: Vascular patterns in cerebral neoplasms and their differential diagnosis. Semin Roentgenol *6*(1):59, 1971.

Schechter MM, Zingesser LH, Rosenbaum A: Tentorial meningiomas. Am J Roentgenol *104*(1):123, 1968.

Sosman MC, Putnam TJ: Roentgenological aspects of brain tumors — meningiomas. Am J Roentgenol *13*:1, 1925.

Stattin S: Meningeal vessels of the internal carotid artery and their angiographic significance. Acta Radiol *55*:329, 1961.

Stattin S: Significance of some angiographic signs of intracranial meningiomas. Acta Radiol (Diag) *5*:530, 1966.

Taveras JM, Wood EH: Diagnostic Neuroradiology. Baltimore, Williams & Wilkins, 1975.

Telenius R: Angiographic appearance of angioblastic meningiomas. Acta Radiol (Diag) *5*:554, 1966.

Traub SP: Roentgenology of Intracranial Meningiomas. Springfield, IL, Charles C Thomas, 1961.

Vassilouthis J, Ambrose J: Computerized tomography scanning appearances of intracranial meningiomas. J Neurosurg *50*:320, 1979.

Wagman AD, Weiss EK, Riggs HE: Hyperplasia of the skull associated with intraosseous meningioma in the absence of gross tumor. J Neuropathol Exper Neurol *19*:111, 1960.

Wilson G, Weidner W, Hanafee W: The demonstration and diagnosis of meningiomas by selective carotid angiography. Am J Roentgenol *95*(4):868, 1965.

Zulch KJ, Eschbach O: Investigation of meningiomas of cerebellar convexities. Neuroradiology *4*(3):179, 1972.

Midline Tumors

Banna M: Arachnoid cysts on computed tomography. Am J Roentgenol *127*:979, 1976.

Bajraktari X et al: Diagnosis of intrasellar cisternal herniation (empty sella) by computer assisted tomography. J Comput Assist Tomography *1*:105, 1977.

Chase NE, Taveras JM: Cerebral angiography in the diagnosis of suprasellar tumors. Am J Roentgenol *84*:154, 1961.

Citrin CM, Davis DO: Computerized tomography in the evaluation of pituitary adenomas. Invest Radiol *12*:27, 1977.

Cummins FM, Taveras JM, Schlesinger EB: Treatment of gliomas of the third ventricle and pinealomas; with special reference to the value of radiotherapy. Neurology *10*:1031, 1960.

Drayer BP et al: Computed tomographic diagnosis of suprasellar masses by intrathecal enhancement. Radiology *123*:339, 1977.

Drayer BP et al: Cerebrospinal fluid rhinorrhea demonstrated by metrizamide CT cisternography. Am J Roentgenol *129*:149, 1977.

Fitz CR et al: Computed tomography in craniopharyngiomas. Radiology *127*:687, 1978.

Gilday DL, Ash J: Accuracy of brain scanning in pediatric craniocerebral neoplasms. Radiology *117*:93, 1975.

Greitz T, Hindmarsh T: Computed assisted tomography of intracranial CSF circulation using a water-soluble contrast medium. Acta Radiol (Diag) *15*:497, 1974.

Grepe A: Cisternography with the non-ionic water-soluble contrast medium metrizamide. A preliminary report. Acta Radiol (Diag), *16*(2):146, 1975.

Harwood-Nash DC: Optic gliomas and pediatric neuroradiology. Radiol Clin North Am *10*:83, 1972.

Horrax G, Wyatt JP: Ectopic pinealomas in the chiasmal region; report of three cases. J Neurosurg *4*:309, 1947.

Kaufman B, Camberlain WB Jr: The ubiquitous "empty" sella turcica. Acta Radiol (Diag) *13*:413, 1972.

Manelfe C, Guiraud B, Tremoulet M: Diagnosis of CSF rhinorrhoea by computerized cisternography using metrizamide (letter). Lancet *2*:1073, 1977.

Naidich TP et al: Evaluation of sellar and parasellar masses by computed tomography. Radiology *120*:91. 1976.

Raymond LA, Tew J: Large suprasellar aneurysms imitating pituitary tumor. J Neurol Neurosurg Psychiatr *41*:83, 1978.

Rozario R et al: Diagnosis of empty sella with CT scan. Neuroradiology *13*:85, 1977.

Segall HD et al: Suprasellar cysts associated with isosexual precocious puberty. Radiology *111*:607, 1974.

Strand RD et al: Metrizamide ventriculography and computed tomography in lesions about the third ventricle. Radiology *128*:405, 1978.

Volpe BT, Foley KM, Howieson J: Normal CAT scans in craniopharyngioma. Ann Neurol *3*:87, 1978.

Hydrocephalus and Porencephaly

Ambrose J: Computerized transverse axial scanning (tomography). II. Clinical application. Br J Radiol *46*:1023, 1973.

Burstein J, Papile L, Burstein R: Intraventricular hemorrhage and hydrocephalus in premature newborns: a prospective study with CT. Am J Roentgenol *132*:631, 1979.

Byrd SE et al: Computed tomography evaluation of holoprosencephaly in infants and children. J Comput Assist Tomography *1*(4):456, 1977.

Carmel PW, Markesbery WR: Early descriptions of the Arnold-Chiari malformation. The contribution of John Cleland. J Neurosurg *37*:543, 1972.

Dandy WE: The diagnosis and treatment of hydrocephalus due to occlusions of the foramina of Magendie and Luschka. Surg Gynecol Obstet *32*:112, 1921.

Dandy WE, Blackfan KD: An experimental and clinical study of internal hydrocephalus. JAMA *61*:2216, 1913.

Davidoff LM, Epstein BS: The Abnormal Pneumoencephalogram. Philadelphia, Lea & Febiger, 1950.

Drayer BP et al: Metrizamide computed tomography cisternography: pediatric applications. Radiology *124*: 349, 1977.

Fitz CR, Harwood-Nash DC: Computed tomography in hydrocephalus. Comput Tomogr *2*:91, 1978.

Heschl R: Gehirndefect und hydrocephalus. Prag Urtijschr F cl prakt. Heilk *61*:59, 1859.

Hounsfield GN: Computerised transverse axial scanning (tomography). I. Description of the system. Br J Radiol *46*:1016, 1973.

Kruyff E, Jeffs R: Skull abnormalities associated with the Arnold-Chiari malformation. Acta Radiol (Diag) *5*:9, 1966.

Kundrat H: Die porencephalie, Eine anatomoische studie. Graz, Leuschner B Tubenski, 1882.

Laurence KM, Coates S: Further thoughts on the natural history of hydrocephalus. Dev Med Child Neurol *4*:263, 1962.

LeCount ER, Semerak CB: Porencephaly. Arch Neurol Psychiatr *14*(3):365, 1925.

Matson DD: Prenatal obstruction of the fourth ventricle. Am J Roentgenol *76*:499, 1956.

Meese W, Lanksch W, Wende S: Diagnosis and postoperative follow-up studies of infantile hydrocephalus using computerized tomography. In: W Lanksch, E Kazner (eds): Cranial Computerized Tomography. New York, Springer Verlag, 1976.

Naidich TP et al: Evaluation of pediatric hydrocephalus by computed tomography. Radiology *119*:337, 1976.

Naidich TP et al: Computed tomographic signs of the Chiari II malformation. I. Skull and dural partitions. Radiology *134*(1):65, 1980; II. Midbrain and cerebellum. Radiology *134*(2):391, 1980; III. Ventricles and cisterns. Radiology *134*(3):657, 1980.

New PFH et al: Computerized axial tomography with the EMI scanner. Radiology *110*:109, 1974.

Newton HT, Potts GD: Radiology of the Skull and Brain, Vol 2. St Louis, CV Mosby, 1974.

Pendergrass EP, Berryman CR: Porencephaly. Am J Roentgenol *56*:441, 1946.

Penfield W, Coburn DF: Arnold-Chiari malformation and its operative treatment. Arch Neurol Psychiatr *40*:328, 1938.

Penfield W, Erickson TC: Epilepsy and Cerebral Localization. Springfield, IL, Charles C Thomas, 1941.

Ramsey RG et al: Computed tomography of porencephaly and other cerebrospinal fluid-containing lesions. Radiology *123*(1):73, 1977.

Robertson EG: Pneumoencephalography. Springfield, IL, Charles C Thomas, 1967.

Schechter MM, Zingesser LH: The radiology of aqueductal stenosis. Radiology *88*:905, 1967.

Skolnick ML et al: Detection of dilated cerebral ventricles in infants: a correlative study between ultrasound and computed tomography. Radiology *131*:447, 1979.

Wagner HN: Principles of Nuclear Medicine. Philadelphia, WB Saunders, 1968.

Walker AE: A case of congenital atresia of the foramina of Luschka and Magendie; surgical cure. J Neuropathol Exp Neurol *3*:368, 1944.

Weinberg PE, Flom RA: Intracranial subarachnoid cysts. Radiology *106*:329, 1973.

Arteriovenous Malformations

Dandy WE: Carotid-cavernous aneurysms (pulsating exophthalmos). Zentralbl Neurochir *2*:77, 1937.

Djindjian R et al: Embolization by superselective arteriography from the femoral route in neuroradiology. Review of 60 cases. I. Technique, indications, complications. Neuroradiology *6*:20, 1973.

Kricheff II, Madayag M, Braunstein P: Transfemoral catheter embolization of cerebral and posterior fossa arteriovenous malformations. Radiology *103*:107, 1972.

Locke CE Jr: Internal intracranial arteriovenous aneurysm or pulsating exophthalmos. Ann Surg *80*:1, 279, 1924.

Luessenhop AJ: Artificial embolization for cerebral arteriovenous malformations. Prog Neurol Surg *3*:320, 1969.

Luessenhop AJ, Spence WT: Artificial embolization of cerebral arteries: report of use in a case of arteriovenous malformation. JAMA *172*:1153, 1960.

Luessenhop AJ, Gibbs M, Velasquez AC: Cerebrovascular response to emboli. Observations in patients with arteriovenous malformations. Arch Neurol *7*:264, 1962.

Luessenhop AJ et al: Clinical evaluation of artificial embolization in the management of large cerebral arteriovenous malformations. J Neurosurg *23*:400, 1965.

Margolis G et al: The role of small angiomatous malformations in the production of intracerebral hematomas. J Neurosurg *8*:564, 1951.

Perret G, Nishioka H: Arteriovenous malformations: an analysis of 545 cases of cranio-cerebral arteriovenous malformations and fistulae reported to the Cooperative Study. J Neurosurg *25*:467, 1966.

Porter AJ, Bull J: Some aspects of the natural history of cerebral arteriovenous malformation. Br J Radiol *42*:667, 1969.

Ramos M, Mount LA: Carotid cavernous fistula with signs on contralateral side. Case report. J Neurosurg *10*:178, 1953.

Rischbieth RHC, Bull JWD: The significance of enlargement of the superior orbital (sphenoidal) fissure. Br J Radiol *31*:125, 1958.

Robles C, Carrasco-Zanini J: Treatment of cerebral arteriovenous malformations by muscle embolization. J Neurosurg *29*:603, 1968.

Serbinenko FA: Balloon catheterization and occlusion of major cerebral vessels. J Neurosurg *41*:125, 1974.

Solis OJ et al: Dural arteriovenous malformation associated with subdural and intracerebral hematoma: a CT scan and angiographic correlation. Comput Tomogr *1*(2):145, 1977.

Wilson CB, Roy M: Calcification within congenital aneurysms of vein of Galen. Am J Roentgenol *91*:1319, 1969.

Zilkha A, Schechter MM: Arteriovenous fistulas of the major vessels of the neck. Acta Radiol (Diag) *9*:560, 1969.

Trauma

Amendola MA, Ostrum BJ: Diagnosis of isodense subdural hematomas by computed tomography. Am J Roentgenol *129*:693, 1977.

Bergstrom M et al: Computed tomography of cranial subdural and epidural hematomas: variation of attenuation related to time and clinical events such as rebleeding. J Comput Assist Tomography *1*:449, 1977.

Briggs M et al: Post-traumatic skull radiographs (letter). Lancet *2*(8086):426, 1978.

Carton CA: Cerebral Angiography in the Management of Head Trauma. Springfield, IL, Charles C Thomas, 1959.

Conqvist S, Köhler R: Angiography in epidural haematomas. Acta Radiol (Diag) *1*:42, 1963.

Cornel SH, Chiu LC, Christie JH: Diagnosis of isodense subdural hematomas by computed tomography. Am J Roentgenol *129*:693, 1977.

Cummins RO et al: Post-traumatic skull radiography (letter). Lancet *2*(8087):471, 1978.

Davis DO, Coxe WS: The angiographic evaluation of anterior polar brain injury. Radiology *93*:1061, 1969.

Davis KR et al: Computed tomography in head trauma. Semin Roentgenol *12*:53, 1977.

Dolinskas CA et al: Computed tomography of intracerebral hematomas. I. Transmission CT observations on hematoma resolution. Am J Roentgenol *129*:681, 1977; II. Radionuclide and transmission CT studies of the perihematoma region. Am J Roentgenol *129*:689, 1977.

Dublin AB, French BN, Rennick JM: Computed tomography in head trauma. Radiology *122*:365, 1977.

Eyes B et al: Post-traumatic skull radiographs. Time for a reappraisal. Lancet *2*(8080):85, 1978.

Feldman RA et al: Perforation of the skull by a Gardner-Wells tong. Case report. J Neurosurg *44*(1):119, 1976.

Ferris EJ, Lehrer H, Shapiro JH: Pseudosubdural hematoma. Radiology *88*:75, 1967.

Forbes GS et al: Computed tomography in the evaluation of subdural hematomas. Radiology *126*:143, 1978.

Gurdjian ES, Webster JE, Lissner HR: The mechanism of skull fracture. J Neurosurg *7*:106, 1950.

Gurdjian ES, Webster JE, Lissner HR: Observations on prediction of fracture site in head injury. Radiology *60*:226, 1953.

Handel SF et al: Subdural hematomas due to ruptured cerebral aneurysms: angiographic diagnosis and potential pitfall for CT. Am J Roentgenol *130*(3):507, 1978.

Haas FL: Complication of linear skull fracture in young children. Am J Dis Child *129*(10):1197, 1975.

Hooper R: Observations on extradural haemorrhage. Br J Surg *47*:71, 1959.

Jennett B et al: Skull x-ray policy (letter). Lancet *2*(8084):312, 1978.

Kim KS, Hemmati M, Weinberg PE: Computed tomography in isodense subdural hematoma. Radiology *128*:71, 1978.

Koo AH, LaRozue RL: Evaluation of head trauma by computed tomography. Radiology *123*:345, 1977.

Luckett WH: Air in the ventricles of the brain following a fracture of the skull: report of a case. Surg Gynecol Obstet *17*:237, 1913.

Lusins J, Nakagawa H, Bender MB: Computed assisted tomography of unoperated subdural hematoma: short and long term follow-up. J Comput Assist Tomography *2*:460, 1978.

Marcu H, Becker H: Computed tomography of bilateral isodense chronic subdural hematomas. Neuroradiology *14*:81, 1977.

Martin G: Skull x-ray policy (letter). Lancet *2*(8089):572, 1978.

Merino-deVillasante J, Taveras JM: Computerized tomography (CT) in acute head trauma. Am J Roentgenol *126*:765, 1976.

Messina AV: Computed tomography contrast media within subdural hematomas. A preliminary report. Radiology *119*:725, 1976.

Munro D, Maltby GL: Extradural hemorrhage: a study of forty-four cases. Ann Surg *113*:192, 1941.

New PFJ, Momose KJ: Traumatic dissection of the internal carotid artery at the atlantoaxial level, secondary to nonpenetrating injury. Radiology *93*:41, 1969.

Norman O: Angiographic differentiation between acute and chronic subdural and extradural haematomas. Acta Radiol *46*:371, 1956.

Rothman L et al: The spectrum of growing skull fracture in children. Pediatrics *57*(1):26, 1976.

Samuelson S, Long DM, Chou SN: Subdural hematoma as a complication of shunting procedures for normal pressure hydrocephalus. J Neurosurg *37*:548, 1972.

Scotti G et al: Evaluation of the age of subdural hematomas by computed tomography. J Neurosurg *47*:311, 1977.

Sones PJ, Hoffman J, Brylski JR: Epidural subtemporal hematoma: angiographic changes involving the meningeal artery. Am J Roentgenol *108*:756, 1970.

Sweet RC et al: Significance of bilateral abnormalities on the CT scan in patients with severe head injury. Neurosurgery *3*(1):16, 1978.

Weinman DF, Jayamanne D: The role of angiography in the diagnosis of extradural haematomas. Br J Radiol *39*:350, 1966.

Wilkins RH, Odom GL: Intracranial arterial spasm associated with craniocerebral trauma. J Neurosurg *32*:626, 1970.

Zimmerman RA et al: Computed tomography of acute intracerebral hemorrhagic contusion. Comput Axial Tomography *1*:271, 1977.

Zimmerman RA et al: Computed tomography of shearing injuries of the cerebral white matter. Radiology *127*(2):393, 1978.

Zimmerman RA et al: Cranial computed tomography in diagnosis and management of acute head trauma. Am J Roentgenol *13*(1):27, 1978.

Zingesser LH, Schechter MM, Rayport M: Truths and untruths concerning the angiographic findings in extracerebral haematomas. Br J Radiol *38*:835, 1965.

Posterior Fossa Lesions

Archer CA et al: Enlarged cisternae magnae and posterior fossa cysts simulating Dandy-Walker syndrome on computed tomography. Radiology *127*:681, 1978.

Baker HI Jr et al: Computed tomography in the diagnosis of posterior fossa lesions. Radiol Clin North Am *14*(1):129, 1976.

Berk ME: Chemodectoma of the glomus intravagale: a case report and review. Clin Radiol *12*:219, 1961.

Braun IF et al: Dense intracranial epidermoid tumors. Radiology *122*:717, 1977.

Bray PF, Carter S, Taveras JM: Brainstem tumors in children. Neurology *8*:1, 1958.

Camp JD, Cilley EIL: The significance of asymmetry of the pori acustici as an aid in diagnosis of eighth nerve tumors. Am J Roentgenol *41*:713, 1939.

Dandy WE: The diagnosis and treatment of hydrocephalus due to occlusions of the foramina of Magendie and Luschka. Surg Gynecol Obstet *32*:112, 1921.

Davis KR et al: CT of acoustic neuromas. Radiology *124*:81, 1977.

Drayer BP et al: Posterior fossa extraaxial cyst: diagnosis with metrizamide CT cisternography. Am J Roentgenol *128*(3):431, 1977.

Fawcitt RA, Isherwood I: Radiodiagnosis of intracranial pearly tumours with particular reference to the value of computer tomography. Neuroradiology *11*:235, 1976.

Gado M, Huete I, Mikhael M: Computerized tomography of infratentorial tumors. Semin Roentgenol *12*:109, 1977.

Greenberger JS, Cassady JR, Levene MB: Radiation therapy of thalamic, midbrain and brain stem gliomas. Radiology *122*:463, 1977.

Greitz T: Evaluation of circulation time in angiography of the vertebral artery. Acta Radiol *9*:300, 1969.

Greitz T, Sjögren SE: The posterior inferior cerebellar artery. Acta Radiol (Diag) *1*:284, 1963.

Gyldensted C, Lester J, Thomsen J: Computer tomography in the diagnosis of cerebellopontine angle tumors. Neuroradiology *11*:191, 1976.

Hammerschlag SB, Wolpert SM, Carter BL: Computed coronal tomography. Radiology *120*:217, 1976.

Hanafee WN, Shiu PC, Dayton GO: Orbital venography. Am J Roentgenol *104*:29, 1968.

Huang YP, Wolf BS: Veins of the white matter of the cerebral hemispheres (the medullary veins). Diagnostic importance in carotid angiography. Am J Roentgenol *92*:739, 1964.

Huang YP, Wolf BS: Angiographic features of the pericallosal cistern. Radiology *82*:14, 1964.

Huang YP, Wolf BS: Angiographic features of unilateral hydrocephalus of obstructive nature. Am J Roentgenol *92*:792, 1964.

Huang YP, Wolf BS: The veins of the posterior fossa — superior or galenic draining group. Am J Roentgenol *95*:808, 1965.

Huang YP, Wolf BS: Precentral cerebellar vein in angiography. Acta Radiol *5*:250, 1966.

Huang YP, Wolf BS: The vein of the lateral recess of the fourth ventricle and its tributaries. Roentgen appearance and anatomic relationships. Am J Roentgenol *101*:1, 1967.

Huang YP et al: Angiographic features of aqueductal stenosis. Am J Roentgenol *104*:90, 1968.

Huang YP et al: The veins of the posterior fossa — anterior or petrosal draining group. Am J Roentgenol *104*:36, 1968.

Huang YP, Wolf BS, Okudera T: Angiographic anatomy of the inferior vermian vein of the cerebellum. Acta Radiol *9*:327, 1969.

Huang YP, Wolf BS: Angiographic features of fourth ventricle tumors with special reference to the posterior inferior cerebellar artery. Am J Roentgenol *107*:543, 1969.

Huang YP, Wolf BS: Angiographic features of brain stem tumors and differential diagnosis from fourth ventricle tumors. Am J Roentgenol *110*:1, 1970.

Huang YP, Wolf BS: Differential diagnosis of fourth ventricle tumors from brain stem tumors in angiography. Neuroradiology *1*:4, 1970.

Kendall BE: Cranial chordomas. Br J Radiol *50*(598):687, 1977.

Kendall BE, Symon L: Investigation of patients presenting with cerebellopontine angle syndromes. Neuroradiology *13*:65, 1977.

Kricheff II et al: CT — air cisternography and canalography in the diagnosis of small acoustic neuromas. Presented at the 17th Annual Meeting of American Society of Neuroradiology, May 1979.

Liliequist B: Encephalography in the Arnold-Chiari malformation. Acta Radiol *53*:17, 1960.

Lindgren E: Encephalographic examination of tumours in the posterior fossa. Acta Radiol *34*:331, 1950.

Mani RL, Newton TH, Glickman MG: The superior cerebellar artery: an anatomic-roentgenographic correlation. Radiology *91*:1102, 1968.

Moller A, Hatem A, Olivecrona H: The differential diagnosis of pontine angle meningioma and acoustic neuroma with computed tomography. Neuroradiology *17*:21, 1978.

Naidich TP et al: The anterior inferior cerebellar artery in mass lesions. Preliminary findings with emphasis on the lateral projection. Radiology *119*(2):375, 1976.

Naidich TP et al: Computed tomography in the diagnosis of extra-axial posterior fossa masses. Radiology *120*:333, 1976.

Naidich TP: Infrantentorial masses. In: D Norman, M Korobkin, TH Newton (eds): Computed Tomography. St Louis, CV Mosby, 1977.

Naidich TP et al: Primary tumors and other masses of the cerebellum and fourth ventricle: differential diagnosis by computed tomography. Neuroradiology *14*:153, 1977.

Olsson O: Vertebral angiography in the diagnosis of acoustic nerve tumours. Acta Radiol *39*:265, 1953.

Olsson O: Vertebral angiography in cerebellar haemangioma. Acta Radiol *40*:9, 1953.

Peeters FL, Westra D, Verbeeten B Jr: Radiological diagnosis of pontine angle tumours. Radiol Clin (Casel) *46*:94, 1977.

Penfield W, Coburn DF: Arnold-Chiari malformation and its operative treatment. Arch Neurol Psychiatr *40*:328, 1938.

Quencer RM et al: Jugular venography for evaluation of abnormalities of the skull base. J Neurosurg *44*(4):485, 1976.

Rice RP, Holman CB: The roentgenographic manifestations of tumors of the glomus jugulare (chemodectoma). Am J Roentgenol *89*:1201, 1963.

Robbins B et al: Computed tomography of acoustic neurinoma. Radiology *128*(2):367, 1978.

Rosenbaum AE et al: Visualization of small extracanalicular neurilemmomas by metrizamide cisternographic enhancement. Arch Otolaryngol *104*(5):239, 1978.

Russell DS, Rubinstein LJ: Pathology of Tumours of the Nervous System. Baltimore, Williams & Wilkins, 1977.

Sortland O: Computed tomography combined with gas cisternography for the diagnosis of expanding lesions in the cerebellopontine angle. Neuroradiology *10*:19, 1979.

Sugar O, Holden LB, Powell CB: Vertebral angiography. Am J Roentgenol *61*:166, 1949.

Sutton D: The radiological assessment of the normal aqueduct and fourth ventricle. Br J Radiol *23*:208, 1950.

Sutton D: Radiologic aspects of pontine gliomata. Acta Radiol *40*:234, 1953.

Taggart JK Jr, Walker AE: Congenital atresia of the foramens of Luschka and Magendie. Arch Neurol Psychiatr *48*:583, 1942.

Takahashi M, Wilson G, Hanafee W: The significance of the petrosal vein in the diagnosis of cerebellopontine angle tumors. Radiology *89*:834, 1967.

Takahashi M, Wilson G, Hanafee W: The anterior inferior cerebellar artery: its radiographic anatomy and significance in the diagnosis of extra-axial tumors of the posterior fossa. Radiology *90*:281, 1968.

Takahashi M, Wilson G, Hanafee W: Catheter vertebral angiography: a review of 300 examinations. J Neurosurg *30*:722, 1969.

Taveras JM: The roentgen diagnosis of intracranial incisural space occupying lesions. Am J Roentgenol *84*:52, 1960.

Twining EW: Radiology of the third and fourth ventricles: Parts I and II. Br J Radiol *12*:385, 569, 1939.

Walker AE: A case of congenital atresia of the foramina of Luschka and Magendie: surgical cure. J Neuropathol Exp Neurol *3*:368, 1944.

Wolf BS, Newman CM, Khilnani MT: The posterior inferior cerebellar artery on vertebral angiography. Am J Roentgenol *87*:322, 1962.

Zimmerman RA et al: Spectrum of medulloblastomas demonstrated by computed tomography. Radiology *126*(1):137, 1978.

Zimmerman RA et al: Computed tomography of cerebellar astrocytoma. Am J Roentgenol *130*:929, 1978.

The Orbit

Baker HL Jr et al: Computerized transaxial tomography in neuro-ophthalmology. Am J Ophthalmol *78*:285, 1974.

Bergström K: Computer tomography of the orbits. Acta Radiol (Suppl)*346*:155, 1975.

Byrd SE et al: Computed tomography of intraorbital optic nerve gliomas in children. Radiology *129*:73, 1978.

Chu FC: Radiological methods of studying the orbit. Comput Tomogr *1*(1):45, 1977.

Daily MJ, Smith JL, Dickens W: Giant drusen (astrocytic hamartoma) of the optic nerve seen with computerized axial tomography. Am J Ophthalmol *81*:100, 1976.

Dallow RL et al: Comparison of ultrasonography, computerized tomography (EMI scan) and radiographic techniques in evaluation of exophthalmos. Tr Am Acad Ophthalmol Otolaryngol *81*:305, 1976.

Drayer BP et al: Ophthalmologic applications of computed tomography in nonhuman primates. J Comput Assist Tomography *1*(3):324, 1977.

Enzmann D et al: Computed tomography in orbital pseudotumor (idiopathic orbital inflammation). Radiology *120*:597, 1976.

Enzmann D et al: Computed tomography in Graves' ophthalmology. Radiology *118*:615, 1976.

Fenton M et al: Computerized axial tomographic scanning in the investigation of orbital lesions. Ir Med J *71*(6):192, 1978.

Forman WH et al: Cosmetic eye shadow mimicking orbital calcification (letter). JAMA *238*(25):2695, 1977.

Gado MH et al: Computerized tomography of the orbit. Int Ophthalmol Clin *18*(1):151, 1978.

Gawler J et al: Computer-assisted tomography in orbital disease. Br J Ophthalmol *58*:571, 1974.

Goldberg L et al: Computed tomographic scanning in the management of retinoblastoma. Am J Ophthalmol *84*(3):380, 1977.

Haverling M et al: Computed sagittal tomography of the orbit. Am J Roentgenol *131*(2):346, 1978.

Hilal SK, Trokel SL, Coleman DJ: High resolution computerized tomography and B-scan ultrasonography of the orbits. Tr Am Acad Ophthalmol Otolaryngol *81*:607, 1976.

Hilal SK, Trokel SL, Kreps SM: Diseases of the orbit: computerized tomography. In: TD Duane (ed): Clinical Ophthalmology, Vol 2. Hagerstown MD, Harper & Row, 1976.

Hilal SK et al: Computerized tomography of the orbit using thin sections. Semin Roentgenol *12*(2):137, 1977.

Kadir S et al: The use of computerized tomography in the detection of intra-orbital foreign bodies. Comput Tomogr *1*(2):151, 1977.

Kennerdell JS et al: CT scan appearance of dysthyroid orbital disease. Ann Ophthalmol *10*(2):153, 1978.

Lampert VL, Zeich JV, Cohen DN: Computed tomography of the orbits. Radiology *113*:351, 1974.

Leonardi M et al: Sagittal computed tomography of the orbit. J Comput Assist Tomography *1*(4):511, 1977.

Leone CR Jr, Wilson FC: Computerized axial tomography of the orbit. Ophthalmic Surg *7*:34, 1976.

Lloyd GA: The impact of CT scanning and ultrasonography on orbital diagnosis. Clin Radiol *28*(6):583, 1977.

Momose KJ, Dallow RL: Comparison in the use of computerized axial tomography with ultrasonography in the investigation of orbital lesions. Presented at the 13th Annual Meeting, American Society of Neuroradiology, June 1975.

Momose KJ et al: The use of computed tomography in ophthalmology. Radiology *115*:361, 1975.

Moseley IF, Bull JWD: Computerized axial tomography, carotid angiography and orbital phlebography in the diagnosis of space-occupying lesions of the orbit. In: G Salamon (ed): Advances in Cerebral Angiography. Berlin, Springer, 1975.

Nikoskelainen E et al: Computerized tomography of the orbits. A report of 196 patients. Acta Ophthalmol (Kbh) *55*(6):885, 1977.

Potter GD: Tomography of the orbit. Radiol Clin North Am *10*:21, 1972.

Salvolini U et al: Computer assisted tomography in 90 cases of exophthalmos. J Comput Assist Tomography *1*(4):511, 1977.

Tadmor R et al: Computed tomography of the orbit with special emphasis on coronal sections. I. Normal anatomy. J Comput Assist Tomography *2*(1):24, 1978.

Tadmor R et al: Computed tomography of the orbit with special emphasis on coronal sections. II. Pathological anatomy. J Comput Assist Tomography *2*(1):35, 1978.

Takahashi M et al: Coronal computed tomography in orbital disease. J Comput Assist Tomography *1*(4):505, 1977.

Vermess M et al: Computer assisted tomography of orbital lesions in Wegener's granulomatosis. J Comput Assist Tomography *2*(1):45, 1978.

Vignaud J, Clay C, Bilaniuk LT: Venography of the orbit; an analytical report of 413 cases. Radiology *110*:373, 1974.

Weinstein MA, Berlin AJ Jr, Duchesneau PM: High resolution computed tomography of the orbit with the Ohio-Nuclear Delta head scanner. Am J Roentgenol *127*:175, 1976.

Wright JE, Lloyd GAS, Ambrose J: Computerized axial tomography in the detection of orbital space-occupying lesions. Am J Ophthalmol *80*:78, 1975.

Myelography

Ahlgren P: Amipaque myelography without late adhesive arachnoid changes. Neuroradiology *14*(5):231, 1978.

Amundsen P et al: Cervical myelography with metrizamide (Amipaque). Acta Neurochir (Wien) *31*(3-4):257, 1975.

Arnell S: Myelography with water-soluble contrast with special regard to the normal roentgen picture. Acta Radiol (Suppl) *75*:70, 1948.

Bailey P, Casamajor L: Osteo-arthritis of the spine as a cause of compression of the spinal cord and its roots, with reports of five cases. J Nerv Ment Dis *38*:588, 1911.

Baker RA et al: Sequelae of metrizamide myelography in 200 examinations. Am J Roentgenol *130*(3):499, 1978.

Benedict KT Jr et al: Respiratory arrest — a fatal complication of myelography. Radiology *122*(2 Suppl):729, 1977.

Brodley PA et al: Nerve rootlet avulsion. A complication of myelography using the Chynn needle. Radiology *125*(3):734, 1977.

Cramer F, Hudson F: Myelographically demonstrated cervical intervertebral discs, coexisting with tumors. Tr Am Neurol Ass *81*:171, 1956.

Chamberlain WE, Young BR: The diagnosis of intervertebral disk protrusion by intraspinal injection of air; air myelography. JAMA *113*:2022, 1939.

Cusick JF, Haughton VM, Williams AL: Radiological assessment of intramedullary spinal cord lesions. J Neurosurg *4*:216, 1979.

Davies ER, Sutton D, Bligh A: Myelography in brachial plexus injury. Br J Radiol *39*:362, 1966.

DiChiro G, Doppman JL: Differential angiographic features of hemangioblastomas and arteriovenous malformations of the spinal cord. Radiology *93*:25, 1969.

DiChiro G et al: Computerized axial tomography in syringohydromyelia. N Engl J Med *292*:13, 1975.

DiChiro G, Schellinger D: Computed tomography of spinal cord after lumbar intrathecal introduction of metrizamide (computer-assisted myelography). Radiology *120*:101, 1976.

Djindian R: Arteriography of the spinal cord. Am J Roentgenol *107*:461, 1969.

Drayer BP et al: Suprasellar masses on computerised tomography with intrathecal metrizamide (letter). Lancet *2*(7988):736, 1976.

Drayer BP et al: Posterior fossa extraaxial cyst: diagnosis with metrizamide CT cisternography. Am J Roentgenol *128*(3):431, 1977.

Eastwood JB et al: Bilateral central fracture-dislocation of hips after myelography with meglumine iocarnate (Dimmer X). Br Med J *1*(6114):692, 1978.

Feinberg SB: The place of diskography in radiology as based on 2,320 cases. Am J Roentgenol *92*:1275, 1964.

Fitz CR et al: The tethered conus. Am J Roentgenol *125*(3):515, 1975.

Forbes WS, Isherwood I: Computed tomography in syringomyelia and the associated Arnold-Chiari type I malformation. Neuroradiology *15*:73, 1978.

Gershater R, Holgate RC: Lumbar epidural venography in the diagnosis of disc herniations. Am J Roentgenol *126*:992, 1976.

Golman K et al: Metrizamide in experimental urography. IV. Effects of bilateral ureteric stasis on urine iodine concentration after intravenous injection of an ionic and a non-ionic contrast medium. Invest Radiol *11*(2):80, 1976.

Grossman ZD et al: Recognition of vertebral abnormalities in computed tomography of the chest and abdomen. Radiology *121*:369, 1976.

Hammerschlag SB, Wolpert SM, Carter BL: Computed tomography of the spinal canal. Radiology *121*:361, 1976.

Harwood-Nash DC, Fitz CR: Myelography and syringohydromyelia in infancy and childhood. Radiology *113*:661, 1974.

Harwood-Nash DC, Barry J: Spinal lesions spotted with metrizamide. JAMA *237*:757, 1977.

Haughton VM et al: Severity of postmyelographic arachnoiditis and concentration of meglumine iocarmate in primates. Am J Roentgenol *130*(2):313, 1978.

Haughton VM et al: Comparison of arachnoiditis produced by meglumine iocarmate and metrizamide myelography in an animal model. Am J Roentgenol *131*(1):129, 1978.

Hinck VC, Clark WM Jr, Hopkins CE: Normal interpediculate distances (minimum and maximum) in children and adults. Am J Roentgenol *97*:141, 1966.

Hindmarsh T et al: Metrizamide-phenothiazine interaction. Report of a case with seizures following myelography. Acta Radiol (Diag) *16*(2):129, 1975.

Horwitz T: The diagnosis of posterior protrusion of the intervertebral disc. With special reference to (1) its differentiation from certain degenerative lesions of the disc and its related structures and (2) the interpretation of contrast myelography. Am J Roentgenol *49*:199, 1943.

Howland WJ, Curry JL, Butler AK: Pantopaque arachnoiditis: experimental study of blood as a potentiating agent. Radiology *80*:489, 1963.

Hungerford GD et al: Avulsion of nerve rootlets with the Cuatico needle during Pantopaque removal after myelography. Am J Roentgenol *129*(3):485, 1977.

Hurteau EF, Baird WC, Sinclair E: Arachnoiditis following the use of iodized oil. J Bone Joint Surg *36A*:393, 1954.

Kaada B: Transient EEG abnormalities following lumbar myelography with metrizamide. Acta Radiol (Suppl) (335):380, 1973.

Kelly DL Jr, Alexander E Jr: Lateral cervical puncture for myelography. J Neurosurg *29*:106, 1968.

Kernohan JW, Woltman HW, Adson AW: Intramedullary tumors of the spinal cord. A review of fifty-one cases, with an attempt at histological classification. Arch Neurol Psychiatr *25*:679, 1931.

Kernohan JW, Woltman HW, Adson AW: Gliomas arising from the region of the cauda equina. Clinical, surgical and histologic considerations. Arch Neurol Psychiatr *29*:287, 1933.

Khilnani MT, Wolf BS: Transverse diameter of cervical spinal cord on Pantopaque myelography. J Neurosurg *20*:660, 1963.

Kwan WW et al: Pantopaque pulmonary embolism during myelography. J Neurosurg *46*(3):391, 1977.

Laasonen EM et al: Gross deformity of the spine; a lumbar myelographic risk with Conray and Dimer X. Neuroradiology *15*(3):175, 1978.

Lee CP, Kazam E, Newman AD: Computed tomography of the spine and spinal cord. Radiology *128*:95, 1978.

Lieberman P et al: Chronic urticaria and intermittent anaphylaxis. Reactions to iophendylate. JAMA *236*:1495, 1976.

McRae DL: Asymptomatic intervertebral disc protrusions. Acta Radiol *46*:9, 1956.

Malis LI: The myelographic examination of the foramen magnum. Radiology *70*:196, 1958.

Margolis MT: A simple myelographic maneuver for the detection of mass lesions at the foramen magnum. Radiology *119*:482, 1976.

Mason MS, Raaf J: Complications of Pantopaque myelography. Case report and review. J Neurosurg *19*:302, 1962.

Mitchell GE, Lourie H, Berne AS: The various causes of scalloped vertebrae with notes on their pathogenesis. Radiology *89*:67, 1967.

Mixter WJ, Barr JS: Rupture of the intervertebral disc with involvement of the spinal canal. N Engl J Med *211*:210, 1934.

Mones R, Werman R: Pantopaque myeloencephalography. Radiology *72*:803, 1959.

Munro D: Lumbar and sacral compression radiculitis (herniated lumbar disk syndrome). N Engl J Med *254*:243, 1956.

Neuhauser EBD, Wittenberg MH, Dehlinger K: Diastematomyelia. Transfixation of the cord or cauda equina with congenital anomalies of the spine. Radiology *54*:659, 1950.

O'Callahan JP et al: Computed tomography of facet distraction in flexion injuries of the thoracolumbar spine: the "naked" facet. Am J Roentgenol *134*:563, 1980.

Pallis C, Jones AM, Spillane JD: Cervical spondylosis; incidence and implications. Brain *77*:274, 1954.

Pool JL: Spinal cord and local signs secondary to occult sacral meningoceles in adults. Bull NY Acad Med *28*:655, 1952.

Post MJD et al: A comparison of radiographic methods of

diagnosing constrictive lesions of the spinal canal. J Neurosurg *48*:360, 1978.

Quencer RM et al: Percutaneous spinal cord puncture and myelocystography. Its role in the diagnosis and treatment of intramedullary neoplasms. Radiology *118*(3):637, 1976.

Resjo IM et al: Computed tomographic metrizamide myelography in spinal dysraphism in infants and children. J Comput Assist Tomography *2*:549, 1978.

Resjo IM et al: Normal cord in infants and children examined with computed metrizamide myelography. Radiology *130*:691, 1979.

Resjo IM et al: Computed tomographic metrizamide myelography in syringohydromyelia. Radiology *131*:405, 1979.

Sackett JF et al: Metrizamide — CSF contrast medium . Analysis of clinical application in 215 patients. Radiology *123*(3):779, 1977.

Sanford H, Doub HP: Epidurography. A method of roentgenologic visualization of protruded intervertebral disks. Radiology *36*:712, 1941.

Schindler E et al: Pantopaque — myelographic findings in brachial plexus root avulsion. Fortschr Geb Roentgenstr Nuklearmed *122*(6):528, 1975.

Schlesinger EB, Taveras JM: Factors in the production of "cauda equina" syndromes in lumbar discs. Tr Am Neurol Ass *78*:263, 1953.

Schwarz GA, Reback S: Compression of the spinal cord in osteitis deformans (Paget's disease) of the vertebrae. Am J Roentgenol *42*:345, 1939.

Skalpe IO, Amundsen P: Lumbar radiculography and metrizamide, a nonionic water-soluble contrast medium. Radiology *115*:91, 1975.

Spangfort EV: Lumbar disc herniation. Acta Orthop Scand (Suppl) *142*:1, 1972.

Speck U et al: The effect of position of patient on the passage of metrizamide (Amipaque), meglumine iocarmate (Dimer X) and ioserinate (Myelografin) into the blood after lumbar myelography. Neuroradiology *14*(5):251, 1978.

Tarlov IM: Sacral Nerve-Root Cysts. Springfield, IL, Charles C Thomas, 1953.

Theron J et al: Lumbar phlebography by catheterization of the lateral sacral and ascending lumbar veins with abdominal compression. Neuroradiology *11*:175, 1976.

Ullrich CG et al: Quantitative measurement of the lumbar spinal canal by computed tomography. Presented at the 16th Annual Meeting of the American Society of Neuroradiology, 1978. Radiology *134*:137, 1980.

Weinstein MA et al: Computed tomography in diastematomyelia. Radiology *118*:609, 1975.

Wolf A: Tumors of the spinal cord, nerve roots, and membranes. In: CA Elsberg: Surgical Diseases of the Spinal Cord, Membranes and Nerve Roots. New York, PB Hoeber, 1941.

Wolf BS, Khilnani M, Malis L: The sagittal diameter of the bony cervical spinal canal and its significance in cervical spondylosis. J Mt Sinai Hosp NY *23*:283, 1956.

Wood EH Jr: The diagnosis of spinal meningiomas and schwannomas by myelography. Am J Roentgenol *61*:683, 1949.

Wood EH Jr, Taveras JM, Pool JL: Myelographic demonstration of spinal cord metastases from primary brain tumors. Am J Roentgenol *69*:221, 1953.

Young DA, Burney RE: Complication of myelography: transection and withdrawal of a nerve filament by the needle. N Engl J Med *285*:156, 1971.

INDEX

(Page numbers in *italic* type refer to illustrations.)

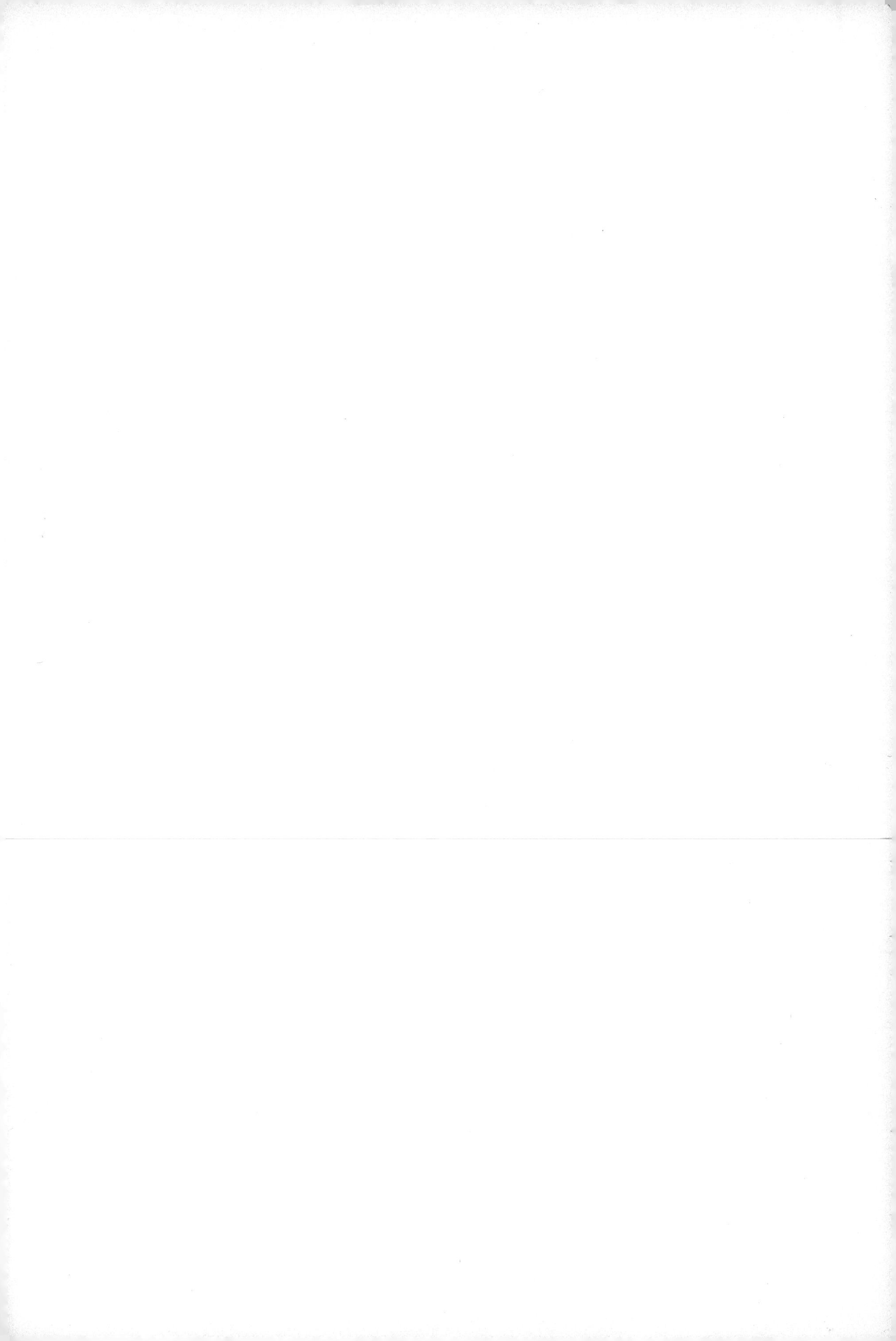